The very best patient care begins wit ... st

CARE PLANNING RESOURCES

...now and throughout your career!

Doenges, Moorhouse & Murr

NURSE'S POCKET GUIDE
Diagnoses, Prioritized Interventions and Rationales

The perfect portable guide for practitioners and nursing students on the go! Here's everything you need to select the appropriate diagnoses for your patients and develop safe and effective care plans.

Doenges & Moorhouse

APPLICATION OF NURSING PROCESS AND NURSING DIAGNOSIS
An Interactive Text for Diagnostic Reasoning

Master the nursing process with this step-by-step approach to the whys and hows, while you develop the diagnostic reasoning and problem-solving skills you need to 'think like a nurse.'

Doenges, Moorhouse & Murr

NURSING DIAGNOSIS MANUAL
Planning, Individualizing, and Documenting Client Care

Rely on this complete reference to identify interventions commonly associated with specific nursing diagnoses across the lifespan, and to help plan, individualize, and document care for more than 800 diseases and disorders.

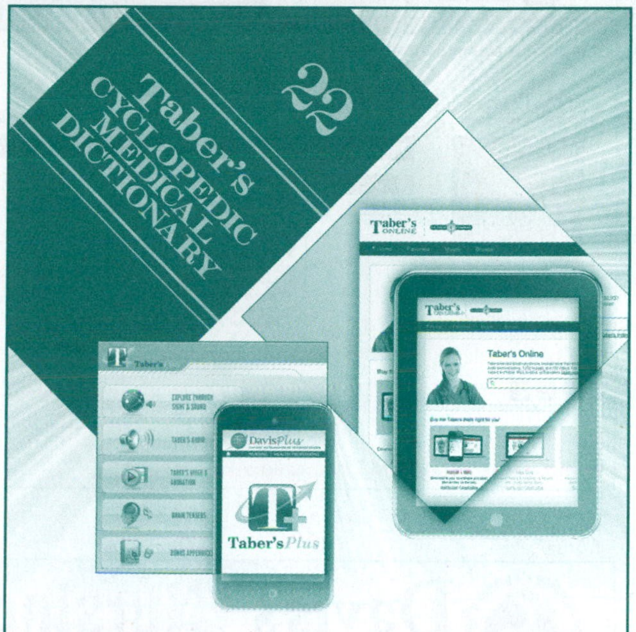

Taber's® 22

brings meanings to life!

TABER'S 22

Edited by Donald Venes, MSJ, MD

Meet the needs of diverse learning styles and today's time-pressed students with FREE mobile and web access, flash-card app, audio pronunciations, interactive learning activities, and more!

WEB. MOBILE. PRINT.
The choice is yours.

www.Tabers.com

ORDER YOUR COPIES TODAY!

www.FADavis.com

F.A. DAVIS COMPANY

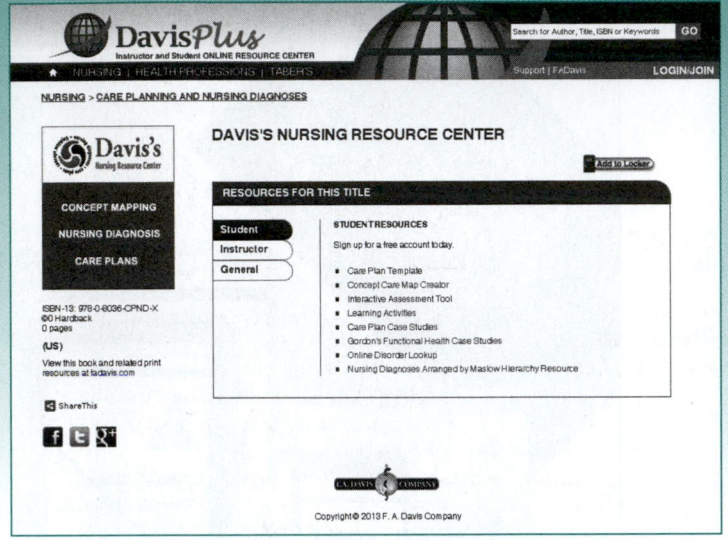

INDEX OF DISEASES/DISORDERS

This is 1 of 2 indexes in the book. It should be compiled by the indexer and only needs to contain the disorder/disease and the page number in which the care plan for that disorder/disease begins.

KEY TO ESSENTIAL TERMINOLOGY

Client Assessment Database

Provides an overview of the more commonly occurring etiology and coexisting factors associated with a specific medical and/or surgical diagnosis or health condition as well as the signs and symptoms and corresponding diagnostic findings.

Nursing Priorities

Establishes a general ranking of needs and concerns on which the Nursing Diagnoses are ordered in constructing the plan of care. This ranking would be altered according to the individual client situation.

Discharge Goals

Identifies generalized statements that could be developed into short-term and intermediate goals to be achieved by the client before being "discharged" from nursing care. They may also provide guidance for creating long-term goals for the client to work on after discharge.

Nursing Diagnosis

The general need or problem (diagnosis) is stated without the distinct cause and signs and symptoms, which would be added to create a client diagnostic statement when specific client information is available. For example, when a client displays increased tension, apprehension, quivering voice, and focus on self, the nursing diagnosis of Anxiety might be stated: severe Anxiety related to unconscious conflict, threat to self-concept as evidenced by statements of increased tension, apprehension; observations of quivering voice, focus on self.

In addition, diagnoses identified within these guides for planning care as actual, risk, or health-promotion can be changed or deleted and new diagnoses added, depending entirely on the specific client situation or available information.

May Be Related to/Possibly Evidenced by

These lists provide the usual or common reasons (etiology) why a particular need or problem may occur with probable signs and symptoms, which would be used to create the "related to" and "evidenced by" portions of the *client diagnostic statement* when the specific situation is known.

When a risk diagnosis has been identified, signs and symptoms have not yet developed and therefore are not included in the nursing diagnosis statement. However, interventions are provided to prevent progression to an actual problem. Furthermore, health-promotion diagnoses (readiness for enhanced) do not contain related factors, but do have defining characteristics for the "evidenced by" segment of the client diagnostic statement.

Desired Outcomes/Evaluation Criteria—Client Will

These give direction to client care as they identify what the client or nurse hopes to achieve. They are stated in general terms to permit the practitioner to modify or individualize them by adding time lines and specific client criteria so they become "measurable." For example, "Client will appear relaxed and report anxiety is reduced to a manageable level within 24 hours."

Nursing Outcomes Classification (NOC) labels are also included. The outcome label is selected from a standardized nursing language and serves as a general header for the outcome indicators that follow.

Actions/Interventions

Nursing Interventions Classification (NIC) labels are drawn from a third standardized nursing language and serve as a general header for the nursing actions that follow.

Nursing actions are divided into independent—those actions that the nurse performs autonomously—and collaborative—those actions that the nurse performs in conjunction with others, such as implementing physician orders. The interventions in this book are generally ranked from most to least common. When creating the individual plan of care, interventions would normally be ranked to reflect the client's specific needs and situation. In addition, the division of independent and collaborative is arbitrary and is actually dependent on the individual nurse's capabilities, agency protocols, and professional standards.

Rationale

Although not commonly appearing in client plans of care, rationale has been included here to provide a pathophysiological basis to assist the nurse in deciding about the relevance of a specific intervention for an individual client situation.

Clinical Pathway

This abbreviated plan of care or care map is event- or task-oriented and provides outcome-based guidelines for goal achievement within a designated length of stay. Several samples have been included to demonstrate alternative planning formats.

NURSING DIAGNOSES ACCEPTED FOR USE AND RESEARCH FOR 2012–2014

Activity Intolerance [specify level]
Activity Intolerance, risk for
Activity Planning, ineffective
Activity Planning, risk for ineffective
Adverse Reaction to Iodinated Contrast Media, risk for
Airway Clearance, ineffective
Allergy Response, risk for
Anxiety [specify level]
Aspiration, risk for
Attachment, risk for impaired
Autonomic Dysreflexia
Autonomic Dysreflexia, risk for
Behavior, disorganized infant
Behavior, readiness for enhanced organized infant
Behavior, risk for disorganized infant
Bleeding, risk for
Blood Glucose Level, risk for unstable
Body Image, disturbed
Body Temperature, risk for imbalanced
Breast Milk, insufficient
Breastfeeding, ineffective
Breastfeeding, interrupted
Breastfeeding, readiness for enhanced
Breathing Pattern, ineffective
Cardiac Output, decreased
Caregiver Role Strain
Caregiver Role Strain, risk for
Childbearing Process, ineffective
Childbearing Process, readiness for enhanced
Childbearing Process, risk for ineffective
Comfort, impaired
Comfort, readiness for enhanced
Communication, impaired verbal
Communication, readiness for enhanced
Confusion, acute
Confusion, chronic
Confusion, risk for acute
Constipation
Constipation, perceived
Constipation, risk for
Contamination
Contamination, risk for
Coping, compromised family
Coping, defensive
Coping, disabled family
Coping, ineffective
Coping, ineffective community
Coping, readiness for enhanced
Coping, readiness for enhanced community
Coping, readiness for enhanced family
Death Anxiety
Decision-Making, readiness for enhanced
Decisional Conflict
Denial, ineffective
Dentition, impaired
Development, risk for delayed
Diarrhea
Dignity, risk for compromised human
Disuse Syndrome, risk for
Diversional Activity, deficient
Dry Eye, risk for
Electrolyte Imbalance, risk for
Energy Field, disturbed
Environmental Interpretation Syndrome, impaired
Failure to Thrive, adult
Falls, risk for
Family Processes, dysfunctional
Family Processes, interrupted
Family Processes, readiness for enhanced
Fatigue
Fear
Feeding Pattern, ineffective infant
Fluid Balance, readiness for enhanced
[Fluid Volume, deficient hyper/hypotonic]
Fluid Volume, deficient [isotonic]
Fluid Volume, excess
Fluid Volume, risk for deficient
Fluid Volume, risk for imbalanced
Gas Exchange, impaired
Gastrointestinal Motility, dysfunctional
Gastrointestinal Motility, risk for dysfunctional
Gastrointestinal Perfusion, risk for ineffective
Grieving
Grieving, complicated
Grieving, risk for complicated
Growth, risk for disproportionate
Growth and Development, delayed
Health, deficient community
Health Behavior, risk-prone
Health Maintenance, ineffective
Home Maintenance, impaired
Hope, readiness for enhanced
Hopelessness
Human Dignity, risk for compromised
Hyperthermia
Hypothermia
Immunization Status, readiness for enhanced
Impulse Control, ineffective
Incontinence, bowel
Incontinence, functional urinary
Incontinence, overflow urinary
Incontinence, reflex urinary
Incontinence, risk for urge urinary
Incontinence, stress urinary
Incontinence, urge urinary
Infection, risk for
Injury, risk for
Insomnia
Intracranial Adaptive Capacity, decreased
Jaundice, neonatal
Jaundice, risk for neonatal
Knowledge, deficient [Learning Need] [specify]
Knowledge [specify], readiness for enhanced
Latex Allergy Response
Latex Allergy Response, risk for
Lifestyle, sedentary
Liver Function, risk for impaired
Loneliness, risk for
Maternal-Fetal Dyad, risk for disturbed
Memory, impaired
Mobility, impaired bed
Mobility, impaired physical
Mobility, impaired wheelchair
Moral Distress
Nausea
Noncompliance [Adherence, ineffective] [specify]
Nutrition: less than body requirements, imbalanced
Nutrition: more than body requirements, imbalanced
Nutrition: more than body requirements, risk for imbalanced
Nutrition, readiness for enhanced
Oral Mucous Membrane, impaired
Pain, acute
Pain, chronic
Parenting, impaired
Parenting, readiness for enhanced
Parenting, risk for impaired
Perioperative Positioning Injury, risk for
Peripheral Neurovascular Dysfunction, risk for
Personal Identity, disturbed
Personal Identity, risk for disturbed
Poisoning, risk for
Post-Trauma Syndrome [specify stage]
Post-Trauma Syndrome, risk for
Power, readiness for enhanced
Powerlessness [specify level]
Powerlessness, risk for
Protection, ineffective
Rape-Trauma Syndrome
Relationship, ineffective
Relationship, readiness for enhanced
Relationship, risk for ineffective
Religiosity, impaired
Religiosity, readiness for enhanced
Religiosity, risk for impaired
Relocation Stress Syndrome
Relocation Stress Syndrome, risk for
Renal Perfusion, risk for ineffective
Resilience, impaired individual
Resilience, readiness for enhanced
Resilience, risk for compromised
Role Conflict, parental
Role Performance, ineffective
Self-Care, readiness for enhanced
Self-Care Deficit: bathing
Self-Care Deficit: dressing
Self-Care Deficit: feeding
Self-Care Deficit: toileting
Self-Concept, readiness for enhanced
Self-Esteem, chronic low
Self-Esteem, risk for chronic low
Self-Esteem, risk for situational low
Self-Esteem, situational low
Self-Health Management, ineffective
Self-Health Management, readiness for enhanced
Self-Mutilation
Self-Mutilation, risk for
Self-Neglect
[Sensory Perception, disturbed (specify: visual, auditory, kinesthetic, gustatory, tactile, olfactory)] (retired 2012)
Sexual Dysfunction
Sexuality Pattern, ineffective
Shock, risk for
Skin Integrity, impaired
Skin Integrity, risk for impaired
Sleep, readiness for enhanced
Sleep Deprivation
Sleep Pattern, disturbed
Social Interaction, impaired
Social Isolation
Sorrow, chronic
Spiritual Distress
Spiritual Distress, risk for
Spiritual Well-Being, readiness for enhanced
Stress Overload
Sudden Infant Death Syndrome, risk for
Suffocation, risk for
Suicide, risk for
Surgical Recovery, delayed
Swallowing, impaired
Therapeutic Regimen Management, ineffective family
Thermal Injury, risk for
Thermoregulation, ineffective
Tissue Integrity, impaired
Tissue Perfusion, ineffective peripheral
Tissue Perfusion, risk for decreased cardiac
Tissue Perfusion, risk for ineffective cerebral
Tissue Perfusion, risk for ineffective peripheral
Transfer Ability, impaired
Trauma, risk for
Trauma, risk for vascular
Unilateral Neglect
Urinary Elimination, impaired
Urinary Elimination, readiness for enhanced
Urinary Retention [acute/chronic]
Vascular Trauma, risk fo
Ventilation, impaired spontaneous
Ventilatory Weaning Response, dysfunctional
Violence, risk for other-directed
Violence, risk for self-directed
Walking, impaired
Wandering [specify sporadic or continual]
[ ] author recommendations

Nursing Care Plans

Guidelines for Individualizing Client Care Across the Life Span

EDITION 9

Nursing Care Plans

Guidelines for Individualizing Client Care Across the Life Span

Marilynn E. Doenges, APRN, BC-Retired
Clinical Specialist, Adult Psychiatric/Mental Health Nursing, Retired
Retired Adjunct Faculty
Beth-El College of Nursing and Health Sciences, UCCS
Colorado Springs, Colorado

Mary Frances Moorhouse, RN, MSN, CRRN
Adjunct Faculty/Clinical Instructor
Pikes Peak Community College
Nurse Consultant/TNT-RN Enterprises
Colorado Springs, Colorado

Alice C. Murr, BSN, RN-Retired
Independence, Missouri

EDITION 9

F.A. Davis Company • Philadelphia

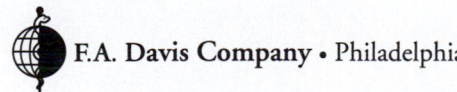

F. A. Davis Company
1915 Arch Street
Philadelphia, PA 19103
www.fadavis.com

Printed in the United States of America

Last digit indicates print number: 10 9 8 7 6 5 4 3 2 1
Publisher, Nursing: Joanne Patzek DaCunha, RN, MSN
Director of Content Development: Darlene Pederson, MSN, APRN, BC
Project Editor: Elizabeth Hart
Art and Design Manager: Carolyn O'Brien
Electronic Project Editor: Tyler Baber

As new scientific information becomes available through basic and clinical research, recommended treatments and drug therapies undergo changes. The authors and publisher have done everything possible to make this book accurate, up-to-date, and in accord with accepted standards at the time of publication. The authors, editors, and publisher are not responsible for errors or omissions or for consequences from application of the book, and make no warranty, expressed or implied, in regard to the contents of the book. Any practice described in this book should be applied by the reader in accordance with professional standards of care used in regard to the unique circumstances that may apply in each situation. The reader is advised always to check product information (package inserts) for changes and new information regarding dose and contraindications before administering any drug. Caution is especially urged when using new or infrequently ordered drugs.

Library of Congress Cataloging-in-Publication Data

Doenges, Marilynn E., 1922– author.
Nursing care plans : guidelines for individualizing client care across the life span / Marilynn E. Doenges, Mary Frances Moorhouse, Alice C. Murr.—Edition 9.
p. ; cm.
Includes bibliographical references and index.
ISBN-13: 978-0-8036-3041-3
ISBN-10: 0-8036-3041-7
I. Moorhouse, Mary Frances, 1947– author. II. Murr, Alice C., 1946– author. III. Title.
[DNLM: 1. Patient Care Planning—Handbooks. 2. Nursing Process—Handbooks. WY 49]
RT49
610.73—dc23
2013041055

To our spouses, children, parents, and friends, who much of the time have had to manage without us while we work as well as having to cope with our struggles and frustrations.

The Doenges families: the late Dean, whose support and encouragement is sorely missed; Jim; Barbara and Bob Lanza; David, Monita, and Tyler; Matthew, Trish, Sara, and Natilia; John, Holly, Nicole, and Kelsey; and the Daigle families: Nancy, Jim; Jennifer, Brandon, Annabelle, Will, and Henry Smith-Daigle, and Jonathan, Kim, and Mandalyn JoAn.

The Moorhouse family: husband Jan, Paul Moorhouse; Jason and Thenderlyn Moorhouse; Alexa, Tanner, and Quinton Plant; and Mary Isabella Moorhouse.

To my Kansas City family, Darin and Ck, Joe and Chelsea-Jane, Maxwell and Eisley: You have given me support, love and joy when I most needed it during this project. Thank you! -Alice Murr (aka Mom/Grammy)

To our F. A. Davis family, especially Robert Allen and Sam Rondinelli, whose support is so vital to the completion of a project of this magnitude. And to Joanne DaCunha, who is not just our acquisitions editor but also a colleague and friend who has seen the project from both sides now. Last but not least, Elizabeth Hart, who supports us on a daily basis and keeps track of all the pieces. Thank you for your support and understanding. We are fortunate to have you working with us.

To the nurses we are writing for, who daily face the challenge of caring for the acutely ill client and are looking for a practical way to organize and document this care. We believe that nursing diagnosis and these guides will help.

To NANDA-I and to the international nurses who are developing and using nursing diagnoses—here we come!

Finally, to the late Mary Lisk Jeffries, who initiated the original project. The memory of our early friendship and struggles remains with us. We miss her and wish she were here to see the growth of the profession and how nursing diagnosis has contributed to the process.

CONTRIBUTORS TO THE 9TH EDITION

Sharon A. Aronovitch, PhD, RN, ACNS-BC, CWOCN-AP
Faculty, Graduate Nursing Program
Excelsior College
Albany, New York

Cathryn Baack, PhD, RN, CPNP
Assistant Professor; Online Faculty Manager
Chamberlain College of Nursing
Columbus, Ohio

Becky Craig, RN, MN, PhD
Georgia Perimeter College
Clarkston, Georgia

Catherine M. Gagnon, RNC-OB, MSN
Nursing Faculty
Pikes Peak Community College
Colorado Springs, Colorado

William H. Loughmiller, CRT
Respiratory Therapist
St. Francis Medical Center
Colorado Springs, Colorado

Maria Mackey, MSN, RN
Instructor
St. Luke's School of Nursing
Bethlehem, Pennsylvania

Margaret (Peggy) Malone, MN, RN, CCRN
Clinical Nurse Specialist
St. John Medical Center
Longview, Washington

Laure Miller, MSN, RN
Associate Professor Nursing
Iowa Lakes Community College
Emmetsburg, Iowa

Ellen Odell, DNP, ACNS, CNE, RN
Assistant Professor
College of Education and Health Professions
Eleanor Mann School of Nursing
University of Arkansas
Fayetteville, Arkansas

Lillian Ostrander, RN, MSN, MALS
Professor
Bergen Community College
Paramus, New Jersey

Nancy E. Rogers, MA, BSN, RN
Professor, Simulation Specialist
Carroll Community College
Westminster, Maryland

Ruth A. Wittmann-Price, PhD, RN, CNS, CNE
Chair, Department of Nursing
Professor of Nursing
Francis Marion University
Florence, South Carolina

David W. Woodruff, MSN, RN-BC, CMSRN, CEN
President
Ed4Nurses, Inc.
Macedonia, Ohio

CONTRIBUTORS TO THE 9TH EDITION

Mope T. Adeola, RN, MSN, CNS, OCN
Jane V. Arndt, MS, RN, CWOCN
Nancy Buttry, MSN, RN
Kathleen A. Curtis, RN, MSN
Rosemary Fliszar, PhD, RN, CNE
Brenda Hicks, RN, OCN
Christie A. Hinds, MSN, APRN-BC
Jennifer Limongiello, MSN, ARNP
Bill Loughmiller, CRT
Larry Manalo, RN, MSN
Julie Matheny, RRT
Kathleen Molden, RN, MSN, CNE
Kimberly Tucker Pfennigs, MA, BAN, RN
Gilda Rolls-Dellinger, RN
Rochelle Salmore, MSN, RN, CGRN, NE, BC
April Sheker, RN, MSN(c), CMSRN
Geri L. Tierney, RN, BSN, ONC
Kathleen H. Winder, RN, BSN
Anne Zobec, MS, RN, CS, NP, AOCN

REVIEWERS FOR THE 9TH EDITION

Mary Brune, RN, MS, CNE, EdD(c)
Instructor
Northwestern Oklahoma State University
Woodward, Oklahoma

Natalie Burkhalter, RN, MSN, CS, FNP-BC, ACNP-BC
Associate Professor
Texas A&M International University
Laredo, Texas

Karen Reilly, ARNP
Nursing Professor
Daytona State College
Daytona Beach, Florida

ACKNOWLEDGMENTS

The late Nancy Lea Carter, RN, MA
Clinical Nurse, Orthopedics
Albuquerque, New Mexico

Special thanks for many hours of research!
Kathe Lynn Ellis
Case Manager
Colorado Springs, Colorado
Statistical Research

Linda R. Renberg, BA
Instructor, Retired
English, Music and Education
Mitchell, South Dakota
Statistical Research

INTRODUCTION

We are often asked how we came to write the Care Plan books. In the late 1970s, we were involved with some publishing efforts that did not come to fruition. In this work we had included care plans, so ensuing discussions revolved around the need for a Care Plan book. We spent a year struggling to write care plans before we realized our major difficulty was the lack of standardized labels for client problems. At that time, we were given a list of nursing diagnoses from the Clearinghouse for Nursing Diagnosis, which became the North American Nursing Diagnosis Association (NANDA) and is now NANDA International (NANDA-I). This work answered our need by providing concise titles that could be used in various plans of care and followed across the spectrum of client care. We believed these nursing diagnosis labels would both define and focus nursing care.

Because we had long been involved in direct client care in our nursing careers, we knew there was a need for guidelines to assist nurses in planning care. As we began to write, our focus was the nurse in a small rural community who at 2 a.m. needed the answer to a burning question for her client and had few resources available. We believed the book would give definition and direction to the development and use of individualized nursing care. Thus, in the first edition, the theory of nursing process, diagnosis, and intervention was brought to the clinical setting for implementation by the nurse. We also anticipated that nursing students would appreciate having access to these guidelines as they struggled to learn how to provide nursing care. Therefore, we did not consider the book to be an end in itself, but rather a vehicle for the continuing growth and development of the profession. Obviously, we struck a chord and met a need because the first edition was an immediate success.

In becoming involved with NANDA, we acknowledged that maintaining a strict adherence to its wording, while adding our own clearly identified recommendations, would help develop this neophyte standardized language and would promote the growth of nursing as a profession. We have continued our involvement with NANDA-I, promoting the use of the language by practicing nurses in the United States and around the world and encouraging them to participate in updating and refining the diagnoses. The wide use of our books within the student population has supported and fostered the acceptance of both the activity of diagnosing client problems or needs and the use of standardized language.

Nursing instructors initially expressed concern that students would simply copy the plans of care and thus limit their learning. However, as students used the plans to individualize care and to develop practice priorities and client care outcomes, the book met with more acceptance. Instructors began not only to recommend the book but also to adopt it as an adjunct text. Today, it remains the best-selling nursing care plan book, recognized as an important adjunct for student learning.

In writing the second edition, we recognized the need for an assessment tool with a nursing focus instead of a medical focus. Not finding one that met our needs, we constructed our own. To facilitate problem identification, we categorized the nursing diagnosis labels and the information obtained in the client assessment database into a framework entitled "Diagnostic Divisions." Our philosophy is to provide a way in which to gather information and to intervene beneficially, while thinking about the rationale for every action we take and the standardized language that best expresses it. When nurses do this they are defining their practice and are able to identify it with a code and charge for it. By doing this, we promote client protection (quality of care issue) and provide for the definition and protection of nursing practice and the protection of the individual (legal implications). The latter is important because we live in a litigation-minded society and the nurse's license and livelihood are at stake.

One of the most significant achievements in the healthcare field over the past 25 or more years has been the emergence of the nurse as an active coordinator and initiator of client care. Although the transition from physician's helpmate to healthcare professional has been painfully slow and is not yet complete, the importance of the nurse within the system can no longer be denied or ignored. Today's nurse designs nursing care interventions that move the total client toward improved health and maximum independence.

Professional care standards and healthcare providers and consumers will continue to increase the expectations for nurses' performance. Each day brings new challenges in client care and the struggle to understand the human responses to actual and potential health problems. To meet these challenges competently, the nurse must have up-to-date assessment skills and a working knowledge of pathophysiological concepts concerning the common diseases and conditions presented. We believe that this book is a tool, providing a means of attaining that competency.

In the past, plans of care were viewed principally as learning tools for students and seemed to have little relevance after graduation. However, the need for a written format to communicate and document client care has been recognized in all care settings. In addition, healthcare policy, governmental regulations, and third-party payor requirements have created the need to validate many things, including appropriateness of care provided, staffing patterns, and monetary charges. Thus, although the student's "case studies" are too cumbersome to be practical in the clinical setting, it has long been recognized that the client plan of care meets certain needs and therefore its appropriate use was validated.

The practicing nurse, as well as the nursing student, can welcome this text as a ready reference in clinical practice. It is designed for use in the acute care, community, and home-care settings. It is organized by systems for easy reference.

Chapter 1 examines current issues and trends and their implications for the nursing profession. An overview of major factors driving changes in healthcare and the challenges and opportunities for nursing to participate and even lead some of the changes is presented. The importance of the nurse's role in collaboration and coordination with other healthcare professionals is integrated throughout the plans of care.

Chapter 2 reviews the historical use of the nursing process in formulating plans of care and the nurse's role in the delivery of that care. Nursing diagnoses, outcomes, and interventions are discussed to assist the nurse in understanding her or his role in the nursing process. In this book, we have also linked NANDA-I diagnoses with Nursing Interventions Classification (NIC) and Nursing Outcomes Classification (NOC) languages.

Chapter 3 discusses care plan construction and describes the use and adaptation of the guides presented in this book. A nursing-based assessment tool is provided to assist the nurse in identifying appropriate nursing diagnoses. A sample client situation with individual database and a corresponding plan of care is included to demonstrate how critical thinking is used to adapt nursing process theory to practice. Finally, a dynamic and creative approach for developing and documenting the planning of care is also included. Mind Mapping is another technique or learning tool provided to assist you in achieving a holistic view of your client, enhance your critical thinking skills, and facilitate the creative process of planning client care.

Chapters 4 through 15 present plans of care that include information from multiple disciplines to assist the nurse in providing holistic care. In addition to the care plans in the textbook, you will also find Psychiatric and Maternal/Newborn care plans on DavisPlus. (To access these, use the Plus Code found in front of your book.)

Each plan includes a Client Assessment Database presented in a nursing format and associated Diagnostic Studies. After the database is collected, Nursing Priorities are sifted from the information to help focus and structure the care. Discharge Goals are created to identify what should be generally accomplished by the time of discharge from the care setting.

Nursing diagnosis labels are then chosen and combined with possible related factors designated by "may be related to," and the signs and symptoms or defining characteristics as "possibly evidenced by," if present, to create Client Diagnostic Statements that provide a clear picture of the client's needs. Next, Desired Client Outcomes are stated in measurable behavioral terms to evaluate both the client's progress and the effectiveness of care provided.

Corresponding actions/interventions are designed to promote resolution of the identified client needs. The nurse acting independently or collaboratively within the health team then uses a decision-making model to organize and prioritize nursing interventions. No attempt is made in this book to indicate whether independent or collaborative actions come first because this must be dictated by the individual situation. We do, however, believe that every collaborative action has a component that the nurse must identify and for which nursing has responsibility and accountability.

Rationales for the nursing actions, which are not required in the customary plan of care, are included to assist the nurse in deciding whether the interventions are appropriate for an individual client. Additional information is provided to further assist the nurse in identifying and planning for rehabilitation as the client progresses toward discharge and across all care settings. Continuing the life span, a plan of care for children (Pediatric Considerations) is included in Chapter 15, and Pediatric Pearls have been added to 11 plans of care common to this population. The Pediatric Pearls are noted by this icon P. Lastly, a bibliography is provided as a reference and to allow further research as desired.

This book is designed for students who will find the plans of care helpful as they learn and develop skills in applying the nursing process and using nursing diagnoses. It will complement their classroom work and support the critical thinking process. The book also provides a ready reference for the practicing nurse as a catalyst for thought in planning, evaluating, and documenting care.

As a final note, this book is not intended to be a procedure manual, and efforts have been made to avoid detailed descriptions of techniques or protocols that might be viewed as individual or regional in nature. Instead, the reader is referred to a procedure manual or text covering Standards of Care if detailed direction is desired.

As we always say when we sign a book, "Use and enjoy."

MD, MFM, and AM

CONTENTS IN BRIEF

A table of contents including nursing diagnoses follows.

DETAILED CONTENTS

CHAPTER 15

CONTENTS ON DAVIS PLUS

CHAPTER 1

Issues and Trends in Nursing and Healthcare Delivery

The Ever-Changing Healthcare Environment

One of the few guarantees in this new millennium is that how we provide and pay for healthcare is going to change. As experts struggle to predict the new face of healthcare, the nursing profession is poised to advance if nurses can navigate the turbulent waters of the impending changes. The leading change agent is the Affordable Care Act (ACA) of 2010. While increased access to care is a major driver, a primary focus of the ACA is preventive healthcare to help individuals stay healthy, avoid onset of disease, lead productive lives, and limit the need for more costly healthcare (Stokowski, 2011).

In addition to mandating that third-party payors provide preventive screenings free of co-pays, billions of dollars will be invested in various programs across the life span. For example, Stokowski (2011) highlights the promotion of Maternal, Infant, and Early Child Home Visitation Programs providing counseling for at-risk prenatal clients and families along with interventions to improve health outcomes for infants, children, and adolescents. There also are initiatives expanding school-based health centers to reach children in disadvantaged neighborhoods and support for public health departments to address obesity and smoking cessation, promote physical activity, and improve nutrition.

The expectation is that use of data-driven approaches and evidenced-based interventions and guidelines will reduce the occurrence of chronic disease and will help accomplish the goals of Healthy People 2020 (U.S. Department of Health & Human Services, no date):

- *Attain high-quality, longer lives free of preventable disease, disability, injury, and premature death.*
- *Achieve health equity, eliminate disparities, and improve the health of all groups.*
- *Create social and physical environments that promote good health for all.*
- *Promote quality of life, healthy development, and healthy behaviors across all life stages.*

Challenges, Trends, and Opportunities

To accomplish this move from acute illness care to a wellness and prevention model, a shift to increased delivery of primary care is required. Nurses can and should play a fundamental role in this transformation of the healthcare system. The Institute of Medicine (IOM) 2010 report *The Future of Nursing* noted that the nursing profession is the largest segment of the healthcare workforce and can play a vital role in accomplishing the outcomes envisioned in the 2010 Affordable Care Act. To this end, the IOM has identified barriers limiting nursing's ability to respond effectively to the coming changes and recommends the following:

- *Nurses should practice to the full extent of their education and training.*
- *Nurses should achieve higher levels of education and training through an improved education system that promotes seamless academic progression.*
- *Nurses should be full partners, with physicians and other health professionals, in redesigning healthcare in the United States.*
- *Effective workforce planning and policy making require better data collection and information infrastructure.*

Strong clinical leadership will be required in order to take risks and innovate to improve the care provided and achieve the shift to a wellness focus. After a decade of research, Peter Buerhaus et al (2012) report that the latest survey results create a picture of nursing's capacity to practice successfully in a care delivery environment that is expected to emphasize teams, care coordination, and become driven by payment incentives that reward quality, safety, and efficiency.

New roles for nurses are being created and tested throughout the country. For example, at Massachusetts General Hospital the concept of the "Attending Nurse" has been introduced for the purpose of coordinating the work of the interdisciplinary team, which addresses overuse, underuse, and misuse of services to improve clinical outcomes, enhance client and staff satisfaction, reduce length of stay for inpatients, and lower costs. The Attending Nurse serves as a consistent contact for client/family and the healthcare team in support of the staff nurse and facilitates consistent use of a comprehensive client plan of care by all members of the healthcare team. The Attending Nurse also works to promote seamless communication between the healthcare team members to identify the next steps to ensure progression of the client's plan of care (Erickson, 2012).

Another role first introduced in oncology care 20 years ago is now expanding to other specialties—Nurse Navigator. The role, title, and description of Nurse Navigator (or Patient Navigator) vary with disease, practice setting, and gaps in care (Desimini, 2011). Various healthcare organizations are now utilizing Nurse Navigators to proactively address clients' and families' psychosocial, information, and care coordination needs (Horner, 2013). Nurse Navigators guide the client and family through healthcare experiences—answering healthcare questions, providing education, helping individuals understand their diagnoses and treatment options, communicating with insurance carriers, and facilitating timely access to appropriate healthcare resources, including appointments and diagnostic testing and support for follow-up care. Nurse Navigators also work in elder care with the goal of maintaining independence and quality of life for their aging clients.

In addition to new roles, nursing is developing innovative care models, such as nurse-managed health clinics, home visitation programs for low-income mothers, and the Transitional Care Model (TCM). By emphasizing the use of master's-prepared nurses to oversee care from the hospital to within the home, this model has reduced readmissions for elderly clients with multiple chronic conditions. In support of these new models and the IOM recommendations, advanced practice nurses (APNs) must be allowed to practice to the full extent of their education and licensure. Working independently or with physicians, they can provide cost-effective care and help address the growing primary care shortage (Hassmiller, 2010).

In the community setting, nurses working in collaboration with physicians can create a patient-centered medical home (PCMH), which is a model of care where individuals have a direct relationship with a provider who coordinates a cooperative team of healthcare professionals, takes collective responsibility for the care provided, and arranges for appropriate care from other qualified providers when needed. This model encourages self-management support, electronic prescribing, test and referral tracking, and advanced electronic communication, resulting in a model that is dependent on information technology and exchange of health data (HIMS & NCQA, no date).

In this new era, nurses must not only embrace technology but become super users. To date, nurses have not necessarily welcomed information technology for a number of reasons, such as complexity of user interface or difficulty of program navigation. More importantly, programs have often been developed for other departments, such as billing, or to promote physician order entry. As a result, nursing's contribution to healthcare is often virtually invisible.

In truth, nursing is a costly yet essential resource whose value is not adequately captured in the healthcare record. There have been no well-received and few successful software programs developed that accurately collect and generate data reflecting the true value of nursing, which is critical to assure adequate investment in the nursing profession (Rutherford, 2012). In fact, with a few exceptions, current billing practices subsume nursing in the room rate much like a hotel includes housekeeping and maintenance services in their room rates. This practice essentially makes nursing invisible and implies that nursing care is static with all clients receiving the same level of care regardless of their diagnosis or individual needs. Harris (2007) further notes "the use of the DRG as the basis for payment suggests that nursing care is wholly linked to the medical diagnosis." The growth of nursing informatics is leading the way in developing and implementing software programs using standardized nursing languages to demonstrate nursing's contribution and provide data to support evidence-based practice.

The rapid growth in information technology has already had a radical impact on healthcare. Advances in digital technology have increased the applications of telehealth and telemedicine, bringing together client and provider without physical proximity (Heller, 2011). Technological advances in the treatment of disease have led to the increased need for ethical, informed decision making by clients and families. The enhanced power of the consumer in the client-provider relationship has created a heightened demand for more sophisticated health education techniques for both the client and the provider. For example, "informational" sites have exploded on the Internet, providing the consumer with both factual resources and misinformation. For the nurse, distance learning modalities link students and faculty from different locales and expand the potential for continuing professional education. And technically sophisticated clinical simulation laboratories have been developed to sharpen critical thinking and client care skills in a safe and user-friendly environment (Hibbard, 2008).

In 2011, an estimated 101.1million Americans were aged 50 years or over, representing more than 32% of the population. This number is predicted to rise to 111.3 million by 2016. Increased U.S. life expectancy has shifted the leading causes of death from infectious diseases and acute illnesses to chronic diseases and degenerative illnesses. Some 80% of older Americans live with at least one chronic condition (Economist Intelligence Unit, 2011). These statistics make two things clear to healthcare providers: (1) More people will receive their health and preventive care in community settings, and (2) people in need of hospital and other facility care will be sicker and in need of a higher level of care. Heller noted that the standard ratio of critical care/specialty beds to general-use beds in hospitals today is close to 1:1, up substantially from a decade ago. Furthermore, expanded life expectancy has led to increases in the number, severity, and duration of chronic conditions, thereby increasing the complexity of the care provided and managed by clinicians (Heller, 2011). Because of this escalating need for healthcare, there is legitimate concern in the healthcare world regarding the impact of potential mass retirements on the supply of nurses available to the workforce.

The discussion of issues and challenges would be incomplete without consideration of the building and retention of the nurse workforce. Literature review confirms the ever-present issues of actual and perceived nursing shortages, financial constraints, and the promotion and funding of nursing education. But there is another issue that feels like the proverbial elephant in the room . . . aging. The average age of nurses today is 46 years. Baby boomers now in their 50s comprise approximately 25% of today's workforce (AACN, 2012). Research does support that, while young people are entering the field of nursing, aging is affecting the current workforce as a whole. Aging nurses are reported to have higher workload demands than other professions, as they struggle with the high demands of caring for an aging population with high-acuity needs. This increases the risk of stress reactions, including fatigue, poor health, injury, and chronic pain (Gabrielle, 2008). The Aging Nurse Project (2007) concluded that older nurses were most concerned about their physical health, particularly their backs, especially since many older nurses are working longer than they expected, reportedly because of changes in their retirement plans or other economic downturns (Restuccia, 2007).

Numerous authors have recently discussed multigenerational conflict in the nursing workforce as one of the challenges nurses face (Kupperschmidt, 2006; Lancaster, 2002). When people born in the year 2000 begin working, the workforce will be composed of four generations, each bringing to the work setting the unique characteristics of their parentage, work ethic, and worldview.

As might be expected, the oldest of the older nurses (so-called Traditionalists) have fewer technology skills, but a strong work ethic (almost a calling), and are dismayed by what they consider unprofessionalism in younger nurses. Baby boomers, who often rejected the conformity of their parents' generation, are considered independent, critical thinkers who view their work as a career. These nurses have not necessarily welcomed information technology into their practice, but have been forced to learn and use technology. The next-generation nurses (often called Gen Xers) entered the workforce in a time of national recession and witnessed their parents losing pensions and job security. They experience more portability and options for the use of their practice skills and have little patience for hierarchical reverence in the workplace. The youngest nurses (and those who will be entering practice in the next few years) grew up enmeshed in digital technology, are not deeply invested in who does the work as long as the work gets done, and may view nursing more as an occupation than a profession.

Finally, the patient population and the nursing workforce are becoming increasingly multicultural. Exactly how this is affecting (and will affect) healthcare in general is not known. What is clear is that there will be change and nursing needs to be an active participant in shaping this change.

In closing, we take an optimistic view. Nursing is a rich and diverse profession practiced by people from many cultural and educational backgrounds and in varied settings, which creates a rich source for innovative thinking. Nurses are in a position—and have the opportunity *and* the challenge—to return to their earlier roots in community-focused nursing as front-line advocates and supporters for improving the health and well-being of clients, families, or populations through cost-effective, culturally appropriate, evidence-based practice.

The future of the profession is in our hands. It's time to step up and demonstrate the real power, creativity, and caring of nursing.

CHAPTER 2

The Nursing Process: Planning Care Using Nursing Diagnoses

Nurses and healthcare consumers agree that nursing care is a key factor in achieving positive outcomes and enhancing client satisfaction. Nursing care is instrumental in all phases of acute care as well as in the maintenance of general well-being, in such areas as prevention of illness, rehabilitation, and maximization of health, or, where a return to health is not possible, the relief of pain and discomfort and a peaceful death. To this end, the nursing profession has identified a problem-solving process that "combines the most desirable elements of the art of nursing with the most relevant elements of systems theory, using the scientific method" (Shore, 1988).

The original concept of the nursing process introduced in the 1950s involved three steps: assessment, planning, and evaluation, based on the scientific method of observing, measuring, gathering data, and analyzing the findings. Over time, this process became part of the conceptual framework of all nursing curricula and is included in the legal definition of nursing in the Nurse Practice Acts of most states. After years of study, use, and refinement, the three-step process was expanded to five steps: (1) assessment (systematic collection of data relating to clients and their problems and needs), (2) diagnosis (analysis and interpretation of data), (3) planning (prioritizing needs, identifying goals, and choosing solutions), (4) implementation (putting the plan into action), and (5) evaluation (assessing the effectiveness of the plan and changing the plan as indicated by current needs). All five steps are central to nursing actions and the delivery of high-quality, individualized client care in any setting.

When a client enters the healthcare system, the nurse uses the steps of the nursing process to work toward achieving desired outcomes and goals identified for the client. The effectiveness of the plan of care is evaluated by ascertaining whether or not the desired outcomes and goals have been attained (client's problems and needs have been resolved) or whether problems remain at the time of discharge. If problems are unresolved, plans need to be made for further follow-up, including assessment, additional problem and need identification, alteration of desired outcomes and goals, and changes in interventions in the next care setting.

Although some nurses view the nursing process as separate, progressive steps, the elements are actually interrelated. Taken together, they form a continuous circle of thought and action throughout the client's contact with the healthcare system. The process combines all the skills of critical thinking and good nursing care because it creates a method of active problem-solving that is both dynamic and cyclic. Figure 2.1 demonstrates the way this cyclic process works.

As we learned more about diagnostic reasoning and critical thinking, some scholars proposed a new model to describe what nurses do, focusing more on consumer outcomes than nursing tasks. With this emphasis in mind, the 1995 Social Policy Statement of the American Nurses Association (ANA) increased the focus on nursing care outcomes. Through ongoing research into the nature of thinking and reasoning, the conception of the nursing process continues to be redefined (Pesut & Herman, 1999).

A number of years ago, implementation of prospective and capitated payment plans moved a greater portion of healthcare delivery away from acute care hospitals into the community, with an emphasis on multifaceted free-standing care centers and home health services. Standards of care such as those published by the American Association of Critical-Care Nurses (AACN) and the Joint Commission (formerly Joint Commission on Accreditation of Healthcare Organizations [JCAHO]) emphasized that in every healthcare environment, nursing must meet standards that specified parameters for client assessment, monitoring, and documentation of care.

It had become apparent that nurses needed a common framework of communication and documentation so that their contribution to healthcare was recognized as essential and remunerated accordingly. At the very least, nursing required a commonality of terms describing practice so that it was visible in healthcare databases (Aquilino, 2000; Delany, 2000).

Through the years, the "what" and "how" of the work of nursing had been partially explained in a number of publications that helped operationalize the work of nursing. The ANA Social Policy Statement (1980) defined nursing as the "diagnosis and treatment of human responses to actual and potential health problems," providing a framework for understanding nursing's relationship with society and nursing's obligations to those receiving nursing care. In 1991, the ANA *Standards of Clinical Nursing Practice* described the client

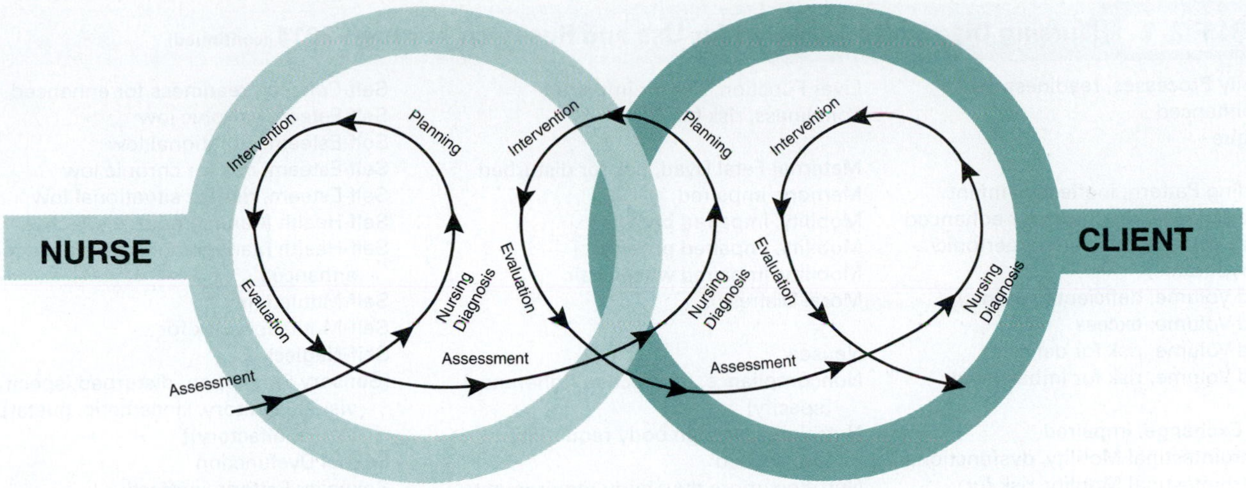

Figure 2.1 Diagram of the nursing process. The steps of the nursing process are interrelated, forming a continuous circle of thought and action that is both dynamic and cyclic.

care process and standards for professional performance, providing impetus and support for the development and use of nursing diagnosis in the practice setting. Finally, NANDA International (formerly North American Nursing Diagnosis Association) initiated research and intensified the work (ongoing for more than 30 years) of identifying client problems and needs for which nurses are accountable.

The linkage of nursing diagnoses to specific nursing interventions and client outcomes led to the development of a number of standardized nursing languages, for instance, the Omaha System, Clinical Care Classification (formerly Home Healthcare Classification), Ozbolt Patient Care Data Set (now retired), and Perioperative Minimum Data Set. The purpose of these languages is to help ensure continuity of appropriate cost-effective nursing care for the client regardless of setting. This is accomplished in part through enhanced communication, standardization of the process of evaluating the care provided, and facilitation of documentation.

Today, NANDA-I continues the development of nursing diagnosis labels (Table 2.1), which are complemented by the Iowa Intervention Project: Nursing Interventions Classification (NIC) and the Iowa Outcomes Project: Nursing Outcomes Classification (NOC). NIC directs our focus to the content and process of nursing care by identifying and standardizing the care activities nurses perform, and NOC describes client outcomes that are responsive to nursing intervention and develops corresponding measurement scales. Combined, these three standardized languages (NNN) form a single language describing client problems or needs, nursing actions, and outcomes for evaluation of the care provided.

TABLE 2.1 Nursing Diagnoses Accepted for Use and Research Through 2014

Activity Intolerance [specify level]
Activity Intolerance, risk for
Activity Planning, ineffective
Activity Planning, risk for ineffective
Adverse Reaction to Iodinated Contrast Media, risk for
Airway Clearance, ineffective
Allergy Response, risk for
Anxiety [specify level]
Aspiration, risk for
Attachment, risk for impaired
Autonomic Dysreflexia
Autonomic Dysreflexia, risk for

Behavior, disorganized infant
Behavior, readiness for enhanced organized infant
Behavior, risk for disorganized infant
Bleeding, risk for
Blood Glucose Level, risk for unstable
Body Image, disturbed
Body Temperature, risk for imbalanced
Breast Milk, insufficient
Breastfeeding, ineffective
Breastfeeding, interrupted
Breastfeeding, readiness for enhanced
Breathing Pattern, ineffective

Cardiac Output, decreased
Caregiver Role Strain
Caregiver Role Strain, risk for
Childbearing Process, ineffective
Childbearing Process, readiness for enhanced
Childbearing Process, risk for ineffective
Comfort, impaired
Comfort, readiness for enhanced
Communication, impaired verbal
Communication, readiness for enhanced
Confusion, acute
Confusion, risk for acute
Confusion, chronic
Constipation
Constipation, perceived
Constipation, risk for
Contamination
Contamination, risk for
Coping, compromised family
Coping, defensive
Coping, disabled family
Coping, ineffective
Coping, ineffective community
Coping, readiness for enhanced
Coping, readiness for enhanced community
Coping, readiness for enhanced family

Death Anxiety
Decision Making, readiness for enhanced
Decisional Conflict (specify)
Denial, ineffective
Dentition, impaired
Development, risk for delayed
Diarrhea
Disuse Syndrome, risk for
Diversional Activity, deficient
Dry Eye, risk for

Electrolyte Imbalance, risk for
Energy Field, disturbed
Environmental Interpretation Syndrome, impaired

Failure to Thrive, adult
Falls, risk for
Family Processes, dysfunctional
Family Processes, interrupted

(continues on page 6)

TABLE 2.1 Nursing Diagnoses Accepted for Use and Research Through 2014 (continued)

Family Processes, readiness for enhanced
Fatigue
Fear
Feeding Pattern, ineffective infant
Fluid Balance, readiness for enhanced
[Fluid Volume, deficient hypertonic/hypotonic]
Fluid Volume, deficient [isotonic]
Fluid Volume, excess
Fluid Volume, risk for deficient
Fluid Volume, risk for imbalanced

Gas Exchange, impaired
Gastrointestinal Motility, dysfunctional
Gastrointestinal Motility, risk for dysfunctional
Gastrointestinal Perfusion, risk for ineffective
Grieving
Grieving, complicated
Grieving, risk for complicated
Growth, risk for disproportionate
Growth and Development, delayed

Health, deficient community
Health Behavior, risk-prone
Health Maintenance, ineffective
Home Maintenance, impaired
Hope, readiness for enhanced
Hopelessness
Human Dignity, risk for compromised
Hyperthermia
Hypothermia

Immunization Status, readiness for enhanced
Impulse Control, ineffective
Incontinence, bowel
Incontinence, functional urinary
Incontinence, overflow urinary
Incontinence, reflex urinary
Incontinence, stress urinary
Incontinence, urge urinary
Incontinence, risk for urge urinary
Infection, risk for
Injury, risk for
Insomnia
Intracranial Adaptive Capacity, decreased

Jaundice, neonatal
Jaundice, risk for neonatal

Knowledge, deficient [Learning Need] [specify]
Knowledge [specify], readiness for enhanced

Latex Allergy Response
Latex Allergy Response, risk for
Lifestyle, sedentary
Liver Function, risk for impaired
Loneliness, risk for

Maternal-Fetal Dyad, risk for disturbed
Memory, impaired
Mobility, impaired bed
Mobility, impaired physical
Mobility, impaired wheelchair
Moral Distress

Nausea
Noncompliance, [ineffective Adherence] [specify]
Nutrition: less than body requirements, imbalanced
Nutrition: more than body requirements, imbalanced
Nutrition: more than body requirements, risk for imbalanced
Nutrition, readiness for enhanced

Oral Mucous Membrane, impaired

Pain, acute
Pain, chronic
Parenting, impaired
Parenting, readiness for enhanced
Parenting, risk for impaired
Perioperative Positioning Injury, risk for
Peripheral Neurovascular Dysfunction, risk for
Personal Identity, disturbed
Personal Identity, risk for disturbed
Poisoning, risk for
Post-Trauma Syndrome [specify stage]
Post-Trauma Syndrome, risk for
Power, readiness for enhanced
Powerlessness [specify level]
Powerlessness, risk for
Protection, ineffective

Rape-Trauma Syndrome
Relationship, ineffective
Relationship, readiness for enhanced
Relationship, risk for ineffective
Religiosity, impaired
Religiosity, readiness for enhanced
Religiosity, risk for impaired
Relocation Stress Syndrome
Relocation Stress Syndrome, risk for
Renal Perfusion, risk for ineffective
Resilience, impaired individual
Resilience, readiness for enhanced
Resilience, risk for compromised
Role Conflict, parental
Role Performance, ineffective

Self-Care, readiness for enhanced
Self-Care Deficit, bathing
Self-Care Deficit, dressing
Self-Care Deficit, feeding
Self-Care Deficit, toileting
Self-Concept, readiness for enhanced
Self-Esteem, chronic low
Self-Esteem, situational low
Self-Esteem, risk for chronic low
Self-Esteem, risk for situational low
Self-Health Management, ineffective
Self-Health Management, readiness for enhanced
Self-Mutilation
Self-Mutilation, risk for
Self-Neglect
[Sensory Perception, disturbed (specify: visual, auditory, kinesthetic, gustatory, tactile, olfactory)]
Sexual Dysfunction
Sexuality Pattern, ineffective
Shock, risk for
Skin Integrity, impaired
Skin Integrity, risk for impaired
Sleep, readiness for enhanced
Sleep Deprivation
Sleep Pattern, disturbed
Social Interaction, impaired
Social Isolation
Sorrow, chronic
Spiritual Distress
Spiritual Distress, risk for
Spiritual Well-Being, readiness for enhanced
Stress Overload
Sudden Infant Death Syndrome, risk for
Suffocation, risk for
Suicide, risk for
Surgical Recovery, delayed
Swallowing, impaired

Therapeutic Regimen Management, ineffective family
Thermal Injury, risk for
Thermoregulation, ineffective
Tissue Integrity, impaired
Tissue Perfusion, ineffective peripheral
Tissue Perfusion, risk for decreased cardiac
Tissue Perfusion, risk for ineffective cerebral
Tissue Perfusion, risk for ineffective peripheral
Transfer Ability, impaired
Trauma, risk for

Unilateral Neglect
Urinary Elimination, impaired
Urinary Elimination, readiness for enhanced
Urinary Retention [acute/chronic]

Vascular Trauma, risk for
Ventilation, impaired spontaneous
Ventilatory Weaning Response, dysfunctional
Violence, risk for other-directed
Violence, risk for self-directed

Walking, impaired
Wandering [specify sporadic or continual]

[ ] author recommendations

Herdman, T.H. (Ed.). Nursing Diagnoses—Definitions and Classification 2012–2014. Copyright © 2012, 1994–2012 NANDA International. Used by arrangement with John Wiley & Sons Limited. In order to make safe and effective judgments using NANDA-I nursing diagnoses it is essential that nurses refer to the definitions and defining characteristics of the diagnoses listed in this work.

Planning Care

Medicine and nursing, as well as other healthcare disciplines, are interrelated, and therefore the developments in each discipline have implications for the others. This interrelationship allows for exchange of information and ideas and for development of plans of care that include all data pertinent to the individual client and family. In this book, the plans of care contain not only the actions initiated by medical and nursing orders but also the coordination of care provided by all related healthcare disciplines. The nurse is often the person responsible for coordinating these various activities into a comprehensive functional plan, which is essential in providing holistic care for the client. Although independent nursing actions are an integral part of this process, collaborative actions are also present based on the medical regimen or orders from other disciplines participating in the care of the client. We believe that nursing is an essential part of collaborative practice, and as such, nursing has a responsibility and accountability in every collaborative problem in which the nurse interacts with the client. The educational background and expertise of the nurse, standing protocols, delegation of tasks, the use of care partners, and the area of practice—for example, rural or urban, acute care or community care settings—influence whether an intervention is actually an independent nursing function or requires collaboration.

The well-developed plan of care communicates the client's past and present health status and current needs to all members of the healthcare team involved in providing care. It identifies problems solved and those yet to be solved, can provide information about approaches that have been successful, and notes patterns of client responses to interventions. In legal terms, the plan of care documents client care in areas of liability, accountability, and quality improvement. It also provides a mechanism to help ensure continuity of care when the client leaves a care setting while still needing services.

Components of the Plan of Care

The critical element for providing effective planned nursing care is its relevance as identified in client assessments. ANA's 2010 *Nursing: Scope and Standards of Practice* determined that client assessment is indicated in, but not limited to, the following areas and abilities: physical, emotional, sexual, psychosocial, cultural, spiritual/transpersonal, cognitive, functional, age-related, economic, and environmental. These assessments, combined with the results of medical findings and diagnostic studies, are documented in the client database and form the foundation for development of the client's plan of care. For each plan of care presented in this book, pathophysiology, etiology, statistics, and a glossary are provided. A client assessment database is then created from information that would likely be obtained from the history and physical examination. A separate table defining diagnostic studies often associated with the condition provides information explaining usual findings. Next, nursing priorities and discharge goals are simply stated and represent a general ranking system for the nursing diagnoses in the plan of care. These can be reworded and reorganized, along with their timelines, to create short- and long-term goals. Nursing diagnosis statements are presented, which include possible related or risk factors (etiology) and corresponding defining characteristics (signs and symptoms or cues) as appropriate. Desired client outcomes are then identified and followed by appropriate independent and collaborative interventions with accompanying rationales.

Client Database

In this book, each selected medical condition has an accompanying client database that includes subjective ("may report") and objective ("may exhibit") data that would likely be collected through the history-taking interview, physical assessment, diagnostic studies, and review of prior records. The client database is organized within the 13 categories of the Diagnostic Divisions. A sample medical/surgical assessment tool, definitions of the Divisions, and a client situation are included in Chapter 3. As the plan of care is developed, the nurse will also individualize it to the client's situation.

Interviewing

Interviewing the client and significant other(s) provides data that the nurse obtains through conversation and observation. This information includes the individual's perceptions, that is, what the client perceives to be a problem or need and typically what he or she wants to share. Data may be collected during one or more contact periods and should include all relevant information. All participants in the interview process need to know that collected data are used in planning the client's care. Organizing and updating the data assists in the ongoing identification of client care needs and nursing diagnoses.

Physical Assessment

During information gathering, the nurse exercises perceptual and observational skills, assessing the client through the senses of sight, hearing, touch, and smell. The duration and depth of any physical assessment depend on the current condition of the client and the urgency of the situation, but it usually includes inspection, palpation, percussion, and auscultation. In this book, the physical assessment data are presented within the client database as objective data.

Diagnostic Studies

A separate section for lab tests and other diagnostic studies describes the test and the usual findings. Some tests are used to diagnose disease, whereas others are useful in following the course of a disease or in adjusting therapies. The nurse needs to be aware of significant test results that require reporting to the physician and/or initiation of specific nursing interventions. In many cases, the relationship of the test to the pathological physiology is clear, but in other cases it is not. This is the result of the interrelationship between various organs and body systems.

Nursing Priorities

In this book, nursing priorities are listed in a certain order to facilitate the linking and ranking of selected associated nursing diagnoses that appear in the plan of care guidelines. In any given client situation, nursing priorities are based on the client's specific needs and can vary from minute to minute. A nursing diagnosis that is a priority today may be less of a priority tomorrow, depending on the fluctuating physical and psychosocial condition of the client or the client's changing responses to the existing condition and/or treatment.

An example of nursing priorities for a client diagnosed with severe hypertension would include the following:

1. Maintain or enhance cardiovascular functioning.
2. Prevent complications.
3. Provide information about disease process, prognosis, and treatment regimen.
4. Support active client control or management of the condition.

Discharge Goals

Once the nursing priorities are determined, the next step is to establish goals of treatment. In this book, each medical condition has established discharge goals that are broadly stated and reflect the desired general status of the client on discharge or transfer to another care setting.

Discharge goals for a client with severe hypertension would include the following:

1. Blood pressure within acceptable limits for individual.
2. Cardiovascular and systemic complications prevented or minimized.
3. Disease process, prognosis, and therapeutic regimen understood.
4. Necessary lifestyle and behavioral changes initiated.
5. Plan in place to meet needs after discharge.

NANDA

Nursing Diagnosis (Problem and Need Identification)

Nursing diagnoses are a uniform way of identifying, focusing on, and dealing with specific client needs and responses to actual or high-risk problems and life processes. Nursing diagnosis labels (see Table 2.1) provide a format for expressing the problem-identification portion of the nursing process. In 1989, NANDA developed a taxonomy, or classification scheme, to categorize and classify nursing diagnostic labels. (This was replaced by a new taxonomy in 2000.) The NANDA definition of nursing diagnosis approved in 1990 further clarified the second step of the nursing process (i.e., diagnosis or problem and need identification). The definition of nursing diagnosis developed by NANDA is presented in Box 2.1.

There are several steps involved in the process of problem and need identification. Integrating these steps provides a systematic approach to accurately identifying nursing diagnoses using the process of critical thinking.

1. Collect a client database (nursing interview, physical assessment, and diagnostic studies) combined with information collected by other healthcare providers.
2. Review and analyze the client data.
3. Synthesize the gathered client data as a whole and then label the clinical judgment about the client's responses to these actual or high-risk problems and life processes.
4. Compare and contrast the relationships of clinical judgments with related factors and defining characteristics for the selected nursing diagnosis. This step is crucial to choosing and validating the appropriate nursing diagnosis label that will be used to create a specific client diagnostic statement.
5. Combine the nursing diagnosis with the related factors and define characteristics, or risk factors, to create the client diagnostic statement. For example, the diagnostic statement for a paraplegic client with a pressure ulcer could read as follows: "impaired Skin Integrity related to mechanical factors (pressure, shearing forces), impaired circulation, and impaired sensation evidenced by destruction of skin layers—sacral area."

Box 2.1 NANDA-I Definition of Nursing Diagnosis

A nursing diagnosis is a clinical judgment about individual, family, or community experiences/responses to actual or potential health problems/life processes. A nursing diagnosis provides the basis for selection of nursing interventions to achieve outcomes for which the nurse is accountable.

The nursing diagnosis is as correct as the present information allows because it is supported by the immediate data collected. It documents the client's situation at the present time and should reflect changes as they occur in the client's condition. Accurate need identification and diagnostic labeling provide the basis for selecting nursing interventions.

The nursing diagnosis may be a physical or a psychosocial response. Physical nursing diagnoses include those that pertain to physical processes, such as "circulation (risk for ineffective Renal Perfusion), ventilation (impaired Gas Exchange), and elimination (Constipation)." Psychosocial nursing diagnoses include those that pertain to the mind ("acute Confusion"), emotions ("Fear"), or lifestyle and relationships ("ineffective Role Performance"). Unlike medical diagnoses, nursing diagnoses change as the client progresses through various stages of illness and/or maladaptation to resolution of the problem or to the conclusion of the condition. Each decision the nurse makes is time dependent, and with additional information gathered at a later time, decisions may change. For example, the initial problems and needs for a client undergoing cardiac surgery may be "acute Pain, decreased Cardiac Output, risk for ineffective Breathing Pattern, and risk for Infection." As the client progresses, problems and needs are likely to shift to "Activity Intolerance, deficient Knowledge, and Self-Care Deficit."

Diagnostic reasoning is used to ensure the accuracy of the client diagnostic statement. The defining characteristics and related factors associated with the chosen nursing diagnosis are reviewed and compared with the client data.

If the diagnosis is not consistent with at least two or more cues, additional data may be required or another nursing diagnosis considered.

Desired Client Outcomes

The nurse identifies expected outcomes for a plan of care individualized for a specific client (ANA, 2010). A desired client outcome is defined as the result of achievable nursing interventions and client responses that is desired by the client or caregiver and attainable within a defined time period, given the current situation and resources. These desired outcomes are the measurable steps toward achieving the previously established discharge goals and are used to evaluate the client's response to nursing interventions. (The fifth step of the nursing process, evaluation, is addressed in the sample client situation provided in Chapter 3.) Useful desired client outcomes must have the following characteristics:

1. Be specific
2. Be realistic or achievable
3. Be measurable
4. Indicate a definite time frame for achievement or review
5. Consider client's desires and resources

Desired client outcomes are created by listing items and behaviors that can be observed or heard. They are monitored to determine whether an acceptable outcome has been achieved within a specified time frame. Action verbs and time frames are used, for example, "client will ambulate, using cane, within 24 hours of surgery." The action verbs describe the client's behavior to be evaluated. Time frames are dependent on the client's projected or anticipated length of stay or period of care, often determined by diagnosis-related group (DRG) classification and considering the presence of complications or extenuating circumstances, such as age, debilitating disease process, and so on. The ongoing work of NOC in identifying 490 outcomes now also addresses client groups or aggregates. When using NOC, the outcomes are listed in general terms such as "Ambulation," and 16 indicators have been identified for this outcome that can be measured by a five-point Likert-type scale, ranging from "severely compromised" to "not compromised." This facilitates tracking clients across care settings and can demonstrate client progress even when outcomes are not met.

When outcomes are properly written, they provide direction for planning and validating the selected nursing interventions. Consider the two following client outcomes: "Client will identify individual nutritional needs within 36 hours" and ". . . formulate a dietary plan based on identified nutritional needs within 72 hours." Based on the clarity of these outcomes, the nurse can select nursing interventions to ensure that the client's dietary knowledge is assessed, individual needs identified, and nutritional education presented. Often, the client outcomes identified are not unique to nursing because care is provided in a team approach with other disciplines. However, the NOC indicators for outcomes are generally more sensitive to nursing interventions. Other team members can use the majority of NOC labels and identify different indicators relative to their specialty focus to demonstrate their contribution to client improvement or to track deterioration. In this book, the identified outcomes in each plan of care are stated in more specific terms but are organized by using possible NOC labels (which are boxed to call attention to this language). The nurse is directed to the NOC work (Morehead, 2013) when choosing to use this specific language.

Planning (Goals and Actions/Interventions)

Once the outcomes are identified, the nurse develops a plan that prescribes strategies and alternatives to achieve the expected outcomes (ANA, 2010). Nursing strategies are interventions and actions to be carried out or facilitated by nurses to achieve specific behaviors expected from the client. These actions and interventions are selected to assist the client in achieving the stated desired client outcomes and discharge goals. The expectation is that the prescribed behavior will benefit the client and family in a predictable way related to the identified problem or need and chosen outcomes. These interventions have the intent of individualizing care by meeting a specific client need and should incorporate identified client strengths when possible.

Nursing interventions should be specific and clearly stated, beginning with an action verb indicating what the nurse is expected to do. Qualifiers expressing how, when, where, time, frequency, and amount provide the content of the planned activity, for example, "Assist as needed with self-care activities each morning"; "Record respiratory and pulse rates before, during, and after activity"; and "Instruct family in postdischarge care."

The NIC project has identified 554 interventions (both direct and indirect) that are stated in general terms, such as "Respiratory Monitoring." Each label has a varied number of activities that may be chosen to accomplish the intervention. The interventions encompass a broad range of nursing practice, with some requiring specialized training or advanced certification. Others may be appropriate for delegation to other care providers (for example, licensed practical nurses [LPNs] or vocational nurses [LVNs], nursing assistants, and unlicensed personnel) but still require planning and evaluation by registered nurses. In this text, these sample NIC labels are boxed to help the user identify how they can be used. As with the NOC labels, the nurse is directed to the NIC work (Bulechek, 2013) when choosing to use the language in planning client care.

This book divides the nursing interventions and actions into independent (nurse initiated) and collaborative (initiated by and/or performed in conjunction with other care providers) under the appropriate NIC labels. Examples of these two different professionally initiated actions are as follows:

- Independent: Provide calm, restful surroundings, minimize environmental activity and noise, and limit numbers of visitors and length of stay.
- Collaborative: Administer anti-anxiety medication as indicated.

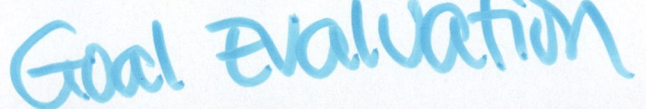

Rationale

Although rationales do not appear on regular plans of care, they are included in this book to assist the student and practicing nurse in associating the pathophysiological and psychological principles with the selected nursing intervention. This will help the nurse determine whether an intervention is appropriate for a specific client.

Conclusion

This book is intended to facilitate the application of the nursing process and the use of nursing diagnosis in medical and surgical clients. (Plan of care guides for maternity, newborn, and psychiatric clients are available on a supporting Web site.) Each plan of care guideline was designed to provide generalized information on the associated medical condition. The guidelines can be modified either by using portions of the information provided or by adding more client care information to the existing guides. The plan of care guidelines were developed using the NANDA-I recommendations, except in a few bracketed examples where the authors believed more clarification and enhancement were required. The ongoing controversy over the validity of the nursing diagnosis of "deficient Knowledge" approved by NANDA-I is one example where further clarification was added. The term "Learning Need" has been added to the nursing diagnosis label. Also, on a few occasions, some diagnoses, such as "Anxiety/Fear," have been combined for convenience; the combination indicates that two or more factors may be involved, and the nurse can then choose the most appropriate diagnosis for a specific client. We recognize that not all of the nursing diagnoses approved by NANDA-I have been used in the plan of care guidelines, but we hope that these guidelines will assist you in determining your clients' needs, outcomes, and nursing interventions.

Next, Chapter 3 will assist you in applying and adapting theory to practice.

CHAPTER 3

Critical Thinking: Adaptation of Theory to Practice

Critical thinking is defined as the "intellectually disciplined process of actively and skillfully conceptualizing, applying, analyzing, synthesizing, and evaluating information gathered from or generated by observation, experience, reflection, reasoning, or communication, as a guide to belief and action" (Scriven, 1987). In short, critical thinking is self-directed, self-disciplined, self-monitored, and self-corrective thinking that also entails effective communication with others in figuring out solutions to complex problems (Paul, 2008). It requires cognitive, psychomotor, and affective skills in order to use the tools of a comprehensive knowledge base, the nursing process, and established standards of care, as well as nursing research, to analyze data and plan a course of action based on new insights and conclusions. To this end, the nurse defines the problem, selects pertinent information for the solution, recognizes stated and unstated assumptions, formulates and selects relevant and promising hypotheses, draws conclusions, and judges the validity of the inferences (Hickman, 1993). Although critical thinking skills are used in all aspects of nursing practice, they are most evident when assessment data are analyzed to identify relevant information, make decisions about client needs, and develop an individualized plan of care. Therefore, client assessment is the foundation on which identification of individual needs, responses, and problems is based. Nurses of the future will still manage and interpret data and evaluate nursing activities and interventions. They will also need competencies in case and financial management, healthcare policy and economics, legislative outcomes, and research methods. Additionally, they will need delegation skills and the ability to think and reason across diverse settings in which they will practice (Pesut & Herman, 1999).

To facilitate the steps of assessing and diagnosing in the nursing process and to aid in the critical thinking process, assessment databases have been developed (Fig. 3.1) that use a nursing focus instead of the traditional medical approach of a review of systems. To achieve this nursing focus, we have grouped NANDA International (NANDA-I) nursing diagnoses into related categories titled Diagnostic Divisions (Box 3.1). These categories reflect a blending of theories, primarily Maslow's Hierarchy of Needs and a self-care philosophy. These divisions serve as the framework or outline for data collection and direct the nurse to the corresponding nursing diagnosis labels.

Because these divisions are based on human responses and needs and are not specific systems, data may be recorded in more than one area. For this reason, the nurse is encouraged to keep an open mind and to collect as much information as possible before choosing the nursing diagnosis label. The results (synthesis) of the collected data are written concisely (client diagnostic statements) to best reflect the client's situation.

From the specific data recorded in the database, the related or risk factors (etiology) and signs and symptoms can be identified, and an individualized client diagnostic statement can be formulated according to the problem, etiology, and signs and symptoms (PES) format to accurately represent the client's situation. For example, the diagnostic statement may read as follows: "ineffective peripheral Tissue Perfusion related to smoking, hypertension, diabetes mellitus, evidenced by diminished pulses, pale and cool feet, paresthesia of feet when walks 1/4 mile."

Outcomes are identified to facilitate choosing appropriate interventions and to serve as evaluators of both nursing care and client response. In addition to being measurable, outcomes must be achievable and desired by the client. These outcomes also form the framework for documentation.

Interventions are designed to specify the action of the nurse, the client, and significant other(s). They are not all-inclusive because such basic nursing actions as "bathe the client" or "notify the physician of changes" have been omitted. It is expected that these actions are included in routine client care. On occasion, controversial issues or treatments are presented for the sake of information and because different therapies may be used in different care settings or geographic locations.

Interventions need to promote the client's movement toward health and independence. This requires involvement of the client in his or her own care, including participation in decisions about the care activities and projected outcomes. This promotes client responsibility, negating the idea that healthcare providers control clients' lives.

(text continues on page 19)

ADULT MEDICAL/SURGICAL ASSESSMENT TOOL

General Information

Name: ____________________

Age: ________ DOB: ________ Gender: ________ Race: ________

Admission Date: ________ Time: ________ From: ________

Reason for this admission (primary concern): ________

Cultural concerns (relating to healthcare decisions, religious concerns, pain, childbirth, family involvement, communication, etc): ________

Source of information: ________ Reliability (1–4 with 4 = very reliable): ________

Activity/Rest

Subjective (Reports)

Occupation: ________

Leisure time/diversional activities: ________

Able to participate in usual activities/hobbies: ________

Ambulatory: ____ Gait (describe): ________

Activity level (sedentary to very active): ________

Daily exercise/type: ________

Muscle mass/tone/strength (e.g., normal, increased, decreased): ________ Change: ________

History of problems/limitations imposed by condition (e.g., immobility, can't transfer, weakness, breathlessness): ________

Feelings (e.g., exhaustion, restlessness, can't concentrate, dissatisfaction): ________

Developmental factors (e.g., delayed/age): ________

Sleep: Hours: ____ Naps: ____ Aids: ____

Insomnia: ____ Related to: ________

Difficulty falling asleep: ________

Difficulty staying asleep: ________

Rested on awakening: ________

Excessive grogginess: ________

Sleeps on more than one pillow: ________

Bedtime rituals: ________

Relaxation techniques: ________

Oxygen use (type): ________ When used: ________

Medications or herbals for/affecting sleep: ________

Objective (Exhibits)

Observed response to activity: Heart rate: ________

Rhythm (reg/irreg): ________

Blood pressure: ________

Respiration rate: ________

Pulse oximetry: ________

Mental status (i.e., cognitive impairment, withdrawn/lethargic): ________

Neuromuscular assessment:

Muscle mass/tone: ________

Posture (e.g., normal, stooped, curved spine): ________

Tremors: ________ (location): ________

ROM: ________

Strength: ________

Deformity: ________

Uses mobility aid (list): ________

Circulation

Subjective (Reports)

History of/treatment for (date): High blood pressure: ________

Brain injury: ________ Stroke: ________

Heart problems/surgery: ________ Palpitations: ________

Syncope: ________ Rheumatic fever: ________

Cough/hemoptysis: ________ Blood clots: ________

Bleeding tendencies/episodes: ________ (location): ________

Pain in legs w/activity ________

Extremities: Numbness: ________ (location): ________

Tingling: ________ (location): ________

Slow healing (describe): ________

Change in frequency/amount of urine: ________

History of spinal cord injury/dysreflexia episodes: ________

Medications/herbals: ________

Objective (Exhibits)

Color (e.g., pale, cyanotic, jaundiced, mottled, ruddy):

Skin: ________ Mucous membranes: ________ Lips: ________

Nail beds: ________ Conjunctiva: ________ Sclera: ________

Skin moisture (e.g., dry, diaphoretic): ________

BP: Lying: R________ L________ Sitting: R________ L________

Standing: R________ L________

Pulse pressure: ________ Auscultatory gap: ________

Pulses (palpated 1–4 strength): Carotid: ________ Temporal: ________

Jugular: ________ Radial: ________ Femoral: ________ Popliteal: ________

Post-tibial: ________ Dorsalis pedis: ________

Cardiac (palpation): Thrill: ________ Heaves: ________

Heart sounds (auscultation): Rate: ________ Rhythm: ________

Quality: ________ Friction rub: ________

Murmur (describe location/sounds): ________

Vascular bruit (location): ________ Jugular vein distention: ________

Breath sounds (location/describe): ________

Extremities: Temperature: ________ Color: ________

Capillary refill (1–3 sec): ________ Homan's sign: ________

Varicosities (location): ________

Distribution/quality of hair: ________

Edema (location/severity +1– +4): ________

Trophic skin changes: ________ Nail abnormalities: ________

Ego Integrity

Subjective (Reports)

Relationship status: ______
Expression of concerns (e.g., financial, lifestyle, relationship, or role changes): ______
Stress factors: ______
Usual ways of handling stress: ______
Expression of feelings: Anger: ______ Anxiety: ______
Fear: ______ Grief: ______ Helplessness: ______
Hopelessness: ______ Powerlessness: ______
Cultural factors/ethnic ties: ______
Religious affiliation: ______ Active/practicing: ______
Practices prayer/meditation: ______
Religious/spiritual concerns: ______
Desires clergy visit: ______
Expression of sense of connectedness/harmony with self and others: ______
Medications/herbals: ______

Objective (Exhibits)

Emotional status (check those that apply):
Calm: ______ Anxious: ______
Angry: ______ Withdrawn: ______
Fearful: ______ Irritable: ______
Restive: ______ Euphoric: ______
Observed body language: ______
Observed physiological responses (e.g., palpitations, crying, change in voice quality/volume): ______
Changes in energy field:
Temperature: ______
Color: ______
Distribution: ______
Movement: ______
Sounds: ______

Elimination

Subjective (Reports)

Usual bowel elimination pattern: ______
Character of stool (e.g., hard, soft, liquid): ______
Stool color (e.g., brown, black, yellow, clay colored, tarry): ______
Date of last BM and character of stool: ______
History of bleeding: ______ Hemorrhoids/fistula: ______
Constipation: acute: ______ or chronic: ______
Diarrhea: acute: ______ or chronic: ______
Bowel incontinence: ______
Laxative: ______ (how often): ______
Enema/suppository: ______ (how often): ______
Usual voiding pattern and character of urine: ______
Difficulty voiding: ______ Urgency: ______
Frequency: ______ Retention: ______
Bladder spasms: ______ Pain/Burning: ______
Urinary incontinence (type/time of day usually occurs): ______
History of kidney/bladder disease: ______
Diuretic use: ______ Other medications: ______
Herbals: ______

Objective (Exhibits)

Abdomen (auscultation): Bowel sounds (location/type): ______
Abdomen (palpation): Soft/firm: ______
Tenderness/pain (quadrant location): ______
Distention: ______ Palpable mass/location: ______
Size/girth: ______ CVA tenderness: ______
Bladder palpable: ______ Overflow voiding: ______
Residual urine per scan: ______
Rectal sphincter tone (describe): ______
Hemorrhoids/fistulas: ______ Stool in rectum: ______
Impaction: ______ Occult blood (+ or −): ______
Presence/use of catheter or continence devices: ______
Ostomy appliances (describe appliance and location): ______

Food/Fluid

Subjective (Reports)

Usual diet (type): ______
Calorie, carbohydrate, protein, fat intake (g/day): ______
# of meals daily: ______ Snacks (number/time consumed): ______
Dietary pattern/content:
B: ______
L: ______
D: ______
Snacks: ______
Last meal consumed/content: ______
Food preferences: ______
Food allergies/intolerances: ______
Cultural or religious food preparation concerns/prohibitions: ______
Usual appetite: ______ Change in appetite: ______
Usual weight: ______
Unexpected/undesired weight loss or gain: ______
Nausea/vomiting: ______ (related to): ______
Heartburn/indigestion: ______
(related to): ______ (relieved by): ______
Chewing/swallowing problems: ______
Gag/swallow reflex present: ______

Objective (Exhibits)

Current weight: ______ Height: ______
Body build: ______ Body fat %: ______
Skin turgor (e.g., firm, supple, dehydrated): ______
Mucous membranes (moist/dry): ______
Edema: Generalized: ______
Dependent: ______
Feet/ankles: ______
Periorbital: ______
Abdominal/ascites: ______
Jugular vein distention: ______
Breath sounds (auscultate)/location: ______
Faint/distant: ______ Crackles: ______ Wheezes: ______
Condition of teeth/gums: ______ Appearance of tongue: ______
Mucous membranes: ______
Abdomen: Bowel sounds (quadrant location/type): ______
Hernia/masses: ______
Urine S/A or Chemstix: ______
Blood glucose (Glucometer): ______

Food/Fluid (continued)

Subjective (Reports)

Facial injury/surgery: ______

Stroke/other neurological deficit: ______

Teeth: Normal: ___ Dentures (full/partial): ______

Loose/absent teeth/poor dental care: ______

Sore mouth/gums: ______

Dental hygiene practices: ______

Professional dental care/frequency: ______

Diabetes/type: _____ Controlled with diet/pills/insulin: ______

Vitamin/food supplements: ______

Medications/herbals: ______

Hygiene

Subjective (Reports)

Ability to carry out activities of daily living: ______

Independent/dependent (level 1 = no assistance needed to level 4 = completely dependent): ______

Mobility: ___ Assistance needed (describe): ______

Assistance provided by: ______

Equipment/prosthetic devices required: ______

Feeding: ___ Help with food preparation: ______

Help with eating utensils: ______

Hygiene: ___ Get supplies: ___ Wash body/body parts: ___

Regulate bath water temperature: ___ Get in/out alone: ___

Preferred time of personal care/bath: ______

Dressing: ___ Can select clothing: ___ Can dress self: ___

Needs assistance with(describe): ______

Toileting: ___ Can get to toilet/commode alone: ______

Needs assistance with (describe): ______

Objective (Exhibits)

General appearance: Manner of dress: ______

Grooming/personal habits: ______

Condition of hair/scalp: ______

Body odor: ______

Presence of vermin (e.g., lice, scabies): ______

Neurosensory

Subjective (Reports)

History of brain injury, trauma, stroke (residual effects): ___

Fainting spells/dizziness: ______

Headaches (location/type/frequency): ______

Tingling/numbness/weakness (location): ______

Seizures: ___ History or new onset: ______

Type (e.g., grand mal, partial): _____ Frequency: ______

Aura: _____ Postictal state: _____ How controlled: ___

Vision: Loss/changes in vision: _____ Date last exam: ___

Glaucoma: ___ Cataract: ___ Eye surgery (type/date): ___

Hearing loss: ___ Sudden or gradual: ______

Date last exam: ______

Sense of smell (changes): ______

Sense of taste (changes): ______

Other: ______

Objective (Exhibits)

Mental status (note duration of change):

Oriented/disoriented: Person: ______ Time: ______

Place: ______ Situation: ______

Check all that apply: Alert: ___ Drowsy: ___ Lethargic: ___

Stupor: __ Comatose: __ Cooperative: __ Agitated/Restless: __

Combative: ___ Follows commands: ______

Delusions (describe): _____ Hallucinations (describe): ______

Affect (describe): ______ Speech Pattern: ______

Memory: Recent: ______ Remote: ______

Pupil shape: ______ Size/reaction: R/L: ______

Facial droop: ______ Swallowing: ______

Hand grasp/release: R: ______ L: ______

Coordination: _____ Balance: _____ Walking: ______

Deep tendon reflexes (present/absent/location): ______

Tremors: _____ Paralysis (R/L): _____ Posturing: ______

Wears glasses: _____ Contacts: _____ Hearing aids: _____

Pain/Discomfort

Subjective (Reports)

Primary focus: ______ Location: ______

Intensity (use pain scale or pictures): ______

Quality (e.g., stabbing, aching, burning): ______

Radiation: _____ Duration: _____ Frequency: _____

Precipitating factors: ______

Relieving factors (including nonpharmaceuticals/therapies):

______

Associated symptoms (e.g., nausea, sleep problems):

______

Effect on daily activities: ______

Relationships: ______

Enjoyment of life: ______

Additional pain focus (describe): ______

Medications: ______ Herbals: ______

Objective (Exhibits)

Facial grimacing: _____ Guarding affected area: ______

Expressive behavior (e.g., crying, withdrawal, anger): ___

Narrowed focus: ______

Vital sign changes (acute pain):

BP: ______

Pulse: ______

Respirations: ______

Photosensitivity: ______

Employment: ______

Respiration

Subjective (Reports)

Dyspnea/related to: ____
Precipitating factors: ____ Relieving factors: ____
Airway clearance (e.g., spontaneous/device): ____
Cough (e.g., hard, persistent, croupy): ____
Produces sputum (describe color/character): ____
Requires suctioning: ____
History of (year): Bronchitis: ____ Asthma: ____
Emphysema: ____ Tuberculosis: ____
Recurrent pneumonia: ____
Exposure to noxious fumes/allergens, infectious agents/diseases, poisons/pesticides: ____
Smoker: ____ packs/day: ____ # pack-years: ____
Cigars: ____ Smokeless tobacoo: ____
Use of respiratory aids: ____ Oxygen (type/frequency): ____
Medications/herbals: ____

Objective (Exhibits)

Respirations (spontaneous/assisted): ____ Rate: ____
Depth: ____ Chest excursion (e.g., equal/unequal): ____
Use of accessory muscles: ____
Nasal flaring: ____ Fremitus: ____
Breath sounds (presence/absence; crackle, wheezes): ____
Egophony: ____
Skin/mucous membrane color (e.g., pale, cyanotic): ____
Clubbing of fingers: ____
Sputum characteristics: ____
Mentation (e.g., calm, anxious, restless): ____
Pulse oximetry: ____

Safety

Subjective (Reports)

Allergies/sensitivity (medications, foods, environment, latex, iodine): ____
Type of reaction: ____
Blood transfusion/number: ____ Date: ____
Reaction (describe): ____
Exposure to infectious diseases (e.g., measles, influenza, pink eye): ____
Exposure to pollution, toxins, poisons/pesticides, radiation: ____
(describe reactions): ____
Geographic areas lived in/recent travel: ____
Immunization history: Tetanus: ____ MMR: ____ Polio: ____
Influenza: ____ Pneumonia: ____ Hepatitis: ____ HPV: ____
Altered/suppressed immune system (infection cause): ____
History of sexually transmitted disease (date/type): ____
Testing: ____
High risk behaviors: ____
Uses seat belt regularly: ____ Helmets: ____
Other safety devices: ____
Workplace safety/health issues (describe): ____
Currently working: ____
Rate working conditions (e.g., safety, noise, heating, water, ventilation): ____
History of accidental injuries: ____
Fractures/dislocations: ____
Arthritis/unstable joints: ____ Back problems: ____
Skin problems (e.g., rashes, lesions, moles, breast lumps, enlarged nodes) (describe): ____
Delayed healing (describe): ____
Cognitive limitations (e.g., disoriented, confusion): ____
Sensory limitations (e.g., impaired vision/hearing, detecting heat/cold, taste, smell, touch): ____
Prostheses: ____ Ambulatory devices: ____
Violence (episodes or tendencies): ____

Objective (Exhibits)

Body temperature/method: (e.g., oral, temporal, tympanic): ____
Skin integrity (mark location on diagram): Scars: ____
Bruises: ____ Rashes: ____ Abrasions: ____
Lacerations: ____ Ulcerations: ____ Blisters: ____
Drainage: ____ Burns [degree/%]: ____

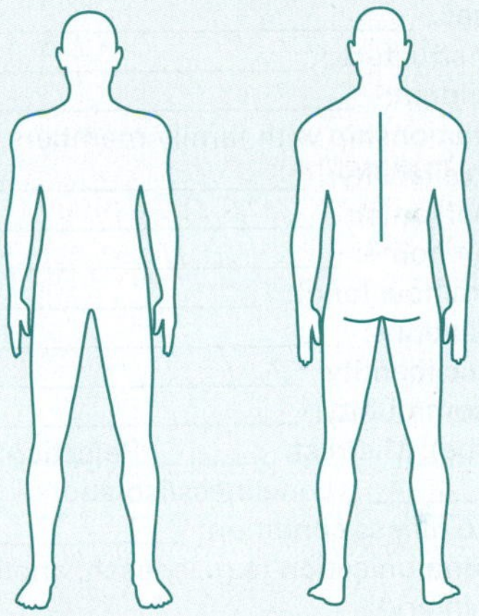

Musculoskeletal: General strength: ____ Muscle tone: ____
Gait: ____ ROM: ____ Paresthesia/paralysis: ____
Results of testing (e.g., cultures, immune function, TB, hepatitis): ____

Sexuality [Component of Social Interaction]

Subjective (Reports)

Sexually active: ____ Monogamous: ____
Birth control method: ____ Use of condoms: ____
Sexual concerns/difficulties (e.g., pain, relationship, role performance): ____
Recent change in frequency/interest: ____

Objective (Exhibits)

Comfort level with subject matter: ____

Male: Subjective (Reports)

Penis: Circumcised: ____ Vasectomy (date): ____
Prostate disorder: ____
Practice self-exam: Breast: ____ Testicles: ____
Last proctoscopic/prostate exam: ____ Last PSA/date: ____
Medications/herbals: ____

Objective (Exhibits)

Genitalia: Penis: Circumcised: ____ Warts/lesions: ____
Bleeding/discharge: ____ Testicles (e.g., lumps): ____
Breasts examination: ____
Test results: PSA: ____ STI: ____

Sexuality [Component of Social Interaction] (continued)

Female: Subjective (Reports)

Menstruation: Age at menarche: ____ Length of cycle: ____
Duration: ____ Number of pads/tampons used/day: ____
Last menstrual period: ____
Bleeding between periods: ____
Reproductive: Infertility concerns: ____
Type of therapy: ____ Pregnant now: ____
Para: ____ Gravida: ____ Due date: ____
Menopause: ____ Last period: ____
Hysterectomy (type/date): ____
Problem with: Hot flashes: ____ Night sweats: ____
Vaginal lubrication: ____ Vaginal discharge: ____
Hormonal therapies: ____
Osteoporosis medications: ____
Breasts: Practices breast self-exam: ____
Last mammogram: ____ Biopsy/surgery: ____
Last PAP smear: ____

Objective (Exhibits)

Breasts examination: ____
Genitalia: Warts/lesions: ____
Vaginal bleeding/discharge: ____
Test results: PAP ____
Mammogram: ____
STI: ____

Social Interactions

Subjective (Reports)

Relationship status (check): Single: ____ Married: ____
Living with partner: ____ Divorced: ____ Widowed: ____
Years in relationship: ____ Perception of relationship: ____
Concerns/stresses: ____
Role within family structure: ____
Number/age of children: ____
Perception of relationship with family members: ____
Extended family/availability: ____
Other support person(s): ____
Individuals living in home: ____
Caregiver (to whom/how long): ____
Ethnic/cultural affiliations: ____
Strength of ethnic identity: ____
Lives in ethnic community: ____
Feelings of (describe): Mistrust: ____ Rejection: ____
Unhappiness: ____ Loneliness/isolation: ____
Problems related to illness/condition: ____
Difficulties with communication (e.g., speech, another language, brain injury): ____
Use of speech/communication aids (list): ____
Interpreter needed: ____ Primary language: ____
Genogram: Diagram on separate page

Objective (Exhibits)

Communication/speech: Clear: ____
Slurred: ____
Unintelligible: ____
Aphasic: ____
Unusual speech pattern/impairment: ____
Laryngectomy present: ____
Verbal/nonverbal communication with family/SO(s): ____
Family interaction (behavioral) pattern: ____

Teaching/Learning

Subjective (Reports)

Communication: Dominant language (specify): ____
Second language: ____ Literate (reading/writing): ____
Education level: ____
Learning disabilities (specify): ____
Cognitive limitations: ____
Culture/ethnicity: Where born: ____
If immigrant, how long in this country: ____
Health and illness beliefs/practices/customs: ____
Which family member makes health care decisions/is spokesperson for client: ____
Presence of Advance Directives: ____ Code status: ____
Durable Medical Power of Attorney: ____
Designee: ____
Health goals: ____
Current health problem: ____
Client understanding of problem: ____
Special health care concerns (e.g., impact of religious/cultural practices): ____
Healthcare decisions: ____
Family involvement: ____

Familial risk factors (indicate relationship):
Diabetes: ____ Thyroid (specify): ____
Tuberculosis: ____ Heart disease: ____ Stroke: ____
Hypertension: ____ Epilepsy/seizures: ____
Kidney disease: ____ Cancer: ____
Mental illness/depression: ____ Other: ____
Prescribed medications: Drug: ____ Dose: ____
Times (circle last dose): ____ Take regularly: ____
Purpose: ____ Side effects/problems: ____
Nonprescription drugs/frequency: OTC drugs: ____
Vitamins: ____ Herbals: ____
Street drugs: ____ Alcohol (amount/frequency): ____
Tobacco: ____ Smokeless tobacco: ____
Admitting diagnosis per provider: ____
Reason for hospitalization/visit per client: ____
History of current concern: ____

Teaching/Learning (continued)

Subjective (Reports)

Expectations of this hospitalization/visit: ______

Will admission cause any lifestyle changes (describe): ______

______

Previous illnesses and/or hospitalizations/surgeries: ______

______

Evidence of failure to improve: ______

Last complete physical exam: ______

Discharge Plan Considerations

Projected length of stay (days or hours): ______

Anticipated date of discharge: ______

Date information obtained: ______

Resources available: Persons: ______

Financial: ______

Groups: ______

Community supports: ______

Areas that may require alteration/assistance

Food preparation: ______ Shopping: ______ Transportation: ______

Ambulation: ______ Medication/IV therapy: ______

Treatments: ______ Wound care: ______

Supplies: ______ Durable medical equip: ______

Self-care (specify): ______

Homemaker/maintenance (specify): ______ Socialization: ______

Physical layout of home (specify): ______

Anticipated changes in living situation after discharge: ______

Living facility other than home (specify): ______

Referrals (date/source/services): Social Services: ______

Rehab services: ______ Dietary: ______ Home care: ______

Resp/O_2: ______ Equipment: ______

Supplies: ______ Other: ______

Hospice: ______

Figure 3.1 Adult medical-surgical assessment tool. This is a suggested guide and tool for creating a database reflecting a nursing focus. Although the diagnostic divisions are alphabetized here for ease of presentation, they can be prioritized or rearranged in any manner to meet individual needs. In addition, this assessment tool can be adapted to meet the needs of specific client populations.

Box 3.1 Nursing Diagnoses Organized According to Diagnostic Divisions

After data are collected and areas of concern or need identified, the nurse is directed to the Diagnostic Divisions to review the list of nursing diagnoses that fall within the individual categories. This will assist the nurse in choosing the specific diagnostic label to accurately describe the data. Then, with the addition of etiology or related/risk factors (when known), and signs and symptoms, or cues (defining characteristics), the client diagnostic statement emerges.

Activity/Rest—ability to engage in necessary or desired activities of life (work and leisure) and to obtain adequate sleep and rest

- Activity Intolerance
- Activity Intolerance, risk for
- Activity Planning, ineffective
- Activity Planning, risk for ineffective
- Disuse Syndrome, risk for
- Diversional Activity, deficient
- Fatigue
- Insomnia
- Lifestyle, sedentary
- Mobility, impaired bed
- Mobility, impaired wheelchair
- Sleep, readiness for enhanced
- Sleep Deprivation
- Sleep Pattern, disturbed
- Transfer Ability, impaired
- Walking, impaired

Circulation—ability to transport oxygen and nutrients necessary to meet cellular needs

- Autonomic Dysreflexia
- Autonomic Dysreflexia, risk for
- Bleeding, risk for
- Cardiac Output, decreased
- Gastrointestinal Perfusion, risk for ineffective
- Intracranial Adaptive Capacity, decreased
- Renal Perfusion, risk for ineffective
- Shock, risk for
- Tissue Perfusion, ineffective peripheral
- Tissue Perfusion, risk for decreased cardiac
- Tissue Perfusion, risk for ineffective cerebral
- Tissue Perfusion, risk for ineffective peripheral

Ego Integrity—ability to develop and use skills and behaviors to integrate and manage life experiences

- Anxiety [specify level]
- Body Image, disturbed
- Coping, defensive
- Coping, ineffective

(continues on page 18)

Box 3.1 Nursing Diagnoses Organized According to Diagnostic Divisions (continued)

- Coping, readiness for enhanced
- Death Anxiety
- Decision-Making, readiness for enhanced
- Decisional Conflict
- Denial, ineffective
- Energy Field, disturbed
- Fear
- Grieving
- Grieving, complicated
- Grieving, risk for complicated
- Health Behavior, risk-prone
- Hope, readiness for enhanced
- Hopelessness
- Human Dignity, risk for compromised
- Impulse Control, ineffective
- Moral Distress
- Personal Identity, disturbed
- Personal Identity, risk for disturbed
- Post-Trauma Syndrome
- Post-Trauma Syndrome, risk for
- Power, readiness for enhanced
- Powerlessness
- Powerlessness, risk for
- Rape-Trauma Syndrome
- Relationships, ineffective
- Relationships, readiness for enhanced
- Relationships, risk for ineffective
- Religiosity, impaired
- Religiosity, readiness for enhanced
- Religiosity, risk for impaired
- Relocation Stress Syndrome
- Relocation Stress Syndrome, risk for
- Resilience, impaired individual
- Resilience, readiness for enhanced
- Resilience, risk for compromised
- Self-Concept, readiness for enhanced
- Self-Esteem, chronic low
- Self-Esteem, risk for chronic low
- Self-Esteem, situational low
- Self-Esteem, risk for situational low
- Sorrow, chronic
- Spiritual Distress
- Spiritual Distress, risk for
- Spiritual Well-Being, readiness for enhanced

Elimination—ability to excrete waste products

- Constipation
- Constipation, perceived
- Constipation, risk for
- Diarrhea
- Gastrointestinal Motility, dysfunctional
- Gastrointestinal Motility, risk for dysfunctional
- Incontinence, bowel
- Incontinence, functional urinary
- Incontinence, overflow urinary
- Incontinence, reflex urinary
- Incontinence, stress urinary
- Incontinence, urge urinary
- Incontinence, risk for urge urinary
- Urinary Elimination, impaired
- Urinary Elimination, readiness for enhanced
- Urinary Retention, [acute/chronic]

Food/Fluid—ability to maintain intake of and utilize nutrients and liquids to meet physiological needs

- Blood Glucose Level, risk for unstable
- Breast Milk, insufficient
- Breastfeeding, ineffective
- Breastfeeding, interrupted
- Breastfeeding, readiness for enhanced
- Dentition, impaired
- Electrolyte Imbalance, risk for
- Failure to Thrive, adult
- Feeding Pattern, ineffective infant
- Fluid Balance, readiness for enhanced
- [Fluid Volume, deficient hypertonic or hypotonic]
- Fluid Volume, deficient [isotonic]
- Fluid Volume excess
- Fluid Volume, risk for deficient
- Fluid Volume, risk for imbalanced
- Liver Function, risk for impaired
- Nausea
- Nutrition: less than body requirements, imbalanced
- Nutrition: more than body requirements, imbalanced
- Nutrition: more than body requirements, risk for imbalanced
- Nutrition, readiness for enhanced
- Oral Mucous Membrane, impaired
- Swallowing, impaired

Hygiene—ability to perform activities of daily living

- Self-Care, readiness for enhanced
- Self-Care Deficit: bathing
- Self-Care Deficit: dressing
- Self-Care Deficit: feeding
- Self-Care Deficit: toileting
- Self-Neglect

Neurosensory—ability to perceive, integrate, and respond to internal and external cues

- Behavior, disorganized infant
- Behavior, risk for disorganized infant
- Behavior, readiness for enhanced organized infant
- Confusion, acute
- Confusion, risk for acute
- Confusion, chronic
- Memory, impaired
- Peripheral Neurovascular Dysfunction, risk for
- [Sensory Perception, disturbed (specify: visual, auditory, kinesthetic, gustatory, tactile, olfactory)]
- Stress Overload
- Unilateral Neglect

Pain/Discomfort—ability to control internal/external environment to maintain comfort

- Comfort, impaired
- Comfort, readiness for enhanced
- Pain, acute
- Pain, chronic

Box 3.1 Nursing Diagnoses Organized According to Diagnostic Divisions (continued)

Respiration—ability to provide and use oxygen to meet physiological needs

- Airway Clearance, ineffective
- Aspiration, risk for
- Breathing Pattern, ineffective
- Gas Exchange, impaired
- Ventilation, impaired spontaneous
- Ventilatory Weaning Response, dysfunctional

Safety—ability to provide safe, growth-promoting environment

- Adverse Reaction to Iodinated Contrast Media, risk for
- Allergy Response, risk for
- Body Temperature, risk for imbalanced
- Contamination
- Contamination, risk for
- Dry Eye, risk for
- Environmental Interpretation Syndrome, impaired
- Falls, risk for
- Health Maintenance, ineffective
- Home Maintenance, impaired
- Hyperthermia
- Hypothermia
- Immunization Status, readiness for enhanced
- Infection, risk for
- Injury, risk for
- Jaundice, neonatal
- Jaundice, risk for neonatal
- Latex Allergy Response
- Latex Allergy Response, risk for
- Maternal-Fetal Dyad, risk for disturbed
- Mobility, impaired physical
- Perioperative Positioning Injury, risk for
- Poisoning, risk for
- Protection, ineffective
- Self-Mutilation
- Self-Mutilation, risk for
- Skin Integrity, impaired
- Skin Integrity, risk for impaired
- Sudden Infant Death Syndrome, risk for
- Suffocation, risk for
- Suicide, risk for
- Surgical Recovery, delayed
- Thermal Injury, risk for
- Thermoregulation, ineffective
- Tissue Integrity, impaired
- Trauma, risk for
- Vascular Trauma, risk for
- Violence, risk for other-directed
- Violence, risk for self-directed
- Wandering [specify sporadic or continual]

Sexuality [Component of Ego Integrity and Social Interaction]—ability to meet requirements/characteristics of male or female role

- Childbearing Process, ineffective
- Childbearing Process, readiness for enhanced
- Childbearing Process, risk for ineffective
- Sexual Dysfunction
- Sexuality Pattern, ineffective

Social Interaction—ability to establish and maintain relationships

- Attachment, risk for impaired
- Caregiver Role Strain
- Caregiver Role Strain, risk for
- Communication, impaired verbal
- Communication, readiness for enhanced
- Coping, compromised family
- Coping, disabled family
- Coping, readiness for enhanced community
- Coping, readiness for enhanced family
- Family Processes, dysfunctional
- Family Processes, interrupted
- Family Processes, readiness for enhanced
- Loneliness, risk for
- Parenting, impaired
- Parenting, risk for impaired
- Parenting, readiness for enhanced
- Role Conflict, parental
- Role Performance, ineffective
- Social Interaction, impaired
- Social Isolation

Teaching/Learning—ability to incorporate and use information to achieve healthy lifestyle and optimal wellness

- Development, risk for delayed
- Growth, risk for disproportionate
- Growth and Development, delayed
- Health, deficient community
- Knowledge, deficient [Learning Need] (specify)
- Knowledge (specify), readiness for enhanced
- Noncompliance [Adherence, ineffective] [specify]
- Self-Health Management, ineffective
- Self-Health Management, readiness for enhanced
- Therapeutic Regimen Management, ineffective family

To assist in visualizing this critical thinking process, a prototype client situation (Fig. 3.2) is provided as an example of data collection and construction of a plan of care. As the client assessment database is reviewed, the nurse can identify the related or risk factors, and defining characteristics (signs and symptoms) if present, that were used to formulate the client diagnostic statements. The addition of timelines to specific client outcomes and goals reflects the anticipated length of stay and individual client-nurse expectations. Interventions are based on concerns and needs identified by the client and nurse during data collection. In addition, physician and other discipline orders are also considered when identifying interventions. Although not normally included in a plan of care, rationales are included in this sample for the purpose of explaining or clarifying the choice of interventions.

(text continues on page 24)

Client Situation: Diabetes Mellitus

Mr. R.S., a client with type 2 diabetes (non–insulin-dependent) for 8 years, presented to his physician's office with a nonhealing ulcer of 3 weeks' duration on his left foot. Screening studies done in the physician's office revealed blood glucose (BG) of 356/fingerstick and urine Chemstix of 2%. Because of distance from medical provider and lack of local community services, he is admitted to the hospital.

Admitting Physician's Orders

Culture/sensitivity and Gram's stain of foot ulcer
Random blood glucose on admission and fingerstick BG qid—call for BG>250
CBC, electrolytes, serum lipid profile, glycosylated Hb in AM
Chest x-ray and ECG in AM
Humulin R 10 units SC on admission
DiaBeta 10 mg, PO bid
Glucophage 500 mg, PO daily to start—will increase gradually
Humulin N 10 U SC q AM. Begin insulin instruction for post-discharge self-care if necessary
Dicloxacillin 500 mg PO q6h, start after culture obtained
Darvocet-N 100 mg PO q4h prn pain
Diet—2400 calories, 3 meals with 2 snacks
Arrange consult with dietician
Up in chair ad lib with feet elevated
Foot cradle for bed
Irrigate lesion L foot with NS tid, then cover with sterile dressing
Vital signs qid

Client Assessment Database

Name: R.S. Informant: Client Reliability (Scale 1–4): 3 Age: 73 DOB: 5/3/39 Race: Caucasian
Gender: M Adm. date: 6/28/2012 Time: 7 PM From: Home

ACTIVITY/REST

Subjective (Reports):
Occupation: Farmer
Usual activities/hobbies: reading, playing cards. "Don't have time to do much. Anyway, I'm too tired most of the time to do anything after the chores."
Limitations imposed by illness: "Have to watch what I order if I eat out."
Sleep: Hours: 6 to 8 hr/night Naps: No Aids: No
Insomnia: "Not unless I drink coffee after supper."
Usually feels rested when awakens at 4:30 AM but feeling fatigued past several weeks

Objective (Exhibits):
Observed response to activity: limps, favors L foot when walking
Mental status: Alert/active
Neuro/muscular assessment: Muscle mass/tone: Bilaterally equal/firm
Posture: Erect ROM: Full all extremities
Strength: Equal 3 extremities/(favors L foot currently)

CIRCULATION

Subjective (Reports):
History of slow healing: Lesion L foot, 3 weeks' duration
Extremities: Numbness/tingling: "My feet feel cold and tingly like sharp pins poking the bottom of my feet when I walk the quarter mile to the mailbox."
Cough/character of sputum: Occ./white
Change in frequency/amount of urine: Yes/voiding more lately

Objective (Exhibits):
Peripheral pulses: Radials 3+; popliteal, dorsalis, post-tibial/pedal, all 1+
BP: R: Lying: 146/90 Sitting: 140/86 Standing: 138/90
L: Lying: 142/88 Sitting: 138/88 Standing: 138/84
Pulse: Apical: 86 Radial: 86 Quality: Strong Rhythm: Regular
Chest auscultation: few wheezes clear with cough, no murmurs/rubs
Jugular vein distention: 0
Extremities: Temperature: Feet cool bilaterally/legs warm
Color: Skin: Legs pale Capillary refill: Slow both feet (approx. 4 seconds)
Homans' sign: 0 Varicosities: Few enlarged superficial veins both calves
Nails: Toenails thickened, yellow, brittle
Distribution and quality of hair: Coarse hair to midcalf, none on ankles/toes
Color: General: Ruddy face/arms Mucous membranes/lips: Pink
Nailbeds: Blanch well Conjunctiva and sclera: White

EGO INTEGRITY

Subjective (Reports):

Report of stress factors: "Normal farmer's problems: weather, pests, bankers, etc."
Ways of handling stress: "I get busy with the chores and talk things over with my livestock. They listen pretty good."
Financial concerns: No supplemental insurance; needs to hire someone to do chores while here
Relationship status: Married
Cultural factors: Rural/agrarian, eastern European descent, "American, no ethnic ties"
Religion: Protestant/practicing
Lifestyle: Middle class/self-sufficient farmer
Recent changes: No
Feelings: "I'm in control of most things, except the weather and this diabetes now."
Concerned re possible therapy change "from pills to shots."

Objective (Exhibits):

Emotional status: generally calm, appears frustrated at times
Observed physiological response(s): occasionally sighs deeply/ frowns, fidgeting with coin, shoulders tense/shrugs shoulders, throws up hands

ELIMINATION

Subjective (Reports):

Usual bowel pattern: almost every PM
Last BM: last night Character of stool: firm/brown
Bleeding: 0 Hemorrhoids: 0 Constipation: occ.
Laxative used: hot prune juice on occ.
Urinary: Voiding more frequently, up 1 or 2 times nightly
Character of urine: pale yellow

Objective (Exhibits):

Abdomen tender: no Soft/firm: soft Palpable mass: 0
Bowel sounds: active all 4 quads

FOOD/FLUID

Subjective (Reports):

Usual diet (type): 2400 calorie (occ. "cheats" with dessert; "My wife watches it pretty closely.")
No. of meals daily: 3/1 snack
Dietary pattern: B: Fruit juice/toast/ham/decaf coffee
L: Meat/potatoes/veg/fruit/milk D: ½ meat sandwich/soup/fruit/decaf coffee
Snack: Milk/crackers at HS. Usual beverage: Skim milk, 2 to 3 cups decaf coffee, drinks "lots of water— several quarts"
Last meal/intake: Dinner: Roast beef sandwich, vegetable soup, pear with cheese, decaf coffee
Loss of appetite: "Never, but lately I don't feel as hungry as usual."
Nausea/vomiting: 0 Food allergies: None
Heartburn/food intolerance: Cabbage causes gas, coffee after supper causes heartburn
Mastication/swallowing problems: 0
Dentures: Partial upper plate—fits well
Usual weight: 175 lb Recent changes: Has lost about 6 lb this month
Diuretic therapy: No

Objective (Exhibits):

Wt: 170 lb Ht: 5 ft 10 in Build: stocky
Skin turgor: Good/leathery
Condition of teeth/gums: Good, no irritation/bleeding noted
Appearance of tongue: Midline, pink
Mucous membranes: Pink, intact, moist
Breath sounds: Few wheezes cleared with cough
Bowel sounds: Active all 4 quads
Urine Chemstix: 2% Fingerstick: 356 (Dr. office) 450 random BG on adm

HYGIENE

Subjective (Reports):

Activities of daily living: Independent in all areas
Preferred time of bath: PM

Objective (Exhibits):

General appearance: Clean, shaven, short-cut hair; hands rough and dry; skin on feet dry, cracked, and scaly
Scalp and eyebrows: Scaly white patches
No body odor

NEUROSENSORY

Subjective (Reports):
Headache: "Occasionally behind my eyes when I worry too much."
Tingling/numbness: Feet, 4 or 5 times/week (as noted)
Eyes: Vision loss, farsighted, "Seems a little blurry now." Examination: 2 yr ago
Ears: Hearing loss R: "Some" L: No (has not been tested)
Nose: Epistaxis: 0 Sense of smell: "No problem."

Objective (Exhibits):
Mental status: Alert, oriented to person, place, time, situation
Affect: Concerned Memory: Remote/recent: Clear and intact
Speech: Clear/coherent, appropriate
Pupil reaction: PERRLA/small
Glasses: Reading Hearing aid: No
Handgrip/release: Strong/equal

PAIN/DISCOMFORT

Subjective (Reports):
Primary focus: L foot Location: Medial aspect, L heel
Intensity (0–10): 4 to 5 Quality: Dull ache with occ. sharp stabbing sensation
Frequency/duration: "Seems like all the time." Radiation: No
Precipitating factors: Shoes, walking How relieved: ASA, not helping
Other concerns: Sometimes has back pain following chores/heavy lifting, relieved by ASA/liniment rubdown; knees ache—uses topical heat ointment

Objective (Exhibits):
Facial grimacing: When lesion border palpated
Guarding affected area: Pulls foot away
Narrowed focus: No
Emotional response: Tense, irritated

RESPIRATION

Subjective (Reports):
Dyspnea: 0 Cough: Occ. morning cough, white sputum
Emphysema: 0 Bronchitis: 0 Asthma: 0 Tuberculosis: 0
Smoker: Filters pk/day: 1/2 No. yrs: 25+
Use of respiratory aids: 0

Objective (Exhibits):
Respiratory rate: 22 Depth: Good Symmetry: Equal, bilateral
Auscultation: Few wheezes, clear with cough
Cyanosis: 0 Clubbing of fingers: 0
Sputum characteristics: None to observe
Mentation/restlessness: Alert/oriented/relaxed

SAFETY

Subjective (Reports):
Allergies: 0 Blood transfusions: 0
Sexually transmitted disease: 0
Risk behaviors: Wears seat belt
Fractures/dislocations: L clavicle, 1960s, fell getting off tractor
Arthritis/unstable joints: "Some in my knees."
Back problems: Lower back pain 2 or 3 times/month
Vision impaired: Requires glasses for reading
Hearing impaired: Slightly (R), compensates by turning "good ear" toward speaker
Immunizations: Current flu/pneumonia 3 yrs ago/tetanus maybe 8 yrs ago

Objective (Exhibits):
Temperature: 99.4°F (37.4°C) tympanic
Skin integrity: Impaired L foot Scars: R inguinal, surgical
Rashes: 0 Bruises: 0 Lacerations: 0 Blisters: 0
Ulcerations: Medial aspect L heel, 2.5-cm diameter, approx. 3 mm deep, wound edges inflamed, draining small amount cream-color/pink-tinged matter, slight musty odor noted
Strength (general): Equal all extremities Muscle tone: firm
ROM: Good Gait: Favors L foot Paresthesia/paralysis: Tingling, prickly sensation in feet after walking ¼ mile

SEXUALITY: MALE

Subjective (Reports):
Sexually active: Yes Use of condoms: No (monogamous)
Recent changes in frequency/interest: "I've been too tired lately."
Penile discharge: 0 Prostate disorder: 0 Vasectomy: 0

SEXUALITY: MALE (continued)

Subjective (Reports): Last proctoscopic examination: 2 yr ago Prostate examination: 1 yr ago
Practice self-examination: Breast/testicles: No
Problems/complaints: "I don't have any problems, but you'd have to ask my wife if there are any complaints."

Objective (Exhibits): Examination: Breast: No masses Testicles: Deferred Prostate: Deferred

SOCIAL INTERACTIONS

Subjective (Reports): Marital status: Married 45 yr Living with: Wife
Report of problems: None
Extended family: 1 daughter lives in town (30 miles away); 1 daughter married/grandson, living out of state
Other: Several couples, he and wife play cards/socialize with 2 to 3 times/mo
Role: Works farm alone; husband/father/grandfather
Report of problems related to illness/condition: None until now
Coping behaviors: "My wife and I have always talked things out. You know the 11th commandment is 'Thou shalt not go to bed angry.'"

Objective (Exhibits): Speech: Clear, intelligible
Verbal/nonverbal communication with family/SO(s): Speaks quietly with wife, looking her in the eye; relaxed posture
Family interaction patterns: Wife sitting at bedside, relaxed, both reading paper, making occasional comments to each other

TEACHING/LEARNING

Subjective (Reports): Dominant language: English Second language: 0 Literate: Yes
Education level: 2-yr college
Health and illness/beliefs/practices/customs: "I take care of the minor problems and see the doctor only when something's broken."
Presence of Advance Directives: Yes—wife to bring in
Durable Medical Power of Attorney: Wife
Familial risk factors/relationship:
- Diabetes: Maternal uncle
- Tuberculosis: Brother died, age 27
- Heart disease: Father died, age 78, heart attack
- Strokes: Mother died, age 81
- High BP: Mother

Prescribed medications:
- Drug: Diabeta Dose: 10 mg bid
- Schedule: 8 AM/6 PM, last dose 6 PM today
- Purpose: Control diabetes
- Takes medications regularly? Yes

Home urine/glucose monitoring: "Only using TesTape, stopped some months ago when I ran out. It was always negative, anyway. Don't like sticking my fingers."
Nonprescription (OTC) drugs: Occ. ASA Herbals/supplements: No
Use of alcohol (amount/frequency): Socially, occ. beer
Tobacco: 1/2 pk/day Smokeless: No
Admitting diagnosis (physician): Hyperglycemia with nonhealing lesion L foot
Reason for hospitalization (client): "Sore on foot and the doctor is concerned about my blood sugar, and says I'm supposed to learn this fingerstick test now."
History of current complaint: "Three weeks ago I got a blister on my foot from breaking in my new boots. It got sore so I lanced it but it isn't getting any better."
Client's expectations of this hospitalization: "Clear up this infection and control my diabetes."
Other relevant illness and/or previous hospitalizations/surgeries:
1960s, R inguinal hernia repair, tonsils age 5 or 6
Evidence of failure to improve: Lesion L foot, 3 wk
Last physical examination: Complete 1 yr ago, office follow-up 5 mo ago

DISCHARGE CONSIDERATIONS (AS OF 6/28)

Anticipated discharge: 7/1/12 (3 days)
Resources: Self, wife

DISCHARGE CONSIDERATIONS (AS OF 6/28) (continued)

Financial: "If this doesn't take too long to heal, we got some savings to cover things."
Community supports: Diabetic support group (has not participated)
Anticipated lifestyle changes: Become more involved in management of condition
Assistance needed: May require farm help for several days
Teaching: Learn new medication regimen and wound care; review diet; encourage smoking cessation
Referral: Supplies: Downtown Pharmacy or AARP
Equipment: Glucometer-AARP
Follow-up: Primary care provider 1 wk after discharge to evaluate wound healing and potential need for additional changes in diabetic regimen

Figure 3.2 Client situation: Diabetes mellitus.

Another way to conceptualize the client's care needs is to create a Mind Map, or Concept Map (Fig. 3.3). This technique and learning tool has been developed to help visualize the linkages or interconnections between various client symptoms, interventions, or problems as they impact each other. The best parts of the traditional care plans (problem-solving and categorizing) are retained, but the linear and columnar nature of the plan is changed to a design that uses the whole brain—a design that brings left-brained, linear problem-solving thinking together with the free-wheeling, interconnected, creative right brain. Joining mind mapping and care planning enables the nurse to create a holistic view of a client, strengthening critical thinking skills and facilitating the creative process of planning client care.

Mind mapping starts in the center of the page with a representation of the main concept—the client. (This helps keep in mind that the client is the focus of the plan, not the medical diagnosis or condition.) From that central thought, other main ideas that relate to the client radiate out from the center similar to spokes of a wheel (however, they do not have to be added in a balanced manner; it does not have to be a round "wheel"). Different concepts can be grouped together by geometric shapes, color coding, or by placement on the page. Connections and interconnections between groups of ideas are represented by the use of arrows or lines, with defining phrases added that explain how the interconnected thoughts relate to one another. In this manner, many different pieces of information *about* the client can be connected directly *to* the client.

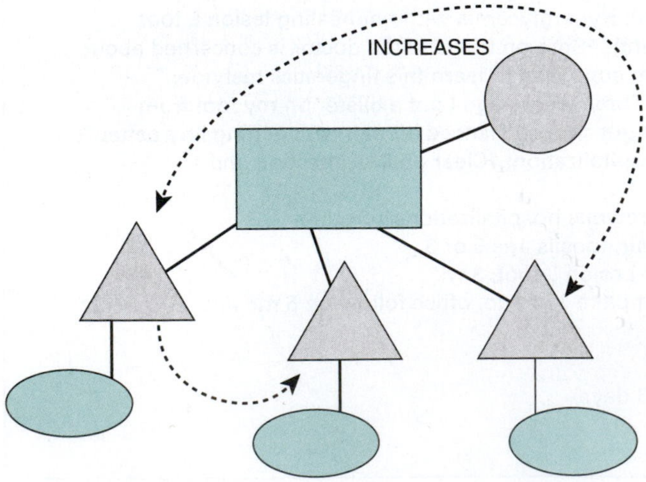

Whichever piece is chosen becomes the first layer of connections—clustered assessment data, nursing diagnoses, or outcomes. For example, a map could start with nursing diagnoses featured as the first "branches," each one being listed separately in some way on the map. Next, the signs and symptoms or data supporting the diagnoses could be added. Or, the plan could begin with the client outcomes to be achieved and then connecting them to nursing diagnoses. When the plan is completed, there should be a nursing diagnosis (supported by subjective and objective assessment data), nursing interventions, desired client outcome(s), and any evaluation data, all connected in a manner that shows there is a relationship between them. It is critical to understand that there is no preset order for the pieces because one cluster is not more or less important than another (or one is not subsumed under another). It is important, however, that those pieces within a branch be in the same order in each branch.

Finally, to complete the learning experience, samples of the evaluation step based on the client situation are presented.

Evaluation

As nursing care is provided, ongoing assessment evaluates the client's response to therapy and progress toward accomplishing the desired outcomes. This activity serves as the feedback and control part of the nursing process through which the status of the individual client diagnostic statement is judged to be resolved, continuing, or requiring revision.

This process is visualized in Figure 3.4. Observation of Mr. R.S.'s wound reveals that edges are clean and pink and drainage is scant. Therefore, he is progressing toward achieving wound healing; this problem will continue to be addressed, although no revision in the treatment plan is required at this time.

Documentation

To date, a number of charting formats have been used for documentation. These include block notes, with a single entry covering an entire shift (e.g., 7 to 3 p.m.); narrative

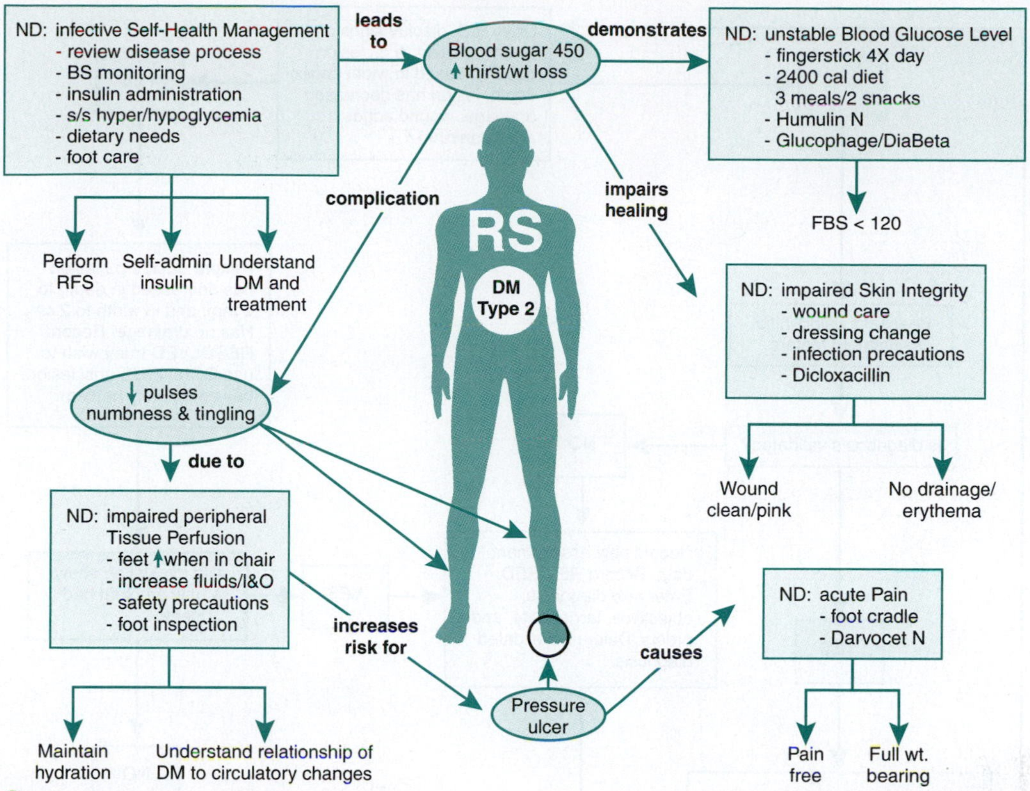

Figure 3.3 Mind map for Mr. R.S.

timed notes (e.g., 8:30 a.m., ate 100% of breakfast); the problem-oriented medical record system (POMR) to record the **s**ubjective and **o**bjective data, **a**nalysis of the data, and the resulting **p**lan (SOAP); and flow sheets with charting by exception, to name a few. The POMR can provide thorough documentation, but it was designed by physicians for episodic care and requires that the entries be tied to a problem identified from a problem list.

A charting system format created by nurses for documentation of frequent or repetitive care is Focus Charting®. It was designed to encourage looking at the client from a positive rather than a negative (or problem-oriented) perspective by using precise documentation to record the nursing process. Recording of assessment, interventions, and evaluation information in *data, action,* and *response* (DAR) categories facilitates tracking and following what is happening to the client at any given moment. Charting focuses on client and nursing concerns, with the focal point being client status and the associated nursing care. The focus is always stated in a way that reflects the client's concerns or needs rather than a nursing task or medical diagnosis. Thus, the focus can be a client's problems or concerns or nursing diagnosis; signs and symptoms of potential importance, for instance, fever, dysrhythmia, and edema; a significant event or change in status; or a specific standard of care or hospital policy. An expansion of this format is DATRP: data, action, teaching, response, and plan.

A more recent way to evaluate and document the client's progress (response to care) is by using clinical pathways. These pathways were originally developed as tools for providing care in case management systems and are now used in many settings. A clinical pathway is a type of abbreviated plan of care that is event oriented (task oriented) and provides outcome-based guidelines for goal achievement within a designated length of stay. The pathway incorporates agency and professional standards of care and may be interdisciplinary, depending on the care setting. As a rule, however, the standardized clinical pathways address a specific diagnosis, condition, or procedure, such as myocardial infarction, total hip replacement, or chemotherapy, and do not provide for inclusion of secondary diagnoses or complications, such as an asthmatic client in alcohol withdrawal. In short, if the client does not achieve the daily outcomes or goals of care, the variance is identified and a separate plan of care must be developed to meet the client's individual needs. Therefore, although clinical pathways are becoming more common in the clinical setting, they have limited value (in place of more individualized plans of care) as learning tools for students who are working to practice the nursing process, critical thinking, and a holistic approach to meeting client needs. A sample clinical pathway (Fig. 3.5) reflects Mr. R.S.'s primary diagnostic problem: nonhealing wound, diabetic.

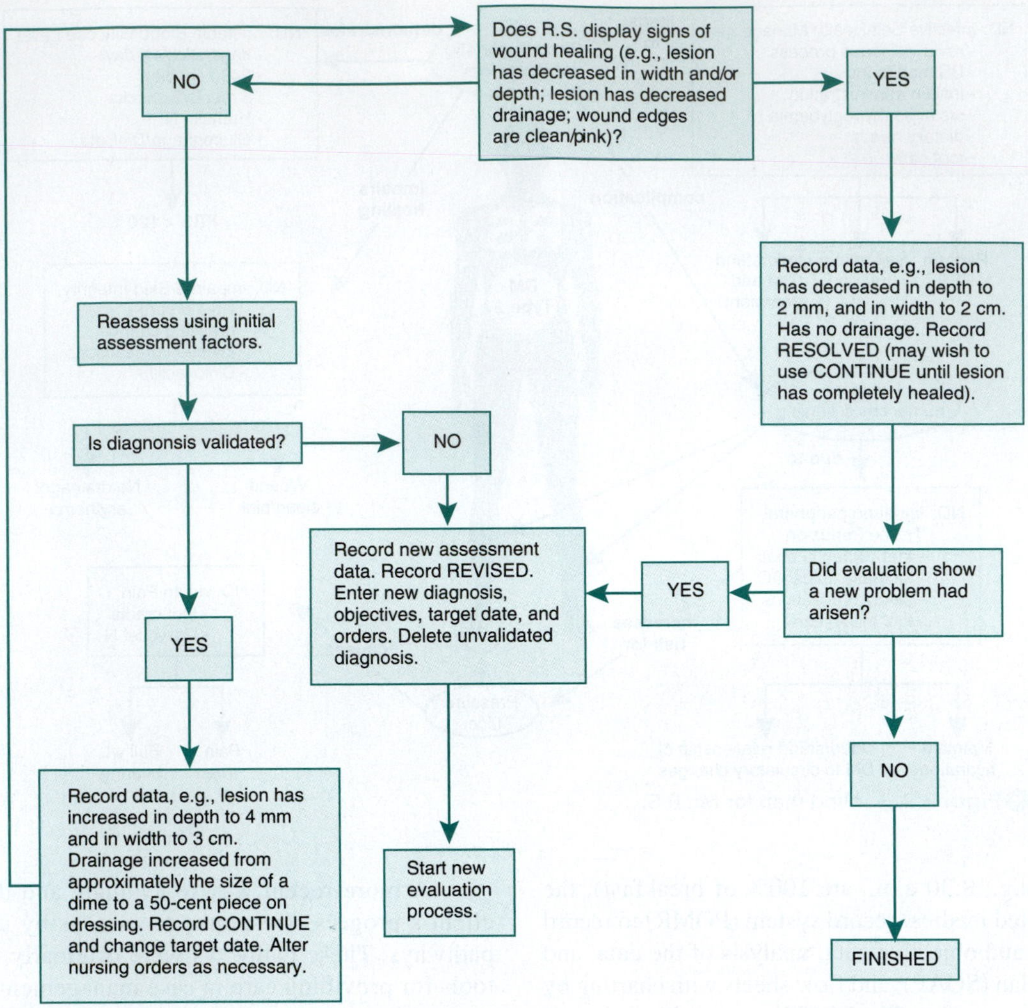
Does R.S. display signs of wound healing (e.g., lesion has decreased in width and/or depth; lesion has decreased drainage; wound edges are clean/pink)?
NO
YES
Reassess using initial assessment factors.
Is diagnosis validated?
NO
YES
Record new assessment data. Record REVISED. Enter new diagnosis, objectives, target date, and orders. Delete unvalidated diagnosis.
Record data, e.g., lesion has increased in depth to 4 mm and in width to 3 cm. Drainage increased from approximately the size of a dime to a 50-cent piece on dressing. Record CONTINUE and change target date. Alter nursing orders as necessary.
Start new evaluation process.
Record data, e.g., lesion has decreased in depth to 2 mm, and in width to 2 cm. Has no drainage. Record RESOLVED (may wish to use CONTINUE until lesion has completely healed).
Did evaluation show a new problem had arisen?
YES
NO
FINISHED

Figure 3.4 Outcome-based evaluation of the client's response to therapy. (Adapted from Newfield, SA, et al: *Cox's Clinical Applications of Nursing Diagnosis,* ed 5. FA Davis, Philadelphia, 2007.)

CP: Non-healing Lesion—Diabetic. ELOS: 3 Days—Variations from Designated Pathway Should Be Documented in Progress Notes

ND and Categories of Care	Adm Day 1 6/28 7pm	Day 2 6/29	Day 3 6/30	Discharge 7/1
impaired Skin/ Tissue Integrity	Actions/Goals:	Actions/Goals: Verbalize understanding of condition Display blood glucose WNL (ongoing)	Actions/Goals: Be free of signs of dehydration Wound free of purulent drainage Verbalize understanding of treatment needs Perform self-care tasks No. 1 and 3 correctly Explain reasons for actions	Actions/Goals: Wound edges show signs of healing process Perform self-care task No. 2 correctly Explain reason for actions Plan in place to meet discharge needs
Referrals		Dietician & determine need for: Home care Physical therapy Visiting nurse		
Diagnostic studies	Wound culture/sensitivity Gram's stain Random blood glucose Fingerstick BG hs	CBC, electrolytes Glycosylated Hb, Serum lipid profile →Fingerstick BG qid/call>250 Chest x-ray (if indicated) ECG (if indicated)	→	Fingerstick BG bid if stable
Additional assessments	VS qid I&O/level of hydration qd Character of wound tid Level of knowledge and priorities of learning needs Observe for signs of antibiotic hypersensitivity reaction	→ → → Anticipated discharge needs	→ VS each shift → →	→ →D/C →
Medications	Antibiotic: *Dicloxacillin 500 mg PO q6h* Antidiabetic: *Humulin R insulin 10 units SC on adm*	Antibiotic: same Antidiabetic: *Humulin N insulin 10 U SC q AM* *DiaBeta 10 mg PO bid* *Glucophage 500 mg PO daily*	Antibiotic: same Antidiabetic: same	Antibiotic: same Antidiabetic: same
Client education	Provide: *Understanding Your Diabetes*	Film *Living with Diabetes* Demonstrate and practice tasks: 1. Fingerstick BG 2. Insulin administration 3. Wound care 4. Routine foot care	Group sessions: *Diabetic management*	Practice self-care task No. 2: *insulin administration* Review discharge instructions
Additional nursing actions	Up ad lib NS soaks/dressing change tid	→ →	→ →	→ →

CP: Non-healing Lesion—Diabetic. ELOS: 3 Days—Variations from Designated Pathway Should Be Documented in Progress Notes
(Continued)

ND and Categories of Care	Adm Day 1 6/28 7pm	Day 2 6/29	Day 3 6/30	Discharge 7/1
acute Pain	Actions/Goals State pain relieved or minimized with 1 hr of analgesic administration (ongoing) Verbalize understanding of when to report pain and rating scale used Verbalize understanding of self-care measures No. 1 and 2 Explain reason for actions	Actions/Goals Verbalize understanding of self-care test No. 3 Explain reason for actions	Actions/Goals Able to participate in usual level: *ambulate full weight bearing*	Actions/Goals State pain-free/ controlled with medication Verbalize understanding of correct medication use
Additional assessments	Characteristics of pain Level of participation activities Individual analgesic needs	→ → →	→ → →	→ → →
Medications Allergies: -0-	Analgesic: Darvocet-N 100 mg PO q4h PRN	Analgesic: same	Analgesic: same	Analgesic: same
Client education	Orient to unit/room Guidelines for self-report of pain and rating scale *0–10* Safety/comfort measures: *1 elevation of feet* *2 proper footwear*	Safety/comfort measures: *3 prevention of injury*		Review discharge medication instructions: dosage, route, frequency, side effects
Additional nursing actions	Bed cradle as indicated			

Figure 3.5 Sample Clinical Pathway.

PLAN OF CARE: Mr. R.S.

Client Diagnostic Statement

impaired Skin Integrity related to pressure, imbalanced nutritional state, impaired circulation, and impaired sensation, as evidenced by destruction of skin layers—draining wound L foot.

Outcome

Wound Healing: Secondary Intention (NOC) Indicators:

Client Will

Be free of purulent drainage within 48 hours (6/30, 7 p.m.).
Display signs of healing with wound edges clean and pink within 60 hours (7/1, 7 a.m.).

ACTIONS/INTERVENTIONS	RATIONALE
Wound Care (NIC)	
Irrigate wound with room-temperature sterile normal saline (NS) tid.	Cleans wound without harming delicate tissues.
Assess wound with each dressing change. Obtain wound tracing on admission and at discharge.	Provides information about effectiveness of therapy and identifies additional needs.
Apply sterile dressing using paper tape.	Keeps wound clean, minimizes cross-contamination. *Note:* Adhesive tape may be abrasive to fragile tissues.
Infection Control (NIC)	
Follow wound precautions.	Use of gloves and proper handling of contaminated dressings reduces likelihood of spread of infection.
Obtain sterile specimen of wound drainage on admission.	Culture/sensitivity identifies pathogens and therapy of choice.
Administer dicloxacillin 500 mg PO q6h, starting at 10 p.m.	Treatment of infection and prevention of complications. Food interferes with drug absorption, requiring scheduling around meals.
Observe for signs of hypersensitivity: pruritus, urticaria, rash.	Although no prior history of penicillin reaction, it may occur at any time.

PLAN OF CARE:

Client Diagnostic Statement

risk for unstable Blood Glucose Level related to lack of adherence to diabetes management and inadequate blood glucose monitoring with fingerstick 450/adm.

Outcome

Blood Glucose Level (NOC) Indicators:

Client Will

Demonstrate correction of metabolic state as evidenced by fasting blood sugar (FBS) less than 170 mg/dL within 36 hours (6/30, 7 a.m.).

ACTIONS/INTERVENTIONS	RATIONALE
Hyperglycemia Management (NIC)	
Perform fingerstick BG qid. Call for BG >250.	Bedside analysis of blood glucose levels is a more timely method for monitoring effectiveness of therapy and provides direction for alteration of medications such as additional regular insulin.
Administer antidiabetic medications:	Treats underlying metabolic dysfunction, reducing hyperglycemia and promoting healing.
10 units Humulin N insulin SC q AM after fingerstick BG	Intermediate-acting preparation with onset of 2 to 4 hr, peak 6 to 12 hr, with a duration of 18 to 24 hr. Increases transport of glucose into cells and promotes the conversion of glucose to glycogen.
DiaBeta 10 mg PO bid	Lowers blood glucose by stimulating the release of insulin from the pancreas and increasing the sensitivity to insulin at the receptor sites.

(continues on page 30)

ACTIONS/INTERVENTIONS (continued) / RATIONALE (continued)

Glucophage 500 mg PO daily. Note onset of side effects.

Glucophage lowers serum glucose levels by decreasing hepatic glucose production and intestinal glucose absorption and increasing sensitivity to insulin. By using in conjunction with DiaBeta, client may be able to discontinue insulin once target dosage is achieved (e.g., 2000 mg/d). An increase of 1 tablet per week is necessary to limit side effects of diarrhea, abdominal cramping, and vomiting, possibly leading to dehydration and prerenal azotemia.

Provide diet 2400 cal—three meals/two snacks.

Proper diet decreases glucose levels and insulin needs, prevents hyperglycemic episodes, can reduce serum cholesterol levels, and promotes satiation.

Schedule consultation with dietitian to restructure meal plan and evaluate food choices.

Calories are unchanged on new orders but have been redistributed to three meals and two snacks. Dietary choices (e.g., increased vitamin C) may enhance healing.

PLAN OF CARE:

Client Diagnostic Statement

acute Pain related to physical agent (open wound L foot) as evidenced by coded report of pain (4–5/10) and guarding behavior.

Outcome

Pain Level (NOC) Indicators:

Client Will

Report pain is minimized or relieved within 1 hr of analgesic administration (ongoing).
Report absence or effective control of pain by discharge (7/1).

Outcome

Pain: Disruptive Effects (NOC) Indicators:

Client Will

Ambulate normally, full weight-bearing by discharge (7/1).

ACTIONS/INTERVENTIONS / RATIONALE

Pain Management (NIC)

Determine pain characteristics through client's description.

Establishes baseline for assessing improvement and changes.

Place foot cradle on bed; encourage use of loose-fitting slipper when up.

Avoids direct pressure to area of injury, which could result in vasoconstriction and increased pain.

Administer Darvocet-N 100 mg PO every 4 hr as needed. Document effectiveness.

Provides relief of discomfort when unrelieved by other measures.

PLAN OF CARE:

Client Diagnostic Statement

ineffective peripheral Tissue Perfusion related to deficient knowledge of disease process and aggravating factors, diabetes mellitus as evidenced by diminished pulses, pale/cool feet, capillary refill 4 sec, paresthesia of feet "when walks 1/4 mile."

Outcomes

Knowledge: Diabetes Management (NOC) Indicators:

Client Will

Verbalize understanding of relationship between chronic disease (diabetes mellitus) and circulatory changes within 48 hr (6/30, 7 p.m.).
Demonstrate awareness of safety factors and proper foot care within 48 hr (6/30, 7 p.m.).
Maintain adequate level of hydration to maximize perfusion (ongoing), as evidenced by balanced intake/output, moist skin and mucous membranes, and capillary refill less than 3 sec (daily; ongoing).

ACTIONS/INTERVENTIONS	RATIONALE
Circulatory Care: Arterial Insufficiency (NIC)	
Elevate feet when up in chair. Avoid long periods with feet in dependent position.	Minimizes interruption of blood flow and reduces venous pooling.
Assess for signs of dehydration. Monitor intake/output. Encourage oral fluids.	Glycosuria may result in dehydration with consequent reduction of circulating volume and further impairment of peripheral circulation.
Instruct client to avoid constricting clothing and socks and ill-fitting shoes.	Compromised circulation and decreased pain sensation may precipitate or aggravate tissue breakdown.
Reinforce safety precautions regarding use of heating pads, hot water bottles, or soaks.	Heat increases metabolic demands on compromised tissues. Vascular insufficiency alters pain sensation, increasing risk of injury.
Recommend cessation of smoking.	Vascular constriction associated with smoking and diabetes impairs peripheral circulation.
Discuss complications of disease that result from vascular changes: ulceration, gangrene, and muscle or bony structure changes.	Although proper control of diabetes mellitus may not prevent complications, severity of effects may be minimized. Diabetic foot complications are the leading cause of nontraumatic lower-extremity amputations. *Note:* Skin dry, cracked, scaly; feet cool; and pain when walking a distance suggest mild to moderate vascular disease (autonomic neuropathy) that can limit response to infection, impair wound healing, and increase risk of bony deformities.
Review proper foot care as outlined in teaching plan.	Altered perfusion of lower extremities may lead to serious or persistent complications at the cellular level.

PLAN OF CARE:

Client Diagnostic Statement

deficient Knowledge/Learning Need regarding diabetic condition, related to misinterpretation of information and/or lack of recall as evidenced by inaccurate follow-through of instructions regarding home glucose monitoring and foot care and failure to recognize signs and symptoms of hyperglycemia.

Outcomes

Knowledge: Diabetes Management (NOC) Indicators:

Client Will

Perform procedure of home glucose monitoring correctly within 36 hr (6/30, 7 a.m.).
Verbalize basic understanding of disease process and treatment within 38 hr (6/30, 9 a.m.).
Explain reasons for actions within 38 hr (6/30, 9 a.m.).
Perform insulin administration correctly within 60 hr (7/1, 7 a.m.).

ACTIONS/INTERVENTIONS	RATIONALE
Teaching: Disease Process (NIC)	
Determine client's level of knowledge, priorities of learning needs, and desire/need for including wife in instruction.	Establishes baseline and direction for teaching and planning. Involvement of wife, if desired, will provide additional resource for recall and understanding and may enhance client's follow-through.
Provide teaching guide, "Understanding Your Diabetes," 6/28 p.m. Show film *Living With Diabetes,* 6/29, 4 p.m., when wife is visiting. Include in group teaching session, 6/30 a.m. Review information and obtain feedback from client and wife.	Provides different methods for accessing and reinforcing information and enhances opportunity for learning and understanding.
Discuss factors related to and altering diabetic control, such as stress, illness, and exercise.	Drug therapy and diet may need to be altered in response to both short- and long-term stressors and changes in activity level.
Review signs and symptoms of hyperglycemia (e.g., fatigue, nausea, vomiting, polyuria, polydipsia). Discuss how to prevent and evaluate this situation and when to seek medical care. Have client identify appropriate interventions.	Recognition and understanding of these signs and symptoms and timely intervention will aid client in avoiding recurrences and preventing complications.

(continues on page 32)

ACTIONS/INTERVENTIONS (continued)	RATIONALE (continued)
Review and provide information about necessity for routine examination of feet and proper foot care (e.g., daily inspection for injuries, pressure areas, corns, calluses; proper nail care; daily washing; application of good moisturizing lotion such as Eucerin, Keri, or Nivea bid). Recommend loose-fitting socks and properly fitting shoes (break new shoes in gradually), and avoid going barefoot. If foot injury or skin break occurs, wash with soap or dermal cleanser and water, cover with sterile dressing, inspect wound and change dressing daily; report redness, swelling, or presence of drainage.	Reduces risk of tissue injury; promotes understanding and prevention of pressure ulcer formation and wound healing difficulties.
Teaching: Prescribed Medication (NIC)	
Instruct regarding prescribed insulin therapy:	May be a temporary treatment of hyperglycemia with infection or may be permanent combination with oral hypoglycemic agent.
Humulin N insulin, SC	Intermediate-acting insulin generally lasts 18 to 28 hr, with peak effect 6 to 12 hr.
Keep vial in current use at room temperature (if used within 30 days).	Cold insulin is poorly absorbed.
Store extra vials in refrigerator.	Refrigeration prolongs the drug shelf-life by preventing wide fluctuations in temperature.
Roll bottle and invert to mix, or shake gently, avoiding bubbles.	Vigorous shaking may create foam, which can interfere with accurate dose withdrawal and damage the insulin molecule. *Note:* New research suggests that gently shaking the vial may be more effective in mixing suspension. (Refer to Procedure Manual.)
Choice of injection sites (e.g., across lower abdomen in Z pattern).	Provides for steady absorption of medication. Site is easily visualized and accessible by client, and Z pattern minimizes tissue damage.
Demonstrate, then observe client in drawing insulin into syringe, reading syringe markings, and administering dose. Assess for accuracy.	May require several instruction sessions and practice before client and wife feel comfortable drawing up and injecting medication.
Instruct in signs and symptoms of insulin reaction or hypoglycemia: fatigue, nausea, headache, hunger, sweating, irritability, shakiness, anxiety, or difficulty concentrating.	Knowing what to watch for and appropriate treatment such as $^{1}/_{2}$ cup grape juice for immediate response and snack within 30 min (e.g., one slice bread with peanut butter or cheese, or fruit and slice of cheese for sustained effect) may prevent or minimize complications.
Review "sick day rules," for example, call doctor if too sick to eat normally or stay active; take insulin as ordered. Keep record as noted in Sick Day Guide.	Understanding of necessary actions in the event of mild-to-severe illness promotes competent self-care and reduces risk of hyperglycemia or hypoglycemia.
Instruct client and wife in fingerstick glucose monitoring to be done four times per day until stable, then twice a day at rotating times, such as FBS and before dinner, or before lunch and at bedtime. Observe return demonstrations of the procedure.	Fingerstick monitoring provides accurate and timely information regarding diabetic control. Return demonstration verifies correct learning.
Recommend client maintain record or log of fingerstick testing, antidiabetic medication and insulin dosage/site, unusual physiological response, and dietary intake. Outline desired goals, for example, FBS 80 to 110, pre-meal 80 to 120.	Provides accurate record for review by caregivers for assessment of therapy effectiveness and needs.
Discuss other healthcare issues, such as smoking habits, self-monitoring for cancer (breasts and testicles), and reporting changes in general well-being.	Encourages client involvement, awareness, and responsibility for own health; promotes wellness. *Note:* Smoking tends to increase client's resistance to insulin.

CHAPTER 4

Cardiovascular

HYPERTENSION: SEVERE

I. Pathophysiology
- **a.** Multifactoral
  - **i.** Complex interactions between the vasculature, kidneys, sympathetic nervous system, baroreceptors, ennin-angiotensin-aldosterone system, and insulin resistance
- **b.** Mosaic theory
  - **i.** Genetic disposition
  - **ii.** Environmental: dietary Na^+/fat intake, trace metals, stress, smoking
  - **iii.** Anatomical: abnormalities of vascular system
  - **iv.** Adaptive: e.g., regulation of intracellular Na^+ and Ca^{++} by cell membrane ion pumps
  - **v.** Neural: variety of complex nerve mechanisms
  - **vi.** Endocrine: pheochromocytoma, primary aldosteronism
  - **vii.** Humoral: varied agents that constrict and dilate blood vessels
  - **viii.** Hemodynamic: blood volume or viscosity, intrarenal hemodynamics

II. Classification—2003 Guidelines National Heart, Lung, and Blood Institute (NHLBI)
- **a.** Normal blood pressure (BP)—less than 120/80 mm Hg
- **b.** Prehypertension—120/80 to 139/89 mm Hg
- **c.** Hypertension—greater than 140/90 mm Hg

III. Degree of Severity
- **a.** Stage I (mild)—140/90 to 159/99 mm Hg
- **b.** Stage II (moderate)—160/100 mm Hg or greater
- **c.** Stage III (severe)—systolic pressure greater than 180 and diastolic pressure greater than 110
- **d.** Stage IV (very severe)—systolic pressure 210 or greater with diastolic pressure greater than 120

IV. Etiology
- **a.** Primary (essential), which accounts for approximately 85% to 95% of all cases, has no identifiable cause
- **b.** Secondary, which occurs as a result of an identifiable, sometimes correctable, pathological condition, such as kidney disorders, adrenal gland tumors, or primary aldosteronism, medications, drugs, or other chemicals

V. Statistics (MMWR, 2011; Roger, 2012)
- **a.** Morbidity:
  - **i.** 68 million Americans are hypertensive (nearly 1 in 3).
  - **ii.** More than 66% of men and 78% of women over age 75 are hypertensive.
  - **iii.** Approximately 20% are undiagnosed.
  - **iv.** Prevalence: African Americans 43%, Caucasians 34%, Hispanics 28%.
- **b.** Mortality (MMWR, 2011; Roger, 2012): High blood pressure was a primary or contributing cause of death for 348,000 Americans in 2008.
- **c.** Cost: Direct economic costs $47.5 billion in 2009 (NHLBI, 2012).

GLOSSARY

Atrial hypertrophy: Increased atrial volume and pressure.

Hyperglycemia: Increased serum glucose.

Hypertension: Blood pressure (BP) greater than 140/90 mm Hg.

Hypokalemia: Low serum potassium.

Prehypertension: BP in range of 120/80 to 139/89 mm Hg.

Stroke: Cellular death of cerebral tissue caused by obstruction of blood flow to sections of the brain, which results in neurological deficits.

Systemic vascular resistance (SVR): An index of arterial compliance or constriction throughout the body; equal to BP divided by cardiac output.

Target organ disease or damage (TOD): Organ or system of organs that are primarily affected by hypertension, such as the heart, kidneys, and brain.

Transient ischemic attack (TIA): Brief periods of confusion or difficulty with speech caused by an intermittent reduction in blood flow to the brain.

Care Setting

Although hypertension is usually treated in a community setting, management of stages III and IV with symptoms of complications or compromise may require inpatient care, especially when target organ disease (TOD) is present. The majority of interventions included here can be used in either setting.

Related Concerns

Cerebrovascular accident (CVA)/stroke, page 214
Myocardial infarction, page 75
Psychosocial aspects of care, page 729
Kidney injury: acute, page 505
Renal failure: chronic, page 517

Client Assessment Database

DIAGNOSTIC DIVISION MAY REPORT	MAY EXHIBIT
ACTIVITY/REST	
• Sedentary lifestyle, which is a major risk factor for hypertension • Weakness, fatigue • Shortness of breath	• Elevated heart rate • Change in heart rhythm • Tachypnea • Dyspnea with exertion
CIRCULATION	
• History of elevated BP over time • Presence of TOD, such as atherosclerotic, valvular, or coronary artery heart disease, including myocardial infarction (MI), angina, heart failure (HF), and cerebrovascular disease • Episodes of palpitations, diaphoresis	• *Pulses:* Bounding carotid, jugular, radial pulsations • Pulse disparities, particularly femoral delay as compared with radial or brachial pulsation and absence of or diminished popliteal, posterior tibial, pedal pulses • *Apical pulse:* Point of maximal impulse (PMI) possibly displaced or forceful • *Heart rate and rhythm:* Tachycardia, various dysrhythmias • *Heart sounds:* Accentuated S_2 at base; S_3 in early HF; S_4, which reflects rigid left ventricle and left ventricular hypertrophy; murmurs of valvular stenosis; vascular bruits audible over carotid, femoral, or epigastrium • Jugular vein distension (JVD) • *Extremities:* Discoloration of skin; cool temperature, indicating peripheral vasoconstriction; and slow or delayed capillary refill, indicating vasoconstriction • *Skin:* Pallor, cyanosis, and diaphoresis, suggesting pulmonary congestion and hypoxemia, or flushing, suggesting pheochromocytoma
EGO INTEGRITY	
• History of personality changes, anxiety, depression, euphoria, or chronic anger that may indicate cerebral impairment • Multiple stress factors, such as relationship, financial, or job-related concerns	• Mood swings, restlessness, irritability • Narrowed focus
ELIMINATION	
• Past or present renal insult, such as kidney infection, renovascular obstruction, or past history of kidney disease	• May have decreased urinary output, if kidney failure is present, or increased output, if taking diuretics
FOOD/FLUID	
• Food preferences that are high-calorie, high-salt, high-fat, and high-cholesterol, such as fried foods, cheese, eggs, or licorice • Low dietary intake of potassium, calcium, and magnesium • Nausea, vomiting • Recent weight changes • Current or history of diuretic use	• Normal weight or obesity • Presence of edema • Venous congestion, JVD • Glycosuria—almost 10% of hypertensive clients are diabetic, reflecting renal TOD

DIAGNOSTIC DIVISION MAY REPORT (continued)	MAY EXHIBIT (continued)
NEUROSENSORY • History of numbness or weakness on one side of the body; TIA or stroke • Fainting spells or dizziness • Throbbing, suboccipital headaches, usually present on awakening and disappearing spontaneously after several hours • Visual disturbances, such as diplopia and blurred vision • Episodes of epistaxis	• *Mental status:* Changes in alertness, orientation, speech pattern and content, affect, thought process, or memory • *Motor responses:* Decreased strength, hand grip, and deep tendon reflexes • *Optic retinal changes:* From mild sclerosis and arterial narrowing to marked retinal and sclerotic changes with edema or papilledema, exudates, hemorrhages, and arterial nicking, although dependent on severity and duration of hypertension and resulting TOD
PAIN/DISCOMFORT • Severe, throbbing occipital headaches located in suboccipital region, present on awakening, and disappearing spontaneously after several hours • Stiffness of neck, dizziness, and blurred vision • Abdominal pain or masses, suggesting pheochromocytoma	• Reluctance to move head, rubbing head, avoidance of bright lights and noise, wrinkled brow, clenched fists; grimacing and guarding behaviors
RESPIRATION • Dyspnea associated with activity or exertion • Tachypnea, orthopnea, paroxysmal nocturnal dyspnea • Cough with or without sputum production • Smoking history, which is a major risk factor	• Respiratory distress or use of accessory muscles • Adventitious breath sounds, such as crackles or wheezes • Pallor or cyanosis generally associated with advanced cardiopulmonary effects of sustained or severe hypertension
SAFETY • Transient episodes of numbness, unilateral paresthesias • Light-headedness with position change	• Impaired coordination or gait
SEXUALITY • Postmenopausal, which is a major risk factor • Erectile dysfunction (ED), which may be associated with hypertension or antihypertensive medications	
TEACHING/LEARNING • Familial risk factors, including hypertension, atherosclerosis, heart disease, diabetes mellitus, and cerebrovascular or kidney disease • Ethnic or racial risk factors, such as increased prevalence in African American and Southeast Asian populations • Use of birth control pills or other hormone replacement therapy • Drug and alcohol use • Use of herbal supplements to manage BP, such as garlic, hawthorn, black cohash, celery seed, coleus, and evening primrose	
DISCHARGE PLAN CONSIDERATIONS • May require assistance with self-monitoring of BP as well as periodic evaluation of and alterations in medication therapy ➧ Refer to section at end of plan for postdischarge considerations.	

Diagnostic Studies

TEST WHY IT IS DONE	WHAT IT TELLS ME
BLOOD TESTS	
• ***Blood urea nitrogen (BUN) and creatinine (Cr):*** BUN measures the amount of urea nitrogen in the blood. Cr measures the amount of creatinine in blood or urine.	Provides information about renal perfusion and function and can reveal cause if hypertension is related to kidney dysfunction.
• ***Glucose:*** Measures the amount of glucose in the blood at the time of sample collection.	Hyperglycemia may result from elevated catecholamine levels, which increases BP, and use of thiazide diuretics. Also, diabetes mellitus can be associated with hypertension.
• ***Serum potassium:*** Potassium is an electrolyte that helps regulate the amount of fluid in the body, stimulate muscle contraction, and maintain a stable acid-base balance.	Hypokalemia may indicate the presence of primary aldosteronism as a possible cause of hypertension or it may be a side effect of diuretic therapy.
• ***Lipid panel, including total lipids, high-density lipoprotein (HDL) cholesterol, low-density lipoprotein (LDL) cholesterol, total cholesterol, triglycerides:*** The group of tests that make up a lipid profile have been shown to be good indicators of risk for heart attack or stroke.	A predisposition for or presence of atheromatous plaque is indicated by the following: HDL levels that are less than 40 mg/dL in men and less than 50 mg/dL in women, triglycerides that are more than 150 mg/dL, and an increase in small-particle LDL.
• ***Thyroid studies:*** Blood test and scan to evaluate thyroid function; most commonly used laboratory test is the measurement of thyroid-stimulating hormone (TSH).	Hypertension is present in approximately 3% of clients with hypothyroidism and 20% to 30% in those with thyrotoxicosis (Vidt, 2004).
• ***Serum/urine aldosterone level:*** May be done to assess for primary aldosteronism as cause of hypertension.	Elevated in primary aldosteronism.
• ***Renin:*** An enzyme that activates the renin-angiotensin system and screens for essential, renal, or renovascular hypertension.	Elevated in renovascular and malignant hypertension and salt-wasting disorders.
• ***C-reactive protein (CRP):*** A member of the class of acute phase reactants. Serum levels rise dramatically during inflammatory processes occurring in the body. Monitoring serial CRP values can help determine disease progress or the effectiveness of treatment.	CRP is an indicator of vascular inflammation and can indicate athlerosclerotic disease that causes renal artery disease and hypertension.
OTHER DIAGNOSTIC STUDIES	
Electrocardiogram (ECG): Record of the electrical activity of the heart that can demonstrate conduction disturbances, enlarged heart, and chamber strain patterns.	Broad, notched P wave is one of the earliest signs of hypertensive heart disease.
• ***Kidney and renography nuclear scan (also called renogram):*** Assists in diagnosing renal disorders.	Determines if hypertension is due to kidney disease.
• ***Urine creatinine clearance:*** Determines extent of nephron damage in known kidney disease.	Reduced in hypertensive patient with renal damage.
• ***Uric acid:*** Measures end product of purine metabolism, providing one index of renal function.	Hyperuricemia has been implicated as a risk factor for the development of hypertension.

Nursing Priorities

1. Maintain or enhance cardiovascular functioning.
2. Prevent complications.
3. Provide information about disease process, prognosis, and treatment regimen.
4. Support active client control of condition.

Discharge Goals

1. BP within acceptable limits for individual.
2. Cardiovascular and systemic complications prevented or minimized.
3. Disease process, prognosis, and therapeutic regimen understood.
4. Necessary lifestyle or behavioral changes initiated.
5. Plan in place to meet needs after discharge.

NURSING DIAGNOSIS: risk for decreased Cardiac Output

Risk Factors May Include

Altered afterload [e.g., increased systemic vascular resistance, vasoconstriction]
Altered contractility [e.g., ventricular hypertrophy or rigidity; myocardial ischemia]

Possibly Evidenced By

(Not applicable; presence of signs and symptoms establishes an *actual* diagnosis)

Desired Outcomes/Evaluation Criteria—Client Will

Circulation Status (NOC)

Participate in activities that reduce BP and cardiac workload.
Maintain BP within individually acceptable range.
Demonstrate stable cardiac rhythm and rate within normal range.

ACTIONS/INTERVENTIONS — RATIONALE

Hemodynamic Regulation (NIC)

Independent

Measure BP in both arms or thighs. Take three readings, 3 to 5 minutes apart while client is at rest, then sitting, and then standing for initial evaluation. Use correct cuff size and accurate technique. Take note of elevations in systolic as well as diastolic readings.

Rationale: Serial measurements using correct equipment provide a more complete picture of vascular involvement and scope of problem. Progressive diastolic readings above 120 mm Hg are considered first accelerated, then malignant (very severe). Systolic hypertension also is an established risk factor for cerebrovascular disease and ischemic heart disease even when diastolic pressure is not elevated. In younger client with normal systolic readings, elevated diastolic numbers may indicate prehypertension.

Note presence and quality of central and peripheral pulses.

Rationale: Bounding carotid, jugular, radial, and femoral pulses may be observed and palpated. Pulses in the legs and feet may be diminished, reflecting effects of vasoconstriction and venous congestion.

Auscultate heart tones and breath sounds.

Rationale: S_4 is commonly heard in severely hypertensive clients because of the presence of atrial hypertrophy. Development of S_3 indicates ventricular hypertrophy and impaired cardiac functioning. Presence of crackles or wheezes may indicate pulmonary congestion secondary to developing or chronic heart failure.

Observe skin color, moisture, temperature, and capillary refill time.

Rationale: Presence of pallor; cool, moist skin; and delayed capillary refill time may be due to peripheral vasoconstriction or reflect cardiac decompensation and decreased output.

Note dependent and generalized edema.

Rationale: Indicates heart or kidney failure or vascular impairment.

Provide calm, restful surroundings, minimize environmental activity and noise. Consider limiting the number of visitors or length of visitation.

Rationale: Helps reduce sympathetic stimulation and promotes relaxation.

Maintain activity restrictions during crisis situation such as bedrest or chair rest and schedule periods of uninterrupted rest; assist client with self-care activities as needed.

Rationale: Reduces physical stress and tension that affect BP and the course of hypertension.

Provide comfort measures, such as back and neck massage or elevation of head.

Rationale: Decreases discomfort and may reduce sympathetic stimulation.

Instruct in relaxation techniques, guided imagery, and distractions.

Rationale: Can reduce stressful stimuli and produce calming effect, thereby reducing BP.

Monitor response to medications that control BP.

Rationale: Response to drug therapy is dependent on both the individual drugs and their synergistic effects. Because of potential side effects and drug interactions, it is important to use the smallest number and lowest dosage of medications possible.

Collaborative

Administer medications, as indicated:

Diuretics, for example, thiazide, such as hydrochlorothiazide with triamterene (Maxide), metatolazone (Zaroxolyn), indapamide (Lozol); and loop diuretics, such as furosemide (Lasix), bumetanide (Bumex), and torsemide (Demadex).

Rationale: Diuretics are considered first-line medications for uncomplicated hypertension and may be used alone or in association with other drugs, such as beta blockers, to reduce BP in clients with relatively normal renal function. These diuretics also potentiate the effects of other antihypertensive agents by limiting fluid retention and may reduce the incidence of stroke and heart failure. *Note*: Loop diuretics are less commonly used for treatment of hypertension.

(continues on page 38)

ACTIONS/INTERVENTIONS (continued)	RATIONALE (continued)
Beta blockers, such as acebutolol (Sectral), atenolol (Tenormin), metoprolol (Lopressor), bisoprolol (Zibeta), nadolol (Corgard), carvedilol (Coreg), propranolol (Inderal), labatolol (Tandate), timolol (Blocarden)	Beta blockers are recommended for BP control in clients with heart failure and cardiovascular disease. Cardioselective beta blockers, such as acebutolol, atenolol, and metroprolol, primarily affect β-1 receptors in the heart, slowing heart rate and decreasing the heart's workload. Nonselective beta blockers, such as propranolol and timolol, also decrease the heart's workload and promote vasodilation, but they exert effects on the beta-2 receptors of the bronchioles as well, causing bronchoconstriction and potentially increasing symptoms of reactive airway disease and chronic obstructive pulmonary disease. Cardioselective beta blockers are safer choices for patients with pulmonary disorders (Woods & Moshang, 2006).
Angiotensin-converting enzyme (ACE) inhibitors, such as captopril (Capoten), enalapril (Vasotec), benazepril (Lotensin), lisinopril (Zestril), fosinopril (Monopril), ramipril (Altace), moexipril (Univasc), and trandolapril (Mavik)	ACE inhibitors are generally considered first-line drugs for clients with documented congestive heart failure (CHF), diabetes, and those at risk for renal failure.
Angiotensin II receptor blockers (ARBs), such as candesartan (Atacand), valsartan (Diovan), losartan (Cozaar), and irbesartan (Avapro)	ARBs block the action of angiotensin II. As a result, blood vessels dilate and BP is reduced.
Calcium channel blockers, such as nifedipine (Adalat), diltiazem (Cardizem), amlodipine (Norvasc), nicardipine (Cardene)	Calcium channel blockers primarily affect blood vessels and can be used to treat severe hypertension when a combination of a diuretic and a sympathetic inhibitor does not sufficiently control BP.
Combination drugs, such as amlodipine and benazepril (Lotrel), hydralazine and hydrochlorothiazide (Vaseretic), nadolol and bendroflumethiazide (Corzide), hydralazine and hydrochlothiazide (Apresazide)	Combination antihypertensives include combined agents from the following pharmacologic classes: diuretics and potassium-sparing diuretics, beta blockers and diuretics, angiotensin-converting enzyme (ACE) inhibitors and diuretics, angiotensin-II antagonists and diuretics, and calcium channel blockers and ACE inhibitors. *Note*: Single-dose combination antihypertension therapy is an important option that combines efficacy of blood pressure reduction and a low side-effect profile with convenient once-daily dosing to enhance compliance (Skolnik, 2000).
Direct-acting parenteral vasodilators, such as diazoxide (Hyperstat), nitroprusside (Nitropress), and labetalol (Normodyne)	These are given intravenously (IV) for management of hypertensive emergencies.
Implement dietary restrictions, as indicated, such as reducing calories and avoiding refined carbohydrates, sodium, fat, and cholesterol. (Refer to ND: imbalanced Nutrition.)	Limiting sodium and sodium-rich processed foods can help manage fluid retention and, with associated hypertensive response, decrease myocardial workload. A diet rich in calcium, potassium, and magnesium may help lower BP.
Prepare for surgery when indicated.	When hypertension is due to pheochromocytoma, removing the tumor corrects the condition.

NURSING DIAGNOSIS: Activity Intolerance

May Be Related To

Generalized weakness

Imbalance between oxygen supply and demand

Possibly Evidenced By

Reports fatigue; feeling weak

Abnormal heart rate or BP response to activity

Exertional discomfort or dyspnea

ECG changes reflecting ischemia, arrhythmias

Desired Outcomes/Evaluation Criteria—Client Will

Endurance (NOC)

Participate in necessary and desired activities.

Report a measurable increase in activity tolerance.

Demonstrate a decrease in physiological signs of intolerance.

ACTIONS/INTERVENTIONS	RATIONALE
Energy Management (NIC)	
Independent	
Assess the client's response to activity, noting pulse rate more than 20 beats per minute faster than resting rate; marked increase in BP (systolic increases more than 40 mm Hg or diastolic increases more than 20 mm Hg) during and after activity, dyspnea or chest pain, excessive fatigue and weakness, and diaphoresis, dizziness, and syncope.	Changes in baseline are helpful in assessing physiological responses to the stress of activity and, if present, are indicators of overexertion.
Instruct client in energy-conserving techniques, such as using chair when showering, sitting to brush teeth or comb hair, and carrying out activities at a slower pace.	Energy-saving techniques reduce the energy expenditure, thereby assisting in equalization of oxygen supply and demand.
Encourage progressive activity and self-care when tolerated. Provide assistance as needed.	Gradual activity progression prevents a sudden increase in cardiac workload. Provide assistance only as needed, which encourages independence in performing activities.

NURSING DIAGNOSIS: acute Pain

May Be Related To

Physical agent [increased cerebral vascular pressure]

Possibly Evidenced By

Verbal/coded report
Positioning to avoid pain
Self-focus

Desired Outcomes/Evaluation Criteria—Client Will

Pain Control (NOC)

Report pain or discomfort is relieved or controlled.
Verbalize methods that provide relief.
Follow prescribed pharmacological regimen.

ACTIONS/INTERVENTIONS	RATIONALE
Pain Management (NIC)	
Independent	
Determine specifics of pain—location (e.g., suboccipital region), characteristics (e.g., throbbing, neck stiffness, blurred vision), intensity (0 to 10, or similar scale), onset (e.g., present on awakening), and duration (e.g., disappears spontaneously after being up and about). Note nonverbal cues (e.g., reluctance to move head, rubbing head, avoidance of bright lights/noise).	Facilitates diagnosis of problem and initiation of appropriate therapy. Helpful in evaluating effectiveness of therapy.
Encourage and maintain bedrest during acute phase, if indicated.	Minimizes stimulation and promotes relaxation.
Provide or recommend nonpharmacological measures for relief of headache, such as placing a cool cloth to forehead; back and neck rubs; quiet, dimly lit room; relaxation techniques, such as guided imagery and distraction; and diversional activities.	Measures that reduce cerebral vascular pressure and that slow or block sympathetic response are effective in relieving headache and associated complications.
Eliminate or minimize vasoconstricting activities that may aggravate headache, such as straining at stool, prolonged coughing, and bending over.	Activities that increase vasoconstriction accentuate the headache in the presence of increased cerebral vascular pressure.
Assist client with ambulation, as needed.	Dizziness and blurred vision frequently are associated with vascular headache. Client may also experience episodes of postural hypotension, causing weakness when ambulating.
Collaborative	
Administer analgesics, as indicated.	Reduce or control pain and decrease stimulation of the sympathetic nervous system.
Administer anti-anxiety agents, such as lorazepam (Ativan), alprazolam (Xanax), and diazepam (Valium).	May aid in the reduction of tension and discomfort that is intensified by stress.

NURSING DIAGNOSIS: imbalanced Nutrition: more than body requirements

May Be Related To

Excessive intake in relation to metabolic need or physical activity (caloric expenditure)

Possibly Evidenced By

Weight 20% over ideal for height and frame
Triceps skinfold >15 mm in men or >25 mm in women
Sedentary lifestyle
Dysfunctional eating patterns

Desired Outcomes/Evaluation Criteria—Client Will

Knowledge: Treatment Regimen (NOC)

Identify correlation between hypertension and obesity.

Weight-Loss Behavior (NOC)

Demonstrate change in eating patterns, such as food choices and quantity, to attain desirable body weight with optimal maintenance of health.

Initiate and maintain individually appropriate exercise program.

ACTIONS/INTERVENTIONS	RATIONALE
Weight-Reduction Assistance (NIC)	
Independent	
Assess client's understanding of direct relationship between hypertension and obesity.	Obesity is an added risk with hypertension because of the disproportion between fixed aortic capacity and increased cardiac output associated with increased body mass. Reduction in weight may reduce or eliminate the need for drug therapy needed to control BP. *Note:* Research suggests that bringing weight within 15% of ideal weight can result in a drop of 10 mm Hg in both systolic and diastolic BP (Khan et al, 2004).
Discuss necessity for decreased caloric intake and limited intake of fats, salt, and sugar, as indicated.	Faulty eating habits contribute to atherosclerosis and obesity that can predispose to hypertension and subsequent complications, such as stroke, kidney disease, and heart failure. Excessive salt intake expands the intravascular fluid volume and may damage kidneys, which can further aggravate hypertension.
Determine client's desire to lose weight.	Motivation for weight reduction is internal. The individual must want to lose weight or the program most likely will not succeed.
Review usual daily caloric intake and dietary choices.	Identifies current strengths and weaknesses in dietary program. Aids in determining individual need for adjustment and teaching.
Establish a realistic weight-reduction plan with the client, such as weight loss of 1 pound per week.	Slow reduction in weight is associated with fat loss with muscle sparing and generally reflects a change in eating habits.
Encourage client to maintain a diary of food intake, including when and where eating takes place and the circumstances and feelings around which the food was eaten.	Provides a database for both the adequacy of nutrients eaten and the relationship of emotion to eating. Helps focus attention on factors that client can control or change.
Instruct and assist client in appropriate food selections, such as implementing a diet rich in fruits, vegetables, and low-fat dairy foods referred to as the Dietary Approaches to Stop Hypertension (DASH) diet. Help the client identify—and thus avoid—foods high in saturated fat, such as butter, cheese, eggs, ice cream, and meat, and those that are high in cholesterol, such as whole dairy products, shrimp, and organ meats.	Moderation and use of low-fat products in place of total abstinence from certain food items may prevent client's sense of deprivation and enhance commitment to achieving health goals. Avoiding foods high in saturated fat and cholesterol is important in preventing progressing atherogenesis. The DASH diet, in conjunction with exercise, weight loss, and limits on salt intake, may reduce or even eliminate the need for drug therapy in early stages of hypertension (Elmer et al, 2006).
Collaborative	
Refer to dietitian or weight management programs, as indicated.	Can provide additional counseling and assistance with meeting individual dietary needs.

NURSING DIAGNOSIS: ineffective Coping

May Be Related To
Situational crisis
Inadequate level of perception of control
Inadequate resources available
Inadequate level of confidence in ability to cope

Possibly Evidenced By
Reports inability to cope, or ask for help
Inability to meet role expectations, basic needs, or
Inadequate problem-solving
Destructive behavior toward self [overeating], or use of forms of coping that impedes adaptive behavior

Desired Outcomes/Evaluation Criteria—Client Will

Coping (NOC)
Identify ineffective coping behaviors and consequences.
Verbalize awareness of own coping abilities and strengths.
Identify potential stressful situations and steps to avoid or modify them.
Demonstrate the use of effective coping skills.

ACTIONS/INTERVENTIONS	RATIONALE
Coping Enhancement (NIC)	
Independent	
Assess effectiveness of coping strategies by observing behaviors, such as ability to verbalize feelings and concerns, and willingness to participate in the treatment plan.	Adaptive mechanisms are necessary to appropriately alter one's lifestyle, deal with the chronicity of hypertension, and integrate prescribed therapies into daily living.
Note reports of sleep disturbances, increasing fatigue, impaired concentration, irritability, decreased tolerance of headache, and inability to cope or problem-solve.	Manifestations of maladaptive coping mechanisms may be indicators of repressed anger and may contribute to hypertension.
Assist client to identify specific stressors and possible strategies for coping with them.	Recognition of stressors is often the first step in altering one's response to the stressor.
Include client in planning of care and encourage maximum participation in treatment plan and with the multidisciplinary team.	Involvement provides client with an ongoing sense of control, improves coping skills, and enhances commitment to achieving health goals. Ongoing intensive assessment and management by a team can promote timely adjustments to therapeutic regimen.
Encourage client to evaluate life priorities and personal goals. Ask questions such as, "Is what you are doing getting you what you want?"	Focuses client's attention on reality of present situation relative to client's goals. Strong work ethic, need for "control," and outward focus may have led to lack of attention to personal needs.
Assist client to identify and begin planning for necessary lifestyle changes. Assist to adjust, rather than abandon, personal and family goals.	Necessary changes should be realistically prioritized so client can avoid being overwhelmed and feeling powerless.

NURSING DIAGNOSIS: ineffective Self-Health Management

May Be Related To
Complexity of therapeutic regimen
Economic difficulties
Perceived seriousness
Deficient knowledge

Possibly Evidenced By
Failure to take action to reduce risk factors
Failure to include treatment regimen in daily living
Ineffective choices in daily living for meeting health goals

Desired Outcomes/Evaluation Criteria—Client Will

Self-Management: Hypertension (NOC)
Verbalize understanding of disease process and treatment regimen.
Identify drug side effects and possible complications that necessitate medical attention.
Maintain BP within individually acceptable parameters.
Describe reasons for therapeutic actions and treatment regimen.

ACTIONS/INTERVENTIONS	RATIONALE
Teaching: Disease Process (NIC) *Independent*	
Assist client in identifying modifiable risk factors, such as obesity; diet high in sodium, saturated fats, and cholesterol; sedentary lifestyle; smoking; alcohol intake of more than 2 ounces per day on a regular basis; and a stressful lifestyle.	These risk factors contribute to hypertension and cardiovascular and renal disease.
Problem-solve with client to identify ways in which appropriate lifestyle changes can be made to reduce modifiable risk factors.	Changing "comfortable or usual" behavior patterns can be very difficult and stressful. Support, guidance, and empathy can enhance client's success in accomplishing his or her health goals.
Discuss importance of eliminating smoking, and assist client in formulating a plan to quit smoking. Refer to smoking cessation program or healthcare provider for helpful medications.	Nicotine increases catecholamine discharge, resulting in increased heart rate, BP, vasoconstriction, and myocardial workload, and reduces tissue oxygenation.
Reinforce the importance of adhering to treatment regimen and keeping follow-up appointments.	Lack of engagement in the treatment plan is a common reason for failure of antihypertensive therapy. Therefore, ongoing evaluation for client participation is critical to successful treatment. When client understands causative factors and consequences of inadequate intervention and is motivated to achieve health, the client typically participates in treatment interventions.
Instruct and demonstrate BP self-monitoring technique. Evaluate client's hearing, visual acuity, manual dexterity, and coordination.	Monitoring BP at home is reassuring to client because it provides visual feedback to determine treatment outcomes and helps promote early detection of deleterious changes.
Help client develop a simple, convenient schedule for taking medications.	Individualizing schedule to fit client's personal habits may make it easier to get in the habit of including antihypertensives in healthcare management activities.
Explain prescribed medications along with their rationale, dosage, expected and adverse side effects, and particular traits, such as the following:	Adequate information and understanding about side effects can enhance client's commitment to the treatment plan. For instance, mood changes, initial weight gain, and dry mouth are common and often subside with time.
Diuretics:	
Take daily or larger dose in the early morning.	Scheduling doses early in the day minimizes nighttime urination.
Weigh self on a regular schedule and record.	Primary indicator of effectiveness of diuretic therapy.
Avoid or limit alcohol intake.	The combined vasodilating effect of alcohol and the volume-depleting effect of a diuretic greatly increase the risk of orthostatic hypotension.
Notify physician if unable to tolerate food or fluid.	Dehydration can develop rapidly if intake is poor and client continues to take a diuretic.
Antihypertensives:	
Take prescribed dose on a regular schedule; avoid skipping, altering, or making up doses; and do not discontinue without notifying the healthcare provider. Review potential side effects and drug interactions, and discuss need for informing healthcare provider about onset of adverse effects such as erectile dysfunction (ED).	Because clients often cannot feel the difference the medication is making in BP, it is critical that there be understanding about the medication's actions and side effects. For example, abruptly discontinuing a drug may cause rebound hypertension, leading to severe complications, or medication may need to be altered to reduce adverse effects. *Note:* Many drugs used to treat hypertension have been linked to ED. Drugs may need to be changed or dose adjusted.
Rise slowly from a lying to standing position, sitting for a few minutes before standing. Sleep with the head slightly elevated. Suggest frequent position changes and leg exercises when lying down.	Measures reduce potential for orthostatic hypotension associated with the use of vasodilators and diuretics.
Recommend avoiding hot baths, steam rooms, and saunas, especially with concomitant use of alcoholic beverages.	Prevents vasodilation with potential for dangerous side effects of syncope and hypotension.
Instruct client to consult healthcare provider before taking other prescription or over-the-counter (OTC) medications.	Any drug that contains a sympathetic nervous stimulant may increase BP or counteract effects of antihypertensive medications.
Instruct client, as indicated, about increasing intake of foods and fluids high in potassium, such as oranges, bananas, figs, dates, tomatoes, potatoes, raisins, apricots, Gatorade, and fruit juices; and foods and fluids high in calcium, such as low-fat milk, yogurt, or calcium supplements.	Some diuretics can deplete potassium levels. Dietary potassium is desirable means of correcting deficits and may be more palatable to the client than drug supplements. Correcting mineral deficiencies can also affect BP.
Review the signs and symptoms that require the client to notify the healthcare provider, such as headache present on awakening that does not abate; sudden and continued increase of BP; chest pain; shortness of breath; irregular or increased pulse rate; significant weight gain (2 lb/day or 5 lb/wk); peripheral or abdominal swelling; visual disturbances; frequent, uncontrollable nosebleeds; depression or emotional lability;	Early detection and reporting of developing complications, decreased effectiveness of drug regimen, or adverse reactions allow for timely intervention.

ACTIONS/INTERVENTIONS (continued)	RATIONALE (continued)
severe dizziness or episodes of fainting; muscle weakness or cramping; nausea or vomiting; or excessive thirst.	
Explain rationale for prescribed dietary regimen—usually a diet low in sodium, saturated fat, and cholesterol.	Excess saturated fats, cholesterol, sodium, alcohol, and calories have been defined as nutritional risks in hypertension. A diet low in fat and high in polyunsaturated fat reduces BP, possibly through prostaglandin balance in both normotensive and hypertensive people.
Help client identify sources of sodium intake, such as table salt, salty snacks, processed meats and cheeses, sauerkraut, sauces, canned soups and vegetables, baking soda, baking powder, and monosodium glutamate. Emphasize the importance of reading ingredient labels of foods and OTC drugs.	A moderately low-salt diet may be sufficient to control mild hypertension or reduce or eliminate the need for drug therapy to control BP.
Encourage foods rich in essential fatty acids, such as salmon, cod, mackerel, and tuna.	Omega-3 fatty acids in fish tend to relax artery walls, reducing blood pressure. They also make blood thinner and less likely to clot.
Encourage client to establish a regular exercise program, incorporating aerobic exercise within client's capabilities. Stress the importance of avoiding isometric activity.	Besides helping to lower BP, aerobic activity aids in toning the cardiovascular system. Isometric exercise can increase serum catecholamine levels, further elevating BP.
Demonstrate application of ice pack to the back of the neck and pressure over the distal third of nose, and recommend that client lean head forward if nosebleed occurs.	Nasal capillaries may rupture as a result of excessive vascular pressure. Cold temperature and pressure constrict capillaries to slow or halt bleeding. Leaning forward reduces the amount of blood that is swallowed.
Provide information regarding community resources, and support client in making lifestyle changes. Initiate referrals, as indicated.	Community resources, such as the American Heart Association, "coronary clubs," stop smoking clinics, alcohol or drug rehabilitation, weight-loss programs, stress management classes, and counseling services may be helpful in client's efforts to initiate and maintain lifestyle changes.

POTENTIAL CONSIDERATIONS following acute hospitalization (dependent on client's age, physical condition and presence of complications, personal resources, and life responsibilities)

- ***Activity Intolerance***—imbalance between oxygen supply and demand
- ***imbalanced Nutrition: more than body requirements***—excessive intake in relation to metabolic needs/physical activity; sedentary lifestyle
- ***ineffective Self-Health Management***—complexity of therapeutic regimen, economic difficulties, perceived seriousness
- ***Sexual Dysfunction***—altered body function (activity intolerance, side effects of medication)
- ***readiness for enhanced family Coping***—SO(s) moves in direction of health promotion

HEART FAILURE: CHRONIC

I. Pathophysiology

- **a.** Remodeling of the myocardium (as a structural response to injury) changes the heart from an efficient football shape to an inefficient basketball shape, making coordinated contractility difficult.
  - **i.** Ventricular dilation (systolic dysfunction) results in poor contractility and inadequate emptying of chamber.
  - **ii.** Ventricular stiffening (diastolic dysfunction) impairs ability of chamber to relax and receive and eject blood.
- **b.** Failure of the left and/or right chambers of the heart results in insufficient output to meet metabolic needs of organ and tissues.
- **c.** Cardiac-related elevation of pulmonary or systemic venous pressures leads to organ congestion.
- **d.** Backward heart failure (HF): passive engorgement of the veins caused by elevated systemic venous pressure or a "backward" rise in pressure proximal to the failing cardiac chambers (right ventricular failure)
- **e.** Forward HF: decreased cardiac output with reduced forward flow into the aorta, systemic circulation (inadequate renal blood flow leads to sodium and water retention), and increasing pulmonary venous pressure results in fluid accumulation in alveoli (left ventricular failure)
- **f.** Myocardial muscle dysfunction associated with left ventricular hypertrophy (LVH) causes decreased cardiac output, activating neurohormones.
- **g.** Elevated circulating or tissue levels of neurohormones, norepinephrine, angiotensin II, aldosterone, endothelin, vasopressin, and cytokines causes sodium retention and peripheral vasoconstriction, increasing hemodynamic stresses on the ventricle.

II. Classification

- **a.** Stages (American College of Cardiology/American Heart Association (ACC/AHA) 2009 Guidelines include specific recommendations for each stage [Jessup et al, 2009]).
  - **i.** Stage A—high risk for HF associated with such conditions as hypertension, diabetes, and obesity. Treatment is focused on comorbidity.
  - **ii.** Stage B—presence of structural heart disease, such as left ventricular remodeling (LVH, or previous myocardial

(continues on page 44)

infarction (MI) but is asymptomatic. Treatment is focused on retarding the progression of ventricular remodeling and delaying the onset of HF symptoms.

iii. Stage C—clients with past or current HF symptoms associated with structural heart disease, such as advanced ventricular remodeling. Treatment is focused on modifying fluid and dietary intake and drug therapies as well as nonpharmacological measures, such as biventricular pacing and valvular or revascularization surgery.

iv. Stage D—refractory advanced HF symptoms at rest or with minimal exertion and frequently requiring intervention in the acute setting. Treatment is focused on promoting clinical stability, including supportive therapy to sustain life, such as left ventricular assist device, continuous intravenous (IV) inotropic therapy, experimental surgery or drugs, a heart transplant, or end-of-life or hospice care.

III. Etiology

a. Multifactoral

i. Complex clinical syndrome resulting from any structural or functional cardiac disorder that impairs the ability of the ventricle to fill with or eject blood (ACC/AHA 2009 Guidelines; Jessup et al, 2009).

ii. Risk factors and co-morbidities—hypertension; obesity; diabetes; coronary artery disease (CAD); peripheral and cerebrovascular disease; valvular heart disease with onset of atrial fibrillation (AF); sleep disorders such as sleep apnea; history of exposure to cardiotoxins, for example, chemotherapy, alcohol, and cocaine; family history of cardiomyopathy

IV. Statistics

a. High morbidity and mortality, particularly in stage D clients. (Jessup et al, 2009)

b. Morbidity: 5.7 million Americans have HF. (Roger, 2012; Centers for Disease Control and Prevention [CDC], 2012)

c. Mortality: Heart failure was listed as a contributing cause of 280,000 deaths in 2008 and was listed at number 4 in leading causes of death in 2009. (Roger, 2012; Kochanek, 2011).

d. Cost: Direct costs projected to be $24.7 billion in 2010. (Heidenriech, 2011)

GLOSSARY

Angiotensin converting enzyme inhibitor (ACEI) (also called ACE inhibitors): Medication that blocks the action of the angiotensin-converting enzyme in the lungs so that angiotensin I is not converted into angiotensin II. The production of this powerful blood vessel constrictor is thereby prevented and blood vessels remain dilated, which results in lower blood pressure.

Angiotensin receptor blocker (ARB): Medication that blocks the chemical receptors for angiotensin II on the small arteries. Therefore, the angiotensin cannot cause these arteries to constrict, which lowers blood pressure.

Ascites: Accumulation of fluid in the abdominal cavity can be associated with increased blood pressure in the veins draining the liver, with impaired drainage in the lymph system, and with low levels of albumin and other proteins in the blood.

Cardiac remodeling: The left ventricular chamber dilates and becomes more spherical. This condition increases the stress on the myocardial walls and depresses cardiac performance. Remodeling often precedes symptoms and may contribute to worsening of symptoms despite treatment (Jessup et al, 2009).

Heart failure (HF): A clinical syndrome characterized by inadequate systemic perfusion to meet the body's metabolic demands as a result of impaired cardiac pump function (McCance & Heuther, 2009).

Heart sounds: S_1 corresponds to the closure of mitral and tricuspid valves. S_2 corresponds to closure of the aortic and pulmonary valves. S_3, heard mid-diastolic at the apex, is a low-pitched gallop or blowing sound sometimes called a ventricular gallop and is a common sign of left ventricular failure or distension in adults (Karmath & Thornton, 2002).

Positive hepatojugular reflex: An elevation of venous pressure, visible in the jugular veins and measurable in the veins of the arm, which is produced by firm pressure with the flat hand over the abdomen in active or impending congestive heart failure.

Pulsas alternans: Alternating weak and strong beats of the pulse associated with weak left ventricular function.

Pulse pressure: Difference between systolic and diastolic blood pressures.

Care Setting

Although generally managed at the community level, an inclient stay may be required for periodic exacerbation of failure or development of complications.

Related Concerns

Myocardial infarction, page 75
Hypertension: severe, page 33
Cardiac surgery, page 98
Dysrhythmias, page 87
Psychosocial aspects of care, page 729

Client Assessment Database

DIAGNOSTIC DIVISION MAY REPORT	MAY EXHIBIT
ACTIVITY/REST • Fatigue, exhaustion progressing throughout the day • Inability to perform normal daily activities, such as making bed, climbing stairs, and so on • Exercise intolerance • Dyspnea at rest or with exertion • Insomnia, inability to sleep flat	• Limited exercise tolerance • Fatigue • Restlessness, mental status changes, such as anxiety and lethargy • Vital sign changes with activity
CIRCULATION • History of hypertension, recent or past MIs, multiple MIs, previous episodes of HF, valvular heart disease, cardiac surgery, endocarditis, systemic lupus erythematosus, anemia, septic shock • Swelling of feet, legs, abdomen, or "belt too tight"	• Blood pressure (BP) may be low with cardiac pump failure; in normal range with mild or chronic HF; or high with fluid overload, left-sided HF, and increased systemic vascular resistance (SVR) • Pulse pressure narrow, reflecting reduced ventricular stroke volume • ***Heart rate and rhythm:*** Tachycardia; dysrhythmias such as atrial fibrillation, premature ventricular contractions, heart blocks • ***Apical pulse:*** Point of maximal intensity (PMI) diffuse and displaced to the left • ***Heart sounds:*** S_1 and S_2 possibly softened; S_3 gallop rhythm diagnostic of congestive HF; S_4 occurring with hypertension; systolic and diastolic murmurs indicating the presence of valvular stenosis or insufficiency, causing or exacerbating heart failure • ***Pulses:*** Peripheral pulses diminished; central pulses may be bounding, for example, visible jugular, carotid, abdominal pulsations • Pulsus alternans may be noted • Skin tissue color pale, ashen, dusky, or cyanotic • Nail beds pale or cyanotic, with slow capillary refill • Liver enlarged and palpable; positive hepatojugular reflex may be present in right-sided HF • Edema dependent, generalized, or pitting, especially in extremities • Bulging neck veins (jugular vein distention [JVD])
EGO INTEGRITY • Anxiety, apprehension, fear • Stress related to illness or financial concerns (job, cost of medical care)	• Various behavioral manifestations, for example, anxiety, anger, fear, irritability
ELIMINATION • Decreased voiding, dark urine • Night voiding	• Decreased daytime urination and increased nighttime urination (nocturia)
FOOD/FLUID • History of diet high in salt and processed foods, fat, sugar, and caffeine • Loss of appetite, anorexia • Nausea, vomiting • Significant weight gain (may not respond to diuretic use) • Tight clothing or shoes • Use of diuretics	• Rapid or continuous weight gain • Generalized edema, including whole body or lower extremity swelling—edema generalized, dependent, pitting, brawny • Abdominal distention, suggesting ascites or liver engorgement
HYGIENE • Fatigue, weakness, exhaustion during self-care activities	• Appearance indicative of neglect of personal care

(continues on page 46)

DIAGNOSTIC DIVISION MAY REPORT (continued)	MAY EXHIBIT (continued)
NEUROSENSORY • Weakness • Dizziness • Fainting episodes	• Lethargy, confusion, disorientation • Behavior changes, irritability
PAIN/DISCOMFORT • Chest pain • Chronic or acute angina • Right upper abdominal pain (right-sided HF) • Generalized muscle aches and pains	• Restlessness • Narrowed focus and withdrawal • Guarding behavior
RESPIRATION • Dyspnea with exertion or rest • Nocturnal dyspnea that interrupts sleep • Sleeping sitting up or with several pillows • Cough with or without sputum production, especially when recumbent • Use of respiratory aids, for example, oxygen or medications	• Tachypnea • Shallow, labored breathing • Use of accessory muscles, nasal flaring • Moist cough with left-sided HF • Sputum may be blood-tinged, pink, and frothy (pulmonary edema) • Breath sounds may be diminished, with bibasilar crackles and wheezes • Mentation may be diminished; lethargy, restlessness present • Pallor or cyanosis
SAFETY	• Changes in mentation and confusion • Loss of strength or muscle tone • Increasing risk for falls • Skin excoriations, rashes
SOCIAL INTERACTION • Decreased participation in usual social activities	
TEACHING/LEARNING • Family history of developing HF at young age (genetic form) • Family risk factors, such as heart disease, hypertension, diabetes • Use or misuse of cardiac medications • Use of vitamins, herbal supplements, for example, niacin, coenzyme Q10, garlic, ginkgo, black hellebore, dandelion, or aspirin • Recent or recurrent hospitalizations • Evidence of failure to improve	
DISCHARGE PLAN CONSIDERATIONS • Assistance with shopping, transportation, self-care needs, homemaker and maintenance tasks • Alteration in medication use or therapy • Changes in physical layout of home • May need oxygen at home ➧ Refer to section at end of plan for postdischarge considerations.	

Diagnostic Studies

TEST WHY IT IS DONE	WHAT IT TELLS ME
BLOOD TESTS	
• *Atrial natriuretic peptide (ANP):* Hormone secreted from right atrial cells when pressure increases.	Increased in congestive HF.
• *Beta-type natriuretic peptide (BNP):* Neurohormone secreted from the cardiac ventricles as a response to ventricular volume and fluid overload.	The level of BNP in the blood increases when symptoms of HF worsen and decreases when symptoms of HF improve to stable condition. Elevation of BNP correlates with both the severity of symptoms and the prognosis in congestive HF. A level of BNP that is greater than 100 pg/mL is predictive of HF and increased risk of sudden death and 1-year mortality (Kociol et al, 2011).
• *Liver enzyme tests, alanine aminotransferase (ALT) and aspartate aminotransferase (AST) (formally referred to as SPGT and SGOT):* To determine degree of end-organ involvement.	Elevated in liver congestion, which may be present in right-sided HF.
• *Erythrocyte sedimentation rate (ESR):* Shows the alteration of blood proteins caused by inflammatory and necrotic processes.	May be elevated, indicating acute systemic inflammatory reaction, especially if viral infection is cause of HF.
• *Bleeding and clotting times:* Clotting factors, prothrombin time (PT), partial thromboplastin time (PTT), platelets.	Identifies those at risk for excessive clot formation and identifies therapeutic range for anticoagulant therapy.
• *Electrolytes (sodium, potassium, chloride, magnesium, calcium):* Elements or chemicals needed for the body and heart to work properly.	Electrolytes may be altered because of fluid shifts and decreased renal function associated with HF and medications (e.g., diuretics, ACE inhibitors) used in HF treatment.
• *Arterial blood gas (ABG):* Measures arterial pH, PCO_2, and PO_2. Evaluates respiratory function and provides a measure for determining acid-base balance.	Left ventricular failure is characterized by mild respiratory alkalosis (early); respiratory acidosis, with hypoxemia; and increased PCO_2, with decompensated HF.
• *Albumin and transferrin, total protein:* Plasma proteins exert oncotic pressure needed to keep fluid in the capillaries.	May be decreased as a result of reduced protein intake (nutritional) or reduced protein synthesis (congested liver associated with HF).
• *Thyroid studies:* Blood test and scan to evaluate thyroid function. The most commonly used laboratory screening test is the measurement of thyroid-stimulating hormone (TSH).	Increased thyroid activity suggests thyroid hyperactivity as precipitator of HF. Hypothyroidism can also cause or exacerbate HF.
• *Blood urea nitrogen (BUN) and creatinine:* BUN levels reflect the balance between production and excretion of urea. Creatine is end product of creatinine metabolism and must be cleared from blood via the kidneys.	Elevated BUN suggests decreased renal perfusion as may occur with HF or as a side effect of prescribed medications (e.g., diuretics and ACE inhibitors). Elevation of both BUN and creatinine is typical in HF.
OTHER DIAGNOSTIC STUDIES	
• *Chest x-ray:* Evaluates organs and structures within the chest.	May demonstrate calcification in valve areas or aorta, causing blood flow obstruction, or cardiac enlargement, indicating HF.
• *Electrocardiogram (ECG):* Record of the electrical activity of the heart.	An abnormal ECG can point out the underlying cause of HF, such as ventricular hypertrophy, valvular dysfunction, ischemia, and myocardial damage patterns.
• *Echocardiography (also called two-dimensional echocardiogram or Doppler ultrasound):* Evaluates the left ventricle, including size, valvular function, wall thickness, and pumping action as measured by the ejection fraction (EF).	May reveal enlarged chamber dimensions or alterations in valvular and ventricular function and structure. EF is reduced (less than 50%), indicating systolic dysfunction, or "preserved" (normal is 50% to 65%), indicating diastolic dysfunction (Cunningham, 2006).
• *Stress test (also called exercise treadmill or exercise ECG):* Raises heart rate and BP by means of exercise; heart rate can also be raised pharmacologically through the use of such drugs as dobutamine or dipyridamol.	Helps detect valvular heart disease ventricular remodeling and structural anomalies and problems with coronary circulation affecting heart function.
• *Cardiac angiography (also called cardiac catheterization):* Assesses patency of coronary arteries, reveals abnormal heart and valve size or shape, and evaluates ventricular contractility. Pressures can be measured within each chamber of the heart and across the valves.	Abnormal pressures indicate problems with ventricular function, helping to identify valvular stenosis or insufficiency and differentiating right-sided versus left-sided HF.

Nursing Priorities

1. Improve myocardial contractility and systemic perfusion.
2. Reduce fluid volume overload.
3. Prevent complications.
4. Provide information about disease and prognosis, therapy needs, and prevention of recurrences.

Discharge Goals

1. Cardiac output adequate for individual needs.
2. Complications prevented or resolved.
3. Optimum level of activity and functioning attained.
4. Disease process, prognosis, and therapeutic regimen understood.
5. Plan in place to meet needs after discharge.

NURSING DIAGNOSIS: decreased Cardiac Output

May Be Related To

Altered contractility (such as valvular defects and ventricular aneurysm)
Altered heart rate, rhythm
Altered afterload (vascular resistence)

Possibly Evidenced By

Tachycardia, arrhythmias, ECG changes
Variations in blood pressure readings (hypotension, hypertension)
Decreased peripheral pulses
S_3, S_4 heart sounds
Orthopnea, crackles, jugular vein distension, edema, weight gain
Skin color changes, clammy skin
Oliguria

Desired Outcomes/Evaluation Criteria—Client Will

Cardiac Pump Effectiveness (NOC)

Display vital signs within acceptable limits, dysrhythmias absent or controlled, and no symptoms of failure, for example, hemodynamic parameters within acceptable limits and urinary output adequate.
Report decreased episodes of dyspnea and angina.

Cardiac Disease Self-Management (NOC)

Participate in activities that reduce cardiac workload.

ACTIONS/INTERVENTIONS	RATIONALE
Hemodynamic Regulation (NIC)	
Independent	
Auscultate apical pulse; assess heart rate, rhythm, and document dysrhythmia if telemetry available.	Tachycardia is usually present, even at rest, to compensate for decreased ventricular contractility. Premature atrial contractions (PACs), paroxysmal atrial tachycardia (PAT), PVCs, multifocal atrial tachycardia (MAT), and AF are common dysrhythmias associated with HF, although others may also occur. *Note:* Intractable ventricular dysrhythmias unresponsive to medication suggest ventricular aneurysm.
Note heart sounds.	S_1 and S_2 may be weak because of diminished pumping action. Gallop rhythms are common (S_3 and S_4), produced as blood flows into noncompliant, distended chambers. Murmurs may reflect valvular incompetence and stenosis.
Palpate peripheral pulses.	Decreased cardiac output may be reflected in diminished radial, popliteal, dorsalis pedis, and post-tibial pulses. Pulses may be fleeting or irregular to palpation, and pulsus alternans may be present.
Monitor BP.	In early, moderate, or chronic HF, BP may be elevated because of increased SVR. In advanced HF, the body may no longer be able to compensate, and profound or irreversible hypotension may occur. *Note:* Many clients with HF have consistently low systolic BP (80 to 100 mm Hg) due to their disease process and the medications they take. Most tolerate these BPs without incident (Wingate, 2007).
Inspect skin for pallor and cyanosis.	Pallor is indicative of diminished peripheral perfusion secondary to inadequate cardiac output, vasoconstriction, and anemia. Cyanosis may develop in refractory HF. Dependent areas are often blue or mottled as venous congestion increases.

ACTIONS/INTERVENTIONS (continued)	RATIONALE (continued)
Monitor urine output, noting decreasing output and dark or concentrated urine.	Kidneys respond to reduced cardiac output by retaining water and sodium. Urine output is usually decreased during the day because of fluid shifts into tissues but may be increased at night because fluid returns to circulation when client is recumbent.
Note changes in sensorium, for example, lethargy, confusion, disorientation, anxiety, and depression.	May indicate inadequate cerebral perfusion secondary to decreased cardiac output.
Encourage rest, semirecumbent in bed or chair. Assist with physical care, as indicated.	Physical rest should be maintained during acute or refractory HF to improve efficiency of cardiac contraction and to decrease myocardial oxygen consumption and workload.
Provide quiet environment, explain medical and nursing management, help client avoid stressful situations, listen and respond to expressions of feelings or fears.	Physical and psychological rest helps reduce stress, which can produce vasoconstriction, elevating BP and increasing heart rate and work.
Provide bedside commode. Have client avoid activities eliciting a vasovagal response, for instance, straining during defecation and holding breath during position changes.	Commode use decreases work of getting to bathroom or struggling to use bedpan. Vasovagal maneuver causes vagal stimulation followed by rebound tachycardia, which further compromises cardiac function and output.
Elevate legs, avoiding pressure under knee. Encourage active and passive exercises. Increase ambulation and activity as tolerated.	Decreases venous stasis and may reduce incidence of thrombus and embolus formation.
Check for calf tenderness; diminished pedal pulse; and swelling, local redness, or pallor of extremity.	Reduced cardiac output, venous pooling and stasis, and enforced bedrest increases risk of thrombophlebitis.
Withhold digoxin, as indicated, and notify physician if marked changes occur in cardiac rate or rhythm or signs of digoxin toxicity occur.	Incidence of toxicity is high (20%) because of narrow margin between therapeutic and toxic ranges. Digoxin may have to be discontinued in the presence of toxic drug levels, a slow heart rate, or low potassium level. (Refer to CP: Dysrhythmias; ND: risk for Poisoning [Digoxin Toxicity].)
Collaborative	
Administer supplemental oxygen, as indicated.	Increases available oxygen for myocardial uptake to combat effects of hypoxia and ischemia.
Administer medications, as indicated, for example:	A variety of medications (usually a combination of a diuretic, an ACEI, or ARB and beta blocker) may be used to increase stroke volume, improve contractility, and reduce congestion.
Loop diuretics, such as furosemide (Lasix), ethacrynic acid (Edecrin), and bumetanide (Bumex); thiazide and thiazide-like diuretics, such as hydrochlorothiazide (HCTZ) and metolazone (Zaroxolyn)	Diuretics, in conjunction with restriction of dietary sodium and fluids, often lead to clinical improvement in clients with stages I and II HF. In general, type and dosage of diuretic depend on cause and degree of HF and state of renal function. Preload reduction is most useful in treating clients with a relatively normal cardiac output accompanied by congestive symptoms. Loop diuretics block chloride reabsorption, thus interfering with the reabsorption of sodium and water.
ACE inhibitors, such as elanopril (Vasotec), captopril (Capoten), lisinopril (Prinivil), quinapril (Accupril), ramipril (Altace), and moexipril (Univasc)	ACE inhibitors represent first-line therapy to control HF by decreasing ventricular filling pressures and SVR, while increasing cardiac output with little or no change in BP and heart rate.
ARBs (also known as angiotensin II receptor antagonists), such as candesartan (Atacand), losartan (Cozaar), eprosartan (Teveten), ibesartan (Avapro), and valsartan (Diovan)	Antihypertensive and cardioprotective effects are attributable to selective blockade of AT_1 (angiotensin II) receptors and angiotensin II synthesis. *Note:* ARBs used in combination with ACE inhibitors and beta blockers are thought to have decreased hospitalizations for HF clients.
Vasodilators, such as nitrates (Nitro-Dur, Isordil); arteriodilators such as hydralazine (Apresoline); combination drugs, such as prazosin (Minipress) and nesiritide (Natrecor)	Vasodilators are used to increase cardiac and renal output, reducing circulating volume (preload and afterload), and decreasing SVR, thereby reducing ventricular workload. *Note:* Nesiritide is used in acutely decompensated congestive HF and has been used with digoxin, diuretics, and ACE inhibitors. Parenteral vasodilators are reserved for clients with severe HF or those unable to take oral medications.
β-adrenergic receptor antagonists (also called beta blockers), such as carvedilol (Coreg), bisoprolol (Zebeta), and metoprolol (Lopressor)	Useful in the treatment of HF by blocking the cardiac effects of chronic adrenergic stimulation. Many clients experience improved activity tolerance and EF.
Inotropic agents, such as amrinone (Inocor), milrinone (Primacor), and vesnarinone (Arkin-Z)	These medications are useful for short-term treatment of HF unresponsive to cardiac glycosides, vasodilators, and diuretics in order to increase myocardial contractility and produce vasodilation.

(continues on page 50)

ACTIONS/INTERVENTIONS (continued)	RATIONALE (continued)
Digoxin (Lanoxin)	Digoxin is no longer used routinely in HF but may be prescribed for symptomatic individuals with late-stage HF on maximal medication therapy (Suter, 2012). Digoxin may be added in low doses (0.125) to the client's medication regimen to improve symptoms and is also used to treat atrial fibrillation.
Anti-anxiety agents and sedatives	Allays anxiety and breaks the feedback cycle of anxiety to catecholamine release to anxiety. Promotes rest and relaxation, reducing oxygen demand and myocardial workload.
Anticoagulants, such as low-dose heparin, and warfarin (Coumadin); or antiplatelet agents, for example, low-dose aspirin, clopidogrel (Plavix), tirofiban (Aggrastat)	May be used prophylactically to prevent thrombus and embolus formation in the presence of risk factors, such as venous stasis, enforced bedrest, cardiac dysrhythmias, and history of previous thrombolic episodes.
Administer IV solutions, restricting total amount, as indicated. Avoid saline solutions.	Because of existing elevated left ventricular pressure, client may not tolerate increased fluid volume (preload). Clients with HF also excrete less sodium, which causes fluid retention and increases myocardial workload.
Monitor and replace electrolytes, as indicated.	Fluid shifts and use of diuretics can alter electrolytes (especially potassium and chloride), which affect cardiac rhythm and contractility.
Monitor serial ECG and chest x-ray changes.	ST-segment depression and T-wave flattening can develop because of increased myocardial oxygen demand, even if no CAD is present. Chest x-ray may show enlarged heart and changes of pulmonary congestion.
Measure cardiac output and other functional parameters, as indicated.	Cardiac index, preload and afterload, contractility, and cardiac work can be measured noninvasively by using thoracic electrical bioimpedance (TEB) technique. TEB is useful in determining effectiveness of therapeutic interventions and response to activity.
Prepare for insertion and maintain pacemaker or pacemaker/defibrillator, if indicated.	May be necessary to correct bradydysrhythmias unresponsive to drug intervention, which can aggravate congestive failure and produce pulmonary edema. *Note:* Biventricular pacemaker and cardiac defibrillators are designed to provide resynchronization for the heart by simultaneous electrical activation of both the right and left sides of the heart, thereby creating a more effective and efficient pump.
Prepare for surgery, such as valve replacement, angioplasty, coronary artery bypass grafting (CABG), as indicated:	HF due to ventricular aneurysm or valvular dysfunction may require aneurysmectomy or valve replacement to improve myocardial contractility and function. Revascularization of cardiac muscle by CABG may be done to improve cardiac function.
Cardiomyoplasty	Cardiomyoplasty, an experimental procedure in which the latissimus dorsi muscle is wrapped around the heart and electrically stimulated to contract with each heartbeat, may be done to augment ventricular function while the client is awaiting cardiac transplantation or when transplantation is not an option. *Note*: Despite all basic research and various clinical investigations, the role of cardiomyoplasty in the treatment of heart failure remains unclear (Bocchi, 2001).
Assist with and maintain mechanical circulatory support system, such as intra-aortic balloon pump (IABP) or left-ventricular assist device (LVAD), when indicated.	An IABP may be inserted into the aorta as a temporary support to the failing heart in the critically ill client with potentially reversible HF. A short (external) or long-term (implanted) LVAD may also be used, sometimes as a bridge to transplantation. A growing use of the LVAD is in so-called destination therapy (DT). The DT population typically includes individuals with end-stage heart failure and poor predictive survival in their current medical state. These people are also noneligible for transplantation, usually due to advanced age, significant comorbidities, or psychosocial issues contraindicating transplant. Clients who undergo LVAD implantation live the rest of their lives with the device permanently in place.

NURSING DIAGNOSIS: Activity Intolerance

May Be Related To

Imbalance between oxygen supply and demand
Generalized weakness
Sedentary lifestyle

Possibly Evidenced By

Reports fatigue, feeling weak
Abnormal blood pressure/heart rate in response to activity
Exertional dyspnea

Desired Outcomes/Evaluation Criteria—Client Will

Endurance (NOC)

Participate in desired activities; meet own self-care needs.
Achieve measurable increase in activity tolerance, evidenced by reduced fatigue and weakness and by vital signs within acceptable limits during activity.

ACTIONS/INTERVENTIONS / RATIONALE

Energy Management (NIC)

Independent

Check vital signs before and immediately after activity during acute episode or exacerbation of HF, especially if client is receiving vasodilators, diuretics, or beta blockers.

Orthostatic hypotension can occur with activity because of medication effect (vasodilation), fluid shifts (diuresis), or compromised cardiac pumping function.

Document cardiopulmonary response to activity. Note tachycardia, dysrhythmias, dyspnea, diaphoresis, and pallor.

Compromised myocardium and inability to increase stroke volume during activity may cause an immediate increase in heart rate and oxygen demands, thereby aggravating weakness and fatigue.

Assess level of fatigue, and evaluate for other precipitators and causes of fatigue, for example, HF treatments, pain, cachexia, anemia, and depression.

Fatigue because of advanced HF can be profound and is related to hemodynamic, respiratory, and peripheral muscle abnormalities. Fatigue is also a side effect of some medications (e.g., beta blockers). Other key causes of fatigue should be evaluated and treated as appropriate and desired.

Evaluate accelerating activity intolerance.

May denote increasing cardiac decompensation rather than overactivity.

Provide assistance with self-care activities, as indicated. Intersperse activity with rest periods.

Meets client's personal care needs without undue myocardial stress or excessive oxygen demand.

Collaborative

Implement graded cardiac rehabilitation and activity program.

Strengthens and improves cardiac function under stress if cardiac dysfunction is not irreversible. Gradual increase in activity avoids excessive myocardial workload and oxygen consumption.

NURSING DIAGNOSIS: excess Fluid Volume

May Be Related To

Compromised regulatory mechanism (reduced glomerular filtration rate, increased antidiuretic hormone [ADH] production, and sodium and water retention)
Excess sodium intake

Possibly Evidenced By

Orthopnea, S_3 heart sound
Oliguria, edema, JVD, positive hepatojugular reflex
Weight gain over short period of time
Blood pressure changes
Pulmonary congestion, adventitious breath sounds

Desired Outcomes/Evaluation Criteria—Client Will

Fluid Overload Severity (NOC)

Demonstrate stabilized fluid volume with balanced intake and output, breath sounds clear or clearing, vital signs within acceptable range, stable weight, and absence of edema.
Verbalize understanding of individual dietary and fluid restrictions.

ACTIONS/INTERVENTIONS	RATIONALE
Fluid Management (NIC)	
Independent	
Monitor urine output, noting amount and color, as well as time of day when diuresis occurs.	Urine output may be scanty and concentrated (especially during the day) because of reduced renal perfusion. Recumbency favors diuresis; therefore, urine output may be increased at night or during bedrest.
Monitor 24-hour intake and output (I&O) balance.	Diuretic therapy may result in sudden or excessive fluid loss, creating a circulating hypovolemia, even though edema and ascites remain in the client with advanced HF or CHF.
Maintain chair rest or bedrest in semi-Fowler's position during acute phase.	Recumbency increases glomerular filtration and decreases production of ADH, thereby enhancing diuresis.
Establish fluid intake schedule if fluids are medically restricted, incorporating beverage preferences when possible. Give frequent mouth care and ice chips as part of fluid allotment.	Involving client in therapy regimen may enhance sense of control and cooperation with restrictions.
Weigh daily.	Documents changes in or resolution of edema in response to therapy. A gain of 5 lb represents approximately 2 L of fluid. Conversely, diuretics can result in rapid and excessive fluid shifts and weight loss.
Assess for distended neck and peripheral vessels. Inspect dependent body areas for edema with and without pitting; note presence of generalized body edema (anasarca).	Excessive fluid retention may be manifested by venous engorgement and edema formation. Peripheral edema begins in feet and ankles, or dependent areas, and ascends as failure worsens. Pitting edema is generally obvious only after retention of at least 10 lb of fluid. Increased vascular congestion—associated with right-sided HF—eventually results in systemic tissue edema.
Change position frequently. Elevate feet when sitting. Inspect skin surface, keep dry, and provide padding, as indicated. (Refer to ND: risk for impaired Skin Integrity.)	Edema formation, slowed circulation, altered nutritional intake, and prolonged immobility or bedrest are cumulative stressors that affect skin integrity and require close supervision and preventive interventions.
Auscultate breath sounds, noting decreased and adventitious sounds, for example, crackles and wheezes. Note presence of increased dyspnea, tachypnea, orthopnea, paroxysmal nocturnal dyspnea, and persistent cough.	Excess fluid volume often leads to pulmonary congestion. Symptoms of pulmonary edema may reflect acute left-sided HF. With right-sided HF, respiratory symptoms of dyspnea, cough, and orthopnea may have slower onset but are more difficult to reverse.
Investigate reports of sudden extreme dyspnea and air hunger, need to sit straight up, sensation of suffocation, feelings of panic or impending doom.	May indicate development of complications, such as pulmonary edema or embolus, which differs from orthopnea or paroxysmal nocturnal dyspnea in that it develops much more rapidly and requires immediate intervention.
Monitor BP and central venous pressure (CVP) (if available).	Hypertension and elevated CVP suggest fluid volume excess and may reflect developing or increasing pulmonary congestion, HF.
Assess bowel sounds. Note complaints of anorexia, nausea, abdominal distention, and constipation.	Visceral congestion, occurring in progressive HF, can alter gastrointestinal function.
Provide small, frequent, easily digestible meals.	Reduced gastric motility can adversely affect digestion and absorption. Small, frequent meals may enhance digestion and prevent abdominal discomfort.
Measure abdominal girth, as indicated.	In progressive right-sided HF, fluid may shift into the peritoneal space, causing increasing abdominal girth (ascites).
Palpate abdomen. Note reports of right upper-quadrant pain or tenderness.	Advancing HF leads to venous congestion, resulting in abdominal distention, liver engorgement (hepatomegaly), and pain. This can alter liver function and impair or prolong drug metabolism.
Note increased lethargy, hypotension, and muscle cramping.	These are signs of potassium and sodium deficits that may occur because of fluid shifts and diuretic therapy.
Fluid/Electrolyte Management (NIC)	
Collaborative	
Administer medications, as indicated, for example:	
Diuretics, such as furosemide (Lasix) and bumetanide (Bumex), toresemide (Demadex)	Increases rate of urine flow and may inhibit reabsorption of sodium and chloride in the renal tubules.
Potassium-sparing thiazides such as spironolactone (Aldactone), amiloride (Midamor), triamterene (Direnium)	Promotes diuresis without excessive potassium losses.
Potassium supplements, such as K-Dur, K-Lor, Micro-K	Replaces potassium that is lost as a common side effect of diuretic therapy, which can adversely affect cardiac function.
Maintain fluid and sodium restrictions, as indicated.	Fluid restriction is not a general recommendation, but fluids should be restricted to less than 2 L/day in patients who have significant hyponatremia (<130 mEq/L). Fluid restriction may also be considered when patients have difficulty

ACTIONS/INTERVENTIONS (continued)	RATIONALE (continued)
	controlling fluid retention despite high diuretic doses and sodium restriction (HFSA, 2010).
Consult with dietitian.	May be necessary to provide diet acceptable to client that meets caloric needs within sodium restriction.
Monitor chest x-ray.	Reveals changes indicative of increase or resolution of pulmonary congestion.
Monitor CBC and electrolytes, especially potassium and sodium.	Hyponatremia and anemia may be signs of disease progression. Hypokalemia is a common adverse effect of diuretic treatment, and hyperkalemia may complicate therapy with ACE inhibitors, ARBs, and aldosterone antagonists (Suter, 2012).
Assist with other therapies such as dialysis, or ultrafiltration, as indicated.	Although not frequently used, mechanical fluid removal rapidly reduces circulating volume, especially in pulmonary edema refractory to other therapies.

NURSING DIAGNOSIS: risk for impaired Gas Exchange

Risk Factors May Include

Alveolar-capillary membrane changes such as fluid collection and shifts into interstitial space or alveoli

Possibly Evidenced By

(Not applicable; presence of signs and symptoms establishes an *actual* diagnosis)

Desired Outcomes/Evaluation Criteria—Client Will

Respiratory Status: Gas Exchange (NOC)

Demonstrate adequate ventilation and oxygenation of tissues by ABG values and oximetry within client's normal ranges and be free of symptoms of respiratory distress.

Participate in treatment regimen within level of ability and situation.

ACTIONS/INTERVENTIONS	RATIONALE
Airway Management (NIC)	
Independent	
Auscultate breath sounds, noting crackles and wheezes.	Reveals presence of pulmonary congestion or collection of secretions, indicating need for further intervention.
Instruct client in effective coughing and deep breathing.	Clears airways and facilitates oxygen delivery.
Encourage frequent position changes.	Helps prevent atelectasis and pneumonia.
Maintain chair rest and bedrest in a semi-Fowler's position, with head of bed elevated 20 to 30 degrees.	Reduces oxygen consumption and demands and promotes maximal lung inflation.
Collaborative	
Monitor and graph serial ABG values and pulse oximetry.	Hypoxemia can be severe during pulmonary edema. Compensatory acid-base changes are usually present in chronic HF.
Administer supplemental oxygen, as indicated.	Increases alveolar oxygen concentration, which may correct or reduce tissue hypoxemia.
Administer medications, as indicated, such as the following:	
Diuretics, such as furosemide (Lasix)	Reduce pulmonary congestion, enhancing gas exchange.

NURSING DIAGNOSIS: risk for chronic Pain

Risk Factors May Include

Chronic physical disease or condition

Altered ability to continue previous activities

Possibly Evidenced By

(Not applicable; presence of signs and symptoms establishes an *actual* diagnosis)

Desired Outcomes/Evaluation Criteria—Client Will

Pain Control (NOC)

Verbalize and demonstrate relief or control of pain or discomfort.

Demonstrate and initiate behavioral modifications of lifestyle and appropriate use of therapeutic interventions.

ACTIONS/INTERVENTIONS	RATIONALE
Pain Management (NIC)	
Independent	
Assess for presence of pain.	Pain, physical discomfort, or both are reported by 30% to 80% of clients with advanced HF (Walke et al, 2004). It is unknown whether pain occurs because of the HF itself, due to edema, chest fullness, and underperfused organs (Wingate, 2007), or whether it is related to myocardial stress.
Note coexisting condition(s).	Many HF clients are elderly and have multiple chronic conditions, such as angina, arthritis, gout, back pain, claudication, and neuropathies.
Assess for lifestyle effects of pain, such as deconditioning, severe fatigue, weight loss or gain, sleep difficulties, and depression.	Pain issues should be addressed and managed, when present, even though it may not be possible to determine if pain is a result of the HF itself (associated with underperfused organs) or be related to other conditions.
Provide anticipatory guidance.	In client with HF in which pain is common, educating client and significant other (SO) about when, where, and how to seek interventions or treatment may reduce limitations imposed by pain. If pain is present, pain management should be initiated.
Collaborative	
Assist with treatment of underlying or coexisting conditions.	Promotes general well-being.
Administer analgesics, as indicated.	Promotes rest and relaxation and may enhance ability to engage in desired activities.

NURSING DIAGNOSIS: risk for Impaired Skin Integrity

Risk Factors May Include

Impaired circulation

Possibly Evidenced By

(Not applicable; presence of signs and symptoms establishes an *actual* diagnosis)

Desired Outcomes/Evaluation Criteria—Client Will

Tissue Perfusion: Peripheral (NOC)

Maintain skin integrity.

Demonstrate behaviors or techniques to prevent skin breakdown.

ACTIONS/INTERVENTIONS	RATIONALE
Pressure Management (NIC)	
Independent	
Inspect skin, noting skeletal prominences, presence of edema, and areas of altered circulation and pigmentation.	Skin is at risk because of impaired peripheral circulation, obesity or emaciation, edema, physical immobility, and alterations in nutritional status.
Provide gentle massage around reddened or blanched areas.	Improves blood flow, minimizing tissue hypoxia. *Note:* Direct massage of compromised area may cause tissue injury.
Encourage frequent position changes in bed and chair. Assist with active or passive range of motion (ROM) exercises.	Reduces pressure on tissues, improving circulation and reducing time any one area is deprived of full blood flow.
Provide frequent skin care; minimize contact with moisture or excretions.	Excessive dryness or moisture damages skin and hastens breakdown.
Check fit of shoes or slippers and change as needed.	Dependent edema may cause shoes to fit poorly, thereby increasing risk of pressure and skin breakdown on feet.
Avoid intramuscular route for medication administration.	Interstitial edema and impaired circulation impede drug absorption and predispose to tissue breakdown and development of infection.
Collaborative	
Provide alternating pressure, air- or water-filled mattress, and elbow and heel protectors.	Reduces pressure to skin and may improve circulation.

NURSING DIAGNOSIS: ineffective Self-Health Management

May Be Related To

Complexity of therapeutic regimen
Perceived seriousness/susceptibility
Deficient knowledge
Economic difficulties

Possibly Evidenced By

Reports difficulty with prescribed regimen
Failure to include treatment regimen in daily living
Failure to take action to reduce risk factors
Unexpected acceleration of illness symptoms

Desired Outcomes/Evaluation Criteria—Client Will

Self-Management: Heart Failure (NOC)

Identify relationship of ongoing therapies (treatment program) to reduction of recurrent episodes and prevention of complications.
List signs and symptoms that require immediate intervention.
Identify own stress and risk factors and some techniques for handling them.
Initiate necessary lifestyle and behavioral changes.

ACTIONS/INTERVENTIONS	RATIONALE
Teaching: Disease Process (NIC)	
Independent	
Discuss normal heart function. Include information regarding client's variance from normal function. Explain difference between heart attack and HF.	Knowledge of disease process and expectations can facilitate client's participation in management of HF, including prescribed treatment regimen if teaching is individualized to the client (Fredericks, 2009).
Reinforce treatment rationale. Include SO and family members in teaching as appropriate, especially for complicated regimens such as management of technology, for example, implantable cardioverter-defibrillator (ICD) or LVAD, dobutamine infusion home therapy when client does not respond to customary combination therapy or cannot be weaned from dobutamine, or in those awaiting heart transplant.	Client may believe it is acceptable to alter postdischarge regimen when feeling well and symptom-free or when feeling below par, which can increase the risk of exacerbation of symptoms. Understanding of regimen, medications, technology, and restrictions may augment cooperation with control of symptoms. Home IV therapy requires a significant commitment by caregivers to operate and troubleshoot infusion pump, change dressing for peripherally inserted central catheter (PICC) line, and monitor I&O and signs and symptoms of HF.
Encourage developing a regular home exercise program and provide guidelines for sexual activity.	Promotes maintenance of muscle tone and organ function for overall sense of well-being. Changing sexual habits, for example, sex in morning when well rested, client on top, inclusion of other physical expressions of affection, may be difficult but provides opportunity for continuing satisfying sexual relationship.
Discuss importance of being as active as possible without becoming exhausted and need for rest between activities.	Excessive physical activity or overexertion can further weaken the heart, exacerbating failure, and necessitates adjustment of exercise program.
Discuss importance of sodium limitation. Provide list of sodium content of common foods that are to be avoided or limited. Encourage reading of labels on food and drug packages.	Dietary intake of sodium of more than 2 g/day can offset effect of diuretic. Most common source of sodium is table salt and obviously salty foods, although canned soups and vegetables, luncheon meats, and dairy products also may contain high levels of sodium.
Refer to dietitian for counseling specific to individual needs and dietary customs.	May be helpful in meeting client's nutrition needs, especially in presence of obesity (major risk factor for developing HF), diabetes, or presence of nausea and vomiting and resulting wasting syndrome (cardiac cachexia). Eating six small meals and using liquid dietary supplements and vitamin supplements can limit inappropriate weight loss.
Review medications, purpose, and side effects. Provide both oral and written instructions.	Understanding therapeutic needs and importance of prompt reporting of side effects can prevent occurrence of drug-related complications. Anxiety may block comprehension of input or details, and client and SO may refer to written material at later date to refresh memory.

(continues on page 56)

ACTIONS/INTERVENTIONS (continued)	RATIONALE (continued)
Recommend taking diuretic early in morning.	Provides adequate time for drug effect before bedtime to prevent or limit interruption of sleep.
Instruct and receive return demonstration of ability to take and record daily pulse and BP and when to notify healthcare provider, for example, parameters above or below preset rate and changes in rhythm or regularity.	Promotes self-monitoring of condition and response to therapies. Early detection of changes allows for timely intervention and may prevent complications, such as digoxin toxicity.
Explain and discuss client's role in control of risk factors, such as smoking and alcohol abuse, and precipitating or aggravating factors, such as high-salt diet, inactivity or overexertion, and exposure to extremes in temperature.	Adds to body of knowledge and permits client to make informed decisions regarding control of condition and prevention of recurrence or complications. Smoking potentiates vasoconstriction; sodium intake promotes water retention and edema formation. Improper balance between activity and rest and exposure to temperature extremes may result in exhaustion, increased myocardial workload, and increased risk of respiratory infections. Alcohol can depress cardiac contractility. Limitation of alcohol use to social occasions or maximum of one drink per day may be tolerated unless cardiomyopathy is alcohol induced, which requires complete abstinence.
Review signs and symptoms that require immediate medical attention, such as rapid and significant weight gain, edema, shortness of breath, increased fatigue, cough, hemoptysis, and fever.	Self-monitoring increases client responsibility in health maintenance and aids in prevention of complications such as pulmonary edema, pneumonia. Weight gain of more than 3 lb in 1 week requires medical evaluation or adjustment of diuretic therapy. *Note:* Client should weigh self daily in morning without clothing, after voiding and before eating.
Provide opportunities for client and SO to ask questions, discuss concerns, and make necessary lifestyle changes.	Chronicity and recurrent, debilitating nature of HF often exhausts coping abilities and supportive capacity of both client and SO, leading to depression.
Address caregiver's concerns and needs. Refer for support, assistance, and resources, as indicated.	Caregiver burden can exhaust SO's coping capabilities and health, especially when client has advanced HF, has a ventricular assist device, or is awaiting heart transplantation. (Refer to CP: Multiple Sclerosis; ND: risk for Caregiver Role Strain.)
Discuss general health risks, such as infection, and recommend avoidance of crowds and individuals with respiratory infections and obtaining yearly influenza immunization and one-time pneumonia immunization.	This population is at increased risk for infection because of circulatory compromise, potential immunosuppression, and chronicity of disease.
Emphasize importance of reporting signs and symptoms of digoxin toxicity (as indicated): development of gastrointestinal and visual disturbances, changes in pulse rate and rhythm, and worsening of HF.	Early recognition of developing complications and involvement of healthcare provider may prevent toxicity and hospitalization.
Identify community resources or support groups and visiting home health nurse, as indicated.	May need additional assistance with self-monitoring and home management, especially when HF is progressive.
Discuss importance of advance directives and of communicating plan and wishes to family and primary care providers.	Up to 50% of all deaths from HF are sudden, with many occurring at home, possibly without significant worsening of symptoms. The presumption is that sudden cardiac death is produced by a lethal cardiac arrhythmia, as well as structural and functional changes in the heart (Tomaselli, 2004). If client chooses to refuse life-support measures, an alternative contact person (rather than 911) needs to be designated, should cardiac arrest occur.

POTENTIAL CONSIDERATIONS following discharge from care setting (dependent on client's age, physical condition and presence of complications, personal resources, and life responsibilities)

- ***Activity Intolerance***—imbalance between oxygen supply and demand, generalized weakness
- ***excess or deficient Fluid Volume***—compromised regulatory mechanism, diuretic use, individual fluid and salt intake
- ***risk for impaired Skin Integrity***—physical immobilization, changes in skin turgor, impaired circulation, edema
- ***ineffective Self-Health Management***—complexity of therapeutic regimen, economic difficulties, perceived seriousness
- ***impaired Home Maintenance***—disease (chronic, debilitating condition), insufficient finances, inadequate support systems
- ***Self-Care Deficit***—weakness, fatigue, decreased motivation

Sample clinical pathway follows in Table 4.1.

TABLE 4.1 Sample CP: Heart Failure, Hospital. ELOS 3 Days Cardiology or Medical Unit

ND and Categories of Care	Day 1 ___	Day 2 ___	Day 3 ___	Day 4 Discharge
decreased Cardiac Output R/T altered contractility, altered heart rate/rhythm, altered preload	Goals Participate in actions to reduce cardiac workload	Display VS within acceptable limits; dysrhythmias controlled; pulse oximetry within acceptable range Meets own self-care needs with assistance as necessary	→ Dysrhythmias controlled or absent Free of signs of respiratory distress Demonstrate measurable increase in activity tolerance	→ → →
excess Fluid Volume R/T compromised regulatory mechanisms (sodium/water retention), excess fluid/sodium intake	Verbalize understanding of fluid/food restrictions	Verbalize understanding of general condition and healthcare needs Breath sounds clearing Urinary output adequate Weight loss (reflecting fluid loss)	Plan for lifestyle/behavior changes Breath sounds clear Balanced I&O Edema resolving	Plan in place to meet postdischarge needs Weight stable or continued loss if edema present
Referrals	Cardiology Dietitian	Cardiac rehabilitation Occupational therapist (for ADLs) Social services Home care	Community resources	
Diagnostic studies	ECG, echo-Doppler ultrasound, stress test, cardiac scan	Echo-Doppler (if not done day 1) or other cardiac scans	CXR	
	CXR			
	ABGs/pulse oximetry	Cardiac enzymes (if ↑)		
	Cardiac enzymes; ANP, BNP			
	BUN/Cr	BUN/Cr	BUN/Cr	
	CBC/electrolytes, MG++	Electrolytes	Electrolytes	
	PT/aPTT	PT/aPTT (if taking anticoagulants)	PT/aPTT (as indicated)	
	Liver function studies			
	Serum glucose			
	Albumin/total protein			
	Thyroid studies			
	Digoxin level (as indicated)		Repeat digoxin level (if indicated)	
	UA			
Additional assessments	Apical pulse, heart/breath sounds q8h	→	→ bid	→
	Cardiac rhythm (telemetry) q4h	→	→ D/C	
	BP, P, R q2h until stable, q4h	→ q8h	→	→ D/C
	Temp q8h	→	→	→ qd
	I&O q8h	→	→	→ D/C
	Weight qAM	→	→	→
	Peripheral edema q8h	→	→ bid	→ qd
	Peripheral pulses q8h	→	→ bid	→ D/C
	Sensorium q8h	→	→ bid	→D/C
	DVT check qd	→	→	→
	Response to activity	→	→	→
	Response to therapeutic interventions	→	→	→

(continues on page 58)

TABLE 4.1 Sample CP: Heart Failure, Hospital. ELOS 3 Days Cardiology or Medical Unit (continued)

ND and Categories of Care	Day 1 _____	Day 2 _____	Day 3 _____	Day 4 Discharge
Medications	IV diuretic	→ PO	→	→
Allergies:	ACEI, ARB, vasodilators, beta blocker	→	→	→
___________				
___________	IV/PO potassium	→	→ D/C	→
	Digoxin	→	→	→
	PO/cutaneous nitrates	→	→	→
	Morphine sulfate	→	→	→
	Daytime hours sedation	→	→	→ D/C
	PO/low-dose anticoagulant	→	→ PO or D/C	→
	Stool softener/laxative	→	→	→
Client education	Orient to unit/room	Cardiac education per protocol	Signs/symptoms to report to health-care provider	Provide written instructions for homecare
	Review advance directives	Review medications: dose, times, route, purpose, side effects	Plan for home-care needs	Schedule for follow-up appointments
	Discuss expected outcomes, diagnostic tests/results	Progressive activity program		
	Fluid/nutritional restrictions/needs	Skin care		
Additional nursing actions	Bedrest/chair rest	→ BPR/Ambulate as tolerated, cardiac program	→ Up ad lib/ graded program	→
	Assist with physical care	→	→	→
	Pressure-relieving mattress	→	→	→(send home)
	Dysrhythmia/angina care per protocol	→	→	→
	Supplemental O_2	→	→ D/C if able	
	Cardiac diet	→	→	→

Key: ABG, arterial blood gas; ACEI, angiotensin converting enzyme inhibitor; ad lib, as needed; ADLs, activities of daily living; ANP, atrial natriuretic peptide; aPTT, activated prothrombin time; ARB, angiotensin II receptor blockers; bid, twice a day; BNP, beta-type natriuretic peptide; BP, blood pressure; BRP, bathroom privileges; BUN, blood urea nitrogen; CBC, complete blood count; Cr, creatinine; CXR, chest x-ray; D/C, discontinue; ECG, electrocardiogram; ELOS, estimated length of stay; I&O, intake and output; MG++, magnesium; P, pulse; PO, by mouth; PT, prothrombin time; q2h, every 2 hours; q4h, every 4 hours; q8h, every 8 hours; qAM, every morning; qd, every day; R, respirations; R/T, related to; UA, urinalysis; VS, vital signs.

ACUTE CORONARY SYNDROME (ACS)

"Acute coronary syndrome" refers to a group of clinical symptoms compatible with myocardial ischemia and includes (1) unstable angina (UA), (2) non-ST-segment elevation myocardial infarction (NSTEMI), and (3) ST-segment elevation myocardial infarction (STEMI).

I. Pathophysiology (Overbaugh, 2009; Kumar, 2009; Dechant, 2012)

- **a.** The disorder is characterized by a narrowing of coronary arteries due to atherosclerosloritc plaque, damaging the internal linings of coronary arteries. This condition is known as coronary artery disease (CAD).
- **b.** As the process progresses, oxygen transport to the heart muscle is restricted, resulting in myocardial ischemia and pain.
- **c.** Hard plaque causes hardened arteries, whereas soft plaque can cause formation of blood clots, either of which can restrict blood flow. There can be plaque rupture or clot formation causing a sudden reduction of blood flow and a partial or complete occlusion of the coronary artery.
- **d.** Angina (chest pain) is characterstic of ACS. Pain may or may not radiate to jaw, neck, back, or arm. Angina equivents may include dyspnea, diaphoresis, nausea, and lightheadedness. Pain may be accompanied by changes in vital signs, decreased oxygen saturation (SaO_2), or cardiac dysrhythmias.
- **e.** Women often present with atypical symptoms, such as "indigestion," palpitations, nausea, fatigue, numbness in the hands, and discomfort (not necessarily pain) and not necessarily in the chest (Pilote, 2007).

II. Types of ACS (Overbaugh, 2009; Kumar, 2009; Dechant, 2012)

- **a.** Unstable angina (UA)
  - **i.** May be new onset of pain with exertion or at rest, or acceleration in frequency, duration, or intensity of chest pain.
  - **ii.** Occurs in no regular pattern, usually lasts longer (15 minutes), not generally relieved with rest or medications.

iii. Electrocardiographic (ECG) manifestations include ST-segment depression and inverted T waves. These changes are transient and not always detected.
iv. Cardiac biomarkers are not elevated.

b. Non-ST-segment elevation myocardial infarction (NSTEMI)
i. Pain and angina equivalents may be much the same as in UA or may be of longer duration and more intense.
ii. Electrocardiographic (ECG) manifestations include ST-segment depression and inverted T waves, which may persist after resolution of ischemia and pain.
iii. Cardiac biomarkers are elevated.

c. ST-segment elevation myocardial infarction (STEMI)
i. Electrocardiographic (ECG) manifestations include ST-segment elevation in two contiguous leads (diagnostic of STEMI), and abnormal Q waves appear as a result of alterations in electrical conductivity of the infracted myocardial cells.
ii. The imbalance between oxygen supply and demand is severe enough to cause tissue necrosis and the client requires emergency revascularization.

III. Etiology (Go et al, 2012; Mayo Clinic, 2010)

a. Coronary artery disease (CAD) common cause with plaque formation narrowing vessels and pieces of plaque breaking off, creating emboli, and coronary artery obstruction.
b. Risk factors—age (older than 45 for men, and 55 for women).
c. Presence of "metabolic syndrome" (e.g., fasting plasma glucose ≥100 mg/dL or undergoing drug treatment for elevated glucose; HDL cholesterol <40 mg/dL in men or <50 mg/dL in women or undergoing drug treatment for reduced HDL cholesterol; triglycerides ≥150 mg/dL or undergoing drug treatment for elevated triglycerides; waist circumference ≥102 cm in men or ≥88 cm in women; BP ≥130 mm Hg systolic or ≥85 mm Hg diastolic or undergoing drug treatment for hypertension.
d. Being overweight or obese, lack of physical activity, smoking.
e. Type 2 diabetes and family history of chest pain, heart disease, or stroke.

IV. Statistics (National Heart, Lung and Blood Institute [NHLBI], 2011; Centers for Disease Control and Prevention [CDC], 2012)

a. Morbidity: There are an estimated 82.6 million Americans with some form of cardiovascular disease.
b. Coronary artery disease (CAD) accounts for 16.3 million; angina, approximately 9 million.
c. 400,000 new cases annually, most are over age 65.
d. Mortality: There were 812,000 deaths from cardiovascular disease in 2008; accounts for approximately 33% of total deaths.
e. Cost: Inpatient cardiovascular procedures and operations in 2009—echocardiogram $2.3 billion, diagnostic cardiac catheterization/coronary angiography $5.9 billion, angioplasty (PTCA) $11 billion, pacemaker procedures $8.2 billion (Pfunter, 2012).

GLOSSARY

Angioplasty: See Percutaneous coronary interventions (PCIs), below.

Cardiac biomarkers: Substances that are released into the blood when the heart is damaged or stressed. Measurement of these biomarkers is used to help diagnose, monitor, and manage people with suspected ACS and cardiac ischemia. The current biomarker test of choice for detecting heart damage is troponin (see below). Other cardiac biomarkers (e.g, CK, CK-MB, myoglobin) are less specific for the heart and may also be elevated in skeletal muscle injury, liver disease, or kidney disease (Lab Tests Online, 2012).

Coronary artery disease (CAD): Disease in which there is a narrowing or blockage of the coronary arteries that carry blood and oxygen to the heart muscle.

Myocardial infarction (MI): An occlusion or blockage of arteries supplying the muscles of the heart, resulting in injury or necrosis of the heart muscle (heart attack).

Occlusive thrombus: Blood clot which completely blocks a coronary artery.

Percutaneous coronary interventions (PCIs), also known as angioplasty: A nonsurgical procedure used to treat stenotic coronary arteries of the heart found in coronary heart disease. During PCI, a cardiologist feeds a deflated balloon or other device on a catheter from the inguinal femoral artery or radial artery up through blood vessels until they reach the site of blockage in the heart. X-ray imaging is used to guide the catheter threading. At the blockage, the balloon is inflated to open the artery, allowing blood to flow. A stent is often placed at the site of blockage to permanently open the artery.

Non-ST-segment elevation myocardial infarction (NSTEMI): Partial block of coronary arteries (nonocclusive thrombus). There will be no ST elevation or Q waves on ECG, as transmural infarction is not seen. The main difference between NSTEMI and unstable angina is that in NSTEMI the severity of ischemia is sufficient to cause cardiac enzyme elevation. Fibrolynics are not beneficial in NSTEMI due to increased risk of bleeding complications.

ST-segment elevation myocardial infarction (STEMI): A transmural infarction of the myocardium where the entire thickness of the myocardium has undergone necrosis. Usually due to an occlusive thrombus. This requires the use of thrombolytics to lyse the thrombus.

Troponin (also known as Cardiac-specific Troponin I and Troponin T): Blood test used to help diagnose a heart attack, to detect and evaluate mild to severe heart injury, and to distinguish chest pain that may be due to other causes. Troponins are the preferred tests for a suspected heart attack because they are more specific for heart injury than other tests and remain elevated for a longer period of time (Lab Tests Online, 2012).

Unstable angina (UA): Chest pain produced when the heart muscle is not getting enough blood flow is considered "unstable" when it no longer follows the predictable patterns typical of "stable angina." Unstable angina is called "unstable" for two reasons: (1) symptoms occur in a more random and unpredictable fashion, and (2) it is most often caused by the actual rupture of a plaque in a coronary artery resulting in clot formation, with impairment of free blood flow to tissues. The imminent risk of a complete myocardial infarction is very high in unstable angina. Such a condition is quite "unstable," and for this reason is a medical emergency (Fogoros, 2011).

Care Setting

Client may have a short hospitalization during acute stage for stabilization and possible cardiac revascularization. The client who has sustained a STEMI or is judged to be at intermediate or high risk for MI will be hospitalized for further evaluation and therapeutic intervention.

Related Concerns

Angina, page 67
Dysrrhythmias, page 87
Myocardial infarction, page 75
Psychosocial aspects of care, page 729

Client Assessment Database

DIAGNOSTIC DIVISION MAY REPORT	MAY EXHIBIT
ACTIVITY/REST	
• Sedentary lifestyle • Weakness, feeling incapacitated after exercise • Fatigue • Activities and sleep disrupted by pain	• Exertional dyspnea
CIRCULATION	
• History of heart disease, hypertension in self or family • Palpitations	• Tachycardia, dysrhythmias • Blood pressure (BP) may be normal, elevated, or decreased • ***Heart sounds:*** May be normal, late S_4 or transient late systolic murmur may be evident during pain • Moist, cool, pale skin, mucous membranes in presence of vasoconstriction • Orthostatic blood pressure changes
EGO INTEGRITY	
• Stressors of work, family, others, and financial concerns	• Apprehension, uneasiness
FOOD/FLUID	
• Nausea, "heartburn," or epigastric distress • Diet high in cholesterol and fats, salt, caffeine, liquor	• Belching, gastric distention
NEUROSENSORY	
• History of dizziness, fainting spells, transient numbness, tingling in extremities (ischemia anywhere in the body can produce transient neurological symptoms)	
PAIN	
Note: Reports of pain location and severity differ between men and women. • Substernal or anterior chest pain that may radiate to jaw, neck, shoulders, and upper extremities, often to left side more than right. Women may report pain between shoulder blades, back pain. • ***Quality:*** Varies from transient and mild to moderate, heavy pressure, tightness, squeezing, burning. Women may report dull aching pain. • ***Duration:*** Usually more than 15 minutes • ***Precipitating factors:*** May be unpredictable or occur during rest or sleep • ***Relieving factors:*** Pain may not be responsive to particular relief mechanisms, such as rest and anti-anginal medications	• Facial grimacing, restlessness • Placing fist over midsternum • Rubbing left arm, muscle tension • Autonomic responses, for example, tachycardia, blood pressure changes
RESPIRATION	
• Exertional dyspnea, which may resolve with rest or pain relief • Smoking history	Increased rate and rhythm, alteration in depth

DIAGNOSTIC DIVISION MAY REPORT (continued)	MAY EXHIBIT (continued)
TEACHING/LEARNING • Family history or risk factors of CAD: obesity, sedentary lifestyle, HTN, stroke, diabetes, smoking, hyperlipidemia • Use or misuse of cardiac, antihypertensive, and over-the-counter (OTC) drugs **DISCHARGE PLAN CONSIDERATIONS** • Assistance with homemaker or maintenance tasks • Changes in physical layout of home	

Diagnostic Studies

TEST WHY IT IS DONE	WHAT IT TELLS ME
DIAGNOSTIC STUDIES	
• *Electrocardiogram (ECG):* Record of the electrical activity of the heart to detect dysrhythmias, to identify any myocardial ischemia present, or any damage to myocardial tissue from the past	In the emergency setting, ECG is the most important diagnostic test. It may show changes during symptoms and in response to treatment; confirm a cardiac basis for symptoms. It also may demonstrate preexisting structural or ischemic heart disease (left ventricular hypertrophy, Q waves). ECG changes associated with unstable angina (UA) include ST-segment depression, transient ST-segment elevation, and T-wave inversion or some combination of these factors (Kumar, 2009; Coven, 2013). An ST-wave elevation of 0.1 mV or more, if present in at least two leads, indicates acute MI in 90% of people, as confirmed by serial measurements of cariac biomarkers (Kumar, 2009).
• *Echocardiography (also called two-dimensional echocardiogram and Doppler ultrasound):* Provides visual of working heart and structures	May play an important role in the setting of ACS as it identifies regional wall-motion abnormalities associated with myocardial ischemia. An echocardiogram can also help in defining the extent of an infarction when muscle damage occurs.
• *Cardiac catheterization with angiography:* Assesses patency of coronary arteries, reveals abnormal heart and valve size or shape, and evaluates ventricular contractility	Cardiac catheterization defines coronary anatomy and the extent of a client's disease. Client with intractable angina (despite medication) should immediately undergo cardiac catheterization (Coven, 2013). For high-risk patients with ACS without persistent ST elevation, angiography with glycoprotein IIb/IIIa inhibition has been recommended (Katritsis et al, 2011). Most individuals with UA and NSTEMI benefit from angiography when they have a TIMI (Thrombolysis in Myocardial Infarction) risk score of less than 3 points (Antman et al, 2000).
• *Coronary computed tomography angiography (CTA):* High-resolution, three-dimensional pictures of the moving heart and great vessels	Scanners can do a full scan in 10 seconds and produce high-resolution images that allow fine details of coronary arteries to be seen. This technology allows for noninvasive and early diagnosis of CAD and thus earlier treatment before the coronary arteries become more or completely occluded.
• *Chest x-ray:* Visualize any infiltrates that may be present in the lung	Helps in assessing cardiomegaly and pulmonary edema, or it may reveal complications of ischemia, such as pulmonary edema.
BLOOD TESTS	
• *Cardiac enzymes, including troponin I and troponin T. Also possibly CPK, CK, and CK-MB:* Substances released from heart muscle when it is damaged	Cardiac-specific troponins are not detectable in the blood of healthy individuals; therefore, they provide high specificity for detecting injury to cardiac myocytes. These molecules are also more sensitive than CK-MB for myocardial necrosis and therefore improve early detection of small myocardial infarctions. NSTEMI is distinguished from unstable angina by elevated cardiac enzymes and biomarkers of myocyte

(continues on page 62)

Diagnostic Studies (continued)

TEST WHY IT IS DONE (continued)	WHAT IT TELLS ME (continued)
	necrosis. Differentiation is generally based on three sets of tests measured at 6- to 8-hour intervals after the client's presentation to the emergency depertment. The current definition of NSTEMI requires a typical clinical syndrome plus elevated troponin (or creatine kinase isoenzyme MB [CK-MB]) levels to over 99% of the normal reference. Given this definition, nearly 25% of individuals who were previously classified as having unstable angina now fulfill the criteria for NSTEMI (Coven, 2013; Lab Tests Online, 2011).
• *Complete blood count (CBC)*	The CBC count helps in ruling out anemia as a secondary cause of ACS. Leukocytosis has prognostic value in the setting of acute myocardial infarction.
• *C-reactive protein (CRP):* A marker for inflammation	CRP levels have been shown to predict risk of both recurrent ischemia and death among those with stable and unstable angina (Jiang, 2011).
• *Metabolic profile, including blood glucose electrolytes BUN/Cr*	Important for client with new-onset angina. Close monitoring of potassium and magnesium levels is important in client with ACS because low levels may predispose to ventricular dysrhythmias. Creatinine levels must be considered before using an angiotensin-converting enzyme (ACE) inhibitor and particularly if cardiac catheterization is considered.
• *Serum lipids, including total lipids, lipoprotein electrophoresis, isoenzymes, cholesterols (HDL, LDL, very low density lipoprotein [VLDL]), triglycerides, phospholipids:* A group of tests that make up a lipid profile	The presence of lipid abnormalities increases the risk of CAD.
• *Coagulation studies, including partial thromboplastin time (PTT), activated partial thromboplastin time (aPPT), and platelets:* Injury to a vessel wall or the tissue initiates the coagulation cascade and formation of a thrombus.	Thrombus formation can potentiate ischemic damage to the myocardium as blood flow is blocked.

Nursing Priorities

1. Relieve or control pain.
2. Prevent or minimize development of myocardial complications.
3. Provide information about disease process, prognosis, and treatment.
4. Support client or significant other (SO) in initiating necessary lifestyle or behavioral changes.

Discharge Goals

1. Desired activity level achieved, with return to activity baseline, and self-care needs met with minimal or no pain.
2. Remains free of complications.
3. Disease process, prognosis, and therapeutic regimen understood.
4. Participates in treatment program and behavioral changes.
5. Plan in place to meet needs after discharge.

NURSING DIAGNOSIS: acute Pain

May Be Related To

Physical agents (increased cardiac workload and oxygen consumption, decreased myocardial blood flow, tissue ischemia)

Possibly Evidenced By

Verbal/coded reports of pain
Expressive behaviors (such as moaning, crying, pacing, or restlessness)
Diaphoresis; changes in blood pressure, heart rate, respiratory rate, pupillary dilation
Self-focus

Desired Outcomes/Evaluation Criteria—Client Will

Pain Level (NOC)

Report anginal episodes decreased in frequency, duration, and severity.
Demonstrate relief of pain as evidenced by stable vital signs and absence of muscle tension and restlessness.

ACTIONS/INTERVENTIONS	RATIONALE
Pain Management (NIC)	
Independent	
Instruct client to notify nurse immediately when chest pain occurs.	Pain and decreased cardiac output may stimulate the sympathetic nervous system to release excessive amounts of norepinephrine, which increases platelet aggregation, and release of thromboxane A2. This potent vasoconstrictor causes coronary artery spasm, which can precipitate, complicate, and prolong an anginal attack. Unbearable pain may cause vasovagal response, thus decreasing BP and heart rate.
Assess and document client response and effects of medication.	Provides information about disease progression. Aids in evaluating effectiveness of interventions and may indicate need for change in therapeutic regimen.
Identify precipitating event, if any; identify frequency, duration, intensity, and location of pain.	Helps differentiate chest pain and aids in evaluating possible progression or process. Stable angina usually lasts 3 to 15 minutes and is often relieved by rest and sublingual nitroglycerin (NTG); UA, NSTEMI, and STEMI pain is more intense, occurs unpredictably, may last longer, and is not usually relieved by NTG or rest.
Evaluate reports of pain in jaw, neck, shoulder, arm, or hand (typically on left side).	Cardiac pain may radiate; for example, pain is often referred to more superficial sites served by the same spinal cord nerve level.
Monitor vital signs every 5 minutes during initial anginal attack.	BP may initially rise because of sympathetic stimulation and then fall if cardiac output is compromised. Tachycardia also develops in response to sympathetic stimulation and may be sustained as a compensatory response if cardiac output falls.
Monitor heart rate and rhythm.	Clients with unstable angina have an increased risk of acute life-threatening dysrhythmias, which occur in response to ischemic changes and stress hormones. (Refer to ND: risk for decreased Cardiac Output.)
Place client at complete rest during anginal episodes.	Reduces myocardial oxygen demand to minimize risk of tissue injury and necrosis.
Elevate head of bed if client is short of breath.	Facilitates gas exchange to decrease hypoxia and resultant shortness of breath.
Observe for associated symptoms, such as dyspnea, nausea, vomiting, dizziness, palpitations, and desire to urinate.	Decreased cardiac output, which may occur during ischemic myocardial episode, stimulates sympathetic or parasympathetic nervous system, causing a variety of vague sensations that client may not identify as related to anginal episode.
Stay with client who is experiencing pain or appears anxious.	Anxiety releases catecholamines, which increase myocardial workload and can escalate or prolong ischemic pain. Presence of nurse can reduce feelings of fear and helplessness.
Maintain quiet, comfortable environment; restrict visitors as necessary.	Mental or emotional stress increases myocardial workload.
Collaborative	
Collaborate in treatment of condition.	Initial therapy for ACS should focus on stabilizing the client's condition, relieving ischemic pain, and providing antithrombotic therapy to reduce myocardial damage and prevent further ischemia. (Refer to NDs: risk for decreased cardiac Tissue Perfusion, and risk for decreased Cardiac Output, following, for discussion of additional medications.)
Provide supplemental oxygen.	Increases oxygen available for myocardial uptake to relieve ischemic pain.
Adminster analgesics, such as morphine sulfate (MS) or fentanyl (Duragesic) by appropriate route, for example, IV, oral, patch, etc.	Potent opioid analgesic may be used in acute angina because of its beneficial side effects. Such effects include peripheral vasodilatation and reduced myocardial workload; sedation, which produces relaxation; and interrupted flow of vasoconstricting catecholamines, thereby effectively relieving severe chest pain.
Administer anti-anginal medication(s) promptly, as indicated, for example:	
Sublingual and/or IV nitroglycerin.	Nitrates do not improve mortality. However, they provide symptomatic relief by means of several mechanisms, including coronary vasodilation, improved collateral blood flow, decrease in preload (venodilation and reduced venous

(continues on page 64)

ACTIONS/INTERVENTIONS	RATIONALE
	return), and decrease in afterload (arterial vasodilation) (Thandani, 1994). Care should be taken to avoid hypotension, because this can potentially reduce coronary perfusion pressure.
Calcium channel blockers, such as bepridil (Vascor), amlodipine (Norvasc), nicardipine (Cardene), nifedipine (Procardia), felodipine (Plendil), isradipine (DynaCirc), and diltiazem (Cardizem).	Produce relaxation of coronary vascular smooth muscle, dilate coronary arteries, and decrease peripheral vascular resistance.
Monitor serial ECG changes.	Ischemia during anginal attack may cause transient ST-segment depression or elevation, and T-wave inversion. Serial tracings verify ischemic changes, which may disappear when client is pain-free. They also provide a baseline against which to compare later pattern changes.

NURSING DIAGNOSIS: risk for decreased Cardiac Tissue Perfusion

Risk Factors May Include

Coronary artery spasm
Hypertension, hypoxemia
Elevated C-reactive protein; hypelipdemia
Family history of cardiac disease

Possibly Evidenced By

(Not applicable; presence of signs and symptoms establishes an *actual* diagnosis)

Desired Outcomes/Evaluation Criteria—Client Will

Cardiac Pump Effectiveness (NOC)

Report or display decreased episodes of angina.
Participate in behaviors and activities that reduce the workload of the heart.

ACTIONS/INTERVENTIONS	RATIONALE
Hemodynamic Regulation (NIC)	
Independent	
Maintain bedrest or chair rest in position of comfort during acute episode.	Decreases oxygen consumption and demand, reducing myocardial workload and risk of decompensation.
Monitor vital signs and cardiac rhythm.	Tachycardia and changes in blood pressure (hypotension or hypertension) may be present because of pain, anxiety, hypoxemia, and circulating stress hormones. ECG changes reflecting ischemia and dysrhythmias indicate need for additional evaluation and therapeutic intervention.
Auscultate breath sounds and heart sounds.	S_3, S_4, may occur with cardiac decompensation, or pulmonary complication.
Monitor for and document effects of and adverse response to medications, noting BP, heart rate, and rhythm (especially when giving combination of calcium antagonists, beta blockers, and nitrates).	Desired effect is to decrease myocardial oxygen demand by decreasing cardiac stress. Drugs with negative inotropic properties can decrease perfusion to an already ischemic myocardium.
Encourage immediate reporting of pain for prompt administration of medications, as indicated.	Timely interventions can reduce oxygen consumption and myocardial workload and may prevent or minimize cardiac complications.
Assess for signs and symptoms of heart failure.	Angina is only a symptom of underlying pathology causing myocardial ischemia. Progressionof disorder may compromise cardiac function to point of decompensation.
Collaborative	
Administer supplemental oxygen as needed.	Increases oxygen available for myocardial uptake to improve contractility and reduce ischemia.
Monitor pulse oximetry or arterial blood gases (ABGs), as indicated.	Oxygen saturation may decrease as oxygen demands increase for heart muscle and systemic circulation. Monitoring determines adequacy of respiratory function and O_2 therapy.
Administer medications, as indicated, for example:	
Beta blockers, such as metaprolol (Lopressor), esmilol (Brevibloc)	Beta blockers have anti-arrhythmic and anti-hypertensive properties, as well as the ability to reduce ischemia. They minimize

ACTIONS/INTERVENTIONS	RATIONALE
	the imbalance between myocardial supply and demand by reducing afterload and wall stress (Coven, 2013). *Note*: Beta blockers are indicated in all clients unless they have the following contraindications: systolic blood pressure less than 90 mm Hg, cardiogenic shock, severe bradycardia, second- or third-degree heart block, asthma or emphysema that is sensitive to beta agonists.
Antithrombotic therapy, including antiplatelet agents, such as aspirin (Anacin, Bayer aspirin)	Antiplatelet therapy reduces mortality by reducing the risk of fatal myocardial infarctions. Aspirin permanently impairs the cyclooxygenase pathway of thromboxane A2 production in platelets, in this way inhibiting platelet function.
Clopidogrel (Plavix), prasugre (Effient)	Inhibits activation of the glycoprotein IIb/IIIa complex, a necessary step for platelet aggregation. This process results in intense inhibition of platelet function, particularly in combination with aspirin. Effient is an oral antiplatelet (OAP) medicine that, when taken with aspirin, has been shown in clinical studies to help reduce the risk of a future heart-related event, such as a heart attack or blood clot in a stent, in clients with an ACS event that was treated with angioplasty (Medlineplus, 2009).
Glycoprotein IIb/IIIa receptor antagonists such as abciximab (ReoPro), eptifibatid (Integrilin), tirofiban (Aggrastat)	These agents prevent the binding of fibrinogen, thereby blocking platelet aggregation, and in combination with aspirin are considered standard antiplatelet therapy for client at high risk for unstable angina. Tirofiban has been approved for use in combination with heparin for patients with unstable angina who are being treated medically and for patients undergoing percutaneous coronary intervention (Coven, 2013).
Anticoagulants, such as heparin, low-molecular weight heparin (LMWH)	An IV bolus of heparin, followed by continuous infusion, is recommended to help reduce risk of subsequent MI by reducing the thrombotic complications of plaque rupture for clients diagnosed with intermediate or high-risk UA. Use of low-molecular-weight heparin is increasing because it is more predictable and has fewer adverse effects. It also does not require anticoagulation monitoring. *Note*: One study found that unfractionated heparin was associated with a 33% reduction in the risk of myocardial infarction or death in individuals who were treated with aspirin plus heparin, compared with those who were treated with aspirin alone (Oler, 1996).
Prepare for interventions such as angioplasty with or without intracoronary stent placement, as indicated.	Angioplasty, also called percutaneous transluminal coronary angioplasty (PTCA), increases coronary blood flow by compression of atheromatous lesions and dilation of the vessel lumen in an occluded coronary artery. Intracoronary stents may be placed to provide structural support within the coronary artery and improve the odds of long-term patency. Drug-eluting stents may be considered for clients at high risk for thrombosis or acute closure. Stent placement may also be effective for the variant form of angina where periodic vasospasms impair arterial flow.

NURSING DIAGNOSIS: risk for decreased Cardiac Output

Risk Factors May Include

Altered contractility, stroke volume
Altered preload

Possibly Evidenced By

(Not applicable; presence of signs and symptoms establishes *actual* diagnosis)

Desired Outcomes/Evaluation Criteria—Client Will

Cardiac Pump Effectiveness (NOC)

Maintain hemodynamic stability, such as BP, cardiac output within normal range, adequate urinary output, decreased frequency or absence of dysrhythmias.
Report decreased episodes of dyspnea and angina.
Demonstrate an increase in activity tolerance.

ACTIONS/INTERVENTIONS	RATIONALE
Cardiac Care: Acute (NIC)	
Independent	
Obtain BP readings. Compare both arms and obtain lying, sitting, and standing pressures when able.	Hypotension may occur related to ventricular dysfunction, hypoperfusion of the myocardium, and vagal stimulation. However, hypertension is also a common phenomenon, possibly related to pain, anxiety, catecholamine release, and preexisting vascular problems.
Monitor heart rate and rhythm. Document dysrhythmias.	Dysrhythmias, especially premature ventricular contractions or heart blocks, can compromise cardiac function or increase ischemic damage. Acute or chronic atrial flutter or fibrillation may be seen with coronary artery involvement and may or may not be pathological.
Auscultate heart sounds. Note development of S_3 and S_4.	S_3 is usually associated with heart failure, but it may also be noted with left ventricular overload that can accompany infarction in STEMI. S_4 may be associated with myocardial ischemia, ventricular stiffening, and pulmonary or systemic hypertension.
Auscultate breath sounds.	Crackles reflect pulmonary congestion; may develop because of depressed myocardial function.
Have emergency equipment and medications available.	Sudden coronary occlusion, lethal dysrhythmias, extension of infarct, and unrelenting pain are situations that may precipitate cardiac arrest, requiring immediate life-saving therapies or transfer to CCU.
Collaborative	
Administer supplemental oxygen, as indicated.	Increases amount of oxygen available for myocardial uptake, reducing ischemia and resultant cellular irritation and dysrhythmias.
Review serial ECGs.	Provides information regarding progression or resolution of ischemia, status of ventricular function, electrolyte balance, and effect of drug therapies.
Review chest x-ray.	May reflect pulmonary edema related to ischemia and ventricular dysfunction.
Monitor laboratory data, such as cardiac enzymes, arterial blood gases (ABGs), and electrolytes.	Enzymes monitor resolution or extension of infarction. Presence of hypoxia indicates need for supplemental oxygen. Electrolyte imbalances, such as hypo- or hyperkalemia, adversely affect cardiac rhythm and contractility.
Maintain IV or saline-lock access, as indicated.	Patent line is important for administration of fluids to support circulation and to administer emergency drugs in presence of persistent lethal dysrhythmias or chest pain.
Administer medications, as indicated: Antidysrhythmic drugs (refer to CP: Dysrhythmias)	Dysrhythmias are usually treated symptomatically, but have the potential for becoming lethal; therefore must be monitored diligently and treated promptly.
Assist with insertion and maintain pacemaker or automatic internal cardiac defibrillator (AICD) when used (refer to CP: Dysrhythmias)	Pacing may be a temporary support measure during acute phase or may be needed permanently if infarction severely damages conduction system.
Refer to CP: Myocardial Infarction for additional interventions.	If STEMI is occurring, many more supportive interventions may be needed.

NURSING DIAGNOSIS: deficient Knowledge [Learning Need] regarding condition, postprodecure care, potential complications

May Be Related To

Lack of exposure or recall
Unfamiliarity with information resources

Possibly Evidenced By

Reports the problem

Desired Outcomes/Evaluation Criteria—Client Will

Self-Management: Coronary Artery Disease (NOC)

Verbalize understanding of condition, postprocedure needs, and potential complications.
Identify individual risk factors.
Initiate necessary lifestyle changes.

ACTIONS/INTERVENTIONS	RATIONALE
Teaching: Disease Process (NIC)	
Independent	
Reinforce explanation of particular procedure/treatment provided and self-care needs.	Individually specific information creates knowledge base for management of condition.
Encourage identification and reduction of individual risk factors such as smoking, alcohol consumption, and obesity.	These behaviors and substances have direct adverse effects on cardiovascular function and may impede recovery, increase risk for complications.
Reinforce explanations of dietary and activity restrictions and routine and prophylactic medications.	Provides opportunity for client to retain information and to assume control and participate in wellness program.
Review appropriate exercise program and encourage client to set realistic goals.	Individual capabilities and expectations depend on type of procedure performed, underlying cardiac function, and prior physical conditioning.
Stress importance of checking with physician before taking OTC drugs.	OTC drugs may potentiate or negate effects of prescribed medications.
Discuss use of herbals such as ginseng, garlic, ginkgo, hawthorn, and bromelain, as indicated.	Some herbals can affect bleeding and clotting, especially when added to medications such as Plavix or Coumadin, which increase bleeding. Others, such as hawthorn, can increase the effects of certain heart medications.
Review symptoms to be reported to physician, particularly recurrence of chest pain and changes in response to medications.	Knowledge of expectations can avoid undue concern for insignificant events or prevent delay in treatment of worrisome symptoms.
Identify services and resources available after discharge.	Provides for ongoing monitoring, continutation of prescribed therapies, and support for lifestyle changes.

POTENTIAL CONSIDERATIONS following discharge from care setting (dependent on client's age, physical condition and presence of complications, personal resources, and life responsibilities)
- ***acute Pain***—physical agents (decreased myocardial blood flow, tissue ischemia)
- ***Activity Intolerance***—imbalance between oxygen supply and demand, sedentary lifestyle
- ***risk for ineffective Self-Health Management***—complexity of therapeutic regimen, perceived barriers, economic difficulties

ANGINA: CHRONIC/STABLE

I. Pathophysiology

a. Chronic/stable angina is an episodic clinical manifestation of ischemic heart disease due to transient myocardial ischemia. May be called "stable ischemic heart disease" (SIHD) or "ischemic heart disease" (IHD) (Fihn et al, 2012; Snow, 2004).
b. Stable means no increase in frequency or severity of attacks over a prolonged period of time.
c. Most commonly caused by atherosclerotic coronary artery disease (CAD).
d. Atypical presentations of angina are more common in women than in men (Abrams, 2007).
e. Many people experience anginal attacks despite revascularization and pharmacological anti-anginal treatments (Khan, 2011).
f. Usually presents as chest discomfort precipitated by stress or exertion that rapidly resolves with rest or nitrates.
g. If symptoms occur at rest, or if severity or frequency of attacks increases, the individual is said to have unstable angina.

II. Etiology (Snow et al, 2004)

a. Conditions that create increased myocardial oxygen demand (including hyperthyroidism, hyperthermia, cocaine use, valvular disease such as aortic stenosis, and severe uncontrolled hypertension)
b. Conditions that create decreased myocardial oxygen supply, such as anemia, or hypoxemia secondary to pulmonary disease
c. Risk factors: being overweight and obese, smoking, sedentary lifestyle, diabetes, family history of early heart disease, metabolic syndrome (fasting hyperglycemia and insulin resistance, hypertension, central obesity, decreased high-density lipoprotein [HDL] and elevated low-density lipoprotein [LDL] cholesterol, elevated triglycerides)

III. Statistics (National Heart, Lung and Blood Institute [NHLBI], 2011; Centers for Disease Control and Prevention [CDC], 2012)

a. Morbidity: There are an estimated 82.6 million Americans with some form of cardiovascular disease.
   i. Coronary artery disease (CAD) accounts for 16.3 million; angina, approximately 9 million.
   ii. 400,000 new cases annually; most are over age 65
b. Mortality: There were 812,000 deaths from cardiovascular disease in 2008; accounts for approximately 33% of total deaths.
c. Cost: Estimates of direct care cost for chronic angina vary from $17 billion to $49 billion annually (Reynolds, 2004).

GLOSSARY

Angioplasty (also called percutaneous transluminal coronary angioplasty or PTCA): Procedure that increases coronary blood flow by compression of atheromatous lesions and dilation of the vessel lumen in an occluded coronary artery.

Cardiovascular disease (CVD): Diseases of the heart and blood vessels.

Coronary artery disease (CAD): A disease in which there is a narrowing or blockage of the coronary arteries that carry blood and oxygen to the heart muscle.

Hypertension (HTN): High blood pressure.

Care Setting

Client may be seen in community physician offices or emergency department. Clients judged to be at intermediate or high risk for MI are often hospitalized for further evaluation and therapeutic intervention.

Related Concerns

Acute coronary syndrome, page 58
Cardiac surgery: postoperative care, page 98
Dysrhythmias, page 87
Myocardial infarction, page 75
Psychosocial aspects of care, page 729

Client Assessment Database

DIAGNOSTIC DIVISION MAY REPORT	MAY EXHIBIT
ACTIVITY/REST	
• Sedentary lifestyle • Weakness, feeling incapacitated after exercise • Fatigue • Activities and sleep disrupted by pain	• Exertional dyspnea
CIRCULATION	
• History of heart disease in self or family (especially early-age onset) • Hypertension in self or family • History of prior MI or revascularization procedure	• Tachycardia, dysrhythmias • Blood pressure (BP) normal, elevated, or decreased • *Heart sounds:* May be normal, late S_4, or transient late systolic murmur—that may be evident during pain • Moist, cool, pale skin, mucous membranes in presence of vasoconstriction
EGO INTEGRITY	
• Stressors of work, family, others, and financial concerns	• Apprehension, uneasiness
FOOD/FLUID	
• Nausea, "heartburn," or epigastric distress with eating, bloating, gas • Diet high in cholesterol and fats, salt, caffeine, liquor	• Belching, gastric distention
NEUROSENSORY	
• History of dizziness, fainting spells, transient numbness, tingling in extremities (ischemia anywhere in the body can produce transient neurological symptoms)	
PAIN	
Note: Reports of pain location and severity differ between men and women. • Substernal or anterior chest pain that may radiate to jaw, neck, shoulders, and upper extremities, often to left side more than right. Women may report pain between shoulder blades, back pain.	• Facial grimacing, restlessness • Placing fist over midsternum • Rubbing left arm, muscle tension • Autonomic responses; for example, tachycardia, blood pressure changes

DIAGNOSTIC DIVISION MAY REPORT (continued)	MAY EXHIBIT (continued)
• *Quality:* Varies from transient and mild to moderate; may describe heavy pressure, tightness, squeezing, burning. Women may report dull aching pain. • *Duration:* Usually less than 15 minutes • *Precipitating factors:* Physical exertion or great emotion, such as anger or sexual arousal; exercise in weather extremes • *Relieving factors:* Pain usually responsive to particular relief mechanisms, such as rest and anti-anginal medications.	
RESPIRATION • Dyspnea associated with activity or rest • Smoking history	• Increased rate and rhythm, alteration in depth
SAFETY • History of falls, fainting spells, or light-headedness	
SEXUALITY • Chest pain during sex	
TEACHING/LEARNING • Family history or risk factors of CAD: obesity, sedentary lifestyle, hypertension, stroke, diabetes, smoking, hyperlipidemia • Use or misuse of cardiac, antihypertensive, and over-the-counter (OTC) drugs • History of hormone replacement therapy (HRT) in postmenopausal women • Use of vitamins or herbal supplements, such as niacin, coenzyme Q10, ginger, bilberry, comfrey, garlic, or L-carnitine • Use or misuse of alcohol or illicit drug use, such as cocaine or amphetamines	
DISCHARGE PLAN CONSIDERATIONS • Assistance with homemaker or maintenance tasks • Changes in physical layout of home ➧ Refer to section at end of plan for postdischarge considerations.	

Diagnostic Studies

TEST WHY IT IS DONE	WHAT IT TELLS ME
BLOOD TESTS • ***Cardiac enzymes, including troponin I and cardiac troponin T, CPK, CK and CK-MB, LDH and isoenzymes*** LD_1, LD_2: Substances released from heart muscle when it is damaged.	Usually within normal limits. Any elevation indicates myocardial damage.
• ***Serum lipids, including total lipids, lipoprotein electrophoresis, isoenzymes, cholesterols (HDL, LDL, very low density lipoprotein [VLDL]), triglycerides, phospholipids:*** A group of tests that make up a lipid profile.	The presence of lipid abnormalities can increase the risk of CAD.
• ***C-reactive protein (CRP):*** A marker for inflammation.	CRP levels have been shown to predict risk of both recurrent ischemia and death among those with stable and unstable angina (Jiang, 2011).

(continues on page 70)

Diagnostic Studies (continued)

TEST WHY IT IS DONE (continued)	WHAT IT TELLS ME (continued)
• *Electrocardiogram (ECG):* Record of the electrical activity of the heart to detect dysrhythmias, to identify electrolyte imbalance, to identify any myocardial ischemia present or any damage to myocardial tissue from the past.	Resting ECG has been found to be normal in more than 50% of individuals with chronic stable angina. Findings on resting ECG that favor the diagnosis of CAD are evidence of left ventricular hypertrophy or ST–T-wave changes consistent with ischemia and evidence of previous Q-wave MI. Many dysrhythmias are also nonspecific indicators of CAD (Snow et al, 2004).
• *Exercise or pharmacological stress electrocardiography (also called stress test, exercise treadmill, or exercise ECG):* Raises heart rate and blood pressure by means of exercise. Heart can also be stressed with drugs such as dobutamine or persantine.	Can determine whether pain episodes correlate to ECG with or change during exercise or activity. *Note:* Stress imaging (not exercise ECG) is recommended in (1) client with previous cardiac catheterization, to identify ischemia in the distribution of a coronary lesion of borderline severity, and (2) client with previous revascularization now showing significant change in anginal pattern suggestive of ischemia (Snow et al, 2004).
• *Echocardiography (also called two-dimensional echocardiogram and Doppler ultrasound):* Evaluates structures and function of the heart.	Visualizes changes in heart wall motion that occur during myocardial ischemia; identifies areas of decreased myocardial perfusion as might occur with coronary artery occlusion; reveals function of structures of the heart (e.g., valves and chambers); and measures cardiac output.
• *Risk-Assessment Studies (not recommended for client with known CAD):*	
• *Myocardial perfusion imaging (MPI) scans, which may include stress MPI and single-photon emission computed tomography (SPECT):* Scans the heart using radioactive dyes to show areas of increased metabolic activity and decreased blood flow.	MPI is the most widely used imaging test for the evaluation of suspected myocardial ischemia. SPECT is capable of assessing cardiovascular risk with a high degree of accuracy, measuring both ventricular function and relative regional perfusion at rest and with stress.
• *Calcium scoring (also called coronary artery calcium scoring computed tomography, or CT, scan):* Ultrafast CT scan that measures the amount of calcium in the coronary arteries.	Elevated calcium scoring in client with other risk factors, such as family history, hypertension, diabetes, or hypercholesterolemia, is an indication of some level of CAD.

Nursing Priorities

1. Relieve or control pain.
2. Prevent or minimize development of myocardial complications.
3. Provide information about disease process, prognosis, and treatment.
4. Support client or significant other (SO) in initiating necessary lifestyle or behavioral changes.

Discharge Goals

1. Desired activity level achieved, with return to activity baseline, and self-care needs met with minimal or no pain.
2. Remains free of complications.
3. Disease process, prognosis, and therapeutic regimen understood.
4. Participates in treatment program and behavioral changes.
5. Plan in place to meet needs after discharge.

NURSING DIAGNOSIS: risk for acute Pain

Risk Factors May Include

Physical agents (increased cardiac workload and oxygen consumption, tissue ischemia)

Possibly Evidenced By

(Not applicable; presence of signs and symptoms establishes an *actual* diagnosis)

Desired Outcomes/Evaluation Criteria—Client Will

Pain Level (NOC)

Report anginal episodes decreased in frequency, duration, and severity.

Demonstrate relief of pain as evidenced by stable vital signs and absence of muscle tension and restlessness.

ACTIONS/INTERVENTIONS	RATIONALE
Pain Management (NIC)	
Independent	
Perform thorough pain assessment with each reported pain episode, using appropriate pain scale. Instruct client to notify nurse immediately when chest pain occurs.	Helpful in identifying changes from client's usual angina discomfort, which may have certain charactistics in location, duration, or intensity. If nature of angina is changing, or there is a new-onset coronary occlusion occurring, pain and decreased cardiac output may stimulate the sympathetic nervous system to release excessive amounts of norepinephrine, which increases platelet aggregation and release of thromboxane A2. This potent vasoconstrictor causes coronary artery spasm, which can precipitate, complicate, and prolong an anginal attack.
Identify precipitating event, if any; identify frequency, duration, intensity, and location of pain.	Helps differentiate chest pain and aids in evaluating possible progression to unstable angina. Stable angina usually lasts 3 to 15 minutes and is often relieved by rest and sublingual nitroglycerin (NTG); unstable angina is more intense, occurs unpredictably, may last longer, and is not usually relieved by NTG or rest. (Refer to CP: Acute Coronary Syndromes for assessments and interventions related to unstable angina.)
Monitor for changes in vital signs during pain episode if it is different from usual pattern of angina.	BP may initially rise because of sympathetic stimulation and then fall if cardiac output is compromised. Tachycardia also develops in response to sympathetic stimulation and may be sustained as a compensatory response if cardiac output falls.
Evaluate heart rate and rhythm, as indicated.	Client with changes may now have unstable angina, with an increased risk of acute life-threatening dysrhythmias, which occur in response to ischemic changes and stress.
Assess and document client response to and effects of usual medication. Evaluate need for change in medication regimen.	Client with established CAD and/or history of cardiac reperfusion procedures will likely be on a regimen of various medications, including beta blockers, ACE inhiitors, and other drugs including nitrates for control of persistent angina discomfort.
Collaborative	
Provide supplemental oxygen, as indicated.	Increases oxygen available for myocardial uptake and reversal of ischemia.
Administer anti-anginal medication(s) promptly, as indicated; for example:	Three categories of drugs are commonly used to lower the oxygen demand of the heart muscle and to treat or prevent episodes of stable angina. These categories are nitrates, beta blockers, and calcium channel blockers.
Nitrates: NTG sublingual (Nitrostat, NitroQuick); metered-dose spray (Nitrolingual); transdermal patch (Minitran, Nitrodisc); isosorbide (Isordil, Imdur)	Nitrate can be used as chronic therapy to help prevent episodes of angina. The biggest problem is "tolerance," where chronic exposure to nitrates causes a diminished effect and the anti-anginal effect of the drug disappears. Nitrate tolerance can be prevented by scheduling dosing in such a way as to guarantee daily nitrate-free intervals. If client is still experiencing pain after following prescribed nitrate use, further assessment of chest pain and additional interventions may be required.
Beta blockers, such as atenolol (Tenormin), carteolol (Cartrol), labetalol (Tropol, Lopressor), bisoprolol (Zebta)	The benefits provided by beta blockers have made them the drugs of first choice in treating patients with CAD and angina. In client with angina, beta blockers are effective in improving the amount of exercise that can be performed without developing ischemia or angina. In addition, beta blockers are the only anti-angina drugs that have been shown to lower the risk of having another myocardial infarction in patients who have already had a heart attack (Fogoros, 2011).
Calcium channel blockers, such as diltiazem (Cardizem), amlodipine (Norvasc), verapamil (Tarka), felodipine (Plendil)	By reducing calcium influx into muscle cells, calcium channel blockers cause the muscle cells to "relax." This relaxing effect results in the dilation of blood vessels and a reduced force of contraction of the heart muscle. In treating angina, the most commonly used calcium blockers are the longer-acting forms of diltiazem and verapamil, norvasc, or plendil.
Review ECG, if indicated.	Ischemia during anginal attack may cause transient ST-segment depression or elevation and T-wave inversion. Serial tracings verify ischemic changes, which may disappear when client is pain-free, or may reveal a new-onset cardiac blockage.

(continues on page 72)

ACTIONS/INTERVENTIONS (continued)	RATIONALE (continued)
Prepare for/assist with additional diagnostic studies, procedures, or interventions, as indicated. (Refer to CP: Acute Coronary Syndrome.)	If angina is atypical or unrelenting, complications may be occurring, such as MI, new-onset occlusion or coronary artery or restenosis, or blockage of stent in client who has had past revascularization procedures.

NURSING DIAGNOSIS: risk for decreased Cardiac Output

Risk Factors May Include

Altered contractility

Altered heart rate, rhythm

Possibly Evidenced By

(Not applicable; presence of signs and symptoms establishes an *actual* diagnosis)

Desired Outcomes/Evaluation Criteria—Client Will

Cardiac Pump Effectiveness (NOC)

Demonstrate increased activity tolerance.

Report or display decreased episodes of dyspnea, angina, and dysrhythmias.

Participate in behaviors and activities that reduce the workload of the heart.

ACTIONS/INTERVENTIONS	RATIONALE
Hemodynamic Regulation (NIC)	
Independent	
Maintain bedrest or chair rest in position of comfort during acute angina episodes.	Decreases oxygen consumption and demand, reducing myocardial workload and risk of decompensation.
Monitor vital signs and cardiac rhythm.	Tachycardia and changes in blood pressure (hypotension or hypertension) may be present because of pain, anxiety, hypoxemia, and reduced cardiac output. ECG changes reflecting ischemia and dysrhythmias indicate need for additional evaluation and therapeutic intervention.
Auscultate breath sounds and heart sounds.	S_3, S_4, or crackles may occur with cardiac decompensation or some medication.
Listen for murmurs.	Development of murmurs may reveal a valvular cause for chest pain, such as aortic or mitral stenosis or papillary muscle rupture.
Provide for adequate rest periods. Assist with or perform self-care activities, as indicated.	Conserves energy and reduces cardiac workload.
Encourage immediate reporting of pain for prompt administration of medications, as indicated.	Timely interventions can reduce oxygen consumption and myocardial workload and may prevent or minimize cardiac complications.
Assess for signs and symptoms of heart failure.	Angina is only a symptom of underlying pathology causing myocardial ischemia. Disease may compromise cardiac function to point of decompensation.
Evaluate mental status, noting development of confusion and disorientation.	Reduced perfusion of the brain can produce observable changes in sensorium.
Note skin color and presence and quality of pulses.	Peripheral circulation is reduced when cardiac output falls, giving the skin a pale or gray color depending on level of hypoxia and diminishing the strength of peripheral pulses.
Assess lung for adventitious sounds, such as crackles.	Respiratory system may become decompensated with anginal attack.
Collaborative	
Administer supplemental oxygen as needed.	Increases oxygen available for myocardial uptake to improve contractility and reduce ischemia.
Monitor chest x-ray.	Identifies new or worsening congestive heart failure.
Monitor pulse oximetry or arterial blood gases (ABGs), as indicated.	Oxygen saturation may decrease as oxygen demands increase for heart muscle and systemic circulation. Monitoring determines adequacy of respiratory function and O_2 therapy.
Administer medications, as indicated; for example:	
Calcium channel blockers, such as diltiazem (Cardizem), felodipine (Plendil)	Although differing in mode of action, calcium channel blockers play a major role in preventing and terminating ischemia induced by coronary artery spasm and in reducing vascular resistance, thereby decreasing BP and cardiac workload.

ACTIONS/INTERVENTIONS (continued)	RATIONALE (continued)
Beta blockers, such as atenolol (Tenormin) and esmolol (Brevibloc)	These medications decrease cardiac workload by reducing heart rate and systolic BP. *Note:* Overdose produces bradycardia and hypotension.
Angiotension-converting-enzyme (ACE) inhibitors, for example, elanapril (Vasotec), benazepril (Lotensin)	These agents are used in the prevention of cardiovascular events in clients with chronic stable angina and in those with CAD who also have diabetes, systolic dysfunction, or both
Antiplatelets agents, such as aspirin (ASA), clopidogrel (Plavix), ticlopidine (Ticlid), tirofiban (Aggrastat), and eptifibatide (Integrilin)	Aspirin is proven beneficial in primary and secondary prevention of coronary artery disease. For clients with major gastrointestinal intolerance, alternative drugs may be indicated. Newer antiplatelets, especially Plavix, are frequently used in conjunction with angioplasty and stent placement for relief of angina and prevention of reocclusion.
Lipid-lowering agents, for example, cholestyramine (Questran), atorvastatin (Lipitor), lovastatin (Mevacor), gemfibrozil (Lopid), fenofibrate (Tricor), and niacin.	These agents are comprised of four different classes of pharmaceuticals (e.g., bile acid sequestrants, statins, fibric acid derivatives, and niacin) that are used in the treatment of hyperlipidemias. These agents work in various ways to minimize deleterious effects of cholesterol in the cardiovascular system. While one group of drugs, statins, lowers cholesterol, the other group, fibrates, is known to take care of fatty acids and triglycerides. As lipids are critical in the progression of cardiovascular diseases, these drugs have been shown to reduce fatal and nonfatal cardiovascular events in the general population (Pahan, 2006).
Discuss purpose and prepare for additional testing, when indicated.	Stress radionuclide imaging or stress echocardiography and/or coronary angiography may be required for client who has a significant change in clinical status despite medical management of angina (Snow et al, 2004).
Prepare for interventions such as angioplasty with or without intracoronary stent placement, valve replacement, and coronary artery bypass grafting (CABG), if indicated. (Refer to CPs: Acute Coronary Syndrome; Cardiac Surgery, as indicated.)	Revascularization procedures may be required to enhance coronary blood flow and cardiac function. CABG is the recommended treatment when testing confirms myocardial ischemia due to left main coronary artery disease or symptomatic three-vessel disease, especially in those with left ventricular dysfunction.

NURSING DIAGNOSIS: ineffective Self-Health Management

May Be Related To
Complexity of therapeutic regimen
Perceived barriers, economic difficulties
Family patterns of healthcare

Possibly Evidenced By
Reports difficulty with prescribed regimen
Failure to take action to reduce risk factors
Ineffective choices in daily living for meeting health goals
Unexpected acceleration of illness symptoms

Desired Outcomes/Evaluation Criteria—Client Will

Participate in learning process.
Assume responsibility for own learning, looking for information and asking questions.

Knowledge: Coronary Artery Disease Management (NOC)
Verbalize understanding of condition, disease process, and potential complications.
Verbalize understanding of and participate in therapeutic regimen.
Initiate necessary lifestyle changes.

ACTIONS/INTERVENTIONS	RATIONALE
Cardiac Risk Management (NIC) ***Independent***	
Discuss pathophysiology of condition. Emphasize need for preventing and managing anginal attacks.	Clients with angina need to learn why it occurs and what they can do to manage it. This focus of therapeutic management aims to reduce the likelihood of MI, heart failure, and sudden death, and to promote heart-healthy lifestyle.
Encourage avoidance of factors or situations that may precipitate anginal episode, such as emotional stress, extensive or intense physical exertion, use of recreational drugs, ingestion of large or heavy meal (especially close to bedtime), and exposure to extremes in environmental temperature.	This is a crucial step in limiting or preventing anginal attacks.
Review importance of cessation of smoking, weight control, dietary changes, and exercise.	Knowledge of the significance of risk factors provides client with opportunity to make needed changes. Clients with high cholesterol who do not respond to a 6-month program of low-fat diet and regular exercise will require medication.
Review significance of cholesterol levels and differentiate between LDL and HDL factors. Emphasize importance of periodic laboratory measurements and use of cholesterol-lowering drugs.	Client should seek to maintain total cholesterol less than 200 mg/dL. Client with two or more risk factors, including smoking, hypertension, diabetes mellitus, and positive family history, should seek to maintain LDL (also called "bad" cholesterol) around 115 mg/dL; and those with diagnosis of CAD should seek to maintain LDL below 100 mg/dL. HDL (also called "good" cholesterol) below 35 to 45 is considered a risk factor; a level above 60 mg/dL is considered protective against cardiac disease (American Heart Association [AHA], 2013).
Encourage client to follow prescribed reconditioning program.	Fear of triggering attacks may cause client to avoid participation in activity that has been prescribed to enhance recovery. Cardiac rehabilitation programs provide a phased approach to increasing client's activity and exercise tolerance.
Demonstrate how and encourage client to monitor own pulse and BP during and after activities, when appropriate, and to schedule and simplify activities and take rest periods.	Allows client to identify those activities that can be modified to avoid cardiac stress and stay below the anginal threshold.
Discuss impact of condition on desired lifestyle and activities, including work, driving, sexual activity, and hobbies. Provide information, privacy, or consultation, as indicated.	Client may be reluctant to resume or continue certain activities because of fear of anginal attack or death. If symptoms have worsened or the client has decreased physical activity to avoid precipitating angina, then he/she should be reevaluated and treated accordingly. *Note:* Erectile dysfunction (ED) can be a sign of CAD or diabetes in men. Use of Viagra, or similar drugs, is contraindicated with nitrates, which are usually used with angina.
Review prescribed medications for control and prevention of anginal attacks. Refer to NDs: risk for acute Pain, and risk for decreased cardiac Tissue Perfusion (above) for discussion of drugs.	Angina is a complicated condition that often requires the use of many drugs to decrease myocardial workload, improve coronary circulation, and control the occurrence of attacks.
Stress importance of checking with physician before taking OTC drugs.	OTC drugs may potentiate or negate effects of prescribed medications.
Discuss use of herbals such as ginseng, garlic, ginkgo, hawthorn, and bromelain, as indicated.	Some herbals, such as ginkgo, ginseng, and bromelain can affect bleeding and clotting, especially when added to medications such as Plavix or Coumadin, which increase bleeding. Others, such as hawthorn, can increase the effects of certain heart medications.
Review symptoms to be reported to physician, particularly an increase in frequency and duration of attacks and changes in response to medications.	Knowledge of expectations can avoid undue concern for insignificant events or prevent delay in treatment of worrisome symptoms.
Discuss importance of follow-up appointments (e.g., physician evaluation, laboratory monitoring, etc.)	Angina is a symptom of CAD that can be progressive, should be monitored, and may require occasional adjustment of treatment regimen.
Encourage client to wear medical alert bracelet or necklace.	Alerts care providers of client's diagnosis when emergency occurs.
Recommend that SO/caregivers have ready access to emergency phone numbers and encourage them to take CPR classes.	Helps family to be prepared for emergency actions when needed.

POTENTIAL CONSIDERATIONS following discharge from care setting (dependent on client's age, physical condition and presence of complications, personal resources, and life responsibilities)

- ***risk for decreased cardiac Tissue Perfusion***—coronary artery spasm
- ***Activity Intolerance***—imbalance between oxygen supply and demand, sedentary lifestyle
- ***ineffective Denial***—lack of control of life situation, anxiety
- ***interrupted Family Processes***—situational transition or crisis, shift in health status of family member
- ***impaired Home Maintenance***—impaired functioning, inadequate support systems, unfamiliarity with neighborhood resources

MYOCARDIAL INFARCTION

I. Pathophysiology

a. Marked reduction or loss of blood flow through one or more of the coronary arteries, resulting in cardiac muscle ischemia, and over a finite period, resulting in necrosis
b. Occurs most often due to coronary artery disease (CAD)
c. Cellular ischemia and necrosis can affect the heart's rhythm, pumping action, and blood circulation.
d. Other problems may also ensue, such as heart failure, life-threatening arrhythmias, and death.
e. Delay in seeking treatment is the largest barrier to receiving therapy quickly.

II. Classification

a. Types of myocardial infarction (MI) can be identified on the electrocardiogram (ECG).
  i. ST-segment elevation (also called STEMI)
  ii. Non-ST elevation (NSTEMI)
b. Location of MI can be identified on the ECG.
  i. Anterior wall of the ventricle
  ii. Inferior wall of the ventricle
  iii. Posterior wall of the ventricle
  iv. Lateral wall of the ventricle
c. Infarcts are usually classified by size.
  i. Microscopic (focal necrosis)
  ii. Small (<10% of the left ventricle)
  iii. Medium (10% to 30% of the left ventricle)
  iv. Large (>30% of the left ventricle)
d. Point of time can be identified on the ECG by the Q wave and the client's history.
  i. Acute or evolving infarction is characterized by the presence of polymorphonuclear leukocytes unless the interval between the onset of infarction and death is brief (e.g., 6 hours), minimal, or no polymorphonuclear leukocytes may be seen.
  ii. Old or healed infarction is manifested as scar tissue without cellular infiltration, a process usually requiring 5 to 6 weeks or more.

III. Etiology

a. CAD common cause with plaque formation narrowing vessels and pieces of plaque breaking off, creating emboli
b. Severe spasm of a coronary artery is less common cause.
c. Risk factors—age, being overweight or obese, smoking, hyperlipidemia, family history
d. Greater risk in presence of kidney problems, peripheral arterial disease, or prior MI

IV. Statistics (Centers for Disease Control and Prevention [CDC], 2012; National Heart, Lung and Blood Institute [NHLBI], 2009)

a. Morbidity: Approximately 935,000 people in the United States suffer from MI annually.
b. Mortality: Almost 50% die, approximately 460,000 annually.
c. CAD is leading killer of both men and women in the United States.
d. Leading cause of death for American Indians, Alaskan Natives, African Americans, Hispanics, and whites, and second leading cause of death for Asians and Pacific Islanders
e. Cost: Inpatient hospital costs for AMI estimated at $5.3 billion in 2009 (Stranges, 2011).

GLOSSARY

Atherosclerosis: Abnormal accumulation of lipid deposits and fibrous tissue within the arterial walls and lumen.

Coronary artery disease (CAD): Narrowing or blockage of the arteries and vessels that provide oxygen and nutrients to the heart, caused by atherosclerosis. The resulting blockage restricts blood flow to the heart. When the blood flow is completely cut off, the result is a heart attack (also called a myocardial infarction, MI).

Coronary artery bypass graft (CABG): Surgical procedure in which a blood vessel from another part of the body is grafted onto the occluded coronary artery above and below the occlusion in such a way that blood flow bypasses the blockage.

Creatine kinase (CK): Enzyme found in human tissues. One of the three types of CK is specific to the heart muscle and may be used as an indicator of heart muscle injury.

Myocardial infarction (MI, also called acute MI or AMI): Reduced myocardial perfusion and death of heart tissue caused by lack of oxygenated blood flow.

NSTEMI: Non-ST elevation myocardial infarction

Percutaneous coronary interventions (PCIs): A nonsurgical procedure used to treat the stenotic coronary arteries found in coronary heart disease. During PCI, a cardiologist feeds a deflated balloon or other device on a catheter from the femoral artery or radial artery up through blood vessels until they

(continues on page 76)

GLOSSARY (continued)

reach the site of blockage in the heart. X-ray imaging is used to guide the catheter threading. At the blockage, the balloon is inflated to open the artery, allowing blood to flow. A stent is often placed at the site of blockage to permanently open the artery

STEMI: ST-segment elevation myocardial infarction

Stent: Woven mesh that provides structural support to a coronary vessel, preventing its closure.

Thrombolytic: Agent or process that breaks down blood clots.

Troponin: A cardiac-specific biomarker used to assess heart muscle injury.

Care Setting

Myocardial infarctions are treated in the emergency room, inpatient acute hospital, critical care unit (CCU), intensive care unit (ICU), step-down unit, or medical unit.

Related Concerns

Acute coronary syndrome, page 58
Angina, page 67
Dysrhythmias, page 87
Heart failure: chronic, page 43
Psychosocial aspects of care, page 729
Thrombophlebitis: deep vein thrombosis, page 109

Client Assessment Database

DIAGNOSTIC DIVISION MAY REPORT	MAY EXHIBIT
ACTIVITY/REST	
• History of sedentary lifestyle, sporadic exercise schedule • Weakness, fatigue, intolerance to usual activities. • Women often report unusual fatigue (67% in one study; McSweeney, 2003)	• Chest pain with activity or rest • Tachycardia, dyspnea with rest or activity • Fatigue with normal daily activities
CIRCULATION	
• History of previous MI, CAD, heart failure, hypertension, diabetes mellitus, hypercholesterolemia	• *Color:* Pallor or cyanosis; mottling of the skin, nail beds, mucous membranes, and lips • Blood pressure (BP) may be increased or decreased; orthostatic changes may occur • Pulse normal, full, bounding, or having a weak or thready quality with delayed capillary refill • Dysrhythmias, tachycardia, or bradycardia • *Heart sounds:* S_3 and S_4, reflecting a pathological condition such as cardiac failure, decreased ventricular contractility, or compliance • Murmurs reflecting valvular insufficiency or papillary muscle dysfunction • Friction rub suggests pericarditis • *Edema:* Signs of jugular vein distention (JVD), peripheral edema, dependent edema, generalized edema
EGO INTEGRITY	
• Denial of significance of symptoms and presence of condition • Fear of dying, feelings of impending doom • Anger at inconvenience of illness and the "unnecessary" attention and hospitalization • Worry about family, employment, finances, childcare, elders at home, and pets at home	• Withdrawal, anxiety, lack of eye movements • Irritability, anger, combative behavior; may refuse emergent care • Focus on self and pain
ELIMINATION	
• History of straining with bowel movements • Syncopal events with bowel movements	• Normal or decreased bowel sounds

DIAGNOSTIC DIVISION

MAY REPORT (continued)	MAY EXHIBIT (continued)
FOOD/FLUID • History of/current obesity • Nausea, vomiting, belching, heartburn • Recent history of eating large, fatty meals; alcohol consumption	• Vomiting • Poor skin turgor, dry or diaphoretic skin • Decreased urine output
NEUROSENSORY • History of dizziness, fainting spells, falling	• Mentation changes such as disorientation, poor memory, changes in thought processes • Weakness
PAIN/DISCOMFORT • Sudden onset of chest pain unrelieved by rest or nitroglycerin • *Location:* Typically, anterior chest including substernal and precordium pain that may radiate to arms, jaw, face • May have atypical location, such as pain in epigastric or abdominal area, elbow, jaw, back, neck, between shoulder blades, or throat • Women may report absence of pain or pain between shoulder blades or back (McSweeney, 2003) • *Quality:* Crushing, constricting, squeezing, heavy, steady pain. Women may report dull aching pain. • *Intensity:* Usually a 10 on a scale of 0 to 10 or the "worst pain ever experienced" • Pain sometimes absent in postoperative clients, those with prior stroke or heart failure, diabetes, hypertension, or an older person • *Precipitating factors:* May or may not be associated with activity or increased stress	• Facial grimacing, changes in body posture; may place clenched fist on midsternum when describing pain • Crying, groaning, squirming, stretching • Withdrawal, lack of eye contact • *Autonomic responses:* Changes in heart rate and rhythm, blood pressure, respirations, skin color and moisture, and level of consciousness
RESPIRATION • Recent history of dyspnea with or without exertion, nocturnal dyspnea, unable to sleep flat • Recent history of cough with or without sputum production • History of smoking, chronic respiratory disease	• Increased respiratory rate, shallow and labored breathing • *Color:* Pallor or cyanosis • Decreased oxygen saturation on pulse oximetry • *Breath sounds:* May be clear or crackles and wheezes present • *Sputum:* Clear, possibly pink-tinged
SOCIAL INTERACTION • Recent history of stressors such as work, family, financial, caretaking • Difficulty coping with recent or current stressors • May be worried about current hospitalization's effect on self and family and question coping abilities	• Difficulty resting quietly • Overemotional responses such as intense anger or fear • Withdrawal from family • Not willing to cooperate with treatment recommendations; not responsive to teaching
SEXUALITY • Postmenopausal; past history of hormone replacement therapy • Erectile dysfunction (ED): May be associated with hypertension or antihypertensive medications	
TEACHING/LEARNING • Family history of heart disease, MI, diabetes, stroke, hypertension, peripheral vascular disease, hypercholesterolemia • Use of tobacco; may express desire or attempts at smoking cessation • Use of alcohol or other drugs • Use or misuse of cardiac medications, over-the-counter (OTC) preparations • Use of vitamins and herbal supplements such as vitamin E, ginseng, garlic, ginkgo, hawthorn, bromelain	

(continues on page 78)

Client Assessment Database (continued)

DIAGNOSTIC DIVISION MAY REPORT (continued)	MAY EXHIBIT (continued)
DISCHARGE PLAN CONSIDERATIONS • May require assistance with activities of daily living (ADLs), food preparation, shopping, transportation, homemaking or maintenance tasks, modifications of physical layout of home ➧ Refer to section at end of plan for postdischarge considerations	

Diagnostic Studies

TEST WHY IT IS DONE	WHAT IT TELLS ME
DIAGNOSTIC STUDIES	
• *Electrocardiogram (ECG):* Record of the electrical activity of the heart to detect dysrhythmias, to identify any myocardial ischemia present, or any damage to myocardial tissue from the past.	In the emergency setting, the ECG is the most important diagnostic test. High probability of myocardial infarction is indicated by ST-segment elevation greater than 1 mm in two anatomically contiguous leads (indicates acute MI in 90% of people, as confirmed by serial measurements of cardiac biomarkers) or by the presence of new Q waves (Kumar, 2009). Results that indicate intermediate probability of myocardial infarction are ST-segment depression, T-wave inversion, and other nonspecific ST–T-wave abnormalities. *Note*: Some emergency departments use an 80-lead ECG that enhances the ability to detect acute MI in the right ventricle, posterior, and high left lateral regions of the myocardium (Franks, 2012).
• *Cardiac catheterization with angiography:* Assesses patency of coronary arteries; reveals abnormal heart size, valvular function by measuring chamber pressures; and evaluates ventricular contractility by measuring ejection fraction (EF).	Cardiac catheterization defines coronary anatomy and the extent of a client's disease. Client with intractable angina (despite medication) should immediately undergo cardiac catheterization (Coven, 2013). Most individuals with UA and NSTEMI benefit from angiography when they have a TIMI (Thrombolysis in Myocardial Infarction) risk score of less than 3 points (Antman et al, 2000).
• *Chest x-ray:* Procedure used to evaluate organs and structures within the chest	Visualize changes in heart size and any infiltrates that may be present in the lung.
BLOOD TESTS	
• *Cardiac enzymes, including troponin I and troponin T. Also possibly CPK, CK, and CK-MB:* Substances released from heart muscle when it is damaged.	Troponin levels are now considered to be the criterion standard for defining and diagnosing myocardial infarction, according to the American College of Cardiology (ACC)/American Heart Association (AHA) (Zafari, 2013). Cardiac-specific troponins are not detectable in the blood of healthy individuals; therefore, they provide high specificity for detecting injury to cardiac myocytes. These molecules are also more sensitive than CK-MB for myocardial necrosis and therefore improve early detection of small myocardial infarctions. Differentiation is generally based on three sets of tests measured at 6- to 8-hour intervals after the client's presentation to the emergency department. The current definition of NSTEMI requires a typical clinical syndrome plus elevated troponin (or creatine kinase isoenzyme MB [CK-MB]) levels to over 99% of the normal reference. Given this definition, nearly 25% of individuals who were previously classified as having unstable angina now fulfill the criteria for NSTEMI (Coven, 2013; Lab Tests Online, 2011).

TEST WHY IT IS DONE (continued)	WHAT IT TELLS ME (continued)
• *Complete blood count (CBC), including red (RBC) and white blood cell (WBC) counts, hemoglobin/hematocrit (Hgb/Hct), platelets*	May be done if MI is suspected in order to rule out anemia as a cause of decreased oxygen supply and prior to giving thrombolytics. Leukocytosis is also common, but not universal, signifying an acute inflammatory state. The platelet count is necessary if a IIb/IIIa agent is considered or may become dangerously low after the use of heparin (Zafari, 2013).
• *Metabolic profile, including blood glucose electrolytes (BUN/Cr)*	Important for client with new-onset angina. Close monitoring of potassium and magnesium levels is important because low levels may predispose to dysrhythmias. Creatinine levels must be considered before using an angiotensin-converting enzyme (ACE) inhibitor and particularly if cardiac catheterization is considered
• *Serum lipids, including total lipids, lipoprotein electrophoresis, isoenzymes, cholesterols (HDL, LDL, very low density lipoprotein [VLDL]), triglycerides, phospholipids:* A group of tests that make up a lipid profile.	The lipid profile numbers may be low during an acute MI; therefore, it is important to follow up. It may show that the client has hyperlipidemia that was not identified or was uncontrolled in the past, (a risk factor for CAD and MI).
• *Coagulation studies, including partial thromboplastin time (PTT), activated partial thromboplastin time (aPPT), and platelets:* Injury to a vessel wall or the tissue initiates the coagulation cascade and formation of a thrombus.	Thrombus formation can potentiate ischemic damage to the myocardium as blood flow is blocked.
• *Arterial blood gases (ABG):* Assessment of levels of oxygen (PaO_2) and carbon dioxide ($PaCO_2$).	Should be checked and repeatedly corrected if clinical findings suggest hypoxemia, which may result from pulmonary congestion, atelectasis, or ventilatory impairment secondary to complications of MI.

Nursing Priorities

1. Relieve pain and anxiety.
2. Reduce myocardial workload.
3. Prevent, detect, and assist in treatment of life-threatening dysrhythmias or complications.
4. Promote cardiac health and self-care.

Discharge Goals

1. Chest pain absent or controlled.
2. Heart rate and rhythm sufficient to sustain adequate cardiac output and tissue perfusion.
3. Achievement of activity level sufficient for basic self-care.
4. Anxiety reduced and managed.
5. Disease process, treatment plan, and prognosis understood.
6. Plan in place to meet needs after discharge, including follow-up appointments.

NURSING DIAGNOSIS: acute Pain

May Be Related To

Physical agent (tissue ischemia)

Possibly Evidenced By

Verbal/coded reports of pain
Facial mask (grimacing)
Restlessness
Changes in heart rate, blood pressure

Desired Outcomes/Evaluation Criteria—Client Will

Pain Level (NOC)

Verbalize relief or control of chest pain within appropriate period for administered medications.
Display reduced tension, relaxed manner, and ease of movement.

Pain Control (NOC)

Demonstrate use of relaxation techniques.

ACTIONS/INTERVENTIONS	RATIONALE
Pain Management (NIC)	
Independent	
Monitor and document characteristics of pain, noting verbal reports, nonverbal cues, for example, moaning, crying, restlessness, diaphoresis, clutching chest, rapid breathing, and hemodynamic response (BP and heart rate changes).	Variation of appearance and behavior of clients in pain may present a challenge in assessment. For example, men and women consistently present differently (McSweeney, 2003), or an individual may present differently from one episode to another. However, most clients with an acute MI appear ill, distracted, and focused on pain. Verbal history and deeper investigation of precipitating factors should be postponed until pain is relieved. Respirations may be increased as a result of pain and associated anxiety; release of stress-induced catecholamines increases heart rate and BP.
Obtain full description of pain from client including location, intensity (using 0 to 10 or similar scale), duration, characteristics (dull or crushing), and radiation. Assist client to quantify pain by comparing it to other experiences.	Pain is a subjective experience and must be described by client. Provides baseline for comparison to aid in determining effectiveness of therapy, resolution or progression of problem.
Note history of previous angina, anginal equivalent, or MI pain. Discuss family history if pertinent.	May differentiate current pain from preexisting patterns as well as identify complications, such as extension of infarction, pulmonary embolus, or pericarditis.
Instruct client to report pain immediately.	Delays in reporting pain hinders pain relief and may necessitate increased dosage of medication to achieve relief. In addition, severe pain may induce shock by stimulating the sympathetic nervous system, thereby creating further damage and interfering with diagnostics and relief of pain.
Assist or instruct in relaxation techniques, such as deep, slow breathing and distraction.	Helpful in decreasing perception of or response to pain. Provides a sense of having some control over the situation, increase in positive attitude.
Check vital signs before and after administration of opioid medication.	Hypotension and respiratory depression can occur as a result of opioid administration. These problems may increase myocardial damage in presence of ventricular insufficiency.
Collaborative	
Administer supplemental oxygen by appropriate route.	Increases amount of oxygen available for myocardial uptake and thereby may relieve discomfort associated with tissue ischemia.
Administer medications, as indicated; for example:	
Anti-anginals, such as nitroglycerin (Nitro-Bid, Nitrostat, Nitro-Dur), isosorbide dinitrate (Isordil), and mononitrate (Imdur)	Nitrates are useful for pain control by coronary vasodilating effects, which increase coronary blood flow and myocardial perfusion. Peripheral vasodilation effects reduce the volume of blood returning to the heart (preload), thereby decreasing myocardial workload and oxygen demand.
Analgesics, such as morphine sulfate	Although intravenous (IV) morphine is the usual drug of choice, other injectable opioids may be used in acute-phase or recurrent chest pain (unrelieved by nitroglycerin) to reduce severe pain, provide sedation, and decrease myocardial workload. IM injections should be avoided, if possible, because they can alter the CPK diagnostic indicator and are not well absorbed in underperfused tissue.

NURSING DIAGNOSIS: risk for decreased Cardiac Output

Risk Factors May Include

Altered heart rate/rhythm
Reduced preload—increased systemic vascular resistance (SVR)
Altered contractility—infarcted or dyskinetic muscle

Possibly Evidenced By

(Not applicable; presence of signs and symptoms establishes *actual* diagnosis)

Desired Outcomes/Evaluation Criteria—Client Will

Cardiac Pump Effectiveness (NOC)

Maintain hemodynamic stability, such as BP, cardiac output within normal range, adequate urinary output, decreased frequency or absence of dysrhythmias.
Report decreased episodes of dyspnea and angina.
Demonstrate an increase in activity tolerance.

ACTIONS/INTERVENTIONS	RATIONALE
Cardiac Care: Acute (NIC)	
Independent	
Monitor mental status. Investigate sudden changes or continued alterations in mentation, such as anxiety, confusion, lethargy, and stupor.	Cerebral perfusion is directly related to cardiac output and is influenced by electrolyte and acid-base variations, hypoxia, and systemic emboli.
Inspect for pallor, cyanosis, mottling, and cool or clammy skin.	Systemic vasoconstriction resulting from diminished cardiac output may be evidenced by decreased skin perfusion and diminished pulses.
Monitor respirations, noting work of breathing.	Cardiac pump failure and ischemic pain may precipitate respiratory distress.
Auscultate breath sounds.	Crackles reflect pulmonary congestion; may develop because of depressed myocardial function.
Evaluate quality and equality of pulses.	Decreased cardiac output results in diminished, weak, or thready pulses. Irregularities suggest dysrhythmias, which may require further evaluation and monitoring.
Auscultate heart sounds:	
Note development of S_3 and S_4.	S_3 is usually associated with heart failure, but it may also be noted with the mitral insufficiency (regurgitation) and left ventricular overload that can accompany severe infarction. S_4 is an almost universal finding during the early stages of acute MI if the patient has sinus rhythm. A fourth heart sound can occur with or without signs of heart failure (Williams, 1990).
Note presence of murmurs and rubs.	Indicates disturbances of normal blood flow within the heart, such as incompetent valve, septal defect, or vibration of papillary muscle and chordae tendineae (complication of MI). Presence of rub with an infarction is also associated with inflammation, such as pericardial effusion and pericarditis.
Obtain frequent BP readings. Monitor hemodynamic pressures when invasive lines/devices are available.	Hypotension may occur related to ventricular dysfunction, hypoperfusion of the myocardium, and vagal stimulation. However, hypertension is also a common phenomenon, possibly related to pain, anxiety, catecholamine release, and preexisting vascular problems.
Monitor heart rate and rhythm. Document dysrhythmias via telemetry.	Heart rate and rhythm can be affected by presence of coronary artery blockage, myocardial necrosis, and impairment of ventricular contractility, electrolyte and acid-base imbalances, and circulating catecholamines. Dysrhythmias, especially premature ventricular contractions or progressive heart blocks, can compromise cardiac and become lethal. Acute or chronic atrial flutter or fibrillation may be seen with coronary artery or valvular involvement and may or may not be pathological. (Refer to CP: Dysrhythmias.)
Monitor output, noting changes in urine output. Record urine specific gravity, as indicated. Calculate fluid balance.	Decreased output may reflect systemic perfusion problems and may reflect heart failure. Inotropic drugs may be needed for support of circulation or additional fluids to enhance circulating volume and kidney function. *Note:* Specific gravity measurements reflect hydration status and renal function.
Note jugular vein distention (JVD) and development of dependent edema.	Suggests developing congestive failure or fluid volume excess.
Weigh daily at the same time on the same scale.	Sudden changes in weight reflect alterations in fluid balance.
Have emergency equipment and medications available.	Sudden coronary occlusion, lethal dysrhythmias, extension of infarct, and unrelenting pain are situations that may precipitate cardiac arrest, requiring immediate life-saving therapies or transfer to CCU.
Collaborative	
Administer supplemental oxygen, as indicated.	Supplemental oxygen should be given to maintain oxygen saturation >90% to prevent hypoxemia and resultant depression of myocardial function and dysrhythmias (Zafari, 2013).
Measure cardiac output and other functional parameters as appropriate.	Cardiac index, preload and afterload, contractility, and cardiac work can be measured noninvasively with thoracic electrical bioimpedance (TEB) technique. Useful in evaluating response to therapeutic interventions and identifying need for more aggressive or emergency care.
Review serial ECGs.	Provides information regarding progression or resolution of infarction, status of ventricular function, electrolyte balance, and effect of drug therapies.

(continues on page 82)

ACTIONS/INTERVENTIONS (continued)	RATIONALE (continued)
Monitor laboratory data, such as cardiac enzymes, arterial blood gases (ABGs), and electrolytes.	Enzymes monitor resolution or extension of infarction. Presence of hypoxia indicates need for supplemental oxygen. Electrolyte imbalances, such as hypo- or hyperkalemia, adversely affect cardiac rhythm and contractility.
Assist with medical or surgical interventions, as indicated:	As a general rule, initial therapy for acute MI is directed toward restoration of perfusion as soon as possible to salvage as much myocardium as possible. This may be accomplished through thrombolytic therapy, angiography with percutaneous coronary interventions (PCIs), which may include percutaneous transluminal coronary angioplasty (PTCA) or surgery, such as coronary artery bypass graft—CABG (Zafari, 2013).
Administer medications as indicated:	
Antidysrhythmic drugs (Refer to CP: Dysrhythmias)	Dysrhythmias are usually treated symptomatically. Early inclusion of ACE inhibitor therapy, especially in presence of large anterior MI, ventricular aneurysm, or heart failure, enhances ventricular output, increases survival, and may slow progression of heart failure.
Beta blockers	Beta-adrenergic blockers are of benefit when given intravenously within 4 hours of the onset of pain and continued on a long-term basis. The American Heart Association (AHA) recommends the initiation of beta blockers to all patients with STEMI, unless beta blockers are contraindicated (Zafari, 2013).
Angiotensin-converting enzyme (ACE) inhibitors	ACE inhibitors are useful for long-term therapy and also appear to benefit client who has no evidence of hypotension if administration is begun within the first 24 hours after the onset of MI. May be given to reduce risk of developing heart failure in client with diminished ventricular EF and in those with hypertension, diabetes, or chronic kidney disease, unless contraindicated (Smith et al, 2006; Zafari, 2013).
Angiotensin receptor blockers (ARBs)	May be used in client intolerant to ACE inhibitors or if client has had an MI with left ventricular EF ≤40%. *Note:* Research has shown that ARBs are beneficial in women after an MI or those in heart failure, but beta blockers should not be used universally. This research supports the fact that men and women not only show different symptoms during an evolving MI but respond differently to medicines given for treatment of MI (Mosca, 2011).
Aspirin (ASA)	Giving aspirin as soon as possible (unless contraindicated) inhibits platelet activity, interrupting platelet aggregation at the site of plaque rupture—a key mechanism in the unfolding acute MI. Clients who receive aspirin in the acute phase have a 15% lower mortality rate than those who don't (Lackey, 2006).
Thrombolytic agents, for example, second-generation drugs (including agents such as tenecteplase)	Thrombolytic therapy prevents the formation of thrombi associated with myocardial infarction and has been shown to improve survival rates in STEMI. Second-generation drugs have clot sensitivity without causing a systemic lytic state and should be administered as soon as possible after onset of acute MI (Zafari, 2013).
Percutaneous coronary interventions (PCIs), including percutaneous transluminal coronary angioplasty (PTCA), with or without stenting	A group of catheter-based technologies used to establish coronary reperfusion. Angiography, which provides essential knowledge of the extent of coronary disease, is performed prior to PCI. In regard to STEMI, PCI may be performed either as a primary intervention or after thrombolysis failure. The advantage of performing primary PTCA in MI is the ability to achieve reperfusion of the infarcted vessel with a lower risk of bleeding than that associated with thrombolytic therapy (Zafari, 2013).
Prepare for surgery, as indicated. (Refer to CP: Cardiac Surgery.)	Emergent or urgent CABG surgery may be indicated if angioplasty fails or client develops mechanical complications, such as a ventricular septal defect or left ventricular or papillary muscle rupture.
Assist with insertion and maintain pacemaker or automatic internal cardiac defibrillator (AICD) when used. (Refer to CP: Dysrhythmias.)	Pacing may be a temporary support measure during acute phase or may be needed permanently if infarction severely damages conduction system, impairing systolic function. Use of AICD is currently advocated in client who had ventricular fibrillation or tachycardia resulting in arrest.

NURSING DIAGNOSIS: Activity Intolerance

May Be Related To

Imbalance between oxygen supply and demand

Possibly Evidenced By

Abnormal heart rate and BP response to activity
Reports fatigue; exertional discomfort
ECG changes reflecting arrhythmias or ischemia

Desired Outcomes/Evaluation Criteria—Client Will

Activity Tolerance (NOC)

Demonstrate measurable, progressive increase in tolerance for activity with heart rate and rhythm, BP within client's normal limits, and skin warm, pink, and dry.

Report absence of angina with activity.

ACTIONS/INTERVENTIONS	RATIONALE
Energy Management (NIC)	
Independent	
Record and document heart rate and rhythm and BP changes before, during, and after activity, as indicated. Correlate with reports of chest pain or shortness of breath. (Refer to ND: risk for decreased Cardiac Output, and CP: Dysrhythmias.)	Trends determine client's response to activity and may indicate myocardial oxygen deprivation that may require short-term reduction of activities, changes in medication regimen, or use of supplemental oxygen.
Encourage bedrest to chair rest initially. Thereafter, limit activity on basis of pain or adverse cardiac response. Provide nonstress diversional activities.	Reduces myocardial workload and oxygen consumption, reducing risk of complications, such as extension of MI. Clients with uncomplicated MI are encouraged to engage in mild activity out of bed, including short walks 12 hours after incident.
Instruct client to avoid actions that raise abdominal pressure, such as straining during defecation.	Activities that require holding the breath and bearing down, such as Valsalva's maneuver, can result in bradycardia with temporarily reduced cardiac output and rebound tachycardia with elevated BP.
Explain pattern of graded increase of activity level, such as getting up to commode or sitting in chair, progressive ambulation, and resting after meals.	Progressive activity provides a controlled demand on the heart, increasing strength and preventing overexertion.
Review signs and symptoms reflecting intolerance of present activity level or requiring notification of nurse or physician.	Palpitations, pulse irregularities, development of chest pain, or dyspnea may indicate need for changes in exercise regimen or medication.
Collaborative	
Refer to cardiac rehabilitation program.	Provides continued support and additional supervision and promotes participation in recovery and wellness process.

NURSING DIAGNOSIS: [moderate/severe] Anxiety

May Be Related To

Situational crisis
Threat to or change in health, economic status; threat of death
Unconscious conflict about essential values, goals of life
Interpersonal transmission

Possibly Evidenced By

Fearful attitude
Apprehension, increased tension, restlessness, facial tension
Uncertainty, feelings of inadequacy
Reports concern due to change in life events
Focus on self, worried

Desired Outcomes/Evaluation Criteria—Client Will

Anxiety Self-Control (NOC)

Recognize and verbalize feelings.
Identify causes and contributing factors.
Verbalize reduction of anxiety or fear.
Demonstrate positive problem-solving skills.
Identify and use resources appropriately.

ACTIONS/INTERVENTIONS	RATIONALE
Anxiety Reduction (NIC)	
Independent	
Identify and acknowledge client's perception of threat or situation. Encourage expressions of, and avoid denying feelings of, anger grief, sadness, and fear.	Coping with the pain and emotional trauma of an MI is difficult. Client may fear death or be anxious about immediate environment. Ongoing anxiety related to concerns about impact of heart attack on future lifestyle, matters left unattended or unresolved, and effects of illness on family may be present in varying degrees for some time and may be manifested by symptoms of depression.
Note presence of hostility, withdrawal, and denial—inappropriate affect or refusal to comply with medical regimen.	Research into survival rates between personality types in individuals and the impact of denial has been ambiguous; however, studies show some correlation between degree and expression of anger or hostility and an increased risk for MI.
Maintain confident manner, without false reassurance.	Client and SO may be affected by the anxiety or uneasiness displayed by health team members. Honest explanations can alleviate anxiety.
Orient client and SO to routine procedures and expected activities. Promote participation when possible.	Predictability and information can decrease anxiety for client.
Observe for verbal and nonverbal signs of anxiety, and stay with client. Intervene if client displays destructive behavior.	Client may not express concern directly, but words or actions may convey sense of agitation, aggression, and hostility. Intervention can help client regain control of own behavior.
Accept but do not reinforce use of denial. Avoid confrontations.	Denial can be beneficial in decreasing anxiety but can postpone dealing with the reality of the current situation. Confrontation can promote anger and increase use of denial, reducing cooperation and possibly impeding recovery.
Answer all questions factually. Provide consistent information; repeat as indicated.	Accurate information about the situation reduces fear, strengthens nurse-client relationship, and assists client and SO to deal realistically with situation. Attention span may be short, and repetition of information helps with retention.
Encourage client and SO to communicate with one another, sharing questions and concerns.	Sharing information elicits support and comfort and can relieve tension of unexpressed worries.
Provide privacy for client and SO.	Allows needed time for personal expression of feelings; may enhance mutual support and promote more adaptive behaviors.
Provide rest periods and uninterrupted sleep time and quiet surroundings, with client controlling type and amount of external stimuli.	Conserves energy and enhances coping abilities.
Support normality of grieving process, including time necessary for resolution.	Can provide reassurance that feelings are normal response to situation and perceived changes. Helps client and SO identify realistic goals, thereby reducing risk of discouragement in face of the reality of limitations of condition and pace of recuperation.
Encourage independence, self-care, and decision making within accepted treatment plan.	Increased independence from staff promotes self-confidence and reduces feelings of abandonment that can accompany transfer from coronary unit and discharge from hospital.
Encourage discussion about postdischarge expectations.	Helps client and SO identify realistic goals, thereby reducing risk of discouragement in face of the reality of limitations of condition and pace of recuperation.
Collaborative	
Administer anti-anxiety or hypnotics, as indicated, such as alprazolam (Xanax) and lorazepam (Ativan).	Promotes relaxation and rest and reduces feelings of anxiety.

NURSING DIAGNOSIS: risk for ineffective Tissue Perfusion [specify]

May Be Related To

Coronary artery spasm, recent myocardial infarction
Hypertension
Treatment-related side effects; thrombolytic therapy

Possibly Evidenced By

(Not applicable; presence of signs and symptoms establishes an *actual* diagnosis)

Desired Outcomes/Evaluation Criteria—Client Will

Cardiac Pump Effectiveness (NOC)

Demonstrate adequate perfusion as individually appropriate, such as skin warm and dry, peripheral pulses present and strong, vital signs within client's normal range, client alert or oriented, balanced intake and output (I&O), absence of edema, free of pain or discomfort, stable, improving ECG, vitals, and mentation.

ACTIONS/INTERVENTIONS	RATIONALE
Hemodynamic Regulation (NIC)	
Independent	
Investigate sudden changes or continued alterations in mentation, such as confusion, irritability, lethargy, and stupor.	Cerebral perfusion is directly related to cardiac output but is also influenced by electrolyte and acid-base variations, hypoxia, and systemic emboli.
Monitor respirations, noting work of breathing.	Sudden or continued dyspnea when pain is relieved may indicate thromboembolic pulmonary complications.
Monitor output, noting changes in urine color and output.	May reflect poor kidney perfusion.
Assess gastrointestinal function, noting anorexia, decreased or absent bowel sounds, nausea and vomiting, abdominal distention, and constipation.	Reduced blood flow to mesentery can produce gastrointestinal dysfunction, such as loss of peristalsis. Problems may be potentiated or aggravated by use of analgesics, decreased activity, and dietary changes.
Circulatory Care: Venous Insufficiency (NIC)	
Encourage active or assist with passive leg exercises.	Enhances venous return, reduces venous stasis, and decreases risk of thrombophlebitis.
Assess for pain in lower extremity and Homans' sign, erythema, and edema.	Indicators of deep vein thrombosis (DVT), although calf pain is not always present and absence of Homans' sign does not rule out DVT.
Instruct client in application and periodic removal of antiembolic hose, when used.	Limits venous stasis, improves venous return, and reduces risk of thrombophlebitis in client who is limited in activity.
Collaborative	
Apply sequential compression devices (SCDs), as indicated.	May be desired to prevent DVT, especially in client who is unable to be out of bed or cannot ambulate freely.
Cardiac Care: Acute (NIC)	
Provide supplemental oxygen as prescribed.	Increases oxygen supply to the myocardium.
Monitor laboratory data, such as ABGs, blood urea nitrogen (BUN), creatinine, electrolytes, and coagulation studies (prothrombin time [PT], activated prothrombin time [aPTT], clotting times).	Indicators of organ perfusion and function. Abnormalities in coagulation may occur as a result of therapeutic measures, such as heparin or Coumadin use and some cardiac drugs.
Administer medications as indicated:	
Antiplatelet agents, such as aspirin, abciximab (ReoPro), clopidogrel (Plavix), and eptifibatide (Integrilin)	Reduces mortality in MI clients and is taken daily. Aspirin also reduces coronary reocclusion after percutaneous transluminal coronary angioplasty (PTCA). IV antiplatelet drugs such as ReoPro and Integrilin are used as adjuncts to PTCA to decrease complication of platelet clumping within stent when placed.
Anticoagulants, such as heparin/enoxaparin (Lovenox)	Low-dose heparin is given during PTCA and may be given prophylactically in high-risk clients, such as those with atrial fibrillation, obesity, ventricular aneurysm, or history of thrombophlebitis, to reduce risk of thrombophlebitis or mural thrombus formation.
Cimetidine (Tagamet), ranitidine (Zantac), and antacids	May occasionally be used to reduce or neutralize gastric acid, preventing discomfort and gastric irritation, especially in presence of reduced mucosal circulation.

NURSING DIAGNOSIS: deficient Knowledge [Learning Need] regarding cause and treatment of condition, self-care, and discharge needs

May Be Related To
Lack of information, information misperception
Unfamiliarity with information resources
Lack of recall

Possibly Evidenced By
Reports the problem
Inaccurate follow-through of instructions

Desired Outcomes/Evaluation Criteria—Client Will

Knowledge: Cardiac Disease Management (NOC)
Verbalize understanding of condition, potential complications, individual risk factors, and function of pacemaker (if used).
Relate signs of pacemaker failure.
Verbalize understanding of therapeutic regimen.
List desired action and possible adverse side effects of medications.

Self-Management: Cardiac Disease (NOC)
Correctly perform necessary procedures and explain reasons for actions.
Keep follow-up appointments.

ACTIONS/INTERVENTIONS	RATIONALE
Teaching: Individual (NIC)	
Independent	
Assess client and SO level of knowledge and ability or desire to learn.	Necessary for creation of individual instruction plan. Reinforces expectation that this will be a "learning experience." Verbalization identifies misunderstandings and allows for clarification.
Be alert to signs of avoidance, such as changing subject away from information being presented or extremes of behavior, such as withdrawal or euphoria.	Natural defense mechanisms, such as anger or denial of significance of situation, can block learning, affecting client's response and ability to assimilate information. Changing to a less formal or structured style may be more effective until client and SO are ready to accept or deal with current situation.
Present information in varied learning formats, such as programmed books, audiovisual tapes, question-and-answer sessions, and group activities.	Using multiple learning methods enhances retention of material.
Cardiac Care: Rehabilitation (NIC)	
Reinforce explanations of risk factors, dietary and activity restrictions, medications, and symptoms requiring immediate medical attention.	Provides opportunity for client to retain information and to assume control and participate in rehabilitation program.
Review activity limitations, such as refraining from strenuous activities until first checking with provider. Avoid exertion in extreme heat or cold. Stop any activity if chest pain, unusual shortness of breath, dizziness, light-headedness, or nausea occurs.	During healing phase, restrictions may be needed to limit amount of myocardial workload and oxygen consumption.
Explain rationale of dietary regimen, diet low in sodium, saturated fats, and cholesterol.	Excess saturated fats, cholesterol, calories, and sodium increases BP and risk for heart disease. Excess of cholesterol builds plaque in arteries.
Instruct client to consult healthcare provider before taking other prescription or OTC medications.	Many drugs may contain sympathetic nervous stimulants and may increase BP or counteract other medications.
Discuss use of herbals, such as ginseng, garlic, ginkgo, hawthorn, and bromelain, as indicated.	Use of supplements or herbal remedies can result in alterations in blood clotting, especially when anticoagulant therapy, such as Plavix or ASA, is prescribed. Hawthorn can increase the effect of certain cardiac medications.
Encourage identification and reduction of individual risk factors, such as smoking and alcohol consumption and obesity.	These behaviors and chemicals have direct adverse effects on cardiovascular function and may impede recovery and increase risk for complications.
Warn against isometric activity, Valsalva's maneuver, and activities requiring arms positioned above head.	These activities greatly increase cardiac workload and myocardial oxygen consumption and may adversely affect myocardial contractility and output.
Review programmed increases in levels of activity. Educate client regarding resumption of activities, such as walking, work, and recreational and sexual activity. Provide guidelines for gradually increasing activity and instruction regarding target heart rate and pulse taking, as appropriate.	Gradual increase in activity increases strength and prevents overexertion, may enhance collateral circulation, and promotes return to normal lifestyle. *Note:* Sexual activity can be safely resumed once client can accomplish activity equivalent to climbing two flights of stairs without adverse cardiac effects.
Identify alternative activities for "bad weather" days, such as measured walking in house or shopping mall.	Provides for continuing daily activity program.
Review signs and symptoms requiring reduction in activity and notification of healthcare provider. Differentiate between increased heart rate that normally occurs during various activities and worsening signs of cardiac stress: chest pain, dyspnea, palpitations, increased heart rate lasting more than 15 minutes after cessation of activity, and excessive fatigue the following day.	Pulse elevations beyond established limits, development of chest pain, or dyspnea may require changes in exercise and medication regimen.
Emphasize importance of follow-up care, and identify community resources and support groups, such as cardiac rehabilitation programs, "coronary clubs," and smoking cessation clinics.	Reinforces that this is an ongoing or continuing health condition for which support and assistance is available after discharge. *Note:* After discharge, client may encounter limitations in physical functioning and often incur difficulty with emotional, social, and role functioning, requiring ongoing support.
Recommend client receive annual influenza and periodic pneumonia vaccination unless otherwise contraindicated.	Helps protect against viral and bacterial cardiorespiratory illnesses that can negatively impact client's heart health.
Emphasize importance of contacting physician if chest pain, change in anginal pattern, or other symptoms recur.	Timely evaluation and intervention may prevent complications.
Stress importance of reporting development of fever in association with diffuse or atypical chest pain (pleural, pericardial) and joint pain.	Post-MI complication of pericardial inflammation (Dressler's syndrome) requires further medical evaluation and intervention.

ACTIONS/INTERVENTIONS (continued)	RATIONALE (continued)
Encourage client and SO to share concerns and feelings. Discuss signs of pathological depression versus transient feelings frequently associated with major life events. Recommend seeking professional help if feelings of depression persist.	Depressed clients have a greater risk of dying 6 to 18 months following a heart attack (Glassman, 2007). Timely intervention may be beneficial. *Note:* Selective serotonin reuptake inhibitors (SSRIs), such as paroxetine (Paxil), have been found to be as effective as tricyclic antidepressants but with significantly fewer adverse cardiac complications.

POTENTIAL CONSIDERATIONS following discharge from care setting (dependent on client's age, physical condition and presence of complications, personal resources, and life responsibilities)

- ***Activity Intolerance***—imbalance between oxygen supply and demand
- ***Grieving***—loss of significant object (e.g., general well-being, required changes in lifestyle)
- ***Decisional Conflict***—multiple or divergent sources of information; support system deficit
- ***interrupted Family Processes***—situational transition or crisis; shift in health status of a family member
- ***impaired Home Maintenance***—disease/illness, impaired functioning, inadequate support systems, unfamiliarity with neighborhood resources

DYSRHYTHMIAS

I. Pathophysiology

a. Abnormal formation or conduction of the electrical impulses within the heart

b. Bradyarrhythmias: decreased intrinsic pacemaker function or block in conduction, often at atrioventricular (AV) junction or His-Purkinje system

c. Tachyarrhythmias: caused by reentry, often due to enhanced or abnormal automaticity

i. Causes abnormalities of the heart rate, rhythm, or both

ii. Change in conduction may alter pumping action of heart, affecting blood pressure and perfusion of body organs.

II. Classification: Types of Dysrhythmias (Wedro, 2007)

a. Named according to the site of origination and the mechanism of conduction involved:

i. Sinus or sinoatrial (SA) node

ii. AV node

iii. Involved heart chamber—atrial or ventricular

iv. Between the atria and ventricles—supraventricular or junctional dysrhythmias

b. Differentiated by rate

i. Slow: bradycardia, pulse below 60 in adult

ii. Fast: tachycardia, pulse above 100 in adult

c. Rhythm disturbances can be regular (e.g., sinus tachycardia) or irregular (e.g., atrial fibrillation).

III. Etiology

a. Primary cardiac disorder: coronary artery disease (CAD), myocardial infarction (MI), heart valve dysfunction, coronary artery bypass (CABG) surgery, or valve replacement surgery

b. Systemic conditions: hypothyroidism and hyperthyroidism; fever and dehydration; sepsis; shock states (hypovolemic, cardiogenic); anemia; pulmonary diseases; brain injury; catecholamine release, such as occurs in intense emotional stress or vigorous exercise; anxiety disorders and panic attacks

c. Electrolyte imbalances, such as with potassium

d. Effects of drugs and drug toxicity, such as with digoxin, aminophylline, atropine, and caffeine

e. Illicit drug use, such as cocaine, methamphetamines

IV. Statistics

a. Atrial fibrillation (AF) occurs in approximately 2.2 million people in the United States (Fuster et al, 2006).

b. Hospital admissions for AF have increased 66% in the past 20 years (Fuster et al, 2006).

COMMON DYSRHYTHMIAS

Tachycardias

I. Sinus Tachycardia

a. Sinus node creates rate that is faster than normal (greater than 100).

b. Associated with physiological or psychological stress; medications, such as catecholamines, aminophylline, atropine, stimulants, and illicit drugs; enhanced automaticity; and autonomic dysfunction

II. Atrial Flutter

a. Occurs in the atrium and creates regular atrial rates between 250 and 400. Because AV node cannot keep up with conduction of all these impulses, not all atrial impulses are conducted into the ventricle, causing a therapeutic block at the AV node.

III. Atrial Fibrillation (AF)

a. Rapid, irregular twitching of the atrial musculature with an atrial rate of 300 to 600 and a ventricular rate of 120 to 200 if untreated

b. Associated with advanced age, valvular heart disease, hyperthyroidism, pulmonary disorder, pulmonary disease, alcohol ingestion ("holiday heart syndrome"), hypertension, diabetes, CAD, or after open-heart surgery

IV. Paroxysmal Supraventricular Tachycardia (PSVT, also called SVT)

a. Pathways in the AV node or atrium allow an altered conduction of electricity, causing a regular and fast rate of sometimes more than 150 to 200.

(continues on page 88)

b. Ventricle, sensing the electrical activity coming through the AV node, beats along with each stimulation.
c. Rarely a life-threatening event, but most people feel uncomfortable when PSVT occurs.

V. Ventricular Tachycardia (VT)

a. Rapid heartbeat initiated within the ventricles, characterized by three or more consecutive premature ventricular beats with elevated and regular heart rate (such as 160 to 240 beats per minute).
b. Heart rate sustained at a high rate causes symptoms such as weakness, fatigue, dizziness, fainting, or palpitations.
c. Potentially lethal disruption of normal heartbeat that can degenerate to ventricular fibrillation.

VI. Ventricular Fibrillation (VF)

a. Aside from myocardial ischemia, other causes of ventricular fibrillation may include severe weakness of the heart muscle, electrolyte disturbances, drug overdose, and poisoning.
b. Electrical signal is sent from the ventricles at a very fast and erratic rate, impairing the ability of ventricles to fill with blood and pump it out, markedly decreasing cardiac output and resulting in very low blood pressure and loss of consciousness.
c. Sudden death will occur if VF not corrected.

Bradycardias

I. Sinus Bradycardia

a. Rarely symptomatic until heart rate drops below 50, then fainting or syncope may be reported.
b. Causes include hypothyroidism, athletic training, sleep, vagal stimulation, increased intracranial pressure, MI, hypovolemia, hypoxia, acidosis, hypokalemia and hyperkalemia, hyperglycemia, hypothermia, toxins, tamponade, tension pneumothorax, thrombosis (cardiac or pulmonary), and trauma.
c. Medications, such as beta blockers, calcium channel blockers, and amiodarone, also slow the heart.

II. Sick Sinus Syndrome (SSS)

a. Variety of conditions affecting SA node function, including bradycardia, sinus arrest, sinoatrial block, episodes of tachycardia, and carotid hypersensitivity.
b. Signs and symptoms related to cerebral hypoperfusion.
c. May be associated with rapid rate (tachycardia) or alternate between too fast and too slow (bradycardia-tachycardia syndrome). A long pause (asystole) may occur between heartbeats, especially after an episode of tachycardia.

III. Heart Blocks

a. First-degree AV block
   i. Asymptomatic; usually an incidental finding on electrocardiogram (ECG)
b. Second-degree AV (type I and type II)
   i. Usually asymptomatic, although some clients can feel irregularities (palpitations) of the heartbeat, or syncope may occur, which usually is observed in more advanced conduction disturbances such as Mobitz II AV block.
   ii. Medications affecting AV node function, such as digoxin, beta blockers, calcium channel blockers, may contribute.
c. Third-degree AV block (also called complete heart block)
   i. May be associated with acute MI, either causing the block or related to reduced cardiac output from bradycardia in the setting of advanced atherosclerotic CAD.
   ii. Symptomatic with fatigue, dizziness, and syncope and possible loss of consciousness
   iii. Can be life-threatening, especially if associated with heart failure

Other Dysrhythmias

I. Premature Atrial Complex (PAC)

a. Electrical impulse starts in the atrium before the next normal impulse of the sinus node.
b. Causes include caffeine, alcohol, and nicotine use; stretched atrial myocardium; anxiety; hypokalemia; and hypermetabolic states (pregnancy); or may be related to atrial ischemia, injury, or infarction.

II. Premature Ventricular Contraction (PVC)

a. Electrical signal originates in the ventricles, causing them to contract before receiving the electrical signal from the atria.
b. PVCs not uncommon and are often asymptomatic.
c. Increase to several per minute may cause symptoms such as weakness, fatigue, dizziness, fainting, or palpitations.
d. Irritability of the heart demonstrated by frequent and or multiple back-to-back PVCs can lead to VF.

III. Long QT Syndrome (LQTS) (National Heart, Lung, and Blood Institute [NHLB], 2011; Mayo Clinic, 2011)

a. May be inherited or acquired
b. Of the seven types of inherited; three are common:
   i. In types 1 and 2, the flow of potassium through ion channels in heart cells is abnormal. This may occur when client exercises or experiences strong emotions and can cause a rapid, uncontrollable heart rhythm that can be fatal if it's not quickly brought under control.
   ii. In type 3, problems usually occur when the heart beats slower than normal, such as during sleep.
c. Aquired types may be medication-induced or have other causes:
   i. Medications may include (or are not limited to) antihistamines, diuretics, some antiarrhythmia agents, certain antidepressants, cholesterol-lowering drugs.
   ii. Other causes include severe vomiting and diarrhea, eating disorders (e.g., bulimia), where sodium or potassium losses affect electrical activity of the heart.

GLOSSARY

Arrhythmias (also called dysrhythmias): Heart rhythm disturbances classified by rate (normal, tachycardia, bradycardia); mechanism (automaticity, reentry, fibrillation); and by site of origin (atrial, ventricular, junctional).

AV node: The electrical relay station between the atria (the upper) and the ventricles (the lower chambers of the heart).

Bigeminal pulse: Irregular strong beat alternating with weak beat.

Bradycardias: Abnormally slow rhythms may be ascribed to two general mechanisms—failure of the sinoatrial (SA) node to generate impulses, such as in sinus bradycardia, or failure of the impulses to conduct normally to the ventricles, such as in heart blocks.

Pacemaker: A system that sends electrical impulses to the heart in order to set the heart rhythm. The pacemaker can be the natural pacemaker of the heart or it can be an artificial electronic device.

Palpitations: An increased awareness of the heartbeat and palpitations can result from many dysrhythmias, including any bradycardia and tachycardia, premature ventricular and atrial contractions, sick sinus syndrome (SSS), advanced arteriovenous block, or ventricular tachycardia (VT). Palpitations associated with dizziness, near-syncope, or syncope suggest tachyarrhythmia and are potentially more serious.

Pulse deficit: Difference between apical pulse and radial pulse.

Pulsus alternans: Regular strong beat, alternating with weak beat.

Sinoatrial (SA) node: One of the major elements in the cardiac conduction system that controls the heart rate. The SA node generates electrical impulses and conducts them throughout the muscle of the heart, stimulating the heart to contract and pump blood.

Sudden cardiac death (also known as sudden cardiac arrest [SCA]): A sudden, unexpected death caused by loss of heart function. Most sudden cardiac deaths are caused by dysrhythmias, such as ventricular fibrillation (VF). The only treatment is defibrillation with an electrical shock.

Tachycardias: Rapid heart rates originating from either the atrium or the ventricle.

Care Settings

Generally, minor dysrhythmias are monitored and treated in the community setting; however, potential life-threatening situations (including heart rates above 150 beats per minute) may require a short inpatient stay.

Related Concerns

Acute coronary syndrome, page 58
Angina, page 67
Heart failure: chronic, page 43
Myocardial infarction, page 75
Psychosocial aspects of care, page 729

Client Assessment Database

DIAGNOSTIC DIVISION MAY REPORT	MAY EXHIBIT
ACTIVITY/REST	
• Generalized weakness • Exertional fatigue	• Changes in heart rate/blood pressure (BP) with activity or exercise
CIRCULATION	
• History of previous or acute MI (90% to 95% experience dysrhythmias), cardiac surgery, cardiomyopathy, rheumatic heart disease and heart failure (HF), valvular heart disease, long-standing hypertension, use of pacemaker • *Pulse:* Fast, slow, or irregular; palpitations, skipped beats	• BP changes (hypertension or hypotension) during episodes of dysrhythmia • Pulses may be irregular, for example, skipped beats; pulsus alternans, bigeminal pulse • Pulse deficit • *Heart sounds:* irregular rhythm, extra sounds, dropped beats • Skin color and moisture changes, such as pallor, cyanosis, diaphoresis (HF, shock) • Edema dependent, generalized, jugular vein distention (JVD) (in presence of HF) • Urine output decreased if cardiac output is severely diminished
EGO INTEGRITY	
• Feeling nervous (certain tachydysrhythmias), sense of impending doom • Stressors related to current medical problems	• Anxiety, fear, withdrawal, anger, irritability, crying • Denial of health problems

(continues on page 90)

Client Assessment Database (continued)

DIAGNOSTIC DIVISION MAY REPORT (continued)	MAY EXHIBIT (continued)
FOOD/FLUID • Loss of appetite, anorexia • Food intolerance (with certain medications) • Nausea or vomiting • Changes in weight	• Weight gain or loss • Edema • Changes in skin moisture or turgor • Lung sounds have crackles
NEUROSENSORY • Dizzy spells, sudden fainting • Headaches • Numbness or tingling of fingers or toes	• Mental status or sensorium changes, such as disorientation, confusion, loss of memory; changes in usual speech pattern and consciousness, stupor, coma • Behavioral changes, such as combativeness, lethargy, hallucinations • Pupil changes (equality and reaction to light) • Loss of deep tendon reflexes with life-threatening dysrhythmias (VT, severe bradycardia)
PAIN/DISCOMFORT • Chest pain (mild to severe) that may or may not be relieved by anti-anginal medication	• Distraction behaviors, such as restlessness
RESPIRATION • Chronic lung disease • History of or current tobacco use • Shortness of breath • Coughing with or without sputum production	• Changes in respiratory rate and depth during dysrhythmia episode • ***Breath sounds:*** Adventitious sounds such as crackles, rhonchi, or wheezing, indicating respiratory complications, such as left-sided heart failure (pulmonary edema) or pulmonary thromboembolic phenomena • Hemoptysis • Abnormal pulse oximetry or blood gases
SAFETY	• Fever • ***Skin:*** Rashes (medication reaction) • Loss of muscle tone and strength
TEACHING/LEARNING • Familial risk factors, such as heart disease, stroke • Use or misuse of prescribed medications, such as heart medications, anticoagulants, or over-the-counter (OTC) medications, for example, cough syrup, analgesics containing aspirin (ASA), and decongestants • Use of vitamins and herbal supplements for heart rhythm, such as belladonna, camphor, dong quai, ginseng, goldenseal • Stimulant abuse, including caffeine and nicotine; street drugs, including cocaine derivatives, methamphetamines, ecstasy, inhalants • Lack of understanding about disease process and therapeutic regimen • Evidence of failure to improve, such as recurrent or intractable dysrhythmias that are life-threatening	
DISCHARGE PLAN CONSIDERATIONS • Alteration of medication use and therapy • Coumadin precautions • Teaching regarding pacemaker or other device ➧ Refer to section at end of plan for postdischarge considerations.	

Diagnostic Studies

TEST WHY IT IS DONE	WHAT IT TELLS ME
• *Electrocardiogram (ECG):* Records electrical activity of the heart.	Measures how long it takes for impulses to travel through the atria, the conduction system, and the ventricles. Identifies when hypoxia (e.g., due to coronary artery obstruction or myocardial muscle damage) and imbalance of electrolytes (e.g., potassium, magnesium, and calcium) are affecting cardiac rhythm and contractility (American Heart Association [AHA], 2012). *Note:* Exercise ECG reveals dysrhythmias occurring only when client is not at rest (can be diagnostic for cardiac cause of syncope).
• *Extended or event monitoring (Holter monitor):* Extended ECG tracing (24 hours to weeks).	May be used to determine which dysrhythmias occur intermittently or may be causing specific symptoms (e.g., sudden fainting [syncope] or bradycardia only when client is at rest). May also be used to evaluate pacemaker function, antidysrhythmic drug effect, or effectiveness of cardiac rehabilitation.
• *Signal-averaged ECG (SAE):* May be used to screen high-risk clients especially, with post-MI or unexplained syncope.	May reveal ventricular dysrhythmias, presence of delayed conduction, and late potentials—as occurs with sustained ventricular tachycardia.
STUDIES THAT MAY BE USED TO PROVOKE/ REPRODUCE DYSRHYTHMIAS	
• *Electrophysiological (EP) mapping:* Test that records the electrical activity and maps the electrical pathways of the heart by means of electrode catheters placed in the heart.	Valuable for provoking known but infrequent dysrhythmias and for unmasking suspected dysrhythmias. Electrodes may stimulate heart to beat at rates that may trigger—or halt—dysrhythmia.
• *Stress tests (e.g., treadmill exercise or pharmacological-induced stress test)*	Provokes dysrhythmias and makes diagnosis (and, thus, treatment) easier. A treadmill test may be used for stable client whose suspected dysrhythmias are clearly exercise-related. Drug-induced testing helps identify dysrhythmias that may be from ischemia in client who cannot physically perform treadmill.
• *Tilt test:* Shows heart rate and blood pressure response to change in position from lying down to standing up.	
BLOOD TESTS	
• *Electrolytes:* Substances that, in solution, conduct an electric current and are decomposed by its passage. Sodium, potassium, calcium, and magnesium are common electrolytes.	Imbalance of electrolytes, such as potassium, magnesium, and calcium, adversely affects cardiac rhythm and contractility
• *Drug screen:* Laboratory procedure that checks blood or urine sample for presence of certain medications or drugs of abuse.	May reveal therapeutic or toxic levels of prescription medications; suggest interaction of drugs, such as digoxin and quinidine; or detect presence of street drugs that can affect or contribute to dysrhythmias.

Nursing Priorities

1. Prevent or treat life-threatening dysrhythmias.
2. Support client and significant other (SO) in dealing with anxiety and fear of potentially life-threatening situation.
3. Assist in identification of cause or precipitating factors.
4. Review information regarding condition, prognosis, and treatment regimen.

Discharge Goals

1. Free of life-threatening dysrhythmias and complications of impaired cardiac output and tissue perfusion.
2. Anxiety reduced and managed.
3. Disease process, therapy needs, and prevention of complications understood.
4. Plan in place to meet needs after discharge.

NURSING DIAGNOSIS: risk for decreased Cardiac Output

Risk Factors May Include

Altered heart rate/rhythm
Altered contractility

Possibly Evidenced By

(Not applicable; presence of signs and symptoms establishes an *actual* diagnosis)

Desired Outcomes/Evaluation Criteria—Client Will

Cardiac Pump Effectiveness (NOC)

Maintain or achieve adequate cardiac output as evidenced by BP and pulse within normal range, adequate urinary output, palpable pulses of equal quality, and usual level of mentation.
Display reduced frequency or absence of dysrhythmia(s).
Participate in activities that reduce myocardial workload.

ACTIONS/INTERVENTIONS	RATIONALE
Dysrhythmia Management (NIC)	
Independent	
Palpate radial, carotid, femoral, and dorsalis pedis pulses, noting rate, regularity, amplitude (full or thready), and symmetry. Document presence of pulsus alternans, bigeminal pulse, or pulse deficit.	Differences in equality, rate, and regularity of pulses are indicative of the effect of altered cardiac output on systemic and peripheral circulation.
Auscultate heart sounds, noting rate, rhythm, presence of extra heartbeats, and dropped beats.	Specific dysrhythmias are more clearly detected audibly than by palpation. Hearing extra heartbeats or dropped beats helps identify dysrhythmias in the unmonitored client.
Monitor vital signs. Assess adequacy of cardiac output and tissue perfusion, noting significant variations in BP, pulse rate equality, respirations, changes in skin color and temperature, level of consciousness and sensorium, and urine output during episodes of dysrhythmias.	Although not all dysrhythmias are life-threatening, immediate treatment may be required to terminate dysrhythmia in the presence of alterations in cardiac output and tissue perfusion.
Determine type of dysrhythmia and document with rhythm strip if cardiac or telemetry monitoring is available:	Useful in determining need and type of intervention required.
Sinus tachycardia	Tachycardia can occur in response to stress, pain, fever, infection, coronary artery blockage, valvular dysfunction, hypovolemia, hypoxia, or as a result of decreased vagal tone or of increased sympathetic nervous system activity associated with the release of catecholamines. Although it generally does not require treatment, persistent tachycardia may worsen underlying pathology in clients with ischemic heart disease because of shortened diastolic filling time and increased oxygen demands. These clients may require medications.
Sinus bradycardia	Bradycardia is common in clients with acute MI (especially anterior and inferior) and is the result of excessive parasympathetic activity, blocks in conduction to the SA or AV nodes, or loss of automaticity of the heart muscle. Clients with severe heart disease may not be able to compensate for a slow rate by increasing stroke volume; therefore, decreased cardiac output, HF, and potentially lethal ventricular dysrhythmias may occur.
Atrial dysrhythmias, such as PACs, atrial flutter, AF, and atrial supraventricular tachycardias (SVT) (i.e., paroxysmal atrial tachycardia [PAT], multifocal atrial tachycardia [MAT])	PACs can occur as a response to ischemia and are normally harmless but can precede or precipitate AF. Acute and chronic atrial flutter or fibrillation (the most common dysrhythmia) can occur with coronary artery or valvular disease and may or may not be pathological. Rapid atrial flutter or fibrillation reduces cardiac output as a result of incomplete ventricular filling (shortened cardiac cycle) and increased oxygen demand.
Ventricular dysrhythmias, such as PVCs and ventricular premature beats (VPBs), ventricular tachycardia (VT), and ventricular flutter and fibrillation (VF)	PVCs or VPBs reflect cardiac irritability and are commonly associated with MI, digoxin toxicity, coronary vasospasm, and misplaced temporary pacemaker leads. Frequent, multiple, or multifocal PVCs result in diminished cardiac output and may lead to potentially lethal dysrhythmias, such as VT or sudden death or cardiac arrest from ventricular flutter or VF. *Note:* Intractable ventricular dysrhythmias unresponsive to

medication may reflect ventricular aneurysm. Polymorphic VT (torsades de pointes) is recognized by inconsistent shape of QRS complexes and is often related to use of drugs such as procainamide (Pronestyl), quinidine (Quinaglute), disopyramide (Norpace), and sotalol (Betapace).

Heart blocks — Reflect altered transmission of impulses through normal conduction channels (slowed, altered) and may be the result of MI or CAD with reduced blood supply to SA or AV nodes, drug toxicity, and sometimes cardiac surgery. Progressing heart block is associated with slowed ventricular rates, decreased cardiac output, and potentially lethal ventricular dysrhythmias or cardiac standstill.

Provide calm and quiet environment. Review reasons for limitation of activities during acute phase. — Reduces stimulation and release of stress-related catecholamines, which can cause or aggravate dysrhythmias and vasoconstriction, increasing myocardial workload.

Demonstrate and encourage use of stress management behaviors such as relaxation techniques; guided imagery; and slow, deep breathing. — Promotes client participation in exerting some sense of control in a stressful situation.

Investigate reports of chest pain, documenting location, duration, intensity (0 to 10 scale), and relieving or aggravating factors. Note nonverbal pain cues, such as facial grimacing, crying, changes in BP and heart rate. — Reasons for chest pain are variable and depend on underlying cause. However, chest pain may indicate ischemia due to altered electrical conduction, decreased myocardial perfusion, or increased oxygen need, such as impending or evolving MI.

Be prepared to initiate cardiopulmonary resuscitation (CPR), as indicated. — Development of life-threatening dysrhythmias requires prompt intervention to prevent ischemic damage or death.

Collaborative

Monitor laboratory studies, such as the following:

Electrolytes — Imbalance of electrolytes, such as potassium, magnesium, and calcium, adversely affects cardiac rhythm and contractility.

Medication and drug levels — Reveal therapeutic and toxic level of prescription medications or street drugs that may affect or contribute to presence of dysrhythmias.

Administer supplemental oxygen, as indicated. — Increases amount of oxygen available for myocardial uptake, reducing irritability caused by hypoxia.

Prepare for and assist with diagnostic and treatment procedures such as EP studies, radiofrequency ablation (RFA), and cryoablation (CA). — Treatment for several tachycardia dysrhythmias, including SVT, atrial flutter, Wolf-Parkinson-White (WPW) syndrome, AF, and VT, is often carried out as first-line treatment via heart catheterization or angiographic procedures. After rhythm is confirmed with EP study, the client will then often have either an RFA or CA to terminate or disrupt the dysfunctional pattern. Medications may be tried first or added after ablation for increased treatment success.

Insert and maintain intravenous (IV) access. — Patent access line may be required for administration of emergency drugs.

Administer medications, as indicated, for example:

Potassium — Correction of hypokalemia may be sufficient to terminate some ventricular dysrhythmias. *Note:* Potassium imbalance is the number one cause of AF.

Antidysrhythmics (Vaughn's Summaries, 2012), such as the following: — Class I drugs block sodium (Na+) channels and are subdivided.

Class I drugs

Class Ia, such as disopyramide (Norpace), procainamide (Procanabid), quinidine (Cardioquin) — These drugs increase action potential, duration, and effective refractory period and decrease membrane responsiveness, prolonging both QRS complex and QT interval. This also results in decreasing myocardial conduction velocity and excitability in the atria, ventricles, and accessory pathways. They suppress ectopic focal activity. Useful for treatment of atrial and ventricular premature beats and repetitive dysrhythmias, such as atrial tachycardias and atrial flutter and AF. *Note:* Myocardial depressant effects may be potentiated when class Ia drugs are used in conjunction with any drugs possessing similar properties.

Class Ib, such as lidocaine (Xylocaine), phenytoin (Dilantin, Phenytek), tocainide (Tonocard) — These drugs slow conduction by depressing SA node automaticity and decreasing conduction velocity through the atria, ventricles, and Purkinje's fibers. The result is prolongation of the PR interval and lengthening of the QRS complex. They suppress and prevent all types of ventricular dysrhythmias.

(continues on page 94)

ACTIONS/INTERVENTIONS (continued)	RATIONALE (continued)
Class Ic, such as flecainide (Tambocor), encainide (Enkaid), propafenone (Rhythmol)	These drugs inhibit the voltage-dependent sodium channels and prolong the depolarization phase, thus increasing conduction velocity, and have little effect on the repolarization phase. This makes them useful in the treatment of atrial flutter or fibrillation in clients with structurally normal hearts. *Note:* Flecainide increases risk of drug-induced dysrhythmias post-MI. Propafenone can worsen or cause new dysrhythmias, a tendency called the "pro-arrhythmic effect."
Class II drugs, (most used) such as atenolol (Tenormin), carvedilol (Coreg), propranolol (Inderal), nadolol (Corgard), acebutolol (Sectral), esmolol (Brevibloc)	Beta-adrenergic blockers have anti-adrenergic properties and decrease automaticity. They reduce the rate and force of cardiac contractions, which in turn decrease cardiac output, blood pressure, and peripheral vascular resistance. Therefore, they are useful in the treatment of dysrhythmias caused by SA and AV node dysfunction, including SVTs, atrial flutter, and AF. *Note:* These drugs may exacerbate bradycardia and cause myocardial depression, especially when combined with drugs that have similar properties.
Class III drugs, such as bretylium tosylate (Bretylol), amiodarone (Cordarone), sotalol (Betapace), ibutilide (Corvert), and dofetilide (Tikosyn)	These drugs are potassium channel blockers; they prolong the refractory period and action potential duration, consequently prolonging the QT interval. They decrease peripheral resistance and increase coronary blood flow. They have anti-anginal and anti-adrenergic properties. They are used to terminate VF and other life-threatening ventricular dysrhythmias and sustained ventricular tachyarrhythmias, especially when lidocaine and procainamide are not effective.
Class IV drugs, such as amlodipine (Norvasc), verapamil (Adalat, Calan), diltiazem (Cardizem, Tiazac)	Calcium channel blockers slow conduction time through the AV node, prolonging PR interval to decrease ventricular response in SVTs, atrial flutter, and AF. Calan and Cardizem may be used for bedside conversion of acute AF.
Class V drugs, such as atropine sulfate, isoproterenol (Isuprel), and cardiac glycosides (digoxin [Lanoxin]; digitoxin Tardigal].	Miscellaneous drugs useful in treating bradycardia by increasing SA and AV conduction and enhancing automaticity. Cardiac glycosides may be used alone or in combination with other antidysrhythmic drugs to reduce ventricular rate in presence of uncontrolled or poorly tolerated atrial tachycardias or atrial flutter and AF.
Prepare for and assist with elective cardioversion.	May be used in AF after trials of first-line drugs—such as atenolol, metoprolol, diltiazem, and verapamil—have failed to control heart rate or in certain unstable dysrhythmias to restore normal heart rate or relieve symptoms of heart failure.
Assist with insertion and maintain pacemaker (external or temporary, internal or permanent) function.	Temporary pacing may be necessary to accelerate impulse formation in bradydysrhythmias, synchronize electrical impulsivity, or override tachydysrhythmias and ectopic activity to maintain cardiovascular function until spontaneous pacing is restored or permanent pacing is initiated. These devices may include atrial and ventricular pacemakers and may provide single-chamber or dual-chamber pacing.
Prepare for precedures, such as PCIs, including angiography with possible angioplasty and stent placement; catheter or surgical ablation; or surgery, such as aneurysmectomy or CABG, as indicated.	Treatment may include revascularization procedures such as stenting or CABG, indicated to enhance circulation to myocardium and conduction system. Ablation therapy destroys a small spot of heart tissue and creates an electrical block along the pathway that stops the dysrhythmia and redirects electrical conduction pathways. Resection of ventricular aneurysm may be required to correct intractable ventricular dysrhythmias unresponsive to medical therapy.
Prepare for placement of ICD when indicated.	This device may be surgically implanted in those clients with recurrent, life-threatening ventricular dysrhythmias (such as might occur with Long QT Syndrome [LQTS]), or other dysrhythmias unresponsive to tailored drug therapy (NHLB, 2011). The latest generation of devices can provide multilevel or "tiered" therapy, that is, antitachycardia and antibradycardia pacing, cardioversion, or defibrillation, depending on how each device is programmed.

NURSING DIAGNOSIS: risk for Poisoning [Digitalis toxicity]

Risk Factors May Include

Deficient knowledge regarding pharmaceutical agents; lack of proper precautions
Reduced vision, cognitive limitations
[Limited range of therapeutic effectiveness]

Possibly Evidenced By

(Not applicable; presence of signs and symptoms establishes an *actual* diagnosis)

Desired Outcomes/Evaluation Criteria—Client Will

Knowledge: Medication

Verbalize understanding of individual prescription, how it interacts with other drugs or substances, and importance of maintaining prescribed regimen.
Recognize signs of digoxin overdose and developing heart failure, and identify what to report to physician.

Cardiac Pump Effectiveness

Be free of signs of toxicity; display serum drug level within individually acceptable range.

ACTIONS/INTERVENTIONS	RATIONALE
Medication Management (NIC) *Independent*	
Evaluate client for need for digitalis.	Incidence of digitalis toxicity has declined because of a decrease in digitalis usage, improvement in digoxin formulation, increased awareness in drug-to-drug interactions, increased availability of other drugs to treat heart failure and techniques like catheter ablation therapy for supraventricular tachycardias. However, digitalis toxicity rates remain relatively stable. *Note:* Approximately 1.1% of outpatients on digoxin and 10% to18% of people in nursing homes develop digitalis toxicity (Patel, 2011).
Explain client's specific type of digoxin preparation and its specific therapeutic use.	Reduces confusion due to digoxin preparations varying in name (although they may be similar), dosage strength, and onset and duration of action. The most common precipitating cause of digitalis intoxication is depletion of potassium stores, which occurs often in clients with heart failure (may be the result of diuretic therapy and secondary hyperaldosteronism).
Instruct client not to change dose for any reason, not to omit dose—unless instructed to, based on pulse rate—not to increase dose or take extra doses, and to contact physician if more than one dose is omitted.	Alterations in drug regimen can reduce therapeutic effects, result in toxicity, and cause complications.
Advise client that digoxin may interact with many other drugs, such as barbiturates, neomycin, cholestyramine, quinidine, and antacids, and that physician should be informed that digoxin is taken whenever new medications are prescribed. Advise client not to use OTC drugs, such as laxatives, antidiarrheals, antacids, cold remedies, diuretics, and herbals, without first checking with the pharmacist or healthcare provider.	Knowledge may help prevent dangerous drug interactions.
Review importance of dietary and supplemental intake of potassium, calcium, and magnesium.	Maintaining electrolytes at normal ranges may prevent or limit development of toxicity and correct many associated dysrhythmias.
Provide information and have the client and SO verbalize understanding of toxic signs and symptoms to report to the healthcare provider.	Nausea, vomiting, diarrhea, unusual drowsiness, confusion, very slow or very fast irregular pulse, thumping in chest, double or blurred vision, yellow or green tint or halos around objects, flickering color forms or dots, altered color perception, and worsening HF—such as dependent or generalized edema, dyspnea, decreased amount or frequency of voiding—indicate need for prompt evaluation and intervention. Mild symptoms of toxicity may be managed with a brief drug holiday. *Note:* In severe or refractory heart failure, altered cardiac binding of digoxin may result in toxicity even with previously appropriate drug doses.

(continues on page 96)

ACTIONS/INTERVENTIONS (continued)

Discuss necessity of periodic laboratory evaluations, as indicated:

Serum digoxin (Lanoxin) or digitoxin (Crystodigin) level

Electrolytes, blood urea nitrogen (BUN), creatinine, and liver function studies

Collaborative

Provide supportive therapy, as indicated.

Administer medications, as appropriate, for example:

Digoxin immune Fab (Digibind)

Prepare client for transfer to critical care unit (CCU), as indicated, such as for dangerous dysrhythmias, exacerbation of heart failure.

RATIONALE (continued)

Drug levels are evaluated in conjunction with clinical manifestations and ECG to determine individual's response.

Digoxin has a narrow therapeutic serum range, with toxicity occurring at levels that are dependent on individual response.

Abnormal levels of potassium, calcium, or magnesium increase the heart's sensitivity to digoxin. Impaired kidney function can cause digoxin (mainly excreted by the kidney) to accumulate to toxic levels. Digitoxin levels (mainly excreted by the bowel) are affected by impaired liver function.

Depending on the severity of the toxicity, treatment ranges from simply holding digitalis preparations for a period of time to treatment with IV fluids, oxygenation and support of ventilatory function, discontinuation of the drug, and correction of electrolyte imbalances. Effective management also relies on early recognition that a dysrhythmia and/or noncardiac manifestation may be related to digitalis intoxication.

A first-line treatment for toxicity, Digibind is a relatively pure Fab product that is safe and effective. Onset of action ranges from 20 to 90 minutes, and digoxin is removed irreversibly from the myocardium and other specific binding sites. A complete response generally occurs within 4 hours (Smith, 1982).

In the presence of digoxin toxicity, clients frequently require intensive monitoring until therapeutic levels have been restored. Because all digoxin preparations have long serum half-lives, stabilization can take several days.

NURSING DIAGNOSIS: ineffective Self-Health Management

May Be Related To

Complexity of therapeutic regimen
Deficient knowledge

Possibly Evidenced By

Reports difficulty with prescribed regimen
Failure to take action to reduce risk factors

Desired Outcomes/Evaluation Criteria—Client Will

Self-Management: Dysrhythmias (NOC)

Verbalize understanding of condition, prognosis, and function of pacemaker (if used).
Relate signs of pacemaker failure.
Verbalize understanding of therapeutic regimen.
List desired action and possible adverse side effects of medications.
Correctly perform necessary procedures and explain reasons for actions.

ACTIONS/INTERVENTIONS

Teaching: Individual (NIC)

Independent

Assess client and SO level of knowledge and ability and desire to learn.

Be alert to signs of avoidance, such as changing subject away from information being presented or extremes of behavior (withdrawal or euphoria).

Present information in varied learning formats, for example, programmed books, audiovisual tapes, question-and-answer sessions, and group activities.

RATIONALE

Necessary for creation of individual instruction plan. Reinforces expectation that this will be a "learning experience." Verbalization identifies misunderstandings and allows for clarification.

Natural defense mechanisms, such as anger or denial of significance of situation, can block learning, affecting client's response and ability to assimilate information. Changing to a less formal or structured style may be more effective until client and SO are ready to accept and deal with current situation.

Multiple learning methods may enhance retention of material.

ACTIONS/INTERVENTIONS (continued)	RATIONALE (continued)
Provide information in written form for client and SO to take home.	Follow-up reminders may enhance client's understanding and cooperation with the desired regimen. Written instructions are a helpful resource when client is not in direct contact with healthcare team.
Teaching: Disease Process	
Reinforce explanations of risk factors, dietary and activity restrictions, medications, and symptoms requiring immediate medical attention.	Provides opportunity for client to retain information and to assume control and participate in rehabilitation program.
Encourage identification and reduction of individual risk factors, such as smoking and alcohol consumption and obesity.	These behaviors and chemicals have direct adverse effect on cardiovascular function and may impede recovery and increase risk for complications.
Review normal cardiac function and electrical conduction.	Provides a knowledge base to understand individual variations and reasons for therapeutic interventions.
Explain and reinforce specific dysrhythmia problem and therapeutic measures to client and SO.	Ongoing and updated information, such as whether the problem is resolving or may require long-term control measures, can decrease anxiety associated with the unknown and prepare client and SO to make necessary lifestyle adaptations. Educating the SO may be especially important if client is elderly, visually or hearing impaired, or unable or even unwilling to learn or follow instructions. Repeated explanations may be needed because anxiety and bulk of new information can block or limit learning.
Identify adverse effects and complications of specific dysrhythmias, such as fatigue, dependent edema, progressive changes in mentation, vertigo, and psychological manifestations.	Dysrhythmias may decrease cardiac output, manifested by symptoms of developing cardiac failure and altered cerebral perfusion. Tachydysrhythmias may also be accompanied by debilitating anxiety and feelings of impending doom.
Instruct and document teaching regarding medications. Include the desired action, how and when to take the drug, what to do if a dose is forgotten (dosage and usage information), and expected side effects or possible adverse reactions or interactions with other prescribed and OTC drugs or substances (alcohol, tobacco, herbal remedies), as well as what and when to report to the healthcare provider.	Information necessary for client to make informed choices and to manage medication regimen. *Note:* Use of herbal remedies in conjunction with drug regimen may result in adverse effects, for example, cardiac stimulation and impaired clotting, necessitating evaluation of product for safe use.
Encourage development of regular exercise routine, avoiding overexertion. Identify signs and symptoms requiring immediate cessation of activities, such as dizziness, lightheadedness, dyspnea, and chest pain.	When dysrhythmias are properly managed, normal activity should not be affected. Exercise program is useful in improving overall cardiovascular well-being.
Review individual dietary needs and restrictions, such as potassium and caffeine.	Depending on specific problem, client may need to increase dietary potassium, such as when potassium-depleting diuretics are used. Caffeine may be limited to prevent cardiac excitation.
Demonstrate proper pulse-taking technique. Recommend weekly checking of pulse for 1 full minute or daily recording of pulse before medication and during exercise as appropriate. Identify situations requiring immediate medical intervention, for example, dizziness or irregular heartbeat, fainting, and chest pain.	Continued self-observation or monitoring provides for timely intervention to avoid complications. Medication regimen may be altered or further evaluation may be required when heart rate varies from desired rate or pacemaker's preset rate.
Review safety precautions, techniques to evaluate and maintain pacemaker or ICD function, and symptoms requiring medical intervention; for example, report pulse rate below set limit for demand pacing or less than low-limit rate for rate-adaptive pacers and prolonged hiccups.	Promotes self-care, provides for timely interventions to prevent serious complications. Instructions or concerns depend on function and type of device as well as client's condition and presence or absence of family or caregivers.
Recommend wearing medical alert bracelet or necklace and carrying pacemaker ID card.	Allows for appropriate evaluation and timely intervention, especially if client is unable to respond in an emergency situation.
Discuss monitoring and environmental safety concerns in presence of pacemaker or ICD; for example, microwave ovens and other electrical appliances (including electric blankets, razors, radio/TV) can be safely operated if they are properly grounded and in good repair. There is no problem with metal detectors, although pacemaker may trigger sensitive detectors. Cordless phones are safe, although cellular phones held directly over pacemaker may cause interference; it is recommended that client not carry phone in shirt pocket when phone is on. High-voltage areas, magnetic fields, and radiation can interfere with optimal pacemaker function, so client should avoid high-tension electric wires, arc welding, and large industrial magnets, such as demolition sites and magnetic resonance imaging (MRI).	Aids in clarifying misconceptions and fears and encourages client to be proactive in avoiding potentially harmful situations.

POTENTIAL CONSIDERATIONS following discharge from care setting (dependent on client's age, physical condition and presence of complications, personal resources, and life responsibilities)

- ***Activity Intolerance***—imbalance between oxygen supply and demand
- ***ineffective Self-Health Management***—complexity of therapeutic regimen, decisional conflicts, economic difficulties, inadequate number of cues to action

CARDIAC SURGERY: POSTOPERATIVE CARE—CORONARY ARTERY BYPASS GRAFT (CABG), MINIMALLY INVASIVE DIRECT CORONARY ARTERY BYPASS (MIDCAB), CARDIOMYOPLASTY, VALVE REPLACEMENT

I. Purpose: to maximize cardiac output by improving blood flow and myocardial muscle function

II. Types

- a. Reparative: closure of atrial or ventricular septal defect or repair of stenotic mitral valve; reparative surgeries more likely to produce cure or prolonged improvement
- b. Reconstructive: coronary artery bypass grafting (CABG), restructure of incompetent valve leaflets
- c. Substitutional: valve replacement, cardiac transplant

III. Procedures

- a. Procedures requiring use of cardiopulmonary bypass (CPB)
  - i. CABG has an average patency rate of 20 years and decreased overall mortality from coronary heart disease, relief from angina, improved functional status, and may improve quality of life due to decreased need for pharmacological therapy and a reduction in frequency of interventional procedures (Kark, 2008).
  - ii. Open-heart valve repair or replacement using natural (biological) or artificial (mechanical) valves are the most common minimally invasive heart surgery procedures (Cleveland Clinic, 2007).
  - iii. Port-access coronary artery bypass (PACAB) is a minimally invasive option in certain conditions, such as single bypass from left mammary artery to left anterior descending coronary artery.
- b. Procedures not requiring use of CPB (heart-lung) machine
  - i. Off-pump coronary artery bypass (OPCAB) or beating heart bypass surgery may be an option for client with single-vessel disease, such as the left anterior descending artery or right coronary artery.
  - ii. Minimally invasive direct coronary bypass (MIDCAB)
  - iii. Robotic-assisted coronary artery bypass (RACAB), also called closed-chest heart surgery
  - iv. Totally endoscopic coronary artery bypass (TECAB) using a port access, which may be video and robotic assisted—primarily carried out in large heart centers where specialized equipment and training are available
  - v. Percutaneous mitral, aortic, and pulmonic valvotomy for stenosis; transapical aortic valve implant
  - vi. Transmyocardial laser revascularization (TMR) uses lasers to create channels in heart muscle to improve direct blood flow.
  - vii. Endoscopic pulmonary vein isolation for the treatment of atrial fibrillation, thoracic endografting for the treatment of aortic neurismal disease

IV. Statistics

- a. 397,000 CABG procedures and 106,000 valve replacements were performed in the United States in 2010 (Go et al, 2012).
- b. One-year mortality is similar between CABG and percutaneous coronary interventions (PCI), but five-year survival is significantly better for CABG (Go et al, 2012).
- c. Cost: Annual cost for CABG procedures estimated at $50 billion (Ballard, 2010).

GLOSSARY

Anastomosis: Surgical connection created between tubular structures, such as blood vessels, that are grafted into the coronary arteries to create a bypass channel for circulation around a blocked artery.

Cardiopulmonary bypass (CPB) (also called heart-lung machine): Mechanical means of circulating and oxygenating the blood through the body when it's diverted from the heart and lungs. The heart's beating is stopped so the surgeon can perform the bypass procedure on a still heart.

Coronary artery bypass grafting (CABG): Procedure in which one or more blocked coronary arteries are bypassed by a blood vessel graft to restore normal blood flow to the heart. These grafts usually come from the client's own arteries and veins located in the leg (saphenous vein), internal mammary artery (IMA), or internal thoracic artery (ITA). The graft goes around the blocked artery (or arteries) to create new pathways for oxygen-rich blood to flow to the heart (Cleveland Clinic, 2013).

Minimally invasive direct coronary bypass (MIDCAB): Requires a smaller incision and may be done for CABG and some valve remodeling and replacement procedures.

Off-pump coronary artery bypass (OPCAB) (also called off-pump coronary revascularization): Similar to the conventional CABG procedure. OPCAB still uses a medial sternotomy; however, CPB pump is no longer employed. Off-pump procedures can offer certain advantages in

GLOSSARY (continued)

low-risk populations, such as decreased cost, reduced length of stay, reduced postoperative complications, and avoidance of blood transfusions. They also reduce surgical trauma to the client as well as risk of stroke and kidney failure.

Percutaneous transmyocardial revascularization (PTMR) (also called transmyocardial laser revascularization, or TMR): Laser surgery that opens tiny new pathways within the heart muscle to treat the symptoms of angina in a client who cannot withstand more conventional treatments such as bypass surgery or balloon angioplasty.

Robotic-assisted coronary artery bypass (RACAB): Surgeon views the procedure on a video screen, uses a robot to perform the bypass, and has no direct contact with the client.

Sternotomy: Surgical incision made in the breastbone (mediastinum).

Totally endoscopic coronary artery bypass (TECAB): Robotic-assisted procedure in which small-port incisions are made in intercostal spaces. TECAB is performed on the beating heart using a stabilization device that holds the anastomosis site steady and removes the need for CPB.

Care Setting

Client is cared for at inpatient acute hospital on a surgical or post-intensive care unit (ICU) step-down unit.

Related Concerns

Angina, page 67
Heart failure: chronic, page 43
Dysrhythmias, page 87
Myocardial infarction, page 75
Pneumothorax/hemothorax, page 150
Psychosocial aspects of care, page 729
Surgical intervention, page 762
Transplantation considerations—postoperative and lifelong, page 719

Client Assessment Database

The preoperative data presented here depend on the specific disease process and underlying cardiac condition and reserve.

DIAGNOSTIC DIVISION MAY REPORT	MAY EXHIBIT
ACTIVITY/REST	
• Exercise intolerance • Generalized weakness, fatigue • Inability to perform expected or usual life activities • Insomnia and sleep disturbances	• Abnormal heart rate, blood pressure (BP) changes with activity • Exertional dyspnea • Electrocardiogram (ECG) changes and dysrhythmias with activity
CIRCULATION	
• History of recent or acute MI (three or more), vessel coronary artery disease, valvular heart disease, hypertension • History of inherited clotting disorders, such as hemophilia, and acquired clotting disorders, such as acute lymphocytic leukemia or lupus (which can affect postoperative bleeding) • History of abnormal bleeding with previous surgeries, dental procedures, or childbirth • Current use of antithrombotic drugs, including those that inhibit the production of clotting factors in the liver, such as warfarin (Coumadin); those that interfere with blood clotting by blocking thrombin activity, such as heparin and lepirudin (Refludan); and antiplatelet drugs, such as aspirin, clopidogrel (Plavix), tirofiban (Aggrastat), and eptifibatide (Integrilin), which keep platelets from aggregating into clots. *Note:* Cardiac patients taking these drugs preoperatively require various interventions to ensure their safety for CPB and to reduce postoperative bleeding complications • Recent use of over-the-counter (OTC) drugs, such as ibuprofen, and dietary supplements, such as vitamin E, garlic, ginseng, and ginkgo (can inhibit clotting)	• Variations in BP, heart rate and rhythm • Abnormal heart sounds: S_3/S_4, murmurs • Pallor and cyanosis of skin or mucous membranes • Cool and clammy skin • Edema, jugular vein distention (JVD) • Diminished peripheral pulses • Abnormal breath sounds, such as crackles • Restlessness and other changes in mentation or sensorium (severe cardiac decompensation)

(continues on page 100)

DIAGNOSTIC DIVISION MAY REPORT (continued)	MAY EXHIBIT (continued)
EGO INTEGRITY	
• Feeling frightened, apprehensive, or helpless • Distress over current events • Fear of death or eventual outcome of surgery or possible complications • Fear about changes in lifestyle and role functioning	• Apprehension, restlessness • Facial or general tension • Withdrawal and lack of eye contact • Focus on self, hostility, anger, crying
FOOD/FLUID	
• Change in weight • Loss of appetite • Nausea or vomiting • Change in urine frequency or amount	• Weight gain or loss • Dry skin, poor skin turgor • Postural hypotension • Edema—generalized, dependent, pitting
NEUROSENSORY	
• Fainting spells, vertigo	• Changes in orientation or usual response to stimuli • Restlessness, irritability, apathy
PAIN/DISCOMFORT	
• Chest pain, angina	
RESPIRATION	
• Shortness of breath	• Dyspnea • Abnormal breath sounds, such as crackles • Productive cough
SAFETY	
• Infectious episode with valvular involvement or myopathy	
TEACHING/LEARNING	
• Familial risk factors of diabetes, heart disease, hypertension, strokes • Use of various cardiovascular drugs • Failure to improve	
POSTOPERATIVE ASSESSMENT	
Pain/Discomfort	
• Incisional discomfort • Pain or paresthesia of shoulders, arms, hands, legs	• Guarding of incisional areas • Facial mask of pain, grimacing • Distraction behaviors, moaning, restlessness • Changes in BP, pulse, respiratory rate
• ***Respiration:*** Inability to cough or take a deep breath	• Decreased chest expansion • Splinting or muscle guarding • Dyspnea—normal response to thoracotomy • Areas of diminished or absent breath sounds (atelectasis) • Changes in arterial blood gas (ABG) levels or pulse oximetry
• ***Safety:*** Oozing or bleeding from chest or donor site incisions	
TEACHING/LEARNING	
• Modifiable risk factors for sternal wound infection, such as obesity, diabetes, and smoking • Postoperative incision care to minimize or prevent infection	

DIAGNOSTIC DIVISION MAY REPORT (continued)	MAY EXHIBIT (continued)
DISCHARGE PLAN CONSIDERATIONS • Short-term assistance with food preparation, shopping, transportation, self-care needs, and homemaker and home maintenance tasks ➧ Refer to section at end of plan for postdischarge considerations.	

Diagnostic Studies (Postoperative)

TEST WHY IT IS DONE	WHAT IT TELLS ME
BLOOD TESTS	
• ***Hemoglobin (Hgb) and hematocrit (Hct):*** To identify red blood cell (RBC) and fluid replacement needs.	Whether heart surgery is performed on or off CPB equipment, clients develop moderate hemodilution from the fluids given perioperatively, thus lowering the Hct and platelet count. A low Hgb reduces oxygen-carrying capacity and indicates need for RBC replacement. Elevation of Hct suggests dehydration and need for fluid replacement.
• ***Coagulation studies:*** Various studies may be done, such as platelet count and bleeding and clotting time.	Platelet function and coagulation factors are altered as a result of CPB and don't normalize for up to 12 hours after surgery. Body temperature is also lowered for open heart surgery, which can depress normal platelet function for a time, even after the client is rewarmed, raising the risk of abnormal bleeding (Sorensen et al, 2006).
• ***Electrolytes:*** A substance that, in solution, conducts an electric current and is decomposed by its passage. Sodium (Na), potassium (K^+), and calcium (Ca) are common electrolytes.	Imbalances—hyperkalemia or hypokalemia, hypernatremia or hyponatremia, and hypocalcemia—can affect cardiac function and fluid balance.
• ***Arterial blood gases (ABGs):*** Assessment of levels of oxygen (PaO_2) and carbon dioxide ($PaCO_2$)	Verifies oxygenation status, effectiveness of respiratory function, and acid-base balance.
• ***Blood urea nitrogen (BUN) and creatinine (Cr):*** Elevated BUN can occur with dehydration, shock due to blood loss, or any condition that decreases blood flow to the kidneys.	Provides good evidence of the filtering function of the kidneys and a measure of the degree of systemic hydration.
• ***Glucose:*** Blood glucose levels should be controlled in all patients with diabetes to avoid hyperglycemia perioperatively.	Fluctuations may occur because of preoperative nutritional status, presence of organ dysfunction, and impact of IV infusions.
• ***Cardiac enzyme and isoenzymes Troponin 1 (cTnl) and Troponin T (cTnT):*** Contractile proteins found in the myocardium with nearly absolute myocardial tissue specificity, as well as high sensitivity. Troponins increase within 3 to 4 hours of myocardial injury.	Elevated in the presence of acute, recent, or perioperative myocardial infarction (MI).
OTHER DIAGNOSTIC STUDIES	
• ***Chest x-ray:*** Evaluates organs and structures within the chest.	Reveals heart size and position, pulmonary vasculature, and changes indicative of pulmonary complications, such as atelectasis or pulmonary edema. Verifies condition of valve prosthesis and sternal wires, position of pacing leads, intravascular or cardiac lines.
• ***Electrocardiogram (ECG):*** Record of the electrical activity of the heart.	Identifies changes in electrical and mechanical function such as might occur in immediate postoperative phase, acute or perioperative MI, valve dysfunction, and pericarditis.

Nursing Priorities

1. Support hemodynamic stability and ventilatory function.
2. Promote relief of pain and discomfort.
3. Promote healing.
4. Provide information about postoperative expectations and treatment regimen.

Discharge Goals

1. Activity tolerance adequate to meet self-care needs.
2. Pain alleviated or managed.
3. Complications prevented or minimized.
4. Incisions healing.
5. Postdischarge medications, exercise, diet, and therapy understood.
6. Plan in place to meet needs after discharge.

NURSING DIAGNOSIS: risk for decreased Cardiac Output

Risk Factors May Include

Altered contractility recent
Altered preload—hypovolemia; altered afterload—systemic vascular resistance
Altered heart rate/rhythm

Possibly Evidenced By

(Not applicable; presence of signs and symptoms establishes an *actual* diagnosis)

Desired Outcomes/Evaluation Criteria—Client Will

Tissue Perfusion: Cardiac (NOC)

Display hemodynamic stability, such as stable blood pressure, cardiac output.
Report and display decreased episodes of angina and dysrhythmias.
Demonstrate an increase in activity tolerance.
Participate in activities that maximize and enhance cardiac function.

ACTIONS/INTERVENTIONS	RATIONALE
Hemodynamic Regulation (NIC)	
Independent	
Monitor and document trends in heart rate and BP, especially noting hypertension. Be aware of specific systolic and diastolic limits defined for client.	Tachycardia is a common response to discomfort, inadequate blood or fluid replacement, and the stress of surgery. However, sustained tachycardia increases cardiac workload and can decrease effective cardiac output. Hypotension may result from fluid deficit, dysrhythmias, heart failure, and shock. Hypertension can occur (fluid excess or preexisting condition), placing stress on suture lines of new grafts and changing blood flow or pressure within heart chambers and across valves, with increased risk for various complications.
Monitor and document cardiac dysrhythmias. Observe client response to dysrhythmias, such as drop in BP, chest pain, and dyspnea.	Hypothermia, inhaled anesthetics, electrolyte and metabolic disturbances, manual manipulation of the heart, and myocardial ischemia may be factors in postoperative dysrhythmias. The incidence of atrial fibrillation ranges from 10% to 65% depending on many factors, including preoperative history and medications and type of surgery performed (Kern, 2004). Decreased cardiac output and hemodynamic compromise that occur with dysrhythmias require prompt intervention.
Observe for bleeding from incisions and chest tube (if in place).	Helps identify bleeding complications that can reduce circulating volume, organ perfusion, and cardiac function.
Observe for changes in usual mental status, orientation, and body movement or reflexes, such as onset of confusion, disorientation, restlessness, reduced response to stimuli, and stupor.	May indicate decreased cerebral blood flow or systemic oxygenation as a result of diminished cardiac output—sustained or severe dysrhythmias, low BP, heart failure, or thromboembolic phenomena, including perioperative stroke.
Record skin temperature and color and quality and equality of peripheral pulses.	Warm, pink skin and strong, equal pulses are general indicators of adequate cardiac output.
Measure and document intake and output (I&O) and calculate fluid balance.	Useful in determining fluid needs or identifying fluid excesses, which can compromise cardiac output and oxygen consumption.
Schedule uninterrupted rest and sleep periods. Assist with self-care activities as needed.	Prevents fatigue or exhaustion and excessive cardiovascular stress.

ACTIONS/INTERVENTIONS (continued)	RATIONALE (continued)
Monitor graded activity program. Note client response; vital signs before, during, and after activity; and development of dysrhythmias.	Regular exercise stimulates circulation and promotes feeling of well-being. Progression of activity depends on cardiac tolerance.
Evaluate presence and degree of anxiety or emotional duress. Encourage the use of relaxation techniques such as deep breathing and diversional activities.	Excessive or escalating emotional reactions can negatively affect vital signs and systemic vascular resistance, eventually affecting cardiac function.
Inspect for JVD, peripheral or dependent edema, congestion in lungs, shortness of breath, and change in mental status.	May be indicative of acute or chronic heart failure.
Investigate reports of angina or severe chest pain accompanied by restlessness, diaphoresis, and ECG changes.	Although not a common complication of CABG, perioperative or postoperative MI can occur.
Investigate and report profound hypotension and unresponsiveness to fluid challenge, tachycardia, distant heart sounds, and stupor or coma.	Development of cardiac tamponade can rapidly progress to cardiac arrest because of the heart's inability to fill adequately for effective cardiac output. *Note:* This is a relatively rare, life-threatening complication that usually occurs in the immediate postoperative period but can occur later in the recovery phase.
Collaborative	
Review serial ECGs.	Most frequently done to follow the progress in normalization of electrical conduction patterns and ventricular function after surgery or to identify complications such as perioperative MI.
Measure cardiac output and other functional parameters, as indicated.	Useful in evaluating response to therapeutic interventions and identifying need for more aggressive or emergency care.
Monitor Hgb, Hct, and coagulation studies, such as activated prothrombin time (aPTT), international normalized ratio (INR), activated clotting time (ACT), and platelet count.	Help to identify bleeding or clotting problems associated with the surgery. *Note:* Diverting the client's blood through the CPB machine activates the clotting cascade and decreases the number (as well as the function) of platelets. Hemodilution occurs when the client's blood mixes with the crystalloid solution used to prime the CPB machine. Because blood is being diluted, the Hct drops, as does the concentration of coagulation factors, fibrinogen, and platelets. In addition, the use of hypothermia during surgery to decrease tissue oxygen requirements slows down the process of clotting and decreases platelet function.
Monitor results of thromboelastography (TEG), as indicated.	TEG is a point-of-care test that can rapidly identify whether the client has a normal hemostasis or is bleeding and whether it is due to surgery, coagulopathy, or residual anticoagulation therapy. Results will identify the specific therapy to treat it, whether client needs fresh frozen plasma (FFP), platelets, antifibrinolytic drugs, or thrombolytic drugs (Lab Tests Online, 2012; Sorensen et al, 2006).
Administer intravenous (IV) fluids or blood products as needed.	Clients who have surgery on CPB equipment are more likely to bleed excessively than those who have off-bypass cardiac surgery. RBC replacement is often indicated to restore and maintain adequate circulating volume and enhance oxygen-carrying capacity. IV fluids may be discontinued before discharge from the ICU or may remain in place for fluid replacement and emergency cardiac medications.
Administer supplemental oxygen as appropriate.	Promotes maximal oxygenation to reduce cardiac workload and aid in resolving myocardial irritability and dysrhythmias.
Administer electrolytes and medications, as indicated, such as potassium, antidysrhythmics, digoxin preparations, diuretics, and anticoagulants.	Client needs are variable, depending on type of surgery, client's response to surgical intervention, and preexisting conditions, such as general health, age, and type of heart disease. Electrolytes, antidysrhythmics, and other heart medications may be required on a short-term or long-term basis to maximize cardiac contractility and output.
Maintain surgically placed pacing wires (atrial or ventricular) and initiate pacing if indicated.	May be required to support cardiac output in presence of conduction disturbances (severe dysrhythmias) that compromise cardiac function.

NURSING DIAGNOSIS: acute Pain

May Be Related To

Injuring physical agents—surgical incisions, tissue inflammation, edema formation, intraoperative nerve trauma

Possibly Evidenced By

Verbal/coded reports of pain
Guarding behavior
Expressive behaviors—restlessness, irritability
Changes in heart rate, blood pressure, respiratory rate

Desired Outcomes/Evaluation Criteria—Client Will

Pain Level (NOC)

Verbalize relief or absence of pain.
Demonstrate relaxed body posture and ability to rest and sleep appropriately.

Pain Control (NOC)

Differentiate surgical discomfort from angina or preoperative heart pain.

ACTIONS/INTERVENTIONS	RATIONALE
Pain Management (NIC) *Independent*	
Note type and location of incision(s).	Newer procedures, such as MIDCAB, require smaller chest and leg incisions, with less significant pain. Many CABG clients do not experience severe discomfort in chest incision and may complain more often of donor site incision discomfort. Severe pain in either area should be investigated further for possible complications.
Encourage client to report type, location, and intensity of pain, rating it on a scale. Note associated symptoms. Ascertain how this compares with preoperative chest pain.	Pain is perceived, manifested, and tolerated individually. It is important for client to differentiate incisional pain from other types of chest pain, such as angina or discomfort from chest tubes.
Observe for anxiety, irritability, crying, restlessness, and sleep disturbances.	These nonverbal cues may indicate the presence or degree of pain being experienced.
Monitor vital signs.	Heart rate usually increases with acute pain, although a bradycardic response can occur in a severely diseased heart. BP may be elevated slightly with incisional discomfort but may be decreased or unstable if chest pain is severe or myocardial damage is occurring.
Identify and promote position of comfort, using adjuncts as necessary.	Pillows or blanket rolls are useful in supporting extremities, maintaining body alignment, and splinting incisions to reduce muscle tension and promote comfort.
Provide comfort measures, such as back rubs and position changes, assist with self-care activities, and encourage diversional activities, as indicated.	May promote relaxation, redirect attention, and reduce analgesic dosage or frequency.
Schedule care activities to balance with adequate periods of sleep and rest.	Rest and sleep are vital for cardiac healing (balance between oxygen demand and consumption) and can enhance coping with stress and discomfort.
Identify and encourage use of behaviors such as guided imagery, distractions, visualizations, and deep breathing.	Relaxation techniques aid in management of stress, promote sense of well-being, may reduce analgesic needs, and promote healing.
Tell client that it is acceptable, even preferable, to request analgesics as soon as discomfort becomes noticeable.	Presence of pain causes muscle tension, which can impair circulation, slow healing process, and intensify pain.
Medicate before procedures and activities, as indicated.	Client participation in respiratory treatments, ambulation, and procedures, such as removal of chest tubes, pacemaker wires, and sutures, are facilitated by maximum analgesic blood level.
Investigate reports of pain in unusual areas, for instance, calf of leg or abdomen—or vague complaints of discomfort, especially when accompanied by changes in mentation, vital signs, and respiratory rate.	May be an early manifestation of developing complication, such as thrombophlebitis, infection, and gastrointestinal dysfunction.
Note reports of pain or numbness in ulnar area (fourth and fifth digits) of the hand, often accompanied by pain and discomfort of the arms and shoulders. Tell client that the problem usually resolves with time.	Indicative of a stretch injury of the brachial plexus as a result of the position of the arms during surgery. No specific treatment is currently useful.

Collaborative

Administer analgesics medications—(e.g., opioids, nonsteroidal anti-inflammatory drugs [NSAIDs]) by appropriate route (e.g., IV, patch, by mouth) as indicated

Provides for control of pain and inflammation and reduces muscle tension, which improves client comfort and promotes healing. *Note:* IV narcotics will be used during the immediate postoperative period, while client is intubated. Oral narcotics will most likely still be required for some time after extubation. Narcotic-induced respiratory depression is a risk during this time, requiring vigilant monitoring of client's respiratory status.

NURSING DIAGNOSIS: risk for ineffective Breathing Pattern

Risk Factors May Include

Pain

Musculoskeletal impairment

Possibly Evidenced By

(Not applicable; presence of signs and symptoms establishes an *actual* diagnosis)

Desired Outcomes/Evaluation Criteria—Client Will

Respiratory Status: Ventilation (NOC)

Maintain an effective respiratory pattern free of cyanosis and other signs and symptoms of hypoxia, with breath sounds equal bilaterally, lung fields clearing.

Display complete reexpansion of lungs with absence of pneumothorax and hemothorax.

ACTIONS/INTERVENTIONS — RATIONALE

Respiratory Monitoring (NIC)

Independent

Evaluate respiratory rate and depth. Note respiratory effort; for example, presence of dyspnea, use of accessory muscles, and nasal flaring.

Client responses are variable. Rate and effort may be increased by pain, fear, fever, diminished circulating volume due to blood or fluid loss, accumulation of secretions, hypoxia, or gastric distention. Respiratory suppression can occur from long time period under anesthesia or heavy use of opioid analgesics. Early recognition and treatment of abnormal ventilation may prevent complications.

Auscultate breath sounds. Note areas of diminished or absent breath sounds and presence of adventitious sounds, such as crackles or rhonchi.

Breath sounds are often diminished in lung bases for a period of time after surgery because of normally occurring atelectasis. Loss of active breath sounds in an area of previous ventilation may reflect collapse of the lung segment, especially if chest tubes have recently been removed. Crackles or rhonchi may be indicative of fluid accumulation due to interstitial edema, pulmonary edema, or infection, or partial airway obstruction with pooling of secretions.

Observe chest excursion. Investigate decreased expansion or lack of symmetry in chest movement.

Air or fluid in the pleural space prevents complete expansion (usually on one side) and requires further assessment of ventilation status.

Observe character of cough and sputum production.

Frequent coughing may simply be throat irritation from operative endotracheal tube (ET) placement or can reflect pulmonary congestion. Purulent sputum suggests onset of pulmonary infection.

Inspect skin and mucous membranes for cyanosis.

Cyanosis of lips, nail beds, or earlobes or general duskiness may indicate a hypoxic condition due to heart failure or pulmonary complications. General pallor, commonly present in immediate postoperative period, may indicate anemia from blood loss or insufficient blood replacement or RBC destruction from CPB pump.

Elevate head of bed, place in upright or semi-Fowler's position. Assist with early ambulation and increased time out of bed.

Enhances respiratory function and lung expansion. Effective in preventing and resolving pulmonary congestion.

Encourage client participation in and responsibility for deep-breathing exercises, use of adjuncts (e.g., incentive spirometer), and coughing, as indicated.

Aids in lung reexpansion and maintaining patency of small airways, especially after removal of chest tubes. Coughing is not necessary unless wheezes and rhonchi are present, indicating retention of secretions.

(continues on page 106)

ACTIONS/INTERVENTIONS (continued)	RATIONALE (continued)
Demonstrate and reinforce splinting chest with pillows during deep breathing or coughing.	Reduces incisional tension, promotes maximal lung expansion, and may enhance effectiveness of cough effort.
Explain that coughing and respiratory treatments will not loosen or damage grafts or reopen chest incision.	Provides reassurance that injury will not occur and may enhance cooperation with therapeutic regimen.
Encourage maximal fluid intake within cardiac reserves.	Adequate hydration helps liquefy secretions, facilitating expectoration.
Medicate with analgesic before respiratory treatments, as indicated.	Allows for easier chest movement and reduces discomfort related to incisional pain, facilitating client cooperation with and effectiveness of respiratory treatments.
Record response to deep-breathing exercises or other respiratory treatment, noting breath sounds before and after treatment, as well as cough and sputum production.	Documents effectiveness of therapy or need for more aggressive interventions.
Investigate and report respiratory distress, diminished or absent breath sounds, tachycardia, severe agitation, and drop in BP.	Although not a common complication, hemothorax or pneumothorax may occur following removal of chest tubes and requires prompt intervention.
Collaborative	
Review chest x-ray reports and laboratory studies (such as ABGs, Hgb), as indicated.	Monitors effectiveness of respiratory therapy and documents developing complications. A blood transfusion may be needed if blood loss is the reason for respiratory hypoxemia.
Instruct in and assist with use of incentive spirometer.	Maximizes lung inflation, reduces atelectasis, and prevents pulmonary complications.
Administer supplemental oxygen by cannula or mask, as indicated.	Enhances oxygen delivery to the lungs for circulatory uptake, especially in presence of reduced and altered ventilation.
Assist with reinsertion of chest tubes or thoracentesis if indicated.	Reexpands lung by removal of accumulated blood and air and restoration of negative pleural pressure.

NURSING DIAGNOSIS: impaired Skin/Tissue Integrity

May Be Related To

Mechanical factors (e.g., surgery)

Possibly Evidenced By

Disruption of skin surface/damaged tissue [surgical incisions, puncture wounds]

Desired Outcomes/Evaluation Criteria—Client Will

Wound Healing: Primary Intention (NOC)

Demonstrate behaviors and techniques to promote healing and prevent complications.

Display timely wound healing.

ACTIONS/INTERVENTIONS	RATIONALE
Incision Site Care (NIC)	
Independent	
Inspect all incisions. Evaluate healing progress. Review expectations for healing with client.	Healing begins immediately, but complete healing takes time. Chest incision heals first (minimal muscle tissue), but donor site incision requires more time (more muscle tissue, longer incision, slower circulation). As healing progresses, the incision lines may appear dry, with crusty scabs. Underlying tissue may look bruised and feel tense, warm, and lumpy, suggesting resolving hematoma.
Suggest wearing soft cotton shirts and loose-fitting clothing, leaving incisions open to air as much as possible, covering and padding portion of incisions as necessary.	Reduces suture line irritation and pressure from clothing. Leaving incisions open to air promotes healing process and may reduce risk of infection.
Have client shower in warm water, washing incisions gently. Instruct client to avoid tub baths until approved by physician.	Keeps incision clean and promotes circulation and healing. *Note:* Climbing out of tub requires use of arms and pectoral muscles, which can put undue stress on sternotomy.
Encourage ankle exercises and elevation of legs when sitting in chair.	Promotes circulation and reduces edema to improve tissue healing.
Review normal signs of healing, such as itching along wound line, bruising, slight redness, and scabbing.	Helps client understand expected progression of healing and recognize signs of complications or nonhealing requiring further evaluation and intervention.
Instruct to watch for and report to physician places in incision that do not heal; reopening of healed incision; bloody or	Incisional problems rank second behind chest pain as cause of readmission after CABG. The incidence of deep sternal

ACTIONS/INTERVENTIONS (continued)	RATIONALE (continued)
purulent drainage; localized area that is swollen with redness, feels increasingly painful, and is hot to touch; and temperature greater than 101.5(F (38.6°C) for longer than 24 hours.	wound infection (mediastinitis) following coronary artery bypass graft surgery has decreased from 1.57% to 0.88% in last 5 years (Matros, 2010); however, this devastating complication occurs more in clients with comorbidities (e.g., diabetes, obesity, and advanced age) and can result in higher mortality rates and significant financial and care burden.
Promote adequate nutritional and fluid intake.	Helps maintain good circulating volume for tissue perfusion and meets cellular energy requirements to facilitate tissue regeneration and healing process.
Collaborative	
Obtain specimen of wound drainage, as indicated. Administer antimicrobials and local treatments, as indicated.	If infection occurs, local and systemic treatments may be required.

NURSING DIAGNOSIS: deficient Knowledge [Learning Need] regarding condition, postoperative care, self-care, and discharge needs

May Be Related To

Lack of exposure or recall

Information misinterpretation

Possibly Evidenced By

Reports the problem

Inaccurate follow-through of instructions

Desired Outcomes/Evaluation Criteria—Client Will

Self-Management: Cardiac Disease (NOC)

Participate in learning process.

Assume responsibility for own learning.

Begin to ask questions and look for information.

Knowledge: Treatment Regimen (NOC)

Verbalize understanding of condition, prognosis, and potential complications.

Describe reasons for therapeutic actions.

ACTIONS/INTERVENTIONS	RATIONALE
Teaching: Disease Process (NIC)	
Independent	
Reinforce surgeon's explanation of particular surgical procedure, providing diagram as appropriate.	Provides individually specific information, creating knowledge base for subsequent learning regarding home management. Length of rehabilitation and prognosis are dependent on type of surgical procedure, preoperative physical condition, and duration and severity of any complications.
Discuss importance of changes in memory or mentation and plans for follow-up with appropriate healthcare providers if client has long-term mental status changes.	Mental status changes after heart surgery have long been reported, including confusion, delirium, seizures, coma, prolonged alteration in mental status, combativeness, and agitation. Many of these changes are transient, occurring in the immediate postoperative period, and client's recovery is complete. Some clients may have slower recovery time or have new onset and/or worsening mental status. It is believed that some changes can be associated with preexisting cerebrovascular disease and other comorbidities. However, other factors may be involved, including length of time on cardiopulmonary bypass (CPB). Cerebral dysfunction associated with CPB may present from 1 to several days after the procedure, thus affecting length of stay and mortality rates (McKhann et al, 2006).
Cardiac Care: Rehabilitation (NIC)	
Reinforce continuation of breathing exercises, incentive spirometry, and coughing with splinting incision.	Promotes alveolar ventilation, reducing risk of lung congestion.
Discuss routine and prophylactic medications and OTC drug use. Stress importance of checking with physician before	Depending on type of valve replacement (i.e., synthetic), lifelong anticoagulant therapy may be indicated. Potential for

(continues on page 108)

ACTIONS/INTERVENTIONS (continued)	RATIONALE (continued)
taking any drugs. Reinforce need for routine laboratory tests, outpatient education, and community resources when client with valve replacement will be taking warfarin (Coumadin).	drug interactions must be considered before adding therapeutic agents to regimen. *Note:* Using herbal products, such as ginkgo, garlic, and vitamins, can alter coagulation and have an adverse effect when taken with anticoagulants.
Review prescribed cardiac rehabilitation or exercise program and progress to date. Assist client and significant other (SO) to set realistic goals.	Individual capabilities and expectations depend on type of surgery, underlying cardiac function, and prior physical conditioning. *Note:* Obesity is a predictor of hospital readmission and may require additional interventions.
Encourage participation in home routines, such as self-care and cooking. Suggest alternating rest periods with activity and light tasks with heavy tasks. Avoid heavy lifting and isometric and strenuous upper-body exercise.	Prevents excessive fatigue and exhaustion. Scheduling rest periods and short naps several times a day enhances coping abilities, reduces nervousness (common in this phase), and promotes healing. *Note:* Strenuous use of arms can place undue stress on sternotomy.
Problem-solve with client and SO ways to continue progressive activity program during temperature extremes and high wind or pollution days, such as walking predetermined distance within own house, in local indoor shopping mall, or on exercise track.	Having a plan forestalls giving up exercise because of interferences such as weather.
Reinforce physician's time limitations about lifting, driving, returning to work, resuming sexual activity, and exercising that involves upper extremities.	These restrictions are present until after the first postoperative office visit for assessment of sternum healing.
Assist client and SO to develop strategies for dealing with changes during recovery period, such as shifting responsibilities to other family members, friends, or neighbors; acquiring temporary assistance for housekeeping; and investigating avenues for financial assistance.	Planning for changes that may occur or be required promotes sense of control and accomplishment without loss of self-esteem.
Discuss issues concerning resumption of sexual activity, such as comparison of stress of sexual intercourse with other activities:	Concerns about sexual activity often go unexpressed, but clients usually desire information about what to expect. In general, client can safely engage in sex when activity level has advanced to point at which client can climb two flights of stairs, which is about the same amount of energy expenditure.
Position recommendations	Client should avoid positions that restrict breathing (sexual activity increases oxygen demand and consumption). Client with sternotomy should not support self or partner with arms (breast bone healing, support muscles stretched).
Expectations of sexual performance	Impotence appears to occur with some regularity in postoperative cardiac surgery clients. Although etiology is unknown, condition usually resolves in time without specific intervention. If situation persists, it may require further evaluation.
Appropriate timing; for example, avoid sexual intercourse following heavy meal, during periods of emotional distress, when client is fatigued or exhausted.	Timing of activity may reduce occurrence of complications or angina.
Pharmacological considerations.	Some clients may benefit from prophylactic use of anti-anginal medications for sexual activity.
Identify services and resources available after discharge. Provide telephone contact number or schedule follow-up calls as appropriate. Include referral names for home-care services, as indicated.	Facilitates transition to home and provides for ongoing monitoring, continuation of prescribed therapies, and opportunity to discuss concerns and alleviate anxiety.

POTENTIAL CONSIDERATIONS following discharge from care setting (dependent on client's age, physical condition and presence of complications, personal resources, and life responsibilities)

- ***Activity Intolerance***—generalized weakness, sedentary lifestyle
- ***impaired Skin/Tissue Integrity***—mechanical factors (surgical incisions, puncture wounds)
- ***impaired Home Maintenance***—illness, impaired functioning, inadequate support systems, unfamiliarity with neighborhood resources
- ***risk for Infection***—broken skin, traumatized tissue, invasive procedures, decreased hemoglobin
- ***Self-Care deficit***—discomfort, weakness, fatigue
- ***risk for ineffective Role Performance***—physical illness, body image alteration, fatigue, pain

THROMBOPHLEBITIS: VENOUS THROMBOEMBOLISM (INCLUDING PULMONARY EMBOLI CONSIDERATIONS)

I. Pathophysiology: Related to three factors known as the Virchow triad—stasis of blood flow, vessel wall injury, and alterations in the clotting mechanism.

a. Mechanical (e.g., trauma, surgery) or physiological (e.g., hypertension, phlebitis) damage to the vessel wall leads to platelet activation, with platelets adhering to one another and clumping together, forming a thrombus.

b. The thrombus either dissolves over time or grows and becomes large enough to occlude a vessel, which causes blood flow to slow, expands the veins to accommodate the increased volume, and causes more clots to form.

c. Proximal venous thromboembolism (VTE) extending to the popliteal, femoral, or iliofemoral vessels—more likely to break away from the vessel and cause pulmonary embolism (PE).

d. Approximately 50% of clients with VTE are asymptomatic.

II. Etiology

a. Thromboembolism can affect superficial or deep veins although VTE is more serious in terms of potential complications, including PE, postphlebotic syndrome, chronic venous insufficiency, and vein valve destruction.

b. Predisposing and risk factors:

i. Major surgery, especially orthopedic; trauma; prolonged immobilization for any cause; spinal cord injury; extended travel

ii. Cardiovascular conditions such as valvular heart disease with dysrhythmias, myocardial infarction (MI), heart failure, stroke

iii. Cancer; central venous catheter use

iv. Obesity; age greater than 40

v. Pregnancy-related complications

vi. Intravenous (IV) drug users, hormone replacement therapy, oral estrogen birth control pills

III. Statistics

a. Morbidity: Approximately 250,000 incidents of VTE occur annually in the United States (Go et al, 2012).

b. Mortality: Thirty-day VTE survival is 75% (DVT, 96%; PE with or without DVT, 59%) (Go et al, 2012).

c. Cost: Estimates vary; Jaffer (2008) suggests $1.5 billion annually for VTE/PE.

GLOSSARY

Coagulation: Complex process or cascade of events involving more than 30 types of cells and substances by which blood cells clump together to form a clot via one of two pathways: extrinsic (blood is exposed to a subendothelial tissue factor) or intrinsic (triggered when the blood is exposed to a foreign substance). Disorders of coagulation can lead to an increased risk of bleeding and clotting or thrombus formation.

Embolus: Something that travels through the bloodstream, lodges in a blood vessel, and blocks it. Examples of emboli are a detached blood clot, a clump of bacteria, and foreign material such as air.

Homans' sign: Deep calf pain in affected leg upon dorsiflexion of foot, which is present in approximately 50% of cases of DVT.

Post-thrombotic syndrome: Occurs when blood can no longer circulate properly because venous circulation is impaired from veins and valves that have been damaged by thrombosis. It can mimic recurrent DVT.

Pulmonary embolism (PE): A thrombus that dislodges from a vessel wall and travels through the right side of the heart into the pulmonary artery, thereby obstructing blood flow.

Recurrent VTE: Occurs within a year after the initial event. Because of persistent abnormalities in affected vasculature after the initial VTE, it can be difficult to clinically differentiate an acute event from an ipsilateral limb recurrence. Diagnosis requires evidence of new clot formation.

Thrombophlebitis: Inflammation of a vein that occurs when a blood clot develops in the vein.

Venous thromboembolism (VTE): A blood clot (thrombus) in a deep vein in the thigh or leg. The clot can break off as an embolus and make its way to the lung, where it can cause respiratory distress and respiratory failure.

Care Settings

Primarily treated at the community level, with short inpatient stay generally indicated in the presence of embolization.

Related Concerns

Cancer, page 827
Fractures, page 601
Spinal cord injury, page 248
Surgical intervention, page 762
Ventilatory assistance (mechanical), page 157

Client Assessment Database

DIAGNOSTIC DIVISION MAY REPORT	MAY EXHIBIT
ACTIVITY/REST	
• Occupation that requires sitting or standing for long periods of time • Prolonged immobility • Leg pain with activity • Fatigue, general malaise • Weakness of affected extremity	• Generalized or extremity weakness
CIRCULATION	
• History of previous peripheral vascular disease, venous thrombosis, varicose veins • Presence of other predisposing factors, such as pregnancy-induced hypertension, diabetes mellitus, MI or valvular heart disease, thrombotic stroke, or blood dyscrasias	• Tachycardia • Peripheral pulse may be diminished in the affected extremity • Varicosities • Hardened, bumpy, or knotty vein • Skin color and temperature in affected extremity pale, cool, edematous (deep vein), pinkish red, warm along the superficial vein • Edema of affected extremity, ankle engorgement • Differences in leg circumferences: (Affected leg may be larger than the unaffected leg, when measured 10 cm [4 inches] below the kneecap [tibial tuberosity])
FOOD/FLUID	
	• Poor skin turgor, dry mucous membranes (dehydration predisposes to hypercoagulability) • Obesity (predisposes to stasis and pelvic vein pressure) Pitting edema may be present on affected leg
PAIN/DISCOMFORT	
• Throbbing, tenderness, aching pain aggravated by standing or movement of affected extremity • Groin tenderness	• Guarding of affected extremity
SAFETY	
• History of direct or indirect injury to extremity or vein, such as major trauma or fractures, orthopedic or pelvic surgery, surgical procedures longer than 2 hours, urologic surgery, pregnancy, prolonged labor with fetal head pressure on pelvic veins, heart failure, venous cannulation or catheterization or IV therapy • Presence of malignancy, particularly neoplasms of the pancreas, lung, gastrointestinal system, prostate • Sepsis	• Fever, chills
TEACHING/LEARNING	
• Use of oral contraceptives and estrogens; recent anticoagulant therapy predisposes to hypercoagulability • Use of vitamins and herbal supplements, such as vitamin B_6, vitamin E, niacin, magnesium, L-carnitine, and bromelain, for heart or blood pressure health • Recurrence and lack of resolution of previous thrombophlebotic episode	
DISCHARGE PLAN CONSIDERATIONS	
• Temporary assistance with shopping, transportation, and homemaker and maintenance tasks • Properly fitted antiembolic hose ➧ Refer to section at end of plan for postdischarge considerations.	

Diagnostic Studies

TEST WHY IT IS DONE	WHAT IT TELLS ME
BLOOD TESTS	
• *Complete blood count (CBC):* Battery of screening tests, which typically includes hemoglobin (Hgb), hematocrit (Hct), red blood cell (RBC) count, morphology, indices, and distribution width index; platelet count and size; and white blood cell (WBC) count and differential.	Hemoconcentration (elevated Hct) potentiates risk of thrombus formation.
• *Coagulation profile:* Tests that measure the speed of blood coagulation at different steps of the coagulation pathway. There are many types of coagulation tests. Some are general and tell only whether a person's blood is clotting normally. Other tests can identify which element within the blood is causing abnormal clotting.	Identifies clotting problems that may increase one's risk of VTE. For example, antithrombin is useful in determining cause of hypercoagulation; inherited biochemical conditions; and deficits in certain other coagulation modulators, such as antithrombin iii, protein s, or protein c, that can predispose client to thrombus formation.
• *D-dimer assay:* Measures fibrin degradation fragments generated by fibrinolysis.	An elevated D-dimer level indicates a thrombotic process but is not specific to DVT. This test is useful as an adjunct to noninvasive testing (Stockman, 2008).
OTHER DIAGNOSTIC STUDIES	
• *Noninvasive flow studies (Doppler ultrasound; compression ultrasongraphy duplex venous ultrasound):* Detect and measure blood flow.	Ultrasound imagery can reveal a thrombus in a deep vein, especially above the knee. The Doppler ultrasound measures the blood flow velocity in veins and can detect flow abnormalities (Stockman, 2008). *Note:* In most circumstances, compression ultrasonography is the test of choice for patients with suspected DVT. When a blood clot is present in a vein, it is relatively difficult to collapse, making compression ultrasound a reliable indicator of DVT, especially in veins of the groin and thigh (Pai, 2013; Fogoros, 2012). Duplex venous ultrasonography appears to be the most accurate noninvasive method for diagnosing multiple proximal VTE in iliac, femoral, and popliteal veins but is less reliable in detecting isolated calf vein thrombi.
• *Impedance plethysmography (IPG):* Noninvasive test that uses a blood pressure cuff and electrodes to assess blood flow and volume of body fluid based on the idea that changes in volume cause electrical resistance.	Abnormal readings coupled with a high clinical suspicion of VTE are sufficient for diagnosis of VTE. *Note:* Abnormal findings include a fully occluded vessel, although IPG does not detect most calf vein thrombi and may not detect partially occlusive thrombi (Crowther & McCourt, 2005).
• *Contrast venography:* A special x-ray of the veins that is performed by first injecting a radiopaque contrast into the vein in question and then taking a conventional x-ray.	Used to demonstrate a vein blockage. Radiographically confirms diagnosis through changes in blood flow and size of channels. *Note:* Although considered the diagnostic gold standard, this study carries a risk of inducing VTE and therefore is reserved for the client with negative or difficult to interpret noninvasive studies.
• *Magnetic resonance imaging (MRI):* Technique that uses the properties of magnetic fields to provide images of the body.	May be done for diagnosis of both proximal and distal VTE and is believed to be superior to other diagnostic tests for detection of pelvic VTE or suspected VTE of the inferior vena cava or pelvic veins (Stockman, 2008).
• *Additional tests might be done if PE is supected:* Could include chest x-ray, ABGs, lung scan.	Diagnostic testing for PE is aimed at confirming the condition, defining the severity of the problem, and ruling out conditions that may mimic PE, such as pneumonia, myocardial infarction, or pneumothorax.

Nursing Priorities

1. Maintain or enhance tissue perfusion and facilitate resolution of thrombus.
2. Promote optimal comfort.
3. Prevent complications.
4. Provide information about disease process, prognosis, and treatment regimen.

Discharge Goals

1. Tissue perfusion improved in affected limb.
2. Pain or discomfort relieved.
3. Complications prevented or resolved.
4. Disease process, prognosis, and therapeutic needs understood.
5. Plan in place to meet needs after discharge.

NURSING DIAGNOSIS: ineffective peripheral tissue Perfusion

May Be Related To

Deficient knowledge of aggravating factors—sedentary lifestyle/immobility, trauma, smoking, obesity

Possibly Evidenced By

Edema, extremity pain

Diminished pulses, capillary refill >3 seconds

Altered skin characteristics—color, temperature

Desired Outcomes/Evaluation Criteria—Client Will

Tissue Perfusion: Peripheral (NOC)

Demonstrate improved perfusion as evidenced by peripheral pulses present, equal skin color, and temperature normal and absence of edema.

Engage in behaviors or actions to enhance tissue perfusion.

Display increasing tolerance to activity.

ACTIONS/INTERVENTIONS	RATIONALE
Embolus Care: Peripheral (NIC)	
Independent	
Evaluate circulatory and neurological studies of involved extremity, both sensory and motor. Inspect legs from groin to foot for skin color and temperature changes as well as edema. Note symmetry of calves; measure and record calf circumference. Report proximal progression of inflammatory process and traveling pain.	Symptoms help distinguish between thrombophlebitis and VTE. Redness, heat, tenderness, and localized edema are characteristic of superficial involvement. *Note:* Unilateral edema is one of the most reliable physical findings in VTE. Calf vein involvement is associated with absence of edema; femoral vein involvement is associated with mild to moderate edema; and iliofemoral vein thrombosis is characterized by severe edema.
Examine extremity for obviously prominent veins. Palpate gently for local tissue tension, stretched skin, and knots or bumps along course of vein.	Distention of superficial veins can occur in VTE because of backflow through communicating veins. Thrombophlebitis in superficial veins may be visible or palpable.
Assess capillary refill.	Diminished capillary refill usually present in VTE.
Evaluate client for Homans' sign (pain in the calf of the leg upon dorsiflexion of the foot with the leg extended) per protocol.	Homans' sign is easily applied at point-of-care and is an assessment that clinicians often perform. However, its use is considered unreliable because Homans' is absent in many clients with VTE and can be positive in several other conditions besides DVT. A negative Homans' sign, on the other hand, doesn't automatically exclude DVT (Rasavong, 2009).
Promote early ambulation.	Short, frequent walks are better for extremities and prevention of pulmonary complications than one long walk. If client is confined to bed, ensure range-of-motion exercises.
Elevate legs when in bed or chair, as indicated.	Reduces tissue swelling and rapidly empties superficial and tibial veins, preventing overdistention and thereby increasing venous return. *Note:* Some physicians believe that elevation may potentiate release of thrombus, thus increasing risk of embolization and decreasing circulation to the most distal portion of the extremity.
Initiate active or passive exercises while in bed; for example, flex, extend, and rotate feet periodically. Assist with gradual resumption of ambulation as soon as client is permitted out of bed.	These measures are designed to increase venous return from lower extremities and reduce venous stasis as well as improve general muscle tone and strength. They also promote normal organ function and enhance general well-being.
Caution client to avoid crossing legs or hyperflex at knee, such as seated position with legs dangling or lying in jackknife position.	Physical restriction of circulation impairs blood flow and increases venous stasis in pelvic, popliteal, and leg vessels, thus increasing swelling and discomfort.
Instruct client to avoid rubbing or massaging the affected extremity.	This activity potentiates risk of fragmenting and dislodging thrombus, causing embolization and increasing risk of complications.
Encourage deep-breathing exercises.	Increases negative pressure in thorax, which assists in emptying large veins.
Increase fluid intake to at least 1500 to 2000 mL/day, within cardiac tolerance.	Dehydration increases blood viscosity and venous stasis, predisposing to thrombus formation.
Collaborative	
Apply warm, moist compresses or heat cradle to affected extremity if indicated.	May be prescribed to promote vasodilation and venous return for resolution of local edema and to enhance comfort (Earhart & Tomlinson, 2007). *Note:* May be contraindicated

in presence of arterial insufficiency, in which heat can increase cellular oxygen consumption and nutritional needs, furthering imbalance between supply and demand.

Administer pharmacological measures, as indicated:

Pharmacological measures involve various types of anticoagulation in order to reduce blood coagulability.

Heparin sodium via continuous or intermittent IV and intermittent subcutaneous (SC) injections

Heparin may be used initially because of its prompt, predictable, antagonistic action on thrombin as it is formed and also because it removes activated coagulation factors XII, XI, IX, and X (intrinsic pathway), preventing further clot formation.

Low-molecular-weight heparin (LMWH) preparations, such as enorxaparin (Lovenox), daltaperin (Fragmin), tenzoparin (Innohep), and fondaparinux (Arixtra) via SC injections

Anticoagulant of choice after major orthopedic surgery and major trauma due to a lower risk of bleeding, more predictable dose response, and longer half-life than heparin sodium. May be used as "bridging" drugs while client starts warfarin therapy.

Vitamin K antagonists, e.g., warfarin (Coumadin) or dicumarol (Sintrom)

Coumadin has a potent depressant effect on liver formation of prothrombin from vitamin K and impairs formation of factors VII, IX, and X (extrinsic pathway). Coumadin is generally used for long-term postdischarge therapy to keep international normalized ratio (INR) at 2 to 3. However, it does have a narrow therapeutic window and requires frequent monitoring. A large number of foods, drugs, and disease processes alter Coumadin's effectiveness, making it difficult to regulate. The elderly client should be started on lower doses and monitored more frequently (Kehl-Pruett, 2006).

Rivaroxaban (Xarelto)

An oral factor Xa inhibitor was approved in November 2012 for treating deep vein thrombosis (DVT) and pulmonary embolism (PE) and for prevention of recurrences. One rivaroxaban pill, on the other hand, metabolizes in about 2 hours. There is no need for IV or subcutaneous injections of heparin for bridging, and the drug can be given in fixed doses without routine coagulation monitoring (Kaiser, 2013; Patel, 2013; Weitz, 2004).

Thrombolytic agents, such as tenecteplase (TNKase), activase (Alteplase), and reteplase (Retavase)

Thrombolytic therapy dissolves thrombi in 50% of patients (Stockman, 2008) if given within first 3 days after acute thrombosis. May be used in hemodynamically unstable client with PE or massive VTE to reduce risk of developing PE or in the presence of valvular damage or chronic venous insufficiency. *Note:* Catheter-directed fibrinolysis may be used to infuse a fibrinolytic agent directly into a thrombus in order to reduce the risks associated with systemic fibrinolytic therapy.

Monitor laboratory studies, as indicated:

Prothrombin time (PT), partial thromboplastin time (PTT), activated prothrombin time (aPTT), international normalized ratio (INR), hemogobin/hematacrit (Hgb/Hct)

Monitors response to anticoagulant therapy, identifies presence of risk factors, such as hemoconcentration and dehydration, which potentiate clot formation. *Note:* Lovenox does not require serial monitoring because PT and aPTT are not affected.

Platelet count, platelet function or aggregation test, and antiheparin antibody assay

On occasion, platelet count may decrease as a result of an immune reaction leading to platelet aggregation or the formation of "white clots." If bacteremia and disseminated intravascular coagulation (DIC) have been ruled out, condition may be the result of heparin-induced thrombocytopenia and thrombosis (HITT), requiring a change to Coumadin or other agents.

Apply and regulate graduated compression stockings and intermittent pneumatic compression if indicated.

Sequential compression devices may be used to improve blood flow velocity and empty vessels by providing artificial muscle-pumping action.

Apply elastic support hose following acute phase. Take care to avoid tourniquet effect.

Properly fitted support hose are useful, once ambulation has begun, to minimize or delay development of postphlebotic syndrome. They must exert a sustained, evenly distributed pressure over entire surface of calves and thighs to reduce the caliber of superficial veins and increase blood flow to deep veins.

Prepare for and assist with procedures, such as the following:

Percutaneous mechanical thrombectomy (PMT)

PMT has generally replaced the open surgical approach. This technology was designed primarily to eliminate the bleeding

(continues on page 114)

ACTIONS/INTERVENTIONS (continued)	RATIONALE (continued)
	risks associated with catheter-directed thrombolysis. As an endovascular technique, PMT employs rotational or hydrodynamic mechanisms to fragment and aspirate thrombi, thus reducing thrombus burden (Marchigiano et al, 2006).
Surgical intervention, such as thrombectomy and vena cava screen, when indicated	Thrombectomy (excision of thrombus) may be done in very rare cases when condition does not respond to typical treatments or circulation is severely restricted. Multiple or recurrent thrombotic episodes unresponsive to medical treatment (or when anticoagulant therapy is contraindicated) may require insertion of a vena cava filter (Siskin, 2011).

NURSING DIAGNOSIS: acute Pain

May Be Related To

Injury agent—physical (inflammatory process); chemical (accumulation of lactic acid in tissues)

Possibly Evidenced By

Reports pain
Guarding behavior
Expressive behaviors—restlessness

Desired Outcomes/Evaluation Criteria—Client Will

Pain Control (NOC)

Report that pain or discomfort is alleviated or controlled.
Verbalize methods that provide relief.
Display relaxed manner; be able to sleep or rest and engage in desired activity.

ACTIONS/INTERVENTIONS	RATIONALE
Pain Management (NIC)	
Independent	
Assess degree and characteristics of discomfort and pain. Note guarding of extremity. Palpate leg with caution.	Degree of pain is directly related to extent of circulatory deficit, inflammatory process, degree of tissue ischemia, and extent of edema associated with thrombus development. Changes in characteristics of pain may indicate development of complications.
Maintain bedrest (if indicated) during acute phase.	Reduces discomfort and may be suggested to prevent dislodging of clot. *Note:* There is lack of consensus in available research regarding bedrest during initial treatment phase. Some studies suggest that individuals with DVT who are receiving appropriate anticoagulant therapy do better with early ambulation (both immediately and later on) provided they have adequate cardiopulmonary reserve and no evidence of PE. Until more definitive evidence becomes available, the appropriate time to begin ambulation will be determined through the clinical judgment of the treating physician (Saab, 2010; Aldrich, 2004).
Elevate affected extremity, as indicated.	May be done to reduce symptoms such as swelling and pain (Smith, 2012).
Monitor vital signs, noting elevated temperature.	Elevations in heart rate may indicate increased discomfort or may occur in response to fever and inflammatory process. Fever can also increase client's discomfort.
Investigate reports of sudden or sharp chest pain, accompanied by dyspnea, tachycardia, and apprehension.	These signs and symptoms suggest the presence of PE as a complication of VTE.
Collaborative	
Administer medications, as indicated; for example, analgesics (opioid and nonopioid) and antipyretics, such as acetaminophen (Tylenol).	Relieves pain and decreases muscle tension. Reduces fever and inflammation. *Note:* Risk of bleeding may be increased by concurrent use of drugs that affect platelet function, such as aspirin and NSAIDs.
Apply moist heat to extremity if indicated.	Often used during early treatment phase, this modality may be continuous or intermittent to improve circulation, relax muscles, and stimulate release of natural endorphins.

NURSING DIAGNOSIS: impaired Gas Exchange (in presence of Pulmonary Embolus)

May Be Related To
Ventilation-perfusion imbalance [altered blood flow to alveoli or to major portions of the lung]
Alveolar-capillary membrane changes

Possibly Evidenced By
Dyspnea, restlessness, [apprehension], somnolence
Abnormal arterial blood gases, hypoxemia, hypercapnia

Desired Outcomes/Evaluation Criteria—Client Will

Respiratory Status: Gas Exchange (NOC)
Demonstrate adequate ventilation and oxygenation by ABGs within client's normal range.
Report or display resolution or absence of symptoms of respiratory distress.

ACTIONS/INTERVENTIONS	RATIONALE
Embolus Care: Pulmonary (NIC) *Independent*	
Note respiratory rate and depth and work of breathing, such as use of accessory muscles or nasal flaring and pursed-lip breathing.	Tachypnea and dyspnea accompany pulmonary obstruction. Dyspnea and increased work of breathing may be first or only sign of subacute PE. Severe respiratory distress and failure accompanies moderate to severe loss of functional lung units.
Auscultate lungs for areas of decreased and absent breath sounds and the presence of adventitious sounds, such as crackles.	Nonventilated areas may be identified by absence of breath sounds. Crackles occur in fluid-filled tissues and airways or may reflect cardiac decompensation.
Observe for generalized duskiness and cyanosis in "warm tissues," such as earlobes, lips, tongue, and buccal membranes.	Indicative of systemic hypoxemia.
Monitor vital signs. Note changes in cardiac rhythm.	Tachycardia, tachypnea, and changes in BP are associated with advancing hypoxemia and acidosis. Rhythm alterations and extra heart sounds may reflect increased cardiac workload related to worsening ventilation imbalance.
Assess level of consciousness and evaluate mentation changes.	Systemic hypoxemia may be demonstrated initially by restlessness and irritability, then by progressively decreased mentation.
Assess activity tolerance, such as reports of weakness and fatigue, vital sign changes, or increased dyspnea during exertion. Encourage rest periods, and limit activities to client tolerance.	These parameters assist in determining client response to resumed activities and ability to participate in self-care.
Airway Management (NIC)	
Institute measures to restore or maintain patent airways, such as deep-breathing exercises, coughing, and suctioning.	Plugged or collapsed airways reduce number of functional alveoli, negatively affecting gas exchange.
Elevate head of bed as client tolerates.	Promotes maximal chest expansion, making it easier to breathe and enhancing physiological and psychological comfort.
Assist with frequent changes of position, and get client out of bed to ambulate as tolerated.	Turning and ambulation enhance aeration of different lung segments, thereby improving oxygen diffusion.
Assist client to deal with fear and anxiety that may be present:	Feelings of fear and severe anxiety are associated with difficulty breathing and may cause increased oxygen consumption.
Encourage expression of feelings and inform client and SOs of normalcy of anxious feelings and sense of impending doom.	Understanding basis of feelings may help client regain some sense of control over emotions.
Provide brief explanations of what is happening and expected effects of interventions.	May allay anxiety related to unknown and help reduce fears concerning personal safety.
Monitor frequently, and arrange for someone to stay with client, as indicated.	Provides assurance that changes in condition will be noted and that assistance is readily available.
Embolus Care: Pulmonary (NIC) *Collaborative*	
Prepare for lung scan.	Reveals pattern of abnormal perfusion in areas of ventilation, reflecting ventilation and perfusion mismatch, confirming diagnosis of PE and degree of obstruction. Absence of both ventilation and perfusion reflects alveolar congestion or airway obstruction.

(continues on page 116)

ACTIONS/INTERVENTIONS (continued)	RATIONALE (continued)
Monitor serial ABGs or pulse oximetry.	Hypoxemia is present in varying degrees, depending on the amount of airway obstruction, usual cardiopulmonary function, and presence and degree of shock. Respiratory alkalosis and metabolic acidosis may also be present.
Airway Management (NIC)	
Administer supplemental oxygen by appropriate method.	Maximizes available oxygen for gas exchange, reducing work of breathing. *Note:* If obstruction is large or hypoxemia does not respond to supplemental oxygenation, it may be necessary to move client to critical care area for intubation and mechanical ventilation.
Administer fluids, IV or by mouth (PO), as indicated.	Increased fluids may be given to reduce hyperviscosity of blood, which can potentiate thrombus formation, or to support circulating volume and tissue perfusion.
Administer medications, as indicated, for example:	
Thrombolytic agents, such as alteplase (Activase, t-PA), reteplase (Retavase), tenecteplase (TNKase)	Indicated in massive pulmonary obstruction when client is seriously hemodynamically threatened. *Note:* These clients will probably be initially cared for in, or transferred to, the critical care setting.
Morphine sulfate and anti-anxiety agents	May be necessary initially to control pain or anxiety and improve work of breathing, maximizing gas exchange.
Provide supplemental humidification, such as ultrasonic nebulizers.	Delivers moisture to mucous membranes and helps liquefy secretions to facilitate airway clearance.
Assist with chest physiotherapy, such as postural drainage and percussion of nonaffected area, blow bottles, and incentive spirometer.	Facilitates deeper respiratory effort and promotes drainage of secretions from lung segments into bronchi, where they may more readily be removed by coughing or suctioning.
Prepare for and assist with bronchoscopy.	May be done to remove blood clots and clear airways.
Prepare for surgical intervention, if indicated.	Vena caval ligation or insertion of an intracaval umbrella may be useful for clients who experience recurrent emboli despite adequate anticoagulation, when anticoagulation is contraindicated, or when septic emboli arising from below the renal veins do not respond to treatment. Additionally, pulmonary embolectomy may be considered in life-threatening situations.

NURSING DIAGNOSIS: deficient Knowledge [Learning Need] regarding condition, treatment program, self-care, and discharge needs

May Be Related To
Lack of exposure or recall
Misinterpretation of information
Unfamiliarity with information resources

Possibly Evidenced By
Reports the problem
Inaccurate follow-through of instructions

Desired Outcomes/Evaluation Criteria—Client Will

Knowledge: Thrombus Prevention (NOC)
Verbalize understanding of disease process, treatment regimen, and limitations.
Participate in learning process.
Identify signs and symptoms requiring medical evaluation.
Correctly perform therapeutic actions and explain reasons for actions.

ACTIONS/INTERVENTIONS	RATIONALE
Teaching: Disease Process (NIC)	
Independent	
Review pathophysiology of condition and signs and symptoms of possible complications, such as PE, chronic venous insufficiency, and venous stasis ulcers (postphlebitic syndrome).	Provides a knowledge base from which client can make informed choices and understand and identify healthcare needs. A significant number of clients experience a recurrence of DVT. *Note:* Genetic blood testing may help identify inherited thrombotic disorders. Screening tests should be done when venous thrombosis occurs in those aged

ACTIONS/INTERVENTIONS (continued)	RATIONALE (continued)
	45 years or younger; when a thrombus occurs at an unusual location such as in gastrointestinal tract, brain, or arm; and when there is an immediate family history of VTE.
Explain purpose of activity restrictions and need for balance between activity and rest.	Rest reduces oxygen and nutrient needs of compromised tissues. Balancing rest with activity prevents exhaustion and further impairment of cellular perfusion.
Establish appropriate exercise and activity program.	Aids in developing collateral circulation, enhances venous return, and prevents recurrence.
Problem-solve solutions to predisposing factors that may be present, such as employment that requires prolonged standing or sitting, wearing restrictive clothing, use of oral contraceptives, obesity, prolonged immobility, and dehydration.	Actively involves client in identifying and initiating lifestyle and behavior changes to promote health and prevent recurrence of condition or development of complications.
Recommend sitting with feet touching the floor, avoiding crossing of legs.	Prevents excess pressure on the popliteal space.
Review purpose and demonstrate correct application and removal of antiembolic hose.	Understanding may enhance cooperation with prescribed therapy and prevent improper or ineffective use.
Instruct in meticulous skin care of lower extremities, such as prevent or promptly treat breaks in skin and report development of ulcers or changes in skin color.	Chronic venous congestion and postphlebitic syndrome may develop, especially in presence of severe vascular involvement and recurrent VTE, potentiating risk of stasis ulcers.
Teaching: Prescribed Medication (NIC)	
Discuss purpose and dosage of anticoagulant. Emphasize importance of taking drug as prescribed.	Promotes client safety by reducing risk of inadequate therapeutic response and deleterious side effects, such as bleeding.
Identify safety precautions, such as use of soft toothbrush, electric razor for shaving, gloves for gardening, avoiding sharp objects (including toothpicks), walking barefoot, engaging in rough sports and activities, or forceful blowing of nose.	Reduces the risk of traumatic injury, which potentiates bleeding or clot formation.
Review client's usual medications and foods (when on oral anticoagulants); emphasize need to read ingredient labels of over-the-counter (OTC) drugs and herbal supplements; and remind client to discuss anticoagulant use with healthcare provider prior to starting new medications.	Warfarin (Coumadin) interacts with many foods, drugs, and herbals either increasing or decreasing the anticoagulant effect.
Identify untoward anticoagulant effects requiring medical attention, such as bleeding from mucous membranes (nose, gums), continued oozing from cuts and punctures, severe bruising after minimal trauma, and development of petechiae.	Early detection of deleterious effects of therapy, such as prolongation of clotting time, allows for timely intervention and may prevent serious complications. *Note:* Even regular use of acetaminophen may prolong clotting times. In addition, use of herbal products, such as ginkgo, garlic, and vitamin E, also impairs clotting and should be avoided during anticoagulant therapy.
Emphasize importance of medical follow-up and laboratory testing.	Understanding that close supervision of anticoagulant therapy is necessary (therapeutic dosage range is narrow and complications may prove fatal) promotes client participation.
Encourage wearing of medical ID bracelet or necklace, as indicated.	Alerts emergency healthcare providers to history of thrombotic problems or current use of or need for anticoagulants, such as prophylactic before and after any procedure or event with an increased risk of venous thromboembolism.

POTENTIAL CONSIDERATIONS following discharge from care setting (dependent on client's age, physical condition and presence of complications, personal resources, and life responsibilities)

- ***ineffective Self-Health Management***—perceived seriousness/benefit

CHAPTER 5

Respiratory

CHRONIC OBSTRUCTIVE PULMONARY DISEASE (COPD) AND ASTHMA

I. Pathophysiology

- a. Chronic obstructive pulmonary disease (COPD): chronic obstructive bronchitis and emphysema
  - i. Chronic airflow limitations (CAL): caused by a mixture of small airway disease (obstructive bronchiolitis) and parenchymal destruction (emphysema)
  - ii. Airway inflammation: causes structural changes, narrowing of lumina, and loss of elastic recoil in parenchyma
- b. Asthma (also called chronic reactive airway disease)
  - i. Chronic inflammatory disorder—episodic exacerbations of reversible inflammation and hyperreactivity and variable constriction of bronchial smooth muscle, hypersecretion of mucus, and edema

II. Spirometric Classification of Severity of COPD—2007 Global Initiative for Chronic Obstructive Lung Disease

- a. Stage I (mild COPD)—mild airflow limitation ($FEV_1/FVC < 0.70$; $FEV_1 \geq$ to 80% predicted)
- b. Stage II (moderate COPD)—worsening airflow limitation ($FEV_1/FVC < 0.70$; 50% $\leq$ to $FEV_1 < 80\%$ predicted); shortness of breath on exertion, and cough and sputum production may be present
- c. Stage III (severe COPD)—continued worsening of airflow limitation ($FEV_1/FVC < 0.70$; 30% $\leq$ to $FEV_1 < 50\%$ predicted); increasing shortness of breath, reduced exercise capacity, fatigue, and repeated exacerbations
- d. Stage IV (very severe COPD)—severe airflow limitation ($FEV_1/FVC < 0.70$; $FEV_1 < 30\%$ predicted or $FEV_1 < 50\%$ predicted plus presence of chronic respiratory failure)

III. Etiology

- a. COPD
  - i. Risk factors: smoking (primary irritant), air pollution, secondhand smoke, history of childhood respiratory infections, heredity—α_1-antitrypsin deficiency
  - ii. Acute exacerbations usually due to pulmonary infections
- b. Asthma
  - i. Tends to be acute and intermittent or episodic
  - ii. Genetic and environmental: household substances (such as dust mites, pets, cockroaches, mold), pollen, foods, latex, emotional upheaval, air pollution, cold weather, exercise, chemicals, medications, viral infections
  - iii. In most children, asthma develops before age 5 years, and, in more than half, asthma develops before age 3 years. Multiple triggers or precipitants as above plus upper respiratory infections (most commonly viral), including respiratory syncytial virus (RSV) bronchiolitis in infancy, irritants such as tobacco smoke, sports and games requiring continuous activity or that are played in cold weather, and changes in atmospheric or barometric pressure (Sharma 2013; Ferki, 2012).

IV. Statistics (American Lung Association, 2011; CDC, 2012)

- a. COPD
  - i. Morbidity: COPD affects more than 15 million people.
  - ii. Mortality: It is the third leading cause of death in the United States with over 124,000 deaths in 2007; women's deaths exceed that of men (64,000 females to 60,000 males).
  - iii. Cost: Projected 2010—$49.9 billion, including $29.5 billion in direct healthcare expenditures, $8.0 billion in indirect morbidity costs, and $12.4 billion in indirect mortality costs.
- b. Asthma (ALA, 2012)
  - i. Morbidity: 2011 estimates are that 25.9 million Americans currently have asthma, including 7.1 million children under 18. (Asthma is the third leading cause for hospitalization of children.)
  - ii. Mortality: In 2009, there were 3,388 deaths attributed to asthma (157 children under 15).
  - iii. Cost: Annual direct healthcare cost is approximately $50.1 billion; indirect costs (e.g., lost productivity) $5.9 billion, totaling $56.0 billion dollars.

GLOSSARY

Asthma: Chronic, reversible inflammation of the airways caused by a reaction of the airways to various stimuli.

BODE Index: A validated grading system designed to predict the risk of death from COPD based on the four factors for which it was named: BMI, obstruction, dyspnea, and exercise. (Celli et al, 2004).

CAT (COPD Assessment Test) Score: Range from 0 to 40. Represents disease impact; score less than 10 equals low impact;

GLOSSARY (continued)

greater than 10 equals high impact A change of score of two or more points is considered clinically significant.

Chronic bronchitis: Inflammation and scarring of the lining of the bronchi.

Chronic obstructive pulmonary disease (COPD): Disease state characterized by an airflow limitation that is not fully reversible. It is usually progressive and associated with an abnormal inflammatory response to noxious particles or gases.

Emphysema: Destruction of the alveoli, which leads to overdistention of the air spaces. Damage is irreversible.

FEV_1: Forced expired volume in 1 second.

FVC: Forced vital capacity.

Care Setting

Primarily community level; however, severe exacerbations may necessitate emergency or inpatient hospital stay.

Related Concerns

Heart failure: chronic, page 43
Pediatric considerations, page 872
Pneumonia, page 129
Psychosocial aspects of care, page 729
Surgical intervention, page 762
Ventilatory assistance (mechanical), page 157

Client Assessment Database

DIAGNOSTIC DIVISION MAY REPORT	MAY EXHIBIT
ACTIVITY/REST	
• Fatigue, exhaustion, malaise • Inability to perform basic activities of daily living (ADLs) because of breathlessness • Inability to sleep, need to sleep sitting up • Dyspnea at rest or in response to activity or exercise	• Fatigue • Restlessness, insomnia • General debilitation or loss of muscle mass
CIRCULATION	
• Swelling of lower extremities	• Elevated blood pressure (BP) • Elevated heart rate or severe tachycardia, dysrhythmias • Distended neck veins, with advanced disease • Dependent edema, which may not be related to heart disease • Faint heart sounds due to increased anteroposterior (AP) chest diameter • Skin color and mucous membranes may be pale or bluish and cyanotic, clubbing of nails and peripheral cyanosis, pallor (can indicate anemia)
EGO INTEGRITY	
• Increased stress factors • Changes in lifestyle • Feelings of hopelessness, loss of interest in life	• Anxious, fearful, irritable behavior, emotional distress • Apathy, change in alertness, dull affect, withdrawal
FOOD/FLUID	
• Nausea—side effect of medication or mucus production • Poor appetite, anorexia (emphysema) • Inability to eat because of respiratory distress • Persistent weight loss, decreased muscle mass or subcutaneous fat (emphysema) • Weight gain reflecting edema (bronchitis, prednisone use)	• Poor skin turgor • Dependent edema • Diaphoresis • Abdominal palpation may reveal hepatomegaly
HYGIENE	
• Decreased ability and increased need for assistance with ADLs	• Poor hygiene

(continues on page 120)

DIAGNOSTIC DIVISION

Respiration

MAY REPORT (continued)

- Variable levels of dyspnea, with insidious and progressive onset (predominant symptom in emphysema), especially on exertion
- Seasonal or episodic occurrence of breathlessness (asthma); sensation of chest tightness, inability to breathe (asthma); chronic "air hunger"
- Persistent cough with sputum production (gray, white, or yellow), which may be copious (chronic bronchitis)
- Intermittent cough episodes, usually nonproductive in early stages, although they may become productive (emphysema)
- Paroxysms of cough (asthma)
- History of recurrent pneumonia; long-term exposure to chemical pollution or respiratory irritants, such as with cigarette smoke, or occupational dust and fumes, such as with cotton, hemp, asbestos, coal dust, sawdust
- Familial and hereditary factors, that is, deficiency of α_1-antitrypsin (emphysema)
- Use of oxygen at night or continuously

MAY EXHIBIT (continued)

- Respirations are usually rapid and may be shallow:
  - Prolonged expiratory phase with grunting, pursed-lip breathing (emphysema)
  - Assumption of three-point ("tripod") position for breathing—especially with acute exacerbation of chronic bronchitis
- Use of accessory muscles for respiration, such as elevated shoulder girdle, retraction of supraclavicular fossae, flaring of nares
- Chest may appear hyperinflated with increased AP diameter (barrel-shaped), minimal diaphragmatic movement
- Breath sounds may be faint with expiratory wheezes (emphysema):
  - Scattered, fine, or coarse moist crackles (bronchitis)
  - Rhonchi, wheezing throughout lung fields on expiration, and possibly during inspiration, progressing to diminished or absent breath sounds (asthma)
- Percussion may reveal hyperresonance over lung fields (air-trapping with emphysema) or dullness over lung fields (consolidation, fluid, mucus)
- Difficulty speaking sentences of more than four or five words at one time, loss of voice
- *Color:* Pallor, with cyanosis of lips, nailbeds; overall duskiness; ruddy color (chronic bronchitis, "blue bloaters"):
  - Normal skin color despite abnormal gas exchange and rapid respiratory rate (moderate emphysema, known as "pink puffers")
- Clubbing of fingernails (not characteristic of emphysema, and if present, should alert clinician to another condition such as pulmonary fibrosis, cystic fibrosis, lung cancer, or asbestosis)

Safety

MAY REPORT

- History of allergic reactions or sensitivity to substances or environmental factors
- Recent or recurrent infections

MAY EXHIBIT

- Flushing, perspiration (asthma)

Sexuality

MAY REPORT

- Decreased libido

Social Interaction

MAY REPORT

- Dependent relationship(s)
- Insufficient support from or to partner or significant other (SO), lack of support systems
- Prolonged disease or disability progression

MAY EXHIBIT

- Inability to converse or maintain voice because of respiratory distress
- Limited physical mobility
- Neglectful relationships with other family members
- Inability to perform or inattention to employment responsibilities, absenteeism, confirmed disability

Teaching/Learning

MAY REPORT

- Use or misuse of respiratory drugs
- Use of herbal supplements, such as astragalus, coleus, Echinacea
- Smoking or difficulty stopping smoking, chronic exposure to secondhand smoke, smoking substances other than tobacco
- Regular use of alcohol
- Failure to improve over long period of time

DIAGNOSTIC DIVISION MAY REPORT (continued)	MAY EXHIBIT (continued)
DISCHARGE PLAN CONSIDERATIONS • Episodic or long-term assistance with shopping, transportation, self-care needs, homemaker or home maintenance tasks • Changes in medication and therapeutic treatments, use of supplemental oxygen, ventilator support; end-of-life issues ➧ Refer to section at end of plan for postdischarge considerations.	

Diagnostic Studies

TEST WHY IT IS DONE	WHAT IT TELLS ME
BLOOD TESTS	
• ***Arterial blood gases (ABGs):*** Measures oxygen and carbon dioxide levels to assess and monitor gas exchange	Abnormalities usually develop late in the disease. Hypoxemia with a PaO_2 <55 mm Hg or SaO_2 < 88% are indications for low-flow oxygen therapy (Kee, 2010). Most often PaO_2 is decreased and $PaCO_2$ is normal or increased in chronic bronchitis and emphysema but is often decreased in asthma; pH normal or acidotic, mild respiratory alkalosis secondary to hyperventilation (moderate emphysema or asthma).
• ***Complete blood count (CBC) and differential:*** Provides baseline data about the hematologic system and yields information related to oxygen-carrying capacity and infection.	Erythropoiesis is stimulated by chronic hypoxemia. Increased hemoglobin (advanced emphysema) and increased eosinophils (asthma); white blood cells (WBCs) can be elevated in severe respiratory infection.
• ***α_1-antitrypsin (AAT):*** A deficiency screening used to verify deficiency of this enzyme and diagnosis of primary emphysema. Performed when COPD develops in patients <45 years old, of Caucasian descent, with strong family history of COPD (Kee, 2010).	A deficiency in AAT is a genetic trait considered to be a risk factor for the development of COPD. Decreased levels are seen in early onset emphysema in adults; increased levels are present in acute and chronic inflammatory disorders.
• ***Pulmonary function tests: (PFTs):*** Numerous specific tests are included as part of the comprehensive PFT and fall within three categories: airway flow rates, lung volumes and capacities, and gas exchange.	Performed to stage or classify the severity of disease process and to assess response to treatment (Daniels, 2012).
• ***Spirometry testing, including FVC and FEV_1:*** Measures the amount of air taken in (volume) and exhaled as a function of time (e.g., after deepest possible inhalation), which is also known as forced vital capacity (FVC).	Used to establish baseline lung function, evaluate dyspnea, detect pulmonary disease, and monitor effects of therapies used to treat respiratory disease. *Note:* The spirometer is also used as an exercise tool for improving lung function, for example, after surgery.
• ***Total lung capacity (TLC):*** Maximum amount of air that lungs can hold, measured at the top of an inhalation.	Increased in obstructive lung disease Decreased in restrictive lung disease
• ***Residual volume (RV):*** Air remaining in the lungs after maximum exhalation	Increased in obstructive lung disease Decreased in restrictive lung disease
• ***Vital capacity (VC):*** Maximum amount of air that can be exhaled during a normal or slow exhalation after fullest possible inhalation. Important measurement in assessing the client's ability to cough and protect airway.	Normal or decreased in obstructive lung disease Decreased in restrictive lung disease
OTHER DIAGNOSTIC STUDIES	
• ***Pulse oximetry:*** Noninvasive measure of arterial blood oxygen diffusion and saturation. Reflects oxygen saturation through measurement of the proportion of light transmitted by oxygenated forms of hemoglobin using finger/earlobe/toe sensor.	Abnormally low levels (<88%) indicate impaired gas exchange and impending respiratory failure. ABG analysis is recommended when SaO_2 <80% (Kee, 2010).
• ***Chest x-ray:*** Evaluates organs or structures within the chest.	May reveal hyperinflation of lungs with increased AP diameter, flattened diaphragm, increased retrosternal air space, decreased vascular markings/bullae (emphysema), increased bronchovascular markings (bronchitis), and normal findings during periods of remission (asthma).

Nursing Priorities

1. Maintain airway patency.
2. Assist with measures to facilitate gas exchange.
3. Enhance nutritional intake.
4. Prevent complications and slow progression of condition.
5. Provide information about disease process, prognosis, and treatment regimen.

Discharge Goals

1. Ventilation/oxygenation adequate to meet self-care needs.
2. Nutritional intake meeting caloric needs.
3. Infection treated or prevented.
4. Disease process, prognosis, and therapeutic regimen understood.
5. Plan in place to meet needs after discharge.

NURSING DIAGNOSIS: ineffective Airway Clearance

May Be Related To

Chronic obstructive pulmonary disease
Airway spasm, allergic airways
Excessive mucus, retained secretions, exudates in the alveoli
Smoking/secondhand smoke

Possibly Evidenced By

Dyspnea, difficulty vocalizing
Changes in depth and rate of respirations
Diminished/adventitious breath [wheezes, rhonchi, crackles]
Absent/ineffective cough
Restlessness, cyanosis

Desired Outcomes/Evaluation Criteria—Client Will

Respiratory Status: Airway Patency (NOC)

Maintain patent airway with breath sounds clear or clearing.
Demonstrate behaviors to improve airway clearance.

ACTIONS/INTERVENTIONS	RATIONALE
Airway Management (NIC) *Independent*	
Auscultate breath sounds. Note adventitious breath sounds such as wheezes, crackles, or rhonchi.	Some degree of bronchospasm is present with obstructions in airway and may or may not be manifested in adventitious breath sounds, such as scattered, moist crackles (bronchitis); faint sounds, with expiratory wheezes (emphysema); or absent breath sounds (severe asthma).
Assess and monitor respiratory rate. Note inspiratory-to-expiratory ratio.	Tachypnea is usually present to some degree and may be pronounced on admission, during stress, or during concurrent acute infectious process. Respirations may be shallow and rapid, with prolonged expiration in comparison to inspiration.
Note presence and degree of dyspnea, for example, reports of "air hunger," restlessness, anxiety, respiratory distress, and use of accessory muscles. Use a 0 to 10 scale or American Thoracic Society's Grade of Breathlessness Scale to rate breathing difficulty. Ascertain precipitating factors when possible. Differentiate acute episode from exacerbation of chronic dyspnea.	Respiratory dysfunction is variable depending on the underlying process, for example, infection, allergic reaction, and the stage of chronicity in a client with established COPD. *Note:* Using a scale to rate dyspnea aids in quantifying and tracking changes in respiratory distress. Rapid onset of acute dyspnea may reflect pulmonary embolus.
(P) Check peak expiratory flow rate (PEFR) before and after treatments using peak flow meter (PFM).	Monitors effectiveness of drug therapy; identifies need for change in regimen in children age 5 and older. *Note:* Although peak flow monitoring in the ER may prove helpful for assessment of lung function and response to treatment, it's usually possible only if client is familiar with the technique because he/she already uses it at home (Volpe, 2011).
Assist client to maintain a comfortable position to facilitate breathing by elevating the head of bed, leaning on over-bed table, or sitting on edge of bed.	Elevation of the head of the bed facilitates respiratory function using gravity; however, client in severe distress will seek the position that most eases breathing. Supporting arms and legs with table, pillows, and so on helps reduce muscle fatigue and can aid chest expansion.
Encourage and assist with abdominal or pursed-lip breathing exercises.	Provides client with some means to cope with and control dyspnea and reduce air-trapping.

ACTIONS/INTERVENTIONS (continued)	RATIONALE (continued)
Observe for persistent, hacking, or moist cough. Assist with measures to improve effectiveness of cough effort.	Cough can be persistent but ineffective, especially if client is elderly, acutely ill, or debilitated. Coughing is most effective in an upright or in a head-down position after chest percussion.
Increase fluid intake to 3000 mL/day within cardiac tolerance. Provide warm or tepid liquids. Recommend intake of fluids between, instead of during, meals.	Hydration helps decrease the viscosity of secretions, facilitating expectoration. Using warm liquids may decrease bronchospasm. Fluids during meals can increase gastric distention and pressure on the diaphragm.
(P) Avoid iced liquids, especially in children.	May trigger bronchospasm.
Limit exposure to environmental pollutants such as dust, smoke, and feather pillows according to individual situation.	Precipitators of allergic type of respiratory reactions that can trigger or exacerbate onset of acute episode.
(P) Use a spacer when administering metered-dose inhaler (MDI); and spacer with mask as indicated.	Most effective way of delivering maximum amount of medication. Mask should be used in child too young to seal lips around mouthpiece. *Note:* Spacer is not to be used with dry powder inhalers.
Collaborative	
Administer medications, as indicated, for example:	
Beta-agonists, such as epinephrine (Adrenalin, AsthmaNefrin, Primatene, Sus-Phrine), albuterol (Proventil, Velmax, Ventolin, AccuNeb, Airet), formoterol (Foradil), levalbuterol (Xopenex), metaproterenol (Alupent), pirbuterol (Maxair), terbutaline (Brethine), and salmeterol (Serevent), Indacterol (Arcapta)	Inhaled β_2-adrenergic agonists are first-line therapies for rapid symptomatic improvement of bronchoconstriction. These medications relax smooth muscles and reduce local congestion, reducing airway spasm, wheezing, and mucus production. Medications may be oral, injected, or inhaled. Inhalation by metered-dose inhaler (MDI) with a spacer is recommended, but medications may be nebulized in the event client has severe coughing or is too dyspneic to puff effectively.
Bronchodilators, such as tiotropium (Spiriva) ipra-tropium (Atrovent), Combivent Respimat	Inhaled anticholinergic agents are now considered the first-line drugs for clients with stable COPD because studies indicate they have a longer duration of action with less toxicity potential, whereas still providing the effective relief of the beta-agonists. Some of these medications are available in combinations; for example, albuterol and Atrovent are available as Combivent.
Leukotriene antagonists, such as montelukast (Singulair), zafirlukast (Accolate), and zileuton (Zyflo)	Reduce leukotriene activity to limit inflammatory response. In mild to moderate asthma, reduces need for inhaled β_2-agonists and systemic corticosteroids. Not effective in acute exacerbations because there is no bronchodilator effect. *Note:* This drug class is not recommended for clients with COPD because of insufficient testing.
Phosphodiesterase type 4 enzyme inhibitors, such as Roflumilast (Daliresp)	Decreases exacerbations in clients with severe COPD associated with chronic bronchitis; acts as a NSAID to decrease number of neutrophils and eosinophils in airway.
Anti-inflammatory drugs: oral, intravenous (IV), and inhaled steroids, such as prednisone (Cordrol, Deltasone, Pred-Pak, Liquid Pred), methylprednisolone (Medrol), dexamethasone (Decadron), beclomethasone (Beclovent, Vanceril), budesonide (Pulmacort), fluticasone (Flovent), and triamcinolone (Azmacort)	Decrease local airway inflammation and edema by inhibiting effects of histamine and other mediators to reduce severity and frequency of airway spasm, respiratory inflammation, and dyspnea. Studies have shown benefits of systemic steroids in the management of COPD exacerbations. Inhaled steroids may serve as a systemic steroid-sparing agent. *Note:* The aim of inhaled corticosteroids is to reduce exacerbation rates and slow decline in health status. Maintenance use of oral corticosteroids is not recommended unless absolutely necessary. Clients must be monitored for osteoporosis as a side effect. Clients over age 65 should be treated prophylactically to prevent osteoporosis.
Antimicrobials	Various antimicrobials may be indicated for control of bacterial exacerbations of COPD, such as pneumonia. (Refer to CP: Pneumonia.)
Methylxanthine derivatives, such as aminophylline, oxtriphylline (Choledyl), and theophylline (Bronkodyl, Theo-Dur, Elixophyllin, Slo-Bid, Slo-Phyllin)	Decrease mucosal edema and smooth muscle spasm (bronchospasm) by indirectly increasing cyclic adenosine monophosphate (AMP). May also reduce muscle fatigue and respiratory failure by increasing diaphragmatic contractility. Use of theophylline may be of little or no benefit in the presence of adequate beta-agonist regimen; however, it may sustain bronchodilation because effect of beta-agonist diminishes between doses. *Note:* Theophylline products are used with less frequency now and are not recommended in older clients because of their potentially adverse cardiovascular effects.

(continues on page 124)

ACTIONS/INTERVENTIONS (continued)	RATIONALE (continued)
Analgesics, cough suppressants, or antitussives, such as codeine and dextromethorphan products (Benylin DM, Comtrex, Novahistine)	Persistent, exhausting cough may need to be suppressed to conserve energy and permit client to rest. *Note:* Regular use of antitussives is not recommended for COPD clients as cough can have a significant protective effect.
Artificial surfactant such as colfosceril palmitate (Exosurf)	Research suggests aerosol administration may enhance expectoration of sputum, improve pulmonary function, and reduce lung volumes (air-trapping).
Provide supplemental humidification, such as ultrasonic nebulizer and aerosol room humidifier.	Humidity helps reduce viscosity of secretions, facilitating expectoration, and may reduce or prevent formation of thick mucous plugs in bronchioles.
Assist with respiratory treatments, such as spirometry and chest physiotherapy.	Breathing exercises help enhance diffusion; aerosol or nebulizer medications can reduce bronchospasm and stimulate expectoration. Postural drainage and percussion enhance removal of excessive and sticky secretions and improve ventilation of bottom lung segments. *Note:* Chest physiotherapy may aggravate bronchospasm in asthmatics.
Monitor and graph serial ABGs, pulse oximetry, and chest x-ray.	Establishes baseline for monitoring progression or regression of disease process and complications. *Note:* Pulse oximetry readings detect changes in saturation as they are happening, helping to identify trends possibly before client is symptomatic. However, studies have shown that the accuracy of pulse oximetry may be questioned if client has severe peripheral vasoconstriction.

NURSING DIAGNOSIS: impaired Gas Exchange

May Be Related To

Ventilation-perfusion imbalance [retained secretions, bronchospasm, air-trapping]
Alveolar-capillary membrane changes

Possibly Evidenced By

Dyspnea
Confusion, restlessness
Abnormal breathing (e.g., rate, rhythm, depth); tachycardia
Abnormal ABGs—hypoxia, hypercapnia
Nasal flaring; abnormal skin color (e.g., pale, dusky)
Reduced tolerance for activity

Desired Outcomes/Evaluation Criteria—Client Will

Respiratory Status: Gas Exchange (NOC)

Demonstrate improved ventilation and adequate oxygenation of tissues by ABGs within client's normal range and be free of symptoms of respiratory distress.
Participate in treatment regimen within level of ability and situation.

ACTIONS/INTERVENTIONS	RATIONALE
Acid-Base Management (NIC)	
Independent	
Assess respiratory rate and depth. Note use of accessory muscles, pursed-lip breathing, and inability to speak or converse.	Useful in evaluating the degree of respiratory distress and chronicity of the disease process
Elevate head of bed and assist client to assume position to ease work of breathing. Include periods of time in prone position as tolerated. Encourage deep, slow, or pursed-lip breathing as individually needed and tolerated.	Oxygen delivery may be improved by upright position and breathing exercises to decrease airway collapse, dyspnea, and work of breathing. *Note:* Recent research supports use of prone position to increase PaO_2.
Assess and routinely monitor skin and mucous membrane color.	Cyanosis may be peripheral (noted in nailbeds) or central (noted around lips or earlobes). Duskiness and central cyanosis indicate advanced hypoxemia.
Encourage expectoration of sputum; suction when indicated.	Thick, tenacious, copious secretions are a major source of impaired gas exchange in small airways. Deep suctioning may be required when cough is ineffective for expectoration of secretions.
Auscultate breath sounds, noting areas of decreased airflow and adventitious sounds.	Breath sounds may be faint because of decreased airflow or areas of consolidation. Presence of wheezes may indicate

bronchospasm or retained secretions. Scattered, moist crackles may indicate interstitial fluid or cardiac decompensation.

Palpate chest for fremitus.

Decrease of vibratory tremors suggests fluid collection or air-trapping.

Monitor level of consciousness and mental status. Investigate changes.

Restlessness and anxiety are common manifestations of hypoxia. Worsening ABGs accompanied by confusion and somnolence are indicative of cerebral dysfunction due to hypoxemia.

Evaluate level of activity tolerance. Provide calm, quiet environment. Limit client's activity or encourage bedrest or chair rest during acute phase. Have client resume activity gradually and increase as individually tolerated.

During severe, acute, or refractory respiratory distress, client may be totally unable to perform basic self-care activities because of hypoxemia and dyspnea. Rest interspersed with care activities remains an important part of treatment regimen. An exercise program is aimed at improving aerobic capacity and functional performance, increasing endurance and strength without causing severe dyspnea, and can enhance sense of well-being.

Evaluate sleep patterns; note reports of difficulties and whether client feels well rested. Provide quiet environment and group care and monitoring activities to allow periods of uninterrupted sleep. Limit stimulants such as caffeine. Encourage position of comfort.

Multiple external stimuli and presence of dyspnea and hypoxemia may prevent relaxation and inhibit sleep. Sleeping difficulties due to hypoxia related to apnea and nocturnal hypopnea may require referral to sleep specialist.

Monitor vital signs and cardiac rhythm.

Tachycardia, dysrhythmias, and changes in BP can reflect effect of systemic hypoxemia on cardiac function.

Collaborative

Monitor and graph serial ABGs and pulse oximetry.

$PaCO_2$ is usually elevated in bronchitis and emphysema, and PaO_2 is generally decreased, so that hypoxia is present in a greater or lesser degree. *Note:* A "normal" or increased $PaCO_2$ signals impending respiratory failure for asthmatics.

Administer supplemental oxygen judiciously via nasal cannula, mask, or mechanical ventilator, and titrate as indicated by ABG results and client tolerance.

Used to correct and prevent worsening of hypoxemia, improve survival and quality of life. Supplemental oxygen can be provided during exacerbations only, or as a long-term therapy. *Note:* Long-term O_2 therapy (greater than 15h/d) has been found to increase long-term survival and improves hemodynamics, hematology, exercise capacity, lung mechanics, mental status, motor speed, and hand strength.

Administer anti-anxiety, sedative, or opioid agents, such as morphine, with caution.

May be used to reduce dyspnea by controlling anxiety and restlessness, which increases oxygen consumption and demand, exacerbating dyspnea. Must be monitored closely because depressive effect may lead to respiratory failure.

Assist with noninvasive (nasal or oronasal) intermittent positive-pressure ventilation (NIPPV) or intubation and institution and maintenance of mechanical ventilation; transfer to critical care unit depending on client directives.

Development of or impending respiratory failure requires prompt life-saving measures. *Note:* NIPPV provides ventilatory support by means of positive pressure, typically through a nasal mask. It may be useful in the home setting as well to treat chronic respiratory failure or limit acute exacerbations in clients who are able to maintain spontaneous respiratory effort.

Prepare for additional referrals and interventions, such as to a pulmonary specialist, to a pulmonary rehabilitation program, or for surgical intervention, as appropriate.

May be indicated to confirm diagnosis and optimize appropriate treatment. A multidisciplinary approach including education and exercise training may be helpful in improving client function and quality of life. Screened candidates—those with severe dyspnea or end-stage emphysema with FEV_1 less than 35% of the predicted value despite maximal medical therapy and with the ability to complete preoperative pulmonary rehabilitation programs—may benefit from lung volume reduction surgery (LVRS) in which hyperinflated giant bullae and cysts are removed. These bullae or cysts may occupy at least one-third of the involved lobe or areas of lung tissue with small cystic disease. In the absence of fibrosis, this procedure removes ineffective lung tissue, allowing for better lung expansion and elastic recoil, enhanced blood flow to healthy tissues (correction of ventilation-perfusion mismatch), improved respiratory muscle efficiency, and increased venous return.

NURSING DIAGNOSIS: imbalanced Nutrition: less than body requirements

May Be Related To

Biological factors—dyspnea; medication side effects; anorexia, nausea or vomiting; fatigue

Possibly Evidenced By

Body weight 20% or more under ideal; poor muscle tone

Reported altered taste sensation, aversion to eating, lack of interest in food

Desired Outcomes/Evaluation Criteria—Client Will

Nutritional Status (NOC)

Display progressive weight gain toward goal as appropriate.

Demonstrate behaviors and lifestyle changes to regain and maintain appropriate weight.

ACTIONS/INTERVENTIONS	RATIONALE
Nutrition Therapy (NIC)	
Independent	
Assess dietary habits, recent food intake. Note degree of difficulty with eating. Evaluate weight and body size or mass.	Client in acute respiratory distress is often anorectic because of dyspnea, sputum production, and medication effects. In addition, many COPD clients habitually eat poorly even though respiratory insufficiency creates a hypermetabolic state with increased caloric needs. As a result, client often is admitted with some degree of malnutrition. People who have emphysema are often thin, with wasted musculature.
Auscultate bowel sounds.	Diminished or hypoactive bowel sounds may reflect decreased gastric motility and constipation (common complication) related to limited fluid intake, poor food choices, decreased activity, and hypoxemia.
Give frequent oral care, remove expectorated secretions promptly, and provide specific container for disposal of secretions and tissues.	Noxious tastes, smells, and sights are prime deterrents to appetite and can produce nausea and vomiting with increased respiratory difficulty.
Encourage a rest period of 1 hour before and after meals. Provide frequent small feedings.	Helps reduce fatigue during mealtime, and provides opportunity to increase total caloric intake.
Avoid gas-producing foods and carbonated beverages.	Can produce abdominal distention, which hampers abdominal breathing and diaphragmatic movement and can increase dyspnea.
Avoid very hot or very cold foods.	Extremes in temperature can precipitate or aggravate coughing spasms.
Weigh, as indicated.	Useful in determining caloric needs, setting weight goal, and evaluating adequacy of nutritional plan. *Note:* Weight loss may continue initially despite adequate intake, as edema is resolving.
Collaborative	
Consult dietitian or nutritional support team to provide easily digested, nutritionally balanced meals by mouth, supplemental or tube feedings, and parenteral nutrition. (Refer to CP: Total Nutritional Support: Parenteral/Enteral Feeding.)	Method of feeding and caloric requirements are based on individual situation and specific needs to provide maximal nutrients with minimal client effort and energy expenditure.
Review serum albumin or prealbumin, transferrin, amino acid profile, iron, nitrogen balance studies, glucose, liver function studies, and electrolyte laboratory values as ordered.	Determines deficits and monitors effectiveness of nutritional therapy.
Administer supplemental oxygen during meals, as indicated.	Decreases dyspnea and increases energy for eating, enhancing intake.

NURSING DIAGNOSIS: ineffective Self-Health Management

May Be Related To

Deficient knowledge; complexity of therapeutic regimen

Economic difficulties

Perceived benefits/seriousness

Possibly Evidenced By

Reports difficulty with prescribed regimen

Failure to include treatment regimens in daily living

Failure to take action to reduce risk factors

NURSING DIAGNOSIS: ineffective Self-Health Management (continued)

Desired Outcomes/Evaluation Criteria—Client Will

Self-Management: Chronic Obstructive Pulmonary Disease/Asthma Management (NOC)

Verbalize understanding of condition and disease process and treatment.
Identify relationship of current signs and symptoms to the disease process and correlate these with causative factors.
Initiate necessary lifestyle changes and participate in treatment regimen.

ACTIONS/INTERVENTIONS	RATIONALE
Teaching: Disease Process (NIC) **Asthma Management (NIC)** ***Independent***	
Explain and reinforce explanations of individual disease process, including factors that lead to exacerbation episodes.	Understanding decreases anxiety and can lead to improved participation in treatment plan.
(P) Review possible disease course as appropriate.	For children with asthma, symptoms may disappear during their teen years but may return in adulthood.
Discuss respiratory medications, side effects, drug interactions, and adverse reactions.	Frequently, these clients are simultaneously on several respiratory drugs that have similar side effects and potential drug interactions. It is important that the client understands the difference between nuisance side effects (medication continued) and untoward or adverse side effects (medication possibly discontinued or dosage changed).
Demonstrate correct technique for using an MDI, such as how to hold it, pausing 2 to 5 minutes between puffs, and cleaning the inhaler.	Proper administration of drug enhances delivery and effectiveness. *Note:* When administering MDI, client begins inhalation and then presses canister. If MDI is used with a spacer, canister is pressed first then client takes two breaths.
Devise system for recording prescribed intermittent drug and inhaler usage.	Reduces risk of improper use or overdosage of prn (as necessary) medications, especially during acute exacerbations, when cognition may be impaired.
Discuss use of herbals, especially when client is on multiple respiratory medications.	Many interactions can occur between herbals and medications used to treat respiratory disorders. Although most herbals do not have dangerous side effects, effects can be dangerous or lethal if combined with other substances or when taken in larger doses. Herbs, such as ephedra, should be used only in very small doses and for a short time. Echinacea can alter the actions of a variety of drugs and is not recommended for persons with HIV infection, multiple sclerosis (MS), and other autoimmune disorders.
Recommend avoidance of sedative anti-anxiety agents unless specifically prescribed and approved by physician treating respiratory condition.	Although client may be nervous and feel the need for sedatives, these can depress respiratory drive and protective cough mechanisms. *Note:* These drugs may be used prophylactically when client is unable to avoid situations known to increase stress and trigger respiratory response.
(P) Instruct asthmatic client/parent in use of peak flow meter (PMF) as appropriate.	Peak flow level can drop before client exhibits any signs and symptoms of asthma after the "first time" the client is exposed to a trigger. Regular use of the peak flow meter may reduce the severity of the attack because of earlier intervention. However, trying to learn to use the PFM during an attack may not be possible.
Encourage client to monitor own status with use of CAT score (evaluates cough, mucus production, chest tightness, ability to rest, activity limitations, confidence and energy levels with a numeric value) and to relay the information to healthcare providers.	This self-administered questionnaire helps the client monitor own respiratory status and changes that may be indicative of improvement or need for prompt medical evaluation.
(P) Recommend client/parent keep a daily or periodic diary of asthma symptoms as indicated.	Helpful in determining effectiveness of treatment plan and need for adjustment as child ages. *Note:* Symptoms at night are an indication of nocturnal asthma or poor control even if condition appears stable during the day (Sawicki, 2012).
Discuss self-management plan:	
(P) Avoidance of triggers and ways to control these factors in and around the home and school/work setting.	Avoiding triggers, such as known allergens, environmental factors, such as excessively dry air, wind, temperature extremes, pollen, chemical products and fumes, tobacco smoke,

(continues on page 128)

ACTIONS/INTERVENTIONS (continued)	RATIONALE (continued)
	aerosol sprays, are important in the self-management of asthma and in the prevention of acute exacerbations.
P Use of asthma symptom zones, as appropriate.	Zones may be divided into green (peak expiratory flow rate [PEFR] 80% to 100% and no breathing difficulty), yellow (PEFR 50% to 80% of baseline and some difficulty breathing, with wheezing and coughing) indicating need for a short-term change or increase in medication, and red (PEFR less than 50% baseline and does not respond to inhaled bronchodilators), which should be evaluated by care provider (Sawicki, 2012).
Review of breathing exercises, coughing effectively, and general conditioning exercises.	Pursed-lip and abdominal or diaphragmatic breathing exercises strengthen muscles of respiration, help minimize collapse of small airways, and provide the individual with means to control dyspnea. General paced conditioning exercises, carried out regularly and perhaps timed with activity soon after taking medication or breathing treatments, can increase activity tolerance, muscle strength, and sense of well-being and quality of life.
Importance of regular oral care and dental hygiene.	Decreases bacterial growth in the mouth, which can lead to pulmonary infections.
Importance of avoiding people with active respiratory infections. Emphasize need for routine influenza and pneumococcal vaccinations.	Decreases exposure to and incidence of acquired acute upper respiratory infections (URIs). *Note:* Studies have shown that in high-risk groups, such as persons with COPD, influenza vaccination alone was associated with a 52% reduction in the risk of hospitalization for pneumonia and a 70% reduction in the risk for death (Nichol, 1999).
P Discuss and encourage family to form a detailed rescue plan for an acute asthmatic episode, including how to identify signs of an acute attack, how to use and monitor effects of rescue medications, and how, when and where to obtain emergent care.	Child (if of age to self-manage) and/or caregiver must have the knowledge and capability of helping child in emergent asthma attack, including medications to use and contact numbers to obtain rapid assistance. Relief medications include short-acting bronchodilators, systemic corticosteroids, and ipratropium (Atrovent) to bring about relaxation of bronchi (Sawicki, 2012; Sharma, 2013).
P Recommend client wear medical identification device at all times.	Provides important information regarding condition, allergies, treatment, emergency contact and provider information during emergencies (Sawicki, 2012).
Review the harmful effects of smoking, and strongly advise cessation of smoking by client and SO. Provide information on QUITLINES, support groups, nicotine substitutes, and other resources that aid in smoking cessation.	Cessation of smoking may slow or halt progression of COPD. Even when client wants to stop smoking, support groups and medical monitoring may be needed. *Note:* Research studies suggest that sidestream or secondhand smoke can be as detrimental as actually smoking (Simon, 2011).
Provide information about benefits of regular exercise while addressing individual activity limitations.	Having this knowledge can enable client and SO to make informed choices and decisions to reduce client's dyspnea, maximize functional level, perform most desired activities, and prevent complications. This may include alternating activities with rest periods to prevent fatigue, conserving energy during activities by pulling instead of pushing articles, sitting instead of standing while performing tasks, using pursed-lip breathing, side-lying position, and possible need for supplemental oxygen during sexual activity.
P Encourage preventive therapy for strenuous play or sports.	Use of a reliever inhaler 10 to 15 minutes before engaging in activities and repeating medication after 2 hours of continuous exercise or conclusion of activity as well as warm-up exercises and appropriate cool-down activities can prevent asthma symptoms.
Discuss importance of regular medical follow-up care, when to notify healthcare professional of changes in condition, and periodic spirometry testing, chest x-rays, and sputum cultures.	Monitoring disease process allows for alterations in therapeutic regimen to meet changing needs and may help prevent complications. P It is recommended that children with asthma see their primary provider every 1 to 6 months, as the choice of medications varies depending on age of child (Sawicki, 2012).
Review oxygen requirements and dosage for client who is discharged on supplemental oxygen. Discuss safe use of oxygen and refer to supplier as indicated.	Reduces risk of misuse—too little or too much—and resultant complications. Promotes environmental and physical safety.
Instruct client and SO in use of NIPPV as appropriate. Problem-solve possible side effects, and identify adverse signs and symptoms such as increased dyspnea, fatigue, daytime drowsiness, or headaches on awakening.	NIPPV may be used at night and periodically during day to decrease CO_2 level, improve quality of sleep, and enhance functional level during the day. Signs of increasing CO_2 level indicate need for more aggressive therapy.

ACTIONS/INTERVENTIONS (continued)	RATIONALE (continued)
Provide information and encourage participation in support groups sponsored by the American Lung Association and public health department.	These clients and their SOs may experience anxiety, depression, and other reactions as they deal with a chronic disease that has an impact on their desired lifestyle. Support groups may be desired or needed to provide assistance, emotional support, and respite care.
Refer for evaluation of home care if indicated. Provide a detailed plan of care and baseline physical assessment to home-care nurse as needed on discharge from acute care.	Provides for continuity of care. May help reduce frequency of hospitalization.
Assist client and SO in making arrangements for access to emergency assistance, such as a buddy system for getting help quickly, special phone numbers, and "panic button."	Client with chronic respiratory condition should have access to prompt assistance when needed. This is both necessary and psychologically comforting for self-management.
Facilitate discussion about healthcare directives and end-of-life wishes as indicated.	Although many clients have an interest in discussing living wills, their wishes may be unspoken. In client with severe pulmonary disease, it is helpful to discuss preferences regarding aggressive treatment, home care only, hospitalization for comfort care, and full life support. It is useful also to discuss the goals of care, such as functional independence or continuation of life support in an extended care nursing facility.

POTENTIAL CONSIDERATIONS following acute hospitalization (dependent on client's age, physical condition and presence of complications, personal resources, and life responsibilities)

- ***Self-Care Deficit, [specify]***—fatigue, weakness, severe anxiety
- ***impaired Home Maintenance***—illness, inadequate support system, insufficient finances, unfamiliarity with neighborhood resources
- ***risk for Infection***—decrease in ciliary action, stasis of body fluids (secretions), tissue destruction, increased environmental exposure, chronic disease, malnutrition

PNEUMONIA

I. Pathophysiology

a. Inflammation of the lung parenchyma associated with alveolar edema and congestion that impairs gas exchange

b. Common pathogens

 i. Viruses (CDC, 2012)

  1. Common causative organisms include respiratory syncytial virus (RSV), influenza, and human parainfluenza viruses (HPIVs)
  2. Account for approximately half of all cases of community-acquired pneumonia (CAP)

 ii. Bacteria

  1. Divided into typical and atypical types
  2. Gram-positive *Streptococcus pneumoniae, Haemophilus,* and *Staphylococcus* most common bacterial causes

 iii. Fungus

  1. Most common causes *Histoplasma capsulatum* and *Coccidioides immitis*
  2. *Pneumocystis jirovecii (formerly carinii)* and cytomegalovirus (CMV) often occur in immunocompromised persons

 iv. Other

  1. Agents include *Mycoplasma, Mycobacterium tuberculosis, Coxiella burnetii, Chlamydia,* and *Legionella*

II. Classification

a. Site and causative agent

 i. Lobar, single lobe; broncho, smaller lung areas in several lobes; interstitial, tissues surrounding the alveoli and bronchi

 ii. Bacteria, viruses, and fungi

b. Distribution

 i. CAP commonly caused by *S. pneumoniae, Chlamydia pneumoniae, Haemophilus influenzae,* RSV, occasionally atypical pathogens

 ii. Nosocomial (now called healthcare-associated pneumonia [HCAP]) develops at least 48 hours after admission to an institution or care center

 iii. HCAP and/or ventilator-associated pneumonia (VAP) is often caused by *Pseudomonas aeruginosa, Klebsiella pneumoniae, Staphylococcus aureus,* and both methicillin-sensitive and methicillin-resistant *S. aureus* (MRSA)

III. Etiology

a. Primary pneumonia is caused by the client's inhalation or aspiration of a pathogen (microaspiration).

b. Secondary pneumonia ensues from lung damage caused by the spread of an infectious agent—bacterial, viral, or fungal—from another site in the body or from various chemical irritants (including gastric reflux and aspiration, smoke inhalation) or radiation therapy.

c. Risk factors: Comorbidities, such as heart or lung disease, compromised immune system, diabetes mellitus, liver or renal failure, malnutrition, smoking, over age 70, previous antibiotic therapy, abdominal or thoracic surgical procedures, endotracheal intubation with mechanical ventilation.

IV. Statistics (American Lung Association, 2010)

a. Morbidity: An estimated 6 million cases are reported annually; hospital discharges attributed to pneumonia in 2009 were 1.1 million (CDC). Respiratory syncytial virus (RSV) is the leading cause of acute lower respiratory infections (ALRI) in children. It is estimated to cause approximately

(continues on page 130)

33.8 million new episodes of ALRI in children annually, 96% of these occurring in developing countries.

b. Mortality: In the United States, deaths attributed to pneumonia in 2006 were over 55,000. Globally, pneumonia kills more than 1.5 million children younger than age 5 years (CDC) and is the leading cause of death in children worldwide (WHO, 2012). RSV is estimated to result in 53,000 to 199,000 deaths annually in young children (WHO, 2012; Nair et al, 2011).

c. Cost:

i. CAP—annual cost exceeds $12.2 billion (Brar, 2011)

ii. HCAP (non-VAP)—estimated $28,008 per incident (Davis, 2012)

iii. VAP—estimated $39,828 per incident (Kollef, 2012)

GLOSSARY

Adventitious breath sounds: Abnormal breath sounds heard when listening to the chest. Adventitious sounds may include crackles or rales, rhonchi or wheezes, or pleural friction rubs.

Bronchial breath sounds: A harsh or blowing quality, made by air moving in the large bronchi and barely, if at all, modified by the intervening lung; may be heard over a consolidated lung.

Community-acquired pneumonia (CAP): Acquired outside healthcare organizations, including hospitals, nursing homes, and other long-term care facilities; includes the first 2 days of hospitalization.

Crackles: An adventitious breath sound produced by air passing over airway secretions; a discontinuous sound, as opposed to a wheeze, which is continuous. Crackles are classified as "fine" or "coarse"; also known as rales.

Empyema: A condition in which pus and fluid from infected tissue collects in a body cavity; most often used to refer to collections of pus in the space around the lungs (pleural cavity).

Fremitus: A palpable vibration, as felt by the hand placed on the chest during coughing or speaking.

Healthcare-associated pneumonia (HAP) (formerly called nosocomial pneumonia): Occurs 48 hours or longer after admission to a facility.

Percussion: An assessment method in which the surface of the body is struck with the fingertips to obtain sounds that can be heard or vibrations that can be felt. It can determine the position, size, and consistency of an internal organ. It is done over the chest to determine the presence of normal air content in the lungs.

Pleural effusion: Accumulation of fluid in the space between the membrane encasing the lung and lining the thoracic cavity.

Pleural friction rub: An abrasive sound that is synchronous with the respiratory movements, made by the rubbing together of two acutely inflamed serous surfaces, as in acute pleurisy.

Respiratory syncytial virus (RSV): A highly contagious virus and the leading cause of lower respiratory disease (e.g., bronchiolitis and pneumonia) in children ages 2 and under. RSV infection is primarily a disease of winter or early spring, with waves of illness sweeping through a community. There is currently no vaccine against RSV.

Care Setting

Most clients are treated as outpatients in community settings; however, persons at higher risk, such as children under 5, those older than 65, and persons with other chronic conditions such as chronic obstructive pulmonary disease (COPD), diabetes, cancer, and congestive heart failure, are treated in the hospital, as are those already hospitalized for other reasons and who have developed nosocomial, or healthcare-acquired, pneumonia.

Related Concerns

Acquired immunodeficiency syndrome (AIDS), page 689
Chronic obstructive pulmonary disease (COPD) and asthma, page 118
Pediatric considerations, page 872
Psychosocial aspects of care, page 729
Sepsis/septicemia, page 665
Surgical intervention, page 762

Client Assessment Database

DIAGNOSTIC DIVISION MAY REPORT	MAY EXHIBIT
ACTIVITY/REST	
• Fatigue, weakness	• Lethargy
• Insomnia	• Decreased tolerance to activity
• Prolonged immobility and bedrest	
CIRCULATION	
• History of recent or chronic heart failure (HF)	• Tachycardia
	• Flushed appearance, pallor, central cyanosis
FOOD/FLUID	
• Loss of appetite	• Distended abdomen
• Nausea, vomiting	• Hyperactive bowel sounds

DIAGNOSTIC DIVISION MAY REPORT (continued)

- May be receiving intestinal, gastric feedings

MAY EXHIBIT (continued)

- Dry skin with poor turgor
- Cachectic appearance (malnutrition)

Neurosensory

May Report:

- Frontal headache (influenza)

May Exhibit:

- Changes in mentation, such as confusion, somnolence
- Changes in behavior, such as irritability, restlessness, lethargy

Pain/Discomfort

May Report:

- Headache
- Chest pain (pleuritic) aggravated by cough
- Substernal chest pain (influenza)
- Myalgia, arthralgia
- Abdominal pain

May Exhibit:

- Splinting, guarding over affected area
- Position—commonly lies on affected side to restrict movement

Respiration

May Report:

- History of recurrent or chronic upper respiratory infections (URIs), tuberculosis, COPD, cigarette smoking
- Progressive shortness of breath
- Presence of tracheostomy, endotracheal tube
- Current treatment with mechanical ventilator
- Cough is dry and hacking (initially), progressing to productive cough

May Exhibit:

- ***Respirations:*** Tachypnea, shallow grunting respirations
- Use of accessory muscles, nasal flaring
- Breath sounds are diminished or absent over involved area
  - Bronchial breath sounds over area(s) of consolidation
  - Coarse inspiratory crackles
- ***Color:*** Pallor or cyanosis of lips or nailbeds
- ***Sputum:*** Scanty or copious; pink, rusty, or purulent (green, yellow, or white)
- ***Percussion:*** Dull over consolidated areas
- ***Fremitus:*** Tactile and vocal, gradually increases with consolidation
- Pleural friction rub
- (P) Signs of respiratory distress (Bradley et al, 2011)
  - Tachypnea—respiratory rate, breaths/min
    - Age 0–2 months: >60
    - Age 2–12 months: >50
    - Age 1–5 years: >40
    - Age 5 years: >20
  - Dyspnea
  - Retractions (suprasternal, intercostals, or subcostal); nasal flaring
  - Grunting
  - Apnea
  - Altered mental status
  - Pulse oximetry measurement 90% room air

Safety

May Report:

- Recurrent chills
- History of altered immune system, such as systemic lupus erythematosus (SLE), AIDS, active malignancies, neurological disease, HF, diabetes, steroid or chemotherapy use; institutionalization, general debilitation

May Exhibit:

- Diaphoresis
- Shaking
- Rash, in cases of rubeola or varicella
- Fever of 102°F to 104°F (39°C to 40°C)

Teaching/Learning

- Recent surgery, chronic alcohol use or long history of alcoholism, intravenous (IV) drug therapy or abuse, chemotherapy or other immunosuppressive therapy
- Use of herbal supplements, such as garlic, ginkgo, licorice, onion, turmeric, horehound, marshmallow, mullein, wild cherry bark, astragalus, echinacea, elderberry, goldenseal, Oregon grape root

Discharge Plan Considerations

- Assistance with self-care, homemaker tasks
- Supplemental oxygen, especially if recovery is prolonged or other predisposing condition exists

➧ Refer to section at end of plan for postdischarge considerations.

Diagnostic Studies

TEST WHY IT IS DONE	WHAT IT TELLS ME
DIAGNOSTIC TESTS	
• *Chest x-ray:* Evaluates organs and structures within the chest. Confirms the diagnosis of pneumonia. • (P) Chest x-rays are not routinely done for children, but should be obtained in child with suspected or documented hypoxemia or significant respiratory distress.	Confirms diagnosis of pneumonia. Identifies structural distribution of pneumonia, such as lobar or bronchial. May show scattered or localized infiltration (bacterial) or diffuse and extensive nodular infiltrates (more often viral). In *Mycoplasma pneumonia*, chest x-ray may be clear.
• *Ultrasongraphy:* Uses ultrasonic waves to visualize internal organs for possible pathology.	(P) Recent studies have found that point-of-care ultrasound imaging can diagnose pneumonia in children and young adults with higher specificity than x-ray (Shah, 2013).
• *Complete blood count (CBC):* Battery of screening tests that typically includes hemoglobin (Hgb); hematocrit (Hct); red blood cell (RBC) count, morphology, indices, and distribution width index; platelet count and size; white blood cell (WBC) count and differential. Provides baseline data about the hematologic system and yields information related to oxygen-carrying capacity and infection.	Leukocytosis with a left shift is usually present in bacterial pneumonia, although a low WBC count may be present in viral infection, immunosuppressed conditions such as AIDS, and overwhelming bacterial pneumonia.
• *Sputum studies:* Collection is often necessary to determine the etiology of disease, type of organisms, and sensitivity to antibiotics. Serial sputum studies may be necessary to determine response to treatment.	More than one type of organism may be present. The bacterium *Streptococcus pneumonia* accounts for 25% to 35% of all community-acquired pneumonias. Fifty percent of pneumonia cases are believed to be caused by viruses and tend to result in less severe illness than pneumonia triggered by bacteria. Viral pneumonia is more commonly seen in the younger population. Mycoplasma pneumonia is one of the most common causes of atypical pneumonia and is caused by an unknown virus. Opportunistic pneumonias (organisms causing disease in a host whose resistance to fight infection is diminished) consists of *Pneumocystis carinii*, cytomegalovirus, and tuberculosis (TB) (Daniels, 2012). *Note:* Sputum cultures may not identify all offending organisms. Blood cultures may show transient bacteremia.
• (P) *RSV washing:* Detects virus that is being shed in the respiratory/nasal secretions of an infected child usually between age 6 months to 2 years.	Rapid results help guide treatment options and possible need for further testing if results are negative in a symptomatic child.
• (P) *Blood cultures:* Determines presence of infection.	Identification of specific organism useful in choice of therapy for child requiring hospitalization for presumed bacterial pneumonia or in outpatient setting for children receiving antibiotic therapy who demonstrate progressive deterioration (Bradley, 2011).
ASSOCIATED TESTS	
• *Serologic studies (viral or Legionella titers, cold agglutinins):* Assist in differential diagnosis of specific organism.	Provide information on the specific organism causing the pneumonia or can rule out other diseases.
• *Arterial blood gases (ABGs):* Measure oxygen and carbon dioxide levels to rule out hypoxemia or hypercapnia.	Abnormalities may be present, depending on extent of lung involvement and underlying lung disease.
• *Bronchoscopy:* Insertion of a flexible scope into the airways allows direct visualization of tracheobronchial tree for abnormalities and to obtain sputum for cytological examination.	May be both diagnostic (qualitative cultures) and therapeutic (reexpansion of lung segment).
• *Pulse oximetry:* Noninvasive measure of arterial blood oxygen diffusion and saturation. • (P) Should be performed in child with pneumonia and suspected hypoxemia.	The percentage expressed is the ratio of oxygen to Hgb. Pulse oximetry less than 90% indicates significant hypoxia. Abnormally low levels (<88%) indicate impaired gas exchange and impending respiratory failure.

Nursing Priorities

1. Maintain or improve respiratory function.
2. Prevent complications.
3. Support recuperative process.
4. Provide information about disease process, prognosis, and treatment.

Discharge Goals

1. Ventilation and oxygenation adequate for individual needs.
2. Complications prevented or minimized.
3. Disease process, prognosis, and therapeutic regimen understood.
4. Lifestyle changes identified and initiated to prevent recurrence.
5. Plan in place to meet needs after discharge.

NURSING DIAGNOSIS: ineffective Airway Clearance

May Be Related To

Infection—[tracheal bronchial inflammation, edema formation]; chronic obstructive pulmonary disease
Exudate in alveoli

Possibly Evidenced By

Changes in respiratory rate
Diminished/adventitious breath sounds
Dyspnea, cyanosis
Ineffective cough

Desired Outcomes/Evaluation Criteria—Client Will

Respiratory Status: Airway Patency (NOC)

Identify and demonstrate behaviors to achieve airway clearance.
Display patent airway with breath sounds clearing and absence of dyspnea and cyanosis.

ACTIONS/INTERVENTIONS	RATIONALE
Airway Management (NIC)	
Independent	
Assess rate and depth of respirations and chest movement. Monitor for signs of respiratory failure, for example, cyanosis and severe tachypnea.	Tachypnea, shallow respirations, and asymmetric chest movement are frequently present because of discomfort of moving chest wall or fluid in lung. When pneumonia is severe, the client may require endotracheal intubation and mechanical ventilation to keep airways clear.
Auscultate lung fields, noting areas of decreased or absent airflow and adventitious breath sounds, such as crackles and wheezes.	Decreased airflow occurs in areas consolidated with fluid. Bronchial breath sounds (normal over bronchus) can also occur in consolidated areas. Crackles, rhonchi, and wheezes are heard on inspiration and expiration in response to fluid accumulation, thick secretions, and airway spasm or obstruction.
Elevate head of bed; change position frequently.	Keeping the head elevated lowers diaphragm, promoting chest expansion, aeration of lung segments, and mobilization and expectoration of secretions to keep the airway clear.
Assist client with frequent deep-breathing exercises. Demonstrate and help client, as needed; learn to perform activity, such as splinting chest and effective coughing while in upright position.	Deep breathing facilitates maximum expansion of the lungs and smaller airways. Coughing is a natural self-cleaning mechanism, assisting the cilia to maintain patent airways. Splinting reduces chest discomfort, and an upright position favors deeper, more forceful cough effort. *Note:* Cough associated with pneumonias may last days, weeks, or even months.
Suction, as indicated, for example, oxygen desaturation related to airway secretions.	Stimulates cough or mechanically clears airway in client who is unable to do so because of ineffective cough or decreased level of consciousness.
Force fluids to at least 2500 mL per day, unless contraindicated, as in HF. Offer warm, rather than cold, fluids.	Fluids, especially warm liquids, aid in mobilization and expectoration of secretions.
Collaborative	
Assist with and monitor effects of nebulizer treatments and other respiratory physiotherapy, such as incentive spirometer, intermittent positive-pressure breathing (IPPB), percussion, and postural drainage. Perform treatments between meals and limit fluids when appropriate.	Facilitates liquefaction and removal of secretions. Postural drainage may not be effective in interstitial pneumonias or those causing alveolar exudates or destruction. Coordination of treatments, schedules, and oral intake reduces likelihood of vomiting with coughing and expectorations.

(continues on page 134)

ACTIONS/INTERVENTIONS (continued) / RATIONALE (continued)

Administer medications, as indicated, for example, mucolytics, expectorants, bronchodilators, and analgesics.

Aids in reduction of bronchospasm and mobilization of secretions. Analgesics are given to improve cough effort by reducing discomfort but should be used cautiously because they can decrease cough effort and depress respirations.

Provide supplemental fluids such as IV, humidified oxygen, and room humidification.

Fluids are required to replace losses, including insensible losses, and aid in mobilization of secretions. *Note:* Some studies indicate that room humidification has been found to provide minimal benefit and is thought to increase the risk of transmitting infection.

Monitor serial chest x-rays, ABGs, and pulse oximetry readings. (Refer to ND: impaired Gas Exchange, following.)

Follows progress and effects of disease process and therapeutic regimen and facilitates necessary alterations in therapy.

NURSING DIAGNOSIS: impaired Gas Exchange

May Be Related To

Alveolar-capillary membrane changes
Ventilation-perfusion imbalance

Possibly Evidenced By

Dyspnea, abnormal skin color (e.g., pale, dusky)
Tachycardia
Restlessness; confusion
Hypoxia

Desired Outcomes/Evaluation Criteria—Client Will

Respiratory Status: Gas Exchange (NOC)

Demonstrate improved ventilation and oxygenation of tissues by ABGs within client's acceptable range and absence of symptoms of respiratory distress.
Participate in actions to maximize oxygenation.

ACTIONS/INTERVENTIONS / RATIONALE

Respiratory Monitoring (NIC)

Independent

Assess respiratory rate, depth, and ease.

Manifestations of respiratory distress are dependent on, and indicative of, the degree of lung involvement and underlying general health status.

Observe color of skin, mucous membranes, and nailbeds, noting presence of peripheral cyanosis (nailbeds) or central cyanosis (circumoral).

Cyanosis of nailbeds may represent vasoconstriction or the body's response to fever or chills; however, cyanosis of earlobes, mucous membranes, and skin around the mouth ("warm membranes") is indicative of systemic hypoxemia.

Assess mental status.

Restlessness, irritation, confusion, and somnolence may reflect hypoxemia or decreased cerebral oxygenation.

Monitor heart rate and rhythm.

Tachycardia is usually present as a result of fever and dehydration, but may represent a response to hypoxemia.

Monitor body temperature, as indicated. Assist with comfort measures to reduce fever and chills, such as addition or removal of bedcovers, comfortable room temperature, and tepid or cool water sponge bath.

High fever, common in bacterial pneumonia and influenza, greatly increases metabolic demands and oxygen consumption and alters cellular oxygenation.

Maintain bedrest. Encourage use of relaxation techniques and diversional activities.

Prevents exhaustion and reduces oxygen consumption and demands to facilitate resolution of infection.

Elevate head and encourage frequent position changes, deep breathing, and effective coughing.

These measures promote maximal inspiration and enhance expectoration of secretions to improve ventilation. (Refer to ND: ineffective Airway Clearance.)

Assess level of anxiety. Encourage verbalization of concerns and feelings. Answer questions honestly. Visit frequently and arrange for significant other (SO) and visitors to stay with client as indicated.

Anxiety is a manifestation of psychological concerns and physiological responses to hypoxia. Providing reassurance and enhancing sense of security can reduce the psychological component, thereby decreasing oxygen demand and adverse physiological responses.

Observe for deterioration in condition, noting hypotension, copious amounts of pink or bloody sputum, pallor, cyanosis, change in level of consciousness, severe dyspnea, and restlessness.

Shock and pulmonary edema are the most common causes of death in pneumonia and require immediate medical intervention.

Collaborative

Monitor ABGs and pulse oximetry.

Identifies problems, such as ventilatory failure; follows progress of disease process or improvement; and facilitates alterations in pulmonary therapy.

Oxygen Therapy (NIC)

Administer oxygen therapy by appropriate means, for example, nasal prongs, mask, Venturi mask.

The purpose of oxygen therapy is to maintain PaO_2 above 60 mm Hg, or greater than 90% O_2 saturation. Oxygen is administered by the method that provides appropriate delivery within the client's tolerance.

Prepare for and transfer to critical care unit if indicated.

Intubation and mechanical ventilation may be required in the event of severe respiratory insufficiency. (Refer to CP: Ventilatory Assistance [Mechanical].)

NURSING DIAGNOSIS: risk for Infection [spread]

Risk Factors May Include

Inadequate primary defenses—decreased ciliary action, stasis of body fluids [respiratory secretions]
Inadequate secondary defenses—[presence of existing infection], immunosuppression; chronic disease, malnutrition

Possibly Evidenced By

(Not applicable; presence of signs and symptoms establishes an *actual* diagnosis)

Desired Outcomes/Evaluation Criteria—Client Will

Infection Severity (NOC)

Achieve timely resolution of current infection without complications.

Risk Control: Infectious Process (NOC)

Identify interventions to prevent and reduce risk and spread of a secondary infection.

ACTIONS/INTERVENTIONS / RATIONALE

Infection Control (NIC)

Independent

Monitor vital signs closely, especially during initiation of therapy.

During this period, potentially fatal complications, such as hypotension or shock, may develop.

Instruct client concerning the disposition of secretions (e.g., raising and expectorating versus swallowing) and reporting changes in color, amount, and odor of secretions.

Although client may find expectoration offensive and attempt to limit or avoid it, it is essential that sputum be disposed of in a safe manner. Changes in characteristics of sputum reflect resolution of pneumonia or development of secondary infection.

Demonstrate and encourage good hand-washing technique.

Effective means of reducing spread or acquisition of infection.

Change position frequently and provide good pulmonary toilet.

Promotes expectoration, clearing of infection.

Perform proper suctioning technique for ventilated clients as appropriate.

Secretions that accumulate below and above the endotracheal (ET) tube cuff are an ideal growth medium for pathogens. The ET tube also prevents normal closure of the epiglottis, resulting in an incomplete seal of the laryngeal structures that normally protect the lungs. This can contribute to aspiration and VAP (Pruitt & Jacobs, 2006).

Limit visitors as indicated.

Reduces likelihood of exposure to other infectious pathogens.

Institute isolation precautions as individually appropriate (e.g, masks and gloves, possibly gowns) during client contact.

Depending on type of infection, response to antibiotics, client's general health, and development of complications, isolation techniques may be instituted to prevent spread and protect client from other infectious processes.

(P) RSV (which is highly contagious) and certain other infective agents that cause pneumonia in children require that caregivers, family, and visitors be protected.

Encourage adequate rest balanced with moderate activity. Promote adequate nutritional intake.

Facilitates healing process and enhances natural resistance.

Monitor effectiveness of antimicrobial therapy.

Signs of improvement in condition should occur within 24 to 48 hours.

Investigate sudden changes or deterioration in condition, such as increasing chest pain, extra heart sounds, altered sensorium, recurring fever, and changes in sputum characteristics.

Delayed recovery or increase in severity of symptoms suggests resistance to antibiotics or secondary infection. Complications affecting any organ system include lung abscess,

(continues on page 136)

ACTIONS/INTERVENTIONS	RATIONALE
	empyema, bacteremia, pericarditis, endocarditis, meningitis, encephalitis, and superinfections.
Collaborative	
Administer antimicrobials, as indicated, by results of sputum and blood cultures, for example, ***macrolides*** such as azithromycin (Zithromax), clarithromycin (Biaxin), erythromycin (E-Mycin); ***penicillin combinations***, for example, amoxicillin (Amoxil) and clavulanate (Augmentin); ***tetracyclines***, for example, doxycycline (Doryx, Bio-Tab), minocycline (Minocin); ***fluoroquinolones***, for example, moxifloxacin (Avelox), levofloxacin (Levaquin), ciprofloxin (Cipro); ***cephalosporins***, for example, cefuroxime (Kefurox, Zinacef), cefaclor (Ceclor), ceftazidime (Ceptax, Fortaz); ***ketolides***, for example, telithromycin (KETEK); ***oxazolidinones***, for example, linezolid (Zyvox).	These drugs are used to combat most of the microbial pneumonias. Combinations of drugs can be used when the pneumonia is a result of mixed organisms. P Amoxicillin is used as first-line therapy for previously healthy, immunized infant and preschool child with mild to moderate CAP suspected to be of bacterial origin (Bradley et al, 2011).
P Provide influenza antiviral therapy (e.g., oseltamivir [Tamiflu]), as indicated.	Should be administered as soon as possible to child with moderate to severe CAP consistent with influenza virus infection during widespread local circulation of influenza viruses (Bradley et al, 2011).
Prepare for and assist with additional diagnostic studies, as indicated.	Fiberoptic bronchoscopy may be done for clients who do not respond in a reasonable amount of time to antimicrobial therapy to clarify diagnosis and therapeutic needs.

NURSING DIAGNOSIS: Activity Intolerance

May Be Related To
Imbalance between oxygen supply and demand
General weakness

Possibly Evidenced By
Report of weakness, fatigue, exertional dyspnea
Tachypnea
Abnormal heart rate response to activity

Desired Outcomes/Evaluation Criteria—Client Will

Activity Tolerance (NOC)
Report and demonstrate a measurable increase in tolerance to activity with absence of dyspnea and excessive fatigue, with vital signs within client's acceptable range.

ACTIONS/INTERVENTIONS	RATIONALE
Energy Management (NIC)	
Independent	
Evaluate client's response to activity. Note reports of dyspnea, increased weakness and fatigue, and changes in vital signs during and after activities.	Establishes client's capabilities and needs and facilitates choice of interventions.
Provide a quiet environment and limit visitors during acute phase, as indicated. Encourage use of stress management and diversional activities as appropriate.	Reduces stress and excess stimulation, promoting rest.
Explain importance of rest in treatment plan and necessity for balancing activities with rest.	Bed and chair rest is maintained during acute phase to decrease metabolic demands, thus conserving energy for healing. Activity restrictions thereafter are determined by individual client response to activity and resolution of respiratory insufficiency.
Assist client to assume comfortable position for rest and sleep.	Client may be comfortable with head of bed elevated, sleeping in a chair, or leaning forward on over-bed table with pillow support.
Assist with self-care activities as necessary. Provide for progressive increase in activities during recovery phase.	Minimizes exhaustion and helps balance oxygen supply and demand.

NURSING DIAGNOSIS: acute Pain

May Be Related To

Injuring agents (e.g., biological—inflammation of lung parenchyma, cellular reactions to circulating toxins; physical—persistent coughing)

Possibly Evidenced By

Verbal/coded report [pleuritic chest pain, headache, muscle or joint pain]
Guarded behavior
Expressive behavior—restlessness

Desired Outcomes/Evaluation Criteria—Client Will

Pain Level (NOC)

Verbalize relief or control of pain.
Demonstrate relaxed manner, resting, sleeping, and engaging in activity appropriately.

ACTIONS/INTERVENTIONS	RATIONALE
Pain Management (NIC)	
Independent	
Determine pain characteristics, such as sharp, constant, and stabbing. Investigate changes in character, location, and intensity of pain.	Chest pain, usually present to some degree with pneumonia, may also herald the onset of complications of pneumonia, such as pericarditis and endocarditis.
Monitor vital signs.	Changes in heart rate or blood pressure (BP) may indicate that client is experiencing pain, especially when other reasons for changes in vital signs have been ruled out.
Provide comfort measures, such as back rubs, change of position, and quiet music or conversation. Encourage use of relaxation and breathing exercises.	Nonanalgesic measures administered with a gentle touch can lessen discomfort and augment therapeutic effects of analgesics. Client involvement in pain control measures promotes independence and enhances sense of well-being.
Offer frequent oral hygiene.	Mouth breathing and oxygen therapy can irritate and dry out mucous membranes, potentiating general discomfort.
Instruct and assist client in chest-splinting techniques during coughing episodes. (Refer to ND: ineffective Airway Clearance.)	Aids in control of chest discomfort while enhancing effectiveness of cough effort.
Collaborative	
Administer analgesics and antitussives, as indicated.	These medications may be used to suppress nonproductive or paroxysmal cough or reduce excess mucus, thereby enhancing general comfort and rest.

NURSING DIAGNOSIS: risk for imbalanced Nutrition: less than body requirements

Risk Factors May Include

Biological factors—increased metabolic needs [fever, infectious process]
[Abdominal distention and gas (swallowing air during dyspneic episodes)]

Possibly Evidenced By

(Not applicable; presence of signs and symptoms establishes an *actual* diagnosis)

Desired Outcomes/Evaluation Criteria—Client Will

Nutritional Status (NOC)

Demonstrate increased appetite.
Maintain or regain desired body weight.

ACTIONS/INTERVENTIONS	RATIONALE
Nutrition Management (NIC)	
Independent	
Identify factors that are contributing to inability to eat, such as severe dyspnea, pain, nausea and vomiting, copious sputum, or respiratory treatments.	Choice of interventions depends on the underlying cause of the problem.

(continues on page 138)

ACTIONS/INTERVENTIONS (continued)	RATIONALE (continued)
Provide covered container for sputum and replace at frequent intervals. Assist with and encourage oral hygiene after emesis, after aerosol and postural drainage treatments, and before meals.	Eliminates noxious sights, tastes, and smells from the client's environment and can reduce nausea.
Schedule respiratory treatments at least 1 hour before meals.	Reduces effects of nausea associated with these treatments.
Auscultate for bowel sounds. Observe and palpate for abdominal distention.	Bowel sounds may be diminished or absent if the infectious process is severe or prolonged. Abdominal distention may occur because of air swallowing or reflect the influence of bacterial toxins on the gastrointestinal (GI) tract.
Provide small, frequent meals, including dry foods, such as toast or crackers, and foods that are appealing to client.	These measures may enhance intake even though appetite may be slow to return.
Evaluate general nutritional state.	Lifestyle, financial, and socioeconomic conditions prior to present illness condition can contribute to malnutrition. Client may present with hypermetabolic state and lowered resistance to infection, which can exacerbate malnutrition and delay response to therapy.
Weigh regularly and graph results.	Monitors effectiveness of nutritional therapy.
Collaborative	
Assist in treatment of underlying condition(s).	May promote healing and strengthen immune system, improve appetite, and enhance general well-being.
Consult dietitian and nutritional team.	To develop dietary plan individualized to client's specific needs and challenges.

NURSING DIAGNOSIS: risk for deficient Fluid Volume

Risk Factors May Include

Excessive losses through normal routes—[e.g., fever, profuse diaphoresis, mouth breathing, hyperventilation]

Deviations affecting intake of fluids

Possibly Evidenced By

(Not applicable; presence of signs and symptoms establishes an *actual* diagnosis)

Desired Outcomes/Evaluation Criteria—Client Will

Fluid Balance (NIC)

Demonstrate fluid balance evidenced by individually appropriate parameters, such as moist mucous membranes, good skin turgor, prompt capillary refill, and stable vital signs.

ACTIONS/INTERVENTIONS	RATIONALE
Fluid Management (NIC)	
Independent	
Assess vital sign changes, such as increased temperature, prolonged fever, tachycardia, and orthostatic hypotension.	Elevated temperature or prolonged fever increases metabolic rate and fluid loss through evaporation. Orthostatic BP changes and increasing tachycardia may indicate systemic fluid deficit.
Assess skin turgor, moisture of mucous membranes—lips and tongue.	Indirect indicators of adequacy of fluid volume, although oral mucous membranes may be dry because of mouth breathing and supplemental oxygen.
Note reports of nausea and vomiting.	Presence of these symptoms reduces oral intake.
Monitor intake and output (I&O), noting color and character of urine. Calculate fluid balance. Be aware of insensible losses. Weigh as indicated.	Provides information about adequacy of fluid volume and replacement needs.
Force fluids to at least 3000 mL per day or as individually appropriate.	Meets basic fluid needs, reducing risk of dehydration.
(P) Ensure child is receiving daily maintenance fluids, in addition to covering fluid losses caused by current conditions (e.g., fever, inability to take oral fluids, vomiting).	Basic fluid needs are determined by child's weight—up to 10 kg: 100 mL/kg/24 hr; 10 to 20 kg: 50 mL/kg/24 hr; more than 20 kg: 20 mL/24 hr. Note that the smaller the child, the greater the percentage of weight is water (Ferki, 2011).
Collaborative	
Administer medications, as indicated, such as antipyretics, antiemetics.	Useful in reducing fluid losses.
Provide supplemental IV fluids as necessary.	In the presence of reduced intake or excessive loss, use of parenteral route may correct or prevent deficiency.

NURSING DIAGNOSIS: deficient Knowledge [Learning Need] regarding condition, treatment, self-care, and discharge needs

May Be Related To

Lack of exposure
Information misinterpretation
Lack of recall

Possibly Evidenced By

Reports the problem
Inaccurate follow-through of instructions

Desired Outcomes/Evaluation Criteria—Client Will

Knowledge: Pneumonia Management (NOC)

Verbalize understanding of condition, disease process, and prognosis.
Verbalize understanding of therapeutic regimen.
Initiate necessary lifestyle changes.
Participate in treatment program.

ACTIONS/INTERVENTIONS	RATIONALE
Teaching: Disease Process (NIC) *Independent*	
Review normal lung function and pathology of condition.	Promotes understanding of current situation and importance of cooperating with treatment regimen.
Discuss debilitating aspects of disease, length of convalescence, and recovery expectations. Identify self-care and homemaker needs and resources.	Information can enhance coping and help reduce anxiety and excessive concern. Respiratory symptoms may be slow to resolve, and fatigue and weakness can persist for an extended period. These factors may be associated with depression and the need for various forms of support and assistance.
Provide information in written and verbal form.	Fatigue and depression can affect ability to assimilate information and follow medical regimen. Having written instructions for later referral may help client/SO in following previous verbal instructions.
Emphasize importance of continuing effective coughing and deep-breathing exercises.	Continuing respiratory exercises may be necessary for an extended period of time while chest is congested and secretions are difficult to manage.
Stress necessity of continuing antimicrobial therapy for prescribed length of time.	Early discontinuation of antibiotics may result in failure to completely resolve infectious process.
Review importance of cessation of smoking. Refer to smoking cessation program, or physician as indicated.	Smoking destroys tracheobronchial ciliary action, irritates bronchial mucosa, and inhibits alveolar macrophages, compromising body's natural defense against infection.
Outline steps to enhance general health and well-being, such as balanced rest and activity, well-rounded diet, program of aerobic exercise or strength training (particularly elderly individuals), and avoidance of crowds during cold and flu season and of persons with upper respiratory infections.	Recent research suggests elderly people with moderate physical limitations can significantly improve immunological defenses through exercise that increases levels of salivary IgA—immunoglobulin that aids in blocking infectious agents entering through mucous membranes.
Stress importance of continuing medical follow-up and obtaining vaccinations and immunizations as appropriate for both children and adults.	May prevent recurrence of pneumonia and related complications. *Note:* In the United States, there are several vaccines that prevent infection by bacteria or viruses that may cause pneumonia. These vaccines include pneumococcal, *Haemophilus influenzae* type b (Hib), pertussis (whooping cough), varicella (chickenpox), measles, and influenza (flu) vaccine (CDC, 2012). (P) *Note:* RSV lower respiratory tract infection has been found to be a risk factor for asthma and wheezing later in childhood (Sorce, 2009).
Identify signs and symptoms requiring notification of healthcare provider, such as increasing dyspnea, chest pain, prolonged fatigue, weight loss, fever or chills, persistence of productive cough, and changes in mentation.	Prompt evaluation and timely intervention may prevent or minimize complications.

POTENTIAL CONSIDERATIONS following acute hospitalization (dependent on client's age, physical condition and presence of complications, personal resources, and life responsibilities)

- ***Fatigue***—disease states, stress
- ***risk for Infection***—inadequate secondary response (e.g., leukopenia, suppressed inflammatory response), chronic disease, malnutrition, [current use of antibiotics]
- ***ineffective Self-Health Management***—complexity of therapeutic regimen, economic difficulties, perceived seriousness and susceptibility.

Sample clinical pathway follows in Table 5.1.

TABLE 5.1 Sample CP: Bacterial Pneumonia, Hospital. ELOS: 5 Days Medical Unit

ND and Categories of Care	Day 1 ADM_____	Day 2 _____	Day 3 _____	Day 4 Discharge_____
impaired Gas Exchange R/T alveolar congestion, inflammation, hypoventilation	Goals: Participate in activities to maximize oxygenation and airway clearance	Demonstrate improving ventilation and oxygenation by lessening symptoms of respiratory distress, ABGs approaching acceptable levels	Verbalize understanding of general healthcare needs Demonstrate ABGs within client's acceptable range and absence of respiratory distress	Initiate activities accepting responsibility for therapeutic regimen within level of ability Plan in place to meet postdischarge needs
Referrals	Pulmonary specialist		Home care Home O_2/Resp. Therapist	
Diagnostic studies	CXR			
	ABGs, CBC, electrolytes		Hb/Hct	
	Sputum C&S/Gram stain			
	Blood culture		Repeat if WBC count elevated, febrile, or ABGs not WNL	
	Pulse oximetry q4h	→ Repeat if pulse ox <87% → D/C if 92%		
Additional assessments	Respiratory rate, rhythm, depth; use of accessory muscles; color of skin and mucous membranes q4h	→	→ q8h	→
	Breath sounds q4h	→	→ q8h	→
	Cough and sputum characteristics	→	→	→
	Vital signs q4h	→	→ q8h	→
	I&O q8h	→	→	→
	Weight qd	→	→	→
Medications	IV antibiotics	→	→ PO	→
Allergies:	Bronchodilator via MDI or nebulizer	→ MDI	→	→
___________	Mucolytic	→	→	→
___________	Antitussives prn	→	→	→
	Acetaminophen if temperature above 101°F	→	→ D/C	
	Analgesics—prn	→ D/C		
Client education	Orient to unit and room Review advance directives Diagnostic tests and results Pulmonary hygiene: T, C, DB, splinting techniques	Adaptive breathing techniques as indicated Pacing of activities Smoking cessation, fluid and nutritional needs, balancing activity and rest	Individual risk factors, prevention of recurrence, vaccinations and immunizations Signs and symptoms to report to healthcare provider	Provide written instructions Medications postdischarge: dose, time, route, purpose, side effects Proper use and care of home-care equipment (e.g., O_2, concentrator, nebulizer)

TABLE 5.1 Sample CP: Bacterial Pneumonia, Hospital. ELOS: 5 Days Medical Unit (continued)

ND and Categories of Care	Day 1 ADM____	Day 2 ____	Day 3 ____	Day 4 Discharge____ Schedule for follow-up appointments
Additional nursing actions	Position for maximal respiratory effort	→ per self	→	→
	Assist with physical care	→	→ as needed	→
	Incentive spirometry q4h	→	→ per self WA	→ D/C
	Supplemental O_2	→	→	→
	Oral care prn	→ per self	→	→ D/C
	Suction as indicated	→	→	→ D/C
	Screen visitors and staff for URI	→	→	
	Encourage fluid to 2500 mL/day as tolerated		→	→ per self

Key: ABG, arterial blood gas; C, cough; CBC, complete blood count; C&S, culture and sensitivity; CXR, chest x-ray; DB, deep breath; D/C, discontinue; ELOS, expected length of stay; Hb/Hct, hemoglobin/hemocrit; I&O, intake and output; qd, every day; MDI, metered-dose inhaler; prn, as necessary; q4h, every 4 hours; q8h, every 8 hours; R/T, related to; T, turn; URI, upper respiratory infection; WA, while awake; WBC, white blood cell; WNL, within normal limits.

LUNG CANCER: POSTOPERATIVE CARE

I. Pathophysiology

a. Usually develops within the wall or epithelium of the bronchial tree

b. Exposure to environmental and occupational carcinogens and an individual's susceptibility to these carcinogens are thought to increase the risk for developing lung cancer. Smoking continues to be the leading cause of lung cancer, accounting for 90% of cases. Tobacco smoke contains more than 40 known carcinogenic agents responsible for DNA mutation. Occupational hazards, including exposure to asbestos and radon, account for about 10% to 15% of cases.

II. Classification (National Cancer Institute, 2010). Cancers of the lung are divided into two major subdivisions:

a. Small cell lung carcinomas (SCLC) and Non-small cell lung carcinomas (NSCLC).

b. SCLC account for approximately 15% of lung cancers, while NSCLC account for approximately 85% of lung cancers.

III. Staging of the tumor is an important prognosticator of the extent of disease. The TNM (tumor-node-metastasis) system, developed by the American Joint Commission for Staging and End Results Reporting, is used to assess the extent of disease.

a. T describes the size and extent of invasion of the cancer into the epithelium;

b. N describes involvement of the lymph nodes; and

c. M describes the extent of metastasis.

d. The system further divides the carcinomas in terms of four stages (I–IV) and two substages (A and B), which have important treatment and prognosis implications.

IV. Etiology (American Cancer Society, 2011)

a. While tobacco smoking is believed to account for 90% of lung cancer cases, not all smokers develop lung cancer and some patients with lung cancer have never smoked. Twenty-five percent of cancers in the non-smoking population may be attributed to inhalation of secondhand smoke.

b. While genetic predisposition can be attributed to all populations, certain other factors, either in conjunction with smoking or independent of smoking, are population-specific, including chronic viral exposure; exposure to arsenic, radon, asbestos; and environmental carcinogens.

V. Statistics

a. Morbidity

i. Lung cancer is the most common cause of cancer worldwide. In the United States, lung cancer is the second most common cancer in women, and second only to prostate cancer in men. Though the rate of lung cancer in men has declined, the incidence in women has risen.

ii. The probability of developing lung cancer increases after age 40 in both sexes and peaks around age 70, especially in men.

iii. African American men who smoke have a 40% increased risk of developing cancer, possibly due to smoking habits and increased susceptibility.

b. Mortality

i. In 2009, 158,081 died of lung cancer in the United States and 1.37 million died worldwide.

ii. Lung cancer has the highest mortality rate in industrialized countries, paralleling trends in smoking, and while the mortality rate for men is higher than for women, the lung cancer mortality rate of women in the United States is the highest in the world.

c. Cost—Annual cost in the United States estimated to be $12.12 billion (Mariotto et al, 2011).

VI. Treatment Options (National Cancer Institute, 2010)

a. Depends upon staging—generally the lower the stage, the more favorable the prognosis

i. Surgery is primary treatment for NSCLC stage I and stage II tumors.

ii. Selected stage III carcinomas may be operable if the tumor is resectable.

(continues on page 142)

b. Surgical procedures for operable tumors of the lung include:
   i. Pneumonectomy—performed for lesions originating in the main-stem bronchus or lobar bronchus
   ii. Lobectomy—preferred for peripheral carcinoma localized in a lobe
   iii. Wedge or segmental resection—performed for lesions that are small and well contained within one segment
   iv. Endoscopic laser resection—may be done on peripheral tumors to reduce the necessity of cutting through ribs
   v. Photodynamic therapy—reduces symptoms such as bleeding or may be used to treat very small tumors
   vi. Cryotherapy—instrument is used to freeze and destroy the tumor
   vii. Electrotherapy—electrical current is used to cauterize (burn) and destroy the tumor

GLOSSARY

Clubbing: Broadening or thickening of the tips of the fingers (and toes) with increased lengthwise curvature of the nail and a decrease in the angle normally seen between the cuticle and the fingernail. Clubbing may be seen in a wide variety of conditions, most of which result in decreased blood oxygen.

Fremitus: Vibration in the chest over areas of consolidation, detectable by palpation.

Hemoptysis: Expectoration of blood or of blood-stained sputum.

Lobectomy: Removal of one lobe.

Photodynamic therapy (PTD): A two-step outpatient procedure where a photosensitizing agent, porfimer sodium (Photofrin), is injected into the bloodstream, specifically targeting cancer cells. The second part of the procedure—24 to 72 hours later—involves inserting a laser light through a scope to the cancerous cells. The light activates the drug, resulting in a chemical reaction that destroys cancerous cells and blood vessels supplying the tumor.

Pneumonectomy: Removal of an entire lung.

Staging: Classification as to the extent of disease, based on pathology report from tissue obtained during bronchoscopy, needle (or other) biopsy, blood work, and imaging studies to rule out distant metastases.

Wedge or segmental resection: Removal of the tumor and a small part of the lung.

Care Setting

Primary Health Care Settings—aimed at health education, prevention (Stop Smoking and Clean Air Campaigns), early diagnosis, and follow-up care

Secondary Health Care Settings—referral to specialists in pulmonology, thoracic surgery, oncology, radiology, nutrition, occupational therapy, outpatient/ambulatory surgery, hospice, home care

Tertiary Health Care Settings—inpatient medical-surgical unit, ICU

Related Concerns

Cancer, page 827
Pneumothorax/hemothorax, page 150
Psychosocial aspects of care, page 729
Radical neck surgery: laryngectomy (postoperative care), see Davis*Plus*
Surgical intervention, page 762

Client Assessment Database (Preoperative)

Findings depend on type, duration of cancer, and extent of metastasis.

DIAGNOSTIC DIVISION MAY REPORT	MAY EXHIBIT
ACTIVITY/REST	
• Fatigue, inability to maintain usual routine • Dyspnea with activity	• Lassitude—usually in advanced stage
CIRCULATION	
• Swelling of extremities • Fast heart rate	• Jugular vein distention (JVD), with vena caval obstruction • *Heart sounds:* Pericardial rub, indicating effusion • Tachycardia and dysrhythmias • Clubbing of fingers
EGO INTEGRITY	
• Frightened feelings, fear of outcome of surgery • Denial of severity of condition and potential for malignancy	• Restlessness • Repetitive questioning

DIAGNOSTIC DIVISION

MAY REPORT (continued)	MAY EXHIBIT (continued)
ELIMINATION • Intermittent diarrhea, due to hormonal imbalance, small cell lung cancer (SCLC) • Increased frequency and amount of urine, due to hormonal imbalance (epidermoid tumor)	
FOOD/FLUID • Weight loss • Poor appetite, decreased food intake • Difficulty swallowing • Thirst, increased fluid intake	• Thin, emaciated, or wasted appearance in late stages • Edema of face or neck, chest, back, due to vena caval obstruction; facial or periorbital edema, due to hormonal imbalance (SCLC) • Glucose in urine, due to hormonal imbalance (epidermoid tumor)
PAIN/DISCOMFORT • Chest pain—not usually present in early stages and not always present in advanced stages • Pain may or may not be affected by position • Shoulder or arm pain, particularly with large cell carcinoma or adenocarcinoma • Bone and joint pain—cartilage erosion secondary to increased growth hormones (large cell carcinoma or adenocarcinoma) • Intermittent abdominal pain	• Distraction behaviors, such as restlessness, withdrawal • Guarding and protective actions
RESPIRATION • History of smoking; occupational exposure to pollutants, industrial dusts, such as asbestos, iron oxides, coal dust, or to radioactive materials • Mild cough or change in usual cough pattern, sputum production • Shortness of breath • Hoarseness or change in voice, such as with vocal cord paralysis	• Dyspnea, aggravated by exertion • Increased tactile fremitus, indicating consolidation • Brief crackles or wheezes on inspiration or expiration • Persistent crackles or wheezes; tracheal shift (space-occupying lesion) • Hemoptysis
SAFETY	• Fever may be present, with large cell carcinoma or adenocarcinoma • Bruising, discoloration of skin, due to hormonal imbalance (SCLC)
SEXUALITY	• Gynecomastia, due to neoplastic hormonal changes (large cell carcinoma) • Amenorrhea, impotence, due to hormonal imbalance (SCLC)
TEACHING/LEARNING • Familial risk factors—cancer, especially lung, tuberculosis • Failure to improve • Use of vitamins or herbal supplements, such as vitamins A, C, E; riboflavin; folic acid; ashwagandha; birch; yellow doc; milk thistle; turmeric; ginger; red clover; echinacea; astragalus; reishi and shiitake mushrooms; zedoary	
DISCHARGE PLAN CONSIDERATIONS • Assistance with transportation, medications, treatments, self-care, homemaker and maintenance tasks ➧ Refer to section at end of plan for postdischarge considerations.	

Diagnostic Studies

TEST	
Note: These tests may be done preoperatively (not necessarily a comprehensive listing)	
WHY IT IS DONE	**WHAT IT TELLS ME**
• *Carcinoembryonic antigen (CEA, also called carcinogenic antigen):* A cancer-specific immune system protein that is present in many adenocarcinomas, including lung adenocarcinoma.	Increased preoperative levels of CEA usually suggest a poor prognosis. A CEA level greater than 50 may indicate advanced-stage lung cancer.
• *Parathyroid hormone protein-related PTHPR):* Measures the release of a protein—similar to parathyroid hormone—produced by some cancers, including all lung cancers.	Blood levels of PTHRP may help to distinguish lung cancer from cancer of the pleura or other diseases, is responsible for the clinical syndrome of hypercalcemia of malignancy, may stimulate proliferation of cancer cells, and is a factor in development of bone metastasis.
• *Lymphocyte count:* Determines number of white blood cells present.	Lymphocytopenia or decreased level of cells can occur with surgical procedures and is associated with shorter survival times for clients with advanced lung cancer. Preoperative treatment with recombinant human interleukin-2 (RHIL-2) may help prevent the lymphocyte decrease.
• *Chest x-ray, posteroanterior (PA) and lateral:* Evaluates organs or structures within the chest.	Lung cancer is often discovered on chest x-ray. Size and location of mass can be determined. Peripheral nodules and hilar and mediastinal changes may suggest lymphadenopathy. Pleural effusions and endobronchial obstruction may be seen.
• *Thoracic CT:* An imaging method that uses x-rays to create cross-sectional pictures of the chest and upper abdomen.	A CT scan is frequently the second step either to follow up on an abnormal chest x-ray finding or to evaluate troublesome symptoms in those with a normal chest x-ray.
• *Positron emission tomography (PET) scan:* Nuclear imaging scan used to evaluate and stage lung cancer.	Identifies occult metastatic disease in the mediastinum and distant sites. More sensitive and specific than CT scan and may be used in combination with, or instead of, CT to determine tumor size and location and for staging.
• *Magnetic resonance imaging (MRI) scan:* Uses magnetic fields to produce two- or three-dimensional images of organs inside the body.	Used to confirm abnormalities seen on chest x-ray, to detect early (<1 cm) lesions not visible on chest x-ray, and to assess spread to the mediastinum. Outlines shape, size, and location of lesion. May reveal erosion of ribs or vertebrae.
• *Pulmonary function studies: including total lung capacity (TLC), functional residual capacity (FRC), and residual volume (RV):* Provide information on the extent of the pulmonary abnormality and if there is air-trapping in the lungs.	Volumes may be increased, indicating air-trapping, especially advanced disease. If airways are blocked by tumor, an obstructive pattern of pulmonary disease may lead to increased or decreased FRC (Schumann, 2005).
• *Biopsy:* May be performed using forceps or needle or may be via open surgical incision. Allows for direct and microscopic examination of tissue for presence of malignant cells.	Needle biopsy may be performed on scalene nodes, hilar lymph nodes, or pleura to establish diagnosis. Tissue biopsy of metastatic sites is used to stage disease and determine prognosis and treatment.
TESTS THAT MAY BE DONE POSTOPERATIVELY	
• *Arterial blood gases (ABGs):* Measures arterial oxygen (PaO_2), carbon dioxide tension ($PaCO_2$), and acidity (pH).	Done to evaluate ventilation and acid-base status to determine treatment needs and response to therapy.
• *Pulse oximetry:* Noninvasive method of measuring arterial oxyhemoglobin saturation (SaO_2) via sensor placed on fingertip or earlobe.	
• *Complete blood count (CBC):* Measures the levels of components in blood, including hemoglobin and hematocrit (Hgb/Hct), red blood cells (RBCs), white blood cells (WBCs) and their components (differential), and platelets.	Identifies presence of anemia (low Hgb/Hct, RBCs) and potential or presence of infection (changes in numbers of WBCs and differential). Altered platelets can cause/exacerbate bleeding and bruising.

Nursing Priorities

1. Maintain or improve respiratory function.
2. Control or alleviate pain.
3. Support efforts to cope with diagnosis and situation.
4. Provide information about disease process, prognosis, and therapeutic regimen.

Discharge Goals

1. Oxygenation and ventilation adequate to meet individual activity needs.
2. Pain controlled.
3. Anxiety and fear decreased to manageable level.
4. Free of preventable complications.
5. Disease process, prognosis, and planned therapies understood.
6. Plan in place to meet needs after discharge.

NURSING DIAGNOSIS: impaired Gas Exchange

May Be Related To

Ventilation-perfusion imbalance [removal of lung tissue, hypoventilation, hypovolemia]

Possibly Evidenced By

Dyspnea
Restlessness
Confusion
Abnormal arterial blood gases—hypoxia, hypercapnia
Abnormal skin color

Desired Outcomes/Evaluation Criteria—Client Will

Respiratory Status: Gas Exchange (NOC)

Demonstrate improved ventilation and adequate oxygenation of tissues by arterial blood gases (ABGs) within client's normal range.
Be free of symptoms of respiratory distress.

ACTIONS/INTERVENTIONS	RATIONALE
Respiratory Monitoring (NIC)	
Independent	
Note respiratory rate, depth, and ease of respirations. Observe for use of accessory muscles, pursed-lip breathing, or changes in skin or mucous membrane color, such as pallor and cyanosis.	Respirations may be increased as a result of pain or as an initial compensatory mechanism to accommodate for loss of lung tissue. However, increased work of breathing and cyanosis may indicate increasing oxygen consumption and energy expenditures or reduced respiratory reserve, for example, in an elderly client or extensive COPD.
Auscultate lungs for air movement and abnormal breath sounds.	Consolidation and lack of air movement on operative side are normal in the client who has had a pneumonectomy; however, a client who has had a lobectomy should demonstrate normal airflow in remaining lobes.
Investigate restlessness and changes in mentation and level of consciousness.	May indicate increased hypoxia or complications such as mediastinal shift in a client who has had a pneumonectomy when accompanied by tachypnea, tachycardia, and tracheal deviation.
Assess client response to activity. Encourage rest periods, limiting activities to client tolerance.	Increased oxygen consumption and demand and stress of surgery may result in increased dyspnea and changes in vital signs with activity; however, early mobilization is desired to help prevent pulmonary complications and to obtain and maintain respiratory and circulatory efficiency. Adequate rest balanced with activity can prevent respiratory compromise.
Note development of fever.	Fever within the first 24 hours after surgery is frequently due to atelectasis. Temperature elevation within postoperative day 5 to 10 usually indicates an infection, such as wound or systemic.
Airway Management (NIC)	
Maintain patent airway by positioning, suctioning, and use of airway adjuncts.	Airway obstruction impedes ventilation, impairing gas exchange. (Refer to ND: ineffective Airway Clearance.)

(continues on page 146)

ACTIONS/INTERVENTIONS (continued) / RATIONALE (continued)

Reposition frequently, placing client in sitting and supine to side positions.
RATIONALE: Maximizes lung expansion and drainage of secretions.

Avoid positioning client with a pneumonectomy on the operative side; instead, favor the "good lung down" position.
RATIONALE: Research shows that positioning clients following lung surgery with their "good lung down" maximizes oxygenation by using gravity to enhance blood flow to the healthy lung, thus creating the best possible match between ventilation and perfusion.

Encourage and assist with deep-breathing exercises and pursed-lip breathing, as appropriate.
RATIONALE: Promotes maximal ventilation and oxygenation and reduces or prevents atelectasis.

Tube Care: Chest (NIC)

Maintain patency of chest drainage system following lobectomy and segmental wedge resection procedures.
RATIONALE: Drains fluid from pleural cavity to promote reexpansion of remaining lung segments.

Note changes in amount or type of chest tube drainage.
RATIONALE: Bloody drainage should decrease in amount and change to a more serous composition as recovery progresses. A sudden increase in amount of bloody drainage or return to frank bleeding suggests thoracic bleeding or a hemothorax; sudden cessation suggests blockage of tube, requiring further evaluation and intervention.

Observe for presence of bubbling in water-seal chamber.
RATIONALE: Air leaks appearing immediately postoperatively are not uncommon, especially following lobectomy or segmental resection; however, this should diminish as healing progresses. Prolonged or new leaks require evaluation to identify problems in client versus a problem in the drainage system.

Airway Management (NIC)

Collaborative

Administer supplemental oxygen via nasal cannula, partial rebreathing mask, or high-humidity face mask, as indicated.
RATIONALE: Maximizes available oxygen, especially while ventilation is reduced because of anesthetic, depression, or pain, and during period of compensatory physiological shift of circulation to remaining functional alveolar units.

Assist with and encourage use of incentive spirometer.
RATIONALE: Prevents or reduces atelectasis and promotes reexpansion of small airways.

Monitor and graph ABGs and pulse oximetry readings.
RATIONALE: Decreasing PaO_2 or increasing $PaCO_2$ may indicate need for ventilatory support.

Note hemoglobin (Hgb) levels.
RATIONALE: Significant blood loss results in decreased oxygen-carrying capacity, reducing PaO_2.

NURSING DIAGNOSIS: ineffective Airway Clearance

May Be Related To

Excessive mucus; retained secretions
[Restricted chest movement—pain, weakness]

Possibly Evidenced By

Changes in respiratory rate
Adventitious breath sounds
Ineffective cough
Dyspnea

Desired Outcomes/Evaluation Criteria—Client Will

Respiratory Status: Airway Patency (NOC)

Demonstrate patent airway, with fluid secretions easily expectorated, clear breath sounds, and noiseless respirations.

ACTIONS/INTERVENTIONS / RATIONALE

Airway Management (NIC)

Independent

Auscultate chest for character of breath sounds and presence of secretions.
RATIONALE: Noisy respirations, rhonchi, and wheezes are indicative of retained secretions or airway obstruction.

Assist client with and provide instruction in effective deep breathing, coughing in upright position (sitting), and splinting of incision.
RATIONALE: Upright position favors maximal lung expansion, and splinting improves force of cough effort to mobilize and remove secretions. Splinting may be done by nurse placing hands anteriorly and posteriorly over chest wall and by client, with pillows, as strength improves.

ACTIONS/INTERVENTIONS (continued)	RATIONALE (continued)
Observe amount and character of sputum and aspirated secretions. Investigate changes, as indicated.	Increased amounts of colorless (or blood-streaked) or watery secretions are normal initially and should decrease as recovery progresses. Presence of thick, tenacious, bloody, or purulent sputum suggests development of secondary problems—for example, dehydration, pulmonary edema, local hemorrhage, or infection—that require correction or treatment.
Suction if cough is weak or breath sounds not cleared by cough effort. Avoid deep endotracheal and nasotracheal suctioning in client who has had pneumonectomy if possible.	"Routine" suctioning increases risk of hypoxemia and mucosal damage. Deep tracheal suctioning is generally contraindicated following pneumonectomy to reduce the risk of rupture of the bronchial stump suture line. If suctioning is unavoidable, it should be done gently and only to induce effective coughing.
Encourage oral fluid intake, at least 2500 mL/day, within cardiac tolerance.	Adequate hydration aids in keeping secretions loose and enhances expectoration.
Assess for pain and discomfort and medicate on a routine basis and before breathing exercises.	Encourages client to move, cough more effectively, and breathe more deeply to prevent respiratory insufficiency.
Collaborative	
Provide and assist client with incentive spirometer and postural drainage and percussion, as indicated.	Improves lung expansion and ventilation and facilitates removal of secretions. *Note:* Postural drainage may be contraindicated in some clients and, in any event, must be performed cautiously to prevent respiratory embarrassment and incisional discomfort.
Use humidified oxygen and ultrasonic nebulizer. Provide additional fluids intravenously (IV), as indicated.	Providing maximal hydration helps loosen and liquefy secretions to promote expectoration. Impaired oral intake necessitates IV supplementation to maintain hydration.
Administer bronchodilators, expectorants, and analgesics, as indicated.	Relieves bronchospasm to improve airflow. Expectorants increase mucus production and liquefy and reduce viscosity of secretions, facilitating removal. Alleviation of chest discomfort promotes cooperation with breathing exercises and enhances effectiveness of respiratory therapies.

NURSING DIAGNOSIS: acute Pain

May Be Related To

Injuring agents—(biological [cancer invasion of pleura, chest wall]; physical [surgical incision, tissue trauma, presence of chest tube])

Possibly Evidenced By

Verbal/coded report
Guarded behavior
Expressive behavior–restlessness
Narrowed focus
Changes in blood pressure (BP), heart, or respiratory rate

Desired Outcomes/Evaluation Criteria—Client Will

Pain Level (NOC)

Report pain relieved or controlled.
Appear relaxed and sleep or rest appropriately.
Participate in desired as well as needed activities.

ACTIONS/INTERVENTIONS	RATIONALE
Pain Management (NIC)	
Independent	
Ask client about pain. Determine pain location and characteristics, for example, continuous, aching, stabbing, or burning. Have client rate intensity on a scale (e.g., numeric, faces, etc.)	Helpful in evaluating cancer-related pain symptoms, which may involve viscera, nerve, or bone tissue. Use of rating scale aids client in assessing level of pain and provides tool for evaluating effectiveness of analgesics, enhancing client control of pain.
Assess client's verbal and nonverbal pain cues.	Discrepancy between verbal and nonverbal cues may provide clues to degree of pain and need for and effectiveness of interventions.

(continues on page 148)

ACTIONS/INTERVENTIONS (continued)	RATIONALE (continued)
Note possible psychological as well as pathophysiological causes of pain.	Fear, distress, anxiety, and grief over confirmed diagnosis of cancer can impair ability to cope. In addition, a posterolateral incision is more uncomfortable for client than an anterolateral incision. The presence of chest tubes can greatly increase discomfort.
Evaluate effectiveness of pain control. Encourage sufficient medication to manage pain; change medication or time span as appropriate.	Pain perception and pain relief are subjective, thus pain management is best left to client's discretion. If client is unable to provide input, the nurse should observe physiological and nonverbal signs of pain and administer medications on a regular basis.
Encourage verbalization of feelings about the pain.	Fears and concerns can increase muscle tension and lower threshold of pain perception. (Refer to ND: Anxiety [specify level], following.)
Provide comfort measures such as frequent changes of position, back rubs, and support with pillows. Encourage use of relaxation techniques, including visualization, guided imagery, and appropriate diversional activities.	Promotes relaxation and redirects attention. Relieves discomfort and augments therapeutic effects of analgesia.
Schedule rest periods; provide quiet environment.	Decreases fatigue and conserves energy, enhancing coping abilities.
Assist with self-care activities, breathing and arm exercises, and ambulation.	Prevents undue fatigue and incisional strain. Encouragement and physical assistance and support may be needed for some time before client is able or confident enough to perform these activities because of pain or fear of pain.
Collaborative	
Assist with patient-controlled analgesia (PCA) or analgesia through epidural catheter. Administer intermittent analgesics routinely, as indicated, especially 45 to 60 minutes before respiratory treatments and deep-breathing and coughing exercises.	Maintaining a constant drug level avoids cyclic periods of pain, aids in muscle healing, and improves respiratory function and emotional comfort and coping.

NURSING DIAGNOSIS: Anxiety [specify level]

May Be Related To

Situational crises
Threat to or change in health status
Threat of death

Possibly Evidenced By

Apprehensive; worried
Poor eye contact
Increased pulse, respiration, blood pressure
Insomnia

Desired Outcomes/Evaluation Criteria—Client Will

Anxiety Level (NOC)

Demonstrate appropriate range of feelings and appear relaxed and resting appropriately.

Anxiety Self-Control (NOC)

Acknowledge and discuss fears and concerns.
Verbalize accurate knowledge of situation.
Report beginning use of individually effective coping strategies.

ACTIONS/INTERVENTIONS	RATIONALE
Anxiety Reduction (NIC)	
Independent	
Evaluate client and significant other (SO) level of understanding of diagnosis.	Client and SO are hearing and assimilating new information that includes changes in self-image and lifestyle. Understanding perceptions of those involved sets the tone for individualizing care and provides information necessary for choosing appropriate interventions.
Acknowledge reality of client's fears and concerns and encourage expression of feelings.	Support may enable client to begin exploring and dealing with the reality of cancer and its treatment. Client may need time to identify feelings and even more time to begin to express them.

ACTIONS/INTERVENTIONS (continued)	RATIONALE (continued)
Provide opportunity for questions and answer them honestly. Be sure that client and care providers have the same understanding of terms used.	Establishes trust and reduces misperceptions or misinterpretation of information.
Accept, but do not reinforce, client's denial of the situation.	When extreme denial or anxiety is interfering with progress of recovery, the issues facing client need to be explained and resolutions explored.
Note comments and behaviors indicative of beginning acceptance or use of effective strategies to deal with situation.	Fear and anxiety will diminish as client begins to accept and deal positively with reality. Indicator of client's readiness to accept responsibility for participation in recovery and to "resume life."
Involve client and SO in care planning. Provide time to prepare for events and treatments	May help restore some feeling of control and independence to client who feels powerless in dealing with diagnosis and treatment.
Provide for client's physical comfort.	It is difficult to deal with emotional issues when experiencing extreme or persistent physical discomfort.

NURSING DIAGNOSIS: deficient Knowledge [Learning Need] regarding condition, treatment, prognosis, self-care, and discharge needs

May Be Related To
Lack of exposure, unfamiliarity with resources
Information misinterpretation
Lack of recall

Possibly Evidenced By
Reports the problem
Inadequate follow-through of instruction
Inappropriate or exaggerated behaviors—agitated, apathetic

Desired Outcomes/Evaluation Criteria—Client Will

Knowledge: Cancer Management (NOC)
Verbalize understanding of ramifications of diagnosis, prognosis, and possible complications.
Participate in learning process.
Verbalize understanding of therapeutic regimen.
Correctly perform necessary procedures and explain reasons for the actions.
Initiate necessary lifestyle changes.

ACTIONS/INTERVENTIONS	RATIONALE
Teaching: Disease Process (NIC)	
Independent	
Discuss diagnosis, current and planned therapies, and expected outcomes.	Provides individually specific information, creating knowledge base for subsequent learning regarding home management. Radiation or chemotherapy may follow surgical intervention, and information is essential to enable the client and SO to make informed decisions.
Reinforce surgeon's explanation of particular surgical procedure, providing diagram as appropriate. Incorporate this information into discussion about short- and long-term recovery expectations.	Length of rehabilitation and prognosis depend on type of surgical procedure, preoperative physical condition, and duration and degree of complications.
Discuss necessity of planning for follow-up care before discharge.	Follow-up assessment of respiratory status and general health is imperative to assure optimal recovery. Also provides opportunity to readdress concerns or questions at a less stressful time.
Identify signs and symptoms requiring medical evaluations, such as changes in appearance of incision, development of respiratory difficulty, fever, increased chest pain, and changes in appearance of sputum.	Early detection and timely intervention may prevent or minimize complications.
Stress importance of avoiding exposure to smoke, air pollution, and contact with individuals with upper respiratory infections (URIs).	Protects lung(s) from irritation and reduces risk of infection.
Review nutritional and fluid needs. Suggest increasing protein and use of high-calorie snacks as appropriate.	Meeting cellular energy requirements and maintaining good circulating volume for tissue perfusion facilitate tissue regeneration and healing process

(continues on page 150)

ACTIONS/INTERVENTIONS (continued)	RATIONALE (continued)
Identify individually appropriate community resources, such as American Cancer Society, visiting nurse, social services, and home care.	Agencies such as these offer a broad range of services that can be tailored to provide support and meet individual needs.
Prescribed Activity/Exercise (NIC)	
Help client determine activity tolerance and set goals.	Weakness and fatigue should decrease as lung heals and respiratory function improves during recovery period, especially if cancer was completely removed. If cancer is advanced, it is emotionally helpful for client to be able to set realistic activity goals to achieve optimal independence.
Evaluate availability and adequacy of support system(s) and necessity for assistance in self-care and home management.	General weakness and activity limitations may reduce individual's ability to meet own needs.
Encourage alternating rest periods with activity and light tasks with heavy tasks. Emphasize avoidance of heavy lifting and isometric or strenuous upper body exercise. Reinforce physician's time limitations about lifting.	Generalized weakness and fatigue are usual in the early recovery period but should diminish as respiratory function improves and healing progresses. Rest and sleep enhance coping abilities, reduce nervousness (common in this phase), and promote healing. *Note:* Strenuous use of arms can place undue stress on incision because chest muscles may be weaker than normal for 3 to 6 months following surgery.
Recommend stopping any activity that causes undue fatigue or increased shortness of breath.	Exhaustion aggravates respiratory insufficiency.
Instruct and provide rationale for arm and shoulder exercises. Have client or SO demonstrate exercises. Encourage following graded increase in number and intensity of routine repetitions.	Simple arm circles and lifting arms over the head or out to the affected side are initiated on the first or second postoperative day to restore normal range of motion (ROM) of shoulder and to prevent ankylosis of the affected shoulder.
Incision Site Care (NIC)	
Encourage inspection of incisions. Review expectations for healing with client.	Healing begins immediately, but complete healing takes time. As healing progresses, incision lines may appear dry with crusty scabs. Underlying tissue may look bruised and feel tense, warm, and lumpy (resolving hematoma).
Instruct client and SO to watch for and report places in incision that do not heal or reopening of healed incision, any drainage (bloody or purulent), and localized area of swelling with redness or increased pain that is hot to touch.	Signs and symptoms indicating failure to heal, development of complications requiring further medical evaluation and intervention.
Suggest wearing soft cotton shirts and loose-fitting clothing; cover portion of incision with pad, as indicated, and leave incision open to air as much as possible, unless compression garment is used.	Reduces suture line irritation and pressure from clothing. Leaving incisions open to air promotes healing process and may reduce risk of infection.
Shower in warm water, washing incision gently. Avoid tub baths until approved by physician.	Keeps incision clean and promotes circulation and healing. *Note:* "Climbing" out of tub requires use of arms and pectoral muscles, which can put undue stress on incision.
Support incision with butterfly bandages as needed when sutures and staples are removed.	Aids in maintaining approximation of wound edges to promote healing.

POTENTIAL CONSIDERATIONS following hospitalization (dependent on client's age, physical condition and presence of complications, personal resources, and life responsibilities)

- ***ineffective Airway Clearance***—excessive mucus, retained secretions, [pain, fatigue]
- ***acute Pain***—physical—surgical incision, tissue trauma, disruption of intercostal nerves, anxiety
- ***Self-Care Deficit***—fatigue, pain/discomfort, weakness

Refer to CP: Cancer for other considerations.

PNEUMOTHORAX/HEMOTHORAX

I. Pathophysiology

a. Partial or complete collapse of lung due to accumulation of air (pneumothorax), blood (hemothorax), or other fluid (pleural effusion) in the pleural space

b. Intrathoracic pressure changes induced by increased pleural space volumes and reduced lung capacity, causing respiratory distress and gas exchange problems and producing tension on mediastinal structures that can impede cardiac and systemic circulation

c. Complications include hypoxemia, respiratory failure, and cardiac arrest.

II. Classification

a. Primary spontaneous pneumothorax

b. Secondary spontaneous pneumothorax

c. Iatrogenic pneumothorax

d. Traumatic pneumothorax

III. Etiology

a. Primary spontaneous: rupture of pleural blebs typically occurs in young people without parenchymal lung disease or occurs in the absence of traumatic injury to the chest or lungs

b. Secondary spontaneous: occurs in the presence of lung disease, primarily emphysema, but can also occur with tuberculosis (TB), sarcoidosis, cystic fibrosis, malignancy, and pulmonary fibrosis

c. Iatrogenic: complication of medical or surgical procedures, such as therapeutic thoracentesis, tracheostomy, pleural biopsy, central venous catheter insertion, positive-pressure mechanical ventilation, inadvertent intubation of right main-stem bronchus

d. Traumatic: most common form of pneumothorax and hemothorax, caused by open or closed chest trauma related to blunt or penetrating injuries

IV. **Statistics** (American Lung Association, June 2005; Schiffman, 2012)

a. Morbidity: Primary spontaneous pneumothorax affects 9000 persons per year and is more common in tall, thin men between 20 and 40 years of age.

b. Recurrence rate is about 40% for both primary and secondary spontaneous pneumothorax, occurring in intervals of 1.5 to 2 years.

c. Mortality: Rate is 15% for those with secondary pneumothorax associated with underlying lung disease.

GLOSSARY

Blunt force chest trauma: Closed trauma to the chest may result in laceration of lung tissue or an artery by a rib, causing blood to collect in the pleural space.

Chest tube drainage unit (CDU): Drainage system that is connected to a chest tube to remove air or fluids from the chest cavity or pleural space. The device consists of a water seal and collection chambers and a suction-control chamber, or a one-way mechanical valve, depending on the amount of drainage anticipated and the client's level of mobility.

Crepitation: A dry, crackling sound or sensation on auscultation or palpation of the skin, indicating the presence of subcutaneous emphysema, or air trapped in the tissues, associated with a pneumothorax.

Empyema: Pus from an infection, such as pneumonia, in the pleural space.

Fremitus: Vibratory sensation or tremors felt through the chest wall during coughing or speaking.

Hemopneumothorax: Both air and blood in the pleural space.

Hemothorax: Collection of blood in the pleural space, which can exert pressure on the lung, causing it to collapse.

Hypercapnia: Increased level of carbon dioxide in the blood.

Hypoxemia: Decreased level of oxygen in the blood.

Penetrating chest trauma: Chest trauma in which a weapon, such as a knife, bullet, or needle, lacerates the lung.

Pleural effusion: Excessive fluid in the pleural space.

Pleural space: Area between the parietal pleura (membrane lining the chest cavity) and the visceral pleura, which surrounds the lungs. Normally, this potential space holds about 50 mL of lubricating fluid that prevents friction between the pleurae as they move during inhalation and exhalation.

Pneumothorax: Buildup of air in the pleural space, exerting pressure against the lung and causing it to collapse.

Tachypnea: Abnormally rapid respirations.

Tension pneumothorax: Unrelieved accumulation of air in the intrapleural space shifts mediastinum to unaffected side, thus impairing ventilation and compromising cardiac function and venous return.

Thoracentesis: Use of a needle to rapidly remove fluid from the pleural space.

Care Setting

Client is treated in inpatient medical or surgical unit. A small pneumothorax without underlying lung disease may resolve on its own.

Related Concerns

Cardiac surgery: postoperative care, page 98
Chronic obstructive pulmonary disease (COPD) and asthma, page 118
Psychosocial aspects of care, page 729
Pulmonary tuberculosis (TB), page 170
Ventilatory assistance (mechanical), page 157

Client Assessment Database

Findings vary depending on the amount of air and/or fluid accumulation, rate of accumulation, and underlying lung function

DIAGNOSTIC DIVISION MAY REPORT	MAY EXHIBIT
ACTIVITY/REST	
• Shortness of breath • Tiredness	• Dyspnea with activity or even at rest

(continues on page 152)

DIAGNOSTIC DIVISION MAY REPORT (continued)	MAY EXHIBIT (continued)
CIRCULATION	• Tachycardia; irregular rate, dysrhythmias • S_3 or S_4 or gallop heart rhythm—heart failure (HF) secondary to effusion • Apical pulse reveals point of maximal impulse (PMI) displaced in presence of mediastinal shift with tension pneumothorax • Homan's sign—crunching sound correlating with heartbeat, reflecting air in mediastinum • *Blood pressure (BP):* Hypertension or hypotension • Jugular vein distention (JVD), especially with tension pneumothorax
EGO INTEGRITY • Anxiety, apprehension	• Restlessness, irritability
PAIN/DISCOMFORT • Unilateral chest pain, aggravated by breathing, coughing, and movement • Sudden onset of symptoms while coughing or straining—spontaneous pneumothorax • Sharp, stabbing pain aggravated by deep breathing, possibly radiating to neck, shoulders, abdomen—pleural effusion	• Guarding affected area • Distraction behaviors • Facial grimacing
RESPIRATION • History of recent chest surgery or trauma; chronic lung disease, lung inflammation or infection (empyema or effusion); diffuse interstitial disease (sarcoidosis); malignancies (e.g., obstructive tumor) • Previous spontaneous pneumothorax; spontaneous rupture of emphysematous bulla, subpleural bleb in COPD • Difficulty breathing, "air hunger" • Coughing, which may be presenting symptom	• *Respirations:* Tachypnea • Increased work of breathing, use of accessory muscles in chest, neck; intercostal retractions; forced abdominal expiration • Breath sounds decreased or absent on involved side • Fremitus decreased on involved site • *Chest percussion:* Hyperresonance over air-filled area—pneumothorax; dullness over fluid-filled area—hemothorax • *Chest observation and palpation:* Unequal or paradoxical chest movement (if trauma, flail), reduced thoracic excursion on affected side • *Skin:* Pallor, cyanosis, diaphoresis, subcutaneous crepitation • *Mentation:* Anxiety, restlessness, confusion, stupor • Use of positive-pressure mechanical ventilation or positive end-expiratory pressure (PEEP) therapy
SAFETY • Recent chest trauma, such as fractured ribs, penetrating wound • Radiation and chemotherapy for malignancy • Presence of central intravenous (IV) line	
TEACHING/LEARNING • History of familial risk factors, such as TB, cancer • Recent intrathoracic surgery or lung biopsy	
DISCHARGE PLAN CONSIDERATIONS • Temporary assistance with self-care, homemaker and maintenance tasks ➧ Refer to section at end of plan for postdischarge considerations.	

Diagnostic Studies

TEST WHY IT IS DONE	WHAT IT TELLS ME
DIAGNOSTIC STUDIES	
• *Chest x-ray:* Evaluates organs or structures within the chest and is the initial study of choice in blunt force chest trauma.	May show chest wall fractures, injuries to the heart or great vessels, and reveal air and fluid accumulation in the pleural space; may show shift of mediastinal structures (heart).
• *Thoracic computed tomography (CT):* Enhances anatomic views of the chest and locates abnormalities. Early CT may influence therapeutic management.	CT is more sensitive than x-ray in detecting thoracic injuries, lung contusion, hemothorax, and pneumothorax.

Nursing Priorities

1. Promote or maintain lung reexpansion for adequate oxygenation and ventilation.
2. Minimize or prevent complications.
3. Reduce discomfort and pain.
4. Provide information about disease process, treatment regimen, and prognosis.

Discharge Goals

1. Adequate ventilation and oxygenation maintained.
2. Complications prevented or resolved.
3. Pain absent or controlled.
4. Disease process, prognosis, and therapy needs understood.
5. Plan in place to meet needs after discharge.

NURSING DIAGNOSIS: ineffective Breathing Pattern

May Be Related To

Musculoskeletal impairment
Pain; anxiety

Possibly Evidenced By

Dyspnea, tachypnea
Alterations in depth of breathing; altered chest excursion
Use of accessory muscles to breath, nasal flaring
Decreased vital capacity

Desired Outcomes/Evaluation Criteria—Client Will

Respiratory Status: Ventilation (NOC)

Establish a normal and effective respiratory pattern with ABGs within client's normal range.
Be free of cyanosis and other signs or symptoms of hypoxia.

ACTIONS/INTERVENTIONS	RATIONALE
Respiratory Monitoring (NIC)	
Independent	
Identify etiology or precipitating factors, such as spontaneous collapse, trauma, malignancy, infection, and complication of mechanical ventilation.	Understanding the cause of lung collapse is necessary for proper chest tube placement and choice of other therapeutic measures.
Evaluate respiratory function, noting rapid or shallow respirations, dyspnea, reports of "air hunger," development of cyanosis, and changes in vital signs.	Respiratory distress and changes in vital signs occur because of physiological stress and pain or may indicate development of shock due to hypoxia or hemorrhage.
Monitor for asynchronous respiratory pattern when using mechanical ventilator. Note changes in airway pressures.	Difficulty breathing with ventilator or increasing airway pressures suggests worsening of condition and development of complications, such as spontaneous rupture of a bleb creating a new pneumothorax.
Auscultate breath sounds.	Breath sounds may be diminished or absent in a lobe, lung segment, or entire lung field (unilateral). Atelectatic area will have no breath sounds, and partially collapsed areas have decreased sounds. Regularly scheduled evaluation also helps determine areas of good air exchange and provides a baseline to evaluate resolution of pneumothorax.

(continues on page 154)

ACTIONS/INTERVENTIONS (continued)	RATIONALE (continued)
Note chest excursion and position of trachea.	Chest excursion is unequal until lung reexpands. Trachea deviates from affected side with tension pneumothorax.
Assess fremitus.	Voice and tactile fremitus (vibration) is reduced in fluid-filled or consolidated tissue.
Ventilation Assistance (NIC)	
Assist client with splinting painful area when coughing or during deep breathing.	Supporting chest and abdominal muscles makes coughing more effective and less traumatic.
Maintain position of comfort, usually with head of bed elevated. Turn to affected side. Encourage client to sit up as much as possible.	Promotes maximal inspiration; enhances lung expansion and ventilation in unaffected side.
Maintain a calm attitude, assisting client to "take control" by using slower, deeper respirations.	Assists client to deal with the physiological effects of hypoxia, which may be manifested as anxiety or fear.
Tube Care: Chest (NIC)	
Ascertain type of client's chest drainage system.	This care plan concerns the hospitalized client whose treatment plan includes use of a traditional chest drainage system. Mobile drains are indicated for those clients who are ambulatory and do not require a suction for reinflation of lungs.
Once chest tube is inserted:	
Determine if dry-seal chest drain or water-seal system is used.	Some chest drains use a mechanical one-way valve in place of a conventional water seal. The one-way valve allows air to escape from the chest and prevents air from entering the chest. Dry suction-control systems regulate suction pressure mechanically rather than with a column of water. Some dry suction systems use a screw-type valve that varies the size of the opening to the vacuum source, thereby limiting the amount of negative pressure that can be transmitted to the chest. These valves narrow the opening of the chest drain in order to adjust the level of negative pressure; therefore, the total amount of air that can flow out of the chest drain is also limited. Thus, this type of dry suction-control mechanism is impractical for clients with significant pleural air leaks (Atrium Product Support, no date given).
If water-seal system is used:	
Check suction-control chamber for correct amount of suction, as determined by water level, wall or table regulator, at correct setting.	Maintains prescribed intrapleural negativity, which promotes optimum lung expansion and fluid drainage. *Note:* Dry-seal setups are also used with an automatic control valve (AVC), which provides a one-way valve seal similar to that achieved with the water-seal system.
Check fluid level in water-seal chamber; maintain at prescribed level.	Water in a sealed chamber serves as a barrier that prevents atmospheric air from entering the pleural space should the suction source be disconnected and aids in evaluating whether the chest drainage system is functioning appropriately. *Note:* Underfilling the water-seal chamber leaves it exposed to air, putting client at risk for pneumothorax or tension pneumothorax. Overfilling, a more common mistake, prevents air from easily exiting the pleural space, thus preventing resolution of pneumothorax and possibly creating a tension pneumothorax.
Observe for bubbling in water-seal chamber.	Bubbling during expiration reflects venting of pneumothorax (desired action). Bubbling usually decreases as the lung expands or may occur only during expiration or coughing as the pleural space diminishes. Absence of bubbling may indicate complete lung reexpansion (normal) or represent complications, such as obstruction, in the tube.
Evaluate for abnormal or continuous water-seal chamber bubbling.	With suction applied, this indicates a persistent air leak that may be from a large pneumothorax at the chest insertion site (client centered) or chest drainage unit (system centered).
Determine location of air leak (client or system centered) by clamping thoracic catheter just distal to exit from chest.	If bubbling stops when catheter is clamped at insertion site, leak is client centered at insertion site or within the client.
Place petrolatum gauze or other appropriate material around the insertion as indicated.	Usually corrects insertion site air leak.
Clamp tubing in stepwise fashion downward toward drainage unit if air leak continues.	Isolates location of a system-centered air leak. *Note:* As a rule, clamping for a suspected leak is the only time that chest tube should be clamped.
Seal drainage tubing connection sites securely with lengthwise tape or bands according to established policy.	Prevents or corrects air leaks at connector sites.

ACTIONS/INTERVENTIONS (continued)	RATIONALE (continued)
Monitor water-seal chamber "tidaling." Note whether change is transient or permanent.	The water-seal chamber serves as an intrapleural manometer (gauges intrapleural pressure); therefore, fluctuation, or tidaling, reflects pressure differences between inspiration and expiration. Tidaling of 2 to 6 cm during inspiration is normal and may increase briefly during coughing episodes. Continuation of excessive tidal fluctuations may indicate existence of airway obstruction or presence of a large pneumothorax.
Position drainage system tubing for optimal function; for example, shorten tubing or coil extra tubing on bed, making sure tubing is not kinked or hanging below entrance to drainage container. Drain accumulated fluid as necessary.	Improper position, kinking, or accumulation of clots and fluid in the tubing changes the desired negative pressure and impedes air or fluid evacuation. *Note:* If a dependent loop in the drainage tube cannot be avoided, lifting and draining it every 15 minutes will maintain adequate drainage in the presence of a hemothorax.
Note character and amount of chest tube drainage, whether tube is warm and full of blood and whether bloody fluid level in water-seal bottle is rising.	Useful in evaluating resolution of pneumothorax or development of hemorrhage requiring prompt intervention. *Note:* Some drainage systems are equipped with an autotransfusion device, which allows for salvage of shed blood.
Evaluate need for gentle "milking" of chest tube per protocol.	May be indicated to maintain drainage in the presence of fresh bleeding, large blood clots, or purulent exudates (empyema). Caution is necessary to prevent undue discomfort or injury, such as invagination of tissue into catheter eyelets and rupture of small blood vessels. *Note:* Although some physicians have expressed concern about this procedure for clot dislodgement, there does not appear to be consensus or guidelines (Hogg et al, 2011).
If thoracic catheter is disconnected or dislodged:	
Observe for signs of respiratory distress. If possible, reconnect thoracic catheter to tubing and suction, using clean technique. If the catheter is dislodged from the chest, cover insertion site immediately with petrolatum dressing and apply firm pressure. Notify physician at once.	Pneumothorax may recur, requiring prompt intervention to prevent fatal pulmonary and circulatory impairment.
After thoracic catheter is removed:	
Cover insertion site with sterile occlusive dressing. Observe for signs or symptoms that may indicate recurrence of pneumothorax, such as shortness of breath and reports of pain. Inspect insertion site, noting character of drainage.	Early detection of a developing complication, such as recurrence of pneumothorax or presence of infection, is essential.
Collaborative	
Assist with and prepare for reinflation procedures; for example, simple aspiration, Heimlich valve, and chest tube placement with chest tube drainage unit (CDU).	Treatment goals include air evacuation, lung reinflation, and prevention of recurrence. Although simple aspiration or Heimlich one-way valve procedures may be useful for small uncomplicated pneumothorax with little or no drainage, chest tube placement is the treatment of choice for traumatic hemopneumothoraces. CDUs include a collection chamber, a water-seal chamber, and a suction-control regulator. A dry suction system can also be used. *Note:* Tension pneumothorax requires immediate needle depression, followed by chest tube placement.
Obtain postplacement x-rays and review serial chest x-rays.	Placement of tube(s) is determined by the cause of the problem; for example, anterior chest near apex of lung, or one tube at the apex and one at posterior fifth to sixth intercostal space. X-rays confirm proper placement and monitor progress of reexpansion of lung.
Ventilation Assistance (NIC)	
Monitor and graph serial ABGs and pulse oximetry. Review vital capacity and tidal volume measurements, where indicated.	Assesses status of gas exchange and ventilation and need for continuation or alterations in therapy.
Administer supplemental oxygen via cannula, mask, or mechanical ventilation, as indicated.	Aids in reducing work of breathing; promotes relief of respiratory distress and cyanosis associated with hypoxemia.
Administer analgesics and sedatives, as indicated.	Given to manage pleuritic pain and reduce anxiety and tachycardia associated with impaired respiratory function, especially when client is on a ventilator.

NURSING DIAGNOSIS: risk for Suffocation

Risk Factors May Include

Disease or injury process—[dependence on external device (chest drainage system)]
Deficient knowledge regarding safety precautions

Possibly Evidenced By

(Not applicable; presence of signs and symptoms establishes an *actual* diagnosis)

Desired Outcomes/Evaluation Criteria—Client Will

Risk Control (NOC)

Recognize need for and seek assistance to prevent complications.

Caregiver Will

Correct and avoid environmental and physical hazards.

ACTIONS/INTERVENTIONS	RATIONALE
Teaching: Procedure/Treatment (NIC)	
Independent	
Review with client purpose and function of CDU, taking note of safety features.	Information on how system works provides reassurance, reducing client anxiety.
Instruct client to refrain from lying or pulling on tubing.	Reduces risk of obstructing drainage or inadvertently disconnecting tubing.
Identify changes and situations that should be reported to caregivers, such as change in sound of bubbling, sudden "air hunger" and chest pain, and disconnection of equipment.	Timely intervention may prevent serious complications.
Tube Care: Chest (NIC)	
Anchor thoracic catheter to chest wall and provide extra length of tubing before turning or moving client.	Prevents thoracic catheter dislodgment or tubing disconnection and reduces pain and discomfort associated with pulling or jarring of tubing.
Secure tubing connection sites.	Prevents tubing disconnection.
Pad banding sites with gauze or tape.	Protects skin from irritation and pressure.
Secure drainage unit to client's bed or on stand or cart placed in low-traffic area.	Maintains upright position and reduces risk of accidental tipping and breaking of unit.
Provide safe transportation if client is sent off unit for diagnostic purposes. Before transporting, check water-seal chamber for correct fluid level; presence or absence of bubbling; and presence, degree, and timing of tidaling. Ascertain whether chest tube can be clamped or disconnected from suction source.	Promotes continuation of optimal evacuation of fluid or air during transport. If client is draining large amounts of chest fluid or air, tube should not be clamped or suction interrupted because of risk of accumulating fluid or air, compromising respiratory status.
Monitor thoracic insertion site, noting condition of skin and presence and characteristics of drainage from around the catheter. Change and reapply sterile occlusive dressing as needed.	Provides for early recognition and treatment of developing skin or tissue erosion or infection.
Observe for signs of respiratory distress if thoracic catheter is disconnected or dislodged. (Refer to ND: ineffective Breathing Pattern.)	Pneumothorax may recur or worsen, compromising respiratory function and requiring emergency intervention.

NURSING DIAGNOSIS: deficient Knowledge [Learning Need] regarding condition, treatment regimen, self-care, and discharge needs

May Be Related To

Lack of exposure

Possibly Evidenced By

Verbalization of problem

Desired Outcomes/Evaluation Criteria—Client Will

Knowledge: Acute Illness Management (NOC)

Verbalize understanding of cause of problem (when known).
Identify signs or symptoms requiring medical follow-up.

Knowledge: Treatment Regimen (NOC)

Follow therapeutic regimen and demonstrate lifestyle changes, if necessary, to prevent recurrence.

ACTIONS/INTERVENTIONS	RATIONALE
Teaching: Disease Process (NIC) *Independent*	
Review pathology of individual problem.	Information reduces fear of unknown. Provides knowledge base for understanding underlying dynamics of condition and significance of therapeutic interventions.
Identify likelihood for recurrence or long-term complications.	Certain underlying lung diseases, such as severe COPD and malignancies, may increase incidence of recurrence. In otherwise healthy clients who suffered a spontaneous pneumothorax, incidence of recurrence is 10% to 50%. Those who have a second spontaneous episode are at high risk for a third incident (60%) (Roman, 2000).
Review signs and symptoms requiring immediate medical evaluation, for example, sudden chest pain, dyspnea, air hunger, and progressive respiratory distress.	Recurrence of pneumothorax and hemothorax requires medical intervention to prevent and reduce potential complications.
Review significance of good health practices, such as adequate nutrition, rest, and exercise.	Maintenance of general well-being promotes healing and may prevent or limit recurrences.
Emphasize need for smoking cessation when indicated.	Prevents respiratory complications, such as fibrotic changes in lung tissue, and may prevent recurrence of collapsed lung.

POTENTIAL CONSIDERATIONS following acute hospitalization (dependent on client's age, physical condition and presence of complications, personal resources, and life responsibilities)

- *risk for Infection*—invasive procedure, traumatized tissue, broken skin, decreased ciliary action
- *ineffective Breathing Pattern*—pain, fatigue, musculoskeletal impairment

VENTILATORY ASSISTANCE (MECHANICAL)

I. Pathophysiology—impairment of respiratory function affecting O_2 uptake and CO_2 elimination, requiring mechanical assist to support or replace spontaneous breathing

- **a.** Inability to maintain adequate oxygenation (hypoxemia)
- **b.** Inability to maintain adequate ventilation due to apnea or alveolar hypoventilation causing a rise in $PaCO_2$ and a fall in serum pH (respiratory acidosis)
- **c.** Inability to continue the work of breathing (respiratory muscle weakness or failure)

II. Mechanical Ventilators

- **a.** Classified by method of *cycling* from the inspiratory phase to the expiratory phase with signal to terminate the inspiratory activity of the machine:
  - **i.** Preset volume (volume-cycled ventilator)
  - **ii.** Preset pressure limit (pressure-cycled ventilator)
  - **iii.** Preset time factor (time-cycled ventilator)
- **b.** Mode of ventilation
  - **i.** Assist control: provides a breath with either a preset volume for ventilator-initiated breaths or peak pressure every time client takes a breath
  - **ii.** Pressure support ventilation: delivers preset level of positive airway pressure, rather than volume, to decrease work of breathing between ventilator-initiated breaths
  - **iii.** Continuous positive airway pressure (CPAP): continuous level of elevated pressure during client-initiated breaths to maintain adequate oxygenation and decrease the work of breathing and the work of the heart
  - **iv.** Positive end-expiratory pressure (PEEP): adjunct to mechanical ventilation using elevated pressure during the expiratory phase of the ventilatory cycle to increase functional residual capacity and surface area for gas exchange and to prevent small airway collapse.
- **c.** Complications
  - **i.** Associated with endotracheal (ET) tube: tissue damage to lips, tongue, throat; mucous plugs impairing ventilation and obstruction caused by client biting tube; auto PEEP; sinusitis or otitis; cuff herniation (rare)
  - **ii.** Associated with the ventilator: infection, hemodynamic instability from positive-pressure ventilation, barotraumas, gastrointestinal (GI) bleeding due to stress ulcer

III. Etiology

- **a.** Acute respiratory hypoxemia: pulmonary edema, severe pneumonia, sepsis, shock, acute respiratory distress syndrome (ARDS), embolism, drug reaction of overdose, lung trauma, high altitude, lung immaturity (neonates)
- **b.** Acute respiratory acidosis: acute exacerbation of chronic emphysema or asthma
- **c.** Respiratory muscle weakness or failure: paralysis of the diaphragm due to Guillain-Barré syndrome, myasthenia gravis, spinal cord injury, or the effects of anesthetic and muscle relaxant drugs; central nervous system (CNS) conditions, such as stroke, brain tumor, infections, sleep apnea; chest trauma, including fractures, pneumothorax

IV. Statistics

- **a.** Morbidity: Acute respiratory failure requiring mechanical ventilation accounts for approximately 30% of admissions to intensive care units (ICUs) (Esteban et al, 2002).
- **b.** Mortality: Prolonged mechanical ventilation has been associated with hospital mortality in the range of 20% to 40%, and overall 1-year mortality for prolonged mechanical ventilation patients ranges from 50% to 60% (Cox, 2012). Other studies showed similar numbers but compared "difficult" vs "simple" weaning in hospital mortality, e.g., ran increased mortality in clients with prolonged weaning (32%) in comparison to those with simple weaning (13%) (Funk et al, 2010; Sellares et al, 2011).
- **c.** Cost: Mean cost of 14.4-day stay in ICU (including treatment for comorbidities) $31,574 (Dasta et al, 2005). Following transfer to long-term care hospitals for weaning, mean cost of care $63,672 (Scheinhorn et al, 2007).

GLOSSARY

Assist-control (AC) ventilation: Ventilator provides full mechanical support, delivering a preset rate and (if the client initiates a breath) a preset tidal volume. If the client fails to initiate a breath, the ventilator delivers the preset ventilator breath.

Assisted breath: Initiated by the client, but controlled and ended by the ventilator.

Auto-positive end-expiratory pressure (PEEP): Complication of mechanical ventilation where gas is trapped in alveoli at end expiration due to inadequate time for expiration, bronchoconstriction, or mucus plugging. It increases the work of breathing.

Barotrauma: Injury to the lungs, airways, or chest wall due to local overinflation caused by high distending pressure in the intrapulmonary airways.

Cycling: Ventilator switches from inspiration to expiration; the flow has been delivered to the volume or pressure target.

Endotracheal (ET) tube: Tube inserted through the mouth into the trachea to facilitate passage of air into and out of the lungs.

Flow: Ventilator delivers a constant flow around the circuit throughout the respiratory cycle (flow-by). A deflection in this flow-by inspiration is monitored by the ventilator and it delivers a breath. This mechanism requires less work by the client than pressure triggering.

Hypercarbia: High level of carbon dioxide in the circulating blood.

Hyperventilation: Fast rate of respiration, which results in loss of carbon dioxide from the blood.

Hypoventilation: High partial pressure of alveolar CO_2 ($PaCO_2$).

Hypoxemia: Low oxygen levels in the blood.

Mandatory breath: Started, controlled, and ended by the ventilator.

Peak inspiratory pressure: Pressure in the lungs at the end of inspiration.

PEEP: Adjuvant to mode of ventilation used to help maintain functional residual capacity (FRC). At the end of expiration, PEEP exerts pressure to oppose passive emptying of lung, opening up collapsed alveoli and increasing surface area for gas exchange.

Positive-pressure ventilation: Increases pressure in airway, thus forcing air into lungs.

Pressure-cycled ventilator: Gas pressure limit is predetermined.

Spontaneous breath: Initiated, controlled, and ended by the client; however, the volume and pressure of the breath delivered by the ventilator are based on client demand.

Ventilation: Ability to remove CO_2 through the lungs.

Volume cycle ventilator: Volume of gas (tidal volume) is predetermined and delivered.

Care Setting

The focus of this plan of care is the client with invasive mechanical ventilation who remains on a ventilator, whether in an acute or postacute care setting. The expectation is that the majority of clients will be weaned before discharge. However, some clients are either unsuccessful at weaning or are not candidates for weaning. For these clients, portions of this plan of care would need to be modified for the discharge care setting, whether it be an extended care facility or home.

Related Concerns

Cardiac surgery: postoperative care, page 98
Chronic obstructive pulmonary disease (COPD) and asthma, page 118
Craniocerebral trauma (acute rehabilitative phase), page 197
Pneumothorax/hemothorax, page 150
Psychosocial aspects of care, page 729
Spinal cord injury (acute rehabilitative phase), page 248
Total nutritional support: parenteral/enteral feeding, page 437

Client Assessment Database

Gathered data depend on the underlying pathophysiology and reason for ventilatory support. Refer to the appropriate plan of care.

Discharge Plan Considerations

If ventilator-dependent, the plan may require changes in physical layout of home, acquisition of equipment and supplies, provision of a backup power source, instruction of significant other (SO) and caregivers, provision for continuation of plan of care, assistance with transportation, and coordination of resources and support systems.

Refer to section at end of plan for postdischarge considerations.

Diagnostic Studies

TEST WHY IT IS DONE	WHAT IT TELLS ME
PULMONARY FUNCTION STUDIES Determine the ability of the lungs to exchange oxygen and carbon dioxide and include, but are not limited to, the following:	
• *Vital capacity (VC):* The total amount of air that can be exhaled after a maximum inspiration; the sum of the inspiratory reserve volume, the tidal volume, and the expiratory reserve volume.	Reduced in restrictive chest or lung conditions; normal or increased in COPD; normal to decreased in neuromuscular diseases, such as Guillain-Barré syndrome; and decreased in conditions limiting thoracic movement, such as kyphoscoliosis. *Note:* Negative inspiratory force (NIF) can be substituted for VC to determine whether client can initiate a breath.
• *Forced vital capacity (FVC):* Total amount of air that can forcibly be blown out after full inspiration.	Reduced in restrictive conditions and in asthma and is normal to reduced in COPD.
• *Tidal volume (V_T):* Specific volume of air that is drawn into and then expired out of the lungs.	May be decreased in both restrictive and obstructive processes.
• *Minute ventilation (V_E):* Measures volume of air inhaled and exhaled in 1 minute of normal breathing.	This reflects muscle endurance and is a major determinant of work of breathing.
• *Inspiratory pressure (Pi_{max}); also called maximum inspiratory force (MIF):* Measures respiratory muscle strength upon inspiration.	Normal values should roughly equal the residual volume. Pi_{max} of less than 20 cm H_2O is considered insufficient for weaning.
• *Forced expiratory volume (FEV_1):* Measures amount of air in liters that a person can forcibly blow out in 1 second. Along with FVC, it is considered one of the primary indicators of lung function.	Usually decreased in obstructive and restrictive lung disorders.
STUDIES THAT MONITOR STATUS, AND HELP DETERMINE READINESS FOR WEANING:	
• *Arterial blood gases (ABGs):* Assesses status of oxygenation, ventilation, and acid-base balance via arterial blood.	ABG results help determine the settings for the ventilator, such as partial pressure of arterial oxygen (PaO_2), arterial oxygen saturation (SaO_2), and partial pressure of arterial carbon dioxide ($PaCO_2$).
• *Chest x-ray:* Procedure used to evaluate organs and structures within the chest.	Monitors resolution and progression of underlying condition, such as ARDS, atelectasis, and pneumonia.
• *Nutritional assessment:* Assesses albumin, prealbumin, serum transferrin, complete blood count (CBC), electrolytes, lipid profile, iron tests, blood urea nitrogen (BUN)/creatinine (Cr), glucose, and so on.	Done to identify nutritional imbalances that might prolong time on ventilator or interfere with successful weaning.

Nursing Priorities

1. Promote adequate ventilation and oxygenation.
2. Prevent complications.
3. Provide emotional support for client and SO.
4. Provide information about disease process, prognosis, and treatment needs.

Discharge Goals

1. Respiratory function maximized and adequate to meet individual needs.
2. Complications prevented or minimized.
3. Effective means of communication established.
4. Disease process, prognosis, and therapeutic regimen understood, including home ventilatory support if indicated.
5. Plan in place to meet needs after discharge.

NURSING DIAGNOSIS: ineffective Breathing Pattern/impaired spontaneous Ventilation

May Be Related To

Neuromuscular dysfunction; spinal cord injury
Respiratory muscle fatigue; musculoskeletal impairment
Metabolic factors

(continues on page 160)

NURSING DIAGNOSIS: ineffective Breathing Pattern/impaired spontaneous Ventilation (continued)

Possibly Evidenced By

Decreased minute volume, vital capacity, tidal volume

Dyspnea; increased use of accessory muscles

Tachypnea or bradypnea or cessation of respirations when off the ventilator

Decreased PO_2 and SaO_2, increased PCO_2

Increased restlessness, apprehension, metabolic rate

Desired Outcomes/Evaluation Criteria—Client Will

Respiratory Status: Ventilation (NOC)

Reestablish and maintain effective respiratory pattern via ventilator with absence of retractions and use of accessory muscles, cyanosis, or other signs of hypoxia; ABGs and oxygen saturation within acceptable range.

Participate in efforts to wean (as appropriate) within individual ability.

Caregiver Will

Demonstrate behaviors necessary to maintain client's respiratory function.

ACTIONS/INTERVENTIONS — RATIONALE

Mechanical Ventilation Management: Invasive (NIC)

Independent

Investigate etiology of respiratory failure.

Understanding the underlying cause of client's particular ventilatory problem is essential to the care of client, for example, decisions about future capabilities and ventilation needs and most appropriate type of ventilatory support.

Observe overall breathing pattern. Note respiratory rate, distinguishing between spontaneous respirations and ventilator breaths.

Client on a ventilator can experience hyperventilation, hypoventilation, or dyspnea and "air hunger" and attempt to correct deficiency by overbreathing.

Auscultate chest periodically, noting presence or absence and equality of breath sounds, adventitious breath sounds, and symmetry of chest movement.

Provides information regarding airflow through the tracheobronchial tree and the presence or absence of fluid, mucous obstruction. *Note:* Frequent crackles or rhonchi that do not clear with coughing or suctioning may indicate developing complications, such as atelectasis, pneumonia, acute bronchospasm, and pulmonary edema. Changes in chest symmetry may indicate improper placement of the ET tube or development of barotrauma.

Count client's respirations for 1 full minute and compare with desired respirations and ventilator set rate.

Respirations vary depending on problem requiring ventilatory assistance; for example, client may be totally ventilator dependent or be able to take breath(s) on own between ventilator-delivered breaths. Rapid client respirations can produce respiratory alkalosis and prevent desired volume from being delivered by ventilator. Slow client respirations and hypoventilation increase $PaCO_2$ levels and may cause acidosis.

Verify that client's respirations are in phase with the ventilator.

Adjustments may be required in flow, tidal volume, respiratory rate, and dead space of the ventilator, or client may need sedation to synchronize respirations and reduce work of breathing and energy expenditure.

Position client by elevating head of bed or chair if possible; place in prone position, as indicated.

Elevating the client's head and helping client get out of bed while still on the ventilator is both physically—helps decrease risk of aspiration—and psychologically beneficial. *Note:* Use of prone position is thought to improve oxygenation in client with severe hypoxic respiratory failure. However, it is not widely used due to the difficulties associated with placing and providing care to the intubated client in prone position as well as lack of studies showing its benefit in reducing mortality or duration of ventilation (Sud et al, 2008).

Inflate tracheal or ET tube cuff properly, using minimal leak and occlusive technique. Check cuff inflation every 4 to 8 hours and whenever cuff is deflated and reinflated.

The cuff must be properly inflated to ensure adequate ventilation and delivery of desired tidal volume and to decrease risk of aspiration. *Note:* In long-term clients, the cuff may be deflated most of the time or a noncuffed tracheostomy tube used if the client's airway is protected.

ACTIONS/INTERVENTIONS (continued)	RATIONALE (continued)
Check tubing for obstruction, such as kinking or accumulation of water. Drain tubing as indicated, avoiding draining toward client or back into the reservoir.	Kinks in tubing prevent adequate volume delivery and increase airway pressure. Condensation in tubing prevents proper gas distribution and predisposes to bacterial growth.
Check ventilator alarms for proper functioning. Do not turn off alarms, even for suctioning. Remove from ventilator and ventilate manually if source of ventilator alarm cannot be quickly identified and rectified. Ascertain that alarms can be heard in the nurses' station.	Ventilators have a series of visual and audible alarms, such as oxygen, low volume or apnea, high pressure, and inspiratory/expiratory (I:E) ratio. Turning off or failure to reset alarms places client at risk for unobserved ventilator failure or respiratory distress or arrest.
Keep resuscitation bag at bedside and ventilate manually whenever indicated.	Provides or restores adequate ventilation when client or equipment problems require client to be temporarily removed from the ventilator.
Assist client in "taking control" of breathing if weaning is attempted or ventilatory support is interrupted during procedure or activity.	Coaching client to take slower, deeper breaths; practice abdominal or pursed-lip breathing; assume position of comfort; and use relaxation techniques can be helpful in maximizing respiratory function.
Collaborative	
Assess ventilator settings routinely and readjust, as indicated:	Controls or settings are adjusted according to client's primary disease and results of diagnostic testing to maintain parameters within appropriate limits.
Note operating mode of ventilation, that is, AC, pressure support (PS), and so on.	Client's respiratory requirements, presence or absence of an underlying disease process, and the extent to which client can participate in ventilatory effort determine parameters of each setting. PS has advantages for client on long-term ventilation because it allows client to strengthen pulmonary musculature without compromising oxygenation and ventilation during the weaning process.
Observe oxygen concentration percentage (FiO_2); verify that oxygen line is in proper outlet or tank; and monitor in-line oxygen analyzer or perform periodic oxygen analysis.	FiO_2 is adjusted (21% to 100%) to maintain an acceptable oxygen percentage and saturation, for example, 90%, for client's condition.
Observe end-tidal CO_2 ($ETCO_2$) values.	Measures the amount of exhaled CO_2 with each breath and is displayed graphically to spot CO_2 exchange problems early before they show up on ABGs. In some cases, a slightly higher level of CO_2 can be beneficial, such as for the client with long-standing emphysema. In this instance, elevated PCO_2 is accepted without correction, leading to the term "permissive hypercapnia" (Byrd, 2012).
Assess set respiratory frequency (f).	Respiratory rate of 10 to 15 per minute may be appropriate except for client with COPD and CO_2 retention. In these individuals, rate and volume should be adjusted to achieve personal baseline $PaCO_2$, not necessarily a "normal" $PaCO_2$.
Assess V_T. Verify proper function of spirometer, bellows, or computer readout of delivered volume; note alterations from desired volume delivery.	Monitors amount of air inspired and expired. Changes may indicate alteration in lung compliance or leakage through machine or around tube cuff. *Note:* For the client without preexisting lung disease, the V_T and rate are traditionally selected by using V_T of 8 to 10 mL/kg delivered 12 times per minute in the AC mode. For clients with COPD, the V_T and rate are slightly reduced to 10 mL/kg at 10 breaths per minute to prevent overinflation and hyperventilation (Girard & Bernard, 2007). Many clinicians now use a smaller V_T (6 to 8 mL/kg), especially in clients with ARDS and sometimes in obstructive and restrictive lung disease, in order to reduce air-trapping and mechanical stress on the lung.
Flow rate	Speed with which the V_T is delivered is usually about 50 L/min, but is variable in order to maintain I:E ratio appropriate for specific situation.
Pressure limit	Regulates the amount of pressure the volume-cycled ventilator can generate to deliver the preset V_T with usual setting at 10 to 20 cm H_2O above the client's peak inspiratory pressure. Airway pressure should remain relatively constant. Increased pressure alarm reading reflects (1) increased airway resistance as may occur with bronchospasm; (2) retained secretions; and (3) decreased lung compliance as may occur with obstruction of the ET tube, development of atelectasis, ARDS, pulmonary edema, worsening COPD, or pneumothorax. Low

(continues on page 162)

ACTIONS/INTERVENTIONS (continued)	RATIONALE (continued)
	airway-pressure alarms may be triggered by pathophysiological conditions causing hypoventilation, such as disconnection from ventilator, low ET cuff pressure, ET tube displaced above the vocal cords, client "overbreathing," or out of phase with the ventilator.
Monitor I:E ratio	Expiratory phase is usually twice the length of the inspiratory rate, but may be longer to compensate for air-trapping to improve gas exchange in the client with COPD.
Set sigh rate, when used	Clinicians once recommended that periodic machine breaths that were 1.5 to 2 times the preset V_T be given 6 to 8 times per hour. At present, accounting for sighs is not recommended if the client is receiving V_T of 8 to 10 mL/kg or if PEEP is required. When a low V_T is used, sighs are preset at 1.5 to 2 times the V_T and delivered 6 to 8 times per hour if the peak and plateau pressures are within acceptable limits (Byrd, 2012).
Note inspired humidity and temperature; use heat moisture exchanger (HME), as indicated.	Usual warming and humidifying function of nasopharynx is bypassed with intubation. Dehydration can dry up normal pulmonary fluids, cause secretions to thicken, and increase risk of infection. Temperature should be maintained at about body temperature to reduce risk of damage to cilia and hyperthermia reactions. The introduction of a heated wire circuit to the traditional system significantly reduces the problem of "rainout" or condensation in the tubing.
Monitor serial ABGs and pulse oximetry.	Adjustments to ventilator settings may be required, depending on client's response and trends in gas exchange parameters.

NURSING DIAGNOSIS: ineffective Airway Clearance

May Be Related To

Presence of artificial airway
Neuromuscular dysfunction

Possibly Evidenced By

Changes in respiratory rate
Ineffective/absent cough
Adventitious breath sounds
Restlessness
Cyanosis

Desired Outcomes/Evaluation Criteria—Client Will

Respiratory Status: Airway Patency (NOC)

Maintain patent airway with breath sounds clear.
Be free of aspiration.

Caregiver Will

Identify potential complications and initiate appropriate actions.

ACTIONS/INTERVENTIONS	RATIONALE
Artificial Airway Management (NIC)	
Independent	
Assess airway patency.	Obstruction may be caused by accumulation of secretions, mucous plugs, hemorrhage, bronchospasm, and problems with the position of tracheostomy or ET tube.
Evaluate chest movement and auscultate for bilateral breath sounds.	Symmetrical chest movement with breath sounds throughout lung fields indicates proper tube placement and unobstructed airflow. Lower airway obstruction, such as pneumonia or atelectasis, produces changes in breath sounds, such as rhonchi and wheezing.
Monitor ET tube placement. Note lip line marking and compare with desired placement. Secure tube carefully with tape or tube holder. Obtain assistance when retaping or repositioning tube.	The ET tube may slip into the right main-stem bronchus, thereby obstructing airflow to the left lung and putting client at risk for a tension pneumothorax.

ACTIONS/INTERVENTIONS (continued)	RATIONALE (continued)
Note excessive coughing, increased dyspnea (using a 0 to 10 [or similar] scale), high-pressure alarm sounding on ventilator, visible secretions in endotracheal or tracheostomy tube, and increased rhonchi.	The intubated client often has an ineffective cough reflex, or client may have neuromuscular or neurosensory impairment, altering ability to cough. Client is usually dependent on suctioning to remove secretions. *Note:* Research supports use of a dyspnea rating scale (like those used to measure pain) to more accurately quantify and measure changes in dyspnea as experienced by client.
Suction as needed when client is coughing or experiencing respiratory distress, limiting duration of suction to 15 seconds or less. Choose appropriate suction catheter. Hyperventilate before and after each catheter pass, using 100% oxygen if appropriate, using vent rather than Ambu bag, which has an increased risk of barotrauma. Suction continuously during withdrawal.	Suctioning should not be routine, and duration should be limited to reduce hazard of hypoxia. Suction catheter diameter should be less than 50% of the internal diameter of the ET or tracheostomy tube for prevention of hypoxia. Hyperoxygenation with ventilator sigh on 100% oxygen may be desired to reduce atelectasis and to reduce accidental hypoxia. *Note:* Instilling normal saline (NS) is no longer recommended (although it persists in practice) because research reveals that the fluid pools at the distal end of the ET or tracheal tube, impairing oxygenation and increasing bronchospasm and the risk of infection.
Use inline catheter suction when available.	Helps maintain oxygen saturation and PEEP when used.
Instruct client in coughing techniques during suctioning, such as splinting, timing of breathing, and "quad cough," as indicated.	Enhances effectiveness of cough effort and secretion clearing.
Reposition or turn periodically.	Promotes drainage of secretions and ventilation to all lung segments, reducing risk of atelectasis.
Encourage the client to drink fluids (if swallowing is possible) and provide fluids within individual capability.	Helps liquefy secretions, enhancing expectoration.
Collaborative	
Provide chest physiotherapy as indicated, such as postural drainage and percussion.	Promotes ventilation of all lung segments and aids drainage of secretions.
Administer intravenous (IV) and aerosol bronchodilators as indicated.	Promotes ventilation and removal of secretions.
Assist with fiber-optic bronchoscopy, if indicated.	May be performed to remove secretions and mucous plugs.

NURSING DIAGNOSIS: impaired verbal Communication

May Be Related To

Physical barrier, tracheostomy intubation

Alteration of central nervous system, [neuromuscular weakness or paralysis]

Possibly Evidenced By

Cannot speak

Desired Outcomes/Evaluation Criteria—Client Will

Communication: Expressive (NOC)

Establish method of communication in which needs can be understood.

ACTIONS/INTERVENTIONS	RATIONALE
Communication Enhancement: Speech Deficit (NIC)	
Independent	
Assess client's ability to communicate by alternative means.	Reasons for long-term ventilatory support are various; client may be alert and be adept at writing (such as chronic COPD with inability to be weaned) or may be lethargic, comatose, or paralyzed. Method of communicating with client is therefore highly individualized. *Note:* The inability to talk while intubated is a primary cause of feelings of fear.
Establish means of communication, for example, maintain eye contact; ask yes/no questions; provide magic slate, paper and pencil, computer, cell phone (if client can text); picture or alphabet board; use sign language as appropriate; and validate meaning of attempted communications.	Eye contact assures client of interest in communicating; if client is able to move head, blink eyes, or is comfortable with simple gestures, a great deal can be done with yes/no questions. Texting, word-processing, writing, or pointing to letter boards is often tiring to client, who can then become frustrated with the process. Use of picture boards that express a concept (e.g., "need pain shot") or routine needs

(continues on page 164)

ACTIONS/INTERVENTIONS (continued)	RATIONALE (continued)
	(e.g., "need bedpan") may simplify communication. Family members and other caregivers may be able to assist and interpret needs.
Consider form of communication when placing IV.	IV positioned in hand or wrist may limit ability to write or sign.
Place call light or bell within reach, making certain client is alert and physically capable of using it. Answer call light or bell immediately. Anticipate needs. Tell client that nurse is immediately available should assistance be required.	Ventilator-dependent client may be better able to relax, feel safe (not abandoned), and breathe with the ventilator knowing that nurse is vigilant and needs will be met.
Place note at central call station informing staff that client is unable to speak.	Alerts all staff members to respond to client at the bedside instead of over the intercom.
Encourage family and SO to talk with client, providing information about family and daily happenings.	SO may feel self-conscious in one-sided conversation, but knowledge that he or she is assisting client to regain or maintain contact with reality and enabling client to feel part of family unit can reduce feelings of awkwardness.
Collaborative	
Evaluate need for or appropriateness of talking tracheostomy tube.	Client with adequate cognitive and muscular skills may have the ability to manipulate talking tracheostomy tube.

NURSING DIAGNOSIS: Anxiety [specify level]

May Be Related To

Situational crises; threat to self-concept
Threat of death
Change in health, economic status, or role functioning
Interpersonal transmission or contagion

Possibly Evidenced By

Increased muscle/facial tension
Insomnia, restlessness
Vigilance
Feelings of inadequacy
Fearful, uncertainty, apprehensive
Focus on self, negative self-talk
Expressed concern due to change in life events

Desired Outcomes/Evaluation Criteria—Client Will

Anxiety Self-Control (NOC)

Verbalize or communicate awareness of feelings and healthy ways to deal with them.
Demonstrate problem-solving skills or behaviors to cope with current situation.

Anxiety Level (NOC)

Report that anxiety is reduced to manageable level.
Appear relaxed and sleeping or resting appropriately.

ACTIONS/INTERVENTIONS	RATIONALE
Anxiety Reduction (NIC)	
Independent	
Identify client's perception of threat represented by situation. Determine current respiratory status and adequacy of ventilation.	Defines scope of individual problem separate from physiological causes, and influences choice of interventions.
Observe and monitor physical responses, such as restlessness, changes in vital signs, and repetitive movements. Note congruency of verbal/nonverbal communication.	Useful in evaluating extent or degree of concerns, especially when compared with "verbal" comments.
Encourage client and SO to acknowledge and express fears.	Provides opportunity for dealing with concerns, clarifies reality of fears, and reduces anxiety to a more manageable level.
Acknowledge the anxiety and fear of the situation. Avoid meaningless reassurance that everything will be all right.	Validates the reality of the situation without minimizing the emotional impact. Provides opportunity for client and SO to accept and begin to deal with what has happened, reducing anxiety.
Identify and review with client and SO the safety precautions being taken, such as backup power and oxygen supplies and emergency equipment at hand for suctioning. Discuss or review the meanings of alarm system.	Provides reassurance to help allay unnecessary anxiety, reduce concerns of the unknown, and preplan for response in emergency situation.
Note reactions of SO. Provide opportunity for discussion of personal feelings, concerns, and future expectations.	Family members have individual responses to what is happening, and their anxiety may be communicated to client, intensifying these emotions.

ACTIONS/INTERVENTIONS (continued)	RATIONALE (continued)
Identify previous coping strengths of client and SO and current areas of control and ability.	Focuses attention on own capabilities, increasing sense of control.
Demonstrate and encourage use of relaxation techniques, such as focused breathing, guided imagery, and progressive relaxation. Provide music therapy and biofeedback as appropriate.	Provides active management of situation to reduce feelings of helplessness.
Provide and encourage sedentary diversional activities within individual capabilities, such as handicrafts, writing, and television.	Although handicapped by dependence on ventilator, activities that are normal or desired by the individual should be encouraged to enhance quality of life.
Collaborative	
Refer to support individuals, groups, and therapy, as needed.	May be necessary to provide additional assistance if client and SO are not managing anxiety or when client is "identified with the machine."

NURSING DIAGNOSIS: impaired Oral Mucous Membrane

Risk Factors May Include

NPO for more than 24 hours
Mechanical factors—tubes [ET, NG]
Decreased salivation
Ineffective oral hygiene

Possibly Evidenced By

(Not applicable; presence of signs and symptoms establishes an *actual* diagnosis)

Desired Outcomes/Evaluation Criteria—Client Will

Tissue Integrity: Skin and Mucous Membrane (NOC)

Report or demonstrate a decrease in symptoms.

Caregiver Will

Identify specific interventions to promote healthy oral mucosa as appropriate.

ACTIONS/INTERVENTIONS	RATIONALE
Oral Health Maintenance (NIC)	
Independent	
Routinely inspect oral cavity, teeth, gums for sores, lesions, and bleeding.	Early identification of problems provides opportunity for appropriate intervention and preventive measures.
Administer mouth care routinely per protocol and as needed, especially in client with an oral intubation tube; for example, cleanse mouth with water, saline, or preferred alcohol-free mouthwash. Brush teeth with soft toothbrush, WaterPik, or moistened swab.	Prevents drying and ulceration of mucous membrane and reduces medium for bacterial growth. Promotes comfort.
Change position of ET tube and airway on a regular and prn (as necessary) schedule as appropriate.	Reduces risk of lip and oral mucous membrane ulceration.
Apply lip balm; administer oral lubricant solution.	Maintains moisture and prevents drying

NURSING DIAGNOSIS: imbalanced Nutrition: less than body requirements

May Be Related To

Inability to ingest/digest food
[Increased metabolic demands]

Possibly Evidenced By

Weight loss; poor muscle tone
Aversion to eating; reported altered taste sensation
Sore buccal cavity
[Hypo-] or hyperactive bowel sounds

Desired Outcomes/Evaluation Criteria—Client Will

Nutritional Status (NOC)

Indicate understanding of individual dietary needs.
Demonstrate progressive weight gain toward goal with normalization of laboratory values.

ACTIONS/INTERVENTIONS | RATIONALE

Nutrition Therapy (NIC)

Independent

Evaluate ability to eat.
Client with a tracheostomy tube may be able to eat, but client with ET tube must have enteral or parenteral nutrition.

Observe and monitor for generalized muscle wasting and loss of subcutaneous fat.
These symptoms are indicative of depletion of muscle energy and can reduce respiratory muscle function.

Weigh, as indicated.
Significant and recent weight loss (7% to 10% body weight) and poor nutritional intake provide clues regarding catabolism, muscle glycogen stores, and ventilatory drive sensitivity.

Document oral intake if and when resumed. Offer foods that client enjoys.
Appetite is usually poor and intake of essential nutrients may be reduced. Offering favorite foods can enhance oral intake.

Provide small, frequent feedings of soft and easily digested foods if able to swallow.
Prevents excessive fatigue, enhances intake, and reduces risk of gastric distress.

Encourage or administer fluid intake of at least 2500 mL/day within cardiac tolerance.
Prevents dehydration that can be exacerbated by increased insensible losses (ventilator or diaphoresis, hypermetabolic state) and reduces risk of constipation.

Assess GI function: presence and quality of bowel sounds and changes in abdominal girth, nausea, and vomiting. Observe and document changes in bowel movements, such as diarrhea and constipation. Test all stools for occult blood.
A functioning GI system is essential for the proper utilization of enteral feedings. Mechanically ventilated clients are at risk of developing abdominal distention (trapped air or ileus) and gastric bleeding (stress ulcers).

Collaborative

Adjust diet to meet respiratory needs, as indicated.
High intake of carbohydrates, protein, and calories may be desired or needed during ventilation to improve respiratory muscle function. Carbohydrates may be reduced and fat somewhat increased just before weaning attempts to prevent excessive CO_2 production and reduced respiratory drive.

Administer tube feeding or hyperalimentation, as needed. (Refer to CP: Total Nutritional Support: Parenteral/Enteral Feeding.)
Provides adequate nutrients to meet individual needs when oral intake is insufficient or not appropriate.

Monitor laboratory studies as indicated, such as prealbumin, serum transferrin, BUN/Cr, and glucose.
Provides information about adequacy of nutritional support or need for change.

NURSING DIAGNOSIS: risk for Infection

Risk Factors May Include

Inadequate primary defenses—traumatized lung tissue, decrease in ciliary action, stasis of body fluids
Inadequate secondary defenses—immunosuppression
Chronic disease, malnutrition
Invasive procedure—intubation

Possibly Evidenced By

(Not applicable; presence of signs and symptoms establishes an *actual* diagnosis)

Desired Outcomes/Evaluation Criteria—Client Will

Risk Control: Infectious Process (NOC)

Indicate understanding of individual risk factors.
Identify interventions to prevent or reduce risk of infection.
Demonstrate techniques to promote safe environment.

ACTIONS/INTERVENTIONS | RATIONALE

Mechanical Ventilation Management: Pneumonia Prevention (NIC)

Independent

Note risk factors for occurrence of infection
Intubation interferes with the normal defense mechanisms that keep microorganisms out of the lungs. ET tubes, especially cuffed ones, interfere with the mucociliary transport system that helps clear airway secretions. Secretions that accumulate below and above the ET tube cuff are an ideal growth medium for pathogens. The ET tube also prevents normal closure of the epiglottis, resulting in an incomplete seal of the laryngeal structures that normally protect the lungs. This can contribute to aspiration, which often leads

to ventilator-associated pneumonia (VAP) (Pruitt & Jacobs, 2006). VAP is the primary cause of hospital-acquired pneumonia (HAP) reportedly occurring in 10% to 25% of individuals receiving mechanical ventilation (Byrd, 2012). Other factors include prolonged mechanical ventilation, trauma, general debilitation, malnutrition, age, and invasive procedures. Awareness of individual risk factors provides opportunity to limit effects and helps prevent VAP.

Observe color, odor, and characteristics of sputum. Note drainage around tracheostomy tube.

Yellow or green, purulent odorous sputum or drainage is indicative of infection; thick, tenacious sputum suggests dehydration.

Engage in proper hand washing or alcohol-based hand rubs, wear gloves when handling respiratory secretions and equipment contaminated with respiratory secretions; maintain sterile techniques when performing arterial punctures (for ABGs) and when suctioning using open system; use closed-system ET tube whenever possible, to allow for continuous removal of secretions.

These factors may be the simplest but are the most important keys to prevention of hospital-acquired infection.

Reduce the number of times the ventilator tubes are open, and provide clean nebulizer and tubing changes per protocol.

The Centers for Disease Control and Prevention's (CDC) guidelines (2005) recommend changing tubing no more often than every 48 hours. Research indicates that frequent changes of the ventilator tubings have not been shown to reduce the risk of VAP and are currently not recommended (Amanullah, 2011).

Auscultate breath sounds.

Presence of rhonchi and wheezes suggests retained secretions requiring expectoration or suctioning.

Monitor for elevation of temperature.

Fever may signal onset of infection, although if client is immunosuppressed fever may not present.

Keep head of bed elevated (if not prohibited by medical conditions such as spinal cord injury) to >30 degrees.

Maximizes lung expansion. It has been suggested that the higher elevation decreases risk of VAP, but studies are not conclusive (Niel-Weise, 2011).

Provide or instruct client and SO in proper oral care and secretion disposal, such as disposing of tissues and soiled tracheostomy dressings.

Reduces risk of pneumonia associated with aspiration of oral bacteria, as well as transmission of fluid-borne organisms. *Note:* Chlorhexidine mouth rinse has been found to reduce plaque and gingival inflammation as a means of preventing VAP (Genuit et al, 2001).

Monitor and screen visitors. Avoid contact with persons with respiratory infections.

Individual is already compromised and is at increased risk with exposure to infections.

Provide respiratory isolation when indicated.

Depending on specific diagnosis, client may require protection from others or must prevent transmission of infection, for example, influenza or tuberculosis (TB) to others.

Maintain adequate hydration and nutrition. Encourage fluids to 2500 mL/day within cardiac tolerance.

Helps improve general resistance to disease and reduces risk of infection from static secretions.

Avoid gastric distention. Check pH of secretions, if indicated. Avoid antacids, as well.

Helps identify presence of gastric secretions in respiratory tract and reduces risk of VAP associated with gastric reflux and aspiration. Although medications may be needed to reduce stress ulcer development, the volume of antacids needed would preclude their use. Although H2 antagonists are useful, their overuse can exacerbate risk for VAP (Myrianthefs, 2004).

Encourage self-care and activities to limit of tolerance. Assist with graded exercise program.

Improves general well-being and muscle strength and may stimulate immune system recovery.

Collaborative

Monitor laboratory tests, e.g., WBCs with differential.

Leukocytosis may indicate presence and severity of infection.

Evaluate period chest x-rays.

Infiltrates may signal presence of pneumonia.

Obtain sputum cultures as indicated.

May be needed to identify pathogens and appropriate antimicrobials. *Note:* Microorganisms implicated in VAP that occurs in the first 48 hours after intubation are those of the upper airway (*Haemophilus influenza* and *Streptococcus pneumonia*). After this early period, gram-negative bacilli (e.g., *Pseudomonas aeruginosa; Escherichia coli;* and *Acinetobacter, Proteus,* and *Klebsiella*) are more predominate. *Staphylococcus aureus,* especially methicillin-resistant *S. aureus* (MRSA), typically becomes a major agent after 7 days of mechanical ventilation (Byrd. 2012).

Administer broad-spectrum antimicrobials, as indicated.

If infection does occur, one or more agents may be used, depending on identified pathogen(s).

NURSING DIAGNOSIS: risk for dysfunctional Ventilatory Weaning Response

Risk Factors May Include

Sleep pattern disturbance
Limited or insufficient energy stores
Uncontrolled pain
Adverse environment—noisy environment, low nurse:patient ratio, inadequate social support
Perceived inefficacy about ability to wean; decreased motivation
History of ventilator dependence >4 days; history of multiple unsuccessful weaning attempts

Possibly Evidenced By

(Not applicable; presence of signs and symptoms establishes an *actual* diagnosis)

Desired Outcomes/Evaluation Criteria—Client Will

Mechanical Ventilation Weaning Response: Adult (NOC)

Actively participate in the weaning process.
Reestablish independent respiration with ABGs within acceptable range and free of signs of respiratory failure.

Activity Tolerance (NOC)

Demonstrate increased tolerance for activity and participate in self-care within level of ability.

ACTIONS/INTERVENTIONS	RATIONALE
Mechanical Ventilatory Weaning (NIC)	
Independent	
Assess physical factors involved in weaning as follows:	
Stable heart rate/rhythm, blood pressure (BP), and clear breath sounds	The heart has to work harder to meet increased energy needs associated with weaning. Weaning may be deferred if tachycardia, pulmonary crackles, or hypertension are present.
Fever	Increase of 1°F (0.6°C) in body temperature raises metabolic rate and oxygen demands by 7%.
Nutritional status and muscle strength	Weaning is hard work. Client not only must be able to withstand the stress of weaning but also must have the stamina to breathe spontaneously for extended periods.
Determine psychological readiness	Weaning provokes anxiety for client regarding concerns about ability to breathe on own and long-term need of ventilator.
Explain weaning techniques, for example, spontaneous breathing trial (SBT), T-piece, pressure support ventilation (PSV), and spontaneous intermittent maximal ventilation (SIMV). Discuss individual plan and expectations.	Assists client to prepare for weaning process, helps limit fear of unknown, promotes cooperation, and enhances likelihood of a successful outcome. *Note:* Current guidelines recommend SBT as the preferred method of weaning as it withdraws ventilatory support while oxygenation is continued. The simplest form of SBT is the T-piece trial. In PSV weaning, all breaths are spontaneous and combined with enough pressure support to ensure that each breath is a reasonable tidal volume. Findings from randomized trials suggest that SIMV weaning delays extubation compared with PSV and SBT and that it should not be the primary mode of weaning in most clients (Byrd et al, 2012).
Provide undisturbed rest and sleep periods. Avoid stressful procedures or situations and nonessential activities.	Maximizes energy for weaning process; limits fatigue and oxygen consumption. *Note:* It takes approximately 12 to 14 hours of respiratory rest to rejuvenate tired respiratory muscles. For clients on AC, raising the rate to 20 breaths per minute can also provide respiratory rest.
Evaluate and document client's progress. Note restlessness; changes in BP, heart rate, and respiratory rate; use of accessory muscles; discoordinated breathing with ventilator; increased concentration on breathing (mild dysfunction); client's concerns about possible machine malfunction; inability to cooperate or respond to coaching; and color changes.	Indicators that client may require slower weaning and an opportunity to stabilize, or may need to stop program. *Note:* Moving from pressure/volume (such as assist/control) ventilator to T-piece may precipitate a "flash" pulmonary edema, requiring prompt intervention (Diel-Oplinger, 2002).
Recognize and provide encouragement for client's efforts.	Positive feedback provides reassurance and support for continuation of weaning process.
Monitor cardiopulmonary response to activity.	Excessive oxygen consumption and demand increases the possibility of failure.
Collaborative	
Consult with dietitian and nutritional support team for adjustments in composition of diet.	Reduction of carbohydrates and fats may be required to prevent excessive production of CO_2, which could alter respiratory drive.

ACTIONS/INTERVENTIONS (continued)	RATIONALE (continued)
Monitor CBC, serum albumin and prealbumin, transferrin, total iron-binding capacity, and electrolytes, especially potassium, calcium, and phosphorus.	Verifies that nutrition is adequate to meet energy requirements for weaning.
Review chest x-ray and ABGs.	Chest x-rays should show clear lungs or marked improvement in pulmonary congestion or infiltrates. ABGs should document satisfactory oxygenation on an FiO_2 of 40% or less.

NURSING DIAGNOSIS: deficient Knowledge [Learning Need] regarding condition, prognosis and therapy, self-care, and discharge needs

May Be Related To

Lack of exposure or recall
Information misinterpretation; unfamiliarity with information resources

Possibly Evidenced By

Reports the problem
Inaccurate performance of skills
Inaccurate follow-through of instructions
Inappropriate behaviors—agitated, apathetic

Desired Outcomes/Evaluation Criteria—Client/SO/Caregiver Will

Health Seeking Behavior (NOC)

Participate in learning process.
Exhibit increased interest, shown by verbal or nonverbal cues.
Assume responsibility for own learning and begin to look for information and to ask questions.

Knowledge: Treatment Regimen (NOC)

Indicate understanding of mechanical ventilation therapy.
Demonstrate behaviors or new skills to meet individual needs and prevent complications.

ACTIONS/INTERVENTIONS	RATIONALE
Learning Facilitation (NIC)	
Independent	
Determine ability and willingness to learn.	Physical condition may preclude client involvement in care before and after discharge. SO/caregiver may feel inadequate, afraid of machinery, and have reservations about ability to learn or deal with overall situation.
Schedule teaching sessions for quiet, nonstressful times when all participants are well rested.	Enhances learners' ability to focus on and absorb content provided.
Arrange information in logical sequence, progressing from simple to more complex material at learners' pace.	Allows learner to build on information learned in previous sessions; is less threatening and overwhelming.
Knowledge: Disease Process	
Provide material in multiple formats, such as books and pamphlets, audiovisuals, hands-on demonstrations, and take-home instruction sheets, as appropriate.	Uses multiple senses to stimulate learning and retention of information. Provides resources for review following discharge.
Discuss specific condition requiring ventilatory support, what measures are being tried for weaning, and short- and long-term goals of treatment.	Provides knowledge base to aid client and SO in making informed decisions. Weaning efforts may continue for several weeks (extended period of time). Dependence is evidenced by repeatedly increased PCO_2 and decline in PaO_2 during weaning attempts, presence of dyspnea, anxiety, tachycardia, perspiration, and cyanosis.
Encourage client and SO to evaluate impact of ventilatory dependence on their lifestyle and what changes they are willing or unwilling to make. Problem-solve solutions to issues raised.	Quality of life must be resolved by the ventilator-dependent client and caregivers who need to understand that home ventilatory support is a 24-hour job that affects everyone.
Promote participation in self-care and diversional activities and socialization, as appropriate.	Refocuses attention toward more normal life activities, increases endurance, and helps prevent depersonalization.
Review issues of general well-being: role of nutrition, assistance with feeding and meal preparation, graded exercise and specific restrictions, and rest periods alternated with activity.	Enhances recuperation and ensures that individual needs will be met.
Recommend that SO and caregivers learn cardiopulmonary resuscitation (CPR).	Provides sense of security about ability to handle emergency situations that might arise until help can be obtained.
Schedule team conference. Establish in-hospital training for caregivers if client is to be discharged home on ventilator.	Team approach is needed to coordinate client's care and teaching program to meet individual needs.

(continues on page 170)

ACTIONS/INTERVENTIONS (continued)	RATIONALE (continued)
Instruct caregiver and client in hand-washing techniques, use of sterile technique for suctioning, tracheostomy or stoma care, and chest physiotherapy.	Reduces risk of infection and promotes optimal respiratory function.
Provide demonstration and "hands-on" sessions, as well as written material, about specific type of ventilator to be used, including function and care of equipment.	Enhances familiarity, reducing anxiety and promoting confidence in implementation of new tasks and skills.
Discuss what and when to report to the healthcare provider, for example, signs of respiratory distress and infection.	Helps reduce general anxiety while promoting timely and appropriate evaluation and intervention to prevent complications.
Ascertain that all needed equipment is in place and that safety concerns have been addressed, such as alternative power source (generator, batteries), backup equipment, and client call and alarm system.	Predischarge preparations can ease the transfer process. Planning for potential problems increases sense of security for client and SO.
Contact community or hospital-based services.	Suppliers of home equipment, physical therapy, care providers, emergency power provider, and social services, such as financial assistance, aid in procuring equipment and personnel and facilitate transition to home.
Refer to vocational or occupational therapist.	Some ventilator-dependent clients are able to resume vocations either while on the ventilator or during the day (while ventilator-dependent at night).

POTENTIAL CONSIDERATIONS following acute hospitalization (dependent on client's age, physical condition and presence of complications, personal resources, and life responsibilities)

If client is discharged on ventilator, the client's needs and concerns remain the same as noted in this plan of care, in addition to the following:

- ***Self-Care Deficit***—musculoskeletal/neuromuscular impairment, weakness, fatigue, pain, environmental barriers
- ***interrupted Family Processes***—situational crisis, shift in family roles, shift in health status of a family member
- ***risk for Relocation Stress Syndrome***—reports powerlessness, decreased health status, lack of predeparture counseling, moderate-to-high degree of environmental change
- ***risk for Caregiver Role Strain***—discharge of family member with significant home-care needs, presence of situational stressors that normally affect families (economic vulnerability, changes in roles and responsibilities), duration of caregiving required, inexperience with caregiving

PULMONARY TUBERCULOSIS (TB)

I. Pathophysiology

a. Bacterial infection by *Mycobacterium tuberculosis* bacilli (TB)
   i. Primarily affects the lungs (70% per Centers for Disease Control and Prevention [CDC], 2004) although it can invade other body systems
   ii. Airborne droplets are inhaled, with the droplet nuclei deposited within the alveoli of the lung.

b. Primary infection followed by a latent or dormant phase, or by active disease in some individuals

c. When the immune system weakens, dormant TB organisms can reactivate and multiply (reactivation TB).

II. Classifications

a. Latent: Body's immune system has encapsulated the bacteria into tiny capsules called tubercles, infection not transmissible to others.

b. Active: Infection is spreading in the body and can be transmitted to others.

III. Etiology

a. Following exposure, the bacilli may (1) be killed by the immune system, (2) multiply and cause primary TB, (3) become dormant and remain asymptomatic, or (4) proliferate after a latency period (reactivation disease) (Herchline & Amorosa, 2007).

b. Multidrug-resistant tuberculosis (MDR-TB)
   i. Primary: caused by person-to-person transmission of a drug-resistant organism
   ii. Secondary: usually the result of nonadherence to therapy or inappropriate treatment
   iii. On the rise especially in large cities, in those previously treated with antitubercular drugs, or in those who failed to follow or complete a drug regimen
   iv. Can progress from diagnosis to death in as little as 4 to 6 weeks

c. Risk factors: individuals with weakened immune systems due to chronic conditions, advanced age, and malnutrition; higher among persons with HIV infection, the homeless, drug-addicted, and impoverished populations, as well as among immigrants from or visitors to countries in which TB is endemic

IV. Statistics (Centers for Disease Control and Prevention [CDC], 2011)

a. Morbidity: In 2010, 11,182 TB cases were reported to CDC, representing a 3.1% decrease from 2009, with foreign-born Hispanics and Asians together accounting for 48% of the national case total.

b. Mortality: No deaths were reported in the United States in 2010 (CDC, 2011). Globally, 1.4 million died from TB in 2011, of which 25% occurred in persons with HIV. The TB death rate dropped 41% between 1990 and 2011 (World Health Organization [WHO], 2013).

c. Costs: 8800 hospitalizations in the United States in 2006 with primary diagnosis of TB at a mean cost of $20,100 per admission. Approximately another 49,000 admitted with TB listed as secondary diagnosis (Holmquist, 2008).

GLOSSARY

Acid-fast bacilli (AFB): Rod-shaped bacteria that can be seen and counted under the microscope on a specially stained sputum sample on a glass slide, called an AFB smear. The most common AFB are members of the genus *Mycobacterium.*

Cavitation: The formation of cavities in a body tissue or an organ, especially those formed in the lung as a result of TB. In cavitary disease, breath sounds are high-pitched and hollow (like blowing over the end of an empty bottle).

Directly observed treatment (DOT): Healthcare worker observes client taking antitubercular medications. DOT provides a mechanism for early detection of adverse medication reactions or nonadherence with medication regimen in high-risk clients or environments, such as jails, homeless shelters, crowded worksites, among others.

Fremitus: Sensation felt by a hand placed on the chest that vibrates during speech.

Multidrug-resistant tuberculosis (MDR-TB): A form of TB caused by bacteria that do not respond to, at least, isoniazid and rifampicin, the two most powerful, first-line (or standard) anti-TB drugs

Tubular breath sounds: Low-pitched and sticky and occur over areas of consolidation.

Whispered pectoriloquies: Transmission of the voice sound through the pulmonary structures so that it is unusually audible on auscultation of the chest, indicating either consolidation of the lung parenchyma or the presence of a large cavity.

Care Setting

Most clients are treated in community clinics but may be hospitalized for diagnostic evaluation or initiation of therapy, adverse drug reactions, or severe illness or debilitation. This plan of care is intended to reflect care of the person with active (rather than latent) TB, although if latent, when TB is diagnosed, treatment will be initiated.

Related Concerns

Extended care, page 781
Pneumonia, page 129
Psychosocial aspects of care, page 729

Client Assessment Database

Data depend on stage of disease and degree of involvement.

DIAGNOSTIC DIVISION MAY REPORT	MAY EXHIBIT
ACTIVITY/REST	
• Generalized weakness and fatigue • Shortness of breath with exertion • Difficulty sleeping, with evening or night fever, chills, and sweats • Nightmares	• Tachycardia, tachypnea/dyspnea on exertion • Muscle wasting, pain, and stiffness (advanced stages)
EGO INTEGRITY	
• Recent or long-standing stress factors • Financial concerns, poverty • Feelings of helplessness and hopelessness	• Denial (especially during early stages) • Anxiety, apprehension, irritability • Inattention, marked irritability, change in mentation (advanced stages)
FOOD/FLUID	
• Loss of appetite • Indigestion • Weight loss • Night sweats	• Poor skin turgor, dry and flaky skin • Muscle wasting and loss of subcutaneous fat
PAIN/DISCOMFORT	
• Chest pain aggravated by recurrent cough	• Guarding of affected area • Distraction behaviors, restlessness
RESPIRATION	
• History of TB or exposure to infected individual • Persistent cough, productive or nonproductive • Shortness of breath	• ***Breath sounds:*** Diminished bilaterally or unilaterally (pleural effusion or pneumothorax); tubular breath sounds and/or whispered pectoriloquies over large lesions; crackles may be noted over apex of lungs during quick inspiration after a short cough (post-tussive crackles).

(continues on page 172)

Client Assessment Database (continued)

DIAGNOSTIC DIVISION MAY REPORT (continued)	MAY EXHIBIT (continued)
	• Increased respiratory rate is associated with extensive disease or fibrosis of the lung parenchyma and pleura. • Asymmetry in respiratory excursion (pleural effusion) • Dullness to percussion and decreased fremitus (pleural fluid or pleural thickening) • ***Sputum characteristics:*** May be green, or purulent, mucoid, or blood-tinged
SAFETY • Presence of immunosuppressed conditions, such as AIDS, cancer • Positive HIV test; HIV infection • Visit to, immigration from, or close contact with persons in areas with high prevalence of TB, such as Southeast Asia, Sub-Saharan Africa (WHO, 2013), the countries of the former Soviet Union, and in prison populations (Schiffman, 2011)	• Low-grade fever or acute febrile illness • Enlarged lymph nodes in neck
SOCIAL INTERACTION • Feelings of isolation and rejection because of communicable disease • Change in usual patterns of responsibility or change in physical capacity to resume role	
TEACHING/LEARNING • Familial history of TB • Person living with HIV • General debilitation and poor health status • Use or abuse of substances such as intravenous (IV) drugs, cocaine, and crack • Failure to improve or reactivation of TB • Nonparticipation in therapy	
DISCHARGE PLAN CONSIDERATIONS • Assistance with or alteration in drug therapy • Temporary assistance in self-care and homemaker and maintenance tasks ➧ Refer to section at end of plan for postdischarge considerations.	

Diagnostic Studies

TEST WHY IT IS DONE	WHAT IT TELLS ME
DIAGNOSTIC TESTS	
• ***Sputum TB culture:*** Acid-fast bacilli (AFB) are rod-shaped bacteria identified through sputum culture and smear. *M. tuberculosis* is the most prevalent species of mycobacteria and the most infectious.	Positive for *M. tuberculosis* in the active stage of the disease. Sputum cultures will be repeated 3 months into therapy to evaluate for possible nonadherence to treatment or to identify drug-resistant bacilli.
• ***Nucleic acid amplification (NAA) test, more commonly referred to as Xpert MTB/RIF:*** Sputum sample assay that can rapidly detect TB and simultaneously detect rifampicin resistance	Recently endorsed by the CDC and the WHO, this test can not only detect *M. tuberculosis* complex but also rifampicin resistance within 2 hours after starting the test. In clinical testing, it outperformed smear microscopy, established a diagnosis in a significant proportion of persons with smear-negative TB,

TEST WHY IT IS DONE (continued)	WHAT IT TELLS ME (continued)
	detected many highly likely TB cases missed by culture, and accurately ruled out rifampicin-resistant TB (Theron et al, 2011). With CDC guidelines recommending the test on at least one sputum sample collected, the test is becoming more widely commercially available, although cost remains an issue (Steingart, 2012; Lin, 2011; CDC MMWR, 2009).
• *Chest x-ray:* Evaluates organs and structures within the chest for evidence of disease.	May show small, patchy infiltrations of early lesions in the upper-lung field, calcium deposits of healed primary lesions, or fluid of an effusion. Changes indicating more advanced TB may include cavitation, scar tissue, and fibrotic areas.
• *TB skin tests (TST), such as purified protein derivative (PPD) administered by single-needle intradermal injection (Mantoux test), multiple-puncture tests (tine, Aplitest):* Determine past or present exposure to TB	A positive reaction—area of induration 10 mm or greater, occurring 48 to 72 hours after intradermal injection of the antigen—indicates past infection and the presence of antibodies but is not necessarily indicative of active disease. Positive results develop 2–10 weeks after exposure. Factors associated with a suppressed response to skin tests include underlying viral or bacterial infections, malnutrition, lymphadenopathy, current use of corticosteroids or other immunosuppressant or exposure to live vaccine viruses, such as measles, mumps, and rubella, within last 4 to 6 weeks. A significant reaction in a client who is clinically ill means that active TB cannot be dismissed as a diagnostic possibility. A significant reaction in healthy persons usually signifies dormant TB or an infection caused by a different mycobacterium.
TESTS ON THE HORIZON	
• *Enzyme-linked immunosorbent spot (ELISpot) and ELISpot Plus:* Newer blood tests to detect the presence of tuberculosis	Research shows that these tests are specific and have high sensitivity in the detection of both active and latent TB, reliability is better, and when combined with the traditional TB skin test, there is a 99% accuracy. Use of this test could shorten diagnosis from weeks to about 48 hours, thereby distinguishing which individuals require further TB testing or intervention, and those who do not (Dosanjh, 2008; Lalvani, n.d.).

Nursing Priorities

1. Achieve and maintain adequate ventilation and oxygenation.
2. Prevent spread of infection.
3. Support behaviors and tasks to maintain health.
4. Promote effective coping strategies.
5. Provide information about disease process, prognosis, and treatment needs.

Discharge Goals

1. Respiratory function adequate to meet individual need.
2. Complications prevented.
3. Lifestyle and behavior changes adopted to prevent spread of infection.
4. Disease process, prognosis, and therapeutic regimen understood.
5. Plan in place to meet needs after discharge.

NURSING DIAGNOSIS: risk for Infection [spread/reactivation]

Risk Factors May Include

Inadequate primary defenses—decreased ciliary action, stasis of body fluids
Tissue destruction, [extension of infection]
Suppressed inflammatory response
Malnutrition
Environmental exposure to pathogens
Deficient knowledge to avoid exposure to pathogens

Possibly Evidenced By

(Not applicable; presence of signs and symptoms establishes an *actual* diagnosis)

(continues on page 174)

NURSING DIAGNOSIS: risk for Infection [spread/reactivation] (continued)

Desired Outcomes/Evaluation Criteria—Client Will

Risk Control: Infectious Process (NOC)
Identify interventions to prevent or reduce risk of spread of infection.
Demonstrate techniques and initiate lifestyle changes to promote safe environment.

ACTIONS/INTERVENTIONS	RATIONALE
Infection Control (NIC)	
Independent	
Review pathology of disease—active or inactive phases, dissemination of infection through bronchi to adjacent tissues or via bloodstream and lymphatic system—and potential spread of infection via airborne droplet during coughing, sneezing, spitting, talking, laughing, and singing.	Helps client realize and accept necessity of adhering to medication regimen to prevent reactivation and complications. Understanding of how the disease is passed and awareness of transmission possibilities help client and significant other (SO) take steps to prevent infection of others.
Identify others at risk, such as household members, close associates, and friends.	Those exposed may require a course of drug therapy to prevent development of infection.
Instruct client to cough, sneeze, and expectorate into tissue and to refrain from spitting. Review proper disposal of tissue and good hand-washing techniques. Request return demonstration.	Behaviors necessary to prevent spread of infection.
Review necessity of infection control measures, such as temporary respiratory isolation.	May help client understand need for protecting others while acknowledging client's sense of isolation and social stigma associated with communicable diseases. *Note:* AFB can pass through standard masks; therefore, particulate respirators are required.
Monitor temperature, as indicated.	Febrile reactions are indicators of continuing presence of infection.
Identify individual risk factors for reactivation of tuberculosis, such as lowered resistance associated with alcoholism, malnutrition, intestinal bypass surgery, use of immunosuppressant drugs, presence of diabetes mellitus or cancer, or postpartum.	Knowledge about these factors helps client alter lifestyle and avoid or reduce incidence of disease reactivation.
Emphasize importance of uninterrupted drug therapy. Evaluate client's potential for cooperation.	Contagious period may last only 2 to 3 days after initiation of drug regimen, but in the presence of cavitation or moderately advanced disease, risk of spread of infection may continue up to 3 months. Compliance with multidrug regimens for prolonged periods is difficult; therefore, DOT should be considered.
Review importance of follow-up and periodic reculturing of sputum for the duration of therapy.	Aids in monitoring the effects of medications and client's response to therapy.
Encourage selection and ingestion of well-balanced meals. Provide frequent small "snacks" in place of large meals as appropriate.	Presence of anorexia or preexisting malnutrition lowers resistance to infectious process and impairs healing. Small snacks may enhance overall intake.
Collaborative	
Administer anti-infective agents, as indicated, for example:	The goals for treatment of TB are to cure the individual and to minimize transmission to other persons. It is essential that treatment be tailored and supervision be based on each client's clinical and social circumstances. DOT may be the most effective way to maximize the completion of therapy.
Primary drugs: isoniazid (INH, Liniazid), rifampin (RIF, Rifadin, Rimactane), pyrazinamide (PZA, Tebrazid), and ethambutol (Etbi, Myambutol)	In active TB, these four drugs will be given together for the initial phase (first 2 months) of therapy, followed by a choice of options (usually two drugs based on drug sensitivity testing (for the continuation phase (usually 4 to 7 months). Although basic TB regimens are broadly applicable, treatment modifications are made in certain circumstances (i.e., HIV infection, drug resistance, pregnancy, or treatment of children) (CDC, 2012; Schiffman, 2011). INH (monotherapy) is the usual drug of choice for those exposed and who are at risk for developing TB. Extended therapy for up to 24 months is indicated for reactivation cases, extrapulmonary reactivated TB, or in the presence of other medical problems, such as diabetes mellitus or silicosis.
rufabutin (Mucobutin)	Therapeutic agent for atypical mycobacterium. May be used in client with advanced HIV disease with TB.

ACTIONS/INTERVENTIONS (continued)	RATIONALE (continued)
Investigational agents such as diarylquinoline (R207910)	Innovative compounds are being developed based on new drug targets and structure to provide shorter and more effective treatment options. This agent, currently in phase II human trials, cuts off the energy supply of the mycobacterium and appears to also be effective against drug-resistant forms of TB (Diacon et al, 2009).
Monitor laboratory studies, such as the following:	
Sputum smear results	Client who has three consecutive negative sputum smears over a 3- to 5-month period, is adhering to drug regimen, and who is asymptomatic will be classified as a nontransmitter.
Liver function studies, such as aspartate aminotransferase (AST), alinine aminotransferase (ALT)	The most common serious adverse effect of drug therapy—particularly RIF, but possibly others as well—is drug-induced hepatitis.
Notify local health department.	Required by law, and should be reported within 1 week of diagnosis. Helpful in identifying contacts to reduce spread of infection. Treatment course is long and usually handled in the community, with public health nurse monitoring.

NURSING DIAGNOSIS: ineffective Airway Clearance

May Be Related To
Infection
Excessive mucus; exudates in the alveoli
[Tracheal or pharyngeal edema]

Possibly Evidenced By
Change in respiratory rate, rhythm
Ineffective cough
Diminished/adventitious breath sounds—[rhonchi, wheezes, stridor]
Dyspnea

Desired Outcomes/Evaluation Criteria—Client Will

Respiratory Status: Airway Patency (NOC)
Maintain patent airway.
Expectorate secretions without assistance.
Demonstrate behaviors to improve or maintain airway clearance.
Participate in treatment regimen, within the level of ability and situation.
Identify potential complications and initiate appropriate actions.

ACTIONS/INTERVENTIONS	RATIONALE
Airway Management (NIC)	
Independent	
Assess respiratory function, such as breath sounds, rate, rhythm, and depth, and use of accessory muscles.	Diminished breath sounds may reflect atelectasis. Rhonchi and wheezes indicate accumulation of secretions and inability to clear airways, which may lead to use of accessory muscles and increased work of breathing.
Note ability to expectorate mucus and cough effectively; document character and amount of sputum and presence of hemoptysis.	Expectoration may be difficult when secretions are very thick as a result of infection or inadequate hydration. Blood-tinged or frankly bloody sputum results from tissue breakdown in the lungs and may require further evaluation and intervention.
Place client in semi- or high-Fowler's position. Assist client with coughing and deep-breathing exercises.	Positioning helps maximize lung expansion and decreases respiratory effort. Maximal ventilation may open atelectatic areas and promote movement of secretions into larger airways for expectoration.
Clear secretions from mouth and trachea; suction as necessary.	Prevents obstruction and aspiration. Suctioning may be necessary if client is unable to expectorate secretions.
Maintain fluid intake of at least 2500 mL/day unless contraindicated.	High fluid intake helps thin secretions, making them easier to expectorate.
Collaborative	
Humidify inspired oxygen.	Prevents drying of mucous membranes and helps thin secretions.

(continues on page 176)

ACTIONS/INTERVENTIONS (continued)	RATIONALE (continued)
Administer medications, as indicated, for example:	
Mucolytic agents, such as acetylcysteine (Mucomyst)	Reduces the thickness and stickiness of pulmonary secretions to facilitate clearance.
Bronchodilators, such as oxtriphylline (Choledyl) and theophylline (Theo-Dur)	Increases lumen size of the tracheobronchial tree, thus decreasing resistance to airflow and improving oxygen delivery.
Corticosteroids (prednisone)	May be useful in the presence of extensive involvement with profound hypoxemia and when inflammatory response is life-threatening.
Be prepared for and assist with emergency intubation.	Intubation may be necessary in rare cases of bronchogenic TB accompanied by laryngeal edema or acute pulmonary bleeding.

NURSING DIAGNOSIS: risk for impaired Gas Exchange

Risk Factors May Include

Ventilation-perfusion imbalance
Alveolar-capillary membrane changes

Possibly Evidenced By

(Not applicable; presence of signs and symptoms establishes an *actual* diagnosis)

Desired Outcomes/Evaluation Criteria—Client Will

Respiratory Status: Gas Exchange (NOC)

Report absence of or decreased dyspnea.
Demonstrate improved ventilation and adequate oxygenation of tissues by ABGs within acceptable ranges.
Be free of symptoms of respiratory distress.

ACTIONS/INTERVENTIONS	RATIONALE
Respiratory Monitoring (NIC)	
Independent	
Assess for dyspnea (using 0 to 10 [or similar] scale), tachypnea, abnormal breath sounds, increased respiratory effort, limited chest wall expansion, and fatigue.	Pulmonary TB can cause a wide range of effects in the lungs, ranging from a small patch of bronchopneumonia to diffuse intense inflammation, caseous necrosis, pleural effusion, and extensive fibrosis.
Evaluate change in level of mentation.	Accumulation of secretions and airway compromise can impair oxygenation of vital organs and tissues, often reflected in change in mental status.
Note cyanosis or change in skin color, including mucous membranes and nailbeds.	Respiratory effects can range from mild dyspnea to profound respiratory distress. *Note:* Using a scale to evaluate dyspnea helps clarify degree of difficulty and changes in condition.
Demonstrate and encourage pursed-lip breathing during exhalation, especially for clients with fibrosis or parenchymal destruction.	Creates resistance against outflowing air to prevent collapse of the airways, thereby helping to distribute air throughout the lungs and relieve or reduce shortness of breath.
Promote bedrest, or limit activity and assist with self-care activities as necessary.	Reducing oxygen consumption and demand during periods of respiratory compromise may reduce severity of symptoms.
Collaborative	
Monitor serial ABGs and pulse oximetry.	Decreased oxygen content (PaO_2) and saturation or increased $PaCO_2$ indicate need for change in therapeutic regimen.
Provide supplemental oxygen as appropriate.	Aids in correcting the hypoxemia that may occur secondary to decreased ventilation and diminished alveolar lung surface.

NURSING DIAGNOSIS: imbalanced Nutrition: less than body requirements

May Be Related To

[Fatigue]
Biological factors—frequent cough and sputum production; dyspnea
Insufficient finances

Possibly Evidenced By

Body weight 20% or more below ideal weight range
Reported lack of interest in food, altered taste sensation
Poor muscle tone

NURSING DIAGNOSIS: imbalanced Nutrition: less than body requirements (continued)

Desired Outcomes/Evaluation Criteria—Client Will

Nutritional Status

Demonstrate progressive weight gain toward goal with normalization of laboratory values and be free of signs of malnutrition.
Initiate behaviors or lifestyle changes to regain and to maintain appropriate weight.

ACTIONS/INTERVENTIONS	RATIONALE
Nutrition Management (NIC)	
Independent	
Document client's nutritional status on admission, noting skin turgor, current weight and degree of weight loss, integrity of oral mucosa, ability to swallow, presence of bowel tones, and history of nausea, vomiting, or diarrhea.	Useful in defining extent of problem and appropriate choice of interventions.
Ascertain client's usual dietary pattern and likes and dislikes.	Helps to identify specific needs or strengths. Consideration of individual preferences may improve dietary intake.
Monitor intake and output (I&O) and weight periodically.	Useful in measuring effectiveness of nutritional and fluid support.
Investigate anorexia, nausea, and vomiting. Note possible correlation to medications. Monitor frequency, volume, and consistency of stools.	Affects dietary choices and can identify areas for problem-solving to enhance intake of nutrients.
Encourage and provide for frequent rest periods.	Helps conserve energy, especially when metabolic requirements are increased by fever.
Provide oral care before and after respiratory treatments.	Reduces bad taste left from sputum or medications used for respiratory treatments that can stimulate the vomiting center.
Encourage small, frequent meals with foods high in protein and carbohydrates.	Maximizes nutrient intake without undue energy expenditure from eating large meals.
Encourage SO to bring foods from home and to share meals with client unless contraindicated.	Creates a more normal social environment during mealtime and helps meet personal and cultural preferences.
Collaborative	
Refer to dietitian/nutritionist for adjustments in dietary composition.	Provides assistance in planning a diet with nutrients adequate to meet client's metabolic requirements, dietary preferences, and financial resources.
Consult with respiratory therapy to schedule treatments 1 to 2 hours before or after meals.	May help reduce the incidence of nausea and vomiting associated with medications or the effects of respiratory treatments on a full stomach.
Monitor laboratory studies, such as blood urea nitrogen (BUN), serum protein, and prealbumin and albumin.	Low values reflect malnutrition and indicate need for change in therapeutic regimen.
Administer antipyretics, as appropriate.	Fever increases metabolic needs and therefore calorie consumption.

NURSING DIAGNOSIS: risk for ineffective Self-Health Management

May Be Related To

Complexity of therapeutic regimen
Deficient knowledge
Economic difficulties
Perceived barriers/seriousness

Possibly Evidenced By

(Not applicable; presence of signs and symptoms establishes an *actual* diagnosis)

Desired Outcomes/Evaluation Criteria—Client Will

Self-Management: Chronic Disease (NOC)

Verbalize understanding of disease process, prognosis, and prevention.
Initiate behaviors or lifestyle changes to improve general well-being and reduce risk of reactivation of TB.
Identify symptoms requiring evaluation and intervention.
Describe a plan for receiving adequate follow-up care.
Verbalize understanding of therapeutic regimen and rationale for actions.

ACTIONS/INTERVENTIONS	RATIONALE
Learning Facilitation (NIC)	
Independent	
Assess client's ability to learn, such as level of fear, concern, fatigue, participation level; best environment in which client can learn; how much content the client can learn; best media and language to teach the client; and determine who should be included.	Learning depends on emotional and physical readiness and is achieved at an individual pace.
Provide instruction and specific written information for client to refer to, such as schedule for medications and follow-up sputum testing for documenting response to therapy.	Written information relieves client of the burden of having to remember large amounts of information. Repetition strengthens learning.
Encourage client and SO to verbalize fears and concerns. Answer questions factually. Note prolonged use of denial.	Provides opportunity to correct misconceptions that may alleviate anxiety. Prolonged denial may affect coping with and managing the tasks necessary to regain health.
Teaching: Disease Process (NIC)	
Identify symptoms that should be reported to healthcare provider, such as hemoptysis, chest pain, fever, difficulty breathing, hearing loss, and vertigo.	May indicate progression or reactivation of disease or side effects of medications, requiring further evaluation.
Emphasize the importance of maintaining high-protein and carbohydrate diet and adequate fluid intake. (Refer to ND: imbalanced Nutrition: less than body requirements.)	Meeting metabolic needs helps minimize fatigue and promotes recovery. Fluids aid in liquefying and expectorating secretions.
Explain medication dosage, frequency of administration, expected action, and the reason for long treatment period. Review potential interactions with other drugs and substances. Emphasize reportable side effects.	Enhances cooperation with therapeutic regimen and may prevent client from discontinuing medication before cure is truly effected. DOT is the treatment of choice when client is unable or unwilling to take medications as prescribed. *Note:* Clients with HIV infection and TB are particularly susceptible to drug interactions because they are typically taking numerous medications, some of which react with antituberculosis medications.
Review potential side effects of treatment, such as dry mouth, gastrointestinal (GI) upset, constipation, visual disturbances, headache, and orthostatic hypertension, and problem-solve solutions.	It is important that antituberculosis drugs not be discontinued because of "nuisance" side effects. Problem-solving, such as taking medication with food and changing the hour of dosing, may reduce discomfort associated with therapy and enhance cooperation with regimen. Severe reactions must be reported to physician.
Emphasize need to abstain from alcohol while on INH.	Combination of INH and alcohol has been linked to increased incidence of hepatitis.
Refer for eye examination after starting and then monthly during the course of ethambutol (EMB).	Major side effect is reduced visual acuity; initial sign may be decreased ability to perceive the color green.
Encourage abstaining from smoking.	Although smoking does not stimulate recurrence of TB, it does increase the likelihood of respiratory dysfunction.
Review that TB is transmitted primarily by inhalation of airborne organisms but may also spread through stools or urine if infection is present in these organ systems; also review hazards of reactivation.	Knowledge may reduce risk of transmission or reactivation. Complications associated with reactivation include cavitation, abscess formation, destructive emphysema, spontaneous pneumothorax, diffuse interstitial fibrosis, serous effusion, empyema, bronchiectasis, hemoptysis, GI ulceration, bronchopleural fistula, tuberculosis laryngitis, and miliary spread.
Discuss and reinforce concerns, such as treatment failure, drug-resistant TB, and relapse.	Treatment failure most often occurs because client is not adhering to treatment regimen, but can also be due to drug resistance, malabsorption of drugs, laboratory error, and extreme biological variation in response. Most relapses or recurrence of positive cultures or radiographic deterioration occur 6 to 12 months after completion of therapy. Continuous monitoring by healthcare providers can identify these concerns early and alter the plan accordingly.
Refer to public health agency as appropriate.	DOT by community nurses is often the most effective way to ensure client adherence to therapy. Monitoring may include pill counts and urine dipstick testing for presence of antitubercular drug. Clients with MDR-TB may be monitored with monthly sputum specimens for AFB smear and culture. *Note:* In some states, there are legal means for involuntary confinement for care if efforts to ensure client adherence are ineffective.

POTENTIAL CONSIDERATIONS following acute hospitalization (dependent on client's age, physical condition and presence of complications, personal resources, and life responsibilities)
- *ineffective Self-Health Management*—complexity of therapeutic regimen, economic difficulties, family patterns of healthcare, perceived seriousness and benefits
- *risk for Infection (secondary)*—decrease in ciliary action, stasis of body fluids (secretions), suppressed inflammatory response, tissue destruction, chronic disease, malnutrition, increased environmental exposure
- *Fatigue*—disease states, malnutrition, discomfort
- *ineffective family Therapeutic Regimen Management*—complexity of therapeutic regimen, decisional conflicts, economic difficulties, family conflict

RESPIRATORY ACID-BASE IMBALANCES

I. Pathophysiology—the body has the remarkable ability to maintain plasma pH within a narrow range of 7.35 to 7.45.

a. Accomplished by chemical buffering mechanisms involving the lungs and kidneys

i. Lungs compensate for acid-base imbalances resulting from altered levels of metabolic acids.

ii. Kidneys compensate for acid-base imbalances resulting from altered levels of carbonic acid.

b. Although simple acid-base imbalances (e.g., respiratory acidosis) do occur, mixed acid-base imbalances are more common (e.g., the respiratory acidosis and metabolic acidosis that occur with cardiac arrest).

RESPIRATORY ACIDOSIS (PRIMARY CARBONIC ACID EXCESS)

I. Types

a. Acute respiratory acidosis: develops when an abrupt failure of ventilation occurs

i. Due to rapid development of problem, metabolic compensation is ineffective.

ii. $PaCO_2$ greater than 47 mm Hg with accompanying acidemia (pH 7.25)

b. Chronic respiratory acidosis: progressive failure of ventilation over time

i. Allows for some degree of compensation through increased renal reabsorption of HCO_3

ii. $PaCO_2$ greater than 47 mm Hg, normal or near normal pH, and elevated serum bicarbonate (HCO_3 greater than 30 mm Hg)

II. Compensatory Mechanisms—occurs over 3 to 5 days

a. Increased respiratory rate

b. Hemoglobin (Hgb) buffering

c. Forming bicarbonate ions and deoxygenated Hgb

d. Increased renal ammonia acid excretions with reabsorption of bicarbonate

III. Etiology

a. Alveolar hypoventilation, reduced CO_2 elimination, excess of carbonic acid (H_2CO_3)

b. Conditions causing a decrease in respiratory rate and volume:

i. Central nervous system (CNS) disorders, such as with depression of the central respiratory center; for example, brainstem disease or trauma, tumors, encephalitis, stroke, or drugs such as use of "downers" or overdose of sedatives or barbiturate poisoning

ii. Pulmonary disorders of the airways or those causing airway obstruction, such as asthma or chronic obstructive pulmonary disease (COPD) exacerbation, bronchiectasis, aspiration of foreign body, acute pulmonary edema, acute laryngospasm, smoke inhalation, excessive CO_2 intake (e.g., use of rebreathing mask, CO_2 therapy)

iii. Neuromuscular disorders restricting chest movement and inability to ventilate adequately, such as myasthenia gravis, amyotrophic lateral sclerosis (ALS), Guillain-Barré syndrome, muscular dystrophy, botulism

iv. Severe restrictive ventilatory defects, such as interstitial fibrosis, thoracic deformities, hemothorax and pneumothorax, atelectasis, acute respiratory distress syndrome (ARDS), spinal cord injuries, anesthesia and surgery, severe obesity (Pickwickian syndrome)

GLOSSARY

Acid: A substance that, when dissolved in water, dissociates and can donate a hydrogen (proton) to another molecule.

Acidosis: Increased acidity (i.e., an increased hydrogen [H^+] ion concentration). If not further qualified, it refers to acidity of the blood plasma. Acidosis is said to occur when arterial pH falls below 7.35.

Alkalosis: A dangerous decrease in the normal acidity of the blood, where there is too much base in the blood.

Base: Chemical opposite of acid.

Base excess/deficit: A calculated number that represents a sum total of the metabolic buffering agents (anions) in the blood; these anions include hemoglobin, proteins, phosphates, and bicarbonate (HCO_3^-, dominant anion); these anions try to compensate for imbalances in the pH caused by diseases or conditions that affect the lungs (respiratory acidosis or alkalosis) or kidneys (metabolic acidosis or alkalosis).

(continues on page 180)

GLOSSARY (continued)

Buffers: Chemicals that help control the pH of body fluids. Each buffer system consists of a weak acid, which releases H^+ when the fluid is too alkaline and a base when the fluid is too acidic. H^+ ions are buffered by extracellular (such as bicarbonate, ammonia) and intracellular buffering agents (including proteins and phosphate).

Carbonic acid (H_2CO_3): If too much acid is present, the bicarbonate ions take up the hydrogen ions and become H_2CO_3, which is then excreted through the lungs in the form of carbon dioxide (CO_2) and water (H_2O^+). Conversely, if too little acid is present in extracellular fluid, the carbonic acid portion of the bicarbonate buffer system releases hydrogen ions. For the pH to remain within normal range (7.35 to 7.45), the ratio of bicarbonate ions to H_2CO_3 must be 20:1 (Felver, 2005).

Circumoral paresthesias: Numbness, stinging, or burning sensation around the mouth.

CO_2: Respiratory acid, which is the only acid that can be exhaled via the lungs.

H^+: The ion that is left when the hydrogen atom loses its electron, forming a proton.

HCO_3^-: Measurement of the metabolic component of the acid-base balance. HCO_3^- is excreted and reabsorbed (conserved) by the kidneys in response to pH imbalances and is directly related to the pH level; as the amount of HCO_3^- rises, so does the pH.

Hypercapnia: Increased amount of CO_2 in the blood.

Hyperventilation: Increased rate and depth of breathing that causes a decrease in CO_2.

Hypoventilation: Reduced rate and depth of breathing that causes an increase in CO_2.

Hypoxemia: Low level of oxygen (O_2) in the blood.

O_2 saturation: Percentage of hemoglobin saturation or how much O_2 is bound to hemoglobin in the red blood cells and available to be carried through the arteries to cells.

Partial pressure of carbon dioxide ($PaCO_2$): Reflects the balance between the production of CO_2 and its elimination. Unless the metabolic rate changes, the amount of CO_2 produced is roughly constant and determines the amount of ventilation required and the level of $PaCO_2$. The normal value in arterial blood is 40 mm Hg. In the healthy, awake individual, the end-exhaled value is usually similar.

Partial pressure of O_2 (PaO_2): Amount of oxygen gas dissolved in blood.

pH: A measure of the level of H^+, which indicates the acid-base status of blood; the pH decreases (becomes more acidic) with increased amounts of $PaCO_2$ and other acids, and the pH increases (blood becomes more alkaline) with decreased $PaCO_2$ or increased amounts of HCO_3^-.

Respiratory acidosis: Acute or chronic condition that occurs when the lungs cannot remove all the CO_2 the body produces.

Respiratory alkalosis: Condition marked by low levels of CO_2 in the blood.

Tachypnea: Rapid, shallow respirations.

Care Setting

This condition does not occur in isolation; rather, it is a complication of a broader health problem, disease, or condition for which the severely compromised client requires admission to a medical-surgical or subacute unit.

Related Concerns

Plans of care specific to predisposing factors and disease or medical condition, such as the following:

Alcohol: acute withdrawal, page 800
Cerebrovascular accident (CVA)/stroke, page 214
Chronic obstructive pulmonary disease (COPD) and asthma, page 118
Craniocerebral trauma (acute rehabilitative phase), page 197
Eating disorders: obesity, page 358
Spinal cord injury (acute rehabilitative phase), page 248
Surgical intervention, page 762
Ventilatory assistance (mechanical), page 157

Other Concerns

Fluid and electrolyte imbalances, page 885
Metabolic acidosis—primary base bicarborate deficiency, page 450
Metabolic alkalosis—primary base bicarborate excess, page 455

Client Assessment Database

DIAGNOSTIC DIVISION MAY REPORT	MAY EXHIBIT
ACTIVITY/REST	
• Fatigue, mild to profound • Sleep disturbances	• Generalized weakness • Ataxia or staggering • Loss of coordination • Stupor

DIAGNOSTIC DIVISION MAY REPORT (continued)	MAY EXHIBIT (continued)
CIRCULATION	• Blood pressure (BP) may be low, with bounding pulses, pinkish color, warm skin • Dilation of conjunctival and superficial facial blood vessels, reflecting vasodilation of severe acidosis • Tachycardia, irregular pulse, various dysrhythmias • Diaphoresis, pallor, and cyanosis—late stage of respiratory failure
FOOD/FLUID • Nausea, vomiting	
NEUROSENSORY • Feeling of fullness in head (acute—associated with vasodilation) • Headache (acute) • Dizziness • Visual disturbances	• Anxiety, confusion, apprehension, agitation, restlessness, delirium, depressed mental status, somnolence (CO_2 narcosis), coma (acute) • Tremors, decreased reflexes, or asterixis, myoclonus, and seizures (severe)

RESPIRATION
• Shortness of breath with exertion
	• Respirations dependent on underlying cause:
	  • Tachypnea can occur often with prolonged expiration.
	  • Hypoventilation can be associated with depression of respiratory center (as in head trauma and respiratory failure), or with muscle paralysis, oversedation, general anesthesia, metabolic alkalosis.
	  • Increased respiratory effort with nasal flaring or yawning, use of neck and upper body muscles
	  • Decreased breath sounds
	  • Hyperresonance on percussion
	  • Adventitious breath sounds—wheezes, stridor, crowing

TEACHING/LEARNING Refer to specific plans of care reflecting individual predisposing or contributing factors.	
DISCHARGE PLAN CONSIDERATIONS May require assistance with changes in therapies for underlying disease process/condition. ➧ Refer to section at end of plan for postdischarge considerations.	

Diagnostic Studies

TEST WHY IT IS DONE	WHAT IT TELLS ME
BLOOD TESTS • Arterial blood gases (ABGs): Measure how much O_2 and CO_2 is in arterial blood. They also look at the acidity (pH) of the blood. *Normal ABGs at sea level:* • PaO_2: 75 to 100 mm Hg • $PaCO_2$: 35 to 45 mm Hg • pH: 7.35 to7.45 • SaO_2: 94 to 100%	*PaO_2:* Normal or low. Oxygen saturation (SaO_2) decreased. *$PaCO_2$:* Increased, greater than 45 mm Hg (primary acidosis) *HCO_3:* Normal or increased, greater than 26 mEq/L (compensated/chronic stage)

(continues on page 182)

Diagnostic Studies (continued)

TEST WHY IT IS DONE (continued)	WHAT IT TELLS ME (continued)
• HCO_3: 22 to 26 mEq/L • Arterial pH: Decreased, less than 7.35	
• *Capnography:* Monitors the concentration or PCO_2 in the respiratory gases.	Provides information about CO_2 production, lung perfusion, alveolar ventilation, respiratory patterns, and elimination of CO_2.
• *Electrolyte tests:* The electrolyte panel is composed of the individual tests for sodium, potassium, chloride, and total carbon dioxide. A related "test" is the anion gap, which is actually a value calculated using the results of an electrolyte panel.	*Serum potassium:* Typically increased *Serum chloride:* Decreased *Serum calcium:* Increased
ASSOCIATED TESTS	
• *Other screening tests:* As indicated by underlying illness or condition, including chest x-ray, chest computed tomography (CT), brain magnetic resonance imaging (MRI), pulmonary function studies, drug and toxicology screens, and tests to measure diaphragmatic function	To determine underlying cause and treatment needs

Nursing Priorities

1. Achieve homeostasis.
2. Prevent or minimize complications.
3. Provide information about condition, prognosis, and treatment needs as appropriate.

Discharge Goals

1. Physiological balance restored.
2. Free of complications.
3. Condition, prognosis, and treatment needs understood.
4. Plan in place to meet needs after discharge.

NURSING DIAGNOSIS: impaired Gas Exchange

May Be Related To

Ventilation-perfusion imbalance
Alveolar-capillary membrane changes

Possibly Evidenced By

Dyspnea, abnormal breathing (tachypnea)
Irritability, confusion
Tachycardia
Hypoxia, hypercapnia

Desired Outcomes/Evaluation Criteria—Client Will

Acute Respiratory Acidosis Severity (NOC)

Demonstrate improved ventilation and adequate oxygenation of tissues as evidenced by ABGs within client's acceptable limits and absence of symptoms of respiratory distress.

Knowledge: Disease Process (NOC)

Verbalize understanding of causative factors and appropriate interventions.
Participate in treatment regimen within level of ability or situation.

ACTIONS/INTERVENTIONS	RATIONALE
Acid-Base Management: Respiratory Acidosis (NIC) ***Independent***	
Monitor respiratory rate, depth, and effort.	Alveolar hypoventilation and associated hypoxemia lead to respiratory failure.
Auscultate breath sounds.	Identifies area(s) of decreased ventilation, such as atelectasis, or airway obstruction and changes as client deteriorates or improves, reflecting effectiveness of treatment and dictating therapy needs.
Note declining level of awareness or consciousness.	Signals severe acidotic state, which requires immediate attention. *Note:* In recovery, sensorium clears slowly because

ACTIONS/INTERVENTIONS (continued)	RATIONALE (continued)
	hydrogen ions are slow to cross the blood-brain barrier and clear from cerebrospinal fluid (CSF) and brain cells.
Monitor heart rate and rhythm.	Tachycardia develops early because the sympathetic nervous system is stimulated, resulting in the release of catecholamines, epinephrine, and norepinephrine in an attempt to increase oxygen delivery to the tissues. Dysrhythmias that may occur are due to hypoxia (myocardial ischemia) and electrolyte imbalances.
Note skin color, temperature, and moisture.	Diaphoresis, pallor, and cool, clammy skin are late changes associated with severe or advancing hypoxemia.
Encourage and assist with deep-breathing exercises, turning, and coughing. Suction as necessary. Provide airway adjunct as indicated. Place in semi-Fowler's position.	These measures improve lung ventilation and reduce or prevent airway obstruction associated with accumulation of mucus.
Restrict use of hypnotic sedatives or tranquilizers.	In the presence of hypoventilation, respiratory depression and CO_2 narcosis may develop.
Discuss cause of chronic condition, when known, and appropriate interventions and self-care activities.	Promotes participation in therapeutic regimen and may reduce recurrence of disorder.
Collaborative	
Assist with identification and treatment of underlying cause.	Treatment of disorder is directed at improving alveolar ventilation. Multiple team management, including physicians, pulmonologist and respiratory therapists, or neurologists, may be required to address the underlying condition, such as oversedation, brain trauma, COPD, pulmonary edema, aspiration, and promote correction of the acid-base disorder.
Monitor and graph serial ABGs and pulse oximetry readings.	Evaluates therapy needs and effectiveness. *Note:* Pulse oximetry monitoring is used to monitor and show early changes in oxygen saturation, which can occur before other signs or symptoms are observed.
Administer oxygen as indicated, using appropriate delivery means—endotracheal (ET) intubation with mechanical ventilation, or nasal continuous positive-pressure ventilation or nasal bi-level ventilation.	Prevents or corrects hypoxemia and pulmonary hypertension, and its use prevents the consequences of long-standing hypoxemia.
Increase respiratory rate or tidal volume of ventilator if used.	Increases lung expansion and opens airways to improve ventilation and gas diffusion, preventing respiratory failure.
Assist with ventilatory aids, such as intermittent positive-pressure breathing (IPPB) in conjunction with bronchodilators. Monitor peak flow pressure.	Assists in correction of acidity and mobilization of respiratory secretions.
Maintain hydration (intravenously [IV]/by mouth [PO]) and provide humidification.	Aids in clearing secretions, which improves ventilation, allowing excess CO_2 to be eliminated.
Administer medications, as indicated, for example:	
Opioid antagonist, such as naloxone hydrochloride (Narcan) and flumazenil (Romazicon)	Useful in reversing the effects of certain opiates and sedative drugs on the respiratory center, stimulating ventilation in presence of drug overdose or sedation, or acidosis resulting from cardiac arrest.
Bronchodilators including beta-agonists, for example, albuterol (Proventil, Ventolin) and salmeterol (Serevent); anticholinergic agents, for example, ipratropium bromide (Atrovent); and methylxanthines, for example, theophylline	Helpful in treating client with acidosis secondary to obstructive lung disease and severe bronchospasm. Theophylline may improve diaphragm muscle contractility and may stimulate the respiratory center.
Electrolytes, as indicated	Respiratory acidosis does not have a great effect on electrolyte levels, although some effects occur on calcium and potassium levels. Acidemia causes an extracellular shift of potassium. Correction of the acidosis may cause a relative serum hypokalemia as potassium shifts back into cells. Potassium imbalance can impair neuromuscular or respiratory function, causing generalized muscle weakness and cardiac dysrhythmias. *Note:* Infusion of sodium bicarbonate is rarely indicated, although it may be considered in cardiopulmonary arrest when pH is less than 7.0.
Provide or refer for pulmonary rehabilitation, as indicated.	Provides restorative and preventative care to reverse respiratory acidosis secondary to underlying conditions, such as bronchial hygiene, breathing retraining, and exercise conditioning. Therapy modalities and length of intervention may vary depending on whether the respiratory acidosis is acute or chronic.
Provide low-carbohydrate, high-fat diet (for example, Pulmocare feedings), if indicated.	Helps reduce CO_2 production and improves respiratory muscle function and metabolic homeostasis.

POTENTIAL CONSIDERATIONS following acute hospitalization (dependent on client's age, physical condition and presence of complications, personal resources, and life responsibilities)

Refer to Potential Considerations relative to underlying cause of acid-base disorder.

RESPIRATORY ALKALOSIS (PRIMARY CARBONIC ACID DEFICIT)

I. Pathophysiology—acute or chronic increase in respiratory rate and volume, primarily triggered by hypoxemia or direct stimulation of the central respiratory center of the brain

- a. Acute: $PaCO_2$ is below lower limit of normal, serum pH is alkalemic due to loss of potassium, and phosphate secondary to cellular uptake.
- b. Chronic: $PaCO_2$ is below the lower limit of normal, but pH is normal or near normal because of renal compensation.

II. Compensatory Mechanisms—occurs over 2 to 3 days

- a. Decreased respiratory rate (if the body is able to respond to the drop in $PaCO_2$)
- b. Increased renal excretion of bicarbonate
- c. Retention of hydrogen

III. Etiology

- a. Alveolar hyperventilation, hypocapnea ($PaCO_2$ less than 35 mm Hg), increased ratio of bicarbonate concentration to $PaCO_2$ (base excess), near-normal or alkaline pH
- b. Most frequently occurring acid-base imbalance in hospitalized clients, with the elderly being at increased risk because of the high incidence of pulmonary disorders and alterations in neurologic status
- c. Conditions or disorders associated with respiratory alkalosis:
  - i. Central nervous system (CNS)—such as stroke, meningitis, encephalitis, brain trauma or tumor, pain, hyperventilation, anxiety, psychosis, fever
  - ii. Hypoxemia—such as severe anemia, any lung disease that leads to shortness of breath, high altitude
  - iii. Drugs—such as salicylates, nicotine, methyxanthines, catecholamines
  - iv. Endocrine—such as hyperthyroidism, pregnancy, increased progesterone levels
  - v. Stimulation of chest receptors—such as pulmonary embolus, pulmonary edema, aspiration, hemopneumothorax
  - vi. Miscellaneous—such as sepsis, liver failure, heat exhaustion, mechanical ventilation (pseudorespiratory alkalosis)

Care Setting

This condition does not occur in isolation, but rather is a complication of a broader problem. Treatment is primarily directed at correcting the underlying disorder causing respiratory alkalosis and is usually found in clients requiring care in a medical-surgical or subacute unit.

Related Concerns

Plans of care specific to predisposing factors, such as:

Anemias—iron deficiency, anemia of chronic disease, pernicious, aplastic, hemolytic, page 459

Cirrhosis of the liver, page 412

Craniocerebral trauma, page 197

Fluid and electrolyte imbalances, page 885

Heart failure: chronic, page 43

Hyperthyroidism (Graves' disease, thyrotoxicosis), page 391

Pneumonia, page 129

Sepsis/septicemia, page 665

Ventilatory assistance (mechanical), page 157

Other Concerns

Metabolic acidosis—primary base bicarbonate deficiency, page 450

Metabolic alkalosis—primary base bicarbonate excess, page 455

Client Assessment Database

Dependent on underlying cause

DIAGNOSTIC DIVISION MAY REPORT	MAY EXHIBIT
CIRCULATION	
• History or presence of anemia • Palpitations	• Hypotension • Tachycardia, irregular pulse and dysrhythmias
EGO INTEGRITY	• Extreme anxiety—most common cause of hyperventilation

DIAGNOSTIC DIVISION MAY REPORT (continued)	MAY EXHIBIT (continued)
FOOD/FLUID	
• Dry mouth • Nausea, vomiting	• Abdominal distention—elevated diaphragm as with ascites, pregnancy • Vomiting
NEUROSENSORY	
• Headache, tinnitus • Numbness or tingling of face, hands, and toes; circumoral numbness and generalized paresthesia • Light-headedness, syncope, vertigo, blurred vision	• Confusion, restlessness, obtunded responses, coma • Hyperactive reflexes, positive Chvostek's and Trousseau signs; tetany, seizures • Heightened sensitivity to environmental noise and activity • Muscle weakness, unsteady gait
PAIN/DISCOMFORT	
• Muscle spasms or cramps • Epigastric pain • Chest tightness	
RESPIRATION	
• Shortness of breath • History of asthma, pulmonary fibrosis	• Tachypnea; rapid, shallow breathing; hyperventilation—often 40 or more respirations per minute • Intermittent periods of apnea
SAFETY	• Fever
DISCHARGE PLAN CONSIDERATIONS	
• May require change in treatment or therapy of underlying disease process or condition ➧ Refer to section at end of plan for postdischarge considerations.	

Diagnostic Studies

TEST WHY IT IS DONE	WHAT IT TELLS ME
BLOOD TESTS	
• ***Arterial blood gases (ABGs):*** Measure how much oxygen and carbon dioxide is in arterial blood. They also look at the acidity (pH) of the blood. ***Normal ABGs at sea level:*** • PaO_2: 75 to 100 mm Hg • $PaCO_2$: 35 to 45 mm Hg • pH: 7.35 to 7.45 • SaO_2: 94 to 100% • HCO_3: 22 to 26 mEq/L *Note:* At altitudes of 3000 feet and above, the oxygen values are lower.	*Arterial pH:* Greater than 7.45 (may be near normal in chronic stage) *HCO_3:* Normal or decreased; less than 25 mEq/L (compensatory mechanism) *$PaCO_2$:* Decreased, less than 35 mm Hg (primary)
• ***Electrolytes:*** The electrolyte panel is composed of the individual tests for sodium, potassium, chloride, and total carbon dioxide. A related "test" is the anion gap, which is actually a value calculated using the results of an electrolyte panel. May be used to detect metabolic disorders causing compensatory respiratory alkalosis.	Minor shifts usually occur, for example, serum sodium, potassium, and phosphate decreased due to intracellular shifts; serum chloride increased; and serum calcium decreased.
• ***Complete blood count (CBC):*** Battery of screening tests, which typically includes hemoglobin (Hgb); hematocrit (Hct); red blood cell (RBC) count, morphology, indices, and distribution	May reveal severe anemia—decreased Hgb and oxygen-carrying capacity; or elevated WBCs (due to, for example, inflammatory process or early sepsis).

(continues on page 186)

Diagnostic Studies (continued)

TEST WHY IT IS DONE (continued)	WHAT IT TELLS ME (continued)
width index; platelet count and size; white blood cell (WBC) count and differential. **Associated Tests** • *Screening tests:* As indicated to determine underlying cause • *Toxicology screening:* To detect common causes such as acute alcohol intoxication or salicylate poisoning	

Nursing Priorities

1. Achieve homeostasis.
2. Prevent or minimize complications.
3. Provide information about condition, prognosis, and treatment needs as appropriate.

Discharge Goals

1. Physiological balance restored.
2. Free of complications.
3. Condition, prognosis, and treatment needs understood.
4. Plan in place to meet needs after discharge.

NURSING DIAGNOSIS: impaired Gas Exchange

May Be Related To

Ventilation-perfusion imbalance
Alveolar-capillary membrane changes

Possibly Evidenced By

Dyspnea, abnormal breathing (tachypnea)
Confusion
Hypocapnia, hypoxia
Tachycardia

Desired Outcomes/Evaluation Criteria—Client Will

Acute Respiratory Alkalosis Severity (NOC)

Demonstrate improved ventilation and adequate oxygenation of tissue as evidenced by ABGs within client's acceptable limits and absence of symptoms of respiratory distress.

Knowledge: Disease Process (NOC)

Verbalize understanding of causative factors and appropriate interventions.
Participate in treatment regimen within level of ability or situation.

ACTIONS/INTERVENTIONS	RATIONALE
Acid-Base Management: Respiratory Alkalosis (NIC)	
Independent	
Monitor respiratory rate, depth, and effort; ascertain cause of hyperventilation if possible, for example, anxiety, pain, and improper ventilator settings.	Identifies alterations from usual breathing pattern and influences choice of intervention.
Assess level of awareness and cognition. Note neuromuscular status—strength, tone, reflexes, sensation, and presence of tremors.	Decreased mentation (mild to severe) and tetany or seizures may occur when alkalosis is severe due to shifts in calcium.
Instruct and encourage client to breathe slowly and deeply. Speak in a low, calm tone of voice. Provide safe environment.	May help reassure and calm the agitated client, thereby aiding the reduction of respiratory rate. Assists client to regain control. *Note:* Clients with hyperventilation syndrome as a cause of their respiratory alkalosis may particularly benefit from reassurance and client education in breathing techniques.
Demonstrate appropriate breathing patterns, if appropriate, and assist with respiratory aids, such as rebreathing mask or bag.	Decreasing the rate of respirations can halt the "blowing off" of CO_2, elevating $PaCO_2$ level and normalizing pH.
Provide comfort measures; encourage use of meditation and visualization. Use tepid sponge bath or cool cloths.	Promotes relaxation and reduces stress. Control and reduction of fever reduces potential for seizures and helps reduce respiration rate.

ACTIONS/INTERVENTIONS (continued)	RATIONALE (continued)
Provide safety and seizure precautions, such as bed in low position, padded side rails, frequent observation.	Changes in mentation and CNS and neuromuscular hyperirritability may result in client harm, especially if tetany or convulsions occur.
Discuss cause of condition, if known, and appropriate interventions and self-care activities.	Promotes participation in therapeutic regimen and may reduce recurrence of disorder.
Collaborative	
Assist with identification and treatment of underlying cause.	Respiratory alkalosis is a complication, not an isolated occurrence, and rarely requires emergent treatment (unless pH is greater than 7.5); thus, correction of alkalosis is undertaken by addressing the primary condition, such as hyperventilation of panic attack, organ failure, severe anemia, and drug effect. Because respiratory alkalosis usually occurs in response to some stimulus, treatment is unsuccessful unless the stimulus is controlled.
Monitor and graph serial ABGs and pulse oximetry.	Identifies therapy needs and effectiveness. *Note:* Rapid correction of $PaCO_2$ in individual with chronic respiratory alkalosis (has a lower serum bicarbonate) may cause metabolic acidosis to develop.
Monitor serum potassium and replace, as indicated.	Hypokalemia may occur as potassium is lost via urine or shifted into the cell in exchange for hydrogen in an attempt to correct alkalosis.
Provide sedation and pain medication, as indicated.	Control of pain and sedation may be needed to reduce cause of hyperventilation if client is not responding to conservative measures.
Administer CO_2 (by rebreathing bag or mask) as indicated. Reduce respiratory rate and tidal volume, or add additional dead space (tubing) to mechanical ventilator.	Increasing CO_2 retention may correct carbonic acid deficit, leading to improvement and resolution of alkalotic state.

POTENTIAL CONSIDERATIONS following acute hospitalization (dependent on client's age, physical condition and presence of complications, personal resources, and life responsibilities)

Refer to Potential Considerations relative to underlying cause of acid-base disorder.

CHAPTER 6

Neurological/Sensory Disorders

SEIZURE DISORDERS

I. Pathophysiology

a. Sudden unregulated electrical discharge within the gray matter of the cortex that temporarily interrupts normal brain activity

b. Genetics plays a role in some cases.

c. May be idiopathic or acquired
  - i. Idiopathic: In approximately 75% of all seizures, which includes epilepsy, no cause is identified (Fagley, 2007).
  - ii. Acquired: Possible causes include acidosis, electrolyte imbalances, hypoglycemia (particularly related to type 1 diabetes), hypoxia, alcohol and drug withdrawal, dehydration, systemic lupus, hypertension, septicemia, tumors, and head trauma (Fagley, 2007).

II. Classification

a. Depends on whether the source of the seizure within the brain is localized (partial or focal onset seizures) or distributed (generalized seizures).

b. In adults, partial seizures are the most common type; can be classified depending on whether consciousness is unaffected (simple-partial seizure) or affected (complex-partial seizure).

c. (P) In children age 10 and younger, generalized seizures are more common while partial seizures are more common in older children (Epilepsy Foundation, 2012).
  - i. Simple (partial motor, partial sensory) seizure may be motor, for example, may manifest as a rhythmic jerking of one hand; sensory, autonomic, or psychic; individual can remember what happens but cannot control what is occurring.
  - ii. Complex seizure lasts 30 seconds to 2 minutes and usually begins in temporal or frontal lobe before affecting other areas of the brain; individual appears dazed and confused with or without motor activity being apparent and may be preceded by an aura.

d. Generalized seizures involve loss of consciousness and are classified according to the effect on the body.
  - i. Absence seizures (petit mal seizures): brief periods of impaired consciousness lasting up to 20 seconds without aura or postictal phase; there are no convulsions.
  - ii. Myoclonic: brief, jerky motor movements lasting more than 1 second that often cluster within several minutes
  - iii. Clonic: rhythmic, jerky motor movements involving upper and lower extremities, with or without impaired consciousness
  - iv. Tonic: sudden tonic extension or flexion of head, trunk, and extremities lasting several seconds
  - v. Tonic-clonic (grand mal seizures): all areas of the cortex are involved, with generalized extension of extremities for several seconds, followed by rhythmic clonic movements and a prolonged postictal phase.
  - vi. Atonic: brief loss of postural tone, often resulting in falls and injury (Cavazos & Lum, 2007)

III. Etiology

a. Major causes in adults include conditions that alter how the brain works or that affect the brain's blood supply (National Institute for Neurological Disorders and Stroke [NINDS], 2008).
  - i. Cerebral pathology: traumatic head injury, stroke, infections, hypoxia, expanding brain lesions, and increased intracranial pressure
  - ii. Toxic agents: poisons, alcohol, overdoses of prescription or nonprescription drugs, and drugs of abuse (with drugs being the leading cause)
  - iii. Chemical imbalances: hypoglycemia, hypokalemia, hyponatremia, hypomagnesemia, and acidosis
  - iv. Fever: acute infections and heatstroke
  - v. Eclampsia: prenatal hypertension and toxemia of pregnancy
  - vi. Idiopathic: unknown origin (also known as epilepsy)

b. Risk factors for seizure by adult age group (Franges, 2006)
  - i. Young adults: trauma, alcohol withdrawal, illicit drug use; brain injury or tumor; cardiovascular disease
  - ii. Adults: brain tumor; cerebrovascular disease, electrolyte and metabolic disorders; alcohol withdrawal
  - iii. Older adults: stroke, brain tumor, Alzheimer's-type dementia

c. (P) In children, febrile seizures are the most common type of seizures and are usually outgrown by the age of 6 (Tejani, 2011). Other common causes in children: infections (e.g., meningitis), brain injury, congenital conditions (e.g., Down syndrome), genetic factors (familial tendencies, primary seizure disorders). Prenatal factors and birth delivery problems are associated with increased risk in infants and toddlers (Epilepsy Foundation, 2012).

IV. Statistics

a. Morbidity: Epilepsy and seizures affect over 3 million Americans of all ages; about 1 in 100 people in the United States have experienced an unprovoked seizure or been diagnosed with epilepsy. For about 80% of those diagnosed with epilepsy, seizures can be controlled with modern medicines and surgical techniques. However, about 25% to 30% of people with epilepsy will continue to experience seizures even with treatment (Epilepsy Foundation, 2012; NINDS, 2012). Incidence of epilepsy is highest in those younger than 2 years and in those older than 65 years. P About 40,000 children diagnosed with epilepsy; most will outgrow condition. Between 70% to 80% of children are well controlled with medication (Benaroch, 2012).

b. Mortality: Seizures can (rarely) result in untimely death, either due to loss of awareness during high-risk activities (swimming, driving), seizure-related injury, status epilepticus, or sudden unexplained death in epilepsy (SUDEP). (Noe, 2011; Cavazos, 2012). Up to 50,000 die annually in the United States due to seizures and related causes (Epilepsy Foundation, 2009).

c. Cost: Estimated $15.5 billion annually for medical costs and lost or reduced earnings and production (Epilepsy Foundation, 2009).

GLOSSARY

Aura: A perceptual disturbance experienced by some people before a seizure in the prodromal phase (see below), often manifesting as the perception of a strange light or an unpleasant smell, but does not ensure the onset of a seizure. The time span between the appearance of the aura and the onset of a seizure can be a few seconds up to an hour.

Epilepsy: Chronic neurological disorder characterized by recurrent seizures.

Ictal phase: Considered to be the seizure itself.

Juvenile Myoclonic Epilepsy (Impulsive Petit Mal): Characterized by generalized seizures (usually tonic-clonic), and sometimes absence seizures. It usually occurs in younger people ages 8 to 20.

Landau-Kleffner Syndrome: Rare epileptic condition that typically affects children ages 3 to 7. It results in the loss of ability to communicate either with speech or by writing (*aphasia*).

Postictal phase: The altered state of consciousness characterized by drowsiness, confusion, nausea, hypertension, headache, and other disorienting symptoms that occurs following a seizure, usually lasting between 5 and 30 minutes, but sometimes longer in the case of larger or more severe seizures.

Prodromal phase: An early symptom indicating the onset of an attack or a disease. Vague changes in emotional reactivity or affective response sometimes preceding aura and lasting minutes to hours, with symptoms such as diminished field of vision, disorientation, aphasia, or photosensitivity.

Progressive Myoclonic Epilepsy: Rare inherited disorder typically occurring in children ages 6 to 15. It usually involves tonic-clonic seizures and marked sensitivity to light flashes.

Seizure: Sudden discharge of electrical activity in the brain.

Care Setting

Seizure disorders are treated in a community setting; however, client with convulsive seizures may require brief inpatient care on a medical or subacute unit for stabilization or for treatment of status epilepticus (a life-threatening emergency).

Related Concerns

Cerebrovascular accident (CVA)/stroke, page 214
Craniocerebral trauma (acute rehabilitative phase), page 197
Pediatric considerations, page 872
Psychosocial aspects of care, page 729
Substance use disorders (SUDs), page 815

Client Assessment Database

DIAGNOSTIC DIVISION MAY REPORT	MAY EXHIBIT
ACTIVITY/REST	
• Fatigue • General weakness • Limitation of activities, occupation imposed by self, significant other (SO), healthcare provider, or others	• Altered muscle tone, strength • Involuntary movement or contractions of muscles or muscle groups—generalized tonic-clonic seizures
CIRCULATION	
	• *Ictal:* Hypertension, increased pulse, cyanosis • *Postictal:* Vital signs normal or depressed with decreased pulse and respiration
EGO INTEGRITY	
• Internal or external stressors related to condition or treatment • Irritability • Fear of death or injury	• Wide range of emotional responses, especially when temporal lobe is involved

(continues on page 190)

DIAGNOSTIC DIVISION MAY REPORT (continued)	MAY EXHIBIT (continued)
• Sense of helplessness, hopelessness • Social embarrassment and isolation • Changes in relationships	
ELIMINATION • Episodic incontinence	• *Ictal:* Increased bladder pressure and sphincter tone • *Postictal:* Muscles relaxed, resulting in urinary or fecal incontinence
FOOD/FLUID • Food sensitivity • Nausea and vomiting correlating with seizure activity	• Dental or soft tissue damage—injury during seizure • Gingival hyperplasia—side effect of long-term Dilantin use
NEUROSENSORY • History of headaches, recurring seizure activity, fainting, dizziness • History of head trauma, stroke, cerebral infections • *Prodromal phase:* Vague changes in emotional reactivity or affective response sometimes preceding aura and lasting minutes to hours • Presence of aura • *Postictal:* Weakness, muscle pain, areas of paresthesias or paralysis	Seizure characteristics are as follows: • ***Convulsive generalized seizures:*** • *Tonic-clonic (grand mal):* Rigidity and jerking, posturing, vocalization, loss of consciousness, dilated pupils, stertorous respiration, excessive salivation (froth), fecal and urinary incontinence, and biting of the tongue may occur and last 2 to 5 minutes • *Tonic phase:* Abrupt increase in muscle tone of torso and face, flexion of arms, extension of legs; lasts seconds • *Clonic phase:* Muscle contraction with relaxation occurring between tonic muscle contractions. Client lies still with flaccid muscles, may have stridorous breathing and excessive salivation. This phase lengthens as tonic muscle activity subsides. • *Postictal:* Client is exhausted, may sleep several hours, then may be weak, confused, and amnesic concerning the episode, with nausea and stiff, sore muscles. • ***Partial seizures:*** • *Complex (psychomotor/temporal lobe)—Ictal:* Consciousness impaired, with reactions such as dream state, staring, wandering, irritability, hallucinations, hostility, or fear. May display involuntary motor symptoms (lip smacking) and behaviors that appear purposeful but are inappropriate (automatism) and include impaired judgment and, on occasion, antisocial acts; lasts 1 to 3 minutes. • *Postictal:* Absence of memory for these events, mild to moderate confusion • *Simple (focal-motor and Jacksonian):* Often preceded by aura—may report déjà vu or fearful feeling • *Ictal:* May experience no loss of consciousness (unilateral) or lose consciousness (bilateral); convulsive movements and temporary disturbance in part controlled by the brain region involved—frontal lobe (motor dysfunction), parietal (numbness, tingling), occipital (bright, flashing lights), posterotemporal (difficulty speaking). Convulsions may march along limb or side of body in orderly progression. If restrained during seizure, client may exhibit combative and uncooperative behavior; lasts seconds to minutes. • *Status epilepticus (SE)—Ictal:* Thirty or more minutes of continuous generalized seizure activity or two or more sequential seizures without full recovery of consciousness in between, possibly related to abrupt withdrawal of anticonvulsants and other metabolic phenomena. If absence seizures are the type of seizure activity, SE may go undetected for a period of time because client does not lose consciousness.

DIAGNOSTIC DIVISION MAY REPORT (continued)	MAY EXHIBIT (continued)
PAIN/DISCOMFORT • Headache • *Ictal:* Paroxysmal abdominal pain may occur during some partial or focal seizures without loss of consciousness • *Postictal:* Muscle, back soreness	• Guarding behavior • Alteration in muscle tone • Distraction behavior, restlessness
RESPIRATION	• *Ictal:* Clenched teeth, cyanosis, decreased or rapid respirations; increased mucous secretions • *Postictal:* Apnea
SAFETY • History of accidental falls, injuries, fractures	• Soft tissue injury, ecchymosis • Decreased general strength and muscle tone
SOCIAL INTERACTION • Problems with interpersonal relationships within family or socially • Limitation or avoidance of social contacts	
TEACHING/LEARNING • Familial history of epilepsy • Drug use or misuse, including alcohol and illicit drugs • Use of herbal supplements, such as aloe, betony, blue cohosh, kava • Increased frequency of episodes, difficulty with learning resulting in failure to improve	
DISCHARGE PLAN CONSIDERATIONS • May require changes in medications, assistance with some homemaker or maintenance tasks relative to issues of safety, and transportation ➧ Refer to section at end of plan for postdischarge considerations.	

Diagnostic Studies

May vary depending upon whether or not the client has a known seizure disorder.

TEST WHY IT IS DONE	WHAT IT TELLS ME
• ***Electroencephalogram (EEG):*** Recording of the electrical activity of the brain by means of electrodes placed on the surface of the scalp.	Definitive test for seizure activity, locating area of cerebral dysfunction and measuring brain activity via waveform. EEGs immediately after a suspected seizure may show nonspecific patterns or may be normal. An EEG within 24 hours is more likely to show an abnormality, and more than one EEG may be necessary to detect seizure activity.
• ***Positron emission tomography (PET) scan:*** Uses radiation, or nuclear medicine imaging, to produce three-dimensional, color images of the functional processes within the body	May be used to locate the part of the brain that is causing seizures
ANCILLARY TESTS	
• ***Serum drug levels:*** To verify and monitor the presence and therapeutic levels of anti-epileptic drugs (AEDs).	Medication dose or schedule may have to be adjusted depending on whether serum drug level is low or high.
• (P) ***Lumbar puncture:*** A procedure in which cerebrospinal fluid (CSF) is removed from the spinal canal for diagnostic testing	(P) May be performed on any child with febrile seizures and meningeal irritation signs to rule out meningitis (Mann, 2011)

Nursing Priorities

1. Prevent or control seizure activity.
2. Protect client from injury.
3. Maintain airway and respiratory function.
4. Promote positive self-esteem.
5. Provide information about disease process, prognosis, and treatment needs.

Discharge Goals

1. Seizure activity controlled.
2. Complications and injury prevented.
3. Capable, competent self-image displayed.
4. Disease process, prognosis, therapeutic regimen, and limitations understood.
5. Plan in place to meet needs after discharge.

NURSING DIAGNOSIS: risk for Trauma/Suffocation

Risk Factors May Include

Weakness, balancing difficulties
Cognitive difficulties, decreased consciousness
Reduced muscle coordination
Emotional difficulties

Possibly Evidenced By

(Not applicable; presence of signs and symptoms establishes an *actual* diagnosis)

Desired Outcomes/Evaluation Criteria—Client Will

Seizure Self-Control (NOC)

Verbalize understanding of factors that contribute to possibility of trauma or suffocation and take steps to correct situation.
Demonstrate behaviors and lifestyle changes to reduce risk factors and protect self from future seizure events and injury.
Modify environment as indicated to enhance safety.
Maintain treatment regimen to control or eliminate seizure activity.

Significant Other [SO]/Caregiver Will

Knowledge: Personal Safety (NOC)

Identify actions or measures to take when seizure activity occurs.

ACTIONS/INTERVENTIONS	RATIONALE
Seizure Precautions (NIC)	
Independent	
Explore with client the various stimuli that may precipitate seizure activity.	Alcohol, various drugs, and other stimuli, such as loss of sleep, flashing lights, and prolonged television viewing, may increase the potential for seizure activity. Client may or may not have control over many precipitating factors, but may benefit from becoming aware of risks.
Discuss seizure warning signs, if appropriate, and usual seizure pattern. Teach SO to recognize warning signs and how to care for client during and after seizure.	Can enable client or SO to protect individual from injury and to recognize changes that require notification of physician and further intervention. Knowing what to do when seizure occurs can prevent injury or complications and decreases SO's feelings of helplessness.
Seizure Management (NIC)	
In hospitalized client:	
Keep padded side rails up with bed in lowest position, or place bed up against wall, and add floor pad if rails are not available or appropriate.	Minimizes injury should frequent or generalized seizures occur while client is in bed.
Maintain strict bedrest if prodromal signs or aura is experienced. Explain necessity for these actions.	Client may feel restless, need to ambulate or even defecate during aural phase, thereby inadvertently removing self from safe environment and easy observation. Understanding importance of providing for own safety needs may enhance client cooperation.
Stay with client during and after seizure.	Promotes client safety and reduces sense of isolation during event.
Turn head to side and suction airway as indicated. Insert soft bite block per facility protocol, only if jaw relaxed.	Helps maintain airway and reduces risk of oral trauma but should not be "forced" or inserted when teeth are clenched because dental and soft tissue damage may result. *Note:* Current practice is mixed regarding the use of airways during seizure activity. (Refer to ND: risk for ineffective Airway Clearance, following.)

ACTIONS/INTERVENTIONS (continued)	RATIONALE (continued)
Cradle head, place on soft area, or assist to floor if out of bed. Do not attempt to restrain.	Gentle guiding of extremities reduces risk of physical injury when client lacks voluntary muscle control. *Note:* If attempt is made to restrain client during seizure, erratic movements may increase, and client may injure self or others.
Perform neurological and vital sign checks after seizure: level of consciousness, orientation, ability to comply with simple commands, ability to speak, memory of incident, weakness or motor deficits, blood pressure (BP), pulse, and respiratory rate.	Documents postictal state and time and completeness of recovery to normal state. May identify additional safety concerns to be addressed.
Reorient client following seizure activity.	Client may be confused, disoriented, and possibly amnesic after the seizure and need help to regain control and alleviate anxiety.
Allow postictal "automatic" behavior without interfering while providing environmental protection.	May display behavior of motor or psychic origin that seems inappropriate or irrelevant for time and place. Attempts to control or prevent activity may result in client becoming aggressive or combative.
Investigate reports of pain.	May be result of repetitive muscle contractions or symptom of injury incurred, requiring further evaluation and intervention.
Observe for SE.	This is a life-threatening emergency that, if left untreated, could cause metabolic acidosis, hyperthermia, hypoglycemia, arrhythmias, hypoxia, increased intracranial pressure, airway obstruction, and respiratory arrest. Immediate intervention is required to control seizure activity and prevent permanent injury or death. *Note:* Although absence seizures may become static, they are not usually life-threatening.
Document preseizure activity, presence of aura or unusual behavior, type of seizure activity, such as location and duration of motor activity, loss of consciousness, incontinence, eye activity, respiratory impairment, and cyanosis, and frequency or recurrence. Note whether client fell, expressed vocalizations, drooled, or had automatisms, such as lip smacking, chewing, and picking at clothes.	Helps localize the cerebral area of involvement and may be useful in chronic conditions in helping client and so prepare for or manage seizure activity.
Collaborative	
Administer medications, as indicated, for example:	
Older, classic medications include: phenytoin (Dilantin); carbamazepine (Tegretol); valproic divalproex (Depakote); diazepam (Valium) and similar tranquilizers such as clonazepam (Klonopin). Newer drugs include: felbamate (Felbatol); tiagabine (Gabitril); levatiracetam (Keppra); pregabalin (Lyrica); gabapentin (Neurontin); zonisamide (Zonegran).	Long-term drug treatment is required for clients who have recurrent seizures, seizure with an unknown cause, or a cause that can't be reversed. Choice of anti-epileptic drugs (AEDs) and route of administration depends on seizure type and current severity. Some clients require multiple medications or frequent medication adjustments to control seizure activity. AEDs treat and/or prevent seizures by raising the seizure threshold, stabilizing nerve cell membranes, reducing the excitability of the neurons, or through direct action on the limbic system, thalamus, and hypothalamus. Goal is optimal suppression of seizure activity with lowest possible dose of drug and with fewest side effects.
Monitor AED drug levels and document corresponding side effects and frequency of seizure activity.	Blood levels of the various AEDs should be evaluated on a regular basis. Blood levels should also be done when breakthrough seizures occur or any change occurs in the client's status. Standard therapeutic level may not be optimal for individual client if untoward side effects develop or seizures are not controlled.
Prepare for/assist with more intensive interventions as indicated.	Vagal nerve stimulation, magnetic beam therapy, electrode implantation, or other surgical interventions, such as temporal lobectomy, may be done for intractable seizures or well-localized epileptogenic lesions when client is disabled and at high risk for serious injury. Success has been reported with gamma ray radiosurgery for the treatment of multiple seizure activity that has otherwise been difficult to control.

NURSING DIAGNOSIS: risk for ineffective Airway Clearance

Risk Factors May Include

Neuromuscular dysfunction
Retained secretions
Airway spasm; foreign body in airway

(continues on page 194)

NURSING DIAGNOSIS: risk for ineffective Airway Clearance (continued)

Possibly Evidenced By

(Not applicable; presence of signs and symptoms establishes an *actual* diagnosis)

Desired Outcomes/Evaluation Criteria—Client Will

Respiratory Status: Airway Patency (NOC)

Maintain effective respiratory pattern with airway patent.
Be free of signs of aspiration.

ACTIONS/INTERVENTIONS	RATIONALE
Airway Management (NIC)	
Independent	
Encourage client to empty mouth of dentures or foreign objects if aura occurs and to avoid chewing gum or sucking lozenges if seizures can occur without warning.	Reduces risk of aspiration or foreign bodies lodging in pharynx.
Place in lying position on a flat surface; turn head to side during seizure activity.	Promotes drainage of secretions; prevents tongue from obstructing airway.
Loosen clothing from neck, chest, and abdominal areas.	Facilitates chest expansion, enhancing breathing.
Insert soft airway as indicated per facility protocol and only if jaw is relaxed.	If inserted before jaw is tightened, these devices may prevent biting of tongue and facilitate suctioning and respiratory support if required. Airway adjunct may be indicated after cessation of seizure activity if client is unconscious and unable to maintain safe position of tongue. *Note:* Current opinion is mixed regarding the use of airways during seizure activity.
Suction as needed.	Reduces risk of aspiration or asphyxiation. *Note:* Risk of aspiration is low unless individual has eaten within the last 40 minutes.
Collaborative	
Administer supplemental oxygen or bag ventilation, as needed postictally.	May reduce cerebral hypoxia resulting from decreased circulation and oxygenation secondary to vascular spasm during seizure. *Note:* Artificial ventilation during general seizure activity is of limited or no benefit because it is not possible to move air in and out of lungs during sustained contraction of respiratory musculature. As seizure abates, respiratory function will return unless a secondary problem exists, such as foreign body or aspiration.
Prepare for and assist with intubation, if indicated.	Presence of prolonged apnea postictally may require ventilatory support.

NURSING DIAGNOSIS: [specify situational or chronic low] Self-Esteem

May Be Related To

Traumatic event (seizure)
Disturbed body image
Perceived lack of respect from others

Possibly Evidenced By

Reports feelings of shame, helplessness; self-negating verbalizations
Exaggerates negative feedback about self; fear of rejection

Desired Outcomes/Evaluation Criteria—Client Will

Self-Esteem (NOC)

Identify feelings and methods for coping with negative perception of self.
Verbalize increased sense of self-esteem in relation to diagnosis.
Verbalize realistic perception and acceptance of self in changed role or lifestyle.

ACTIONS/INTERVENTIONS	RATIONALE
Self-Esteem Enhancement (NIC)	
Independent	
Discuss feelings about diagnosis and perception of threat to self.	Reactions vary among individuals, and previous knowledge or experience with this condition affects acceptance of therapeutic regimen. One recent study indicated that, to patients, the phenomenon of epilepsy is, above all, of a psychosocial nature and in that dimension is closely related to negative emotions, such as shame, fear, and sorrow (Laarson, 2009).
Encourage expression of feelings.	Verbalization of fears, anger, and concerns about future implications can help client begin to accept and deal with situation.
Identify possible or anticipated public reaction to condition. Encourage client to refrain from concealing condition.	Provides opportunity to problem-solve response, and provides measure of control over situation. Concealment is destructive to self-esteem (potentiates denial), blocking progress in dealing with problem, and may actually increase risk of injury or negative response when seizure does occur.
Explore with client current and past successes and strengths.	Focusing on positive aspects can help alleviate feelings of guilt or self-consciousness and help client begin to accept manageability of condition.
Avoid overprotecting client; encourage activities, providing supervision or monitoring when indicated.	Participation in as many experiences as possible can lessen depression about limitations. Observation or supervision may need to be provided for such activities as gymnastics, climbing, and water sports.
Determine attitudes and capabilities of SO. Help individual realize that client's feelings are normal; however, guilt and blame are not helpful.	Negative expectations from SO may affect client's sense of competency and self-esteem and interfere with support received from SO, limiting potential for optimal management and personal growth.
Emphasize importance of staff and SO remaining calm during seizure activity.	Anxiety of caregivers is contagious and can be conveyed to the client, increasing or multiplying individual's own negative perceptions of situation and self.
Refer client/SO to support groups, such as Epilepsy Foundation of America, National Association of Epilepsy Centers, and Delta Society's National Service Dog Center.	Provides opportunity to gain information, support, and ideas for dealing with problems from others who share similar experiences. *Note:* "Seizure dogs" may be trained to bark and alert parent/caregiver when client is seizing. Other dogs (seizure response dog) may help prevent injury by breaking client's fall and staying with client during seizure, and a few may be able to warn of a seizure in advance (seizure predicting dogs), allowing individual to initiate safety measures (Epilepsy Foundation, 2009). Service animals can also increase independence and personal sense of control.
Discuss long-term effects as indicated and possible referral for psychotherapy with client/SO.	Seizures have a profound effect on personal self-esteem, and client/SO may feel guilt over perceived limitations and public stigma. Counseling can help overcome feelings of inferiority and self-consciousness. (P) Emotional and behavioral problems can occur in some children, especially when seizures are not well controlled.

NURSING DIAGNOSIS: ineffective Self-Health Management

May Be Related To

Complexity of therapeutic regimen
Deficient knowledge

Possibly Evidenced By

Reports difficulty with prescribed regimen
Failure to include treatment regimen in daily living
Failure to take action to reduce risk factors (triggers)

Desired Outcomes/Evaluation Criteria—Client Will

Self-Health Management: Chronic Disease (NOC)

Verbalize understanding of disorder and various stimuli that may increase or potentiate seizure activity.
Adhere to prescribed drug regimen.
Initiate necessary lifestyle and behavior changes as indicated.

ACTIONS/INTERVENTIONS	RATIONALE
Teaching: Disease Process NIC	
Independent	
Review pathology and prognosis of condition and lifelong need for treatments as indicated.	Provides opportunity to clarify and dispel misconceptions and present condition as something that is manageable within a normal lifestyle. (P) However, for individuals with long-standing seizure disorder (particularly children), the impact of seizures on memory and learning varies widely and depends on many factors. In general, the earlier a child develops seizures, and the more extensive the area of brain affected, the poorer the outcome. Children with seizures that are not well controlled are at higher risk for intellectual decline and learning and language problems can occur (Miami Children's Hospital, 2010).
Discuss client's particular triggers if known.	The most frequent triggers include missing anti-epilpetic medication doses, taking other drugs that interfere with seizure medications, heavy alcohol use, cocaine or other drug use. (P) As well, flashing lights, hyperventilation, loud noises, video games, TV viewing, and lack of sleep (particularly in teenager) may be problematic.
Review possible effects of female hormonal changes.	Alterations in hormonal levels that occur during menstruation and pregnancy may increase risk of seizure breakthrough.
Discuss significance of maintaining good general health, such as adequate diet; rest; moderate exercise; and avoidance of exhaustion, alcohol, caffeine, and stimulant drugs.	Regularity and moderation in activities may aid in reducing and controlling precipitating factors, enhancing sense of general well-being, and strengthening coping ability and self-esteem. *Note:* Too little sleep or too much alcohol can precipitate seizure activity in some people.
Review importance of good oral hygiene and regular dental care.	Reduces risk of oral infections and gingival hyperplasia.
Encourage client who smokes to refrain from smoking except while supervised.	May cause burns if cigarette is accidentally dropped during aura or seizure activity.
Evaluate need for and provide protective headgear.	Use of helmet may provide added protection for individuals who suffer recurrent and severe seizures.
Identify necessity and promote acceptance of actual limitations; discuss safety measures regarding driving, using mechanical equipment, climbing ladders, swimming, and hobbies.	Reduces risk of injury to self or others, especially if seizures occur without warning.
(P) Recommend parent/caregiver observe child during play and stay with child in unsafe environment (e.g., if falls are risk during seizure activity, or child is bathing or swimming).	(P) Enhances safety, reducing the risk of injury/drowning (Miami Children's Hospital (2010).
Encourage client to wear identification tag or bracelet stating the presence of a seizure disorder.	Expedites treatment and diagnosis in emergency situations.
Stress need for routine follow-up care and laboratory testing as indicated; for example, CBC should be monitored biannually and in presence of sore throat or fever and signs of other infection.	Therapeutic needs may change and serious drug side effects such as agranulocytosis or toxicity may develop.
Discuss local laws or restrictions pertaining to persons with epilepsy or seizure disorder. Encourage awareness but not necessarily acceptance of these policies.	Although legal and civil rights of persons with epilepsy have improved during the past decade, restrictions still exist in some states pertaining to obtaining a driver's license, sterilization, workers' compensation, and required reporting to state agencies.
Teaching: Prescribed Medication NIC	
Review medication regimen, necessity of taking drugs as ordered, and not discontinuing therapy without physician supervision. Include directions for missed dose.	Lack of cooperation with medication regimen is a leading cause of seizure breakthrough. Client needs to know risks of SE resulting from abrupt withdrawal of anticonvulsants. Depending on the drug dose and frequency, client may be instructed to take missed dose if remembered within a predetermined time frame. (P) *Note:* Monotherapy with AED such as Depakote may be preferred for children, as compliance with regimen is enhanced when only taking one pill a day (Senelick, 2012).
Recommend taking drugs with meals if appropriate.	May reduce incidence of gastric irritation, nausea, and vomiting.
Discuss nuisance and adverse side effects of particular drugs, such as drowsiness, fatigue, lethargy, hyperactivity, sleep disturbances, gingival hypertrophy, visual disturbances, nausea or vomiting, rashes, syncope and ataxia, birth defects, and aplastic anemia.	May indicate need for change in dosage or choice of drug therapy. Promotes involvement and participation in decision-making process and awareness of potential long-term effects of drug therapy, and provides opportunity to minimize or prevent complications.
Provide information about potential drug interactions and necessity of notifying other healthcare providers of drug regimen.	Knowledge of anticonvulsant use reduces risk of prescribing drugs that may interact, thus altering seizure threshold or therapeutic effect. For example, phenytoin (Dilantin) potentiates anticoagulant effect of warfarin (Coumadin), whereas

Actions/Interventions	Rationale
	isoniazid (INH) and chloramphenicol (Chloromycetin) increase the effect of Dilantin; and some antibiotics, such as erythromycin, can cause elevation of serum level of carbamazepine (Tegretol), possibly to toxic levels.
Review proper use of diazepam rectal gel (Diastat) with client and SO/caregiver as appropriate.	Useful in controlling serial or cluster seizures. Can be administered in any setting and is effective usually within 15 minutes. May reduce dependence on emergency department visits.
Discuss use of over-the-counter (OTC) medications and supplements and herbals.	Anticonvulsant drugs may interact with many other medications and substances. Some medications can decrease the effectiveness of anticonvulsant drugs, or the client may choose a folk remedy or herbal supplement without being aware of its effect.

POTENTIAL CONSIDERATIONS following acute hospitalization (dependent on client's age, physical condition and presence of complications, personal resources, and life responsibilities)

- ***risk for Injury***—physical (altered consciousness, loss of large or small muscle coordination)
- ***Self-Esteem (specify)***—traumatic situation, disturbed body image, physical illness; ineffective adaptation to loss
- ***ineffective Self-Health Management***—social support deficit, perceived benefit (versus side effects of medication), perceived susceptibility (possible long periods of remission)

CRANIOCEREBRAL TRAUMA—ACUTE REHABILITATIVE PHASE

I. Pathophysiology

a. Craniocerebral trauma, also called traumatic brain injury (TBI), acquired brain injury, head injury—Physical injury to the cranium and intracranial structures with varied outcomes, ranging from no apparent (or a temporary neurological) disturbance to permanent impairment of brain function, including persistent vegetative state or even death depending on the extent of the damage

b. TBI may be open or closed and can include brain concussion, contusion, laceration, hemorrhage, or skull fractures. TBIs are classified as mild, moderate, or severe.

- **i.** Concussion: most minor and most common form of head injury
- **ii.** Intracranial hemorrhage: defined by the region of the brain (intracerebral) or surrounding structures affected, such as subdural, epidural, subarachnoid, brainstem
  1. Intracerebral hemorrhage: may occur along with other brain injuries, particularly contusions, with signs and symptoms dependent on the size and location and may be apparent immediately or develop slowly (Zink, 2005).
  2. Acute subdural hematoma: caused by venous bleeding when bridging veins are torn, occurring in 5% to 25% of all severe head injuries involving a contusion or laceration and often accompanying intracerebral bleeding (Reddy, 2006); signs and symptoms present almost immediately and increase rapidly.
  3. Epidural hematoma: arterial bleeding usually from the middle meningeal artery in the temporal region, typically manifested by a brief loss of consciousness at the time of trauma, then a lucid interval, which may last for several hours; between 30% and 50% of individuals incur neurological deterioration (Reddy, 2006).

II. Etiology

a. Primary injury (Zink, 2005)

- **i.** Penetrating injury: Object forcibly enters the cranial vault, damaging the protective meningeal layers, cerebral blood vessels, and brain tissue.
- **ii.** Contact phenomena injury: Object strikes the head, resulting in concussion, cerebral contusion, skull fracture, or intracranial hemorrhage.
- **iii.** Acceleration-deceleration injury: Brain rapidly accelerates and decelerates within the skull, causing the brain to strike the skull, usually in the front and the back of the skull, causing tearing of neuronal tissue and cerebral blood vessels.
- **iv.** Rotational acceleration-deceleration injury: Forces cause the brain to twist within the skull, resulting in torsion and shearing of nerve tissue and blood vessels.

b. Secondary brain injury (Granacher, 2003)

- **i.** Thought to involve inflammation and the natural process of programmed cell death (apoptosis)
- **ii.** Diffuse axonal injury: shearing injury of large nerve fibers (axons covered with myelin) in many areas of the brain, or stretching or shearing of blood vessels from the same forces, producing hemorrhage
- **iii.** Systemic or neurological complications can also cause or exacerbate secondary brain injury—hypotension, hypoxia, hypercapnia, intracranial hypertension, acid-base imbalance, cerebral vasospasm, electrolyte abnormalities, hyperthermia, infection, cerebral ischemia, seizures, and hypoglycemia or hyperglycemia.

c. Leading mechanism for TBI in the United States (CDC, 2010):

- **i.** Falls: 28%, highest for children aged 0 to 4 and those aged 75 or older
- **ii.** Motor vehicle-traffic crashes: 31.8%

(continues on page 198)

iii. Struck by or against: 19%, which includes assaults, pedestrian/vehicle crashes, and sports-related injuries

iv. Gunshot wounds: 12% of all TBIs are attributed to firearms; in people ages 25 to 34, firearms are a leading cause of TBI. Gunshot wound head trauma is the cause of an estimated 35% of all deaths attributed to TBI (AANS, 2011).

v. Blasts: leading cause of TBI for active duty military personnel in war zones (Congressional Research Service, 2010)

vi. Shaken Baby Syndrome (SBS), a form of abusive head trauma (AHT) and inflicted traumatic brain injury (ITBI), is a leading cause of child maltreatment deaths in the United States.

III. **Statistics** (CDC, 2010; Congressional Research 2011; MMWR, 2011)

a. Morbidity: Traumatic brain injury (TBI) is a leading cause of injury, death, and disability in the United States. During 2002–2006, on average, annually approximately 1.7 million U.S. civilians sustained a TBI. These statistics do not include persons who had a TBI while serving abroad in the U.S. military. TBIs associated with the last decade of wars were reported in 2010 to be greater than 178,000.

b. Mortality: There are approximately 52,000 deaths annually.

c. Cost: TBI costs the country more than $56 billion a year, and more than 5 million Americans alive today have had a TBI resulting in a permanent need for help in performing daily activities (NINDS, 2012).

GLOSSARY

Amnesia: Loss of memory about recent event or a particular period of time, such as events surrounding injury.

Anomia: Inability to remember names of objects; individual may speak fluently but have to use other words to describe familiar objects.

Aphasia: Loss of ability to communicate or express oneself and to understand language due to brain dysfunction.

Apraxia: Inability to perform complex or skilled movement or use objects properly in the absence of sensory or motor impairments.

Ataxia: Loss of muscle control or coordination, especially with voluntary movement, interfering with an individual's ability to walk, talk, and perform activities of daily living (ADLs).

Closed head injury: Blunt trauma to the brain or brain structures by a direct blow or rapid deceleration, such as striking the windshield of a car, without penetration of the skull.

Cognition: The process of knowing, including awareness of thoughts or perceptions, ability to process information, reasoning, and judgment.

Coma: A state of unconsciousness from which the individual cannot be aroused even with stimulation; completely unresponsive to environment.

Concussion: Injury to brain resulting from impact with an object, such as blow to the head or sudden deceleration, causing temporary loss of normal brain function with or without loss of consciousness.

Contusion: Focal brain injury—bruising of brain tissue and damage to blood vessels due to a blow or rapid deceleration.

Deceleration: Rapid decrease in velocity causing injury when a moving body part hits a stationary object, such as the brain hitting the inside of the skull.

Decerebrate posture: Rigid extension of the arms and legs, pronation of forearms, downward pointing of toes, and backward arching of head in response to noxious stimuli when cerebral control of spinal reflexes is lost, as with severe injury at the level of the brainstem.

Decorticate posture: Muscle rigidity with arms flexed toward chest, fists clenched, and legs extended in response to noxious stimuli and associated with brain injury at or above the upper brainstem.

Dystonia: Involuntary prolonged muscle contractions causing twisting of the body, repetitive movements, and abnormal postures.

Glasgow Coma Scale (GCS): Standardized rating scale used to determine an individual's level of consciousness (LOC) and degree of brain impairment by measuring eye opening and verbal and motor response to stimuli. Scores range from a low of 3 to a high of 15, with score of 12 to 15 suggesting mild brain injury; 9 to 11, moderate injury; and 8 or lower, severe brain injury (CNS, 2006).

Hematoma, intracranial: Collection of blood within the skull caused by ruptured blood vessels, which may be localized in one area of the brain (intracerebral), located above the dura mater (epidural), beneath the dura (subdural), or between the arachnoid membrane and the pia mater (subarachnoid).

Hemiparesis: Weakness or partial paralysis of one side of the body.

Mild brain injury (MBI): Accounts for 75% of all diagnosed head injuries (Bazarian, 2005). MBI can be treated in emergency department (ED) settings, yet it is estimated that about 25% of those with MBI fail to seek medical attention. The CDC refers to MBI as a "silent epidemic" because the problems experienced by patients with MBI (e.g., dizziness, headache, and memory disturbance) are often not visible and may result in functional loss and are more difficult for practitioners to detect. Long-term physical, mental, social, or occupational consequences often result (Bay, 2007).

Intracranial pressure (ICP): The pressure exerted by cerebrospinal fluid (CSF) within the cranium is normally 8 to 18 mm Hg in a supine adult at rest. An increase in pressure may be due to an increase in CSF or increased pressure within the brain from a lesion or swelling of the brain itself.

Open head injury: Open fracture of the skull as may occur with high-impact crashes, severe assaults with an object, or gunshot or blast injury to the head.

Post-traumatic amnesia (PTA): A state of agitation, confusion, and memory loss following a traumatic brain injury (TBI), which can last a few days to months and is marked by impaired ability to process information accurately and inability to form new memories. Correlating the length of post-traumatic amnesia (PTA) with time of altered consciousness and Glascow coma score allows for a determination of severity of injury ranging from mild to moderate to severe. For example, a moderate TBI is indicated by loss of consciousness/alteration of consciousness (LOC/AOC) that lasts between

GLOSSARY (continued)

30 minutes and 24 hours, PTA for more than 24 hours or less than 7 days, and a GCS score between 9 and 12. Between 20% to 80% of people with mild injury will continue to experience symptoms 6 months after the injury (de Kruijk, 2002; Meyer, 2008; Bay, 2009).

Posturing: Awkward or unnatural posture maintained for a prolonged period of time that may be associated with brain injury, such as decorticate or decerebrate, suggesting a poor prognosis.

Proprioception: Awareness of posture, movement, equilibrium, and relationship of self and limbs to environment.

Quadriparesis: Muscle weakness or lack of control of all four extremities—also called tetraparesis.

Sympathetic storming (also called storming): Exaggerated stress response in individuals with severe TBI (GCS score 3 to 8), with hypothalamic stimulation of the sympathetic nervous system and adrenal glands, thereby causing an increase in circulating corticoids and catecholamines, which results in increased agitation, extreme posturing, hypertension, tachycardia, tachypnea, diaphoresis, and hyperthermia; episodes occur within first 24 hours of injury or in the weeks following injury (Lemke, 2007).

Care Setting

This plan of care focuses on acute care and acute inpatient rehabilitation. Brain injury care for those experiencing moderate to severe trauma progresses along a continuum of care, beginning with acute hospital care and inpatient rehabilitation to subacute and outpatient rehabilitation, as well as home- and community-based services.

Related Concerns

Brain infections: meningitis and encephalitis, page 229
Cerebrovascular accident (CVA)/stroke, page 214
Psychosocial aspects of care, page 729
Seizure disorders, page 188
Surgical intervention, page 762
Thrombophlebitis: venous thromboembolism (including pulmonary emboli considerations), page 109
Total nutritional support: parenteral/enteral feeding, page 437
Upper gastrointestinal/esophageal bleeding, page 281

Client Assessment Database

Data depend on type, location, and severity of injury and may be complicated by additional injury to other vital organs.

DIAGNOSTIC DIVISION MAY REPORT	MAY EXHIBIT
ACTIVITY/REST • Weakness, fatigue • Sleep problems, insomnia • Clumsiness, loss of balance	• Altered consciousness, lethargy • Hemiparesis, quadriparesis • Unsteady gait (ataxia); balance problems • Orthopedic injuries (trauma) • Loss of muscle tone, muscle spasticity
CIRCULATION	• Normal or altered blood pressure (BP) (hypotension or hypertension); prolonged hypertension and arrhythmias can occur as a result of sympathetic storming (Lemke, 2007). • Changes in heart rate, including bradycardia, tachycardia alternating with bradycardia, other dysrhythmias (not usually associated with hemodynamic instability) • Diaphoresis can be severe with storming (Lemke, 2007).
EGO INTEGRITY • Significant other (SO) may report that client's personality changes and behavioral problems are the most difficult disabilities to handle. • Problems coping • Difficulty making decisions	• Behavior or personality changes (subtle to dramatic) may include depression, apathy, anxiety, irritability, impulsivity, anger, paranoia, confusion, frustration, agitation, and mood swings.
ELIMINATION	• Bowel, bladder incontinence or dysfunction

(continues on page 200)

DIAGNOSTIC DIVISION MAY REPORT (continued)	MAY EXHIBIT (continued)
FOOD/FLUID • Nausea • Changes in appetite	• Vomiting, which may be projectile • Swallowing problems—coughing, drooling, dysphagia • Altered bowel sounds • Inability to eat because of altered awareness or consciousness or traumatic injuries • Weight loss due to increased metabolic rate
HYGIENE	• Problems with bathing, dressing, grooming, feeding, toileting
NEUROSENSORY • Variable levels of awareness at time of impact, such as feeling dazed, confused, "seeing stars" • Amnesia surrounding trauma events • Visual changes, such as double vision, movement of print or stationary objects such as walls and floor; eye strain and visual fatigue • Changes in thinking ability • Vertigo, problems with balance • Ringing in ears, hearing loss • Tingling, numbness in extremities • Loss of or changes in senses of taste or smell	• LOC ranging from lethargy to coma • Pupillary changes—response to light and symmetry; deviation of eyes, inability to follow • Facial asymmetry • Unequal, weak handgrip • Absent or weak deep tendon reflexes • Posturing—decorticate, decerebrate • Seizure activity • Heightened sensitivity to touch and movement—can be painful and/or initiate storming • Apraxia, hemiparesis, quadriparesis • Proprioception • Difficulty with hand-eye coordination • Mental status changes, including altered orientation, alertness or responsiveness, attention, concentration, problem-solving, emotional affect or behavior, and memory. *Note:* The most common impairment among severely head-injured clients is memory loss, characterized by some loss of specific memories and the partial inability to form or store new ones (National Institute for Neurological Disorders and Stroke [NINDS], 2012). • *Vision:* Client may not be able to register what he or she is seeing or may be slow to recognize objects and have difficulty with tracking and hand-eye coordination. • *Language and communication:* Difficulty with understanding and producing spoken and written language, and with the more subtle aspects of communication, such as body language and emotional, nonverbal signals (NINDS, 2012).
PAIN/DISCOMFORT • Headache of variable intensity and location, usually persistent and long-lasting • Other body pain, especially when brain injury is a component of multiple trauma	• Facial grimacing • Withdrawal response to painful stimulus • Restlessness, moaning
RESPIRATION	• Changes in breathing patterns, such as periods of apnea alternating with hyperventilation • Sustained hyperventilation, which may accompany storming • Noisy respirations, stridor, choking • Rhonchi, wheezes (possible aspiration)

DIAGNOSTIC DIVISION MAY REPORT (continued)	MAY EXHIBIT (continued)
SAFETY • History of recent trauma, such as fall, motor vehicle crash, bullet or blast injuries	• Fractures, dislocations • Impaired vision, visual field disturbances, abnormal eye movements • Head or facial lacerations, abrasions, discoloration (raccoon eyes), Battle's sign around ears (trauma signs) • Drainage from ears or nose—CSF • Impaired cognition • Range of motion (ROM) impairment, altered muscle tone, general weakness, incomplete paralysis • Fever, which may be associated with infection or related to hypermetabolic rate or storming; instability in internal regulation of body temperature • Behavioral changes indicative of violence to self or others
SOCIAL INTERACTION • Inability to cope • Relationship problems and role changes • Caregiver/SO has difficulty dealing with caregiver burdens and role	• Expressive or receptive aphasia, unintelligible speech, repetitive speech, dysarthria, anomia • Difficulty dealing with environment, interacting with more than one or two individuals at a time
TEACHING/LEARNING • Use of alcohol, other drugs • Failure to attend to safety issues	
DISCHARGE PLAN CONSIDERATIONS • May require assistance with self-care, ambulation, transportation, food preparation, shopping, treatments, medications, homemaker and maintenance tasks, change in physical layout of home or placement in living facility other than home ➧ Refer to section at end of plan for postdischarge considerations.	

Diagnostic Studies

TEST WHY IT IS DONE	WHAT IT TELLS ME
PRIMARY DIAGNOSTIC STUDIES	
• ***Computed tomography (CT) scan (with/without contrast):*** Uses low radiation x-rays to create a computer-generated, three-dimensional image of the brain tissues at successive layers.	Screening image of choice in acute brain injury. Useful in the differential diagnosis of cerebral infarction, ventricular displacement or enlargement, aneurysms, hemorrhage, hematoma, contusions, and skull fractures. Also identifies brain tissue swelling and shift.
• ***Magnetic resonance imaging (MRI):*** Uses magnetic fields and computer technology to generate images of the internal anatomy of the brain.	More sensitive than CT for detecting cerebral trauma, determining neurological deficits not explained by CT, evaluating prolonged interval of disturbed consciousness, and defining evidence of previous trauma superimposed on acute trauma. *Note:* MRI has limited role in evaluation of acute head injury because of longer procedure time and difficulty obtaining MRI in an acutely injured person.
ANCILLARY TESTS	
• ***Electroencephalogram (EEG):*** Procedure that uses electrodes on the scalp to record electrical activity of the brain.	May reveal presence or development of pathological waves. EEG is not generally indicated in the immediate period of emergency

(continues on page 202)

TEST WHY IT IS DONE (continued)	WHAT IT TELLS ME (continued)
	response, evaluation, and treatment of TBI. If the client fails to improve, EEG may help in diagnostic evaluation for seizures, focal or diffuse encephalopathy, or brain death. With contusions, may reveal progressive abnormalities and lack of tissue repair by the appearance of abnormal waves. *Note:* Continuous EEG monitoring can help clinicians evaluate the effectiveness of high-dose barbiturates in achieving suppression of neuronal activity.
• *Arterial blood gases (ABGs):* Measures oxygen and carbon dioxide levels and pH.	Determines presence of ventilation or oxygenation problems that may exacerbate and increase ICP.
• *Serum chemistry/electrolytes:* Substances that, in solution, conduct an electric current and are decomposed by their passage. Sodium, potassium, calcium, and magnesium are common electrolytes.	May reveal numerous imbalances that contribute to increased ICP and changes in mentation. Increased metabolic rate and diaphoresis can result in elevated sodium (hypernatremia).
• *Blood glucose:* Monitors for fluctuations in serum glucose levels.	Sympathetic storming can result in elevated glucose (hyperglycemia), although hypoglycemia can also occur due to inadequate nutrition.

Nursing Priorities

1. Maximize cerebral perfusion and function.
2. Prevent or minimize complications.
3. Promote optimal functioning/return to preinjury level.
4. Support coping process and family recovery.
5. Provide information about condition, prognosis, potential complications, treatment plan, and resources.

Discharge Goals

1. Cerebral function improved; neurological deficits resolving or stabilized.
2. Complications prevented or minimized.
3. Activities of daily living (ADLs) met by self or with assistance of other(s).
4. Family acknowledges reality of situation and involved in recovery program.
5. Condition, prognosis, complications, and treatment regimen understood and available resources identified.
6. Plan in place to meet needs after discharge.

NURSING DIAGNOSIS: risk for ineffective cerebral Tissue Perfusion

May Be Related To
Head trauma

Possibly Evidenced By
(Not applicable; presence of signs and symptoms establishes an *actual* diagnosis)

Desired Outcomes/Evaluation Criteria—Client Will

Tissue Perfusion: Cerebral (NOC)
Maintain usual or improved LOC, cognition, and motor or sensory function.
Demonstrate stable vital signs and absence of signs of increased ICP.

ACTIONS/INTERVENTIONS	RATIONALE
Neurologic Monitoring (NIC) *Independent*	
Determine factors related to individual situation, cause for coma or decreased cerebral perfusion and potential for increased ICP.	Influences choice of interventions. Deterioration in neurological signs and symptoms or failure to improve after initial insult may reflect decreased intracranial adaptive capacity, requiring the client be transferred to critical care for monitoring of ICP or surgical intervention.

ACTIONS/INTERVENTIONS (continued)	RATIONALE (continued)
Monitor and document neurological status frequently and compare with baseline:	
GCS during first 48 hours.	GCS assesses trends and potential for increased ICP and is useful in determining location, extent, and progression or resolution of CNS) damage. *Note:* The Rancho Los Amigos Scale (or Rancho Levels) may also be used. These levels do not require cooperation from the client and are based on client's response to environmental stimuli and a range of behavioral responses, including no response, confused-agitated, and purposeful-appropriate.
Evaluate eye opening—spontaneous (awake), opens only to painful stimuli, keeps eyes closed (coma).	Determines arousability and LOC.
Assess verbal response; note whether client is alert, oriented to person, place, and time, or is confused, uses inappropriate words and phrases that make little sense.	Measures appropriateness of speech and content of consciousness. If minimal damage has occurred in the cerebral cortex, client may be aroused by verbal stimuli but may appear drowsy or uncooperative. More extensive damage to the cerebral cortex may be displayed by slow response to commands, lapsing into sleep when not stimulated, disorientation, and stupor. Damage to midbrain, pons, and medulla is manifested by lack of appropriate responses to stimuli.
Assess motor response to simple commands, noting purposeful (obeys command, attempts to push stimulus away) and nonpurposeful (posturing) movement. Note limb movement and document right and left sides separately.	Measures overall awareness and ability to respond to external stimuli. Best indicator of state of consciousness in a client whose eyes are closed because of trauma or who is aphasic. Consciousness and involuntary movement are integrated if client can both grasp and release the tester's hand or hold up two fingers on command. Purposeful movement can include grimacing or withdrawing from painful stimuli or movements that the client desires, such as sitting up. Other movements (posturing and abnormal flexion of extremities) usually indicate diffuse cortical damage. Absence of spontaneous movement on one side of the body indicates damage to the motor tracts in the opposite cerebral hemisphere.
Monitor vital signs:	
BP, noting onset of and continuing systolic hypertension and widening pulse pressure; observe for hypotension in multiple trauma client.	Normally, autoregulation maintains constant cerebral blood flow despite fluctuations in systemic BP. Loss of autoregulation may follow local or diffuse cerebrovascular damage. Increasing systolic BP accompanied by decreasing diastolic BP (widening pulse pressure) is an ominous sign of increased ICP when accompanied by decreased LOC. Hypovolemia or hypotension associated with multiple trauma may also result in cerebral ischemia and damage.
Heart rate and rhythm, noting bradycardia, alternating bradycardia and tachycardia, and other dysrhythmias	Changes in rate (most often bradycardia) and dysrhythmias may develop without impacting hemodynamic stability. However, dysrhythmias can reflect brainstem pressure or injury in the absence of underlying cardiac disease. Tachycardia can reflect hydration status, fever or hypermetabolic state, and sympathetic storming.
Respirations, noting patterns and rhythm, including periods of apnea after hyperventilation and Cheyne-Stokes respiration	Irregularities can suggest location of cerebral insult, increasing ICP, and need for further intervention, including possible respiratory support. (Refer to ND: risk for ineffective Breathing Pattern, following.)
Evaluate pupils, noting size, shape, equality, and light reactivity.	Pupil reactions are regulated by the oculomotor (III) cranial nerve and are useful in determining whether the brainstem is intact. Pupil size and equality is determined by balance between parasympathetic and sympathetic innervation. Response to light reflects combined function of optic (II) and oculomotor (III) cranial nerves.
Assess position and movement of eyes, noting whether in midposition or deviated to side or downward. Note loss of doll's eyes or oculocephalic reflex.	Position and movement of eyes help localize area of brain involvement. An early sign of increased ICP is impaired abduction of eyes, indicating pressure or injury to the fifth cranial nerve. Loss of doll's eyes indicates deterioration in brainstem function and poor prognosis.
Note presence or absence of reflexes—blink, cough, gag, and Babinski.	Altered reflexes reflect injury at level of midbrain or brainstem and have direct implications for client safety. Loss of blink reflex suggests damage to the pons and medulla. Absence of cough and gag reflexes reflects damage to medulla. Presence of Babinski reflex indicates injury along pyramidal pathways in the brain.

(continues on page 204)

ACTIONS/INTERVENTIONS (continued)	RATIONALE (continued)
Cerebral Perfusion Promotion (NIC)	
Monitor temperature and regulate environmental temperature, as indicated. Limit use of blankets; administer tepid sponge bath in presence of fever. Wrap extremities in blankets when hypothermia blanket is used.	Fever may reflect damage to hypothalamus. Increased metabolic needs and oxygen consumption occur (especially with fever and shivering), which can further increase ICP.
Monitor intake and output (I&O). Weigh, as indicated. Note skin turgor and status of mucous membranes.	Useful indicators of total body water, which is an integral part of tissue perfusion. Cerebral trauma and ischemia can result in diabetes insipidus (DI) or syndrome of inappropriate antidiuretic hormone (SIADH). Alterations may lead to hypovolemia or vascular engorgement, either of which can negatively affect cerebral pressure.
Maintain head and neck in midline or neutral position. Support with small towel rolls and pillows. Avoid placing head on large pillows. Periodically check position and fit of cervical collar or tracheostomy ties when used.	Turning head to one side compresses the jugular veins and inhibits cerebral venous drainage, thereby increasing ICP. Tight-fitting collar and ties can also limit jugular venous drainage.
Provide rest periods between care activities and limit duration of procedures.	Continual activity can increase ICP and contribute to storming by producing a cumulative stimulant effect.
Decrease extraneous stimuli and provide comfort measures, such as back massage, quiet environment, soft voice, and gentle touch.	Provides calming effect, reduces adverse physiological response, and promotes rest to maintain or lower ICP.
Help client avoid or limit coughing, vomiting, and straining at stool or bearing down, when possible. Reposition client slowly; prevent client from bending knees and pushing heels against mattress to move up in bed.	These activities increase intrathoracic and intra-abdominal pressures, which can increase ICP.
Avoid or limit use of restraints.	Mechanical restraints may enhance fight response, increasing ICP. *Note:* Cautious use may be indicated to prevent injury to client when other measures, including medications, are ineffective.
Limit number and duration of suctioning passes, for example, two passes less than 10 seconds each. Hyperventilate only when indicated.	Prevents hypoxia and associated vasoconstriction that can impair cerebral perfusion. *Note:* The use of prophylactic hyperventilation prior to suctioning or as a stand-alone treatment should be avoided, as it can compromise cerebral perfusion. It may be used episodically for brief periods when there is sudden neurological deterioration and ICP is refractory to sedation.
Encourage SO to talk to client.	Familiar voices of family and SO appear to have a relaxing effect on many comatose clients, which can reduce ICP.
Investigate increasing restlessness, moaning, and guarding behaviors.	These nonverbal cues may indicate increasing ICP or reflect presence of pain when client is unable to verbalize complaints. Unrelieved pain can in turn aggravate or potentiate increased ICP.
Palpate for bladder distention; maintain patency of urinary drainage if used. Monitor for constipation.	May trigger autonomic responses, potentiating elevation of ICP.
Observe for seizure activity and protect client from injury.	Seizures can occur as a result of cerebral irritation, hypoxia, or increased ICP; additionally, seizures can further elevate ICP, compounding cerebral damage.
Assess for nuchal rigidity, twitching, increased restlessness, irritability, and onset of seizure activity.	Indicative of meningeal irritation, which may occur because of interruption of dura or development of infection during acute or recovery period of brain injury. (Refer to Care Plan, Brain Infections: Meningitis, Encephalitis, if indicated)
Collaborative	
Elevate head of bed gradually to 20 to 30 degrees, as tolerated or indicated. Avoid hip flexion greater than 90 degrees.	Promotes venous drainage from head, thereby reducing cerebral congestion and edema, and risk of increased ICP. *Note:* Presence of hypotension can compromise cerebral perfusion pressure, negating beneficial effect of elevating head of bed.
Administer isotonic intravenous (IV) fluids, such as 0.9% sodium chloride, with control device.	Fluids should not be routinely restricted, but should be administered to maintain normal intravascular volume, systemic blood pressure, and cardiac output in order to maintain brain perfusion and decrease risk of cerebral edema and elevated ICP.
Administer supplemental oxygen via appropriate route, such as mechanical ventilator and mask, to maintain appropriate O_2 saturation, as indicated.	Reduces hypoxemia, which is known to increase cerebral vasodilation and blood volume, elevating ICP.
Monitor ABGs or pulse oximetry.	Determines respiratory sufficiency (presence of hypoxia and acidosis) and indicates therapy needs.

ACTIONS/INTERVENTIONS (continued)	RATIONALE (continued)
Administer medications, as indicated, for example:	
Diuretics, such as mannitol (Osmitrol) and furosemide (Lasix)	Diuretics may be used in acute phase to draw water from brain cells into the intravascular space, reducing cerebral edema and ICP. *Note:* Loop diuretics such as Lasix also reduce production of CSF, which can contribute to increased ICP when cerebral edema impairs CSF circulation. Mannitol usually lowers ICP within a few minutes of IV administration. Individuals being treated with mannitol must receive adequate fluid resuscitation to prevent hypovolemia and hypotension.
Barbiturates, such as pentobarbital	Barbiturates are the most common class of drugs used to produce deep sedation in the early phase of TBI treatment. The purpose of the therapy is to protect neurons by decreasing the cerebral metabolic rate, altering vascular tone, and inhibiting some of the biochemical intracellular events known to cause secondary brain injury. Because this therapy causes respiratory depression, it should only be used while client is on a ventilator. *Note:* Use of sedatives and opioids for cerebral protection can suppress signs and symptoms of sympathetic storming. The onset of storming episodes frequently coincides with being weaned off these medications. Oral or enteric medications may then be initiated to reduce the adverse effects of sympathetic storming (Zink, 2005).
Steroids, such as dexamethasone (Decadron) and methylprednisolone (Medrol)	May be effective for treating vasogenic edema—decreasing inflammation, reducing tissue edema. *Note:* Use and efficacy of steroids continues to be debated in this condition.
Anticonvulsant, such as phenytoin (Dilantin)	Dilantin is the drug of choice for treatment and prevention of seizure activity in immediate post-traumatic period to reduce risk of secondary injury from associated increased ICP. Prophylactic anticonvulsive therapy may be continued for an indeterminate period of time.
Analgesics and sedatives, such as lorazepam (Ativan), benzodiazepines, and propofol	May be indicated to relieve pain and agitation and their negative effects on ICP. Client on ventilator will be sedated and possibly require deep sedation (Lettieri, 2006).
Antipyretics, such as acetaminophen (Tylenol)	Reduces or controls fever and its deleterious effect on cerebral metabolism and oxygen needs and insensible fluid losses.
Initiate cooling measures, as indicated.	May be needed to regain or maintain normal core body temperature—hyperthermia exacerbates a hypermetabolic state.
Prepare for surgical intervention, such as craniotomy or insertion of ventricular drain or ICP pressure monitor, if indicated, and transfer to higher level of care.	Client may require decompressive craniotomy to remove a section of the skull and make an incision in the dura so that the brain can expand, relieving pressure. Craniotomy may also be performed to remove bone fragments, elevate depressed fractures, evacuate hematoma, control hemorrhage, and debride necrotic tissue. One way to monitor ICP is by placing a catheter in one of the brain's lateral ventricles. This device can also be used to drain CSF from the brain, reducing intracranial volume and decreasing ICP. When an intraventricular catheter is in place, draining CSF is the first recommended intervention on the critical pathway for reducing ICP. *Note:* Intracranial pressure monitoring devices are usually placed in conjunction with other cranial surgery procedures but may be placed in any client with a GCS score less than 9, with an abnormal CT scan. Monitoring of ICP requires more intensive care and complex therapies.

NURSING DIAGNOSIS: risk for ineffective Breathing Pattern

Risk Factors May Include

Neuromuscular damage

Possibly Evidenced By

(Not applicable; presence of signs and symptoms establishes an *actual* diagnosis)

Desired Outcomes/Evaluation Criteria—Client Will

Respiratory Status: Ventilation (NOC)

Maintain a normal or effective respiratory pattern, free of cyanosis, with ABGs or pulse oximetry within client's acceptable range.

ACTIONS/INTERVENTIONS	RATIONALE
Respiratory Monitoring (NIC)	
Independent	
Monitor rate, rhythm, and depth of respiration. Note breathing irregularities, for example, apneustic, ataxic, or cluster breathing.	Changes may indicate onset of pulmonary complications, common following brain injury, or indicate location and extent of brain involvement. Slow respiration and periods of apnea (apneustic, ataxic, or cluster breathing patterns) are signs of brainstem injury and warn of impending respiratory arrest.
Note competence of gag and swallow reflexes and client's ability to protect own airway. Insert airway adjunct as indicated.	Ability to mobilize or clear secretions is important to airway maintenance. Loss of swallow or cough reflex may indicate need for artificial airway or intubation. Thickening of pulmonary secretions may occur due to diaphoresis, dehydration, or renal insufficiency. *Note:* Soft nasopharyngeal airways may be preferred to prevent stimulation of the gag reflex caused by hard oropharyngeal airway, which can lead to excessive coughing and increased ICP.
Elevate head of bed as permitted and position on sides, as indicated.	Facilitates lung expansion and ventilation, and reduces risk of airway obstruction by tongue.
Encourage deep breathing if client is conscious.	Prevents or reduces atelectasis.
Suction with extreme caution, no longer than 10 to 15 seconds. Note character, color, and odor of secretions.	Suctioning is usually required if client is comatose or immobile and unable to clear own airway. Deep tracheal suctioning should be done with caution because it can cause or aggravate hypoxia, which produces vasoconstriction, adversely affecting cerebral perfusion.
Auscultate breath sounds, noting areas of hypoventilation and presence of adventitious sounds—crackles, rhonchi, and wheezes.	Identifies pulmonary problems such as atelectasis, congestion, and airway obstruction, which may jeopardize cerebral oxygenation or indicate onset of pulmonary infection, a common complication of head injury.
Monitor use of respiratory depressant drugs, such as sedatives.	Can increase respiratory embarrassment and complications.
Collaborative	
Monitor serial ABGs and pulse oximetry.	Determines respiratory sufficiency, acid-base balance, and therapy needs.
Review chest x-rays.	Reveals ventilatory state and signs of developing complications such as atelectasis and pneumonia.
Administer supplemental oxygen by appropriate means.	Maximizes arterial oxygenation and aids in prevention of cerebral hypoxia. If respiratory center is depressed, mechanical ventilation may be required.
Assist with chest physiotherapy when indicated.	Although contraindicated in client with acutely elevated ICP, these measures are often necessary in acute rehabilitation phase to mobilize and clear lung fields and reduce atelectasis or pulmonary complications.

NURSING DIAGNOSIS: [disturbed Sensory Perception (specify)]

May Be Related To
Altered sensory reception, transmission, and integration—neurological trauma or deficit

Possibly Evidenced By
Disorientation; change in usual response to stimuli
Impaired communication patterns
Poor concentration
Change in behavior pattern

Desired Outcomes/Evaluation Criteria—Client Will

Cognition (NOC)
Regain or maintain usual LOC and perceptual functioning.

Knowledge: Stroke Management (NOC)
Acknowledge changes in ability and presence of residual involvement.
Demonstrate behaviors and lifestyle changes to compensate for, or overcome, deficit.

ACTIONS/INTERVENTIONS	RATIONALE
Reality Orientation (NIC)	
Independent	
Evaluate and continually monitor changes in orientation, ability to speak, mood and affect, sensorium, and thought processes.	Upper cerebral functions are often the first to be affected by altered circulation and oxygenation. Damage may occur at time of initial injury or develop later because of swelling or bleeding. Motor, perceptual, cognitive, and personality changes may develop and persist, with gradual normalization of responses, or changes may remain permanently to some degree.
Assess sensory awareness, including response to touch, hot/cold, dull/sharp, and awareness of motion and location of body parts. Note problems with vision and other senses.	Information is essential to client safety. All sensory systems may be affected, with changes involving increased or decreased sensitivity or loss of sensation and the ability to perceive and respond appropriately to stimuli.
Observe behavioral responses—hostility, crying, inappropriate affect, agitation, and hallucinations.	Individual responses may be variable, but commonalities, such as emotional lability, increased irritability or frustration, apathy, and impulsiveness, exist during recovery from brain injury. Documentation of behavior provides information needed for development of structured rehabilitation.
Document specific changes in abilities, such as focusing and tracking with both eyes, following simple verbal instructions, answering "yes" or "no" to questions, and feeding self with dominant hand.	Helps localize areas of cerebral dysfunction, and identifies signs of progress toward improved neurological function.
Eliminate extraneous noise and stimuli, as necessary.	Reduces anxiety, exaggerated emotional responses, and confusion associated with sensory overload.
Speak in calm, quiet voice. Use short, simple sentences. Maintain eye contact.	Client may have limited attention span or understanding during acute and recovery stages, and these measures can help client attend to communication.
Ascertain and validate client's perceptions and provide feedback. Reorient client frequently to environment, staff, and procedures, especially if vision is impaired.	Assists client to differentiate reality in the presence of altered perceptions. Cognitive dysfunction and visual deficits potentiate disorientation and anxiety.
Provide meaningful stimulation: verbal (talk to client), olfactory (e.g., oil of clove, coffee), tactile (touch, hand holding), and auditory (tapes, television, radio, visitors). Avoid physical or emotional isolation of client.	Carefully selected sensory input may be useful for coma stimulation as well as for documenting progress during cognitive retraining.
Provide structured therapies, activities, and environment. Provide written schedule for client to refer to on a regular basis.	Promotes consistency and reassurance, reducing anxiety associated with the unknown. Promotes sense of control and cognitive retraining.
Schedule adequate rest and uninterrupted sleep periods.	Reduces fatigue, prevents exhaustion, and improves sleep. *Note:* Absence of rapid eye movement (REM) sleep is known to aggravate sensory perception deficits.
Use day/night lighting.	Provides for normal sense of passage of time and sleep-wake pattern.
Allow adequate time for communication and performance of activities.	Reduces frustration associated with altered abilities and delayed response pattern.
Provide for client's safety, such as padded side rails or bed enclosed with safety netting, assistance with ambulation, and protection from hot or sharp objects. Document perceptual deficit and compensatory activities on chart and at bedside.	Agitation, impaired judgment, poor balance, and sensory deficits increase risk of client injury.
Identify alternative ways of dealing with perceptual deficits, such as arrange bed, personal articles, and food to take advantage of functional vision; describe where affected body parts are located.	Enables client to progress toward independence, enhancing sense of control, while compensating for neurological deficits.
Collaborative	
Refer to physical, occupational, speech, and cognitive therapists.	Interdisciplinary approach can create an integrated treatment plan based on the individual's unique combination of abilities and disabilities with focus on evaluation and functional improvement in physical, cognitive, and perceptual skills.

NURSING DIAGNOSIS: risk for chronic Confusion

Risk Factors May Include

Head injury

Possibly Evidenced By

(Not applicable; presence of signs and symptoms establishes an *actual* diagnosis)

Desired Outcomes/Evaluation Criteria—Client Will

Cognition (NOC)

Maintain or regain usual mentation and reality orientation.

Distorted Thought Self-Control (NOC)

Recognize changes in thinking and behavior.

Participate in therapeutic regimen and cognitive retraining.

ACTIONS/INTERVENTIONS	RATIONALE
Cognitive Stimulation (NIC)	
Independent	
Assess attention span and distractibility. Note level of anxiety.	Attention span and ability to attend or concentrate may be severely shortened, which both causes and potentiates anxiety, affecting thought processes.
Confer with SO to compare past behaviors and preinjury personality with current responses.	Recovery from head injury often includes a prolonged phase of agitation, angry responses, and disordered thought sequences. It is helpful to know about client's past behaviors in order to determine if current behaviors can be attributed solely to the brain injury. *Note:* SOs often have difficulty accepting and dealing with client's aberrant behavior and may require assistance in coping with situation.
Maintain consistency in staff assigned to client to the extent possible.	Provides client with feelings of stability, familiarity, and control of situation.
Present reality concisely and briefly; avoid challenging illogical thinking.	Client may be totally unaware of injury (amnesic) or of extent of injury and therefore deny reality of injury. Structured reality orientation can reduce defensive reactions.
Provide information about injury process in relationship to symptoms. Explain procedures and reinforce explanations given by others.	Loss of internal structure (changes in memory, reasoning, and ability to conceptualize) and fear of the unknown affect processing and retention of information and can compound anxiety, confusion, and disorientation.
Review necessity of recurrent neurological evaluations.	Understanding that assessments are done frequently to prevent or limit complications and that they do not necessarily reflect seriousness of client's condition may help reduce anxiety.
Reduce provocative stimuli, negative criticism, arguments, and confrontations.	Reduces risk of triggering fight-or-flight response. Aggression, anger, and self-control are common problems in brain-injured clients, who may become violent or physically or verbally abusive.
Listen with regard to client's verbalizations in spite of speech pattern or content.	Conveys interest and worth to individual, enhancing self-esteem and encouraging continued efforts.
Promote socialization within individual limitations.	Reinforcement of positive behaviors, such as appropriate interaction with others, may be helpful in relearning internal structure.
Encourage SO to provide current news and family happenings.	Promotes maintenance of contact with usual events, enhancing reality orientation and normalization of thinking.
Instruct in relaxation techniques. Provide diversional activities.	Can help refocus attention and reduce anxiety to manageable levels.
Maintain realistic expectations of client's ability to control own behavior, comprehend, and remember information.	It is important to maintain an expectation of the ability to improve and progress to a higher level of functioning, to maintain hope, and promote continued work of rehabilitation.
Avoid leaving client alone when agitated or frightened.	Anxiety can lead to loss of control and escalate to panic. Support may provide calming effect, reducing anxiety and risk of injury.
Implement measures to control emotional outbursts or aggressive behavior if needed—speak in a calm voice, tell client to "stop," remove client from the situation, provide distraction, and restrain for brief periods of time, as appropriate.	Client may need help or external control to protect self or others from harm until internal control is regained. Restraints (physical holding, mechanical, and pharmacological) should be used judiciously to avoid escalating violent, irrational behavior.

ACTIONS/INTERVENTIONS (continued)	RATIONALE (continued)
Inform client and SO that intellectual function, behavior, and emotional functioning will gradually improve, but that some effects may persist for months or even be permanent.	Most brain-injured clients have persistent problems with concentration, memory, and problem-solving. If brain injury was moderate to severe, recovery may be complete or residual effects may remain.
Collaborative	
Refer for neuropsychological evaluation as indicated.	Useful for determining therapeutic interventions for cognitive and neurobehavioral disturbances.
Coordinate participation in cognitive retraining or rehabilitation program, as indicated.	Assists client with learning methods to compensate for disruption of cognitive skills. Addresses problems in concentration, memory, judgment, sequencing, and problem-solving. *Note:* New developments in technology and computer software allow for the creation of interactive sensory-motor virtual reality environments. This provides an opportunity for safe interaction between client and naturalistic environments for the purpose of practicing or establishing effective behavioral responses.
Refer to support groups, such as Brain Injury Association, and social services, visiting nurse, and counseling or therapy, as needed.	Additional long-term assistance may be helpful in supporting and sustaining recovery.

NURSING DIAGNOSIS: impaired physical Mobility

May Be Related To
Cognitive impairment
Decreased muscle strength or control
Sensoriperceptual impairment

Possibly Evidenced By
Slowed/uncoordinated movements
Limited ROM; postural instability; gait changes

Desired Outcomes/Evaluation Criteria—Client Will

Immobility Consequences: Physiological (NOC)
Maintain or increase strength and function of affected or compensatory body part(s).
Regain or maintain optimal position of function, as evidenced by absence of contractures and footdrop.

Mobility (NOC)
Demonstrate techniques or behaviors that enable resumption of activities.
Maintain skin integrity and bladder and bowel function.

ACTIONS/INTERVENTIONS	RATIONALE
Exercise Therapy: Muscle Control (NIC)	
Independent	
Review functional ability and reasons for impairment.	Identifies probable functional impairments and influences choice of interventions.
Assess degree of immobility, using a scale to rate dependence (0 to 4).	The client may be completely independent (0), may require minimal assistance or equipment (1), moderate assistance or supervision and teaching (2), extensive assistance or equipment and devices (3), or be completely dependent on caregivers (4). Persons in all categories are at risk for injury, but those in categories 2 to 4 are at greatest risk.
Provide or assist with ROM exercises.	Helps in maintaining movement and functional alignment of joints and extremities.
Instruct and assist client with exercise program and use of mobility aids. Increase activity and participation in self-care as tolerated.	Lengthy convalescence often follows brain injury, and physical reconditioning is an essential part of the program.
Bed Rest Care (NIC)	
Position client to avoid skin and tissue pressure damage. Turn at regular intervals, and make small position changes between turns.	Regular turning more normally distributes body weight and promotes circulation to all areas. If paralysis or limited cognition is present, client should be repositioned frequently.
Provide meticulous skin care, massaging with emollients. Remove wet linen and clothing, and keep bedding free of wrinkles.	Promotes circulation and skin elasticity and reduces risk of skin excoriation.

(continues on page 210)

ACTIONS/INTERVENTIONS (continued)	RATIONALE (continued)
Maintain functional body alignment—hips, feet, and hands. Monitor for proper placement of devices and signs of pressure from devices.	Use of high-top tennis shoes, "space boots," and T-bar sheepskin devices can help prevent footdrop. Hand splints are variable and designed to prevent hand deformities and promote optimal function. Use of pillows, bedrolls, and sandbags can help prevent abnormal hip rotation.
Support head and trunk, arms and shoulders, and feet and legs when client is in wheelchair or recliner. Pad chair seat with foam or water-filled cushion, and assist client to shift weight at frequent intervals.	Maintains comfortable, safe, and functional posture, and prevents or reduces risk of skin breakdown.
Provide eye care with artificial tears and eye patches, as indicated.	Protects delicate eye tissues from drying. Client may require patches during sleep to protect eyes from trauma if unable to keep eyes closed.
Monitor urinary output. Note color and odor of urine. Assist with bladder retraining when appropriate.	Indwelling catheter used during the acute phase of injury may be needed for an extended period of time before bladder retraining is possible. Once the catheter is removed, several methods of continence control may be tried, such as intermittent catheterization for residual and complete emptying, external catheter, planned intervals on commode, and incontinence pads.
Provide fluids within individual tolerance (that is, regarding neurological and cardiac concerns), as indicated.	Once past the acute phase of head injury, and if client has no other contraindicating factors, forcing fluids decreases risk of urinary tract infections and bladder or kidney stone formation. Good hydration provides other positive effects such as normal stool consistency and optimal skin turgor.
Monitor bowel elimination and provide for or assist with a regular bowel routine. Check for impacted stool; use digital stimulation, as indicated. Sit client upright on commode or stool at regular intervals. Add fiber, bulk, and fruit juice to diet, as appropriate.	A regular bowel routine requires simple but diligent measures to prevent complications. Stimulation of the internal rectal sphincter stimulates the bowel to empty automatically if stool is soft enough to do so. Upright position aids evacuation.
Inspect for localized tenderness, redness, skin warmth, muscle tension, or ropy veins in calves of legs. Observe for sudden dyspnea, tachypnea, fever, respiratory distress, and chest pain.	Client is at risk for development of deep vein thrombosis (DVT) and pulmonary embolus (PE), requiring prompt medical evaluation and intervention to prevent serious complications.
Collaborative	
Provide flotation mattress and kinetic therapy, as appropriate.	Equalizes tissue pressure, enhances circulation, and helps reduce venous stasis to decrease risk of tissue injury.
Apply and monitor use of sequential compression devices (SCDs) to legs.	SCD may be used to reduce risk of DVT associated with bedrest and limited mobility.
Exercise Therapy: Muscle Control (NIC)	
Refer to physical and occupational therapists, as indicated.	Useful in determining individual needs, therapeutic activities, and assistive devices.

NURSING DIAGNOSIS: risk for Infection

Risk Factors May Include

Traumatized tissues, broken skin, invasive procedures, CSF leak
Decreased ciliary action, stasis of body fluids
Malnutrition
Suppressed inflammatory response—steroid use

Possibly Evidenced By

(Not applicable; presence of signs and symptoms establishes an *actual* diagnosis)

Desired Outcomes/Evaluation Criteria—Client Will

Infection Severity (NOC)

Maintain normothermia, free of signs of infection.
Achieve timely wound healing when present.

ACTIONS/INTERVENTIONS	RATIONALE
Infection Protection (NIC)	
Independent	
Provide meticulous, clean, or aseptic care; maintain good hand-washing techniques.	First-line defense against nosocomial infections.
Observe areas of impaired skin integrity (wounds, suture lines, invasive line insertion sites), noting drainage characteristics and presence of inflammation.	Early identification of developing infection permits prompt intervention and prevention of further complications.
Monitor temperature routinely. Note presence of chills, diaphoresis, and changes in mentation.	May indicate developing sepsis requiring further evaluation and intervention.
Encourage deep breathing and aggressive pulmonary toilet. Observe sputum characteristics.	Enhances mobilization and clearing of pulmonary secretions to reduce risk of pneumonia and atelectasis. *Note:* Postural drainage should be used with caution if risk of increased ICP exists.
Provide perineal care. Maintain integrity of closed urinary drainage system if used. Encourage adequate fluid intake.	Reduces potential for bacterial growth and ascending infection.
Observe color and clarity of urine. Note presence of foul odor.	Indicators of developing urinary tract infection (UTI) requiring prompt intervention.
Screen and restrict access of visitors or caregivers with upper respiratory infections (URIs).	Reduces risk to "compromised host."
Collaborative	
Obtain specimens, as indicated.	Culture with sensitivities may be done to verify presence of infection and identify causative organism and appropriate treatment choices.

NURSING DIAGNOSIS: risk for imbalanced Nutrition: less than body requirements

Risk Factors May Include

Inability to ingest nutrients—LOC

Biological factors—hypermetabolic state

Possibly Evidenced By

(Not applicable; presence of signs and symptoms establishes an *actual* diagnosis)

Desired Outcomes/Evaluation Criteria—Client Will

Nutritional Status (NOC)

Demonstrate maintenance of desired weight or progressive weight gain toward goal.

Experience no signs of malnutrition, with laboratory values within normal range.

ACTIONS/INTERVENTIONS	RATIONALE
Nutrition Therapy (NIC)	
Independent	
Assess ability to chew, swallow, cough, and handle secretions.	These factors determine choice of feeding options because client must be protected from aspiration.
Auscultate bowel sounds, noting decreased or absent or hyperactive sounds.	Gastrointestinal (GI) functioning is usually preserved in brain-injured clients, so bowel sounds help in determining response to feeding or development of complications, such as ileus.
Weigh, as indicated.	Evaluates effectiveness or need for changes in nutritional therapy.
Provide for feeding safety, such as elevate head of bed while eating or during tube feeding.	Reduces risk of regurgitation and aspiration.
Divide feedings into small amounts and give frequently.	Enhances digestion and client's tolerance of nutrients and can improve client cooperation in eating.
Promote pleasant, relaxing environment, including socialization during meals. Encourage SO to bring in food that client enjoys.	Although the recovering client may require assistance with feeding and use of assistive devices, mealtime socialization with SO or friends can improve intake and normalize the life function of eating.
Check stools, gastric aspirant, and vomitus for blood.	Acute or subacute bleeding may occur (Cushing's ulcer), requiring intervention and alternative method of providing nutrition.

(continues on page 212)

ACTIONS/INTERVENTIONS (continued)	RATIONALE (continued)
Collaborative	
Consult with dietitian or nutritional support team.	Helps determine the client's requirements for energy and to provide needed nutrients. Careful monitoring of nutrition indicators, such as weight and blood tests, are necessary to prevent problems associated with malnutrition—muscle wasting, pressure sores and decubitus ulcers, renal failure, atelectasis, and pneumonia.
Monitor laboratory studies, for example, prealbumin or albumin, transferrin, amino acid profile, iron, blood urea nitrogen (BUN), nitrogen balance studies, glucose, aspartate aminotransferase (AST) and alanine aminotransferase (ALT), and electrolytes.	Identifies nutritional deficiencies, organ function, and response to nutritional therapy.
Administer feedings by appropriate means—IV, tube feeding, or oral feedings with soft foods and thick liquids. (Refer to CP: Total Nutritional Support: Parenteral/Enteral Feeding.)	Choice of route depends on client needs and capabilities. Tube feedings (nasogastric, jejunostomy) may be required initially, or parenteral route may be indicated in presence of gastric or intestinal pathology. If client is able to swallow, soft foods or semiliquid foods may be more easily managed without aspiration.
Involve speech, occupational, and physical therapists when mechanical problem exists, such as impaired swallow reflexes, wired jaws, contractures of hands, and paralysis.	Individual strategies and devices may be needed to improve ability to eat.

NURSING DIAGNOSIS: interrupted Family Processes

May Be Related To

Situational crisis

Shift in health status of a family member; shift in family roles

Possibly Evidenced By

Changes in participation in problem-solving or decision making

[Expressed confusion about what to do, difficulty responding to change]

Desired Outcomes/Evaluation Criteria—Family/Client Will

Family Coping (NOC)

Begin to express feelings freely and appropriately.

Identify internal and external resources to deal with the situation.

Direct energies in a purposeful manner to plan for resolution of crisis.

Encourage and allow injured member to progress toward independence.

ACTIONS/INTERVENTIONS	RATIONALE
Family Integrity Promotion (NIC)	
Independent	
Note components of family unit, availability, and involvement of support systems.	Defines family resources and identifies areas of need.
Encourage expression of concerns about seriousness of condition, possibility of death, or incapacitation.	Verbalization of fears gets concerns out in the open and can decrease anxiety and enhance coping with reality.
Listen for expressions of helplessness and hopelessness.	Joy of survival of victim is often quickly replaced by grief and anger at "loss" of the preinjury person and the necessity of dealing with new person that family does not know and may not even like. Prolongation of these feelings may result in depression.
Encourage expression and acknowledgment of feelings. Do not deny or reassure client/SO that everything will be all right.	Because it is not possible to predict the outcome, it is more helpful to assist the person to deal with feelings about what is happening instead of giving false reassurance.
Support family grieving for "loss" of member. Acknowledge normality of wide range of feelings and ongoing nature of process.	Although grief may never be fully resolved and family may vacillate among various stages, understanding that this is typical may help members accept and cope with the situation.
Emphasize importance of continuous open dialogue between family members.	Provides opportunity to get feelings out in the open. Recognition and awareness promotes resolution of guilt and anger.

ACTIONS/INTERVENTIONS (continued) | RATIONALE (continued)

Help family recognize needs of all members.

Attention may be so focused on injured member that other members feel isolated or abandoned, which can compromise family growth and unity.

Family Mobilization (NIC)

Evaluate and discuss family goals and expectations.

Family may believe that if client is going to live, rehabilitation will bring about a cure. Despite accurate information, expectations may be unrealistic. Also, client's early recovery may be rapid, then plateau, resulting in disappointment and frustration.

Reinforce previous explanations about extent of injury, treatment plan, and prognosis. Provide accurate information at current level of understanding and ability to accept.

Client and SO are unable to absorb or recall all information, and blocking can occur because of emotional trauma. As time goes by, reinforcement of information can help reduce misconceptions, fear about the unknown, and future expectations.

Identify individual roles and anticipated and perceived changes.

Responsibilities and roles may have to be partially or completely assumed by others, which can further complicate family coping.

Assess energy direction, whether efforts at problem-solving are purposeful or scattered.

May need assistance to focus energies in an effective way to enhance coping.

Identify and encourage use of previously successful coping behaviors.

Focuses on strengths and reaffirms individual's ability to deal with current crisis.

Demonstrate and encourage use of stress management skills—relaxation techniques, breathing exercises, visualization, and music.

Helps redirect attention toward revitalizing self to enhance coping ability.

Collaborative

Include family in rehabilitation team meetings, care planning, and placement decisions.

Facilitates communication, enables family to be an integral part of the rehabilitation, and provides sense of control.

Identify community resources, such as visiting nurse, homemaker service, day-care program, respite facility, and legal and financial counselors.

Provides assistance with problems that may arise because of altered role function. Also, as family structure changes over time and client's needs increase with age, additional resources and support are often required.

Refer to family therapy and support groups.

Cognitive and personality changes are usually very difficult for family to deal with. Decreased impulse control, emotional lability, and inappropriate sexual or aggressive and violent behavior can disrupt family functioning and integrity. Trained therapists and peer role models may assist family to deal with feelings and reality of situation and provide support for decisions that are made.

NURSING DIAGNOSIS: deficient Knowledge [Learning Need] regarding condition, prognosis, potential complications, treatment, self-care, and discharge needs

May Be Related To

Lack of exposure, unfamiliarity with information resources
Lack of recall, cognitive limitation

Possibly Evidenced By

Reports the problem
Inaccurate follow-through of instructions

Desired Outcomes/Evaluation Criteria—Client/SO Will

Knowledge: Chronic Disease Management (NOC)

Participate in learning process.
Verbalize understanding of condition, prognosis, and potential complications.
Verbalize understanding of therapeutic regimen and rationale for actions.
Initiate necessary lifestyle changes and involvement in rehabilitation program.
Correctly perform necessary procedures.

ACTIONS/INTERVENTIONS	RATIONALE
Teaching: Disease Process (NIC)	
Independent	
Evaluate capabilities and readiness to learn for both client and SO.	Permits presentation of material based on individual needs. *Note:* Client may not be emotionally or mentally capable of assimilating information.
Review information regarding injury process and aftereffects.	Aids in establishing realistic expectations and promotes understanding of current situation and needs.
Review and reinforce current therapeutic regimen. Identify ways of continuing program after discharge.	Recommended activities, limitations, medications, and therapy needs have been established on the basis of a coordinated interdisciplinary approach, and follow-through is essential to progression of recovery and prevention of complications.
Discuss plans for meeting self-care needs.	Varying levels of assistance may be required, based on individual situation.
Provide written instructions and schedules for activity, medication, and important facts.	Provides visual reinforcement and reference source after discharge.
Identify signs and symptoms of individual risks, such as delayed CSF leak, post-traumatic seizures, headache, and chronic pain.	Recognizing developing problems provides opportunity for prompt evaluation and intervention to prevent serious complications.
Discuss with client/SO development of symptoms, such as reexperiencing traumatic event (flashbacks, intrusive thoughts, repetitive dreams or nightmares); psychic or emotional numbness; and changes in lifestyle, including adoption of self-destructive behaviors.	May indicate occurrence or exacerbation of post-trauma response, which can occur months to years after injury, requiring further evaluation and supportive interventions.
Identify community resources, including head injury support groups, social services, rehabilitation facilities, outpatient programs, and home care or visiting nurse.	May be needed to provide assistance with physical care, home management, adjustment to lifestyle changes, and emotional and financial concerns. *Note:* Studies suggest an increased risk of developing Alzheimer's disease and the possibility of acceleration of the aging process in brain injury survivors. SO and families will require continued support to meet these challenges.
Refer for, and reinforce importance of, follow-up care by rehabilitation team.	With diligent work (often for several years with these providers), the client may eventually overcome residual neurological deficits and be able to resume desired and productive lifestyle.

POTENTIAL CONSIDERATIONS following acute hospitalization (dependent on client's age, physical condition and presence of complications, personal resources, and life responsibilities)

- ***impaired Memory***—neurological disturbances, anemia, hypoxia
- ***ineffective Health Maintenance***—perceptual or cognitive impairment, deficient communication skills, inability to make appropriate judgments, insufficient resources
- ***impaired Home Maintenance***—injury/impaired functioning, insufficient finances, unfamiliarity with neighborhood resources, inadequate support systems
- ***acute/chronic Pain***—physical (tissue injury and neuronal damage), psychological (stress and anxiety); chronic physical disability
- ***chronic Confusion***—head injury

CEREBROVASCULAR ACCIDENT (CVA)/ STROKE

I. Pathophysiology—Cerebrovascular accident (CVA, "stroke" or "brain attack") is injury or death to parts of the brain caused by an interruption in the blood supply to that area causing disability, such as paralysis or speech impairment.

II. Types

a. Ischemic stroke: Impaired cerebral circulation caused by a partial or complete occlusion of a blood vessel with transient or permanent effects

i. Accounts for 87% of all strokes (Morrison, 2007; American Stroke Association [ASA], 2012), with carotid stenosis as the leading cause (Phillips, 2007)

ii. Subdivided based on the underlying cause

1. Large-vessel thrombotic and embolic strokes
2. Small-vessel thrombotic stroke
3. Cardioembolic stroke
4. Other

iii. Ischemia may be transient and resolve within 24 hours, be reversible with resolution of symptoms over a period of 1 week (reversible ischemic neurological deficit [RIND]), or progress to cerebral infarction with variable effects and degrees of recovery.

b. Hemorrhagic stroke: Result of a vessel wall rupture with bleeding into the brain, compressing brain tissue

i. Accounts for approximately 13% of cerebrovascular accidents (Morrison, 2007; ASA, 2012)

III. Etiology

a. Ischemic stroke

i. Large-vessel thrombotic and embolic strokes result from hypoperfusion, hypertension, and emboli traveling from large arteries to distal branches.

ii. Small-vessel thrombotic stroke typically stems from plaque, diabetes mellitus, or hypertension.

iii. Cardioembolic stroke results from atrial fibrillation, valve disease, or ventricular thrombi.

iv. Other types of ischemic stroke are caused by hyperglycemia and hyperinsulinemia, arterial dissection, arteritis, and drug abuse.

b. Hemorrhagic stroke

i. Caused by hemorrhage—subarachnoid or intracerebral—from such conditions as a ruptured aneurysm, arteriovenous malformation (AVM), trauma, infections, tumors, or blood clotting deficiencies

ii. Major risk factor: hypertension (60% [Liebeskind, 2011])

IV. Statistics

a. Morbidity: In 2005, prevalence of stroke was estimated at 2.3 million males and 3.4 million females; many of the approximately 5.7 million U.S. stroke survivors have permanent stroke-related disabilities.

b. Mortality: In 2008, stroke ranked fourth as the cause of death for those aged 65 years or older, with 134,000 deaths (ASA, 2012; National Heart, Lung and Blood Institute [NHLBI], 2012). Hemorrhagic strokes are more severe, and mortality rates are higher than ischemic strokes. Intracerebral hemorrhage accounts for 10% to 15% of strokes and is associated with a 30-day mortality rate near 50% (Kase, 2011).

c. Cost: Estimated direct and indirect cost for 2008 was $65.5 billion (American Heart Association and American Stroke Association, 2008).

GLOSSARY

Agnosia: Impairment of the ability to recognize or comprehend the meaning of various sensory stimuli.

Apraxia: Disorder of voluntary movement consisting of impairment of the performance of skilled or purposeful movements despite physical ability and willingness to move.

Atrial fibrillation: Most common form of irregular heartbeat and a risk factor for embolic ischemic stroke. The condition can cause a pooling of blood in the heart, which can make it easier for clots to form.

Carotid stenosis: Buildup of hardened plaque on the carotid artery wall. This is the leading cause of ischemic stroke.

Cerebral edema: Swelling of the brain.

Contralateral: Refers to the other side. Stroke affecting the *right* side of the brain may cause paralysis, affecting the *left* arm and leg.

Dysarthria: Difficulty in articulating words due to disease of the central nervous system (CNS).

Dysphagia: Difficulty in swallowing.

Embolic stroke: Occurs when a clot is carried into cerebral circulation and causes a localized cerebral infarct.

Embolus: Blood clot that forms in one area of the body and moves to another.

Hemiplegia: One-sided paralysis.

Ipsilateral: Refers to the same side. A stroke on the right side of the brain causes some symptoms on the right side of the body, as opposed to contralateral (the other side).

Thrombosis: Obstruction of a blood vessel by a clot formed at the site of obstruction.

Thrombotic stroke: Type of ischemic stroke usually seen in aging population. It is due to atherosclerosis (plaque buildup), eventually narrowing the lumen of the artery. The symptoms are much more gradual and less dramatic than other strokes due to the slow, ongoing process that produces it. The stroke is "completed" when the condition stabilizes.

Transient ischemic attack (TIA): Temporary lack of adequate blood and oxygen to the brain that causes stroke warning signs but no permanent damage. Generally lasts about 1 minute but can last up to 5 minutes.

Care Setting

Although the client may initially be cared for in the intensive care unit (ICU) for severe or evolving deficits, this plan of care focuses on the step down from medical unit and subacute and rehabilitation units to the community level.

Related Concerns

Hypertension: severe, page 33
Craniocerebral trauma (acute rehabilitative phase), page 197
Psychosocial aspects of care, page 729
Seizure disorders, page 188
Total nutritional support: parenteral/enteral feeding, page 437

Client Assessment Database

Collected data are determined by location, severity, and duration of pathology.

DIAGNOSTIC DIVISION MAY REPORT	MAY EXHIBIT
ACTIVITY/REST	
• Difficulty with activity due to weakness, loss of sensation, or paralysis (hemiplegia) • Tires easily • Difficulty resting, pain or muscle twitching	• Altered muscle tone—flaccid or spastic; generalized weakness • One-sided paralysis • Altered level of consciousness (LOC)
CIRCULATORY	
• History of cardiac disease—myocardial infarction (MI), rheumatic and valvular heart disease, heart failure (HF), bacterial endocarditis, polycythemia	• Arterial hypertension, which is common unless CVA is due to embolism or vascular malformation • Pulse rate may vary due to various factors, such as preexisting heart conditions, medications, effect of stroke on vasomotor center. • Dysrhythmias, electrocardiographic (ECG) changes • Bruit in carotid, femoral, or iliac arteries, or abdominal aorta may or may not be present.
EGO INTEGRITY	
• Feelings of helplessness, hopelessness	• Emotional lability • Exaggerated or inappropriate responses to anger, sadness, happiness • Difficulty expressing self
ELIMINATION	
	• Change in voiding patterns—incontinence, anuria • Distended abdomen • Distended bladder • May have absent or diminished bowel sounds if neurogenic paralytic ileus present
FOOD/FLUID	
• History of diabetes, elevated serum lipids (risk factors) • Lack of appetite • Nausea or vomiting during acute event (increased intracranial pressure [ICP]) • Loss of sensation in tongue, cheek, and throat • Dysphagia	• Obesity (risk factor) • Chewing and swallowing problems
NEUROSENSORY	
• History of TIA, RIND • Dizziness or syncope before stroke or transient during TIA • Severe headache can accompany intracerebral or subarachnoid hemorrhage • Tingling, numbness, and weakness commonly reported during TIAs, found in varying degrees in other types of stroke; involved side seems "dead" • Visual deficits—blurred vision, partial loss of vision (monocular blindness), double vision (diplopia), or other disturbances in visual fields • Sensory loss on contralateral side in extremities and sometimes in ipsilateral side of face • Disturbance in senses of taste, smell	• Mental status/LOC: Coma usually presents in the initial stages of hemorrhagic disturbances; consciousness is usually preserved when the etiology is thrombotic in nature. • Altered behavior—lethargy, apathy, combativeness • Altered cognitive function—memory, problem-solving, sequencing • Extremities: Weakness and paralysis contralateral with all kinds of stroke; unequal hand grasp; diminished deep tendon reflexes (contralateral) • Facial paralysis or paresis (ipsilateral) • Speech: Aphasia: May be expressive (difficulty producing speech), receptive (difficulty comprehending speech), or global (combination of the two) • Agnosia • Altered body image awareness, neglect or denial of contralateral side of body (unilateral neglect); disturbances in perception

DIAGNOSTIC DIVISION MAY REPORT (continued)	MAY EXHIBIT (continued)
	• Apraxia • Pupil size and reaction: May be unequal; dilated and fixed pupil on the ipsilateral side may be present with hemorrhage or herniation. • Seizures—common in hemorrhagic stroke
PAIN/DISCOMFORT • Headache of varying intensity	• Guarding, distraction behaviors • Restlessness • Muscle or facial tension; nuchal rigidity (common in hemorrhagic stroke)
RESPIRATION • Smoking (risk factor)	• Inability to swallow, cough, or protect airway • Labored and irregular respirations • Noisy respirations, rhonchi (aspiration of secretions)
SAFETY	• Problems with vision • Changes in perception of body spatial orientation (right CVA), neglect • Difficulty seeing objects on left side (right CVA) • Being unaware of affected side • Inability to recognize familiar objects, colors, words, faces • Diminished response to heat and cold, altered body temperature regulation • Swallowing difficulty, inability to meet own nutritional needs • Impaired judgment, little concern for safety, impatience, lack of insight (right CVA)
SOCIAL INTERACTION	• Speech problems • Inability to communicate • Inappropriate behavior
TEACHING/LEARNING • Family history of hypertension, stroke, diabetes • African American heritage (higher risk factor) • Use of oral contraceptives • Smoking, alcohol abuse (risk factors) • Obesity **DISCHARGE PLAN CONSIDERATIONS** • Medication regimen and therapeutic treatments • Assistance with transportation, shopping, food preparation, self-care, and homemaker or maintenance tasks • Changes in physical layout of home • Transition placement before return to home setting ➧ Refer to section at end of plan for postdischarge considerations.	

Diagnostic Studies

TEST WHY IT IS DONE	WHAT IT TELLS ME
• *Computed tomography (CT) scan with or without enhancement:* Demonstrates structural abnormalities and presence of edema, hematoma, ischemia, and infarction.	Ischemic infarction may not be evident for 8 to 12 hours after event. Hemorrhagic events are evident immediately; therefore, emergency CT scan is done prior to administration of thrombolytics. Patients experiencing a TIA will have a normal CT scan.
• *CT angiography (CTA):* Similar to a CT scan, but contrast dye is injected into a vein shortly before x-ray image is performed.	CT angiography gives superior views of vessels in the head and neck; therefore it's useful for spotting narrowing there. Because the dye is injected into a vein rather than into an artery CT angiography could be considered less invasive.
• *Magnetic resonance imaging (MRI):* Demonstrates structural abnormalities and presence of edema, hematoma, ischemia, and infarction.	Evaluates the lesion's location and size. May show evidence of stroke within minutes of occurrence and is especially beneficial for assessing smaller strokes deep within the brain.
• *Positron emission tomography (PET) scan:* Provides data on cerebral metabolism and on cerebral blood flow changes.	Abnormal in ischemic event.
• *Cerebral angiography:* Procedure that uses x-ray and opaque dye to help identify abnormalities of the blood vessels within the brain.	Helps determine specific cause of stroke, such as hemorrhage or obstructed artery, and pinpoints site of occlusion or rupture (Springhouse, 2008).
• *Transcranial Doppler ultrasonography:* Evaluates the velocity of blood flow through major intracranial vessels.	Identifies problems with circulation, such as diminished blood flow or presence of atherosclerotic plaques.
• *Stroke scale:* A standardized instrument used to detect/diagnose acute strokes. Some scales (Cincinnati or Los Angeles) are used pre-hospital as a quick screening tool. Others, such as the NIH Stroke Scale, are lengthy and are measured repeatedly over time, using a numeric scale to document trends (National Institutes of Health [NIH], 2003).	If patients have 1 of 3 abnormal findings on the Cincinnati Stroke Scale, there is a 72% probability of an ischemic stroke. If all 3 findings are present, the probability of an acute stroke is more than 85%. For the NIH scale, the higher the score, the more severe the stroke symptoms.

Nursing Priorities

1. Promote adequate cerebral perfusion and oxygenation.
2. Prevent or minimize complications and permanent disabilities.
3. Assist client to gain independence in activities of daily living (ADLs).
4. Support coping process and integration of changes into self-concept.
5. Provide information about disease process, prognosis, and treatment and rehabilitation needs.

Discharge Goals

1. Cerebral function improved and neurological deficits resolving or stabilized.
2. Complications prevented or minimized.
3. ADL needs met by self or with assistance of other(s).
4. Coping with situation in positive manner and planning for the future.
5. Disease process, prognosis, and therapeutic regimen understood.
6. Plan in place to meet needs after discharge.

NURSING DIAGNOSIS: ineffective cerebral Tissue Perfusion

May Be Related To
Embolism, cerebral aneurysm, hypertension, brain tumor, abnormal prothrombin/partial thromboplastin time

Possibly Evidenced By
[Altered LOC; memory loss; sensory, language, intellectual, or emotional deficits]
[Changes in motor or sensory responses]

Desired Outcomes/Evaluation Criteria—Client Will

Tissue Perfusion: Cerebral (NOC)
Maintain usual or improved LOC, cognition, and motor and sensory function.
Demonstrate stable vital signs and absence of signs of increased ICP.
Display no further deterioration or recurrence of deficits.

ACTIONS/INTERVENTIONS	RATIONALE
Cerebral Perfusion Promotion (NIC)	
Independent	
Determine factors related to individual situation, cause for coma, decreased cerebral perfusion, and potential for increased ICP.	Influences choice of interventions. Deterioration in neurological signs and symptoms or failure to improve after initial insult may reflect decreased intracranial adaptive capacity, which requires that client be admitted to critical care area for monitoring of ICP and for specific therapies geared to maintaining ICP within a specified range. If the stroke is evolving, client can deteriorate quickly and require repeated assessment and progressive treatment. If the stroke is "completed," the neurological deficit is nonprogressive, and treatment is geared toward rehabilitation and preventing recurrence.
Monitor and document neurological status frequently and compare with baseline. (Refer to CP: Craniocerebral Trauma—Acute Rehabilitative Phase, ND: ineffective cerebral Tissue Perfusion for complete neurological evaluation.)	Assesses trends in LOC and potential for increased ICP and is useful in determining location, extent, and progression or resolution of CNS damage. May also reveal TIA, which may resolve with no further symptoms or may precede thrombotic CVA.
Monitor vital signs noting:	
Hypertension or hypotension; compare blood pressure (BP) readings in both arms.	Fluctuations in pressure may occur because of cerebral pressure or injury in vasomotor area of the brain. Hypertension or hypotension may have been a precipitating factor. Hypotension may follow stroke because of circulatory collapse. *Note:* Current recommendations for treating hypertension include avoiding more than 10% reduction in blood pressure during first 24 hours after stroke event (Liebeskind, 2011).
Heart rate and rhythm; auscultate for murmurs.	Changes in rate, especially bradycardia, can occur because of the brain damage. Dysrhythmias and murmurs may reflect cardiac disease, which may have precipitated CVA, for example, stroke after MI or from valve dysfunction.
Respirations, noting patterns and rhythm—periods of apnea after hyperventilation, Cheyne-Stokes respiration	Irregularities can suggest location of cerebral insult or increased ICP and need for further intervention, including possible respiratory support. (Refer to CP: Craniocerebral Trauma—Acute Rehabilitative Phase, ND: risk for ineffective Breathing Pattern.)
Evaluate pupils, noting size, shape, equality, and light reactivity.	Pupil reactions are regulated by the oculomotor (III) cranial nerve and are useful in determining whether the brainstem is intact. Pupil size and equality is determined by balance between parasympathetic and sympathetic enervation. Response to light reflects combined function of the optic (II) and oculomotor (III) cranial nerves.
Document changes in vision, such as reports of blurred vision and alterations in visual field or depth perception.	Specific visual alterations reflect area of brain involved, indicate safety concerns, and influence choice of interventions.
Assess higher functions, including speech, if client is alert. (Refer to ND: impaired verbal [and/or written] Communication.)	Changes in cognition and speech content are an indicator of location and degree of cerebral involvement and may indicate increased ICP.
Assess for nuchal rigidity, twitching, increased restlessness, irritability, and onset of seizure activity.	Indicative of meningeal irritation, especially in hemorrhagic disorders. Seizures may reflect increased ICP or reflect location and severity of cerebral injury, requiring further evaluation and intervention.
Position with head slightly elevated and in neutral position.	Reduces arterial pressure by promoting venous drainage and may improve cerebral circulation and perfusion.
Maintain bedrest, provide quiet environment, and restrict visitors or activities, as indicated. Provide rest periods between care activities, limiting duration of procedures.	Continual stimulation can increase ICP. Absolute rest and quiet may be needed to prevent recurrence of bleeding, in the case of hemorrhagic stroke.
Prevent straining at stool or holding breath.	Valsalva's maneuver increases ICP and potentiates risk of bleeding.
Collaborative	
Administer supplemental oxygen, as indicated.	Reduces hypoxemia.
Administer medications, as indicated, for example:	
Intravenous thrombolytics, such as tissue plasminogen activator (tPA), alteplase (Activase), and recombinant prourokinase (Prourokinase)	As the only proven therapy for early acute ischemic stroke, tPA is useful in minimizing the size of the infarcted area by opening blocked vessels that are occluded with clot. Treatment must be started within 3 hours of initial symptoms to improve outcomes. tPA remains the only treatment shown in numerous studies to reduce disability 3 months after

(continues on page 220)

ACTIONS/INTERVENTIONS (continued)	RATIONALE (continued)
	stroke with no increase in the risk of death and a relatively minor rate of symptomatic intracerebral hemorrhage complications (Brethour, 2012). *Note:* These agents are contraindicated in several instances—intracranial hemorrhage as diagnosed by CT scan, recent intracranial surgery, serious head trauma, and uncontrolled hypertension.
Anticoagulants, such as warfarin sodium (Coumadin); low-molecular-weight heparin, for example, enoxaparin (Lovenox) and dalteparin (Fragmin); and direct thrombin inhibitor, such as ximelagatran (Exanta)	May be used to improve cerebral blood flow and prevent further clotting in ischemic stroke (such as when embolus arises from atrial fibrillation, or there is a large cerebral sinus thrombus). *Note:* Anticoagulant therapy carries with it the risk for causing intracranial hemorrhage.
Antiplatelet agents, such as aspirin (ASA), aspirin with extended-release dipyridamole (Aggrenox), ticlopidine (Ticlid), and clopidogrel (Plavix)	Antiplatelet agents may be used following an ischemic stroke or TIA, or to prevent stroke associated with cardiac events, or blood dyscrasias such as sickle cell anemia.
Antihypertensives, such as beta blockers (e.g., labetalol [Trandate]) and angiotensin-converting enzyme inhibitors (ACEIs) (e.g., enalapril [Vasotec]). Nicardipine (Cardene), nitroprusside (Nitopress), and hydralazine (Apressoline) (may be used for more refractory hypertension)	Transient hypertension often occurs during acute stroke and usually resolves without therapeutic intervention. Preexisting or chronic hypertension requires cautious treatment because aggressive management increases the risk of extension of tissue damage during an evolving stroke.
Anticonvulsants: e.g., lorazapem (Ativan), diazepam (Valium), Phenytoin (Dilantin), and phenobarbital	May be used to control seizures and for sedative action. *Note:* Early seizure activity occurs in 4% to 28% of clients with intracerebral hemorrhage, and may be of the nonconvulsive kind (Liebeskind, 2011).
Prepare for surgery, as appropriate—carotid endarterectomy, microvascular bypass, clot evacuation, endovascular treatment of aneurysm or cerebral angioplasty.	May be necessary to resolve current situation, to reduce neurological symptoms or risk of recurrent stroke.
Monitor laboratory studies as indicated, such as prothrombin time (PT), activated partial thromboplastin time (aPTT).	Provides information about effectiveness and therapeutic level of anticoagulants when used.

NURSING DIAGNOSIS: impaired physical Mobility

May Be Related To

Neuromuscular impairment; decreased muscle strength/control; decreased endurance
Sensoriperceptual or cognitive impairment

Possibly Evidenced By

Uncoordinated movements, limited range of motion (ROM)
Postural instability, gait changes

Desired Outcomes/Evaluation Criteria—Client Will

Immobility Consequences: Physiologic (NOC)

Maintain or increase strength and function of affected or compensatory body part.
Maintain optimal position of function as evidenced by absence of contractures and footdrop.
Demonstrate techniques and behaviors that enable resumption of activities.
Maintain skin integrity.

ACTIONS/INTERVENTIONS	RATIONALE
Positioning (NIC)	
Independent	
Assess functional ability and extent of impairment initially and on a regular basis. Classify according to a 0 to 4 scale. (Refer to CP: Craniocerebral Trauma—Acute Rehabilitative Phase, ND: impaired physical Mobility.)	Identifies strengths and deficiencies and may provide information regarding recovery. Assists in choice of interventions because different techniques are used for flaccid and spastic types of paralysis.
Change positions at least every 2 hours (supine, side lying) and possibly more often if placed on affected side.	Reduces risk of tissue ischemia and injury. Affected side has poorer circulation and reduced sensation and is more predisposed to skin breakdown and pressure ulcers.
Position in prone position once or twice a day if client can tolerate.	Helps maintain functional hip extension; however, may increase anxiety, especially about ability to breathe.
Prop extremities in functional position; use footboard during the period of flaccid paralysis. Maintain neutral position of head.	Prevents contractures and footdrop and facilitates use when or if function returns. Flaccid paralysis may interfere with ability to support head, whereas spastic paralysis may lead to deviation of head to one side.
Use arm sling when client is in upright position, as indicated.	During flaccid paralysis, use of sling may reduce risk of shoulder subluxation and shoulder-hand syndrome.

ACTIONS/INTERVENTIONS (continued)	RATIONALE (continued)
Evaluate use of and need for positional aids and splints during spastic paralysis:	Flexion contractures occur because flexor muscles are stronger than extensors.
Place pillow under axilla to abduct arm.	Prevents adduction of shoulder and flexion of elbow.
Elevate arm and hand.	Promotes venous return and helps prevent edema formation.
Place hard hand-rolls in the palm with fingers and thumb opposed.	Hard cones decrease the stimulation of finger flexion, maintaining finger and thumb in a functional position.
Place knee and hip in extended position.	Maintains functional position.
Maintain leg in neutral position with a trochanter roll.	Prevents external hip rotation.
Discontinue use of footboard, when appropriate.	Continued use after change from flaccid to spastic paralysis can cause excessive pressure on the ball of the foot, enhance spasticity, and actually increase plantar flexion.
Observe affected side for color, edema, or other signs of compromised circulation.	Edematous tissue is more easily traumatized and heals more slowly.
Inspect skin regularly, particularly over bony prominences. Gently massage any reddened areas and provide aids such as sheepskin pads, as necessary.	Pressure points over bony prominences are most at risk for decreased perfusion and ischemia. Circulatory stimulation and padding help prevent skin breakdown and decubitus ulcer development.
Exercise Therapy: Muscle Control (NIC)	
Begin active or passive ROM to all extremities (including splinted) on admission. Encourage exercises, such as quadriceps or gluteal exercise, squeezing rubber ball, and extension of fingers and legs and feet.	Minimizes muscle atrophy, promotes circulation, and helps prevent contractures. Reduces risk of hypercalciuria and osteoporosis if underlying problem is hemorrhage. *Note:* Excessive and imprudent stimulation can predispose to recurrence of bleeding.
Assist client to develop sitting balance (such as raise head of bed; assist to sit on edge of bed, having client use the strong arm to support body weight and strong leg to move affected leg; increase sitting time) and standing balance—put flat walking shoes on client, support client's lower back with hands while positioning own knees outside client's knees, and assist in using parallel bars and walker.	Aids in retraining neuronal pathways, enhancing proprioception and motor response.
Get client up in chair as soon as vital signs are stable.	Helps stabilize BP, restoring vasomotor tone, and promotes maintenance of extremities in a functional position and emptying of bladder and kidneys, reducing risk of urinary stones and infections from stasis.
Pad chair seat with foam, gel, or water-filled cushion, and assist client to shift weight at frequent intervals.	Reduces pressure on the coccyx and prevents skin breakdown.
Set goals with client/significant other (SO) for increasing participation in activities, exercise, and position changes.	Promotes sense of expectation of progress and improvement, and provides some sense of control and independence.
Encourage client to assist with movement and exercises using unaffected extremity to support and move weaker side.	May respond as if affected side is no longer part of body and need encouragement and active training to "reincorporate" it as a part of own body. (Refer to ND: Unilateral Neglect.)
Positioning (NIC) *Collaborative*	
Provide egg-crate mattress, water bed, flotation device, or specialized bed, such as kinetic, as indicated.	Promotes even weight distribution, decreasing pressure on bony points and helping to prevent skin breakdown and pressure ulcer formation. Specialized beds help with positioning, enhance circulation, and reduce venous stasis to decrease risk of tissue injury and complications such as orthostatic pneumonia.
Exercise Therapy: Muscle Control (NIC)	
Consult with physical therapist regarding active, resistive exercises and client ambulation.	Individualized program can be developed to meet particular needs and deal with deficits in balance, coordination, and strength.
Assist with electrical stimulation—transcutaneous electrical nerve stimulator (TENS) unit, as indicated.	May assist with muscle strengthening and increase voluntary muscle control, as well as pain control.
Administer muscle relaxants and antispasmodics as indicated, such as baclofen (Lioresal) and dantrolene (Dantrium).	May be required to relieve spasticity in affected extremities.

NURSING DIAGNOSIS: impaired verbal [and/or written] Communication

May Be Related To

Decreased circulation to brain, alteration of central nervous system (CNS)
Weakened musculoskeletal system

Possibly Evidenced By

Does not or cannot speak, verbalizes with difficulty
Difficulty forming words or sentences; difficulty expressing thoughts verbally—aphasia
Inability to use facial expressions
Difficulty in comprehending or maintaining usual communication pattern [oral or written]

Desired Outcomes/Evaluation Criteria—Client Will

Communication (NOC)

Indicate understanding of the communication problems.
Establish method of communication in which needs can be expressed.
Use resources appropriately.

ACTIONS/INTERVENTIONS	RATIONALE
Communication Enhancement: Speech Deficit (NIC)	
Independent	
Assess type and degree of dysfunction, such as receptive aphasia—client does not seem to understand words, or expressive aphasia—client has trouble speaking or making self understood:	Helps determine area and degree of brain involvement and difficulty client has with any or all steps of the communication process. Client may have trouble understanding spoken words (damage to Wernicke's speech area), speaking words correctly (damage to Broca's speech areas), or may experience damage to both areas.
Differentiate aphasia from dysarthria.	Choice of interventions depends on type of impairment. Aphasia is a defect in using and interpreting symbols of language and may involve sensory and/or motor components, such as inability to comprehend written or spoken words or to write, make signs, and speak. A dysarthric person can understand, read, and write language, but has difficulty forming or pronouncing words because of weakness and paralysis of oral musculature, resulting in softly spoken speech.
Listen for errors in conversation and provide feedback.	Client may lose ability to monitor verbal output and be unaware that communication is not sensible. Feedback helps client realize why caregivers are not understanding and responding appropriately and provides opportunity to clarify content and meaning.
Ask client to follow simple commands, such as "Shut your eyes," "Point to the door"; repeat simple words or sentences.	Tests for receptive aphasia.
Point to objects and ask client to name them.	Tests for expressive aphasia—client may recognize item but not be able to name it.
Have client produce simple sounds, such as "sh," "cat."	Identifies dysarthria because motor components of speech (tongue, lip movement, breath control) can affect articulation and may or may not be accompanied by expressive aphasia.
Ask client to write name and/or a short sentence. If unable to write, have client read a short sentence.	Tests for writing disability (agraphia) and deficits in reading comprehension (alexia), which are also part of receptive and expressive aphasia.
Post notice at nurses' station and client's room about speech impairment. Provide special call bell if necessary.	Allays anxiety related to inability to communicate and fear that needs will not be met promptly. Call bell that is activated by minimal pressure is useful when client is unable to use regular call system.
Provide alternative methods of communication, such as writing or felt board and pictures. Provide visual clues—gestures, pictures—"needs" list, and demonstration.	Provides for communication of needs or desires based on individual situation or underlying deficit.
Anticipate and provide for client's needs.	Helpful in decreasing frustration when dependent on others and unable to communicate desires.
Talk directly to client, speaking slowly and distinctly. Use yes/no questions to start, progressing in complexity as client responds.	Reduces confusion and anxiety at having to process and respond to large amount of information at one time. As retraining progresses, advancing complexity of communication stimulates memory and further enhances word and idea association.

ACTIONS/INTERVENTIONS (continued)	RATIONALE (continued)
Speak with normal volume and avoid talking too fast. Give client ample time to respond. Talk without pressing for a response.	Client is not necessarily hearing impaired and raising voice may irritate or anger client. Forcing responses can result in frustration and may cause client to resort to "automatic" speech, such as garbled speech and obscenities.
Encourage SO and visitors to persist in efforts to communicate with client, such as reading mail and discussing family happenings even if client is unable to respond appropriately.	It is important for family members to continue talking to client to reduce client's isolation, promote establishment of effective communication, and maintain sense of connectedness with family.
Discuss familiar topics—job, family, hobbies, and current events.	Promotes meaningful conversation and provides opportunity to practice skills.
Respect client's preinjury capabilities; avoid speaking down to client or making patronizing remarks.	Enables client to feel esteemed because intellectual abilities often remain intact.
Collaborative	
Consult with or refer to speech therapist.	Assesses individual verbal capabilities and sensory, motor, and cognitive functioning to identify deficits and therapy needs.

NURSING DIAGNOSIS: [disturbed Sensory Perception (specify)]

May Be Related To

Altered sensory reception, transmission, integration—neurological trauma or deficit
Psychological stress

Possibly Evidenced By

Disorientation; poor concentration; impaired communication
Change in behavior pattern or usual response to stimuli
Reported or measured change in sensory acuity; sensory distortions
Inability to tell position of body parts (proprioception)

Desired Outcomes/Evaluation Criteria—Client Will

Cognition (NOC)

Regain and maintain usual LOC and perceptual functioning.

Knowledge: Stroke Management (NOC)

Acknowledge changes in ability and presence of residual involvement.
Demonstrate behaviors to compensate for or overcome deficits.

ACTIONS/INTERVENTIONS	RATIONALE
Environmental Management (NIC)	
Independent	
Review pathology of individual condition.	Awareness of type and area of involvement aids in assessing for and anticipating specific deficits and planning care.
Observe behavioral responses such as hostility, crying, inappropriate affect, agitation, and hallucination by using Los Ranchos (or similar) stroke scale, as appropriate.	Individual responses are variable, but commonalities, such as emotional lability, lowered frustration threshold, apathy, and impulsiveness, may complicate care. Use of a stroke scale aids in documenting progress during initial weeks following insult.
Eliminate extraneous noise and stimuli as necessary. Speak in calm, quiet voice, using short sentences. Maintain eye contact.	Reduces anxiety and exaggerated emotional responses and confusion associated with sensory overload.
Ascertain and validate client's perceptions. Reorient client frequently to environment, staff, and procedures.	Client may have limited attention span or problems with comprehension. These measures can help client attend to communication.
Evaluate for visual deficits. Note loss of visual field, changes in depth perception (horizontal or vertical planes), and presence of diplopia.	Assists client to identify inconsistencies in reception and integration of stimuli and may reduce perceptual distortion of reality.
Approach client from visually intact side.	Presence of visual disorders can negatively affect client's ability to perceive environment and relearn motor skills and increases risk of accident and injury.
Leave light on; position objects to take advantage of intact visual fields. Patch affected eye or encourage wearing of prism glasses if indicated.	Provides for recognition of the presence of persons or objects; may help with depth perception problems; and prevents client from being startled. Patching may decrease the sensory confusion of double vision, and prism glasses may enhance vision across midline, decreasing neglect of affected side. (Refer to ND: Unilateral Neglect.)

(continues on page 224)

ACTIONS/INTERVENTIONS (continued)	RATIONALE (continued)
Peripheral Sensation Management (NIC)	
Assess sensory awareness, such as differentiation of hot and cold, dull or sharp, position of body parts, and muscle and joint sense.	Diminished sensory awareness and impairment of kinesthetic sense negatively affects balance and positioning (proprioception) and appropriateness of movement, which interferes with ambulation, increasing risk of trauma.
Stimulate sense of touch—give client objects to touch and grasp. Have client practice touching walls or other boundaries.	Aids in retraining sensory pathways to integrate reception and interpretation of stimuli. Helps client orient self spatially and strengthens use of affected side.
Protect from temperature extremes; assess environment for hazards. Recommend testing warm water with unaffected hand.	Promotes client safety, reducing risk of injury.
Note inattention to body parts and segments of environment and lack of recognition of familiar objects or persons.	Presence of agnosia (loss of comprehension of auditory, visual, or other sensations, although sensory sphere is intact) may result in inability to recognize environmental cues, and considerable self-care deficits.

NURSING DIAGNOSIS: Self-Care Deficit (specify)

May Be Related To

Neuromuscular impairment, weakness, impaired mobility status
Perceptual or cognitive impairment
Pain, discomfort

Possibly Evidenced By

Impaired ability to perform ADLs, such as inability to bring food from receptacle to mouth; inability to wash body part(s) or regulate temperature of water; impaired ability to put on and take off clothing; difficulty completing toileting tasks

Desired Outcomes/Evaluation Criteria—Client Will

Self-Care: Status (NOC)

Demonstrate techniques and lifestyle changes to meet self-care needs.
Perform self-care activities within level of own ability.
Identify personal and community resources that can provide assistance as needed.

ACTIONS/INTERVENTIONS	RATIONALE
Self-Care Assistance (NIC)	
Independent	
Assess abilities and level of deficit (0 to 4 scale) for performing ADLs.	Aids in anticipating and planning for meeting individual needs.
Avoid doing things for client that client can do for self, providing assistance as necessary.	These clients may become fearful and dependent, and although assistance is helpful in preventing frustration, it is important for client to do as much as possible for self to maintain self-esteem and promote recovery.
Be aware of impulsive behavior or actions suggestive of impaired judgment.	May indicate need for additional interventions and supervision to promote client safety.
Maintain a supportive, firm attitude. Allow client sufficient time to accomplish tasks.	Clients need empathy and to know caregivers will be consistent in their assistance.
Provide positive feedback for efforts and accomplishments.	Enhances sense of self-worth, promotes independence, and encourages client to continue endeavors.
Create plan for visual deficits that are present, such as the following:	
Place food and utensils on the tray related to client's unaffected side.	Client will be able to see to eat the food.
Situate the bed so that client's unaffected side is facing the room with the affected side to the wall.	Will be able to see when getting in or out of bed and observe anyone who comes into the room.
Position furniture against wall, out of travel path.	Provides for safety when client is able to move around the room, reducing risk of tripping and falling over furniture.
Provide self-help devices, such as button or zipper hook, knife-fork combinations, long-handled brushes, extensions for picking things up from floor, toilet riser, leg bag for catheter, and shower chair. Assist and encourage good grooming and makeup habits.	Enables client to manage for self, enhancing independence and self-esteem; reduces reliance on others for meeting own needs; and enables client to be more socially active.
Encourage SO to allow client to do as much as possible for self.	Reestablishes sense of independence and fosters self-worth and enhances rehabilitation process. *Note:* This may be

ACTIONS/INTERVENTIONS	RATIONALE
	very difficult and frustrating for the SO/caregiver, depending on degree of disability and time required for client to complete activity.
Assess client's ability to communicate the need to void and ability to use urinal or bedpan. Take client to the bathroom at frequent and scheduled intervals for voiding if appropriate.	Client may have neurogenic bladder, be inattentive, or be unable to communicate needs in acute recovery phase, but usually is able to regain independent control of this function as recovery progresses.
Identify previous bowel habits and reestablish normal regimen. Increase bulk in diet. Encourage fluid intake and increased activity.	Assists in development of retraining program (independence) and aids in preventing constipation and impaction (long-term effects).
Collaborative	
Administer suppositories and stool softeners.	May be necessary to aid in establishing regular bowel function.
Consult with rehabilitation team, such as physical or occupational therapist.	Provides assistance in developing a comprehensive therapy program and identifying special equipment needs that can increase client's participation in self-care.

NURSING DIAGNOSIS: ineffective Coping

May Be Related To
Situational crises, inadequate level of perception of control
Inadequate level of confidence in ability to cope

Possibly Evidenced By
Reports inability to cope or ask for help
Poor concentration; inadequate problem-solving
Inability to meet basic needs or role expectations
Change in usual communication patterns

Desired Outcomes/Evaluation Criteria—Client Will

Coping (NOC)
Verbalize acceptance of self in situation.
Talk or communicate with SO about situation and changes that have occurred.
Verbalize awareness of own coping abilities.
Meet psychological needs as evidenced by appropriate expression of feelings, identification of options, and use of resources.

ACTIONS/INTERVENTIONS	RATIONALE
Coping Enhancement (NIC)	
Independent	
Assess extent of altered perception and related degree of disability. Use measurement scale (e.g., Functional Independence Measure [FIM] score), if appropriate (Hamilton, 1987).	Determination of individual factors aids in developing plan of care, choice of interventions, and discharge expectations.
Identify meaning of the loss and dysfunction or change to client. Note ability to understand events and provide realistic appraisal of situation.	Independence is highly valued in American society, but is not as significant in some other cultures. Some clients accept and manage altered function effectively with little adjustment, whereas others have considerable difficulty recognizing and adjusting to deficits. In order to provide meaningful support and appropriate problem-solving, healthcare providers need to understand the meaning of the stroke and limitations to the client.
Determine outside stressors, including family, work, social, and future nursing and healthcare needs.	Helps identify specific needs, provides opportunity to offer information and support and begin problem-solving. Consideration of social factors, in addition to functional status, is important in determining appropriate discharge destination.
Encourage client to express feelings, including hostility or anger, denial, depression, and sense of disconnectedness.	Demonstrates acceptance of and assists client in recognizing and beginning to deal with these feelings.
Note whether client refers to affected side as "it" or denies affected side and says it is "dead."	Suggests rejection of body part or negative feelings about body image and abilities, indicating need for intervention and emotional support.
Acknowledge statement of feelings about betrayal of body; remain matter-of-fact about reality that client can still use unaffected side and learn to control affected side. Use words	Helps client see that the nurse accepts both sides as part of the whole individual. Allows client to feel hopeful and begin to accept current situation.

(continues on page 226)

such as weak, affected, and right-left, that incorporate that side as part of the whole body.

Identify previous methods of dealing with life problems. Determine presence and quality of support systems. — Provides opportunity to use behaviors previously effective, build on past successes, and mobilize resources.

Emphasize and provide positive I-messages for small gains either in recovery of function or independence. — Consolidates gains, helps reduce feelings of anger and helplessness, and conveys sense of progress.

Support behaviors or efforts such as increased interest and participation in rehabilitation activities. — Suggests possible adaptation to changes and understanding about own role in future lifestyle.

Monitor for sleep disturbance, increased difficulty concentrating, statements of inability to cope, lethargy, and withdrawal. — May indicate onset of depression (common aftereffect of stroke), which may require further evaluation and intervention.

Collaborative

Refer for neuropsychological evaluation and counseling, if indicated. — May facilitate adaptation to role changes that are necessary for a sense of feeling and being a productive person. *Note:* Depression is common in stroke survivors and may be a direct result of the brain damage or an emotional reaction to sudden-onset disability.

NURSING DIAGNOSIS: risk for impaired Swallowing

Risk Factors May Include

Neuromuscular impairment—decreased gag reflex, facial paralysis, perceptual impairment

Cranial nerve involvement

Possibly Evidenced By

(Not applicable; presence of signs and symptoms establishes an *actual* diagnosis)

Desired Outcomes/Evaluation Criteria—Client Will

Swallowing Status (NOC)

Demonstrate feeding methods appropriate to individual situation, with aspiration prevented.

Maintain desired body weight.

ACTIONS/INTERVENTIONS — RATIONALE

Swallowing Therapy (NIC)

Independent

Review individual pathology and ability to swallow, noting extent of paralysis, clarity of speech, facial and tongue involvement, ability to protect airway and episodes of coughing or choking; presence of adventitious breath sounds and amount and character of oral secretions. Weigh periodically, as indicated. — Nutritional interventions, including choice of feeding route, are determined by these factors.

Have suction equipment available at bedside, especially during early feeding efforts. — Timely intervention may limit amount and untoward effect of aspiration.

Promote effective swallowing using methods such as the following:

- Schedule activities and medications to provide a minimum of 30 minutes of rest before eating. — Promotes optimal muscle function and helps to limit fatigue.
- Provide pleasant environment free of distractions, such as TV. — Promotes relaxation and allows client to focus on task of eating and swallowing.
- Assist client with head control or support, and position based on specific dysfunction. — Counteracts hyperextension, aiding in prevention of aspiration and enhancing ability to swallow. Optimal positioning can facilitate intake and reduce risk of aspiration—head back for decreased posterior propulsion of tongue, head turned to weak side for unilateral pharyngeal paralysis, and lying down on either side for reduced pharyngeal contraction.
- Place client in upright position during and after feeding, as appropriate. — Uses gravity to facilitate swallowing and reduces risk of aspiration.
- Provide oral care based on individual need prior to meal. — Clients with dry mouth require a moisturizing agent, such as artificial saliva or alcohol-free mouthwash, before and after eating; clients with excess saliva will benefit from use of a drying agent, such as lemon or glycerin swabs, before meal and a moisturizing agent afterward.
- Season food with herbs, spices, and lemon juice according to client's preference, within dietary restrictions. — Increases salivation, improving bolus formation and swallowing effort.

ACTIONS/INTERVENTIONS (continued)	RATIONALE (continued)
Serve foods at customary temperature and water always chilled.	Lukewarm temperatures are less likely to stimulate salivation, so foods and fluids should be served cold or warm as appropriate. *Note:* Water is the most difficult to swallow.
Stimulate lips to close or manually open mouth by light pressure on lips or under chin, if needed.	Aids in sensory retraining and promotes muscular control.
Place food of appropriate consistency in unaffected side of mouth.	Provides sensory stimulation (including taste), which may increase salivation and trigger swallowing efforts, enhancing intake. Food consistency is determined by individual deficit. *For example:* Clients with decreased range of tongue motion require thick liquids initially, progressing to thin liquids, whereas clients with delayed pharyngeal swallow will handle thick liquids and thicker foods better. *Note:* Pureed food is not recommended because client may not be able to recognize what is being eaten. Most milk products, peanut butter, syrup, and bananas are avoided because they produce mucus and are sticky.
Touch parts of the cheek with tongue blade or apply ice to weak tongue.	Can improve tongue movement and control necessary for swallowing and inhibits tongue protrusion.
Feed slowly, allowing 30 to 45 minutes for meals.	Feeling rushed can increase stress and level of frustration, may increase risk of aspiration, and may result in client's terminating meal early.
Offer solid foods and liquids at different times.	Prevents client from swallowing food before it is thoroughly chewed. In general, liquids should be offered only after client has finished eating solids.
Limit or avoid use of drinking straw for liquids.	Although use may strengthen facial and swallowing muscles, if client lacks tight lip closure to accommodate straw or if liquid is deposited too far back in mouth, risk of aspiration may be increased.
Encourage SO to bring favorite foods.	Provides familiar tastes and preferences. Stimulates feeding efforts and may enhance swallowing and intake.
Maintain upright position for 45 to 60 minutes after eating.	Helps client manage oral secretions and reduces risk of regurgitation.
Maintain accurate record of food and fluid intake; record calorie count if indicated.	If swallowing efforts are not sufficient to meet fluid and nutrition needs, alternative methods of feeding must be pursued.
Encourage participation in exercise or activity program.	May increase release of endorphins in the brain, promoting a sense of general well-being and increasing appetite.
Collaborative	
Review results of radiographic studies, such as video fluoroscopy.	Aids in determining phase of swallowing difficulties—oral preparatory, oral, pharyngeal, or esophageal phase.
Administer intravenous (IV) fluids, parenteral nutrition, or tube feedings.	May be necessary for fluid replacement and nutrition if client is unable to take anything orally.
Coordinate multidisciplinary approach to develop treatment plan that meets individual needs.	Inclusion of dietitian and speech and occupational therapists can increase effectiveness of long-term plan and significantly reduce risk of silent aspiration.

NURSING DIAGNOSIS: Unilateral Neglect

May Be Related To

Left hemiplegia from CVA of right hemisphere; hemianopsis

Possibly Evidenced By

Failure to move eyes, head, limbs, trunk in the neglected hemisphere despite being aware of a stimulus in that space
Appears unaware of positioning of neglected limb
Lack of safety precautions with regard to the neglected side
Failure to eat food from left side of plate and dress or groom neglected side
Failure to notice people approaching from neglected side

Desired Outcomes/Evaluation Criteria—Client Will

Heedfulness of Affected Side (NOC)

Acknowledge presence of impairment.
Incorporate affected body part(s) into self.

Client/Caregiver Will

Adaptation to Physical Disability (NOC)

Identify adaptive or protective measures for individual situation.
Demonstrate behaviors, lifestyle changes necessary to promote physical safety.

ACTIONS/INTERVENTIONS — RATIONALE

Unilateral Neglect Management (NIC)

Independent

Reinforce to client the reality of the dysfunction and need to compensate, avoiding participation in client's use of denial.
— Enhances dealing with reality of situation, thus avoiding scenarios (denial) that can limit progress and attainment of goals.

Instruct client and SO/caregiver in treatment strategies focused on training attention on the neglected side:
— Promotes involvement of all individuals in addressing problem, which may enhance recovery.

- Approach client from unaffected side. — Enhances client's awareness and promotes interaction.
- Encourage client to turn head and eyes to "scan" the environment. — Helps client compensate for visual field loss, increasing awareness of environment.
- Discuss affected side while touching, manipulating, and stroking affected side; provide items of varied size, weight, and texture for client to hold. — Focuses client's attention, and limb activation treatment provides tactile stimuli to promote use of affected limb in neglected hemisphere.
- Have client look at and handle affected side, bring across midline during care activities. — Encourages client to accept affected limb or side as part of self even though it does not feel like it belongs.
- Assist client to position affected extremity carefully and to routinely visualize placement or use a mirror to adjust placement. — Promotes safety awareness, reducing risk of injury.

Instruct SO/caregiver to monitor alignment of limbs and to inspect skin regularly.
— Decreased sensation and positional awareness may result in pressure injuries.

Discuss environmental safety concerns and assist in developing plan to correct risk factors.
— Client may continue to have some ongoing degree of functional impairment, including difficulty with navigating in familiar environments (Barrett & John, 2007).

Reinforce continuation of prescribed rehabilitation activities and neuropsychological therapies, as indicated.
— Maximizes recovery and enhances independence. *Note:* Research indicates that most clients with neglect show early recovery, particularly within the first month, and marked improvement within 3 months (Barrett & John, 2012).

NURSING DIAGNOSIS: deficient Knowledge [Learning Need] regarding condition, prognosis, treatment, self-care, and discharge needs

May Be Related To

Lack of exposure, unfamiliarity with information resources

Cognitive limitation, information misinterpretation, lack of recall

Possibly Evidenced By

Report of problem

Inaccurate follow-through of instructions

Desired Outcomes/Evaluation Criteria—Client/SO Will

Knowledge: Stroke Management (NOC)

Participate in learning process.

Verbalize understanding of condition, prognosis, and potential complications.

Verbalize understanding of therapeutic regimen and rationale for actions.

Initiate necessary lifestyle changes.

ACTIONS/INTERVENTIONS — RATIONALE

Teaching: Disease Process (NIC)

Independent

Evaluate type and degree of sensory-perceptual involvement.
— Deficits affect the choice of teaching methods and content and complexity of instruction.

Include SO and family in discussions and teaching.
— These individuals will be providing support and care and have great impact on client's quality of life.

Discuss specific pathology and individual potentials.
— Aids in establishing realistic expectations and promotes understanding of current situation and needs.

Identify signs and symptoms requiring further follow-up, such as changes or decline in visual, motor, sensory functions; alteration in mentation or behavioral responses; and severe headache.
— Prompt evaluation and intervention reduces risk of complications and further loss of function.

Review current restrictions or limitations and discuss planned or potential resumption of activities, including sexual relations.
— Promotes understanding, provides hope for future, and creates expectation of resumption of more "normal" life.

ACTIONS/INTERVENTIONS (continued)	RATIONALE (continued)
Review and reinforce current therapeutic regimen, including use of medications to control hypertension, hypercholesterolemia, and diabetes, as indicated, and use of aspirin or similar-acting drug, such as ticlopidine (Ticlid) and warfarin sodium (Coumadin). Identify ways of continuing program after discharge.	Recommended activities, limitations, and medication and therapy needs are established on the basis of a coordinated interdisciplinary approach. Follow-through is essential to progression of recovery and prevention of complications. *Note:* Long-term anticoagulation may be beneficial for clients prone to clot formation; however, these drugs are contraindicated for CVA resulting from hemorrhage.
Provide written instructions and schedules for activity, medication, and important facts.	Provides visual reinforcement and reference source after discharge.
Encourage client to refer to lists, written communications or notes, and memory book.	Provides aids to support memory and promotes improvement in cognitive skills.
Discuss plans for meeting self-care needs.	Varying levels of assistance may be required and need to be planned for based on individual situation.
Refer to discharge planner or home-care supervisor and visiting nurse.	Home environment may require evaluation and modifications to meet individual needs.
Identify community resources, such as National Stroke Association, American Heart Association's Stroke Connection, stroke support clubs, senior services, Meals on Wheels, adult day care or respite program, and visiting nurse.	Enhances coping abilities and promotes home management and adjustment to impairments for both stroke survivors and caregivers. *Note:* Recent innovations include such programs as Menu-Direct, which provides fully prepared meal programs with nutrition-rich foods. Some entrees have soufflé-like consistency to help trigger swallowing response.
Suggest client reduce or limit environmental stimuli, especially during cognitive activities.	Multiple or concomitant stimuli may aggravate confusion and impair mental abilities.
Recommend client seek assistance in problem-solving process and validate decisions as indicated.	Some clients, especially those with right CVA, may display impaired judgment and impulsive behavior, compromising ability to make sound decisions.
Identify individual risk factors—hypertension, cardiac dysrhythmias, obesity, smoking, heavy alcohol use, atherosclerosis, poor control of diabetes, and use of oral contraceptives—and discuss necessary lifestyle changes.	Promotes general well-being and may reduce risk of recurrence. *Note:* Obesity in women has been found to have a high correlation with ischemic stroke.
Review importance of a balanced diet, low in cholesterol and sodium, if indicated. Discuss role of vitamins and other supplements.	Improves general health and well-being and provides energy for life activities.
Refer to and reinforce importance of follow-up care by rehabilitation team, such as physical, occupational, speech, and vocational therapists.	Diligent work may eventually overcome or minimize residual deficits.

POTENTIAL CONSIDERATIONS following acute hospitalization (dependent on client's age, physical condition and presence of complications, personal resources, and life responsibilities)

- ***risk for Injury***—physical (general weakness, altered mobility, visual deficits)
- ***imbalanced Nutrition: less than body requirements***—inability to prepare or ingest food; lack of food
- ***Self-Care Deficit***—weakness; perceptual or cognitive impairment; impaired mobility status; pain/discomfort
- ***impaired Home Maintenance***—impaired functioning; inadequate support systems; insufficient finances; unfamiliarity with neighborhood resources
- ***situational low Self-Esteem***—functional impairment
- ***risk for Caregiver Role Strain***—illness severity of/cognitive problems in care receiver; discharge of family member with significant home-care needs; duration of caregiving required; complexity or amount of caregiving tasks, caregiver isolation

BRAIN INFECTIONS: MENINGITIS AND ENCEPHALITIS

Meningitis is an inflammation of the linings of the brain and spinal cord. Encephalitis is an inflammation of the brain.

I. Pathophysiology (Balentine, 2012)

a. Meningitis (indicated by "m" in tables in this section)

i. The brain is normally protected from bloodstream infections by the blood-brain barrier. However, once bacteria or other organisms get into the brain, they are somewhat isolated from the immune system. Replicating bacteria, toxins, and exudates can rapidly spread through the cerebral spinal fluid (CSF), damaging systems such as cranial nerves or obliterating CSF pathways, resulting in cerebral edema and increased intracranial pressure.

ii. The syndrome is most often acute, but may become chronic.

iii. Risk factors include (1) age: can occur at any age, but is more common under 5 years and over 60 years;

(continues on page 230)

(2) certain disorders (e.g., diabetes, renal or adrenal insufficiency; sickle cell disease, bacterial endocarditis); (3) weakened immune system or immunosuppression (increases risk of opportunistic infections and acute bacterial meningitis); (4) crowded living spaces (e.g., college dormitories, military barracks) increase risk for person-to-person contagion; (5) brain defects such as might occur with trauma or surgery; (6) travel to areas known for meningococcal disease (e.g., sub-Saharan Africa); (7) history of/current injected drug use.

b. **Encephalitis** (indicated by "e" in tables in this section)
   i. There are two types of encephalitis—primary and secondary forms. Primary encephalitis is directly due to a new viral infection. Secondary encephalitis, or postinfective encephalitis, arises as a consequence of an ongoing viral infection or from an immunization procedure that utilizes a virus. The latter uses a virus that has been altered to be incapable of causing harm. However, in rare cases, the vaccine itself becomes harmful.
   ii. Encephalitis is classified as either viral or bacterial, with viral being more common.
   iii. Encephalitis can be life-threatening and create lifelong neurological problems, such as learning disabilities, seizures, and memory or motor deficits.
   iv. West Nile encephalitis (NSE) is also a common form and poses the greatest risk to older adults and those with compromised immune systems.
   v. Other, rarer types of encephalitis include Equine, La Crosse, and St. Louis encephalitis (Matthews, 2007).

II. Etiology

a. Meningitis
   i. Causative agents are most commonly bacterial or viral and usually affect the meninges in the frontal portion of the brain. Less common causative agents (e.g., fungus or tubercular) may be concentrated at the base of the brain.
   ii. Common bacteria associated with acute meningitis include *Pneumococcus* and *Haemophilus influenza* (*H. influenzae*), possibly arising from sinus or ear infections or CSF leak following head trauma. *Streptococcus* (*S. pneumoniae*) is the most common bacterial cause and may arise from infections such as pneumonia or endocarditis or can be associated with many high-risk conditions such as hyposplenism, multiple myeloma, or chronic liver disease.
   iii. *Escherichia coli (E. coli)* is the most common agent in neonates, and *H. influenzae* primarily affects infants younger than 2 years of age.
   iv. Less common causative agents include parasites (e.g., *Acanthamoeba* species), and fungi (e.g., *Cryptococcus neoformans, Candida*).
   v. In persons with HIV, meningitis is multifactorial and includes several etiologic agents (e.g., cryptococcal, tubercular, syphilitic).
   vi. Most viral meningitis in America, especially in summer months, is caused by enteroviruses. Other viral causes of meningitis include mumps, herpes viruses (e.g., Epstein-Barr, herpes simplex, varicella-zoster, measles, and influenza).

b. Encephalitis
   i. In the United States, most encephalitis is caused by (1) enteroviruses (e.g., *Herpes simplex 1* and 2; *coxsackievirus, echovirus*, and *poliovirus*); (2) arboviruses (from tick or mosquito bites) and Lyme disease.
   ii. Encephalitis due to *Herpes simplex type 1* virus is most prevalent in people under 20 years of age and older than 40. The disease is contagious, being spread most often by inhalation of water droplets. Encephalitis due to *herpes simplex type 2* is typically spread through sexual contact or, less commonly, a newborn can contract the virus from infected mother during birth.
   iii. In the United States, the four types of mosquito-borne viral encephalitis are equine, lacrosse, St. Louis, and West Nile.
   iv. Other, less common viruses include mumps, HIV, varicella, rubella.
   v. In the United States and Canada, Powassan encephalitis is transmitted to humans by ticks, which have previously acquired the virus from infected deer.

III. Statistics

a. Morbidity
   i. The rate of bacterial meningitis (caused by *H. influenzae, S. pneumoniae,* and *N. meningitidis*) declined by 55% in the United States in the early 1990s when the *Haemophilus influenzae type b (Hib)* conjugate vaccine for infants was introduced. The advent of universal Hib vaccination in developed countries has led to the reduction of more than 99% of invasive disease in the pediatric population (Horn & Felter, 2012).
   ii. Up to 30% of children have neurological sequelae. This varies by organism, with *S. pneumoniae* having the highest rate of complications (Horn & Felter, 2012).
   iii. In Western countries, Herpes simplex virus (HSV) can cause life-threatening encephalitis, with a 50% to 75% mortality (Tyler, 2004; Lawes, 2007). Worldwide, encephalitis due to infections by the herpes simplex viruses causes only about 10% of all cases of the disease.
   iv. About 50% of those who contract Powassan encephalitis will have permanent brain damage.

b. Mortality
   i. While the incidence of bacterial infection has dropped, the case fatality rate has remained relatively stable. In 1998–1999, the fatality rate was 15.7% and was still 14.3% in 2006–2007. Of the 1670 cases reported from 2003 to 2007, *S. pneumoniae* was the predominant infective species (58.0%) (Thigpen, 2011).
   ii. Over half the cases of herpes simplex encephalitis result in death, and more than 15% of those who become infected with Powassan encephalitis die of the infection.

c. Cost: In 2006, costs for meningitis-related hospitalizations in the United States totaled $1.2 billion (Holmquist, 2008).

GLOSSARY

Arbovirus: Any of a large group of viruses that develop in arthropods (chiefly mosquitoes and ticks) and can be transmitted to humans.

Arthropod: A disease caused by one of a phylum of organisms characterized by exoskeletons and segmented bodies.

Encephalitis: Inflammation of the brain, which may be caused by a bacterium, a virus, or an allergic reaction.

Lumbar puncture (LP): A procedure in which cerebrospinal fluid (CSF) is removed from the spinal canal for diagnostic testing or treatment.

Meninges: The three membranes that cover the brain and spinal cord.

Meningitis: Inflammation of the meninges, which can be caused by infection by bacteria or viruses, cancer (metastasis to the meninges), inflammatory diseases, and drugs.

Vector: Any agent, living or otherwise, that carries and transmits diseases.

Viruses: Small living particles that can infect cells and change how the cells function. Infection with a virus can cause a person to develop symptoms. The disease and symptoms that are caused depend on the type of virus and the type of cells that are infected.

Care Setting

Depends on type of infection and severity of symptoms—for example, acute bacterial meningitis, especially meningococcal, is a medical emergency requiring prompt intervention/hospitalization.

Related Concerns

Seizures disorders, page 188
Total nutritional support, page 437

Client Assessment Database

DIAGNOSTIC DIVISION MAY REPORT	MAY EXHIBIT
ACTIVITY/REST	
• Fatigue	
FOOD/FLUID	
• Nausea, vomiting	• Poor feeding (infants [m]); loss of appetite • Nausea, vomiting
NEUROSENSORY	
• Stiff neck (adults and older children in meningitis [m])	• Confusion, altered mental status (mental status changes in encephalitis are usually more severe than in meningitis and range from confusion to delirium to coma). • Irritability (especially infants); poor responsiveness • Sleepiness, difficulty waking up (infants/children [e]) • Nuchal rigidity (m) • Unsteady gait; muscle weakness (e) • Paralysis (e) • Seizures ([e or m], when severe) • Memory loss (e) • Sudden severe dementia (e)
PAIN/DISCOMFORT	
• Headache (m and e)	
SAFETY	
• Fever (sudden onset) (m and e) • Skin rash (West Nile virus m or e) • Spread of infection (bacterial m) • Seizure precautions • Fall prevention	• Fever

(continues on page 232)

Client Assessment Database (continued)

DIAGNOSTIC DIVISION MAY REPORT (continued)	MAY EXHIBIT (continued)
TEACHING/LEARNING • Modes of transmission • Vector safety • Vaccines • Travel information	Vaccines are available for *Neisseria meningitidis* (meningococcus); *Streptococcus pneumoniae* (pneumococcus), *Haemophilus influenzae (H. influenzae)* type b also known as Hib. One recent vaccine (researched and released by the FDA) combines Hib and *Neisseria meningitidis serogroups Y* and *C* for infants and children.
DISCHARGE PLAN CONSIDERATIONS • Medication regimen and therapeutic treatments • Assistance with transportation, shopping, food preparation, self-care, and homemaker or maintenance tasks ➧ Refer to section at end of plan for postdischarge considerations.	

Diagnostic Studies

TEST WHY IT IS DONE	WHAT IT TELLS ME
• ***Lumbar puncture (LP):*** Spinal tap test performed to determine if CSF fluid is consistent with clinical diagnosis.	Primary diagnostic tool for encephalitis and meningitis. The initial tests that are often performed with suspected infections of the central nervous system include: • Protein: Increases in protein are commonly seen with meningitis. • Glucose: May decrease when cells that are not normally present metabolize the glucose. These may include bacteria or cells present due to inflammation (WBCs). • CSF total cell counts: WBCs may be increased with central nervous system infections. • CSF WBC differential: There may be an increase in neutrophils with a bacterial infection, an increase in lymphocytes with a viral infection. • Gram stain may be done for direct observation of microorganisms. • Culture and sensitivity may be done for bacteria, fungi, and viruses.
• ***Computed tomography (CT) scan:*** Uses low radiation x-rays to create a computer-generated, three-dimensional image of the brain.	May be done after CSF evaluation in some populations (e.g., new onset seizures, signs suspicious for space-occupying lesions such as papilledema; prolonged fever; evidence of increased intracranial pressure [ICP]). CT is much less sensitive than MRI for HSV encephalitis but can help because it is rapidly available and can exclude disorders that make lumbar puncture risky.
• ***Magnetic resonance imaging (MRI):*** Uses magnetic fields and computer technology to generate images of the internal anatomy of the brain.	Sensitive for early HSV encephalitis, showing edema in the orbitofrontal and temporal areas, which HSV typically infects. May show basal ganglia and thalamic abnormalities in West Nile and eastern equine encephalitis. MRI can also exclude lesions that mimic viral encephalitis (e.g., brain abscess, sagittal sinus thrombosis).
ANCILLARY TESTS • ***Blood cultures***	• Determines presence of blood-borne infection and agent responsible. Gram stain may be positive or negative. • Cultures may be positive with *H. influenzae, S. pneumoniae, or N. menigitidis,* especially when those agents are also present in nasopharyx, respiratory secretions, skin lesions. • Viral cultures may be done to isolate type and appropriate treating agent.

Nursing Priorities

1. Maximize cerebral perfusion and neurological function.
2. Prevent or minimize complications.
3. Promote optimal functioning.
4. Minimize discomfort.
5. Provide information about condition, prognosis, potential complications, treatment plan, and resources.

Discharge Goals

1. Cerebral and neurological function normal or resolving.
2. Complications prevented or minimized.
3. Activities of daily living (ADLs) met by self or with assistance of others.
4. Condition, prognosis, complications, and treatment regimen understood and available resources identified.

NURSING DIAGNOSIS: risk for Infection [spread]

Risk Factors May Include

Hematogenous dissemination of pathogen, stasis of body fluids, suppressed immune response; exposure of others to pathogens

Possibly Evidenced By

(Not applicable; presence of signs and symptoms establishes an *actual* diagnosis)

Desired Outcomes/Evaluation Criteria—Client Will

Infection Severity (NOC)

Be afebrile, free of malaise/lethargy, and demonstrate negative cultures as appropriate.

Risk Control: Infectious Process (NOC)

Verbalize understanding of individual risk factors.

ACTIONS/INTERVENTIONS	RATIONALE
Infection Control (NIC)	
Independent	
Note client's age.	In infections of the brain and meninges, certain age groups are more susceptible to certain types, e.g., *E. coli* infection is more common in infants, while bacterial meningitis can be more common in college-age students living in a dorm.
Note presence or new onset of fever, chills, diaphoresis, altered level of consciousness.	Systemic infection may already be present when brain infection is diagnosed, requiring immediate and intensive medical treatment, especially in the setting of altered consciousness.
Assess for host-specific factors that affect immunity (e.g., presence of underlying disease process; presence or absence of healthy immune functioning).	Persons with systemic infections are at risk for infection of the brain, although some protection is afforded by the blood-brain barrier. Persons with suppressed immune systems (e.g., HIV, liver diseases) are also at risk for opportunistic infections of the brain.
Implement isolation as indicated:	
Emphasize and model proper hand hygiene techniques, using antibacterial soap and running water.	These first-line defenses are for the client, healthcare providers, and the public.
Use gloves as indicated.	
Provide clean, well-ventilated environment.	
Provide for respiratory isolation as indicated.	Respiratory isolation (e.g., wearing of mask) may be implemented and continued for 24 hours after antibiotics are started.
Use proper protective equipment as dictated by agency policy for particular exposure risk.	
Post visual alerts instructing clients/SO/visitors to inform healthcare providers of respiratory infections or influenza-like symptoms.	
Assist with and encourage regular position changes, early ambulation; deep breathing and coughing exercises, especially after removal from ventilator.	Reduces risk of aspiration and respiratory infection, or helps promote recovery, if respiratory infection is already present (possible source of brain/meninges infections).
Maintain sterile precautions for invasive procedures (e.g., IV insertion and routine care; urinary catheter, tracheostomy, pulmonary suctioning, etc.). Provide site care and promote early removal of devices.	Reduces risk of cross-contamination and device-related infections.
Collaborative	
Assist with and review diagnostic studies, including blood studies and other diagnostic procedures.	Meningitis and encephalitis are most often diagnosed by a combination of interventions, i.e., clinical evaluation, blood work, lumbar puncture, and possibly imaging studies. A series of

(continues on page 234)

ACTIONS/INTERVENTIONS (continued)	RATIONALE (continued)
	tests performed sequentially may be needed to confirm certain pathology.
Administer appropriate antimicrobials:	Most medications are administered IV, initially, and may continue for a lengthy period of time.
antibiotics (such as penicillin [Penicillin G], cefotaxime [Claforan], vancoymicin [Vancomycin])	Bacterial infections are frequently treated with a broad-spectrum antibiotic as soon as, or even before, the cause is positively identified. This therapy may then need to be modified once culture results identify the specific bacteria and its susceptibility to antimicrobial agents. Antibiotics chosen must be able to pass through the blood-brain barrier and reach sufficient concentration in the CSF.
antivirals (e.g., acyclovir [Zovorax] or ganciclovir [Cytovene])	For viral encephalitis or meningitis due to herpes or varicella-zoster viruses, an antiviral drug such as acyclovir may be prescribed. For infections due to HIV, highly active antiretroviral therapy may be required.
antifungals, such as fluconazole (Diflucan), ketoconazole (Nizoral), and miconazole (Monista)	Other antimicrobials (e.g., for fungus or parasites) are determined by the causative agent.
Administer balanced nutrition, including vitamins and trace minerals, using appropriate feeding route (e.g., oral, tube feeding, TPN).	The body is in a hypermetabolic state when severe infection is present. Balanced nutrients are needed to prevent a catabolic state, and to promote healing.

NURSING DIAGNOSIS: risk for decreased Intracranial Adaptive Capacity

Risk Factors May Include

Systemic hypotension with intracranial hypertension; brain infection

Possibly Evidenced By

(Not applicable; presence of signs and symptoms establishes an *actual* diagnosis)

Desired Outcomes/Evaluation Criteria—Client Will

Tissue Perfusion: Cerebral (NOC)

Display blood pressure, neurological signs within client's normal range.

ACTIONS/INTERVENTIONS	RATIONALE
Neurological Monitoring (NIC)	
Independent	
Ascertain presence of acute neurological condition, such as toxic bacterial or viral sepsis and potential for increased intracranial pressure (ICP).	These conditions alter the relationship between intracranial volume and pressure, potentially increasing ICP and decreasing cerebral perfusion.
Investigate changes in neurological status, noting changes in client symptom reports and/or deterioration in neurological findings.	If client is awake and able to report symptoms, attention must be given to reports of worsening headache, particularly when accompanied by loss of coordination, confusion, visual disturbances, difficulty understanding or using language. Client may not be able to report symptoms but may display a range of progressive neurological deficits.
Monitor vital signs:	
Blood pressure	Hypotension may be present because of severe infection (sepsis), dehydration, or effects of circulating toxins. Low blood pressure or severe hypotension causes inadequate perfusion of brain, with adverse changes in consciousness/mentation.
Temperature	Fever is often present, associated with inflammation or systemic infection, and detrimental to cerebral perfusion.
Respirations	Respirations are often rapid and shallow, reflecting presence of infection, fever, hypermetabolic state, or hypoxemia.
Monitor and record cardiac rhythm as indicated.	Cardiac dysrhythmias can occur due to stimulation of the sympathetic nervous system. Bradycardia may occur with high intracranial pressure.
Observe for elevating arterial blood pressure, if hemodynamic monitoring is available.	May indicate rising intracranial pressure with need for more intensive interventions/transfer to critical care unit.
Maintain optimal head of bed (HOB) placement (e.g., 0, 15, 30 degrees).	Various studies demonstrate different perfusion responses to HOB placement, but indicate reduced cerebral perfusion when HOB elevated greater than 30 degrees.

ACTIONS/INTERVENTIONS (continued)	RATIONALE (continued)
Observe client frequently and take safety precautions such as raising the side rails and keeping the bed in low position when the client is alone.	May have a range of altered mentation, varying from confusion to coma. Risk of injury varies also, from falls due to unsteady gait if client is ambulatory, to potential injury during seizure activity.
Provide darkened room and quiet, calm environment.	Client may be hypersensitive to light and sound.
Protect from injury and falls.	Client may be prone to seizure activity, and/or may have balance disturbances, when able to resume walking.
Collaborative	
Monitor pulse oximetry and/or arterial blood gases (ABGs).	$PaCO_2$ level of 28 to 30 mm Hg decreases cerebral blood flow while maintaining adequate cerebral oxygenation, while a PaO_2 of less than 65 mm Hg may cause or exacerbate cerebral edema.
Prepare for/review results of diagnostic imaging (e.g., cerebral CT scans).	To determine severity of condition, which can cause/exacerbate cerebral perfusion problems.
Cerebral Perfusion Promotion (NIC)	
Administer oxygen by appropriate route (e.g., mask, cannula, mechanical ventilation).	Improves cerebral and systemic oxygenation in the setting of hypoxia circulating toxins and hypermetabolic state.
Administer medications as indicated (e.g., diuretics, corticosteroids, anticonvulsants).	In addition to treatment of the underlying infective cause, other medications may be given to reduce inflammatory processes, manage risk of cerebral edema and neurological sequelae.
Administer or restrict fluids as indicated.	Fluids are needed to prevent decreased cerebral perfusion associated with hypovolemia. However, fluids may be restricted if hypertension occurs in order to prevent decreased cerebral perfusion associated with cerebral edema.
Provide hypothermia therapy as indicated.	To reduce effects of hypermetabolic state and risk of cerebral edema.

NURSING DIAGNOSIS: impaired Comfort

May Be Related To
Illness-related symptoms (e.g., meningeal irritation, fever)

Possibly Evidenced By
Reports being uncomfortable, hot
Disturbed sleep pattern; crying; moaning; irritability; restlessness

Desired Outcomes/Evaluation Criteria—Client Will

Discomfort Level (NOC)
Verbalize sense of comfort.
Demonstrate relief of discomfort—appear relaxed, rest/sleep quietly.

ACTIONS/INTERVENTIONS	RATIONALE
Calming Technique (NIC)	
Independent	
Note client's age, developmental level, and current condition (e.g., infant/child/obtunded adult), critically ill, ventilated, sedated.	Affects ability to report symptoms and choice of interventions.
Provide and promote quiet environment, gentle massage, change of position, passive range of motion [ROM] movements; parent holding child, restriction of visitors.	Makes use of therapeutic measures to relieve discomforts, and support relaxation and rest. *Note:* Touch is not always tolerated in client with severe meningeal irritation.
Provide periods of undisturbed rest. Avoid overstimulation and consolidate care activities, where possible.	Client is in a hyperirritable state.
Maintain position of comfort. Raise head of bed as needed. Place client on side if seizures or vomiting occur or are anticipated.	Client often assumes a position with head extended back slightly and body curled (possibly associated with meningeal irritation, and neck pain). Keeping head of bed elevated can improve breathing and reduce risk of aspiration if client vomits.
Assist with, encourage use of relaxation techniques (e.g., focused breathing, guided imagery) when client is able. Provide diversional or distraction activities (e.g., TV, radio, socialization with others).	May help client to focus on something other than pain/other discomforts.

(continues on page 236)

ACTIONS/INTERVENTIONS (continued) | RATIONALE (continued)

Encourage verbalization of feelings, where possible, about discomforts, including pain, nausea, light and touch sensitivity, etc.

Evaluates coping abilities and may identify additional areas of concern.

Pain Management (NIC)

Independent

Obtain client's assessment of pain to include location, characteristics, onset, duration, where possible. Encourage client to report changes in pain. Use pain-rating scale appropriate for age and cognition (e.g., 0 to 10 scale, facial expressions [or similar] scale).

Headache may be first (and most severe pain) at onset of either encephalitis or meningitis. Neck pain and stiffness may also be severe, causing client to be unable to touch chin to chest or turn head. Other discomforts, including body pain, may have slower onset and be more difficult to resolve. *Note:* It is probable that the client recovering from neuroinvasive meningitis will experience some degree of overall body pain for quite some time following the acute phase. Pain may become chronic in nature.

Pay attention to nonverbal cues.

Infant may have a shrill cry or be lethargic and refusing to eat. Older children and adults may withdraw from touch or stimulation, be lethargic or restless and uncommunicative. All clients with meningeal irritation may be highly sensitive to touch, to light, and to loud sounds.

Evaluate and document client's response to medications.

Helps determine effectiveness of interventions and need for change in treatment options.

Collaborative

Assist with treatment of underlying cause.

Treatment of the agent causing the brain and/or meningeal inflammation, as well as supportive therapies including nutrition and fluid, will help in reducing the severity of pain and other discomforts.

Administer medications, as needed, by appropriate route and optimal dosage.

Medications may include analgesics, sedatives, antiemetics, and antipyretics to manage client's pain, relieve nausea and fever, and promote rest.

Administer IV fluids and electrolytes as indicated.

Needed to support body functions, improve circulation, reduce fever, and provide needed protection from electrolyte imbalances that may be contributing to meningeal irritability.

Administer nutrition by appropriate route, including parenteral.

Client is in hypermetabolic state due to sepsis (offending agent and fever), and may or may not be able to consume food. Nutritional support may be required for some time.

NURSING DIAGNOSIS: deficient Knowledge [Learning Need] regarding condition, treatment plan, self-care, and discharge needs

May Be Related To

Cognitive limitation [mental fatigue], lack of exposure or recall, information misinterpretation

Possibly Evidenced By

Reports the problem

Inaccurate follow-through of instruction or performance of activity

Desired Outcomes/Evaluation Criteria—Client/Caregiver Will

Knowledge: Infection Management (NOC)

Identify relationship of signs/symptoms to the disease process.

Initiate necessary lifestyle changes and participate in treatment regimen.

ACTIONS/INTERVENTIONS | RATIONALE

Teaching: Disease Process (NIC)

Independent

Ascertain client/SO level of knowledge, including anticipatory needs.

Learning needs may include disease cause and process, factors contributing to symptoms and behavior (especially in neuroinvasive disease), treatments for symptom control, and prevention of complications.

Note client's age, developmental level, social and cultural influences, as well as effects of current disease process.

These factors affect ability and desire to learn, assimilate new information, and assume responsibility for self-care.

Include family/caregivers in assessment of needs and planning for care after discharge.

If neurological effects persist, the client may need complete care for a period of time, or require assistance with care activities or tasks requiring mental acuity.

ACTIONS/INTERVENTIONS (continued)	RATIONALE (continued)
Emphasize necessity of taking antimicrobial medications as directed (e.g., dose and length of therapy).	Medications may be required for an extended period of time. Premature discontinuation of treatment may result in return of infection or potentiate a drug-resistant strain.
Review individual nutritional needs, appropriate exercise, and need for rest.	Enhances immune system function and promotes healing.
Discuss physical and mental fatigue, and problem-solve ways to manage fatigue (e.g., starting with tasks requiring shorter time of concentration, using memory joggers, planning for longer rest periods for several months).	Fatigue, especially mental fatigue, is common after infection or inflammation in the central nervous system (CNS). This fatigue may remain over months or years, even after recovery from the infection. It may be difficult for the person to go back to school or work, as our high-technology society with its increasing demands on peoples' mental capacity does not accept anything but full engagement, even over time (Schmidt et al., 2006; Berg et al., 2010).
Encourage individuals in close contact with client to seek medical evaluation if they develop symptoms (e.g., headache, fever, neck stiffness, change in mental status); or if they are at high risk because of fragile health status.	Family, friends, roommates of infected persons can contract the disease (if the client has a contagious form) or may need prophylactic therapy.
Discuss vaccination recommendations such as meningococcal polysaccharide vaccine (MPSV4); meningococcal conjugate vaccine (MCV4).	The CDC recommends a meningococcal vaccine for: all children ages 11 to 18, certain younger high-risk children; anyone who has been exposed to meningitis during an outbreak; anyone traveling to or living where meningitis is common; military recruits; people with certain immune system disorders or a damaged or missing spleen (CDC, 2011).
Emphasize need for long-term medical and rehabilitation follow-up.	Although most people will recover without permanent neurological deficits, the client can be left with long-term conditions, including balance problems, chronic pain, epilepsy, learning difficulties, behavioral disorders, speech problems, and hearing loss. The disease can also affect long- and short-term memory (Schmidt et al, 2005; Matthews, 2007; Berg, 2010).

POTENTIAL CONSIDERATIONS following acute hospitalization (dependent on client's age, physical condition and presence of complications, personal resources, and life responsibilities)

- ***Fatigue***—[aftereffects of] disease state, poor physical condition
- ***risk for Injury***—general weakness, balancing difficulties, cognitive impairment
- ***Self-Care Deficit (specify)***—decreased strength and endurance, perceptual and cognitive impairment, muscular pain
- ***risk for ineffective Role Performance***—cognitive changes in one partner, stressful life events; unrealistic expectations

DISC SURGERY

I. Procedure—Laminectomy is the surgical excision of a vertebral posterior arch performed in the presence of a herniated disc for the purpose of relieving pressure on the spinal cord nerve roots and removing a source of pain.

II. Types

a. *Open laminectomy* is performed under general anesthesia; skin, muscles, and ligaments are cut, bone may be permanently removed. Procedures include combinations of disc excision, nerve decompression, and bone fusion—with or without spinal instrumentation, such as pedicle screws, plates, rods, fusion cages, bone grafts, or synthetic disc materials. Spinal fusion may be performed along with disc removal procedures (Rutherford, 2007). Inpatient stay of several days may be required.

b. *Minimally invasive* procedures performed without anesthesia, under brief anesthesia, cause minimal damage to muscles; no bone is removed, and no large incisions are made. Client may go home on day of surgery.

i. Endoscopic surgery—surgical tools are inserted into a small incision and the herniated disc is removed or remodeled.

ii. Percutaneous or endoscopic microdiscectomy—disc material is removed through a small puncture in the skin, using a microscope for guidance.

iii. Damaged discs are replaced with the goal of preserving vertebral height and providing some flexibility and movement.

iv. Artificial Disc Replacement (ADR) substitutes an intervertebral disc with a synthetic one. By doing so, the height of the previously collapsed intervertebral space is restored, alleviating subsequent nerve compression. Implants may be compressible or noncompressible fusion (Bitan, 2013).

III. Statistics

a. Morbidity: Approximately 450 cases of herniated disc per 100,000 require surgery; 150,000 cases annually in the United States, with the average age for surgery at 40 to 45 years.

b. Mortality: Rate is between 0.8% and 1%, approximately 1,000 yearly depending on whether a fusion is included with laminectomy and presence of comorbidities.

c. Cost: More than $20 billion annually (*ScienceDaily*, 2008).

GLOSSARY

Bone-graft substitutes: A large number of bone-graft substitutes are available, including allograft bone preparations such as demineralized bone matrix and calcium-based materials. More and more replacement materials consist of one or more components: an osteoconductive matrix, which supports the ingrowth of new bone; and osteoinductive proteins, which sustain mitogenesis of undifferentiated cells; and osteogenic cells (osteoblasts or osteoblast precursors), which are capable of forming bone in the proper environment. All substitutes can either replace autologous bone or expand an existing amount of autologous bone graft (Kolk, 2012).

Discectomy: Surgical removal of a herniated disc. Discectomy can be performed in a number of different ways, including open surgery or through less-invasive procedures using microscopes, x-rays, small tools, and lasers.

Laminectomy: Surgical removal of the lamina (back of spinal canal) and spurs inside the canal that are causing spinal nerve compression.

Laminotomy: Endoscopic, outpatient procedure to remove the ligamentum flavum, a ligament in the spinal canal that can thicken to the point that it compresses the spinal cord, contributing to spinal stenosis. Spinal fusion often is performed in conjunction with a laminotomy. In more involved cases, a laminectomy may be performed.

Minimally Invasive Spine (MIS) surgery: Developed to treat disorders of the spine with less disruption to the muscles and less damage to nerves, blood vessels, and bone. In MIS approaches, also called "keyhole surgeries," surgeons use a tiny endoscope with a camera on the end, which is inserted through a small incision in the skin. The camera provides surgeons with an inside view, enabling surgical access to the affected area of the spine

Percutaneous endoscopic laser discectomy: X-ray monitoring and fiber optics display images on a monitor, allowing the surgeon to see what is compressing the nerve during the procedure. A laser, camera, suction, irrigation, and other surgical instruments are inserted through a translucent working tube. Once all the tools are in place, the surgeon uses a laser to vaporize the disc material, thus diminishing the pressure on the spinal cord and/or the spinal nerve.

Spinal fusion: Surgical technique in which one or more of the vertebrae of the spine are united together ("fused") so that motion no longer occurs between them. Bone grafts and/or bone-graft substitutes (Kolk, 2012) are placed around the spine during surgery. The body then heals the grafts over several months—similar to healing a fracture —which joins, or "welds," the vertebrae together. There are many potential reasons to consider fusing the vertebrae. These include treatment of a fractured (broken) vertebra; correction of deformity (spinal curves or slippages); elimination of pain from painful motion; treatment of instability; and treatment of some cervical disc herniations.

Care Setting

Inpatient or outpatient surgical or orthopedic unit. This plan of care relates to the open surgical procedures where the client experiences a hospital stay.

Related Concerns

Psychosocial aspects of care, page 729
Surgical intervention, page 762

Client Assessment Database

Refer to CP: Herniated Nucleus Pulposus (Ruptured Intervertebral Disc) for data.

DIAGNOSTIC DIVISION MAY REPORT TEACHING/LEARNING	MAY EXHIBIT
Discharge Plan Considerations May require assistance with activities of daily living (ADLs), transportation, homemaker or maintenance tasks, vocational counseling, and possible changes in layout of home ➧ Refer to section at end of plan for postdischarge considerations.	

Diagnostic Studies

TEST WHY IT IS DONE	WHAT IT TELLS ME
Primary Diagnostic Studies	
• *Spinal x-rays:* Detect serious underlying structural and pathological conditions of the vertebrae and spinal cord.	May show degenerative changes in spine or intravertebral spaces. Can be used to rule out other suspected pathology, such as tumors, osteomyelitis, among others.

TEST WHY IT IS DONE (continued)	WHAT IT TELLS ME (continued)
• *Magnetic resonance imaging (MRI) scan:* Test that uses magnetic fields to produce two- or three-dimensional images of soft tissues and bones.	Diagnostic test of choice for chronic, unremitting back pain due to nerve impingement. Can reveal changes in bone, discs, and soft tissues and can validate disc herniation and surgical considerations. Signal changes on MRI in the vertebral body marrow adjacent to the end plates (also known as Modic changes [MC]) are common in patients with low back pain (LBP) (18% to 58%) and are strongly associated with LBP. In asymptomatic persons the prevalence is 12% to 13%. MC is seen in relation to spondylodiscitis, disc herniation, and severe disc degeneration among other conditions (Albert, 2008).
• *Computed tomography (CT) scan with and without enhancement:* X-ray procedure that combines many x-ray images with the aid of a computer to generate cross-sectional views and, if needed, three-dimensional images of the internal organs and structures of the body.	May reveal spinal canal narrowing or compression and disc protrusion.
• *Myelogram (also called myelography):* Radiopaque contrast dye is injected into the subarachnoid space of the spinal canal. Sometimes performed in conjunction with MRI or used in the client who cannot undergo MRI.	Although rarely performed, the myelogram detects abnormalities of the spinal cord, the spinal canal, the spinal nerve roots, and the blood vessels that supply the spinal cord (Pagana, 2011). Reveals structures causing nerve compression—including narrowing of disc space—and confirms specific location and size of disc herniation and degree of spinal stenosis.
RELATED DIAGNOSTIC STUDIES	
• *Electromyogram (EMG):* Measures the electrical activity of muscles at rest and during contraction.	Identifies diseases that damage muscle tissue, nerves, or neuromuscular junctions. Finds the cause of weakness, paralysis, or muscle twitching. *Note:* EMG and NCS are often done together.
• *Nerve conduction studies (NCS):* Measures how well and how fast the nerves can send electrical signals.	Can identify damage to the peripheral nervous system, including all the nerves that lead away from the spinal cord and the smaller nerves that branch out from those nerves. Can localize lesion to level of particular spinal nerve root involved in impairment and determine the effect on skeletal muscle. *Note:* EMG and NCS are often done together.

Nursing Priorities

1. Maintain tissue perfusion and neurological function.
2. Promote comfort and healing.
3. Prevent or minimize complications.
4. Assist with return to normal mobility.
5. Provide information about condition, prognosis, treatment needs, and limitations.

Discharge Goals

1. Neurological function maintained or improved.
2. Complications prevented.
3. Limited mobility achieved with potential for increasing mobility.
4. Condition, prognosis, therapeutic regimen, and behavior and lifestyle changes are understood.
5. Plan in place to meet needs after discharge.

NURSING DIAGNOSIS: risk for Peripheral Neurovascular Dysfunction

May Be Related To
Orthopedic surgery
Mechanical compression—dressing, edema of operative site, hematoma formation
Vascular obstruction

Possibly Evidenced By
(Not applicable; presence of signs and symptoms establishes an *actual* diagnosis)

Desired Outcomes/Evaluation Criteria—Client Will

Neurological Status: Peripheral (NOC)
Report or demonstrate normal sensations and movement as appropriate.

ACTIONS/INTERVENTIONS	RATIONALE
Peripheral Sensation Management (NIC)	
Independent	
Check neurological signs periodically and compare with baseline. Assess movement and sensation of hands and arms (cervical) and lower extremities and feet (lumbar).	Although some degree of sensory impairment is usually present, changes in neurological assessments may reflect development or resolution of spinal cord edema or tissue inflammation due to damage to motor nerve roots from surgical manipulation. Assessment findings may also indicate tissue hemorrhage that causes spinal cord compression. Spinal cord compression requires prompt medical evaluation and intervention.
Monitor vital signs. Note skin color, warmth, and capillary refill.	Hypotension, especially postural, with corresponding changes in pulse rate may reflect hypovolemia from blood loss, restriction of oral intake, and nausea and vomiting.
Monitor intake and output (I&O) and wound drains, such as Jackson-Pratt or Hemovac, if used.	Fluid balance indicates circulatory status and replacement needs. Excessive or prolonged blood loss requires evaluation and ongoing assessments to continually determine and provide prompt and appropriate intervention.
Visually check and gently palpate operative site for swelling. Inspect dressing for excess drainage. Assess extremities—particularly lower extremities—for redness, swelling, and pain.	Changes in contour of operative site suggest hematoma or edema formation. Inspection may reveal frank bleeding or redness, swelling, and pain in the extremities suggest complications associated with immobility, including deep vein thrombosis (DVT). Refer to CP: Thrombophlebitis.
Collaborative	
Administer intravenous (IV) fluids or blood, as indicated.	Fluid replacement depends on the degree of hypovolemia and duration of oozing or bleeding.
Monitor blood counts—hemoglobin (Hgb), hematocrit (Hct), and red blood cells (RBCs).	These laboratory tests help establish fluid status and the need for fluid and blood product replacement. They also indicate effectiveness of fluid resuscitation interventions.
Apply and maintain schedule for wearing anti-embolic hose or sequential compression devices.	Anti-embolic hose, sequential compression devices, and related products reduce the risk for venous stasis in lower extremities.

NURSING DIAGNOSIS: risk for [spinal] Injury

Risk Factors May Include

Physical—temporary weakness of vertebral column, balancing difficulties, changes in muscle coordination

Possibly Evidenced By

(Not applicable; presence of signs and symptoms establishes an *actual* diagnosis)

Desired Outcomes/Evaluation Criteria—Client Will

Risk Control (NOC)

Maintain proper alignment of spine.

Recognize need for or seek assistance with activity, as appropriate.

ACTIONS/INTERVENTIONS	RATIONALE
Positioning: Neurologic (NIC)	
Independent	
Post sign at bedside regarding prescribed position.	Promotes ongoing communication among the members of the healthcare team and reduces risk of inadvertent strain or flexion of operative area.
Provide bed board or firm mattress.	Aids in stabilizing back.
Maintain brace-wearing schedule, as indicated.	Braces may be used to decrease muscle spasm and support the surrounding structures during healing. Establishing a schedule generally enhances client compliance.
Limit activities such as twisting or bending, as prescribed, when client has had a spinal fusion.	Restricted spinal movement promotes healing of fusion.
Logroll client from side-to-side. Have client fold arms across chest; tighten long back muscles, keeping shoulders and pelvis straight. Use pillows between knees during position change and when on side. Use turning sheet and sufficient personnel when turning, especially on the first postoperative day. Instruct client in these movements as self-care progresses.	Logrolling maintains body alignment. It prevents twisting movements. Twisting movements potentially disrupt alignment, interfering with the overall healing process.

ACTIONS/INTERVENTIONS (continued)	RATIONALE (continued)
Assist out of bed: logroll to side of bed, splint back, and raise to sitting position. Avoid prolonged sitting. Move to standing position in single smooth motion.	Gradual progression of activity with careful consideration of body alignment protects the surgical area. These maneuvers avoid twisting and flexing of back while arising from bed or chair.
Avoid sudden stretching, twisting, flexing, or jarring of spine.	These precautions reinforce the importance of maintaining body alignment. These movements may cause vertebral collapse, shifting of bone graft, delayed hematoma formation, or subcutaneous wound dehiscence.
Monitor blood pressure (BP). Note reports of dizziness or weakness. Recommend client change position slowly.	Presence of postural hypotension may result in fainting, falling, and possible injury to surgical site.
Have client wear firm, flat walking shoes when ambulating.	Such shoes reduce risk of falls.
Collaborative	
Apply lumbar brace or cervical collar, as appropriate.	Braces or corsets may be used in and out of bed during postoperative phase to support spine and surrounding structures until muscle strength improves. Brace is applied while client is supine in bed. Spinal fusion generally requires a lengthy recuperation period in a corset and collar.
Refer to physical therapy. Implement program as outlined.	Body mechanics, range-of-motion, and strengthening exercises may be initiated during the rehabilitative phase to decrease muscle spasm and improve function.

NURSING DIAGNOSIS: risk for ineffective Breathing Pattern

Risk Factors May Include

Neurological damage
Airway obstruction
Pain

Possibly Evidenced By

(Not applicable; presence of signs and symptoms establishes an *actual* diagnosis)

Desired Outcomes/Evaluation Criteria—Client Will

Respiratory Status: Ventilation (NOC)

Maintain a normal, effective respiratory pattern free of cyanosis and other signs of hypoxia, with arterial blood gases (ABGs) within acceptable range.

ACTIONS/INTERVENTIONS	RATIONALE
Respiratory Monitoring (NIC)	
Independent	
Inspect for edema of face and neck (cervical laminectomy), especially first 24 to 48 hours after surgery.	Tracheal edema and compression or nerve injury can compromise respiratory function.
Listen for hoarseness. Encourage voice rest.	Hoarseness may indicate laryngeal nerve injury or edema of surgical area, which can negatively affect cough and ability to clear airway.
Auscultate breath sounds. Note presence of wheezes or rhonchi.	Abnormal breath sounds suggest accumulation of secretions or need to engage in more aggressive therapeutic actions to clear airway.
Instruct in/assist with coughing, turning, and deep breathing. Encourage client's use of incentive spirometry or other devices used to aid deep breathing.	These maneuvers facilitate movement of secretions and clearing of lungs. They also reduce the risk of such respiratory complications (e.g., pneumonia, pulmonary embolus).
Collaborative	
Administer supplemental oxygen, if indicated.	Supplemental oxygen may be necessary for periods of respiratory distress or evidence of hypoxia.
Monitor ABGs or pulse oximetry, as indicated.	Monitors adequacy of respiratory function and oxygen therapy.

NURSING DIAGNOSIS: acute Pain

May Be Related To
Physical agent: surgical manipulation, edema, inflammation, or harvesting of bone graft

Possibly Evidenced By
Verbal/coded reports
Diaphoresis, changes in vital signs, pallor
Alteration in muscle tone
Guarded or expressive behaviors—restlessness

Desired Outcomes/Evaluation Criteria—Client Will

Pain Control (NOC)
Report pain is relieved or controlled.
Verbalize methods that provide relief.
Demonstrate use of relaxation skills and diversional activities.

ACTIONS/INTERVENTIONS	RATIONALE
Pain Management (NIC)	
Independent	
Assess intensity, description, location, radiation of pain, and changes in sensation.	Pain may be mild to severe with radiation to shoulders and occipital area (cervical) or hips and buttocks (lumbar). If bone graft has been taken from the iliac crest, pain may be more severe at the donor site. Numbness or tingling discomfort may reflect return of sensation after nerve root decompression or result from developing edema causing nerve compression.
Instruct in regular use of (a 0–10 or similar) pain-rating scale.	Standardized tool for rating pain helps in assessment and management of pain.
Review expected manifestations or changes in intensity of pain.	Development or resolution of edema and inflammation during the immediate postoperative phase can affect pressure on various nerves and cause changes in degree of pain. Muscle spasms and improved nerve root sensation can intensify pain, especially in early days after procedure.
Encourage client to assume position of comfort, as indicated. Use logrolling for position change.	Positioning is dictated by physical preference and type of operation; for example, head of bed may be slightly elevated after cervical laminectomy. Readjustment of position aids in relieving muscle fatigue and discomfort. Logrolling avoids tension in the operative areas, maintains straight spinal alignment, and reduces risk of displacing epidural patient-controlled analgesia (PCA) when used.
Provide back rub or massage. Avoid the operative site.	Back rubs and massages relieve or reduce pain by alteration of sensory neurons and muscle relaxation.
Demonstrate and encourage use of relaxation skills, such as deep breathing, visualization.	Deep breathing and visualization refocus attention, reduce muscle tension, promote sense of well-being, and control or decrease discomfort.
Provide liquid or soft diet; provide room humidifier; and encourage voice rest.	Following anterior cervical laminectomy, such measures reduce discomfort associated with sore throat and difficulty swallowing.
Investigate client reports of return of radicular pain.	Radicular pain suggests complications, such as collapsing of disc space and shifting of bone graft, which require further medical evaluation and intervention. *Note:* Sciatica and muscle spasms often recur after laminectomy, but should resolve within several days or weeks.
Collaborative	
Administer analgesics, as indicated, for example:	
Opioids, such as morphine sulfate (MS), codeine, meperidine (Demerol), tramadol (Ultram), oxycodone (Percocet), and hydrocodone (Vicodin, Lortab), fentanyl (Duragesic)	Opioids are used during the first few postoperative days. Nonopioid agents are incorporated as intensity of pain diminishes. *Note:* Opioids may be administered via epidural catheter and PCA initially. Some may then be given orally or by patch.
Muscle relaxants, such as cyclobenzaprine (Flexeril) and metaxalone (Skelaxin)	Muscle relaxants may be used to relieve muscle spasms.
Instruct client in use of patient-controlled analgesia (PCA).	PCA gives client control of medication administration (usually opioids) to achieve a more constant level of comfort, which may enhance healing and sense of well-being.

ACTIONS/INTERVENTIONS (continued)	RATIONALE (continued)
Provide throat sprays, lozenges, or viscous lidocaine (Xylocaine).	Sore throat may be a major complaint following cervical laminectomy.
Apply electrical stimulation, as needed.	May be used to block neural transmission of pain by small-diameter nerve fibers.

NURSING DIAGNOSIS: impaired physical Mobility

May Be Related To
Musculoskeletal/neuromuscular impairment
Reluctance to attempt movement; prescribed movement restrictions
Pain; pharmaceutical agents

Possibly Evidenced By
Limited ROM; difficulty turning
Postural instability; slowed movement

Desired Outcomes/Evaluation Criteria—Client Will

Knowledge: Personal Safety (NOC)
Demonstrate techniques or behaviors that enable resumption of activities.

Mobility (NOC)
Maintain or increase strength and function of affected body part.

ACTIONS/INTERVENTIONS	RATIONALE
Body Mechanics Promotion (NIC)	
Independent	
Schedule activity or procedures with rest periods. Encourage participation in ADLs within individual limitations.	Activity and rest enhance healing and build muscle strength and endurance. Client participation promotes sense of independence and control.
Provide or assist with passive and active ROM and core-strengthening exercises, depending on surgical procedure.	Strengthens muscles and promotes good body mechanics.
Assist with activity or progressive ambulation.	Until healing occurs, activity is limited and advanced slowly according to individual tolerance.
Review proper body mechanics or techniques for participation in activities.	Proper body mechanics reduces the risk of muscle strain, injury to the operative area, or pain. It also increases client participation and motivation in progressive activity.

Refer to CP: Herniated Nucleus Pulposus (Ruptured Intervertebral Disc); ND: impaired physical Mobility, for further considerations.

NURSING DIAGNOSIS: Constipation

May Be Related To
Insufficient physical activity
Decreased motility of gastrointestinal tract; opiates, sedatives
Emotional stress
Changes in eating pattern; insufficient fiber/fluid intake

Possibly Evidenced By
Hypoactive bowel sounds
Increased abdominal pressure
Abdominal pain, feeling of rectal fullness, nausea
Decreased frequency, unable to pass stool

Desired Outcomes/Evaluation Criteria—Client Will

Bowel Elimination (NOC)
Reestablish normal patterns of bowel functioning.
Pass stool of soft or semiformed consistency without straining.

ACTIONS/INTERVENTIONS	RATIONALE
Constipation/Impaction Management (NIC)	
Independent	
Note abdominal distention and auscultate bowel sounds.	Abdominal distention and absence of bowel sounds indicate that bowel is not functioning. Possible cause would be the sudden loss of parasympathetic innervation of the gastrointestinal (GI) system.
Provide privacy.	Promotes psychological comfort.
Encourage early ambulation.	Stimulates peristalsis and thereby facilitates passage of flatus.
Collaborative	
Begin progressive diet, as tolerated.	Solid foods are not started until bowel sounds have returned, flatus has been passed, and danger of ileus formation has abated.
Provide rectal tube, suppositories, and enemas, as needed.	May be necessary to relieve abdominal distention and promote resumption of normal bowel habits.
Administer laxatives or stool softeners, as indicated.	Soften stools, promote normal bowel habits or evacuation, and decrease straining.

NURSING DIAGNOSIS: risk for Urinary Retention

Risk Factors May Include

Blockage—swelling in operative area

Possibly Evidenced By

(Not applicable; presence of signs and symptoms establishes an *actual* diagnosis)

Desired Outcomes/Evaluation Criteria—Client Will

Urinary Elimination (NOC)

Empty bladder in sufficient amounts.

Be free of bladder distention, with residuals after voiding within normal limits (WNL).

ACTIONS/INTERVENTIONS	RATIONALE
Urinary Retention Care (NIC)	
Independent	
Observe and record amount and time of voiding.	Determines adequate voiding and bladder function.
Palpate for bladder distention.	May indicate urinary retention.
Force fluids.	Fluid intake helps maintain fluid balance and renal perfusion.
Stimulate bladder emptying by running water, pouring warm water over perineum, or having client put hand in warm water.	These maneuvers relax the urinary sphincter thus stimulating urination.
Collaborative	
Perform ultrasound bladder scan or catheterize for residual after voiding, when indicated. Insert and maintain indwelling catheter as needed.	Helps determine the amount of urine in the bladder. Intermittent or continuous catheterization may be necessary for several days postoperatively until swelling is decreased.

NURSING DIAGNOSIS: deficient Knowledge [Learning Need] regarding condition, prognosis, treatment, self-care, and discharge needs

May Be Related To

Lack of exposure

Information misinterpretation; lack of recall

Unfamiliarity with information resources

Possibly Evidenced By

Reports the problem

Inaccurate follow-through of instruction

Desired Outcomes/Evaluation Criteria—Client Will

Knowledge: Treatment Regimen (NOC)

Verbalize understanding of condition, prognosis, and potential complications.

List signs and symptoms requiring medical follow-up.

Verbalize understanding of therapeutic regimen.

Initiate necessary lifestyle changes.

ACTIONS/INTERVENTIONS	RATIONALE
Teaching: Disease Process (NIC)	
Independent	
Review particular condition or prognosis.	Individual needs dictate tolerance levels and limitations of activity.
Discuss possibility of unrelieved or renewed pain.	Some pain may continue for several months as activity level increases and scar tissue stretches. Pain relief from surgical procedure could be temporary if other discs in the area have similar amount of degeneration.
Discuss safe and appropriate use of heat, such as warm packs and heating pad.	Increased circulation to the back or surgical area transports nutrients needed for healing to the area and aids in removing pathogens or exudates. Decreases muscle spasms that may result from nerve root irritation during healing process.
Discuss judicious use of cold packs before or after stretching activity, if indicated.	Cold packs may decrease muscle spasm in some instances more effectively than heat.
Avoid tub baths per physician recommendation.	Tub baths increase risk of falls and spine twisting or flexing.
Review dietary and fluid needs.	Nutrition should be tailored to reduce risk of constipation, reduce obesity, and avoid weight gain, while meeting nutrient requirements to facilitate healing.
Review or reinforce incisional care.	Correct incisional care promotes healing and reduces risk of wound infection. *Note:* This information is especially critical for the client's significant other (SO)/caregiver. Clients are usually discharged from facility care within 24 hours of surgery.
Identify signs and symptoms requiring notification of healthcare provider, such as fever, increased incisional pain, inflammation, wound drainage, and decreased sensation or motor activity in extremities.	Prompt evaluation and intervention may prevent complications or permanent injury.
Discuss necessity of follow-up care.	Long-term medical supervision may be needed to manage problems or complications and to reincorporate individual into desired or altered lifestyle and activities.
Review need for or use of immobilization device, as indicated.	Correct application and wearing time are important to gaining the most benefit from the brace.
Assess current lifestyle, job, finances, and home and leisure activities.	Knowledge of current situation allows nurse to highlight areas for possible intervention, such as referral for occupational or vocational testing and counseling.
Listen and communicate regarding alternatives and lifestyle changes. Be sensitive to client's needs.	Low-back pain is a frequent cause of long-term disability. According to a recent study, 28% of adults with low-back pain report limited activity due to a chronic condition, as compared to 10% of adults who do not have low-back pain (National Center for Health Statistics, 2006). Many clients may have to stop or modify work and have had long-term or chronic pain, creating relationship and financial crises. Client may be viewed as being a malingerer, which creates further problems in social and work relationships.
Note overt and covert expressions of concern about sexuality.	Although client may not ask directly, there may be concerns about the effect of surgery on both the ability to cope with usual role in the family and community and ability to perform sexually.
Provide written copy of all instructions.	Printed information serves as useful reference after discharge.
Identify community resources as indicated, such as social services and rehabilitation and vocational counseling services.	A team effort can be helpful in providing support during recuperative period.
Recommend counseling, sex therapy, and psychotherapy, as appropriate.	Depression is common in conditions for which a lengthy recuperative time (2 to 9 months) is expected. Therapy may alleviate anxiety, assist client to cope effectively, and enhance healing process. Presence of physical limitations, pain, and depression may negatively affect sexual desire and performance and add additional stress to relationship.
Teaching: Prescribed Activity/Exercise (NIC)	
Discuss return to activities. Stress importance of increasing activities, as tolerated.	Although the recuperative period may be lengthy, following prescribed activity program promotes muscle and tissue circulation, healing, and strengthening.
Encourage development of regular exercise program, such as walking and stretching.	Regular exercise promotes healing, strengthens abdominal and erector muscles to provide support to the spinal column, and enhances general physical and emotional well-being.

(continues on page 246)

ACTIONS/INTERVENTIONS (continued)	RATIONALE (continued)
Discuss importance of good posture and avoidance of prolonged standing or sitting. Recommend sitting in straight-backed chair with feet on a footstool or flat on the floor.	Proper spine alignment prevents further injuries and stress.
Emphasize importance of avoiding activities that increase the flexion of the spine, such as climbing stairs, automobile driving or riding, bending at the waist with knees straight, lifting more than 5 pounds, and engaging in strenuous exercise and sports. Discuss limitations on sexual relations and positions.	Any of these movements, positions, or excess weight potentially can interrupt the healing process and increases risk of injury to spinal cord.
Encourage lying-down rest periods, balanced with activity.	Reduces general and spinal fatigue and assists in the healing and recuperative process.
Explore limitations and abilities.	Placing limitations into perspective with abilities allows client to understand own situation and exercise choice.

POTENTIAL CONSIDERATIONS following acute hospitalization (dependent on client's age, physical condition and presence of complications, personal resources, and life responsibilities)

- ***impaired physical Mobility***—decreased endurance, pain, prescribed movement restrictions, [immobilizing device]; decreased muscle strength
- ***Self-Care Deficit***—weakness, fatigue, pain, environmental barriers—immobilizing device
- ***risk for Falls***—postoperative conditions; impaired balance; narcotics/opiates
- ***compromised family Coping***—temporary family disorganization or role changes

Sample clinical pathway follows in Table 6.1.

TABLE 6.1 Cervical Laminectomy with Fusion. ELOS: 2 Days Orthopedic or Surgical Unit

ND and Categories of Care	Day 1 Day of Surgery____	Day 2 POD #1 ____	Day 3 Discharge____
risk for Peripheral Neurovascular Dysfunction R/T orthopedic surgery, mechanical compression—dressing/ edema, vascular obstruction	Goals: Maintain proper alignment of cervical spine Display stable/improved sensation in affected limbs	Display expected sensory/ motor response Identify appropriate safety measures	
Diagnostic studies		Hb/Hct, RBC Electrolytes	
Additional assessments	VS q1h × 4 then q4h	→ qid	→
	Neurovascular checks UE, q1h × 4 then q4h	→ qid	→ q8h
	Dressings/drainage q4h	→	→ q8h
	I&O q8h	→	→ bid
	Hemovac (if used) q8h	→	→ D/C
	Palpate operative site for swelling, inspect face/neck for edema qh1 × 4	→ q8h	→ D/C
Medications	IV fluids/blood as indicated	→ D/C or convert to NS lock	
Client education	Purpose/necessity of cervical collar Protocol for position change	Cessation of smoking if indicated	Use of heat Signs/symptoms to be reported to health-care provider
Additional nursing actions	Position per protocol/HOB elevated 30°	→	→
	Logroll q2h	→ Ambulate	→
	Cervical collar in place	→	→
	BRP w/assistance—tennis shoes—not slippers	→	→ Per self as tolerated
	Fluids as tolerated	→ Advanced diet as tolerated	→
acute Pain R/T physical agent—surgical intervention	Report pain controlled	→	
		Participate in activities to increase comfort	→ Verbalize understanding of therapeutic interventions

TABLE 6.1 Cervical Laminectomy with Fusion. ELOS: 2 Days Orthopedic or Surgical Unit (continued)

ND and Categories of Care	Day 1 Day of Surgery____	Day 2 POD #1 ____	Day 3 Discharge____
Additional assessments	Pain characteristics/change	→	→
	Response to interventions	→	→
Medications	Analgesics—PCA or IV	→ D/C PCA	
Allergies:______		PO analgesics	→
	Throat spray/lozenges	→	→ D/C
Client education	Orient to unit/room	Relaxation techniques	Use of Tens as indicated
	Reporting of pain/effects of interventions	Medication dose, frequency, purpose, side effects	Signs/symptoms to report to healthcare provider
	Proper use of PCA		
	Recovery/rehabilitation expectations		
	Limitations of movement (e.g., twisting, flexing, pulling)		
	Voice rest (anterior approach)		
Additional nursing actions	Provide firm mattress	→	→
	Comfort measures	→	→
impaired physical Mobility R/T musculoskeletal impairment; pain; therapeutic restriction; pharmaceutical agents		Reestablish normal bowel/bladder elimination	Verbalize understanding of activity program/ restrictions
			Report plan in place to meet needs post-discharge
Referrals	Social Services	Home Care	
Additional assessments	General muscle tone/strength	→ Ability to perform ADLs independently	→
	Level of functional ability	→	→
	Breath sounds q4h	→ q8h	→
	Bowel sounds q4h	→ q8h	→
	Amount/time of voids	→ D/C	
		Edema, pain lower extremities, Homan's sign q8h	→
Medications		Stool softener	→ /enema if no BM
Client education	Activity level/progression	General wellness—diet, exercise, adequate rest	Activity restrictions, e.g., shower instead of tub bath, no lifting, resumption of work, hobbies, sexual activity
	Bed exercises	Home exercise program	
	Skin care needs	Proper body mechanics	
		Use of assistive devices as required	
			Provide written copy of instructions
Additional nursing actions	Perform passive and assist with active ROM exercises	→	→
	Encourage participation of ADLs within level of ability	→	→ Per self
	T, C, DB, q2h	→	→ Per self
	Incentive spirometry q4h	→ q4h while awake	→ D/C
	SCD or thigh-high TEDs	→	→
	Skin care per Risk Protocol	→	→

Key: ADLs, activities of daily life; BRP, bathroom privileges; C, cough; D/C, discontinue; DB, deep breath; ELOS, estimated length of stay; Hb/Hct hemoglobin/hematocrit; HOB, head of bed; I&O, input & output; ND, nursing diagnosis; NS, normal saline; PCA, patient-controlled analgesia; PO, by mouth; POD, postoperative day; q1h, every 1 hour; q4h, every 4 hours; q8h, every 8 hours; qid, 4 times a day; R/T, related to; RBC, red blood cell; ROM, range of motion; T, turn; TEDs, anti-embolism stockings; TENS, transcutaneous electrical nerve stimulator; UE, upper extremities; VS, vital signs.

SPINAL CORD INJURY (ACUTE REHABILITATIVE PHASE)

I. Pathophysiology—injury or insult to spinal cord

a. Primary mechanism of injury (Hausman, 2006)
   i. Hyperflexion (sudden acceleration forward) or hyperextension (sudden acceleration forward, followed by sudden deceleration) of neck
   ii. Compression of spine: as with fall from height landing on feet or buttocks, or blow to top of head as in a diving injury
   iii. Rotation injury: Head is rotated beyond normal range.
   iv. Penetrating injuries
      1. Low-velocity, such as knife causing direct and local injury to site
      2. High-velocity, such as bullet or shrapnel causing both direct and indirect damage

b. Secondary mechanism of injury (NINDS, 2012)
   i. Changes in blood flow in and around the spinal cord
   ii. Highly reactive chemicals called oxidants or "free radicals" attack the body's natural defenses and critical cell structures.
   iii. Release of excess neurotransmitters, leading to secondary damage from overexcited nerve cells
   iv. Neurogenic shock with hypoxemia and ischemia
   v. Fluid and electrolyte imbalances
   vi. Damage to axons—Nerve fibers that signal to other cells
   vii. Nerve cells in the spinal cord below the lesion may die, disrupting spinal cord circuits that help control movement and interpret sensory information.

c. Neurological involvement dependent on level of injury, degree of spinal shock, phase, and degree of recovery
   i. *C1 to C3:* Tetraplegia with total loss of muscular and respiratory function
   ii. *C4 to C5:* Tetraplegia with poor pulmonary capacity, complete dependency for activities of daily living (ADLs)
   iii. *C6 to C7:* Tetraplegia with some arm and hand movement allowing some independence in upper-body ADLs
   iv. *C7 to T1:* Tetraplegia with limited use of fingers and thumbs, increasing independence
   v. *T2 to L1:* Paraplegia with intact arm function, varying function of intercostal and abdominal muscles, and loss of function below level of injury
   vi. *L1 to L2 or below:* Mixed motor-sensory loss and bowel and bladder dysfunction

II. Classifications: (NINDS: American Spinal Injury Association [ASIA] Scale, 2012)

a. Complete: No motor or sensory function is preserved below the level of injury, including the sacral segments S4–S5

b. Incomplete: Sensory, but not motor, function is preserved below the neurologic level and some sensation in the sacral segments S4–S5.

c. Incomplete: Motor function is preserved below the neurologic level; however, more than half of key muscles below the neurologic level have a muscle grade less than 3 (i.e., not strong enough to move against gravity).

d. Incomplete: Motor function is preserved below the neurologic level, and at least half of key muscles below the neurologic level have a muscle grade of 3 or more (i.e., joints can be moved against gravity)..

e. Normal: Motor and sensory functions are normal.

III. Etiology (National Spinal Cord Injury Statistical Center [NSCISC], 2012; Nayduch, 2010)

a. The next most common cause of SCI is falls.

b. Since 2005, motor vehicle crashes account for 39.2% of reported SCI cases.

c. Acts of violence (primarily gunshot wounds) peaked between 1990 and 1999 at 24.8% before declining to 14.6% since 2005.

d. The proportion of injuries due to sports has decreased over time while the proportion of injuries due to falls has increased.

IV. Statistics (NSCISC, 2012)

a. Morbidity: Approximately 12,000 new cases annually and estimated 270,000 individuals living with SCI in 2012; primarily (about 53%) affects adolescents or young adults (aged 16 to 30); however, since 2005, average age of injury has increased to 41 years (may reflect injury to a higher number of persons over 60 and war-related injury statistics); 80.6% are males.

b. Mortality: Rates significantly higher during first year after injury due to pneumonia, pulmonary emboli, sepsis; subsequently, death often related to treatable health problems, such as with cardiovascular and respiratory diseases or diabetes mellitus.

c. Cost: SCI costs are estimated to be $9.7 billion annually in the United States. Reported yearly recurring costs range from $27,568 for paraplegia to $54,400 for low tetraplegia (C5–C8) and up to $132,807 for high tetraplegia (C1– C4) (French, 2007).

GLOSSARY

Alignment: Generally refers to objects being in a straight line or being positioned appropriately in relation to each other. After a spinal injury, the vertebrae may become shifted from their normal position, becoming misaligned. Various forms of surgical or nonsurgical treatment may be required to realign the vertebrae.

Allodynia: Pain caused by something that does not normally cause pain; for example, something cold, warm, or a very light touch to the skin can result in pain.

Atelectasis: Incomplete expansion of a portion of the lung or the whole lung secondary to decreased vital capacity and decreased functional residual capacity due to SCI with dysfunction of respiratory muscles.

Autonomic dysreflexia (AD): Potential complication of SCI; an exaggerated response of the nervous system to a specific trigger, such as an overfull bladder, that occurs because the brain is no longer able to control the body's response to the trigger.

GLOSSARY (continued)

This response leads to a rapid increase in the body's blood pressure, severe headache, and sweating.

Axon: The long, threadlike outgrowth and extension of a nerve cell that carries messages away from the main part of the cell; also referred to as nerve fibers.

Bowel program: The routine that a person uses with regard to emptying his or her bowels.

Cervical vertebrae: The cervical (neck) vertebrae are the upper seven vertebrae in the spinal column, designated C1 through C7 from the top down.

Compression: The act of pressing together, as in a compression fracture, nerve compression, or spinal cord compression.

Flaccid paralysis: Weakness or loss of muscle tone resulting from injury to the nerves innervating the muscles.

Hyperalgesia: An extremely painful response to what is normally only mildly painful.

Hyperextension injury: Occurs when person is struck from behind, or falls striking chin, resulting in a sudden acceleration forward, followed by sudden deceleration.

Hyperflexion injury: Occurs when head is suddenly and forcefully accelerated forward, causing extreme flexion of the neck.

Intercostal muscles: Several groups of muscles that run between the ribs and help form and move the chest wall.

Lumbar vertebrae: The five lumbar vertebrae are situated between the thoracic vertebrae and the sacral vertebrae in the spinal column and are designated as L1 through L5.

Motor: Refers to the activity of the nerves (motor nerves) that send messages away from the brain and spinal cord.

Neurogenic: Starting with or having to do with the nerves or the nervous system, as in neurogenic bladder or bowel, neurogenic shock.

Paralytic ileus: Buildup of pressure in the small intestine that can occur in the early stages after an SCI. Symptoms include absence of normal bowel sounds and visible swelling of the abdomen. It can cause vomiting or force the stomach contents up into the airways.

Paraplegia: Paralysis of the lower part of the body, including the legs.

Phrenic nerve: Nerve that governs movement of the diaphragm during breathing.

Quadriplegia: Complete or incomplete paralysis from the neck downward, affecting all four limbs and the trunk as a result of damage to the spinal cord between C1 and C8. Also called tetraplegia.

Sensory: Relating to sensation, to the perception of a stimulus and the voyage made by incoming (afferent) nerve impulses from the sense organs to the nerve centers.

Spasticity: State of increased tone of a muscle and an increase in the deep tendon reflexes.

Spinal shock: A period of time after an SCI lasting up to 6 weeks when the area around the damaged cord is bruised and swollen. During this time, no messages can pass through the spinal cord below the level of injury, making the loss of function below the injury appear complete. Only when the swelling subsides does the true extent of the damage become clear.

Tetraplegia: Complete or incomplete paralysis from the neck downward, affecting all four limbs and the trunk as a result of damage to the spinal cord between C1 and C8. Also called quadriplegia.

Thoracic vertebrae: The 12 thoracic vertebrae are situated between the cervical (neck) vertebrae and the lumbar vertebrae. The thoracic vertebrae are designated as T1 through T12.

Care Setting

Client is treated in inpatient medical-surgical, subacute, and rehabilitation units.

Related Concerns

Disc surgery, page 237
Fractures, page 601
Pneumonia, page 129
Psychosocial aspects of care, page 729
Thrombophlebitis: venous thromboembolism (including pulmonary emboli considerations), page 109
Total nutritional support: parenteral/enteral feeding, page 437
Upper gastrointestinal/esophageal bleeding, page 281
Ventilatory assistance (mechanical), page 157

Client Assessment Database

Dependent on level of injury.

DIAGNOSTIC DIVISION MAY REPORT	MAY EXHIBIT
ACTIVITY/REST	
	• Paralysis of muscles—flaccid during spinal shock—at or below level of lesion • Muscle or generalized weakness—cord contusion and compression

(continues on page 250)

DIAGNOSTIC DIVISION MAY REPORT (continued)	MAY EXHIBIT (continued)
CIRCULATION	
• Palpitations • Dizziness with position changes	• Low blood pressure (BP) • Postural BP changes, orthostatic hypotension • Tachycardia • Chronic bradycardia—lesions T6 and above • Cool, pale extremities • Absence of perspiration in affected area
ELIMINATION	
	• Bladder and bowel incontinence • Urinary retention • Abdominal distention • Loss of bowel sounds • Melena, coffee-ground emesis or hematemesis
EGO INTEGRITY	
• Denial, disbelief • Sadness, anger	• Fear • Anxiety • Irritability, restlessness • Withdrawal
FOOD/FLUID	
	• Abdominal distention • Loss of bowel sounds—paralytic ileus
HYGIENE	
	• Variable level of dependence in ADLs
NEUROSENSORY	
• Absence of sensation below area of injury or opposite side sensation • Numbness, tingling, burning, twitching of arms or legs	• Flaccid paralysis—spasticity may develop as spinal shock resolves, depending on area of cord involvement. • Loss of sensation—varying degrees may return after spinal shock resolves. • Loss of muscle or vasomotor tone and motor function • Loss of or asymmetrical reflexes, including deep tendon reflexes • Changes in pupil reaction, ptosis of upper eyelid • Loss of sweating in affected area
PAIN/DISCOMFORT	
• Pain or tenderness in muscles • Hyperesthesia immediately above level of injury	• Vertebral tenderness, deformity
RESPIRATION	
• Shortness of breath, "air hunger," inability to breathe	• Shallow or labored respirations • Increased work of breathing and use of accessory muscles • Poor chest wall expansion • Periods of apnea • Diminished breath sounds, rhonchi • Pallor, cyanosis • Decreased coughing
SAFETY	
	• Temperature fluctuations, taking on temperature of environment
SEXUALITY	
• Expressions of concern about return to normal functioning	• Uncontrolled erection (priapism) • Menstrual irregularities

DIAGNOSTIC DIVISION MAY REPORT (continued)	MAY EXHIBIT (continued)
TEACHING/LEARNING	
DISCHARGE PLAN CONSIDERATIONS • Will require varying degrees of assistance with transportation, shopping, food preparation, self-care, finances, medications or treatment, and homemaker and maintenance tasks • May require changes in physical layout of home or placement in a rehabilitative center ➧ Refer to section at end of plan for postdischarge considerations.	

Diagnostic Studies

TEST WHY IT IS DONE	WHAT IT TELLS ME
PRIMARY DIAGNOSTIC STUDIES	
• ***Spinal x-rays:*** The most important diagnostic measure to locate the level and type of bony injury (fracture, dislocation). Determines alignment and reduction after traction or surgery.	Lateral x-rays of the neck can usually detect significant cervical injuries.
• ***Computerized tomography (CT) scan (also known as computerized axial tomography or CAT scan):*** Imaging procedure that uses a combination of x-rays and computer technology to produce cross-sectional images of the body.	Provides images of the fracture, spinal cord edema, and compression.
• ***Magnetic resonance imaging (MRI) scan:*** Noninvasive method of obtaining images of internal soft tissue, such as the spinal cord, through the use of powerful magnets and radio waves.	Can show bruising and other soft tissue damage (such as spinal cord hematoma, hemorrhage or edema, ligament injuries) that might not show up in other studies.
ANCILLARY TESTS	
• ***Arterial blood gases (ABGs):*** Monitors effectiveness of gas exchange and ventilatory effort.	Abnormalities may be present, depending on level of SCI and limitation of chest expansion and muscle involvement.
• ***Pulmonary function studies, such as vital capacity (VC) and tidal volume (VT):*** Measures maximum volume of inspiration and expiration.	Test could be important in client with low cervical lesions, when making decisions about ventilator needs; or in client with thoracic lesions with possible phrenic nerve and intercostal muscle involvement.
• ***Chest x-ray:*** Procedure used to evaluate organs and structures within the chest.	Evaluates for lung injury, such as pneumothorax, or complications associated with SCI, such as atelectasis and pneumonia or changes in level of diaphragm reflecting respiratory muscle paralysis.

Nursing Priorities

1. Maximize respiratory function.
2. Prevent further injury to spinal cord.
3. Promote mobility and independence.
4. Prevent or minimize complications.
5. Support psychological adjustment of client and significant other (SO).
6. Provide information about injury, prognosis and expectations, treatment needs, and possible and preventable complications.

Discharge Goals

1. Ventilatory effort adequate for individual needs.
2. Spinal injury stabilized.
3. Complications prevented or controlled.
4. Self-care needs met by self and with assistance, depending on specific situation.
5. Beginning to cope with current situation and planning for future.
6. Condition, prognosis, therapeutic regimen, and possible complications understood.
7. Plan in place to meet needs after discharge.

NURSING DIAGNOSIS: risk for ineffective Breathing Pattern

Risk Factors May Include

Spinal cord injury

Respiratory muscle fatigue

Possibly Evidenced By

(Not applicable; presence of signs and symptoms establishes an *actual* diagnosis)

Desired Outcomes/Evaluation Criteria—Client Will

Respiratory Status: Ventilation (NOC)

Maintain adequate ventilation as evidenced by absence of respiratory distress and ABGs within acceptable limits and pulse oximetry maintained at 90% or greater.

Demonstrate appropriate behaviors to support respiratory effort.

ACTIONS/INTERVENTIONS	RATIONALE
Respiratory Monitoring (NIC)	
Independent	
Note client's level of injury when assessing respiratory function. Note presence or absence of spontaneous effort and quality of respirations—labored, using accessory muscles.	C1 to C3 injuries result in complete loss of respiratory function. Injuries at C4 or C5 can result in variable loss of respiratory function, depending on phrenic nerve involvement and diaphragmatic function, but generally cause decreased vital capacity and inspiratory effort. For injuries below C6 or C7, respiratory muscle function is preserved; however, weakness and impairment of intercostal muscles may reduce effectiveness of cough, ability to sigh, and deep breaths.
Auscultate breath sounds. Note areas of absent or decreased breath sounds or development of adventitious sounds, such as rhonchi.	Hypoventilation is common and leads to accumulation of secretions, atelectasis, and pneumonia—frequent complications. *Note:* Respiratory complications are among the leading causes of mortality, not only during the acute stage but also later in life.
Note strength and effectiveness of cough.	Level of injury determines function of intercostal muscles and ability to cough spontaneously and move secretions. High-level paraplegics and all tetraplegics lose the ability to cough and are at greatest risk of developing atelectasis and respiratory failure.
Observe skin color for developing cyanosis or duskiness.	Skin color may reveal impending respiratory failure and need for immediate medical evaluation and intervention.
Assess for abdominal distention and muscle spasm.	Abdominal fullness may impede diaphragmatic excursion, thus reducing lung expansion and further compromising respiratory function.
Monitor and limit visitors, as indicated.	General debilitation and respiratory compromise place client at increased risk for acquiring upper respiratory infections (URIs).
Elicit concerns or questions regarding mechanical ventilation devices.	Open discussion acknowledges reality of situation. (Refer to CP: Ventilatory Assistance [Mechanical].)
Provide honest answers.	Future respiratory function and support needs will not be totally known until spinal shock resolves and acute rehabilitative phase is completed. Even though respiratory support may be required, alternative devices and techniques may be used to enhance mobility and promote independence.
Maintain open airway: keep head in neutral position, elevate head of bed slightly if tolerated, and use airway adjuncts, as indicated.	Client with high cervical injury and impaired gag or cough reflex requires assistance in preventing aspiration and maintaining patent airway.
Assist client in "taking control" of respirations as indicated. Encourage deep breathing. Focus attention on the steps of breathing.	Breathing may no longer be an involuntary activity but require conscious effort, depending on level of injury or involvement of respiratory muscles.
Assist with coughing, as indicated for level of injury; for example, have client take a deep breath, hold for 2 seconds before coughing, or inhale deeply, then cough at the end of a slow exhalation. Alternatively, assist by placing hands below diaphragm and pushing upward as client exhales ("quad cough").	Assisted coughing facilitates mobilization of respiratory secretions. *Note:* Quad cough procedure is generally reserved for clients with stable injuries once they are in the rehabilitation stage.
Suction as necessary. Monitor pulse oximetry and heart rate during suctioning. Document quality and quantity of secretions.	Suctioning facilitates removal of respiratory secretions. Routine suctioning increases the risk for bradycardia (heart rate less than 60 beats per minute) and hypoxia, especially with tetraplegia.

ACTIONS/INTERVENTIONS (continued)	RATIONALE (continued)
Reposition and turn periodically. Avoid or limit prone position, as indicated.	Repositioning enhances ventilation of all lung segments and mobilizes secretions. It helps reduce the risks of complications such as atelectasis and pneumonia. *Note:* Prone position significantly decreases vital capacity and increases risk of respiratory compromise and failure.
Provide fluids—at least 1500 to 2000 mL/day, within cardiac tolerance.	Promotes mobilization of secretions.
Collaborative	
Measure and graph:	
Vital capacity (VC), total lung volumes (VT), and inspiratory force	Determines level of respiratory muscle function. Serial measurements may predict impending respiratory failure (acute injury) or determine level of function after spinal shock phase or while weaning from ventilatory support.
Serial ABGs and pulse oximetry	Documents status of ventilation and oxygenation and identifies respiratory problems, such as hypoventilation, hypoxia, acidosis, among others.
Airway Management (NIC)	
Administer oxygen by appropriate method: nasal prongs, mask, intubation, and ventilator.	Oxygen delivery methods are determined by level of injury, degree of respiratory insufficiency, and respiratory muscle function after spinal shock phase.
Assist with use of respiratory adjuncts, such as incentive spirometer or blow bottles, and aggressive chest physiotherapy, such as chest percussion.	Preventing retained secretions is essential to maximize gas diffusion and to reduce risk of pneumonia.
Refer to or consult with respiratory and physical therapists.	Collaboration with respiratory and physical therapists helps identify appropriate therapies that could optimize respiratory function. For example, glossopharyngeal breathing uses muscles of mouth, pharynx, and larynx to swallow air into lungs, thereby increasing vital capicity and chest expansion.

NURSING DIAGNOSIS: risk for [additional spinal] Injury

Risk Factors May Include

Physical (e.g., temporary weakness and instability of spinal column)

Possibly Evidenced By

(Not applicable; presence of signs and symptoms establishes an *actual* diagnosis)

Desired Outcomes/Evaluation Criteria—Client Will

Bone Healing (NOC)

Maintain proper alignment of spine without further spinal cord damage.

ACTIONS/INTERVENTIONS	RATIONALE
Traction/Immobilization Care (NIC)	
Independent	
Maintain bedrest and immobilization device(s)—sandbags, traction, tongs, halo, traction devices; hard or soft cervical collars; vest or brace.	Alignment and stabilization is needed to provide neural decompression of the spinal cord or spinal nerves. *Note:* Traction is used only for cervical spine stabilization.
If traction is used:	
Elevate head of traction frame or bed as indicated. Ensure that traction frames are secured, pulleys are aligned, and weights are hanging free.	Creates safe, effective counterbalance to maintain both client's alignment and proper traction pull.
Check weights for ordered traction pull (usually 10 to 20 lb).	Weight pull depends on client's size and amount of reduction needed to maintain vertebral column alignment.
Reposition at intervals, using adjuncts for turning and support—turn sheets, foam wedges, blanket rolls, and pillows. Use several staff members when turning or logrolling client. Follow special instructions for traction equipment, kinetic bed, and frames once halo is in place.	The use of adjuncts for turning and support maintains proper spinal column alignment and thus reduces the risk of further trauma. *Note:* Grasping the brace or halo vest to turn or reposition client may cause additional injury.
Collaborative	
Prepare for internal stabilization surgery, such as spinal laminectomy or fusion, if indicated.	Surgery may be indicated for vertebral stabilization, spinal cord decompression, nerve decompression, and/or removal of bony fragments.

(continues on page 254)

ACTIONS/INTERVENTIONS (continued)	RATIONALE (continued)
Administer medications as indicated, such as methylprednisolone (Depo-Medrol).	The use of corticosteroids in early treatment to reduce spinal cord edema has long been controversial. Although many national organizations are now changing their recommendations to include this therapy for the improvement of neurological outcome, they are not requiring it, suggesting that its benefits be weighed against the client's potential for developing sepsis (NINDS, 2012).

NURSING DIAGNOSIS: impaired physical Mobility

May Be Related To

Neuromuscular impairment; decreased muscle strength or control
Loss of integrity of bone structure; [immobilization by traction]

Possibly Evidenced By

Limited range of motion; limited ability to perform gross or fine motor skills
Postural instability; difficulty turning

Desired Outcomes/Evaluation Criteria—Client Will

Immobility Consequences: Physiological (NOC)
Maintain position of function as evidenced by absence of contractures and footdrop.

Neurological Status: Spinal Sensory/Motor Function (NOC)
Increase strength of unaffected and compensatory body parts.
Demonstrate techniques or behaviors that enable resumption of activity.

ACTIONS/INTERVENTIONS	RATIONALE
Bed Rest Care (NIC) *Independent*	
Continually assess motor function, as spinal shock and spinal cord edema resolves, by requesting client to perform certain actions, such as shrug shoulders, spread fingers, and squeeze and release examiner's hands.	Continuous motor function assessment helps determine appropriate interventions for the specific motor impairment.
Provide means to summon help, such as special sensitive call light.	Promotes the client's sense of control and reduces fear of being left alone. *Note:* Ventilator-dependent tetraplegic client may require continuous observation for timely interventions.
Perform or assist with full range of motion (ROM) exercises on all extremities using slow, smooth movements. Include periodic hip hyperextension.	ROM exercises enhance circulation, restore or maintain muscle tone and joint mobility, and prevent disuse contractures and muscle atrophy.
Position arms at 90-degree angle for a period of time and at regular intervals.	Appropriate joint positioning prevents frozen shoulder contractures.
Maintain ankles at 90 degrees with footboard. Use high-top tennis shoes. Place trochanter rolls along thighs when in bed.	These measures prevent external rotation of the hip and footdrop.
Elevate lower extremities at regular intervals when seated. Raise foot of the bed when supine, as appropriate. Assess for edema of ankles and feet.	Loss of vascular tone and "muscle action" results in pooling of blood and venous stasis in the lower abdomen and lower extremities, with increased risk of hypotension and thrombus formation. Positioning and frequent assessment is needed to prevent associated complications.
Space periods of rest and activity. Provide uninterrupted rest periods. Encourage client involvement.	Adequate rest and optimal activity prevent fatigue and allows opportunity for maximal efforts and active client participation.
Monitor BP before and after activity in acute phases or until stable. Change position slowly. Use cardiac bed or tilt table or other specialized bed as activity level is advanced.	The loss of sympathetic innervations especially in T6 and higher SCI causes loss of vascular tone, resulting in hypotension and venous pooling. Side-to-side movement or elevation of head can aggravate hypotension and cause syncope.
Reposition periodically even when sitting in chair. Teach client how to use weight-shifting techniques.	Repositioning and weight shifts reduce pressure areas and promote peripheral circulation.
Prepare for weight-bearing activities, such as use of tilt table for upright position and strengthening and conditioning exercises for unaffected body parts.	Early weight bearing reduces osteoporotic changes in long bones and reduces incidence of urinary infections and kidney stones. *Note:* Fifty percent of clients develop heterotopic ossification that can lead to pain and decreased joint flexibility.

ACTIONS/INTERVENTIONS (continued)	RATIONALE (continued)
Encourage use of relaxation techniques.	Relaxation techniques reduce muscle tension and fatigue and may help limit pain of muscle spasms and spasticity.
Inspect skin daily. Observe for pressure areas. Provide meticulous skin care. Teach client to inspect skin surfaces and to use a mirror to look at hard-to-see areas.	Altered circulation, loss of sensation, and paralysis potentiate pressure sore formation. This is a lifelong consideration. (Refer to ND: risk for impaired Skin Integrity.)
Provide, assist with pulmonary hygiene by deep breathing, coughing, and suctioning. (Refer to ND: risk for ineffective Breathing Pattern.)	Immobility and bedrest increase the risk of pulmonary infection.
Assess for redness, swelling, and muscle tension of calf tissues. Record calf and thigh measurements, as indicated.	A high percentage of clients with SCI develop thrombi because of altered peripheral circulation, immobilization, and flaccid paralysis. Refer to CP: Thrombophlebitis: Deep Vain Thrombosis, including Pulmonary Emboli Considerations for related interventions.
Investigate sudden onset of dyspnea, cyanosis, and other signs of respiratory distress.	Development of pulmonary emboli may be "silent" because pain perception is altered or deep vein thrombosis (DVT) is not readily recognized.
Collaborative	
Place client in kinetic therapy bed when appropriate.	Kinetic therapy beds effectively immobilize unstable spinal column and improve systemic circulation. They are thought to decrease complications associated with immobility; however, some research associates kinetic therapy beds with increased rates of infection and respiratory complications in persons with thoracic cord injuries (Chipman, 2006).
Apply anti-embolic hose, leotard, or sequential compression devices (SCDs) to legs, as appropriate.	These devices limit pooling of blood in lower extremities or abdomen, thus improving vasomotor tone and reducing incidence of thrombus formation and pulmonary emboli.
Consult with physical and occupational therapists and rehabilitation team.	Collaboration helps in planning and implementing individualized exercise program. The members of the rehabilitation team identify and develop assistive devices to enhance client's function and overall independence.
Administer medications, as indicated, for example:	
Vasopressors, such as dobutamine (Dobutrex)	Vasopressors may be indicated in acute phase to maintain systolic BP greater than 100 mm Hg. *Note:* The client who requires this level of support will likely be in a critical care unit.
Muscle relaxants and antispasticity agents, as indicated, such as diazepam (Valium), baclofen (Lioresal), and dantrolene (Dantrium)	Muscle relaxants and antispasticity agents may be useful after spinal shock phase in limiting or reducing pain. *Note:* Baclofen may be delivered via implanted intrathecal pump on a long-term basis, as appropriate.
Miscellaneous drugs, e.g., tizanidine (Zanaflex)	Centrally acting α_2-adrenergic agonist reduces spasticity. Short duration of action requires careful dosage monitoring to achieve maximum effect. It may have additive effect with baclofen, but needs to be used with caution because both drugs have similar side effects.

NURSING DIAGNOSIS: [disturbed tactile/proprioception Sensory Perception]

May Be Related To

Altered sensory reception, transmission, or integration
Insufficient environmental stimuli
Psychological stress

Possibly Evidenced By

Change in sensory acuity, sensory distortions
Change in usual response to stimuli
Disorientation

Desired Outcomes/Evaluation Criteria—Client Will

Neurological Status: Spinal Sensory/Motor Function (NOC)

Recognize sensory impairments.

Knowledge: Personal Safety (NOC)

Identify behaviors to compensate for deficits.
Verbalize awareness of sensory needs and potential for deprivation or overload.

ACTIONS/INTERVENTIONS — RATIONALE

Peripheral Sensation Management (NIC)

Independent

Assess and document sensory function or deficit, such as by means of touch, pinprick, or heat and cold, progressing from area of deficit to neurologically intact area.
— Changes may not occur during acute phase, but as spinal shock resolves, dermatome charts or anatomic landmarks should document changes, such as, "2 inches above nipple line."

Protect from bodily harm, such as falls, burns, and improper positioning of body parts.
— The client may not sense pain or be aware of body position.

Assist client to recognize and compensate for alterations in sensation.
— Increased attention to alterations in sensation may help reduce anxiety of the unknown and prevent injury.

Explain procedures before and during care while identifying the involved body part.
— These measures enhance client perception of "whole" body.

Provide tactile stimulation by touching the client in intact sensory areas, such as shoulders, face, and head.
— Touching conveys caring and fulfills normal physiological and psychological needs.

Position client to see surroundings and activities. Provide prism glasses when prone on turning frame. Talk to client frequently.
— These nursing actions provide sensory input, which may be severely limited, especially when client is in prone position.

Provide diversional activities, including television, radio, music, and liberal visitation. Use clocks, calendars, pictures, bulletin boards, and so on. Encourage SO and family to discuss general and personal news.
— The activities aid in maintaining reality orientation and provide some sense of normality in daily passage of time.

Provide uninterrupted sleep and rest periods.
— Adequate sleep and rest reduce sensory overload, enhance orientation and coping abilities, and aid in reestablishing natural sleep patterns.

Note presence of exaggerated emotional responses and altered thought processes, including disorientation and bizarre thinking.
— Exaggerated emotional responses and altered thought processes indicate damage to sensory tracts affecting reception or interpretation of stimuli, or psychological stress, requiring further assessment and intervention.

NURSING DIAGNOSIS: acute Pain

May Be Related To

Physical injury (e.g., damage or dysfunction of nervous system; traction apparatus)

Possibly Evidenced By

Verbal/coded reports
Irritability; restlessness
Self-focus

Desired Outcomes/Evaluation Criteria—Client Will

Pain Control (NOC)

Identify ways to manage pain.
Demonstrate use of relaxation skills and diversional activities as individually indicated.
Report relief or control of pain and discomfort.

ACTIONS/INTERVENTIONS — RATIONALE

Pain Management

Independent

Assess for presence of pain. Help client identify and quantify pain, including location, type of pain, and intensity on a pain-rating scale.
— Pain is a frequent problem in the majority of the SCI population and can occur not only above the level of injury but also at or below the level of injury and in both complete and incomplete injuries. An individual with SCI is likely to experience many types of painful sensations at or below the level of injury that can be troublesome to categorize, making effective treatment difficult. Pain can be neuropathic (resulting from abnormal processing of sensory input); can be due to musculoskeletal disorders caused from injury at the time of SCI; or be associated with organ complications such as ulcers or constipation. Pain can also be "segmental," felt at the level of injury in a bandlike pattern (Turner et al, 2001). Client often reports pain above the level of injury, such as chest, back, or headache, possibly from stabilizer apparatus. After resolution of spinal shock phase, client may also report muscle spasms and radicular pain, described as a

ACTIONS/INTERVENTIONS (continued)	RATIONALE (continued)
	burning or stabbing pain radiating in a dermatomal pattern—associated with injury to peripheral nerves. Onset of this pain is within days to weeks after SCI and may become chronic.
Evaluate increased irritability, muscle tension, restlessness, and unexplained vital sign changes.	Nonverbal cues indicative of pain or discomfort require timely intervention. *Note*: Some people with higher lesions may be unable to show changes in heart rate and blood pressure assessed by the pain score (AHRQ, 2008).
Assist client in identifying precipitating factors.	Burning pain and muscle spasms can be precipitated or aggravated by multiple factors, such as anxiety, tension, external temperature extremes, sitting for long periods, and bladder distention.
Provide comfort measures, such as position changes, massage, ROM exercises, and warm or cold packs, as indicated.	Alternative measures for pain control reduce need for pharmacological agents and provide emotional support.
Encourage use of relaxation techniques, such as guided imagery, visualization, and deep-breathing exercises. Provide diversional activities—television, radio, telephone, and unlimited visitors, as appropriate.	Relaxation and diversional activities refocus attention, promote sense of control, and possibly enhance coping abilities.
Collaborative	
Administer medications, as indicated, for example: muscle relaxants, such as dantrolene (Dantrium) and baclofen (Lioresal); analgesics; anti-anxiety agents, such as alprazalam (Xanax) and diazepam (Valium).	These medications relieve muscle spasm and pain associated with spasticity. They also alleviate anxiety and promote rest.

NURSING DIAGNOSIS: Grieving

May Be Related To

Loss of significant object (e.g., processes of body, job, status)

Possibly Evidenced By

Psychological distress; anger, blame, despair

Disturbed sleep patterns

Desired Outcomes/Evaluation Criteria—Client Will

Grief Resolution (NOC)

Express feelings freely and effectively.

Begin to progress through recognized stages of grief, focusing on 1 day at a time.

ACTIONS/INTERVENTIONS	RATIONALE
Grief Work Facilitation (NIC)	
Independent	
Identify signs of grieving, such as shock, denial, anger, and depression.	Client experiences a wide range of emotional reactions to the injury and its actual and potential impact on life. These stages are not static, and the rate at which client progresses through them is variable.
Shock:	
Note lack of communication or emotional response and absence of questions.	Shock is the initial reaction associated with overwhelming injury. Primary concern is to maintain life. The client may be too ill to express feelings.
Provide simple, accurate information to client and SO regarding diagnosis and care. Be honest; do not give false reassurance while providing emotional support.	Client's awareness of surroundings and activity may be blocked initially, and attention span may be limited. Little is actually known about the outcome of client's injuries during acute phase, and lack of knowledge may add to frustration and grief of family. Therefore, early focus of emotional support may be directed toward SO.
Encourage expressions of sadness, grief, guilt, and fear among client, SO, and friends.	Acknowledging client and SO feelings and encouraging expression could provide appropriate support.
Incorporate SO into problem-solving and planning for client's care.	Shared clinical decision making with the client and SO establishes therapeutic relationships and provides sense of control of the management of current health situation and the subsequent changes.

(continues on page 258)

ACTIONS/INTERVENTIONS	RATIONALE
Denial:	
Assist client and SO to verbalize feelings about situation. Avoid judgment about what is expressed.	Important beginning step to deal with what has happened. Helpful in identifying client's coping mechanisms.
Note comments indicating unrealistic outcomes and bargaining with God. Do not confront these comments in early phases of rehabilitation.	Denial may be a useful coping mechanism during the early phases of rehabilitation. Client may accept disability but may deny uncertainty and permanency of limitations.
Focus on present needs—ROM exercises, skin care, and so on.	Attention on "here and now" reduces frustration and hopelessness of uncertain future and may make dealing with today's problems more manageable.
Anger:	
Identify use of manipulative behavior and reactions to caregivers.	Client may demonstrate manipulative behaviors like spitting, biting, or even pitting caregivers against each other to express anger.
Encourage client to take control when possible—establishing care routines, dietary choices, diversional activities, and so forth.	Encouraging client participation provides a sense of control and responsibility as well as reduces sense of powerlessness.
Accept expressions of anger and hopelessness, such as "let me die." Avoid arguing. Show concern for client.	Nonjudgmental communication of empathy and compassion helps the client regain sense of worth.
Set limits on acting out and unacceptable behaviors when necessary, including abusive language, sexually aggressive or suggestive behavior.	Although it is important to express negative feelings, client and staff need to be protected from violence and embarrassment. Acting out is traumatic for all involved.
Depression:	
Note loss of interest in living, sleep disturbance, suicidal thoughts, and hopelessness. Listen to, but do not confront, these expressions. Let client know nurse is available for support.	Depression may last for weeks, months, or years. Acceptance and support are critical in facilitating resolution. The client may need psychological counseling.
Arrange visit by individual similarly affected, as appropriate.	Talking with another person who has shared similar feelings and fears and survived may help client reach acceptance of reality of condition and deal with perceived and actual losses.
Collaborative	
Consult with and refer to psychiatric nurse, social worker, psychiatrist, and pastor.	Client and SO need assistance to work through feelings of alienation, guilt, and resentment concerning lifestyle and role changes. The family required to make adaptive changes to a member who may be permanently "different" benefits from supportive, long-term assistance and counseling in coping with these changes and the future. Client and SO may suffer great spiritual distress, including feelings of guilt, deprivation of peace, and anger at God, which may interfere with progression through, and resolution of, grief process.

NURSING DIAGNOSIS: situational low Self-Esteem

May Be Related To
Functional impairment; disturbed body image
Loss; social role changes

Possibly Evidenced By
Self-negating verbalizations
Reports uselessness, helplessness
Evaluation of self as unable to deal with situation

Desired Outcomes/Evaluation Criteria—Client Will

Psychosocial Adjustment: Life Change (NOC)
Verbalize acceptance of self in situation.
Recognize and incorporate changes into self-concept in accurate manner without negating self-esteem.
Develop realistic plans for adapting to role changes and new role.

ACTIONS/INTERVENTIONS	RATIONALE
Self-Esteem Enhancement (NIC)	
Independent	
Acknowledge difficulty in determining degree of functional incapacity and chance of functional improvement.	During acute phase of injury, long-term effects are unknown, which delays the client's ability to integrate situation into self-concept.
Listen to client's comments and responses to situation.	Active listening provides clues to client's view of self, role changes, needs, and level of acceptance.
Assess dynamics of client and SOs, including client's role in family and cultural factors.	Client's previous role in family unit is disrupted or altered by injury. Role changes add difficulty in integrating self-concept and level of independence. A person's culture affects role perceptions and performance in the family and community.
Encourage SO to treat client as normally as possible, such as discussing home situations and family news.	Involving client in family unit reduces feelings of social isolation, helplessness, and uselessness and provides opportunity for SO to contribute to client's welfare.
Provide accurate information. Discuss concerns about prognosis and treatment honestly at client's level of acceptance.	Open discussion of treatment and prognosis may focus on current and immediate needs. Ongoing updates enable assimilation.
Discuss meaning of loss or change with client and SO. Assess interactions between client and SO.	Actual change in body image may be different from that perceived by client. Distortions may be unconsciously reinforced by SO.
Accept client and show concern for individual as a person. Identify and build on client's strengths; give positive reinforcement for progress noted.	Genuine concern and regard for the client as an individual establishes therapeutic atmosphere for self-acceptance and encouragement.
Include client and SO in care, allowing client to make decisions and participate in self-care activities, as possible.	Encouraging client participation in care decision making recognizes that client is still responsible for own life and provides some sense of control over situation. It sets the stage for future lifestyle, pattern, and interaction required in daily care. *Note:* Client may reject all help or may be completely dependent during this phase.
Be alert to sexually oriented jokes, flirting, or aggressive behavior. Elicit concerns, fears, and feelings about current situation and future expectations.	Anxiety develops because of perceived loss and change in masculine or feminine self-image and role. Forced dependency is often devastating, especially in light of change in function and appearance.
Be aware of own feelings and reaction to client's sexual anxiety.	Personal reactions to client's sexual anxiety may be as disruptive as the behavior itself, creating conflicts between client and staff, and can potentially eliminate client's willingness to work through situation and participate in rehabilitation.
Arrange visit by similarly affected person, if client desires and situation allows.	Support groups can provide hope and potential future role model. They can be vital resources during difficulties after discharge.
Collaborative	
Refer to counseling or psychotherapy as indicated—psychiatric clinical nurse specialist, psychiatrist, social worker, or sex therapist.	The client may need additional assistance to adjust to change in body image and lifestyle.

NURSING DIAGNOSIS: bowel Incontinence/Constipation

May Be Related To

Neurological impairment; loss of rectal sphincter control; upper or lower motor nerve damage
Abdominal muscle weakness
Change in usual foods or eating patterns; insufficient fiber or fluid intake
Medications

Possibly Evidenced By

Change in bowel pattern, characteristics of stool
Reports inability to feel rectal fullness or recognize urge to defecate
Changes in bowel sounds

Desired Outcomes/Evaluation Criteria—Client Will

Bowel Continence (NOC)

Verbalize behaviors and techniques for individual bowel program.
Reestablish satisfactory bowel elimination pattern.

ACTIONS/INTERVENTIONS	RATIONALE
Bowel Management (NIC)	
Independent	
Auscultate bowel sounds, noting location and characteristics.	Bowel sounds may be absent during spinal shock phase. High tinkling sounds may indicate presence of ileus.
Observe for abdominal distention if bowel sounds are decreased or absent.	Impaired innervation causes paralysis of the bowel (ileus) and bowel distention. *Note:* Overdistention of the bowel is a trigger for AD, once spinal shock subsides. (Refer to ND: risk for Autonomic Dysreflexia.)
Note reports of nausea and onset of vomiting. Check vomitus or gastric secretions (if tube in place) and stools for occult blood.	Gastrointestinal (GI) bleeding may occur in response to injury (Curling's ulcer) or as a side effect of certain therapies—steroids or anticoagulants.
Record frequency, characteristics, and amount of stool.	Assessment of bowel movement helps identify degree of impairment or dysfunction and required level of assistance.
Recognize signs of fecal impaction—no formed stool for several days, semiliquid stool, restlessness, increased feelings of fullness in or distention of abdomen, presence of nausea, vomiting, and possibly urinary retention.	Early intervention is necessary to effectively treat constipation or retained stool and reduce risk of further complications.
Establish regular daily bowel program—digital stimulation, prune juice and warm beverage, and use of stool softeners or suppositories at set intervals. Determine a routine of bowel evacuation.	A lifelong routine bowel program is necessary to control bowel evacuation. Bowel program is important to the client's physical independence and social acceptance. *Note:* Bowel movements in clients with upper motor neuron damage are generally regulated with suppositories or digital stimulation. Lower motor neurogenic bowel is more difficult to regulate and usually requires manual disimpaction. Incorporating elements of client's usual routine may enhance cooperation and success of program. *Note:* Many clients prefer morning program rather than evening schedule often practiced in acute and rehabilitation setting.
Encourage well-balanced diet that includes bulk and roughage and increased fluid intake at least 1500 to 2000 mL/day, including fruit juices.	High fiber and fluid intake improve consistency of stool for transit through the bowel. *Note:* Over-the-counter (OTC) fiber products and cereals, prune juice, applesauce, and bran often provide adequate fiber for effective bowel management.
Observe for incontinence and help client relate incontinence to change in diet or routine.	Client can eventually achieve normal routine bowel habits, which enhance independence, self-esteem, and socialization.
Restrict intake of caffeinated beverages, such as coffee, tea, colas, or energy drinks, if indicated.	Diuretic effect of caffeine can reduce fluid available in the bowel, thus increasing the risk of dry, hard-formed stool.
Provide meticulous skin care.	Loss of sphincter control and innervation in the area potentiates risk of skin irritation and breakdown.
Collaborative	
Insert and maintain nasogastric (NG) tube and attach to suction if appropriate.	The NG tube may be used initially to reduce gastric distention and prevent vomiting.
Consult with dietitian or nutritional support team.	Dietary support team aids in creating dietary plan to meet nutritional needs based on digestive and bowel function.
Administer medications, as indicated:	
Stool softeners, laxatives, suppositories, enemas, such as Therevac-SB	Stool softeners, laxatives, suppositories, and enemas stimulate peristalsis and routine bowel evacuation. Suppositories should be warmed to room temperature and lubricated before insertion. Therevac-SB is a 4 mL enema of docusate and glycerin that may reduce time for bowel care by as much as 1 hour.
Antacids and histamine H_2 antagonists, such as cimetidine (Tagamet) and ranitidine (Zantac)	Antacids and histamine antagonists neutralize gastric acid to lessen gastric irritation and risk of bleeding.

NURSING DIAGNOSIS: impaired Urinary Elimination

May Be Related To

Sensory motor impairment

Urinary tract infection (UTIs)

Possibly Evidenced By

Incontinence

Retention

NURSING DIAGNOSIS: **impaired Urinary Elimination** (continued)

Desired Outcomes/Evaluation Criteria—Client Will

Urinary Continence (NOC)
Verbalize understanding of condition.
Maintain balanced intake and output (I&O), with clear, odor-free urine; free of bladder distention or urinary leakage.
Verbalize or demonstrate behaviors and techniques to prevent retention and urinary infection.

ACTIONS/INTERVENTIONS	RATIONALE
Urinary Elimination Management (NIC)	
Independent	
Assess voiding pattern, including frequency and amount. Compare urine output with fluid intake. Note specific gravity.	Voiding pattern identifies characteristics of bladder function, including effectiveness of bladder emptying, renal function, and fluid balance. *Note:* Urinary complications are a major cause of mortality. Multiple complications can occur when normal innervation to the bladder and urinary sphincter is impaired by urinary incontinence, UTI, upper urinary tract distress, urinary calculi, AD, and bladder cancer (Fonte & Moore, 2008).
Palpate for bladder distention and observe for overflow.	Bladder dysfunction is variable but may include loss of bladder contraction and inability to relax urinary sphincter, resulting in urine retention and reflux incontinence. *Note:* Bladder distention can precipitate AD. (Refer to ND: risk for Autonomic Dysreflexia, following.)
Encourage fluid intake of 1500 to 2000 mL/day, including acid ash juices such as cranberry.	Adequate fluid intake helps maintain renal function. It is thought that fluids (including cranberry juice) can reduce risk of infection by decreasing ability of bacteria to adhere to bladder wall (Santillo & Lowe, 2007). *Note:* Fluid may be restricted for a period during initiation of intermittent catheterization.
Begin bladder retraining per protocol when appropriate, with fluids between certain hours, digital stimulation of trigger area, contraction of abdominal muscles, and so forth.	Timing and type of bladder program depends on type of injury—upper or lower neuron involvement. *Note:* Bladder expression using the Credé maneuver (pushing on the abdomen to forcefully express urine) is included in some programs in an attempt to promote continence and ensure adequate bladder evacuation. Research suggests this maneuver raises intravesical pressures against a closed bladder outlet, raising the risk of vesicoureteral reflux, hernia, rectogenital prolapse, and hemorrhoids (Rigby, 2005).
Observe for changes in urine characteristics—cloudy, bloody, foul odor, and so forth. Test urine with dipstick, as indicated.	Changes in urine characteristics may indicate UTI and increased risk of sepsis. Multistrip dipsticks can provide a quick determination of pH, nitrite, and leukocyte esterase that suggest presence of infection or urinary disease. *Note:* Presence of bacteria in urine is not uncommon if client has indwelling catheter or performs intermittent catheterization. If bacteria are present, the client must be assessed for other signs of developing UTI, and medications may be indicated (Rigby, 2005).
Cleanse perineal area and keep dry. Provide catheter care, as appropriate.	Perineal care decreases risk of skin irritation, breakdown, and development of ascending infection.
Collaborative	
Monitor blood urea nitrogen/creatinine (BUN/Cr), white blood cell (WBC) count, and urinalysis (UA).	These laboratory tests reflect renal function and identify complications.
Administer vitamin C or urinary antiseptics, such as methenamine mandelate (Mandelamine), as indicated.	These medications maintain acidic environment and prevent bacterial growth.
Refer for further evaluation for bladder and bowel stimulation.	Promising clinical research is being conducted on the technology of electronic bladder control. The implantable device sends electrical signals to the spinal nerves that control the bladder and bowel, creating improved bladder capacity and compliance (Vignes, 2003).
Urinary Catheterization (NIC)	
Keep bladder empty by means of indwelling catheter initially. Determine post-void residuals then consider intermittent catheterization program, as appropriate.	Bladder scans are useful in determining post-void residuals. During the acute phase, an indwelling catheter is used to prevent urinary retention and to monitor urinary output. Intermittent

(continues on page 262)

ACTIONS/INTERVENTIONS	RATIONALE
	catheterization may be implemented to reduce complications associated with long-term use of indwelling catheters. A suprapubic catheter may also be inserted for long-term management.
Measure residual urine via post-void catheterization, bladder scan, or ultrasound.	Measuring post-void residual is helpful in detecting urinary retention and effectiveness of bladder training program. *Note:* Use of ultrasound is noninvasive and reduces the risk of bladder colonization.

NURSING DIAGNOSIS: risk for impaired Skin/Tissue Integrity

Risk Factors May Include

Impaired circulation or sensation
Mechanical factors (e.g., pressure, shearing forces)
Impaired physical mobility/immobilization (traction apparatus)
Nutritional factors (e.g., deficit or excess)

Possibly Evidenced By

(Not applicable; presence of signs and symptoms establishes an *actual* diagnosis)

Desired Outcomes/Evaluation Criteria—Client Will

Risk Control (NOC)

Identify individual risk factors.
Verbalize understanding of treatment needs.
Participate to level of ability to prevent skin breakdown.

ACTIONS/INTERVENTIONS	RATIONALE
Skin Surveillance (NIC)	
Independent	
Inspect all skin areas, noting capillary blanching and refill, redness, and swelling. Pay particular attention to back of head, skin under halo frame or vest, and folds where skin continuously touches.	Skin is especially prone to breakdown because of changes in peripheral circulation, inability to sense pressure, immobility, and altered temperature regulation.
Observe halo and tong insertion sites. Note swelling, redness, and drainage.	These sites are prone to inflammation and infection and provide route for pathological microorganisms to enter cranial cavity. *Note:* New style of halo frame does not require screws or pins.
Encourage continuation of regular exercise program.	Exercise stimulates circulation that enhances cellular nutrition and oxygenation.
Elevate lower extremities periodically, if tolerated.	Elevation of lower extremities enhances venous return and reduces edema formation.
Avoid or limit injection of medication below the level of injury.	Areas below the level of injury have reduced circulation and sensation and are at risk for delayed absorption, local reaction, and tissue necrosis.
Skin Care: Topical Treatments (NIC)	
Massage and lubricate skin with bland lotion or oil. Protect pressure points by use of elbow or heel pads, lamb's wool, foam padding, and egg-crate mattress or cushion. Use skin-hardening agents, such as tincture of benzoin, karaya, or Sween cream.	Skin care and massage enhance circulation and protect skin surfaces, thus reducing risk of pressure ulcers. Tetraplegic and paraplegic clients require lifelong protection from decubitus ulcer formation, which can cause extensive tissue necrosis and sepsis.
Reposition frequently, whether in bed or in sitting position. Place in prone position periodically, if not contraindicated by respiratory status.	Repositioning improves skin circulation and reduces pressure on bony prominences.
Wash and dry skin, especially in high-moisture areas such as perineum. Take care to avoid wetting the lining of brace or halo vest.	Clean, dry skin is less prone to excoriation or breakdown.
Keep bedclothes dry and free of wrinkles, crumbs, and creases.	Preventing excessive moisture and friction reduces skin irritation.
Cleanse halo or tong insertion sites routinely and apply antibiotic ointment per protocol.	Halo and tong insertion site care helps prevent local infection and reduces risk of cranial infection.
Collaborative	
Provide kinetic therapy or alternating-pressure mattress as indicated.	Kinetic therapy and alternating-pressure mattress improves systemic and peripheral circulation and reduces pressure on skin and risk for breakdown.

NURSING DIAGNOSIS: deficient Knowledge [Learning Need] regarding condition, prognosis, potential complications, treatment, self-care, and discharge needs

May Be Related To

Lack of exposure or recall
Information misinterpretation
Unfamiliarity with information resources

Possibly Evidenced By

Reports the problem
Inadequate follow-through of instruction
Exaggerated or inappropriate behaviors—hostile, agitated, apathetic

Desired Outcomes/Evaluation Criteria—Client Will

Knowledge: Disease Process (NOC)
Verbalize understanding of condition, prognosis, and treatment.

Adaptation to Physical Disability (NOC)
Correctly perform necessary procedures and explain reasons for the actions.
Initiate necessary lifestyle changes and participate in treatment regimen.

ACTIONS/INTERVENTIONS	RATIONALE
Teaching: Disease Process (NIC) *Independent*	
Discuss injury process, current prognosis, and future expectations.	Open discussion regarding disease process, current prognosis, and future expectations provides common knowledge base necessary for making informed choices and commitment to the therapeutic regimen. *Note:* Improvement in managing effects of SCI has increased life expectancy of clients to only about 5 years below norm for specific age group. Research is ongoing and new treatment options are in clinical trials to determine if they can improve neurological outcomes.
Provide information and demonstrate the following:	
Positioning and weight shifting	Positioning promotes circulation and reduces tissue pressure and risk of complications.
Use of pillows, supports, and splints	Keeps the spine aligned and prevents or limits contractures, thus improving overall function and independence.
Encourage continued participation in daily exercise and conditioning program.	Daily exercise and conditioning programs reduce spasticity complications and risk of thrombogenesis (common complication), as well as increase mobility, muscle strength, and tone for improving organ and body function. Suggested activities are: (1) squeezing rubber ball and arm exercises enhance upper body strength to increase independence in transfers and wheelchair mobility; (2) tightening and contracting rectum or vaginal muscles improves bladder control; and (3) pushing abdomen up, bearing down, and contracting abdomen strengthen trunk and improve GI function in paraplegic clients.
Identify energy conservation techniques and stress importance of pacing activities, having adequate rest, and avoiding fatigue.	Fatigue is common. It limits client's ability to participate in or manage care, decreases quality of life, and increases feelings of helplessness and hopelessness.
Review drug regimen, noting desired effects and expected and adverse side effects, as well as medication interactions.	Medications used to treat spasticity can exacerbate fatigue, necessitating a change in drug choice or dosage. *Note:* Amantadine (Symmetrel) and fluoxetine (Prozac) may be added to decrease sense of fatigue by potentiating the action of dopamine or selectively inhibiting serotonin uptake in the central nervous system (CNS).
Have SO/caregivers participate in client care and demonstrate proper procedures, such as applications of splints, braces, suctioning, positioning, skin care, transfers, bowel and bladder program, checking temperature of bath water, and food.	Participation in client care allows home caregivers to become adept and more comfortable with the care tasks and reduces risk of injury or complications.
Instruct caregiver in techniques to facilitate cough, as appropriate.	Quad coughing is performed to facilitate expectoration of secretions or to move them high enough to be suctioned out.

(continues on page 264)

ACTIONS/INTERVENTIONS (continued)	RATIONALE (continued)
Recommend applying abdominal binder before arising (tetraplegic) and remind to change position slowly.	Appropriate use of abdominal binders reduces pooling of blood in abdomen and pelvis and minimizes postural hypotension.
Use safety belt and adequate number of people during bed-to-wheelchair transfers.	Performing transfers with adequate help prevents falls and related injuries to client and caregivers.
Instruct in proper skin care, inspecting all skin areas daily, using adequate padding—foam, silicone gel, water pads—in bed and chair, and keeping skin dry. Emphasize importance of regularly monitoring condition and positioning of support surfaces, such as cushions, mattresses, and overlays.	Proper skin care reduces skin irritation, thus decreasing incidence of decubitus ulcers. Timely recognition of product fatigue, improper placement, or other misuse can reduce risk of pressure ulcer formation.
Discuss necessity of preventing or managing excessive diaphoresis by using tepid bathwater, providing comfortable environment, such as by using fans, and removing excess clothing.	Management of excessive diaphoresis promotes cooling as well as reduces skin irritation and possible breakdown.
Review nutritional needs, including adequate bulk and roughage. Problem-solve solutions to alterations in muscular strength, tone, and GI function.	Adequate nutrition helps meet the energy needs of the client. Bulk and roughage prevent complications like constipation, abdominal distention, and gas formation.
Review pain-management strategies. Discuss the potential for future pain-management therapies. Recommend avoidance of OTC drugs without approval of healthcare provider.	Review of pain management enhances client safety and may improve cooperation with specific regimen. *Note:* Pain often becomes chronic in clients with SCI and may be mechanical, such as overuse syndrome involving joints; radicular, such as injury to peripheral nerves; or central, with burning and aching just below level of injury. Dysesthetic pain, which is distal to site of injury, is extremely disabling and similar to phantom pain. Treatment for these painful conditions may include a team pain-management approach; medications, such as gabapentin (Neurontin), clonazepam (Klonopin), amitriptyline (Elavil); or electrical stimulation.
Discuss ways to identify and manage AD.	Prompt and appropriate management of AD hinges on client and caregiver identification of signs and symptoms, prevention of precipitating and risk factors, and timely management. (Refer to ND: risk for Autonomic Dysreflexia.)
Identify symptoms to report immediately to healthcare provider, for example, infection, especially urinary and respiratory; skin breakdown; unresolved AD; and suspected pregnancy.	Early identification allows intervention to prevent or minimize complications.
Emphasize importance of continuing with rehabilitation team to achieve specific functional goals and continue long-term monitoring of therapy needs.	No matter what the level of injury, individual may ultimately be able to exercise some independence—manipulating electric wheelchair with mouth stick (C3/C4); being independent for dressing, transfers to bed, car, toilet (C7); or achieving total wheelchair independence (C8 to T4). Over time, new discoveries will continue to modify equipment and therapy needs and increase client's potential.
Evaluate home layout and make recommendations for necessary changes. Identify equipment, medical supply needs, and resources.	Physical changes may be required to accommodate client and support equipment. Prior arrangements facilitate the transfer to the home setting.
Discuss sexual activity and reproductive concerns. Review alternative sexual activities, positions, and spasticity management, as indicated, such as opposing pressure on area of spasm, using pillows for support, regular stretching and ROM exercises, and appropriate medications.	Concerns about individual sexuality or resumption of activity are frequently an unspoken concern that needs to be addressed. SCI affects all areas of sexual functioning. In addition, choice of contraception is impacted by level of SCI and side effects or adverse complications of specific method. Finally, some female clients may develop AD during intercourse or labor and delivery.
Identify community resources and supports, such as health agencies, visiting nurse, financial counselor, service organizations, and Spinal Cord Injury Foundation.	These support resources enhance independence, assist with home management, and provide respite for caregivers.
Coordinate cooperation among community and rehabilitation resources.	Various agencies, therapists, and individuals in community may be involved in the long-term care and safety of client. Coordination can ensure that needs are not overlooked and optimal level of rehabilitation is achieved. *Note:* Individuals with SCI are living longer and more injuries are occurring at advanced ages, creating new challenges in care as SCI clients deal with the effects of aging.
Arrange for transmitter, computer, or other type of emergency call system.	Provides reassurance for safety and prompt assistance.
Plan for alternate caregivers and identify respite services, as needed.	Respite care provides for preventing caregiver strain, illness, and emergencies.

NURSING DIAGNOSIS: risk for Autonomic Dysreflexia

Risk Factors May Include

An injury at T6 or above AND at least one noxious stimulus, e.g., irritating or painful stimuli below level of injury
Bladder (UTI, calculi), bowel (constipation/impaction), cutaneous stimulation—tactile, pain, thermal
Esophageal reflux; gastric ulcers
Sexual intercourse; pregnancy
Extreme environmental temperatures
Deep vein thrombosis; pulmonary emboli

Possibly Evidenced By

(Not applicable; presence of signs and symptoms establishes an *actual* diagnosis)

Desired Outcomes/Evaluation Criteria—Client Will

Symptom Control (NOC)
Recognize signs and symptoms of syndrome.
Identify preventive and corrective measures.

Neurological Status: Autonomic (NOC)
Experience no episodes of dysreflexia.

ACTIONS/INTERVENTIONS — RATIONALE

Dysreflexia Management (NIC)

Independent

Identify and monitor precipitating or risk factors, such as bladder or bowel distention or manipulation; bladder spasms, stones, and infection; skin or tissue-pressure areas and prolonged sitting position; and temperature extremes or drafts.

Visceral distention is the most common cause of AD, which is considered an emergency. Treatment of acute episode must be carried out immediately by removing stimulus or treating unresolved symptoms, then interventions must be geared toward prevention.

Observe for signs and symptoms of syndrome—changes in blood pressure, paroxysmal hypertension, tachycardia or bradycardia, autonomic responses, such as sweating, flushing above level of lesion, pallor below injury, chills, goose flesh, piloerection, nasal stuffiness, and severe pounding headache, especially in occiput and frontal regions. Note associated symptoms, such as chest pains, blurred vision, nausea, metallic taste, Horner's syndrome—contraction of pupil, partial ptosis of eyelid, and sometimes loss of sweating over one side of the face.

Early detection and immediate intervention is essential to prevent serious consequences or complications. *Note:* Average systolic BP in tetraplegic client—after spinal shock has resolved—is 120 mm Hg; therefore, readings greater than 140 mm Hg are considered elevated.

Stay with client during episode.

This is a potentially fatal complication. Continuous monitoring and intervention may reduce client's level of anxiety.

Monitor BP frequently (every 3 to 5 minutes) during acute AD. Take action to eliminate stimulus. Continue to monitor BP at intervals after symptoms subside.

Aggressive therapy and removal of stimulus may drop BP rapidly, resulting in a hypotensive crisis, especially in those clients who routinely have low BP. In addition, AD may recur, particularly if stimulus is not eliminated.

Elevate head of bed to 45-degree angle or place client in sitting position.

Elevation of the head of bed lowers BP to prevent intracranial hemorrhage, seizures, or even death. *Note:* Placing the tetraplegic client in sitting position automatically lowers BP.

Correct or eliminate causative stimulus as able, such as bladder, bowel, and skin pressure, including loosening tight leg bands or clothing; removing abdominal binder and elastic stockings; and temperature extremes.

Removing noxious stimulus usually terminates episode and may prevent more serious AD; for example, in the presence of sunburn, topical anesthetic should be applied. Removal of constrictive clothing or restrictive devices also promotes venous pooling to help lower BP. *Note:* Removal of bowel impaction must be delayed until cardiovascular condition is stabilized.

Inform client and SO of warning signals and how to prevent or limit onset of syndrome.

This lifelong problem can be largely controlled by avoiding pressure from overdistention of visceral organs or pressure on the skin.

Collaborative

Administer medications, as indicated (intravenous [IV], parenteral, oral, or transdermal) and monitor response:

These medications reduce BP if severe or sustained hypertension occurs.

Diazoxide (Hyperstat) and hydralazine (Apresoline), Nifedipine (Procardia) and 2% nitroglycerin ointment (Nitrostat)

Sublingual administration usually effective in absence of IV access for diazoxide (Hyperstat), but may require repeat dose in 30 to 60 minutes. These short-acting drugs may be used in conjunction with topical nitroglycerin.

(continues on page 266)

ACTIONS/INTERVENTIONS (continued)	RATIONALE (continued)
Morphine sulfate	Morphine sulfate relaxes smooth muscle to aid in lowering BP and muscle tension.
Miscellaneous other medications, such as phenoxybenzamine (Dibenzyline) and mecamylamine (Inversine)	Various medications are being used to alleviate symptoms associated with AD (Campagnolo, 2011).
Obtain urinary culture as indicated.	UTI is a common trigger for AD.
Apply local anesthetic ointment to rectum. Remove impaction if indicated after symptoms subside.	Ointment blocks further autonomic stimulation and eases later removal of impaction without aggravating symptoms.
Prepare client for pelvic or pudendal nerve block or posterior rhizotomy if indicated.	Procedures may be considered if AD does not respond to other therapies.
Collaborative	
Provide kinetic therapy or alternating-pressure mattress as indicated.	Kinetic therapy and alternating-pressure mattress improve systemic and peripheral circulation and reduce pressure on skin and risk for breakdown.

POTENTIAL CONSIDERATIONS following acute hospitalization (dependent on client's age, physical condition and presence of complications, personal resources, and life responsibilities)

- ***risk for Disuse Syndrome***—paralysis, mechanical immobilization
- ***Autonomic Dysreflexia***—bladder or bowel distention, skin irritation, deficient caregiver knowledge
- ***Self-Care Deficit***—neuromuscular impairment, weakness, fatigue, pain, depression
- ***risk for imbalanced Nutrition (specify)***—dysfunctional eating pattern, excessive or inadequate intake in relation to metabolic need/physical activity
- ***ineffective Role Performance/Sexual Dysfunction***—neurological deficits, pain, fatigue, depression
- ***interrupted Family Processes***—situational crisis and transition, shift in health status of family member
- ***risk for Caregiver Role Strain***—discharge of family member with significant home-care needs, presence of situational stressors that normally affect families, such as significant loss, economic vulnerability; duration of caregiving required, lack of respite for caregiver, inexperience with caregiving, caregiver's competing role commitments

MULTIPLE SCLEROSIS (MS)

I. Pathophysiology (Luzzio, 2012)

a. Chronic, irregular demyelination of the brain and spinal cord, resulting in varying degrees of cognitive, motor, and sensory dysfunction

b. Often characterized by periods of exacerbations and remissions, but is unrelenting in some individuals

c. Research suggests that in addition to destruction of myelin sheaths, underlying nerve fibers are also damaged or severed, which may account for the permanent neurological impairment.

II. Classification (Fox, 2011)

a. Relapsing-remitting multiple sclerosis (RRMS) is the most common form, wherein symptoms appear for several days to weeks, then resolve spontaneously. Because this may occur many times over years, tissue damage accumulates and client enters next stage.

b. Secondary-progressive multiple sclerosis (SPMS): After a period of time, RRMS may convert to a secondary progressive pattern characterized by continued progression, with increasing disability in approximately 80% of cases. Relapses may be seen in early SPMS but become uncommon as disease progresses (Brodkey, 2011),

c. Primary progressive multiple sclerosis (PPMS): About 15% of clients have manifestations that gradually progress from onset, without ever having remissions. Men and women are almost equally affected in this form (Cottrell, 1999).

III. Etiology

a. An autoimmune inflammatory disease, possibly related to viral infection that produces a limited disruption in the blood-brain barrier, thus allowing beta-lymphocyte clones to colonize the central nervous system (CNS).

b. Genetics may play a role in person's susceptibility.

c. Environmental and geographic factors are being investigated.

d. Predominant CNS disorder among young adults, between the ages of 20 and 40; difficult to diagnose, and cannot be diagnosed after only one presentation of symptoms, but rather over time.

e. Individual prognosis variable and unpredictable, thereby presenting complex physical, psychosocial, and rehabilitative issues.

IV. Statistics

a. Morbidity: Because the Centers for Disease Control and Prevention (CDC) does not require U.S. physicians to report new cases, and because symptoms can be completely invisible, the prevalence of MS in the United States can only be estimated. Approximately 250,000–400,000 people in the United States have been diagnosed with MS (Luzzio, 2012; National MS Society, [no date]; NINDS, 2012). MS affects women twice as often as men (MS Society, National Institute for Neurological Disorders and Stroke [NINDS], 2012).

b. Mortality: Exact figures are difficult to determine, because average life expectancy is 35 years after onset or approximately 95% of normal. Deaths associated with MS are usually due to fulminating MS (rare) or complications of the disease. The cause of death in 50% of a clinic population and in approximately 75% of all multiple sclerosis patients is from complications of multiple sclerosis, usually pneumonia (Reder, 2012). Case fatality ratios are 1:5 for patients with Kurtzke disability scores of less than or equal to 7, but 4:4 for those with scores greater than 7 (Reder, 2012; Sadovnick, 1992).

c. Cost: Because MS is a lifelong, chronic disease—diagnosed primarily in young adults who have an essentially normal life expectancy—estimates place the annual cost in the United States to exceed $10 billion (Fox, 2011).

GLOSSARY

Ataxia: Incoordination and unsteadiness due to the brain's failure to regulate the body's posture and strength and direction of limb movements.

Babinski's sign: Neurological reflex, which constitutes an important part of the medical examination, based upon what the big toe does when the sole of the foot is stroked. The normal, mature Babinski's reflex is characterized by extension of the great toe and also by fanning of the other toes.

Clonus: Sign of spasticity in which involuntary shaking or jerking of the leg occurs when the toe is placed on the floor with the knee slightly bent.

Contracture: Permanent shortening of the muscles and tendons adjacent to a joint that can result from severe, untreated spasticity and that interferes with normal movement around the affected joint.

Demyelination: Destruction, loss, or removal of the protective myelin sheath coating the axons, resulting in their inability to transmit impulses.

Dysarthria: Poorly articulated speech that results from dysfunction of the muscles controlling speech, usually caused by damage to the central nervous system (CNS) or a peripheral motor nerve. The content and meaning of the spoken words remain normal, however.

Intention tremor: Condition where goal-directed movements produce shaking in the moving body parts, most noticeably in the hands. Tremor is more obvious when performing delicate fine movements than broad sweeping ones.

Kurtzke's Expanded Disability Status Scale (EDSS): Scores eight functional systems from 0 for normal to 5 or 6 for maximal impairment. Based on these functional system scores and the person's ability to walk, the EDSS is determined. The EDSS goes in half-point scores from 0.0 for normal to 10.0 for dead from MS. From 0.0 to 4.0, people are able to walk without assistance; from 4.0 to 7.5, the EDSS score comes mainly from how far the person can walk and with what assistance. Essentially, point 6 on the scale represents walking with a cane, and this point is often used as an endpoint in studies looking at progression of disability. From 7.5 to 10.0, the main determinant of EDSS is the person's ability to transfer from wheelchair to bed and to self-care (Kurtzke, 1983).

Neurogenic bladder: Loss of nerve supply to the bladder, which results in an inability to voluntarily control the bladder. It is characterized by a failure to empty, failure to store, or a combination of the two resulting in such symptoms as urinary urgency, frequency, hesitancy, nocturia, and incontinence.

Nystagmus: The jerking to and fro movement of the eyes that occurs when disorder affects the control of eye movement.

Optic neuritis: Inflammation and demyelination of the optic nerve, causing a partial loss of vision.

Paresis: Partial or incomplete paralysis characterized by weakness and reduction in muscular power.

Paresthesia: Abnormal sensations, such as burning, tingling, or a pins and needles feeling.

Scotoma: Blind spot caused by diminished or total lack of function of the retina or optic nerve in a limited area. It may be unnoticed or be seen as a black area in the visual field.

Care Setting

Clients often require community or long-term care with intermittent hospitalization for disease-related exacerbations and complications.

Related Concerns

Extended/Long-term care, page 781
Pneumonia, page 129
Psychosocial aspects of care, page 729
Sepsis/septicemia, page 665

Client Assessment Database

Symptoms depend on the stage, extent of disease, and areas of neuronal involvement. For example, common signs associated with motor systems of the cerebellum include, and are not limited to, ataxia, diplopia, dizziness, dysphagia, fatigability, and tremors. Signs associated with motor systems of the corticospinal tract include, but are not limited to, Babinski's sign, bladder dysfunction, fatigue, heat sensitivity, paralysis, and trigeminal neuralgia. The following range of symptoms may be present at a given time or over time.

DIAGNOSTIC DIVISION MAY REPORT	MAY EXHIBIT
ACTIVITY/REST	
• Extreme fatigue, reported in about 70% of clients (Lazoff, 2008) • Weakness, exaggerated intolerance to activity, needing to rest after even simple activities such as shaving or showering	• Generalized weakness • Decreased muscle tone or mass • Spasticity

(continues on page 268)

DIAGNOSTIC DIVISION MAY REPORT (continued)	MAY EXHIBIT (continued)
• Intolerance of temperature extremes, especially heat, such as with summer weather or hot tubs • Limitation in usual activities, employment, hobbies • Numbness, tingling in the extremities • Sleep disturbances, may awaken early or frequently for multiple reasons	• Tremors • Staggering or dragging of feet • Intention tremors or decreased fine motor skills
CIRCULATION	
• Swelling of feet	• Blue (mottled), puffy extremities • Capillary fragility, especially on face
EGO INTEGRITY	
• Statements reflecting loss of self-esteem or body image • Expressions of grief • Anxiety or fear of exacerbations, progression of symptoms, pain, disability, rejection, or pity • Keeping illness confidential • Feelings of helplessness, hopelessness, or powerlessness (loss of control) • Personal tragedies, such as divorce, abandonment by significant other (SO) or friends	• Denial or rejection • Mood changes, irritability, restlessness, lethargy, euphoria, depression, or anger
ELIMINATION	
• Voiding at night • Urinary or bowel hesitancy or urgency • Incontinence of varying severity • Recurrent urinary tract infections (UTIs)	• Loss of urinary or rectal sphincter control • Kidney stone formation or kidney damage • Incomplete bladder emptying or retention with overflow
FOOD/FLUID	
• Problems getting food to mouth—related to intention tremors of upper extremities • Difficulty chewing or swallowing due to weak throat muscles • Sense of food sticking in throat • Coughing after swallowing • Hiccups, possibly lasting for extended periods	• Difficulty feeding self • Weight loss • Decreased bowel sounds—slowed peristalsis • Abdominal bloating
HYGIENE	
• Use of assistive devices • Need for individual caregiver	• Difficulty with or dependence in some or all activities of daily living (ADLs)
NEUROSENSORY	
• Weakness, dyscoordination, nonsymmetrical paralysis of muscles (may affect one, two, or three limbs, usually worse in lower extremities or may be unilateral) • Paresthesias • Change in visual acuity (diplopia), scotomas (holes in peripheral vision), or eye pain (optic neuritis) • Moving head back and forth while watching television, difficulty driving (distorted visual field), blurred vision (difficulty focusing) • Cognitive changes—attention; comprehension; use of speech; problem-solving; difficulty retrieving or recalling, sorting out information (cerebral involvement) • Difficulty making decisions • Communication difficulties, such as coining words • Seizures	• *Mental status:* Mood swings, depression, euphoria, irritability, apathy, lack of judgment, impairment of short-term memory, disorientation, or confusion • Scanning speech, slow and hesitant speech, poor articulation • Partial or total loss of vision in one eye, vision disturbances • Positional and vibratory senses may be impaired or absent • Impaired touch, pain sensation • Facial or trigeminal nerve involvement, nystagmus, diplopia (brainstem involvement) • Loss of fine or major motor skills • Changes in muscle tone • Spastic paresis or total immobility (advanced stages) • Ataxia, decreased coordination, tremors • Hyperreflexia, positive Babinski's sign, ankle clonus, absent superficial reflexes (especially abdominal)

DIAGNOSTIC DIVISION MAY REPORT (continued)	MAY EXHIBIT (continued)
Pain/Discomfort • Painful muscle cramping, spasms • Burning pain along nerve pathways • May be sporadic, intermittent, or constant • Facial pain • Dull back pain	• Distraction behaviors (restlessness, moaning), guarding • Self-focusing
Safety • Fear of falling because of weakness, decreased vision, slowed reflexes, loss of position sense • History of falls or accidental injuries • Use of ambulation devices • Visual impairment • Suicidal ideation	• Wall, furniture walking
Sexuality • Disturbances in sexual functioning (affected by nerve impairment, fatigue, bowel and bladder control, sense of vulnerability, and effects of medications) • Enhanced or decreased sexual desire • Problems with positioning • Genital anesthesia or hyperesthesia, decreased lubrication (female) • Impotence/nocturnal erections or ejaculatory difficulties (male) • Relationship stresses	
Social Interaction • Feelings of isolation (increased divorce rate and loss of friends) • Difficult time with employment because of excessive fatigue, cognitive dysfunction, physical limitations	• Speech impairment • Lack of social activities and involvement • Withdrawal from interactions with others
Teaching/Learning • Family history of disease, possibly due to common environmental or inherited factors • Use of prescription and over-the-counter (OTC) medications; forgetting to take medication • Difficulty retaining information • Use of complementary and alternative products and practices, trying out cures, or doctor shopping	
Discharge Plan Considerations • May require assistance in ADLs and instrumental activities of daily living (IADLs), depending on individual situation • May eventually need total care or placement in assisted living or extended care facility ➧ Refer to section at end of plan for postdischarge considerations.	

Diagnostic Studies

There are no definitive diagnostic tests for MS. However, tests are indicated to support a clinical diagnosis.

TEST WHY IT IS DONE	WHAT IT TELLS ME
	MS is diagnosed on the basis of clinical findings and supporting evidence from ancillary tests. Clinically, the attack must be compatible with the pattern of neurologic deficits seen in MS,

(continues on page 270)

Diagnostic Studies (continued)

TEST / WHY IT IS DONE (continued)	WHAT IT TELLS ME (continued)
	which typically means that the duration of deficit is days to weeks (Luzzio, 2012).
Ancillary Studies	
• ***Magnetic resonance imaging (MRI) scan:*** Uses a magnetic field to create detailed images of the brain and spinal cord and to detect lesions in the white matter of the brain. May use gadolinium to enhance the images.	MRI is the mainstay in confirming the diagnosis of MS by revealing multifocal white matter lesions (i.e., plaques that are due to nerve sheath demyelination). MRI shows brain abnormalities in 90% to 95% of MS clients and spinal cord lesions in up to 75%, especially in elder clients (Fazekas, 1988).
• ***CT scan with enhancement:*** Demonstrates acute brain lesions and ventricular enlargement or thinning.	Differentiates active or relapsing state versus remission as lesions do not enhance in stable disease.
• ***Evoked potential tests:*** Evoked potentials (visual, brainstem, auditory, and somatosensory) are electrical signals generated by the nervous system in response to stimuli. In these tests, nerves responsible for each type of function are stimulated electronically, and responses are recorded using electrodes placed over the CNS (brain and spine) and peripheral nerves (median nerve in the wrist, peroneal nerve in the knee).	In most cases, persons with MS will demonstrate a slowed conduction of nerve impulses.
• ***Lumbar puncture:*** Needle is inserted between two lower spine (lumbar) vertebrae allowing for the collection and analysis of cerebrospinal fluid (CSF).	Although not used routinely, this test may be of use when MRI is unavailable or MRI findings are nondiagnostic. CSF is evaluated for oligoclonal bands (OCBs) and intrathecal immunoglobulin G (IgG) production, as well as for signs of infection. OCBs are found in 90% to 95% of people with MS, and intrathecal IgG production is found in 70% to 90%. Although these findings are not specific for MS, CSF analysis is the only direct test capable of proving that the patient has a chronic inflammatory CNS condition (Luzzio, 2012; LWW, 2011).

Nursing Priorities

1. Maintain optimal functioning.
2. Assist with or provide for maintenance of ADLs.
3. Support acceptance of changes in body image, self-esteem, and role performance.
4. Provide information about disease process, prognosis, therapeutic needs, and available resources.

Discharge Goals

1. Remain active within limits of individual situation.
2. ADLs are managed by client and caregivers.
3. Changes in self-concept are acknowledged and being dealt with.
4. Disease process, prognosis, and therapeutic regimen are understood and resources identified.
5. Plan in place to meet needs after discharge.

NURSING DIAGNOSIS: Fatigue

May Be Related To

Disease state; poor physical condition
Environmental—humidity, temperature
Stress, depression

Possibly Evidenced By

Reports overwhelming lack of energy, inability to maintain usual routines
Decreased performance
Compromised concentration; disinterest in surroundings
Increase in physical complaints

Desired Outcomes/Evaluation Criteria—Client Will

Energy Conservation (NOC)

Identify risk factors and individual actions affecting fatigue.
Identify alternatives to help maintain desired activity level.
Participate in recommended treatment program.
Report improved sense of energy.

ACTIONS/INTERVENTIONS — RATIONALE

Energy Management (NIC)

Independent

Note and accept presence of fatigue.

Persistent fatigue is the most commonly reported symptom, affecting at least two-thirds of people with MS (Bakshi, 2003). Studies indicate that the fatigue is cognitive as well as physical, occurs with expenditure of minimal energy, is more frequent and severe than "normal" fatigue, has a disproportionate impact on ADLs, has a slower recovery time, and may show no direct relationship between fatigue severity and the clinical neurological status. Studies show a link between MS fatigue and depression independent of physical disability (Bakshi, 2003). Knowledge of these factors provides an opportunity to develop effective measures to maintain or improve mobility.

Identify or review factors affecting ability to be active, such as temperature extremes, inadequate food intake, insomnia, use of medications, or time of day.

Activity intolerance can vary from moment to moment and the precipitating cause is not always apparent, making it difficult to plan and or manage life.

Accept when client is unable to do activities.

Nonjudgmental acceptance of client's evaluation of day-to-day functioning provides opportunity to promote independence and self-esteem.

Determine need for mobility aids, for example, canes, braces, walker, wheelchair, or scooter. Review safety considerations.

Mobility aids can decrease fatigue, enhance independence and comfort, and promote safety.

Schedule ADLs and outside activities in the morning or over time or throughout the course of the day. Investigate use of air-conditioning, cooling vest, light-colored clothing, and wide-brimmed hats, if appropriate.

Fatigue commonly worsens when exposed to high temperatures due to weather, environmental heat, exercise, or fever. Some clients report lessening of fatigue with stabilization of body temperature.

Plan care with consistent rest periods between activities. Encourage afternoon nap.

Consistent rest and activity reduces fatigue and aggravation of muscle weakness.

Emphasize need for stopping exercise or activity before fatigue is unmanageable.

Pushing self beyond individual physical limits can result in excessive or prolonged fatigue and discouragement. In time, client can become very adept at knowing limitations.

Investigate appropriateness of obtaining a service dog.

Service dogs not only can increase client's level of independence, for example, balance and mobility assistance, but also can assist in energy conservation by carrying items in saddlebags, fetching, retrieving, and performing many other tasks.

Collaborative

Recommend participation in support groups that involve fitness, exercise, and other issues related to MS.

Participating can motivate the client to remain at optimal level of activity. Group activities must be carefully selected to meet client's medical needs and prevent discouragement or anxiety.

Administer medications, as indicated, for example:

- Disease-modifying therapies:
  - immunomodulators (e.g., teriflunomide [Augavio]; beta interferons (e.g., interferon beta-1a (Avonex, Rebif); or interferon beta-1b (Betaseron); glatiramer acetate [Copaxone]); immunosuppressant (mitoxantrone [Novantrone]); one monoclonal antibody (natalizumab [Tysabri]); and, most recently, an oral preparation (fingolimod [Gilenya)

All treatments target CNS inflammation with the goal of reducing relapse rates and slowing disease progression by decreasing the formation of new and active lesions as detected on MRI.

- Amantadine (Symmetrel) and pemoline (Cylert)

Amantadine and pemoline help manage fatigue. Common side effects include increased spasticity, insomnia, and paresthesia of hands and feet.

- Tricyclic antidepressants, such as amitriptyline (Elavil) and nortriptyline (Pamelor)

Tricyclic antidepressants help treat emotional lability, neurogenic pain, and associated sleep disorders.

- Steroids, such as prednisone (Deltasone), dexamethasone (Decadron), and methylprednisolone (Solu-Medrol)

Corticosteroids remain the standard in treating MS exacerbations as well as the first acute events that might develop into MS. Corticosteroids are thought to reduce the inflammatory response in the CNS and may also repair a damaged blood-brain barrier or inhibit the synthesis of immunoglobulin G in cerebrospinal fluid.

- Antineoplastic agents, such as mitoxantrone (Novantrone)

Antineoplastic agents may be given to reduce neurological disability and frequency of relapses in clients with SPMS (chronic) or worsening RRMS.

Prepare for plasma exchange treatment as indicated.

While not used as a common form of treatment, research suggests that plasmapheresis may benefit individuals experiencing severe, acute exacerbations not responding to standard high-dose steroid therapy (Cortese, 2011).

NURSING DIAGNOSIS: Self-Care Deficit (specify)

May Be Related To

Neuromuscular or perceptual impairment; impaired mobility
Pain, discomfort, fatigue
Weakness
Decreased motivation

Possibly Evidenced By

Inability to perform tasks of self-care

Desired Outcomes/Evaluation Criteria—Client Will

Self-Care: Status (NOC)

Identify individual areas of weakness, needs.
Demonstrate techniques and lifestyle changes to meet self-care needs.
Perform self-care activities within level of own ability.
Identify personal and community resources that provide assistance.

ACTIONS/INTERVENTIONS	RATIONALE
Self-Care Assistance (NIC)	
Independent	
Determine current activity level or physical condition. Assess degree of functional impairment using a scale of 0 to 4.	Functional assessment provides information to develop plan for rehabilitation. *Note:* Motor symptoms are less likely to improve than sensory ones.
Encourage client to perform at optimal level of function; however, do not rush client.	Encouragement promotes independence and sense of control. It may decrease feelings of helplessness.
Provide assistance with physical limitations. Allow as much autonomy as possible.	Client participation in self-care can ease the frustration over perceived loss of independence.
Encourage client input in planning schedule.	Client's quality of life is enhanced when preferences are considered in daily activities.
Note presence of and accommodate for fatigue.	Fatigue can be very debilitating and greatly impacts ability to participate in ADLs. The subjective nature of reports of fatigue can easily be misinterpreted as manipulative or a form of secondary gain.
Encourage scheduling activities early in the day or during peak energy levels.	Completing ADLs requires high energy expenditure. Poor planning of activities can cause early fatigue, persisting through the rest of the day.
Allow sufficient time to perform task(s). Display patience when movements are slow.	Decreased motor skills and spasticity may interfere with ability to manage simple activities.
Anticipate hygiene and grooming needs. Calmly assist with the care of nails, skin, hair, and mouth, and with shaving (use electric razor), as necessary.	The care provider can model matter-of-fact attitude toward assistance with toileting and grooming activities. This facilitates client and SO to accept changing roles and abilities.
Provide assistive devices as indicated: shower chair, elevated toilet seat with arm supports, and others.	Assistive devices reduce fatigue and enhance participation in care.
Frequently reposition the immobile, bed- or chair-bound client. Provide skin care to pressure points, such as sacrum, ankles, and elbows. Position or encourage sleeping in prone position, as tolerated.	Repositioning reduces pressure on susceptible areas and prevents skin breakdown. It minimizes flexor spasms at knees and hips.
Provide massage, active or passive range of motion (ROM), and stretching and toning exercises on a regular schedule. Encourage use of medications, cold packs, splints, and footboards, as indicated.	These maneuvers prevent problems associated with muscle pain, dysfunction, and disuse. They help maintain muscle tone, muscle strength, joint mobility, and proper body alignment. They decrease spasticity and risk of calcium loss from bones.
Provide strategies to promote independent feeding, such as wrapping fork handle with tape, cutting food, using Sippy cup for fluids.	These strategies promote independence and adequate nutritional intake.
Collaborative	
Consult with physical and occupational therapists.	Interdisciplinary consultations provide appropriate interventions that relieve spastic muscles, improve motor functioning, prevent or reduce muscular atrophy and contractures, and promote optimal level of function, independence, and self-worth.
Administer medications, as indicated, for example:	
Tizanidine (Zanaflex), baclofen (Lioresal), and carbamazepine (Tegretol)	Several drugs are effective for reducing spasticity, promoting muscle relaxation, and inhibiting reflexes at the spinal nerve root level. Tizanidine may have an additive effect

ACTIONS/INTERVENTIONS (continued)	RATIONALE (continued)
	with baclofen, but must be used with caution because both drugs have similar side effects. Short duration of action requires careful dosing to maximize therapeutic effect.
Meclizine (Antivert) and scopolamine patches (Transderm-Scop)	Meclizine and scopolamine patches reduce dizziness, allowing for increased mobility.
Potassium channel blocker, e.g., dalfampridine (Ampyra)	An oral medication for use in people with MS seeking improved mobility, dalfampridine thought to improve conduction in demyelinated nerve fibers.
Prepare for surgical intervention (e.g., deep brain stimulation), as appropriate.	Placement of an electrode—similar to a cardiac pacemaker device—in the region of the thalamus provides for small, adjustable electrical impulses to reduce arm tremors and enhance movement without actually destroying brain tissue.

NURSING DIAGNOSIS: situational low Self-Esteem

May Be Related To

Functional impairment
Ineffective adaptation to loss
Social role changes

Possibly Evidenced By

Evaluation of self as unable to deal with situation
Reports helplessness, uselessness
Self-negating verbalizations

Desired Outcomes/Evaluation Criteria—Client Will

Self-Esteem (NOC)

Verbalize realistic view and acceptance of body.
View self as a capable person.
Participate in and assume responsibility for meeting own needs.
Recognize and incorporate changes in self-concept and role without negating self-esteem.
Develop realistic plans for adapting to role changes.

ACTIONS/INTERVENTIONS	RATIONALE
Self-Esteem Enhancement (NIC)	
Independent	
Establish or maintain a therapeutic nurse-client relationship. Discuss fears and concerns.	Therapeutic nurse-client relationships convey an attitude of caring and develop a sense of trust between client and caregiver. The client is free to express fears of rejection, loss of previous functioning, changes in appearance, feelings of helplessness, and powerlessness. Open communication promotes a sense of support and well-being.
Note withdrawn behaviors, use of denial, or excessive concern with disease process.	These behaviors serve as initial protective responses. If prolonged, these behaviors may impede effective coping.
Support use of defense mechanisms. Allow the client to deal with the information in own time and way.	Confronting client with reality of situation may result in increased anxiety and lessened ability to cope with actual or perceived changes.
Acknowledge reality of grieving process related to actual or perceived changes. Help client deal realistically with feelings of anger and sadness.	The nature of the disease leads to ongoing losses and life changes. It could potentially block resolution of grieving process.
Review information about course of disease, possibility of remissions, and prognosis.	Information regarding the course of the disease helps empower the client to make decisions regarding daily functioning and healthcare decisions.
Provide accurate verbal and written information about what is happening and discuss with client and SO.	Providing current information facilitates client and SO decision making.
Explain that labile emotions are not unusual. Problem-solve ways to deal with these feelings.	Therapeutic communication relieves anxiety and promotes expression and management of emotions.
Note presence of depression, impaired thought processes, and expression of suicidal ideation; evaluate on a scale of 1 to 10.	Adapting to a long-term, progressively debilitating, incurable condition is a difficult emotional adjustment. In addition, cognitive impairment may affect adaptation to life changes. A depressed individual may believe that suicide is the best way to deal with what is happening.

(continues on page 274)

ACTIONS/INTERVENTIONS (continued) / RATIONALE (continued)

Assess interaction between client and SO. Note changes in relationship.
SO may unconsciously or consciously reinforce negative attitudes and beliefs of client, or issues of secondary gain may interfere with progress and ability to manage situation.

Provide an open environment for client and SO to discuss concerns about sexuality, including management of fatigue, spasticity, arousal, and changes in sensation.
Physical and psychological changes often create stress in the relationship, affect usual roles and expectations, and potentially further impair self-concept.

Discuss use of medications and adjuncts to improve sexual function.
Client and partner may want to explore trial of medications, such as papaverine (Pavabid), dinoprostone (Prostin E_2), or other avenues of improving sexual relationship.

Collaborative

Consult with occupational therapist or rehabilitation team.
Identifying assistive devices and equipment enhances level of overall function, participation in activities, and sense of well-being.

Refer to psychiatric clinical nurse specialist, social worker, and psychologist as indicated.
In-depth, supportive counseling may help resolve conflicts and deal with life changes.

NURSING DIAGNOSIS: Powerlessness

May Be Related To
Illness-related regimen—chronic/debilitating condition

Possibly Evidenced By
Reports lack of control, frustration over inability to perform previous activities
Dependence on others, depression over physical deterioration
Lack of involvement/nonparticipation in care

Desired Outcomes/Evaluation Criteria—Client Will

Personal Resiliency (NOC)
Identify and verbalize feelings.
Use coping mechanisms to counteract feelings of hopelessness.
Identify areas over which individual has control.
Participate, monitor, or control self-care and ADLs.

ACTIONS/INTERVENTIONS / RATIONALE

Hope Inspiration (NIC)
Independent

Note behaviors indicative of powerlessness or hopelessness, such as statements of despair, "They don't care" or "It won't make any difference."
These behaviors indicate client's ability to manage life changes.

Acknowledge reality of situation, at the same time expressing hope for client.
Although the prognosis may be discouraging, remissions may occur, and because the future cannot be predicted, hope for some quality of life should be expressed and encouraged. Additionally, research is ongoing, and new treatment options may become available.

Encourage and assist client to identify activities he or she would like to be involved in, such as volunteer work, within the limits of his or her abilities.
Staying active and interacting with others helps counteract feelings of helplessness.

Discuss plans for the future. Suggest visiting alternative care facilities and taking a look at the possibilities for care as condition changes.
Planning promotes sense of control and hope.

Self-Responsibility Facilitation (NIC)

Determine degree of life mastery and locus control.
Life mastery helps determine success in adjusting to the health condition. The locus of control relates to the ability to manage outcomes related to the disease process. An external locus of control would benefit from positive affirmation.

Assist client to identify factors that are under own control, listing things that can or cannot be controlled.
Knowing and accepting what is beyond individual control can reduce helpless and acting-out behaviors and promote focusing on areas individual can control.

Encourage client to assume control over as much of own care as possible.
The client can help plan and supervise own care and participate in health decision making.

Discuss needs openly, and facilitate actions to meet identified needs.
Open discussion empowers the client. It also helps to deal with manipulative behaviors.

ACTIONS/INTERVENTIONS (continued)	RATIONALE (continued)
Incorporate client's daily routine in home-care schedule or hospital stay, as possible	Routines maintain a sense of control, self-determination, and independence.
Collaborative	
Refer to vocational rehabilitation as indicated.	Vocational rehabilitation assists in development and implementation of a vocational plan that incorporates specific interests and abilities.
Identify community resources, such as adult day enrichment program.	Participation in structured activities can reduce sense of isolation and may enhance feeling of self-worth. These resources also provide respite to caregivers.

NURSING DIAGNOSIS: risk for ineffective Coping

Risk Factors May Include

Impairment of nervous system—sensory or perceptual impairment

Inability to conserve adaptive energies

High degree of threat

Possibly Evidenced By

(Not applicable; presence of signs and symptoms establishes an *actual* diagnosis)

Desired Outcomes/Evaluation Criteria—Client Will

Coping (NOC)

Recognize relationship between disease process (cerebral lesions) and emotional responses and changes in thinking and behavior.

Verbalize awareness of own capabilities and strengths.

Display effective problem-solving skills.

Demonstrate behaviors and lifestyle changes to prevent or minimize changes in mentation and maintain reality orientation.

ACTIONS/INTERVENTIONS	RATIONALE
Coping Enhancement (NIC)	
Independent	
Assess current functional capacity and limitations; note presence of distorted thinking processes, labile emotions, and cognitive dissonance. Determine how these affect coping abilities.	Organic or psychological effects may cause client to be easily distracted and to display difficulties with concentration, problem-solving, dealing with what is happening, and being responsible for own care.
Determine client understanding of current situation and previous methods of dealing with life problems.	Client understanding of current health situation provides clues on coping abilities, support system, individual resources, and other needs.
Discuss ability to make decisions, care for children or dependent adults, and handle finances. Identify available options.	Impaired judgment, confusion, and inadequate support systems may interfere with ability to meet own needs and needs of others. Conservatorship, guardianship, or adult protective services may be required until client is able to manage own affairs (if ever).
Maintain an honest, reality-oriented relationship.	Honest, reality-based relationship reduces confusion and minimizes painful, frustrating struggles associated with adaptation to altered environment and lifestyle.
Encourage verbalization of feelings and fears. Accept client statements in a nonjudgmental manner. Note statements reflecting powerlessness and inability to cope. (Refer to ND: Powerlessness.)	Nonjudgmental approach may diminish client's fear, establish trust, provide opportunities to identify problems, and facilitate the problem-solving process.
Observe nonverbal communication—posture, eye contact, movements, gestures, and use of touch. Correlate with verbal content. Clarify meaning, as appropriate.	Careful assessment of both verbal and nonverbal forms of communication provides insight into client response to the health condition and effective coping strategies.
Provide clues for orientation, such as calendars, clocks, note cards, organizers, and date book.	Memory aids facilitate client orientation and coping.
Encourage client to tape-record important information and listen to the recording periodically.	Repetition puts information in long-term memory, where it is more easily retrieved, and can support decision making and problem-solving process.
Collaborative	
Refer to cognitive retraining program.	Improving cognitive abilities can enhance basic thinking skills, including attention span, information processing, learning new skills, insight, judgment, and problem-solving.

(continues on page 276)

ACTIONS/INTERVENTIONS (continued)	RATIONALE (continued)
Refer to counseling, psychiatric clinical nurse specialist, and psychiatrist, as indicated.	Collaboration with psychiatric services may help resolve issues of self-esteem and regain effective coping skills.
Administer medications, as appropriate, such as amitriptyline (Elavil), fluoxetine (Prozac), escitalopram (Lexapro), venlafaxine (Effexor), nefazodone (Serzone®).	These medications improve mood and restful sleep as well as help combat depression and relieve fatigue.

NURSING DIAGNOSIS: risk for disabled family Coping

May Be Related To

Highly ambivalent family relationship; family disorganization/role changes
Prolonged disease that exhausts supportive capacity of significant people
Significant person with chronically unexpressed feelings—guilt, anxiety, hostility, despair

Possibly Evidenced By

(Not applicable; presence of signs and symptoms establishes an *actual* diagnosis)

Desired Outcomes/Evaluation Criteria— Family Will

Family Coping (NOC)

Identify or verbalize resources within themselves to deal with the situation.
Express more realistic understanding and expectations of client.
Interact appropriately with client and healthcare providers providing support and assistance as indicated.
Verbalize knowledge and understanding of disability, disease process, and community resources.

ACTIONS/INTERVENTIONS	RATIONALE
Family Involvement Promotion (NIC)	
Independent	
Note length and severity of illness. Determine client's role in family and how illness has changed the family organization.	Chronic or unresolved illness, accompanied by changes in role performance and responsibility, often exhausts supportive capacity and coping abilities of SO and family.
Determine SO's understanding of disease process and expectations for the future.	Inadequate information or misconception regarding disease process and unrealistic expectations affect ability to cope with current situation. *Note:* A particular area of misconception is the fatigue experienced by clients with MS. Family members may view client's inability to perform activities as manipulative behavior rather than an actual physiological deficit.
Discuss with SO and family members their willingness to be involved in care. Identify other responsibilities and factors impacting participation.	Individuals may not have desire or time to assume responsibility for care. If several family members are available, they may be able to share tasks.
Assess other factors that are affecting abilities of family members to provide needed support, such as own emotional problems and work concerns.	Individual members' preoccupation with own needs and concerns can interfere with providing needed care and support for stresses of long-term illness. Additionally, caregiver(s) may incur decrease or loss of income and risk losing own health insurance if they alter their work hours.
Discuss underlying reasons for client's behaviors.	Helps SO understand and accept and deal with behaviors that may be triggered by emotional or physical effects of MS.
Encourage client and SO to develop and strengthen problem-solving skills to deal with situation.	Family may or may not have handled conflict well before illness. The stress of long-term debilitating condition can create additional problems, including unresolved anger.
Encourage free expression of feelings, including frustration, anger, hostility, and hopelessness.	Individual members may be afraid to express "negative" feelings, believing it will discourage client. Free expression promotes awareness and can help with resolution of feelings and problems (especially when done in a caring manner).
Collaborative	
Identify community resources, such as local MS organization, support groups, home-care agencies, and respite programs.	Community resources provide information, opportunities to share with others who are experiencing similar difficulties, and potential sources of assistance.
Refer to social worker, financial adviser, psychiatric clinical nurse specialist, and psychiatrist, as appropriate.	Client, SO, and family may need more in-depth assistance from professional sources.

NURSING DIAGNOSIS: impaired Urinary Elimination

May Be Related To

Sensory motor impairment

Urinary tract infection (UTI)

Possibly Evidenced By

Incontinence, nocturia, frequency

Retention

Desired Outcomes/Evaluation Criteria—Client Will

Urinary Continence (NOC)

Verbalize understanding of condition.

Demonstrate behaviors and techniques to prevent or minimize infection.

Empty bladder completely and regularly, voluntarily or by catheter, as appropriate.

Be free of urine leakage between voiding.

ACTIONS/INTERVENTIONS	RATIONALE
Urinary Elimination Management (NIC)	
Independent	
Note reports of urinary frequency, urgency, burning, incontinence, nocturia, and size and force of urinary stream. Palpate bladder after voiding.	Urinary habits can help to identify a possible UTI. Bladder fullness after voiding indicates inadequate emptying or retention and requires further evaluation and intervention.
Review drug regimen, including prescribed, OTC, and street drug use.	A number of medications, including some antispasmodics, antidepressants, and opioid analgesics, OTC medications with anticholinergic or alpha-agonist properties, or recreational drugs such as cannabis, may interfere with bladder emptying.
Institute bladder training program or timed voiding, as appropriate.	Bladder training program helps restore bladder functioning and reduces incontinence and bladder infection.
Encourage adequate fluid intake, avoiding caffeine and use of aspartame and limiting intake during late evening and at bedtime. Recommend use of cranberry juice and vitamin C.	Sufficient hydration promotes urinary output and aids in preventing infection. *Note:* When client is taking sulfa drugs, sufficient fluids are necessary to ensure adequate excretion of drug, reducing risk of cumulative effects. *Note:* Aspartame, a sugar substitute (e.g., NutraSweet), may cause bladder irritation leading to bladder dysfunction.
Promote continued mobility.	Continued mobility promotes bladder emptying, thus decreases risk of developing UTI.
Recommend good hand-washing and perineal care.	Reduces risk of ascending infection.
Encourage client to observe for sediment, blood in urine, foul odor, fever, or unexplained increase in MS symptoms, such as spasticity and dysarthria.	Urinary symptoms indicate infection that requires further evaluation and prompt treatment.
Collaborative	
Refer to urinary continence specialist, as indicated.	The continence specialist helps develop individual plan of care to meet client's specific needs using the latest techniques and continence products.
Administer medications, as indicated, such as tolterodine (Detrol), oxybutynin (Ditropan), propantheline (Pro-Banthine), hyoscyamine sulfate (Cytospaz-M), flavoxate (Urispaz).	These medications reduce bladder spasticity and associated urinary symptoms of frequency, urgency, incontinence, and nocturia.
Catheterize, as indicated.	Catheterization may be necessary to relieve or evaluate bladder emptying or urinary retention.
Teach self-catheterization. Instruct in use and care of indwelling catheter.	Self-catheterization helps maintain client autonomy and encourages self-care. Indwelling catheter may be required, depending on client's abilities and degree of urinary problem.
Obtain periodic urinalysis (UA) and urine culture and sensitivity, as indicated.	Monitors kidney and bladder function and identifies presence of UTI. Colony count over 100,000 indicates presence of infection requiring treatment.
Administer anti-infective agents, as necessary, such as co-trimoxazole (Bactrim, Septra), ciprofloxacin (Cipro), norfloxacin (Noroxin).	Bacteriostatic agents inhibit bacterial growth and destroy susceptible bacteria. Prompt treatment of infection is necessary to prevent serious complications of ascending urinary infection, sepsis, and shock.

NURSING DIAGNOSIS: risk for Caregiver Role Strain

Risk Factors May Include

Severity of illness of the care receiver, instability in care receiver's health
Duration of caregiving required, complexity or amount of caregiving tasks
Caregiver is female, spouse
Family/caregiver isolation, lack of respite or recreation for caregiver

Possibly Evidenced By

(Not applicable; presence of signs and symptoms establishes an *actual* diagnosis)

Desired Outcomes/Evaluation Criteria—Caregiver Will

Caregiver Performance: Direct Care (NOC)

Identify individual risk factors and appropriate interventions.
Demonstrate and initiate behaviors or lifestyle changes to prevent development of impaired function.

Caregiver Performance: Indirect Care (NOC)

Use available resources appropriately.
Report satisfaction with plan and support available.

ACTIONS/INTERVENTIONS	RATIONALE
Caregiver Support (NIC)	
Independent	
Note physical and psychosocial condition. Identify client ability to comply with therapeutic regimen.	Careful assessment of physical and psychosocial conditions determines individual needs for planning care and helps identify strengths and needs requiring assistance and accommodation.
Determine caregiver's level of commitment, responsibility, involvement, and anticipated length of care. Use assessment tool, such as Burden Interview, to further determine caregiver's abilities, as appropriate.	Progressive debilitation taxes caregiver and may alter ability to meet client's and own needs. (Refer to ND: compromised/disabled family Coping.)
Discuss caregiver's view of the situation.	Open discussion allows ventilation and clarification of concerns and promotes understanding.
Determine available resources and social support.	Organizations, such as the National MS Society and local support groups, can provide information regarding adequacy of supports and identify needs and possible options.
Facilitate family conference to share information and develop plan for involvement in care activities, as appropriate.	Family conference helps clarify different roles and responsibilities, facilitates coping, and promotes participation and involvement.
Identify additional resources to include financial and legal assistance.	These areas of concern can add to burden of caregiving if not adequately resolved.
Identify adaptive equipment needs, resources for the home, and transportation.	Adaptive devices enhance independence and safety for the client and the caregivers.
Provide information and demonstrate techniques for dealing with acting out, violent, or disoriented behavior.	Information and effective techniques for dealing with such behavior help the caregiver maintain a sense of control and competency and enhances safe care.
Emphasize importance of self-nurturing, such as pursuing self-development interests, personal needs, hobbies, and social activities.	Taking time for self can lessen risk of burnout or being overwhelmed by situation.
Identify alternate care sources, such as sitter or day-care facility, and senior care services, for example, Meals on Wheels, respite care, and home-care agency.	As client's condition worsens, SO may need additional help to maintain client at home.
Assist with short-term and long-term care planning to meet the current and future needs of the recipient of care, including placement in alternative levels of care, extended care, hospice, and so forth.	Short-term and long-term care planning provides ongoing assessment and evaluation of client needs and clinical outcomes and realization of changes in the level of care.
Collaborative	
Refer to supportive services, as indicated.	Medical case manager or social services consultant may be needed to develop ongoing plan to meet changing needs of client and SO/family.

NURSING DIAGNOSIS: ineffective Self-Health Management

May Be Related To

Complexity of therapeutic regimen
Economic difficulties
Perceived benefits/barriers
Social support deficit

Possibly Evidenced By

Ineffective choices in daily living for meeting health goals
Reports difficulty with prescribed regimens
Failure to take action to reduce risk factors

Desired Outcomes/Evaluation Criteria—Client/Caregiver Will

Self-Management: Multiple Sclerosis (NOC)

Participate in learning process.
Assume responsibility for own learning and begin to look for information and to ask questions.
Verbalize understanding of condition, disease process, and treatment.
Initiate necessary lifestyle changes.
Participate in prescribed treatment regimen.

ACTIONS/INTERVENTIONS	RATIONALE
Learning Facilitation (NIC)	
Independent	
Evaluate motivation and readiness to learn of the client, SO, and caregivers.	Motivation and readiness to learn help determine appropriate and pertinent level of information.
Note signs of emotional lability or dissociative states (loss of affect and inappropriate emotional responses).	Client will not process or retain information and has difficulty learning during this time.
Provide information in varied formats based on client perceptual and cognitive abilities and locus of control.	Effective teaching strategies, such as verbal instruction, books, pamphlets, audiovisual and computer materials, are based on understanding the client's attitude toward learning and locus of control.
Encourage active participation of client and SO in learning process, including use of self-paced instruction, as appropriate	Active participation of client and SO enhances sense of independence and control as well as strengthens compliance with therapeutic regimen.
Teaching: Disease Process (NIC)	
Review disease process, prognosis, effects of climate, emotional stress, overexertion, and fatigue.	Clarifies client and SO understanding of current health and living situation.
Identify signs and symptoms that require further evaluation.	Prompt intervention may help limit severity of exacerbation and complications.
Discuss importance of daily routine of rest, exercise, activity, and nutrition. Focus on current capabilities. Instruct in use of appropriate devices to assist with ADLs, such as eating utensils, walking aids, among others.	Discussions on the importance of rest, activity, and nutrition help reduce fatigue and maintain a level of independence.
Emphasize importance of weight control.	Excess weight can interfere with balance and motor abilities and make care more difficult.
Review possible problems such as decreased perception of heat and pain, susceptibility to skin breakdown and infections, especially UTIs, and complications.	These effects of demyelination and associated complications may compromise client's safety and precipitate an exacerbation of signs and symptoms.
Identify measures to promote safety and overall health, such as avoiding exposure to individuals with respiratory infections; avoiding hot baths; regular skin monitoring and care; safe transfers to wheelchair, walker, or scooter; and adequate nutrition and hydration.	Review of safety and preventive measures maintains optimal level of function as well as prevents complications.
Discuss increased risk of osteoporosis and review preventive measures—regular exercise; increased intake of calcium and vitamin D; reduced intake of caffeine; cessation of smoking; hormone replacement therapy (HRT); and fall prevention measures such as wearing low-heeled shoes with nonskid soles, use of handrails and grab bars in bathroom and along stairwells, and removal of small area rugs.	These measures reduce the risk for osteoporosis and complications.
Identify bowel elimination concerns. Recommend adequate hydration and intake of fiber; use of stool softeners, bulking agents, suppositories, or possibly mild laxatives; and bowel training program.	Constipation is common. Bowel urgency and accidents may occur as a result of dietary deficiencies or fecal impaction.

(continues on page 280)

ACTIONS/INTERVENTIONS (continued)	RATIONALE (continued)
Review medications. Recommend avoidance of OTC drugs.	Avoidance of OTC medications reduces likelihood of drug interactions or adverse effects and enhances cooperation with treatment regimen.
Discuss concerns regarding sexual relationships, contraception and reproduction, and effects of pregnancy on the female client. Identify alternative ways to meet individual needs; counsel regarding use of artificial lubrication (females) and provide genitourinary (GU) referral for males regarding available medication and sexual aids.	Pregnancy may be an issue for the young client relative to issues of genetic predisposition and ability to manage pregnancy or parenting. Increased libido is not uncommon and may require adjustments within the existing relationship or in the absence of an acceptable partner. Information about different positions and techniques and other options for sexual fulfillment, such as fondling and cuddling, may enhance personal relationship and feelings of self-worth.
Encourage client to set goals for the future while focusing on the present and what can be done today.	Setting future goals provides opportunity for the client to develop insight and perspective regarding realities of the current situation and uncertainty of the future.
Identify financial concerns.	Loss or change of employment for client or SO impacts income, insurance benefits, and level of independence, requiring additional family or social support.
Refer for vocational rehabilitation, as appropriate.	Assessment of capabilities or job retraining may be indicated due to limitations associated with disease progression.
Recommend contact with local and national MS organizations and other support resources.	Ongoing contact such as mailings informs client of programs and services available and can update client's knowledge base. Support groups can provide role modeling and sharing of information and enhance problem-solving ability and individual and family coping.

POTENTIAL CONSIDERATIONS following acute hospitalization (dependent on client's age, physical condition, presence of complications, personal resources, and life responsibilities)

- ***risk for Trauma***—weakness, poor vision, balancing difficulties, reduced sensation, reduced muscle or hand-eye coordination, cognitive or emotional difficulties, economically disadvantaged
- ***impaired Home Maintenance***—disease, impaired functioning, insufficient finances, unfamiliarity with neighborhood resources, inadequate support systems
- ***risk for Disuse Syndrome***—paralysis, immobilization, severe pain
- ***ineffective Self-Health Management***—economic difficulties, family conflict, social support deficit

CHAPTER 7

Gastrointestinal Disorders

UPPER GASTROINTESTINAL/ESOPHAGEAL BLEEDING

I. Pathophysiology
- **a.** Ulceration and erosion of the mucosa of upper gastrointestinal (GI) organs, including stomach and esophagus, which is indicated by presence of melena, hematemesis, or blood in gastric contents (following lavage)
- **b.** Arises from branches of the celiac artery and superior mesenteric artery
- **c.** Variceal bleeding often arises from esophageal or gastric varices from the coronary vein or short gastric veins in portal hypertension.

II. Etiology
- **a.** Peptic ulcers are localized erosions of the innermost mucosal layer of the digestive tract and remain the most common cause of upper GI bleeding (Cerulli, 2013; Krumberger, 2005).
- **b.** Duodenal ulcer affects the upper part of the small intestine.
- **c.** Gastric ulcer affects the lining of the stomach.
- **d.** With the increased prevalence of bariatric surgery, anastomotic or ischemic ulcers are becoming more common (Chen, GZ, 2011; Levitzky, 2012).
- **e.** Common causes of ulcers include infection with *Helicobacter pylori*; alcohol, aspirin, and aspirin-containing medicines; and various other medicines, such as nonsteroidal anti-inflammatory drugs (NSAIDs).
- **f.** Tear in the mucosa at the gastroesophageal junction (Mallory-Weiss syndrome) can occur as a result of severe vomiting, trauma, or seizures.
- **g.** Hemorrhagic gastritis or stress ulcer can occur as a result of severe physiological stress, such as trauma, burns, surgery, or alcohol abuse (Krumberger, 2005).
- **h.** Esophageal varices are generally associated with alcoholic or posthepatitis cirrhosis of the liver; approximately 30% of such patients experience hemorrhage (Sartin, 2005).
- **i.** Esophageal or gastric cancer
- **j.** Hiatal hernia, hemophilia, leukemia, and disseminated intravascular coagulation (DIC) are less common causes of upper gastrointestinal bleeding (UGIB).

III. Statistics (Varma, 2011)
- **a.** Morbidity: Gross bleeding into the GI tract is responsible for approximately 350,000 hospitalizations annually.
- **b.** Mortality: From 1998 to 2006, the number of inpatient deaths for hospitalizations related to GI bleeding declined from 20,013 in 1998 to 16,344 in 2006. Overall, the inpatient death rate for GI bleeding declined 23% (HCUP, 2008).
- **c.** Cost: Annual direct cost of upper GI bleeding conditions estimated to be $2.5 billion (Kim, 2012).

GLOSSARY

Esophageal varices: Veins in esophagus and stomach become engorged and fragile due to high blood pressure in the portal vein.

Gastrin: Hormone secreted by the stomach into the gastric venous circulation to stimulate the stomach glands to release gastric acid.

Gastroesophageal reflux disease (GERD): Disorder in which there is recurrent backflow of stomach contents into the esophagus, frequently causing heartburn.

***Helicobacter pylori* infection (*H. pylori*):** Most common chronic bacterial infection in humans, and now recognized to be an important cause of gastric and duodenal ulcers.

Hematemesis: Bloody vomitus, whether fresh or partially digested ("coffee-ground" emesis). Hematemesis very strongly suggests an upper GI source of bleeding.

Hematochezia: Sometimes used (incorrectly) as a synonym for lower GI bleeding. The term means literally "to defecate blood" and refers to the passage of blood that still resembles blood—that is, it is red or maroon and recognizable to the person as blood.

Melena: Black, tarry feces due to digestion of blood in stool, and suggests an upper GI source of bleeding.

Peptic ulcer disease: Peptic ulcers are eroded areas that form in the lining of the gastrointestinal tract. They usually occur in the stomach duodenum. The two primary causes of peptic ulcers are infection with specific bacteria (*H. pylori*) and use of nonsteroidal anti-inflammatory (NSAID) medications.

Portal hypertension: Obstruction of portal vein due to hardening of liver from cirrhosis, causing venous blood from intestines and spleen to seek alternate routes to right atrium.

Care Setting

Generally, a client with severe, active bleeding is admitted directly to a critical care unit; however, a client may develop GI bleeding on the medical-surgical unit or be admitted there for evaluation or treatment of subacute bleeding.

Related Concerns

Cirrhosis of the liver, page 412
Fluid and electrolyte imbalances, page 885
Gastrectomy/gastric resection, on Davis*Plus*
Psychosocial aspects of care, page 729
Acute kidney injury (acute renal failure), page 505

Client Assessment Database

DIAGNOSTIC DIVISION MAY REPORT	MAY EXHIBIT
ACTIVITY/REST	
• Weakness, fatigue	• Tachycardia • Tachypnea, hyperventilation in response to activity
CIRCULATION	
• Palpitations • Dizziness with position change	• Hypotension, including postural • Tachycardia, dysrhythmias related to hypovolemia and hypoxemia • Weak and thready peripheral pulse • Capillary refill slow or delayed due to vasoconstriction • ***Skin color:*** Pallor, cyanosis depending on the amount of blood loss • Skin and mucous membrane moisture exhibiting diaphoresis reflecting shock state, acute pain, and possible emotional reactions
EGO INTEGRITY	
• Acute or chronic stress factors due to finances, relationship, or employment • Feelings of helplessness	• Signs of anxiety, such as restlessness, pallor, diaphoresis, narrowed focus, trembling, quivering voice
ELIMINATION	
• Change in usual bowel patterns and characteristics of stool	• Abdominal tenderness, distention • Bowel sounds are often hyperactive during bleeding, hypoactive after bleeding subsides. • ***Character of stool:*** Diarrhea; dark bloody, tarry; constipation may occur due to changes in diet or antacid use. • Urine output may be decreased or concentrated.
NEUROSENSORY	
• Fainting, dizziness, light-headedness, or weakness	• ***Mental status:*** Level of consciousness (LOC) may be altered, ranging from slight drowsiness, disorientation, and confusion to stupor and coma.
PAIN/DISCOMFORT	
• Pain described as sharp, dull, burning, gnawing, sudden, excruciating (perforation) • Nocturnal pain experienced by many • Vague sensation of discomfort or distress following large meals and relieved by food (acute gastritis) • Left to midepigastric pain that can radiate to the back, often accompanied by vomiting after eating and relieved by antacid (gastric ulcers) • Localized right to midepigastric pain, gnawing, burning, occurring about 2 to 3 hours after meals when stomach is empty and relieved by food or antacids (duodenal ulcers) • Midepigastric pain and burning with regurgitation, seen frequently with chronic GERD	• Facial grimacing • Guarding of affected area • Narrowed focus

DIAGNOSTIC DIVISION MAY REPORT (continued)	MAY EXHIBIT (continued)
• Absence of pain seen frequently with esophageal varices • Elderly more likely to be asymptomatic and present with a decreased appetite and weight loss	
SAFETY • History of previous hospitalizations for GI bleeding or related GI problems, such as peptic or gastric ulcer, gastritis, gastric surgery, irradiation of gastric area • Recent, current, or chronic use of prescription or over-the-counter (OTC) drugs containing acetylsalicylic acid (ASA), steroids, or NSAIDs (NSAIDs are leading cause of drug-induced GI bleeding) • Chronic use of alcohol or recreational drugs	
DISCHARGE PLAN CONSIDERATIONS • May require changes in therapeutic and medication regimens ➧ Refer to section at end of plan for postdischarge considerations.	

Diagnostic Studies

TEST WHY IT IS DONE	WHAT IT TELLS ME
DIAGNOSTIC STUDIES	
• ***Esophagogastroduodenoscopy (EGD):*** Allows direct visualization and therapeutic treatment of abnormal conditions of esophagus, stomach, and duodenum.	Procedure of choice for upper GI and allows for the possibility of a therapeutic intervention (biopsy, ligation, or sclerotherapy).
• ***Nasogastric lavage (NGL):*** Insertion of a large-bore flexible tube through the nose down into the stomach, where saline is used to rinse blood from stomach and suction applied to empty stomach contents.	The procedure is performed for both diagnostic and treatment purposes. Once a standard initial procedure for all clients with acute GI bleeding, its use is now under debate. May confirm recent bleeding (coffee ground appearance), possible active bleeding (red blood in the aspirate that does not clear), or a lack of blood in the stomach (active bleeding less likely but does not exclude an upper GI lesion) (Cerulli, 2013).
• ***H. pylori tests:*** Four tests are available: blood antibody test, urea breath test, stool antigen test, and stomach biopsy.	Determines whether an infection with *H. pylori* bacteria may be causing an ulcer or irritation of the stomach lining. *Note:* Fifty to seventy percent of elderly clients with ulcers have been found to have *H. pylori* as an underlying cause. The presence of *H. pylori* increases the risk of peptic ulcer disease 5- to 7-fold, but with the use of NSAIDs, the risk increases 5- to 20-fold.
• ***Occult blood/guaiac testing:*** Used to evaluate the contents of the rectum for occult blood when the presence of melena or hematochezia is in doubt.	The test can be positive for up to two weeks after a bleed, and its lack of specificity for acute bleeding means that it is generally more useful in the diagnosis of chronic occult bleeding. *Note:* The ingestion of some foods (e.g., red meat) may lead to false-positive tests (Westhoff, 2004).
BLOOD TESTS	
• ***Complete blood count (CBC):*** Battery of screening tests that typically includes hemoglobin (Hgb); hematocrit (Hct); red blood cell (RBC) count, morphology, indices, and distribution width index; platelet count and size; white blood cell (WBC) count and differential. Serial CBC or H&H tests should be performed to look at trending of values.	CBC will indicate whether client is anemic (low Hgb) and will also give an idea of the extent of the bleeding (Hgb and Hct) and how chronic it may be. RBC count and platelets may be decreased. WBC count may be elevated, reflecting the body's response to injury. CBC also aids in establishing blood and fluid replacement needs and monitoring effectiveness of therapy. For example, 1 unit of whole blood should raise Hct two to three points. Hct levels may not accurately reflect early or sudden blood loss until 6 to 24 hours after acute bleeding begins.

(continues on page 284)

Diagnostic Studies (continued)

TEST WHY IT IS DONE (continued)	WHAT IT TELLS ME (continued)
• *Blood urea nitrogen (BUN):* Determines presence of end products of breakdown of blood in GI tract.	Elevated within 24 to 48 hours as blood proteins are broken down in the GI tract and kidney filtration is decreased. BUN greater than 40 with normal creatinine level indicates major bleeding. BUN should return to client's normal level approximately 12 hours after bleeding has ceased.

Nursing Priorities

1. Control hemorrhage.
2. Achieve and maintain hemodynamic stability.
3. Promote stress reduction.
4. Provide information about disease process and prognosis, treatment needs, and potential complications.

Discharge Goals

1. Hemorrhage curtailed.
2. Hemodynamically stable.
3. Anxiety and fear reduced to manageable level.
4. Disease process and prognosis, therapeutic regimen, and potential complications understood.
5. Plan in place to meet needs after discharge.

NURSING DIAGNOSIS: risk for Bleeding

May Be Related To

Gastrointestinal disorders (gastric ulcer disease, varicies, etc.)

Possibly Evidenced By

(Not applicable; presence of signs and symptoms establishes an *actual* diagnosis)

Desired Outcomes/Evaluation Criteria—Client Will

Blood Loss Severity (NOC)

Be free of signs of bleeding in GI aspirate or stools, with stabilization of Hgb and Hct.

Hydration (NOC)

Demonstrate improved fluid balance as evidenced by individually adequate urinary output with normal specific gravity, stable vital signs, moist mucous membranes, good skin turgor, and prompt capillary refill.

ACTIONS/INTERVENTIONS	RATIONALE
Bleeding Reduction: Gastrointestinal (NIC) ***Independent***	
Note color and characteristics of vomitus, nasogastric (NG) tube drainage, and stools.	The first step in managing bleeding is to determine its location. Bright red blood that does not clear signals recent or acute arterial bleeding, perhaps caused by gastric ulceration; dark red blood may be old blood that has been retained in intestine or venous bleeding from varices. Coffee-ground appearance is suggestive of partially digested blood from slowly oozing area. Undigested food indicates obstruction or gastric tumor. In a rapid upper GI bleed, stool color may be red or maroon because of rapid transit time through the GI tract.
Monitor vital signs; compare with client's normal and previous readings. Take blood pressure (BP) in lying, sitting, and standing positions when possible.	Changes in BP and pulse may be used for rough estimate of blood loss; BP less than 90 mm Hg and pulse greater than 110 suggest a 15% to 35% decrease in volume, or approximately 1000 mL. Postural hypotension reflects a decrease in circulating volume. *Note:* Heart rate may not rise above normal until up to 30% of total blood volume is lost (Kolecki, 2012).
Note client's individual physiological response to bleeding, such as changes in mentation, weakness, restlessness, anxiety, pallor, diaphoresis, tachypnea, and temperature elevation.	Symptomatology is useful in gauging severity and length of bleeding episode. Worsening of symptoms may reflect continued bleeding, inadequate fluid replacement, and shock.
Measure central venous pressure (CVP) if available.	Reflects circulating volume and cardiac response to bleeding and fluid replacement. CVP values between 5 and 20 cm H_2O usually reflect adequate volume.

ACTIONS/INTERVENTIONS (continued)	RATIONALE (continued)
Monitor intake and output (I&O) and correlate with weight changes. Measure blood and fluid losses via emesis, gastric suction or lavage, and stools.	Provides guidelines for fluid replacement.
Keep accurate record of subtotals of solutions and blood products during replacement therapy.	Potential exists for overtransfusion of fluids, especially when volume expanders are given before blood transfusions.
Maintain bedrest; prevent vomiting and straining at stool. Schedule activities to provide undisturbed rest periods. Eliminate noxious stimuli.	Activity and vomiting increase intra-abdominal pressure and can predispose to further bleeding.
Note signs of renewed bleeding after cessation of initial bleed.	Increased abdominal fullness and distention, nausea or renewed vomiting, and bloody diarrhea may indicate return of bleeding.
Observe for secondary bleeding from nose or gums, oozing from puncture sites, or appearance of ecchymotic areas following minimal trauma.	Loss of or inadequate replacement of clotting factors may precipitate development of DIC.
Collaborative	
Prepare for urgent endoscopy.	Indicated within 24 hours of acute UGIB for diagnosis and intervention when client presents with hematemesis, melena, or postural changes in blood pressure.
Monitor laboratory studies: Hgb, Hct, RBC count, and BUN/Cr levels.	Aids in establishing blood replacement needs and monitoring effectiveness of therapy; for example, 1 unit of whole blood should raise Hct two to three points. Levels may initially remain stable because of loss of both plasma and RBCs. *Note:* Levels may not accurately reflect early or sudden blood loss, and low baseline levels may indicate preexisting anemia. BUN greater than 40 with normal creatinine level indicates major bleeding. BUN should return to client's normal level approximately 12 hours after bleeding has ceased.
Administer intravenous (IV) fluids or volume expanders, as indicated:	
0.9% sodium chloride, lactated Ringer's solution	Fluid replacement with isotonic crystalloid solutions depends on degree of hypovolemia and duration (acute or chronic) of bleeding. *Note:* Use of lactated Ringer's solution may be contraindicated in presence of hepatic failure because metabolism of lactate is impaired and lactic acidosis may develop.
Fresh whole blood or packed RBCs	Other volume expanders, such as albumin, may be infused until type and cross-matching can be completed and blood transfusions begun. The majority of gastric bleeding can be managed without transfusion of blood products. Fresh whole blood is indicated only for acute bleeding with severe volume and RBC depletion because stored blood may be deficient in clotting factors. Packed red blood cells (PRCs) are adequate for stable clients with subacute or chronic bleeding to increase oxygen-carrying capability. *Note:* PRCs are preferred for clients with heart failure (HF) to prevent fluid overload.
Platelets	Platelets are given to correct deficits in platelet number and clotting function. Clotting factors and blood components are depleted by two mechanisms: hemorrhagic loss and the clotting process at the site of bleeding.
Fresh frozen plasma (FFP).	FFP is an excellent source for clotting factors. Administered to clients with coagulation deficiencies who are bleeding or about to undergo an invasive procedure.
Insert and maintain large-bore NG tube in acute bleeding.	Provides route for removing blood and clots; reduces nausea and vomiting; and facilitates diagnostic endoscopy.
Perform gastric lavage with cool or room-temperature saline until aspirate is light pink or clear and free of clots. Simultaneous low-pressure gastric suctioning and continuous saline infusion through the air port of a Salem sump tube may also be used.	Flushes out and breaks up clots and may reduce bleeding by local vasoconstriction. Facilitates visualization by endoscopy to locate bleeding source. *Note:* Research suggests that iced saline is no more effective than room-temperature solution in controlling bleeding, and it may actually damage gastric mucosa and lower client's core temperature, which could prolong bleeding by inhibiting platelet function. Controversy also exists as to whether benefit is obtained from any gastric lavage, whether iced or room temperature.

(continues on page 286)

ACTIONS/INTERVENTIONS (continued)	RATIONALE (continued)
Administer medications, as indicated, such as acid suppressors:	Acid suppression is the general pharmacologic principle of medical management of acute bleeding from a peptic ulcer. Reducing gastric acidity is believed to improve hemostasis primarily through the decreased activity of pepsin in the presence of a more alkaline environment. Two classes of acid-suppressing medications currently in use are proton pump inhibitors and histamine-2 receptor antagonists (Anad, 2012).
Proton pump inhibitors (PPIs), such as omeprazole (Prilosec), lansoprazole (Prevacid), robeprazole (Aciphex), pantoprazole (Protonix), and esomeprasole (Nexium), administered by appropriate route (e.g., may initially be IV followed by oral long-term therapy)	PPIs are highly effective after GI bleed to reduce recurrence of bleeding. For example, an intravenous omeprazole bolus followed by high-dose continuous infusion for 72 h after successful endoscopic therapy can prevent recurrent bleeding (Chen, 2011). PPIs can heal duodenal ulcers in 2 to 4 weeks once severe bleeding is controlled. Typically given with antibiotics when *H. pylori* infection is present (Westhoff, 2004).
Histamine-2 receptor antagonists (H2RAs) such as cimetidine (Tagamet), ranitidine (Zantac), famotidine (Pepcid), nizatidine (Axid)	H2RAs are an older class of medications, and in an actively bleeding ulcer, their use has been largely superseded by the use of intravenous PPIs. Thus, intravenous H2RAs no longer have a role in the management of bleeding peptic ulcers. These drugs may be prescribed later on to reduce recurrence of bleeding in peptic ulcer disease (Anad, 2012).
Somatostatin analogs, e.g., octreotide (Sandostatin), vapreotide (Sanvar)	Helps control esophageal bleeding by decreasing blood flow to the gut, thereby lowering pressure to the portal system. These drugs have been shown to be more useful as adjuncts after endoscopy than gastric acid secretion suppression. Somatostatins have also proven useful in the treatment of nonvariceal bleeding, particularly in the presence of peptic ulcer disease (Bildozala, 2004).
Vasopressin (Pitressin)	Administration of intra-arterial vasoconstrictors may be needed in severe, prolonged bleeding in varices. *Note:* Effects of Pitressin are systemic, whereas octreotide is more regional.
Anti-infectives, such as metronidazole (Flagyl), amoxicillin (Amoxil), and clarithromycin (Biaxin)	Oral antimicrobials are generally combined with PPIs or histamine blockers to treat *H. pylori* infections causing chronic gastritis or peptic ulcers (Anand, 2012).
Assist with and prepare client for GI procedure, such as the following:	
EGD with control of GI bleed, such as:	Hemostasis clips are applied directly to bleeding site, closing bleeding vessel. *Note:* Early endoscopy is associated with an overall lower cost of care, shortened hospital stays, and improved outcomes. In fact, some clients may be discharged directly home after endoscopy is performed in the ED (Westhoff, 2004).
Injection therapies	Epinephrine 1:10,000 causes vasoconstriction when injected directly into bleeding site. Epinephrine injection alone is generally not adequate, but has been shown to be more effective when combined with banding or thermal coagulation (Chen, 2011).
Thermal coagulation	The objective of thermal coagulation is to ablate the bleeding blood vessel while minimizing damage to underlying and surrounding tissues to prevent complications such as perforation (Chen, 2011).
Endoscopic variceal ligation (EVL)	Performed during endoscopy, this banding technique is considered the definitive treatment to control active variceal hemorrhage. Multiple bands may be placed, and the procedure may be repeated several times to ensure that all varices are banded (Smith, 2010).
Endoscopic injection sclerotherapy (EIS)	Performed during endoscopy, an irritating (sclerosing) agent is injected into varices to stop bleeding and prevent recurrence after initial bleeding is controlled. Esophageal varices are most effectively treated with band ligation with small elastic rubber bands or sclerotherapy with agents (e.g., ethanolamine [Ethamolin], sodium tetradecyl sulfate [Sotradecol]). Fundic gastric varices are treated with endoscopic injection of tissue adhesives (e.g., N-butyl-2-cyanoacrylate [Histoacryl]) to close off large variceal complexes, as band ligation is not effective (Anand, 2012; Chen, 2011; Smith, 2010; ASGE, 2007).

Balloon tamponade

Short-term intervention (when endoscopy not available to treat variceal hemorrhage) using Sengstaken-Blakemore tube to compress varices and reduce esophageal blood flow. Although balloon tamponade controls acute hemorrhage in more than 80% of cases, rebleeding upon deflation is common (Garcia-Tsao, 2007).

Electrocoagulation or photocoagulation (laser) therapy

Provides direct coagulation of bleeding sites, such as those due to gastritis, duodenal ulcer, tumor, and esophageal (Mallory-Weiss) tear.

Radiological interventions, such as transjugular intrahepatic portosystemic shunt (TIPS)

Salvage therapy refers to final available treatment for a given condition, when prognosis is poor and the client hasn't responded to or can't tolerate other treatments. For variceal hemorrhage associated with alcoholic liver disease, salvage therapy usually involves placement of a transjugular intrahepatic portosystemic shunt (TIPS).This controls gastric variceal bleeding in 90% of clients. The principle is the same as a surgically placed shunt for bleeding control, but with lower mortality risk (Boyer, 2010; Hegab, 2001).

Surgical intervention (e.g., partial or total gastrectomy; shunt procedures)

When endoscopic therapy fails to stop ongoing ulcer bleeding, emergency surgery may be necessary. Surgery currently is reserved for perforations, clients who have failed nonsurgical treatment, and for those who remain hemodynamically unstable despite aggressive resuscitation (Weskoff, 2004). Shunt procedures (portocaval, splenorenal, mesocaval, or distal splenorenal) may be performed to divert blood flow and reduce pressure within esophageal vessels when other measures fail.

NURSING DIAGNOSIS: risk for Shock

Risk Factors May Include

Hypovolemia

Possibly Evidenced By

(Not applicable; presence of signs and symptoms establishes an *actual* diagnosis)

Desired Outcomes/Evaluation Criteria—Client Will

Circulation Status (NOC)

Maintain and improve tissue perfusion as evidenced by stabilized vital signs, warm skin, palpable peripheral pulses, ABGs within client norms, and adequate urine output.

ACTIONS/INTERVENTIONS — RATIONALE

Shock Prevention (NIC)

Independent

Investigate changes in level of consciousness and reports of dizziness or headache.

Changes may reflect inadequate cerebral perfusion as a result of reduced arterial blood pressure. *Note:* Changes in sensorium may also reflect elevated ammonia levels or hepatic encephalopathy in bleeding client with liver disease.

Investigate reports of chest pain. Note location, quality, duration, and what relieves pain.

May reflect cardiac ischemia related to decreased perfusion. *Note:* Impaired oxygenation status resulting from blood loss can bring on myocardial infarction (MI) in client with cardiac disease.

Auscultate apical pulse. Monitor cardiac rate and rhythm, if continuous electrocardiogram (ECG) available and indicated.

Dysrhythmias and ischemic changes can occur as a result of hypotension, hypoxia, acidosis, electrolyte imbalance, or cooling near the heart if cold saline lavage is used to control bleeding.

Assess skin for coolness; pallor; diaphoresis; delayed capillary refill; and weak, thready peripheral pulses.

Vasoconstriction is a sympathetic response to lowered circulating volume and may occur as a side effect of vasopressin administration.

Note urinary output and specific gravity. Insert Foley catheter to accurately measure urine, as indicated.

Decreased systemic perfusion may cause kidney ischemia and failure, manifested by decreased urine output. Acute tubular necrosis (ATN) may develop if hypovolemic state is prolonged.

(continues on page 288)

ACTIONS/INTERVENTIONS (continued)	RATIONALE (continued)
Note reports of abdominal pain, especially sudden, severe pain or pain radiating to shoulder.	Pain caused by gastric ulcer is often relieved after acute bleeding because of buffering effects of blood. Continued severe or sudden pain may reflect ischemia due to vasoconstrictive therapy, bleeding into biliary tract (hematobilia), or perforation with onset of peritonitis.
Observe skin for pallor and redness. Massage gently with lotion. Change position frequently.	Compromised peripheral circulation increases risk of skin breakdown as demonstrated by redness over bony prominence that does not blanch when digital pressure applied.
Collaborative	
Monitor ABGs and pulse oximetry.	Identifies hypoxemia and effectiveness of and need for therapy.
Provide supplemental oxygen, if indicated.	Treats hypoxemia and lactic acidosis during acute bleed.
Administer IV fluids, as indicated.	Replaces and maintains circulating volume and perfusion. A guideline for fluid replacement is 3 mL of fluid for each 1 mL of blood lost. (Refer to ND: risk for Bleeding.)

NURSING DIAGNOSIS: Anxiety [specify level]

May Be Related To
Change in health status, threat of death

Possibly Evidenced By
Increased tension, restlessness, irritability, fear
Trembling, increased pulse, increased perspiration
Poor eye contact, focus on self
Reports concerns due to change

Desired Outcomes/Evaluation Criteria—Client Will

Anxiety Self-Control (NOC)
Discuss fears and concerns recognizing healthy versus unhealthy fears.
Verbalize appropriate range of feelings.
Appear relaxed and report anxiety is reduced to a manageable level.
Demonstrate problem-solving and effective use of resources.

ACTIONS/INTERVENTIONS	RATIONALE
Anxiety Reduction (NIC)	
Independent	
Monitor physiological responses, such as tachypnea, palpitations, dizziness, headache, tingling sensations, and behavioral cues, such as restlessness, irritability, lack of eye contact, and combativeness or attack behavior.	May be indicative of the degree of fear client is experiencing—client may feel out of control of the situation or reach a state of panic. However, symptoms may also be related to physical condition or shock state.
Encourage verbalization of concerns. Assist client in expressing feelings by active listening.	Establishes a therapeutic relationship. Assists client in dealing with feelings, and provides opportunity to clarify misconceptions.
Acknowledge that this is a fearful situation and that others have expressed similar fears.	When client is expressing own fear, the validation that these feelings are normal can help client to feel less isolated.
Provide accurate, concrete information about what is being done, including sensations to expect and usual procedures undertaken.	Involves client in plan of care and decreases unnecessary anxiety about unknowns.
Provide a calm, restful environment.	Removing client from outside stressors promotes relaxation and may enhance coping skills.
Encourage significant other (SO) to stay with client, as able. Respond to call signal promptly. Use touch and eye contact, as appropriate.	Helps reduce fear of going through a frightening experience alone.
Provide opportunity for SO to express feelings and concerns. Encourage SO to project positive, realistic attitude.	Helps SO to deal with own anxiety and fears that can be transmitted to client. Promotes a supportive attitude that can facilitate recovery.
Demonstrate and encourage relaxation techniques such as visualization, deep-breathing exercises, and guided imagery.	Learning ways to relax can be helpful in reducing fear and anxiety. Because client with GI bleeding may be a person who has difficulty relaxing, learning these skills can be important to recovery and prevention of recurrence.
Help client identify and initiate positive coping behaviors used successfully in the past.	Successful behaviors can be fostered in dealing with current fear, enhancing client's sense of self-control and providing reassurance.

ACTIONS/INTERVENTIONS (continued)	RATIONALE (continued)
Encourage and support client in evaluation of lifestyle.	Changes may be necessary to avoid recurrence of ulcer condition.
Collaborative	
Administer medications, as indicated, such as diazepam (Valium), clorazepate (Tranxene), alprazolam (Xanax).	Sedatives and anti-anxiety agents may be used on occasion to reduce anxiety and promote rest, particularly in client with an ulcer.
Refer to psychiatric clinical nurse specialist, social services, and spiritual advisor.	May need additional assistance during recovery to deal with consequences of emergency situation and adjustments to required and desired changes in lifestyle.

NURSING DIAGNOSIS: acute Pain

May Be Related To
Chemical agent (gastric acid burn of gastric mucosa/oral cavity)
Physical response (such as reflex muscle spasm in the stomach wall)

Possibly Evidenced By
Verbal/coded report of pain
Abdominal guarding, rigid body posture, facial grimacing
Increased blood pressure/pulse/respirations

Desired Outcomes/Evaluation Criteria—Client Will

Pain Level (NOC)
Verbalize relief of pain.
Demonstrate relaxed body posture and be able to sleep or rest appropriately.

ACTIONS/INTERVENTIONS	RATIONALE
Pain Management (NIC)	
Independent	
Note reports of pain, including location, duration, and intensity (0 to 10, or similar coded scale).	Pain is not always present, but if present, should be compared with client's previous pain symptoms. This comparison may assist in diagnosis of etiology of bleeding and development of complications.
Review factors that aggravate or alleviate pain.	Helpful in establishing diagnosis and treatment needs.
Note nonverbal pain cues such as restlessness, reluctance to move, abdominal guarding, tachycardia, and diaphoresis. Investigate discrepancies between verbal and nonverbal cues.	Nonverbal cues may be both physiological and psychological and may be used in conjunction with verbal cues to evaluate extent and severity of the problem.
Provide small, frequent meals, as indicated for individual client.	Food can have an acid-neutralizing effect. Small meals prevent distention and the release of gastrin.
Provide/encourage intake of water, at least 1.5 quarts/day and a glass of water with every pain episode, if possible and not contraindicated.	Helps dilute the acid in the stomach (Kehler, 2008).
Encourage client to avoid smoking.	Besides the fact that smokers have an increased risk of developing peptic ulcers, smoking also interferes with the process of ulcer's lesions healing and increases the chances of infections (Kehler, 2008).
Provide frequent oral care.	Halitosis from bleeding and stagnant oral secretions is unappetizing and can aggravate nausea.
Collaborative	
Provide and implement prescribed dietary modifications.	Client may receive nothing by mouth (NPO) initially. When oral intake is allowed, food choices depend on the diagnosis and etiology of the bleeding. A special diet is not usually indicated for client with ulcers. It is a common-sense approach in the beginning to avoid any food or beverages (e.g., spicy foods, orange juice, tomatoes, coffee) as they increase acid production in the stomach and duodenum, leading to pain (Anand, 2012).
Administer medications, as indicated:	
Analgesics, such as morphine sulfate, ketorolac (Toradol)	Helps relieve acute or severe pain. Morphine also reduces peristaltic activity, and Toradol exerts anti-inflammatory effects.
Antacids	Can reduce epigastric discomfort rapidly.

(continues on page 290)

ACTIONS/INTERVENTIONS (continued)	RATIONALE (continued)
Histamine-2 receptor antagonists (H2RAs) such as cimetidine (Tagamet), ranitidine (Zantac), famotidine (Pepcid), nizatidine (Axid)	These drugs help reduce the production of stomach acids. This helps existent ulcers heal faster and diminishes pain.

NURSING DIAGNOSIS: deficient Knowledge [Learning Need] regarding disease process, prognosis, treatment, self-care, and discharge needs

May Be Related To

Lack of information or recall
Unfamiliarity with information resources
Information misinterpretation

Possibly Evidenced By

Reports the problem
Inaccurate follow-through of instructions

Desired Outcomes/Evaluation Criteria—Client Will

Knowledge: Acute Illness Management (NOC)

Verbalize understanding of cause of own bleeding episode, if known, and treatment modalities used.
Begin to discuss own role in preventing recurrence.
Identify and implement necessary lifestyle changes.
Participate in treatment regimen.

ACTIONS/INTERVENTIONS	RATIONALE
Teaching: Disease Process *Independent*	
Determine client perception of cause of bleeding.	Establishes knowledge base and provides some insight into how the teaching plan needs to be constructed for this individual.
Provide and review information regarding etiology of bleeding, relationship of lifestyle behaviors, and ways to reduce risk and contributing factors. Encourage questions.	Provides knowledge base from which client can make informed choices and decisions about future and control of health problems.
Review drug regimen, possible side effects, and interaction with other drugs, as appropriate.	Helpful to client understanding of reason for taking antiulcer drugs (e.g., PPIs and histamine blockers), and what symptoms are important to report to healthcare provider.
Encourage client to inform all healthcare providers of bleeding history.	Bleeding history may affect future therapy choices and prescriptions.
Emphasize importance of reading labels on OTC drugs and avoiding products containing aspirin. Discuss use of other NSAIDs for pain relief, and recommend alternatives.	Research has shown that NSAID use increases the risk of peptic ulcer disease by 5 times (Huang, 2002). The client must work together with healthcare providers to weigh the benefits and risks of using NSAIDs, even when they have caused an ulcer. Client with a current or resolved NSAID-induced ulcer who needs the benefits of NSAIDs can promote healing and reduce the risk of ulcer recurrence by taking the NSAID with a meal, using the lowest effective dose possible, quitting smoking, and avoiding or limiting alcohol (NDDIC, 2012).
Review significance of signs and symptoms such as coffee-ground emesis, tarry stools, abdominal distention, and severe epigastric and abdominal pain radiating to shoulder or back.	Prompt medical evaluation and intervention is required to prevent more serious complications, such as perforation and severe bleeding.
Discuss importance of cessation of smoking. Refer to support groups and healthcare provider for assistance, as client desires, with treatments such as nicotine replacement gums or antismoking drugs.	Ulcer healing may be delayed in people who smoke, particularly in those who use cimetidine (Tagamet). Smoking stimulates gastric acidity and is associated with increased risk of peptic ulcer development and recurrence. *Note:* Many support services are available to the client who wants to stop smoking.
Refer to support groups or counseling, as indicated.	Client may desire and/or need lifestyle and behavior changes to reduce risk factors (e.g., misuse of alcohol) for ulcer disease and/or life-threatening bleeding.

POTENTIAL CONSIDERATIONS following acute hospitalization (dependent on client's age, physical condition and presence of complications, personal resources, and life responsibilities)

- ***ineffective Self-Health Management***—decisional conflicts (use of NSAIDs for arthritic and chronic pain condition), perceived barriers/benefits, economic difficulties

INFLAMMATORY BOWEL DISEASE (IBD): ULCERATIVE COLITIS, CROHN'S DISEASE

I. Pathophysiolgy—Abnormal response of the immune system, leading to chronic inflammation of various portions of the alimentary tract

a. The peak age of onset for IBD is 15 to 30 years old, although it may occur at any age. About 10% of cases occur in individuals younger than 18 years (CDC, 2012).

b. (P) Pediatric IBD, especially Crohn's disease (CD), is often associated with impaired growth and skeletal development. This is the result of the direct effect of proinflammatory mediators upon growing bone, as well as poor nutritional intake and impaired caloric utilization in the setting of increased metabolic demand (Stephens et al, 2010).

II. Classifications

a. Ulcerative colitis (UC)

i. Four types of UC

1. Ulcerative proctitis: Usually confined to less than the 6 inches of the rectum. Occurring in about 30% of UC clients, it tends to be a milder form associated with fewer complications and a better outlook than more widespread disease (ulcerative proctitis) (Crohn's & Colitis Foundation of America [CCFA], 2013).
2. Proctosigmoiditis: Affects the rectum and sigmoid colon (lower segment of colon located right above the rectum)
3. Left-sided colitis: Continuous inflammation that begins at the rectum and extends as far as a bend in the colon near the spleen
4. Pan-ulcerative colitis: Affects the entire colon. Potentially serious complications include massive bleeding and acute dilation of the colon (toxic megacolon), which may lead to perforation. Serious complications may require surgery.

ii. Affects the innermost layer of the intestinal wall (closest to stool) (Wolf, 2009)

iii. Intermittent, with acute exacerbation and long remissions; however, 30% to 40% of individuals have continuous symptoms.

iv. Tends to run in families

v. Cure is accomplished only by total removal of colon and rectum.

b. Crohn's disease (CD)

i. Five types of Crohn's disease (Seibert, 2011)

1. Ileocolitis, the most common form, affects the lowest part of the small intestine and the large intestine.
2. Ileitis affects the ileum.
3. Gastroduodenal Crohn's disease causes inflammation in the stomach and first part of the small intestine (duodenum).
4. Jejunoileitis causes spotty patches of inflammation in the top half of the small intestine or jejunum.
5. Crohn's granulomatous colitis only affects the colon. However, associated symptoms in other organs include skin lesions, joint pains, and the formation of ulcers, fistulas, and abscesses around the anus.

ii. Affects all layers of the intestinal wall (Wolf, 2009)

iii. Slowly progressive chronic disease, no known cure, and with intermittent acute episodes

III. Etiology (National Digestive Diseases Information Clearinghouse [NDDIC], 2012)

a. Unknown, but may result from a complex interplay between genetic and environmental factors

b. Inability to downregulate immune responses, and consequently, the mucosal immune system remains chronically activated and the intestine chronically inflamed (Hanauer, 2006).

c. Additional risk factors include smoking (in CD) and use of nonsteroidal anti-inflammatory drugs (NSAIDs) or isotretinion (Acutane).

d. Periods of remission are interspersed with episodes of acute inflammation, characterized by frequent episodes of diarrhea, abdominal pain, fever, and weight loss.

e. Extraintestinal manifestations (EMs) include systemic inflammation affecting most of the body's organ systems—internal organs, eyes, blood, skin, and musculoskeletal system.

IV. Statistics (National Digestive Diseases Information Clearinghouse [NDDIC], 2012; Centers for Disease Control and Prevention [CDC], 2012)

a. Morbidity: Each year, in the United States, IBD accounts for over 700,000 physician visits, 100,000 hospitalizations, and disability in 119,000 patients.

b. Mortality: In 2004 in the United States, 933 deaths were attributed to IBD, with Crohn's deaths representing about two-thirds of that number (Everheart, 2008).

c. Cost: IBD is one of the five most prevalent gastrointestinal disease burdens in the United States. This chronic condition is without a medical cure and commonly requires a lifetime of care. Direct care costs for ulcerative colitis in 2008 estimated to be between $3.4 and $8.6 billion, and both direct and indirect costs for Crohn's disease totaled between $10.9 to 15.9 billion (AARDA, 2011).

GLOSSARY

Alimentary tract: Organs comprising the pharynx, esophagus, stomach, small intestine, and large intestine, all of which are involved in digestion and absorption.

(P) **Attenuated vaccine:** A vaccine prepared from live microorganisms or viruses cultured under adverse conditions leading to loss of virulence but retention of ability to induce protective immunity.

Borborygmus: Loud, rumbling bowel sounds caused by peristalsis.

Erythema nodosum: Inflammatory process with raised, tender, red nodules located under the skin, which are 1 to 5 cm in size.

Ileoanal anastomosis, or pull-through operation: Removes the colon and the inside of the rectum, leaving the outer muscles of the rectum. The surgeon then attaches the ileum to the inside of the rectum and the anus, creating a pouch in which waste is stored and passed through the anus in the usual manner.

Ileostomy: Creates a small opening in the abdomen, called a stoma, and attaches the end of the small intestine, called the ileum, to it. Waste travels through the small intestine and exits the body through the stoma. A pouch is worn over the opening to collect waste, and the client empties the pouch as needed.

Inflammatory bowel disease (IBD): Name of a group of disorders in which the intestines (small and large intestines or bowels) become inflamed due to a recurring immune response. The most common forms of IBD are ulcerative colitis (UC), and Crohn's disease.

Peristalsis: Progressive, involuntary rippling motion of muscles in the digestive tract.

Pyoderma gangrenosum: Inflammatory, purulent, pinpoint necrotic papules that can progress to deep ulcers.

Steatorrhea: Foul-smelling and fatty stools seen in some malabsorption syndromes.

Stomatitis: Inflammation or ulceration of the mouth, including the lips, tongue, and mucous membranes.

Care Setting

Care is usually handled at the community level; however, severe exacerbations requiring advanced pain control, nutrition, and rehydration may necessitate short stay in acute care medical unit.

Related Concerns

Fluid and electrolyte imbalances, page 885
Peritonitis, page 320
Psychosocial aspects of care, page 729
Total nutritional support: parenteral/enteral feeding, page 437

Client Assessment Database (Ulcerative Colitis)

DIAGNOSTIC DIVISION MAY REPORT	MAY EXHIBIT
ACTIVITY/REST	
• Weakness, fatigue, malaise, exhaustion, insomnia, not sleeping through the night because of diarrhea • Feeling restless • Restriction of activities or work due to effects of disease process	
CIRCULATION	
	• Tachycardia—response to fever, dehydration, inflammatory process, and pain • *Blood pressure:* Hypotension, including postural changes • Bruising, ecchymotic areas—insufficient vitamin K intake
EGO INTEGRITY	
• Anxiety, apprehension, emotional upsets, such as feelings of helplessness, hopelessness • Acute or chronic stress factors, such as family and job-related, expense of treatment	• Withdrawal, narrowed focus • Depression
ELIMINATION	
• Stool texture varying from soft-formed to mushy or watery. • Constant sense of needing to pass stool (tenesmus, proctosigmoiditis) • Persistent diarrhea accompanied by abdominal pain and blood in the stool • Passing blood, pus, or mucus with or without passing feces	• Diminished or hyperactive bowel sounds, absence of peristalsis or presence of visible peristaltic waves

DIAGNOSTIC DIVISION MAY REPORT (continued)	MAY EXHIBIT (continued)
FOOD/FLUID	
• Anorexia (gastroduodenal and left-side colitis) • Nausea, vomiting (gastroduodenal and left-side colitis) • Weight loss (left-side colitis); and may be significant (pan-ulcerative colitis)	• Mucous membranes pale; sore, dry, inflamed buccal cavity; cracking of tongue due to dehydration or malnutrition
PAIN/DISCOMFORT	
• Moderate lower left abdominal pain (proctosigmoiditis) • Severe left side abdominal pain (left-sided colitis)	• Abdominal tenderness, distention, rigidity
SAFETY	
• History of systemic lupus erythematosus (SLE), hemolytic anemia, vasculitis • Temperature elevation 104°F to 105°F (40°C to 40.6°C) (acute exacerbation) • Blurred vision • Allergies to foods—release of histamine into bowel has an inflammatory effect.	
SEXUALITY	
• Reduced frequency, avoidance of sexual activity	• Loss of normal menstrual cycle
SOCIAL INTERACTION	
• Relationship or role problems related to condition • Inability to be socially active	
TEACHING/LEARNING	
• Family history of inflammatory bowel disease (IBD), immune disorders; increased prevalence in Jewish population • Use of multiple medications or over-the-counter (OTC) medications for bowel health and use of herbal remedies, such as peppermint, psyllium, chamomile	
DISCHARGE PLAN CONSIDERATIONS	
• Assistance with dietary requirements, medication regimen, psychological support ➧ Refer to section at end of plan for postdischarge considerations.	

Diagnostic Studies (Ulcerative Colitis)

TEST WHY IT IS DONE	WHAT IT TELLS ME
DIAGNOSTIC STUDIES	
• ***Endoscopic examinations (proctosigmoidoscopy or colonoscopy):*** Gold standard for diagnosing UC, especially when biopsy is included.	Used to determine the extent of the disease and evaluate structured areas and pseudopolyps. Identifies inflamed and lacerated tissues, deep ulcerations, adhesions, and changes in luminal wall; rules out bowel obstruction.
• ***Computerized axial tomography (CT or CAT scan):*** Combines a series of x-ray views taken from many different angles and computer processing to create cross-sectional images of soft tissues. May be done with or without contrast media.	May reveal signs of ulcerative colitis or complication from the disease. May also reveal how much of the colon is inflamed.
• ***Rectal biopsy and cytology:*** Biopsy removes a small piece of rectal (anal) tissue for examination. Cytology is a study of the cells.	Neoplastic changes can be detected as well as characteristic inflammatory infiltrates, called crypt abscesses.

(continues on page 294)

Diagnostic Studies (Ulcerative Colitis) (continued)

TEST WHY IT IS DONE (continued)	WHAT IT TELLS ME (continued)
• ***Barium enema (also called lower GI series):*** X-ray of the rectum, colon, and lower part of the small intestine. Barium is given rectally to coat the lining of the colon so that abnormal areas will show up on the x-ray.	Assesses the extent of the disease and can detect complications such as strictures and carcinoma. May be performed after visual examination, although rarely done during acute, relapsing stage because it can exacerbate condition.
ASSOCIATED TESTS	
• ***Complete blood count (CBC):*** Battery of screening tests that typically includes hemoglobin (Hgb); hematocrit (Hct); red blood cell (RBC) count, morphology, indices, and distribution width index; platelet count and size; white blood cell (WBC) count and differential.	May show hyperchromic anemia (active disease generally present because of blood loss and iron deficiency); leukocytosis may occur, especially in fulminating or complicated cases and in clients on steroid therapy. Platelets may be increased (thrombocytosis) as a result of inflammatory process.
• ***Serum iron levels:*** Measures the level of iron in the liquid part of client's blood.	May be decreased because of blood loss, poor dietary intake, or malabsorption.
• ***Electrolytes:*** Charged minerals that, in solution, conduct an electric current to transport nutrients and wastes across cell membranes, regulate fluid balance, and help maintain pH level.	Decreased levels of potassium, magnesium, and zinc because of malabsorption; common in severe disease.
• ***Prealbumin/albumin/total proteins:*** Measurement of level of proteins in plasma to determine nutritional status.	Decreased because of loss of plasma proteins, disturbed liver function, and decreased dietary intake.
• ***Stool specimens:*** Used in initial diagnosis and in following disease progression.	Mainly composed of mucus, blood, pus, and intestinal organisms, especially *Entamoeba histolytica* (active stage). Fecal leukocytes and RBCs indicate inflammation of gastrointestinal (GI) tract. Stool that is positive for bacterial pathogens, ova, and parasites or *Clostridium* indicates infection. Stool positive for fat indicates malabsorption.

Client Assessment Database (Crohn's Disease)

DIAGNOSTIC DIVISION MAY REPORT	MAY EXHIBIT
ACTIVITY/REST	
• Weakness, fatigue, malaise, exhaustion • Feelings of restlessness • Restriction of activities or work due to effects of disease process	
EGO INTEGRITY	
• Anxiety, apprehension, emotional upsets, feelings of helplessness, hopelessness • Acute or chronic stress factors, such as family and job-related, expense of treatment	• Withdrawal, narrowed focus, depression
ELIMINATION	
• Unpredictable, intermittent, frequent, uncontrollable episodes of diarrhea (may be bloody) • Sense of urgency and abdominal cramping; sensation of incomplete evacuation • Intermittent constipation, which may lead to bowel obstruction	• Hyperactive bowel sounds with gurgling, splashing sound • Visible peristalsis
FOOD/FLUID	
• Anorexia; nausea, vomiting (gastroduodenal Crohn's) • Weight loss (iliocolitis or gastroduodenal Crohn's) • Failure to grow (when occurs in younger children) • Dietary intolerance, sensitivity, such as to dairy products or fatty foods	• Decreased subcutaneous fat and muscle mass • Weakness, poor muscle tone and skin turgor

DIAGNOSTIC DIVISION MAY REPORT (continued)	MAY EXHIBIT (continued)
PAIN/DISCOMFORT	
• Mild to intense abdominal pain and cramps along with diarrhea following meals (jejunoileitis Crohn's) • Middle or right lower abdomen pain with diarrhea (iliocolitis Crohn's) • Rectal pain • Migratory joint pain, tenderness (arthritis) (granulomatous Crohn's) • Migratory joint pain, tenderness (arthritis) • Eye pain, sensitivity to light (photophobia)	• Abdominal tenderness, distention • Fistulas, or inflammatory abscesses, may form in the lower right section of the abdomen (iliocolitis Crohn's)
SAFETY	
• History of arthritis, SLE, hemolytic anemia, vasculitis • Temperature elevation—low-grade fever • Blurred vision	• Skin lesions may present: erythema nodosum on face, arms; pyoderma gangrenosum on trunk, legs, ankles • Perianal fissures, abscesses, ulcerations (granulomatous Crohn's).
SOCIAL INTERACTION	
• Relationship or role problems related to condition; inability to be active socially	• Loss of normal menstrual cycle
TEACHING/LEARNING	
• Family history of IBD, immune disorders, cultural factor—increased prevalence in Jewish population, northern European, and Anglo-Saxon derivation • Use of multiple medications or OTC medications for bowel health and use of herbal remedies, such as aloe, chamomile, flax, garlic, bosweillia, echinacea, goldenseal	
DISCHARGE PLAN CONSIDERATIONS	
• Assistance with dietary requirements, medication regimen, psychological support ➧ Refer to section at end of plan for postdischarge considerations.	

Diagnostic Studies (Crohn's Disease)

TEST WHY IT IS DONE	WHAT IT TELLS ME
DIAGNOSTIC STUDIES	
• ***Endoscopic examination—colonoscopy with biopsy:*** Gold standard for diagnosis, especially when biopsy included.	May reveal clusters of inflammatory cells called granulomas, which help confirm the diagnosis of Crohn's disease because granulomas don't occur with ulcerative colitis (Mayo Clinic Staff, 2011).
• ***Capsule endoscopy:*** Technology that uses a swallowed video capsule to take photographs of the inside of the esophagus, stomach, and small intestine.	Can diagnose Crohn's disease in the small intestine (Marks, 2008).
• ***Computerized tomography (CT) scan:*** Combines a series of x-ray views taken from many different angles and computer processing to create cross-sectional images of soft tissues. May be done with or without contrast media.	May reveal extent of disease, particularly in the small bowel, or confirm complications such as partial blockages, abscesses, or fistulas.
• ***CT Enterography:*** A special CT scan that provides better images of the small bowel. This test has replaced barium x-rays in many medical centers.	
• ***Magnetic resonance imaging (MRI):*** Scan that uses a magnetic field and radio waves to create detailed images of organs and tissues.	This test is very helpful in diagnosing and managing Crohn's disease, and is particularly useful for evaluating a fistula around the anal area (pelvic MRI) or the small intestine (MRI Enterography) (Mayo Clinic Staff, 2011).

(continues on page 296)

Diagnostic Studies (Ulcerative Colitis) (continued)

TEST WHY IT IS DONE (continued)	WHAT IT TELLS ME (continued)
• ***Double balloon endoscopy:*** For this test, a longer scope is used to look further into the small bowel where standard endoscopes don't reach.	This technique is useful when capsule endoscopy shows abnormalities, but the diagnosis is still in question. It allows for biopsy of the abnormal area.
• ***Barium swallow or barium enema:*** Radiographic studies of the upper GI tract or rectum, colon, and lower part of the small intestine. Barium is given orally or rectally to coat the lining of the GI tract so that abnormal areas will show up on the x-ray.	Barium swallow may demonstrate luminal narrowing in the terminal ileum, stiffening of the bowel wall, mucosal irritability, or ulceration. Fistulas are common and are usually found in the terminal ileum, but may be present in segments throughout the GI tract.
BLOOD TESTS	
• ***Complete blood count (CBC):*** Battery of screening tests that typically includes Hgb; Hct; RBC count, morphology, indices, and distribution width index; platelet count and size; WBC count and differential.	Anemia (low Hgb and hypochromic, occasionally macrocytic RBCs) may occur because of blood loss from the mucosa and iron deficiency. WBCs are usually increased.
• ***ESR and C-reactive protein (CRP):*** Nonspecific test, but measures amount of inflammation in the body.	Increased in client with active inflammation.
• ***Prealbumin/albumin/total proteins:*** Measures levels of protein in plasma to determine nutritional status.	Decreased because of loss of intestinal proteins.
• ***Electrolytes:*** Charged minerals that, in solution, conduct an electric current to transport nutrients and wastes across cell membranes, regulate fluid balance, and help maintain pH level.	Potassium, calcium, and magnesium may be decreased due to malabsorption.

Nursing Priorities

1. Control diarrhea and promote optimal bowel function.
2. Minimize or prevent complications.
3. Promote optimal nutrition.
4. Minimize mental and emotional stress.
5. Provide information about disease process, treatment needs, and long-term aspects and potential complications of recurrent disease.

Discharge Goals

1. Bowel function stabilized.
2. Complications prevented or controlled.
3. Dealing positively with condition.
4. Disease process, prognosis, therapeutic regimen, and potential complications understood.
5. Plan in place to meet needs after discharge.

NURSING DIAGNOSIS: Diarrhea

May Be Related To

Inflammation, irritation, or malabsorption
Anxiety
Presence of toxins

Possibly Evidenced By

Hyperactive bowel sounds
Liquid stools (acute phase)
Abdominal pain; urgency, cramping

Desired Outcomes/Evaluation Criteria—Client Will

Bowel Elimination (NOC)

Report reduction in frequency of stools and return to more normal stool consistency.
Identify and avoid contributing factors.

ACTIONS/INTERVENTIONS	RATIONALE
Diarrhea Management	
Independent	
Observe and document stool frequency, characteristics, amount, and precipitating factors.	Helps differentiate individual disease and assesses severity of episode.

ACTIONS/INTERVENTIONS (continued)	RATIONALE (continued)
Promote bedrest, if indicated, and provide bedside commode.	Rest decreases intestinal motility and reduces the metabolic rate when infection or hemorrhage is a complication. Urge to defecate may occur without warning and be uncontrollable, thus increasing risk of incontinence and falls if facilities are not close at hand.
Remove stool promptly. Provide room deodorizers.	Reduces noxious odors to avoid undue client embarrassment.
Discuss client's usual diet. Have client/SO identify foods and fluids (if any) that precipitate client's diarrhea and/or cramping pain.	There is no one single food or group of foods that precipitates problems for everyone with IBD. Dietary needs and restrictions must be individualized, depending on which disease the client has and what part of the intestine is affected (CCFA, 2013).
Restart oral fluid intake gradually, if client has been on bowel rest (NPO) during treatment. Offer clear liquids hourly and avoid cold fluids.	Provides colon rest by omitting or decreasing the stimulus of foods and fluids. Gradual resumption of liquids may prevent cramping and recurrence of diarrhea; however, cold fluids can increase intestinal motility.
Provide opportunity to vent frustrations related to disease process.	Presence of disease with unknown cause that is difficult to cure and that may require surgical intervention can lead to stress reactions that may aggravate condition.
Observe for fever, tachycardia, lethargy, leukocytosis, decreased serum protein, anxiety, and prostration.	May signify that toxic megacolon or perforation and peritonitis are imminent or have occurred, necessitating immediate medical intervention.
Collaborative	
Administer medications, as indicated:	
Aminosalicylates (5-ASA), such as olsalazine (Dipentum) and balsalazide (Calazal), sulfasalazine (Azulfidine), mesalamine (Asacol), and olsalazine	5-ASA agents work at the level of the lining of the GI tract to decrease inflammation. They are thought to be effective in treating mild-to-moderate episodes of IBD, and are useful in preventing relapses of the disease. They work best in the colon and are not particularly effective if the disease is limited to the small intestine (CCFA, 2013; Allen et al, 2011).
Steroids, such as adrenocorticotropic hormone (ACTH), hydrocortisone (Cortenema, Cortifoam), prednisolone (Delta-Cortef), and prednisone (Deltasone)	Long-term treatment with corticosteroids or use to maintain remission is undesirable, but may be given during acute flares (Allen et al, 2011). Steroids are contraindicated if intra-abdominal abscesses are suspected.
Thiopurines, e.g., azathioprine (Imuran), 6-mercaptopurine (6-MP, Purinethol), thioguanine (Tabloid)	May be given to block inflammatory response, decrease steroid requirements, and promote healing of fistulas (Allen et al, 2011). Thiopurines have not been shown to increase risk of death, as has been associated with long-term steroid use (Lewis et al, 2009).
Biological response modifiers (also called immunomodulators), such as infliximab (Remicade), adalimumab (Humira), certolizumab (Cimzia), natalizumab	These drugs block tissue necrosis factor (TNF), a component of inflammatory response. They help control inflammation, trigger remission, and allow fistulas to close (Allen et al, 2011; Day, 2008).
Anti-infectives, such as metronidazole (Flagyl), ciprofloxacin (Cipro), ampicillin, and others	Used to treat bacterial overgrowth in the small intestine caused by stricture, fistulas, or prior surgery. May be part of a long-term treatment regimen (Allen et al, 2011).
(P) Medication choices for pediatric clients:	
5-ASA agents: balsalazide (Colzal) and sulfasalazine (Alzulfidine)	Approved for use in children over 2 years of age. (Jansen Biotech, 2011; Stephens et al, 2010)
Biologics: infliximab (Remicade)	
Corticosteroids	Should be used as an induction agent only, with weaning to other medications as soon as possible, as they are also implicated in growth disturbances and bone disease, acne, and excess body fat when used long-term.
Budosonide (Entocort EC)	Preferred given the fact that it yields much less systemic steroid exposure.
Methotrexate (MTX)	May be given to child unresponsive to or intolerant of other drugs. *Note*: Determine that client of child-bearing age is tested for pregnancy and is pro-active in pregnancy prevention measures prior to initiation of MTX. Drug is known to cause birth defects (Denson et al, 2007).
Prepare for surgical intervention, such as colectomy, proctocolectomy, or ileostomy.	Two-thirds to three-quarters of patients with Crohn's disease will require surgery at some point during their lives (Allen et al, 2011) if perforation or bowel obstruction occurs or disease is unresponsive to medical treatment. Surgery (a colectomy) can cure UC, and can help, but not cure, Crohn's disease. Surgery to remove the colon and rectum (proctocolectomy) is

(continues on page 298)

followed by ileostomy, or ileoanal anastomosis. If the client isn't critically ill and the anal sphincter is free from lesions, the surgeon may remove the colon and rectum but leave the anus intact. An internal pouch is then formed from the distal ileum and connected to the anal sphincter, allowing the client to have continent bowel movements (Day, 2008). (Refer to CP: Fecal Diversions for additional interventions, as needed.)

NURSING DIAGNOSIS: risk for deficient Fluid Volume

Risk Factors May Include

Excessive losses through normal routes—diarrhea, vomiting
Factors influencing fluid needs (hypermetabolic state—inflammation, fever)
Deviations affecting intake—nausea, anorexia

Possibly Evidenced By

(Not applicable; presence of signs and symptoms establishes an *actual* diagnosis)

Desired Outcomes/Evaluation Criteria—Client Will

Hydration (NOC)

Maintain adequate fluid volume as evidenced by moist mucous membranes, good skin turgor, and capillary refill; stable vital signs; and balanced intake and output (I&O) with urine of normal concentration and amount.

ACTIONS/INTERVENTIONS	RATIONALE
Fluid/Electrolyte Management (NIC)	
Independent	
Monitor I&O. Note number, character, and amount of stools; estimate insensible fluid losses (e.g., diaphoresis). Measure urine specific gravity and observe for oliguria.	Provides information about overall fluid balance, renal function, and bowel disease control, as well as guidelines for fluid replacement.
Assess vital signs (blood pressure [BP], pulse, temperature).	Hypotension (including postural), tachycardia, and fever can indicate response to and effect of fluid loss.
Observe for excessively dry skin and mucous membranes, decreased skin turgor, and slowed capillary refill.	Indicates excessive fluid loss and resultant dehydration.
Weigh daily or per protocol.	Indicator of overall fluid and nutritional status.
Collaborative	
Monitor serial electrolytes and metabolic panel.	Reveals imbalances associated with fluid and electrolyte loss through vomiting and diarrhea.
Adminsiter IV fluids and electrolytes, as indicated.	May be needed to replenish fluid volume and reduce risk of complications associated with electrolyte imbalances.

NURSING DIAGNOSIS: imbalanced Nutrition: less than body requirements

May Be Related To

Altered absorption of nutrients
Inability to ingest food (medically restricted intake)
Biological factors (hypermetabolic state)
Psychological factors (fear that eating may cause diarrhea)

Possibly Evidenced By

Aversion to eating, weight loss
Abdominal pain, cramping
Hyperactive bowel sounds, diarrhea, steatorrhea
Pale mucous membranes

Desired Outcomes/Evaluation Criteria—Client Will

Nutritional Status (NOC)

Demonstrate stable weight or progressive gain toward goal with normalization of laboratory values and absence of signs of malnutrition.

ACTIONS/INTERVENTIONS	RATIONALE
Nutrition Therapy (NIC)	
Independent	
Assess weight, age, body mass, strength, and activity and rest levels. Ascertain stage of disease process and its effects on client's nutritional status.	Provides comparative baseline.
Inspect oral mucosa.	May reveal ulcerations and/or provide information about the integrity of the entire GI tract, affecting ability to eat and absorb nutrients.
Evaluate client's appetite.	Appetite may be suppressed because of altered taste, early satiety, meal-related cramping, diarrhea, or medications, or a combination of these factors.
Weigh frequently.	Provides information about dietary needs and effectiveness of therapy.
Encourage daytime rest periods and limited activity during acute phase of illness.	Decreasing metabolic needs aids in preventing caloric depletion and conserves energy.
Recommend rest before meals.	Quiets peristalsis and increases available energy for eating.
Provide oral hygiene.	A clean mouth can enhance the taste of food.
Serve foods in well-ventilated, pleasant surroundings, with unhurried atmosphere and congenial company.	Pleasant environment aids in reducing stress and is more conducive to eating.
Encourage client to eat a healthy, varied diet as much as possible, incorporating several small meals and snacks per day.	Will promote achieving and maintaining healthy weight and a more strong, active lifestyle.
Encourage client to avoid or limit foods that might cause or exacerbate abdominal cramping and other uncomfortable symptoms, such as dairy products (if client is lactose intolerant), foods high in fiber (e.g., raw vegetables) or fat (e.g., fried foods, nuts, ice cream), alcohol, or foods and drinks containing caffeine (Byer, 2008).	Individual tolerance varies, depending on stage of disease and area of bowel affected.
(P) Discuss special dietary concerns with child/teenager/caregivers. Offer choices, when possible, that child/teenager may find acceptable to personal taste and in social settings.	Children with IBD face special challenges, and finding foods that children and teenagers like to eat is a challenge. A healthy diet is a priority for growth and development, while needing to address food intolerances and those foods that can exacerbate disease symptoms. Parents might think that there's no place in a healthy diet for fast food, but this may not be true. Some of these foods provide a valuable supply of nutrients as well as calories. For example: in pizza the cheese offers calcium, protein, and vitamin D; the tomato sauce provides vitamins A and C; and the crust supplies B vitamins (CCFA, 2013).
Record intake and changes in symptomatology.	Useful in identifying specific deficiencies and determining GI response to foods.
Promote client participation in dietary planning as possible.	Provides sense of control for client and opportunity to select foods desired and enjoyed, which may increase intake.
Encourage client to verbalize feelings concerning resumption of diet, when client has been on bowel rest (NPO).	Hesitation to eat may be the result of fear that food will cause exacerbation of symptoms.
Collaborative	
Keep client on nothing-by-mouth (NPO) status, as indicated.	Resting the bowel decreases peristalsis and diarrhea, limiting malabsorption and loss of nutrients. *Note:* Client with toxic colitis is NPO and placed on parenteral nutrition.
Resume or advance diet as indicated—clear liquids progressing to bland, low-residue, and then high-protein, high-calorie, caffeine-free, nonspicy, and low-fiber, as indicated.	Allows the intestinal tract to readjust to the digestive process. Protein is necessary for tissue healing integrity. Low bulk decreases peristaltic response to meal. *Note:* Dietary measures depend on client's condition; for example, if disease is mild, client may do well on low-residue, low-fat diet high in protein and calories with lactose restriction. In moderate disease, elemental enteral products may be given to provide nutrition without overstimulating the bowel.
Provide nutritional support, for example:	
Enteral feedings, such as Ultra Clear Plus via nasogastric (NG) tube, percutaneous endoscopic gastrostomy (PEG), or J-tube	Many clinical studies have shown early enteral feeding is beneficial in reducing the effects of malabsorption and providing essential nutrients. Although elemental enteral solutions cannot provide all needed nutrients, they can prevent gut atrophy.
Intravenous total parenteral nutrition (TPN)	This regimen rests the GI tract completely while providing essential nutrients. Short-term TPN is indicated during periods of disease exacerbation when bowel rest is needed. The client might also receive enteral nutrition while on TPN in order to provide nutrients directly to the gut (Day, 2008). (Refer to CP: Total Nutritional Support: Parenteral/Enteral Feeding.)

(continues on page 300)

ACTIONS/INTERVENTIONS (continued)	RATIONALE (continued)
Monitor nutritional studies and client's symptoms for deficits and administer vitamins and minerals as individually indicated.	Various supplements may be needed, depending on many factors, such as the client's individual disease, whether disease is active all the time, or in remission at times, or if the client has had surgery that requires life-long supplementation.

NURSING DIAGNOSIS: Anxiety [specify level]

May Be Related To

Stress, situational crises
Threat to self-concept
Threat to, or change in, health status, economic status, role functioning, interaction patterns

Possibly Evidenced By

Abdominal pain; diarrhea
Increased tension, distressed, apprehensive
Reports concerns due to change in life
Awareness of physiological symptoms
Focus on self

Desired Outcomes/Evaluation Criteria—Client Will

Anxiety Control (NOC)

Appear relaxed and report anxiety reduced to a manageable level.
Verbalize awareness of feelings of anxiety and healthy ways to deal with them.

ACTIONS/INTERVENTIONS	RATIONALE
Anxiety Reduction (NIC)	
Independent	
Note behavioral clues—restlessness, irritability, withdrawal, lack of eye contact, and demanding behavior.	Indicators of degree of anxiety or stress; for example, client may feel out of control at home or work managing personal problems. Stress may develop as a result of physical symptoms of condition and the reaction of others.
Encourage verbalization of feelings. Provide feedback.	Establishes a therapeutic relationship. Assists client/significant others (SOs) in identifying problems causing stress. Client with severe diarrhea may hesitate to ask for help for fear of becoming a burden to the staff.
Acknowledge that the anxiety and problems are similar to those expressed by others. Active-listen client's concerns.	Validation that feelings are normal can help reduce stress/isolation and belief that "I am the only one."
Provide accurate, concrete information about what is being done, such as reason for bedrest, restriction of oral intake, and procedures.	Involving client in plan of care provides sense of control and helps decrease anxiety.
Provide a calm, restful environment.	Removing client from outside stressors promotes relaxation and helps reduce anxiety.
Encourage staff/SO to project caring, concerned attitude.	A supportive manner can help client feel less stressed, allowing energy to be directed toward healing and recovery.
Help client identify and initiate positive coping behaviors used in the past.	Successful behaviors can be fostered in dealing with current problems or stress, enhancing client's sense of self-control.
Assist client to learn new coping mechanisms, such as stress management techniques and organizational skills.	Learning new ways to cope can be helpful in reducing stress and anxiety, enhancing disease control.
Collaborative	
Administer medications, as indicated, for example, anti-anxiety agents, such as diazepam (Valium) and alprazolam (Xanax).	May be used to reduce anxiety and to facilitate rest, particularly in the client with UC.
Refer to psychiatric clinical nurse specialist, social services, or spiritual advisor.	May require additional assistance in regaining control and coping with acute episodes or exacerbations, as well as learning to deal with the chronicity and consequences of the disease and therapeutic regimen.

NURSING DIAGNOSIS: acute Pain

May Be Related To

Physical agents—hyperperistalsis, prolonged diarrhea, skin and tissue irritation, perirectal excoriation, fissures, fistulas

Possibly Evidenced By

Verbal/coded reports of pain
Guarding or distraction behaviors, restlessness
Facial mask; self-focusing

Desired Outcomes/Evaluation Criteria—Client Will

Pain Level (NOC)

Report pain is relieved or controlled.
Appear relaxed and able to sleep and rest appropriately.

ACTIONS/INTERVENTIONS	RATIONALE
Pain Management (NIC)	
Independent	
Encourage client to report pain.	May try to tolerate pain rather than request analgesics.
Assess reports of abdominal cramping or pain, noting location, duration, and intensity (using a 0 to 10 or similar coded scale). Investigate and report changes in pain characteristics.	Colicky intermittent pain occurs with Crohn's disease. Predefecation pain frequently occurs in UC with urgency, which may be severe and continuous. Changes in pain characteristics may indicate spread of disease or developing complications, such as bladder fistula, perforation, and toxic megacolon.
Note nonverbal cues, such as restlessness, reluctance to move, abdominal guarding, withdrawal, and depression. Investigate discrepancies between verbal and nonverbal cues.	Body language or nonverbal cues may be both physiological and psychological and may be used in conjunction with verbal cues to determine extent and severity of the problem.
Review factors that aggravate or alleviate pain.	May pinpoint precipitating or aggravating factors (e.g., stressful events, food intolerance) or identify developing complications.
Provide comfort measures (e.g., back rub, reposition) and diversional activities.	Promotes relaxation, refocuses attention, and may enhance coping abilities.
Cleanse rectal area with mild soap and water (or wipes) after each stool and provide skin care with a moisture barrier ointment.	Protects skin from bowel acids, preventing excoriation.
Provide sitz bath, as appropriate.	Enhances cleanliness and comfort in the presence of perianal irritation and fissures.
Observe for perianal ulcerations or fistulas.	Fistulas may develop from erosion and weakening of intestinal wall.
Observe and record abdominal distention, increased temperature, and decreased BP.	May indicate developing intestinal obstruction from inflammation, edema, and scarring.
Collaborative	
Implement prescribed dietary modifications; for example, commence with liquids and increase to solid foods as tolerated.	Bowel rest can reduce pain and cramping.
Administer medications as indicated, for example:	
Analgesics	Pain varies from mild to severe and necessitates management to facilitate adequate rest and recovery. *Note:* Opiates should be used with caution because they may precipitate toxic megacolon.
Anticholinergics	Relieve spasms of GI tract and resultant colicky pain.
Anodyne suppositories	Relax rectal muscle, decreasing painful spasms.

NURSING DIAGNOSIS: ineffective Coping

May Be Related To

Situational crises; inadequate opportunity to prepare for stressors
Uncertainty—unpredictable nature of disease process
Severe/chronic pain
Inadequate level of confidence in ability to cope

(continues on page 302)

NURSING DIAGNOSIS: ineffective Coping (continued)

Possibly Evidenced By

Reports inability to cope
Use of forms of coping that impede adaptive behaviors
Inadequate problem-solving
Sleep pattern disturbance; fatigue

Desired Outcomes/Evaluation Criteria—Client Will

Coping (NOC)

Assess the current situation accurately.
Identify ineffective coping behaviors and consequences.
Acknowledge own coping abilities.
Demonstrate necessary lifestyle changes to limit or prevent recurrent episodes.

ACTIONS/INTERVENTIONS	RATIONALE
Coping Enhancement (NIC)	
Independent	
Assess client's/SO's understanding and previous methods of dealing with disease process.	Enables the nurse to deal more realistically with current problems. Anxiety and other problems may have interfered with previous health teaching and client learning.
Determine outside stressors, such as family, relationships, and social or work environment.	Stress can alter autonomic nervous response, affecting the immune system and contributing to exacerbation of disease. Even the goal of independence in the dependent client can be an added stressor.
Provide opportunity for client to discuss how illness has affected relationships, including sexual concerns.	Stressors of illness affect all areas of life, and client may have difficulty coping with embarrassment, fatigue, and pain in regard to relationship and sexual needs.
(P) Determine child's general well-being regarding social functioning and effects of disease (e.g., is not participating in sports, missing school, declining dates). Refer to appropriate counseling and/or support groups, as indicated.	Child may tend to be tired, underweight, or small, impairing ability to maintain same activity involvement as peers. Adolescent or young adult of dating age may be avoiding relationships and intimacy because of embarrassment over frequent diarrhea or presence of ostomy. Differences in appearance and energy, as well as an overall anxiety over symptoms, can affect the way the child relates to parents, teachers, friends, dates, and coworkers if employed.
Help client identify individually effective coping skills.	Use of previously successful behaviors can help client deal with current situation and plan for the future.
Provide emotional support:	
Active-listen in a nonjudgmental manner.	Aids in communication and understanding client's viewpoint. Can enhance client's feelings of self-worth.
Maintain nonjudgmental body language when caring for client.	Prevents reinforcing client's feelings of being a burden, for example, frequent need to empty bedpan or commode.
Assign same staff as much as possible.	Provides a therapeutic environment and lessens the stress of constant adjustments to different people when client is dealing with embarrassment and depression.
Provide uninterrupted sleep or rest periods.	Exhaustion brought on by the disease tends to magnify problems, interfering with ability to cope.
Encourage use of stress management skills, such as relaxation techniques, visualization, guided imagery, and deep-breathing exercises.	Refocuses attention, promotes relaxation, and enhances coping abilities.
Collaborative	
Include client/SO in team conferences to develop individualized program.	Promotes continuity of care and enables client/SO to feel a part of the plan, imparting a sense of control and increasing cooperation with therapeutic regimen.
Administer medications as indicated, for example, antianxiety agents, such as lorazepam (Ativan) and alprazolam (Xanax).	Aids in psychological and physical rest. Conserves energy and may strengthen coping abilities.
Refer to resources, as indicated, such as local support group, social worker, psychiatric clinical nurse specialist, or spiritual advisor.	Additional support and counseling can assist client/SO in dealing with specific stress or problem areas.

NURSING DIAGNOSIS: ineffective Self-Health Management

May Be Related To

Complexity of therapeutic regimen
Perceived benefits/barriers
Powerlessness; social support deficits

Possibly Evidenced By

Reports desire to manage the illness
Reports difficulty with prescribed regimen
Failure to include treatment regimen in daily living
Unexpected acceleration of illness symptoms

Desired Outcomes/Evaluation Criteria—Client Will

Knowledge: Inflammatory Bowel Disease Management (NOC)

Verbalize understanding of disease processes and possible complications.
Identify stress situations and specific action(s) to deal with them.
Verbalize understanding of therapeutic regimen.
Participate in treatment regimen.
Initiate necessary lifestyle changes.

ACTIONS/INTERVENTIONS	RATIONALE
Teaching: Disease Process (NIC)	
Independent	
Determine client's perception of disease process.	Establishes knowledge base and provides some insight into individual learning needs.
Review disease process, cause-and-effect relationship of factors that precipitate symptoms, and identify ways to reduce contributing factors. Encourage questions.	Precipitating or aggravating factors are individual; therefore, client needs to be aware of what foods, fluids, and lifestyle factors can precipitate symptoms. Accurate knowledge base provides opportunity for client to make informed decisions or choices about future and control of chronic disease. Although most clients know about their own disease process, they may have outdated information or misconceptions.
Review medications, purpose, frequency, dosage, and possible side effects.	Promotes understanding and may enhance cooperation with regimen.
Remind client to observe for side effects of steroids (such as ulcers, facial edema, and muscle weakness) if used on a long-term basis.	Steroids may be used to control inflammation and to effect a remission of the disease; however, drug may lower resistance to infection and cause fluid retention, and increase risk of death when taken over time.
Stress importance of good skin care, including proper hand-washing and perineal skin care.	Reduces spread of bacteria and risk of skin irritation or breakdown and infection.
Recommend cessation of smoking. Refer to antismoking resources, if client is desirous of support and assistance.	Can increase intestinal motility and cause vasoconstriction of intestinal blood vessels, aggravating disease.
Emphasize need for long-term follow-up and periodic reevaluation.	Clients with IBD are at increased risk for colon/rectal cancer, and regular diagnostic evaluations may be required.
(P) Recommend and refer for close monitoring of laboratory studies (e.g., CBC, WBC, platelets, liver enzymes) for adverse effects of drugs on body systems.	Drug interactions and adverse effects of drugs can occur in all populations, but owing to the smaller size of children as well as ongoing changes in their bodies, adverse drug effects can occur more readily and with more harmful long-term consequences. Examples: The known adverse effects of thiopurines include hepatotoxicity, pancreatitis, allergic reactions, fever, rash, infectious complications, and bone marrow suppression, with increased risk for cancer. Corticosteroids increase the risk of infection and may worsen the complications of abscesses and fistulae.
(P) Discuss with client/caregiver use of vaccines in children with IBD. Encourage caregivers to address this issue with healthcare providers ongoing throughout child's appropriate age to receive immunizations.	Depending on age of child at diagnosis and anticipated drug therapy, certain guidelines will be followed. For example: Live vaccines are contraindicated while on some thiopurines (e.g., 6-MP) or immunomodulators (e.g., infliximab). However, immunization guidelines suggest that protection against vaccine-preventable illness is beneficial in immunocompromised IBD patients, and that most attenuated vaccines can be administered. Some immunizations (e.g., HPV, varicella) may be administered prior to initiating thiopurines or immunomodulators (Stevens et al, 2011; Sands et al, 2004).

(continues on page 304)

ACTIONS/INTERVENTIONS (continued)	RATIONALE (continued)
Identify appropriate community resources, such as Crohn's and Colitis Foundation of America (CCFA), United Ostomy Association of America (UOAA), North American Society for Pediatric Gastroenterology, Hepatology and Nutrition (NASPGHN); home healthcare providers and visiting nurse services, nutritionist, and social services.	Client/caregivers may benefit from the services of these agencies in coping with chronicity of the disease and evaluating treatment options.

POTENTIAL CONSIDERATIONS following acute hospitalization (dependent on client's age, physical condition and presence of complications, personal resources, and life responsibilities)

- ***acute Pain***—physical agents (hyperperistalsis, skin and tissue irritation—perirectal excoriation, fissures, fistulas)
- ***ineffective Coping***—uncertainty (unpredictable nature of disease process); severe pain; situational crisis
- ***risk for Infection***—traumatized tissue, change in pH of secretions, altered peristalsis, suppressed inflammatory response, chronic disease, malnutrition
- ***ineffective Self-Health Management***—complexity of therapeutic regimen; perceived benefit; powerlessness; social support deficit

FECAL DIVERSIONS: POSTOPERATIVE CARE OF ILEOSTOMY AND COLOSTOMY

I. Procedures—Incontinent diversions (primary focus of this plan of care), laparoscopic colectomy, and continent diversions, such as the Kock pouch and the ileoanal reservoir

a. Ileostomy

i. Performed when the entire colon, rectum, and anus must be removed, in which case the ileostomy is permanent; or, a temporary ileostomy can be done to provide complete bowel rest in conditions such as with chronic colitis and in some trauma cases, or when ileoanal anastomosis has been preformed

ii. Most frequently performed for complications of inflammatory bowel disease—Crohn's disease and ulcerative colitis—including intestinal perforation or intestinal stricture causing obstruction, abscess, or massive hemorrhage (Gutman, 2011; Boehmke, 2006)

iii. May also be done because of intestinal trauma, polyps, cancer of the bowel, bladder, and reproductive organs, or complications from cancer (Gutman, 2011; Dorman, 2009)

b. Colostomy may be performed at several locations: the ascending, transverse, descending, or sigmoid colon.

i. Ascending colostomy is positioned in the upper right side of the abdomen.

ii. Transverse colostomy is positioned in the mid-to-right upper abdomen.

1. Performed for diverticulitis, bowel obstruction, trauma, or cancer of the descending or sigmoid colon
2. Usually temporary, but can be permanent when the lower portion of the colon must be removed or permanently rested

iii. Descending/sigmoid colostomy is positioned in the lower left side of the abdomen.

1. Most common permanent stoma with opening in the lower end of the colon
2. Performed for cancer of rectum or sigmoid colon as well as for diverticulitis, bowel obstruction, trauma, and paralysis (Gutman, 2011)

II. Etiology—Dependent on underlying pathology requiring procedure

III. Statistics

a. Morbidity: An estimated 42,000 to 65,000 ostomy surgeries are performed each year; about half are temporary (Franz, 2004).

b. Mortality: Deaths associated with ostomies appear to be low (between 0.8% and 3.8%; Franz, 2004) and are dependent on reason for procedure (such as Crohn's disease versus penetrating trauma or cancer) and comorbidities (Bosshardt, 2003).

c. Cost: Direct care costs for cancer cases alone in 2004 estimated at over $4 billion (colorectal) and $1.2 million (small intestines) (Everhart, 2008).

GLOSSARY

Anus: Terminal part of the rectum.

Appliance: Formal term for an ostomy pouch or ostomy bag.

Colectomy: Surgical removal of the colon (also known as the large intestine). Depending on what's necessary, a colectomy can be a partial or a total removal of the colon.

Colon: Part of the intestine that stores digested food and absorbs water. Also referred to as the large intestine or the large bowel.

Colostomy: Surgical opening to bring a portion of the colon (large) intestine through the abdominal wall to form a stoma.

GLOSSARY (continued)

Effluent: Waste from the ostomy.

Ileostomy: Opening that is surgically constructed in the ileum with the intestine brought through the abdominal wall to form a stoma.

Ileum: Lowest part or end of the small intestine.

Irrigation: Enema that is brought through the stoma, used by some colostomates, to regulate the passage of stool.

Ostomy: Umbrella term that refers to the surgically created opening in the body for the discharge of body wastes. Types of ostomies for fecal diversion include colostomy and ileostomy.

Peristalsis: Progressive waves of motion, which occur without voluntary control, to push contents through the intestine.

Pouching system: Device worn over the stoma, which acts as a reservoir for the stool that empties out of the stoma. Pouching systems are made of two primary components: a wafer (also called a skin barrier or faceplate) and a pouch. The pouch can be transparent or opaque, drainable or a "closed end" (disposable), and offered in different sizes and styles (Washuta, 2010).

Prolapse: A "falling out" in which the stoma becomes longer.

Rectum: Lowest portion of the large intestine.

Skin barrier: Solid square or round piece of adhesive material that is used to protect the skin from stool.

Stenosis: Narrowing or tightness of the stoma, which may cause obstruction.

Stoma: Opening at the end of the colon or ileum; this is brought through the surface of the skin. Stomas may protrude above skin level (preferable), be flush at skin level, or retracted below skin level (may be a complication) (Dorman, 2011; Butler, 2009).

Care Settings

Care is handled in an inpatient acute care surgical unit.

Related Concerns

Cancer—general considerations, page 827
Fluid and electrolyte imbalances, page 885
Inflammatory bowel disease (IBD): ulcerative colitis, Crohn's disease, page 291
Psychosocial aspects of care, page 729
Surgical intervention, page 762
Total nutritional support: parenteral/enteral feeding, page 437

Client Assessment Database

Data depend on the underlying problem, duration, and severity (e.g., obstruction, perforation, inflammation, congenital defects).

DIAGNOSTIC DIVISION MAY REPORT	MAY EXHIBIT
TEACHING/LEARNING **DISCHARGE PLAN CONSIDERATIONS:** • Assistance with dietary concerns • Management of ostomy • Acquisition of supplies ➧ Refer to section at end of plan for postdischarge considerations.	

Nursing Priorities

1. Assist client/significant other (SO) in psychosocial adjustment.
2. Prevent complications.
3. Support independence in self-care.
4. Provide information about procedure, prognosis, treatment needs, potential complications, and community resources.

Discharge Goals

1. Adjusting to perceived or actual changes.
2. Complications prevented or minimized.
3. Self-care needs met by self or with assistance depending on specific situation.
4. Procedure, prognosis, therapeutic regimen, and potential complications understood and sources of support identified.
5. Plan in place to meet needs after discharge.

NURSING DIAGNOSIS: risk for impaired Skin Integrity

Risk Factors May Include

Excretions—character and flow of effluent and flatus from stoma; improper fitting or care of appliance/skin
Chemical substance—reaction to product or chemicals used

Possibly Evidenced By

(Not applicable; presence of signs and symptoms establishes an *actual* diagnosis)

Desired Outcomes/Evaluation Criteria—Client Will

Ostomy Self-Care (NOC)

Maintain skin integrity around stoma.
Identify individual risk factors.
Demonstrate behaviors or techniques to promote healing and/or prevent skin breakdown.

ACTIONS/INTERVENTIONS	RATIONALE
Ostomy Care (NIC)	
Independent	
Inspect stoma and peristomal skin area with each pouch change. Note irritation, bruises (dark, bluish color), and rashes.	Identifies areas of concern and need for further evaluation and intervention. Early identification of stomal ischemia or infection (from changes in normal bowel flora) provides for timely interventions to prevent serious complications. Stoma should be red and moist. *Note:* An early postoperative complication (possibly within 24 hours) is stoma ischemia or necrosis due to vascular insufficiency with subsequent retraction and stenosis, with potential early surgical revision (Borwell, 2011; Butler, 2009). Ulcerated areas on stoma may be from a pouch opening that is too small or a faceplate that cuts into stoma. In clients with an ileostomy, the effluent is rich in enzymes, increasing the likelihood of skin excoriation.
Clean with warm water and pat dry. Use soap only if area is covered with sticky stool. If paste has collected on the skin, let it dry, and then peel it off.	Maintaining a clean and dry area helps prevent skin breakdown and increases adherence of appliances.
Measure stoma periodically—at least weekly for first 6 weeks, then once a month for 6 months. Measure both width and length of stoma.	As postoperative edema resolves, the stoma shrinks and the size of the opening in the skin barrier of the appliance must be altered to ensure proper fit so that effluent is collected as it flows from the ostomy and contact with the skin is prevented.
Verify that the opening on the skin barrier is no more than 1/8 inch (2 to 3 mm) larger than the base of the stoma, with adequate adhesive barrier to apply pouch.	Prevents trauma to the stoma tissue and protects the peristomal skin. Adequate adhesive area prevents the skin barrier wafer from being too tight. *Note:* Too tight a fit may cause stomal edema or injure the stoma.
Use a transparent, odor-proof, drainable pouch.	The appliance can be either one-piece (pouch is permanently attached to skin barrier) or two-piece (pouch snaps onto skin barrier). A transparent appliance during the first 4 to 6 weeks allows easy observation of stoma without necessity of removing pouch and irritating skin.
Apply appropriate skin barrier—hydrocolloid wafer, extended-wear skin barrier, or similar products.	Protects skin from pouch adhesive, enhances adhesiveness of pouch, and facilitates removal of pouch when necessary. *Note:* Sigmoid colostomy may not require an appliance if elimination is regulated through irrigation.
Empty, rinse with water, and cleanse ostomy pouch on a routine basis (usually when pouch is half full), using appropriate equipment.	Emptying and rinsing the pouch with the proper solution removes bacteria and odor-causing stool and flatus.
Support surrounding skin when gently removing appliance. Apply adhesive removers as indicated, and then wash thoroughly.	Prevents tissue irritation and destruction associated with "pulling" pouch off.
Investigate reports of burning, itching, or blistering around stoma.	Indicative of effluent leakage with peristomal irritation, or possibly *Candida* infection, requiring intervention.
Evaluate adhesive product and appliance fit on ongoing basis.	Provides opportunity for problem-solving. Determines need for further intervention.
Collaborative	
Consult with certified wound, ostomy, continence (WOC) nurse.	Knowledgeable specialist in the care and teaching of clients with ostomies may be helpful in choosing products appropriate

for client's particular needs (e.g., ostomy appliance and protective barriers); or be able to assist with evaluation and problem-solving in client's physical and emotional needs and capabilities in handling self-care.

Apply corticosteroid aerosol spray and prescribed antifungal powder or other product, as indicated.

Assists in healing if peristomal irritation persists and fungal infection develops. *Note:* These products can have potent side effects and should be used sparingly.

NURSING DIAGNOSIS: disturbed Body Image

May Be Related To

Biophysical—loss of control of bowel elimination
Psychosocial—altered body structure (presence of stoma)
Illness—cancer, colitis, diverticulitis; injury/trauma
Associated treatment regimen

Possibly Evidenced By

Actual change in structure and function—ostomy
Reports feelings that reflect an altered view of one's body (e.g., appearance, structure, function)
Reports negative feelings about body, fear of reaction by others
Not touching or looking at stoma

Desired Outcomes/Evaluation Criteria—Client Will

Body Image (NOC)

Verbalize acceptance of self in situation, incorporating change into self-concept without negating self-esteem.
Demonstrate beginning acceptance by viewing and touching stoma and participating in self-care.
Verbalize feelings about stoma and illness; begin to deal constructively with situation.

ACTIONS/INTERVENTIONS — RATIONALE

Body Image Enhancement (NIC)

Independent

Ascertain whether support and counseling were initiated when the possibility and/or necessity of ostomy was first discussed.

Provides information about client's/SO's level of knowledge and anxiety about individual situation.

Encourage client/SO to verbalize feelings regarding the ostomy. Acknowledge normality of feelings of anger, depression, and grief over loss. Discuss daily "ups and downs" that can occur.

Helps client realize that feelings are not unusual and that feeling guilty about them is not necessary or helpful. Client needs to recognize feelings before they can be dealt with effectively.

Review reason for surgery and future expectations.

Client may find it easier to deal with an ostomy done to correct long-term disease than for traumatic injury or bowel perforation, even if ostomy is only temporary. Also, client who will be undergoing a second procedure to convert ostomy to a continent or anal reservoir may possibly encounter less severe self-image problems because body function eventually will be "more normal."

Be sensitive to client's fears and concerns, noting religious, familial, cultural, relationship and spiritual beliefs that may be impacting the situation.

Recovery from this surgery requires some mental toughness, as well as ongoing support from family/SOs. The client is rallying from surgery and from whatever disease necessitated the ostomy. He/she may be weak and depressed at the same time having to cope with an unpleasant change in body image and function. Concerns can be associated with fear (e.g., of pain, mortality, managing life roles, and sexuality issues). A client's support systems, as well as religious, cultural, and spiritual beliefs impact not only the current situation but also future expectation and outcomes (Borwell, 2011).

Provide opportunities for client/SO to view and touch stoma, using the moment to point out positive signs of healing, normal appearance, and so forth. Remind client that it will take time to adjust, both physically and emotionally.

Although integration of stoma into body image can take months or even years, looking at the stoma and hearing comments made in a normal, matter-of-fact manner can help client with this acceptance. Touching stoma reassures client/SO that it is not fragile and that slight movements of stoma actually reflect normal peristalsis.

(continues on page 308)

ACTIONS/INTERVENTIONS (continued)	RATIONALE (continued)
Provide opportunity for client to deal with ostomy through participation in self-care.	Independence in self-care helps improve self-confidence and acceptance of situation.
Plan care activities with client.	Promotes sense of control and gives message that client can handle situation, enhancing self-concept.
Maintain positive approach during care activities, avoiding expressions of disdain or revulsion. Do not take angry expressions of client/SO personally.	Assists client/SO to accept body changes and feel good about self. Anger is most often directed at the situation and lack of control or powerlessness individual has over what has happened—not with the caregiver.
Note behaviors of withdrawal, increased dependency, manipulation, or noninvolvement in care.	Suggestive of problems in adjustment that may require further evaluation and more intensive interventions.
Ascertain client's desire to visit with a person with an ostomy. Make arrangements for visit, if desired. Refer for psychological interventions, as indicated.	A person who is living with an ostomy can be a good support system and role model for the new ostomate. Shared experiences help reinforce teaching and facilitate acceptance of change as client realizes "life does go on" and can be relatively normal.

NURSING DIAGNOSIS: acute Pain

May Be Related To

Physical factors—disruption of skin or tissues (incisions, drains)
Biological factors—activity of disease process (cancer, trauma)
Psychological factors—fear, anxiety

Possibly Evidenced By

Verbal/coded reports of pain, self-focusing
Guarding and expressive behaviors—restlessness
Changes in vital signs

Desired Outcomes/Evaluation Criteria—Client Will

Pain Level (NOC)
Verbalize that pain is relieved or controlled.
Appear relaxed and able to sleep or rest appropriately.

Pain Control (NOC)
Demonstrate use of relaxation skills and general comfort measures, as indicated for individual situation.

ACTIONS/INTERVENTIONS	RATIONALE
Pain Management (NIC)	
Independent	
Assess pain, noting location, characteristics, and intensity (such as 0 to 10 or similar coded scale).	Helps evaluate degree of discomfort and effectiveness of analgesia or may reveal developing complications. Because abdominal pain usually subsides gradually by the third or fourth postoperative day, continued or increasing pain may reflect delayed healing or peristomal skin irritation. *Note:* Pain in anal area associated with abdominal-perineal resection may persist for months.
Encourage client to verbalize concerns. Active-listen to these concerns, and provide support by acceptance, remaining with client, and giving appropriate information.	Reduction of anxiety and fear can promote relaxation and comfort.
Provide comfort measures, such as back rub, and repositioning. Assure client that position change will not injure stoma.	Reduces muscle tension, promotes relaxation, and may enhance coping abilities.
Encourage use of relaxation techniques such as guided imagery and visualization. Provide diversional activities.	Helps client rest more effectively and refocuses attention, thereby reducing pain and discomfort.
Assist with range-of-motion exercises and encourage early ambulation. Avoid prolonged sitting position.	Reduces muscle and joint stiffness. Ambulation returns organs to normal position and promotes return of usual level of functioning. *Note:* Presence of edema, packing, and drains (if perineal resection has been done) increases discomfort and creates a sense of needing to defecate. Ambulation and frequent position changes reduce perineal pressure.
Investigate and report abdominal muscle rigidity, involuntary guarding, and rebound tenderness.	Suggestive of peritoneal inflammation, which requires prompt medical intervention.

ACTIONS/INTERVENTIONS (continued)	RATIONALE (continued)
Collaborative	
Administer medication, such as opioids, analgesics, and by appropriate route (e.g., IV, patch, oral, patient-controlled analgesia [PCA]), as indicated.	Relieves pain, enhances comfort, and promotes rest. PCA may be more beneficial initially, especially following anal-perineal repair.
Provide sitz baths.	Relieves local discomfort, reduces edema, and promotes healing of perineal wound.

NURSING DIAGNOSIS: impaired Skin/Tissue Integrity

May Be Related To

Mechanical factors—trauma (injury, surgery)
Stasis of secretions or drainage
Impaired circulation
Imbalanced nutritional state—malnutrition, changes in fluid status/turgor

Possibly Evidenced By

Disruption of skin layers—presence of incision and sutures, drains

Desired Outcomes/Evaluation Criteria—Client Will

Wound Healing: Primary Intention (NOC)

Achieve timely wound healing free of signs of infection.

ACTIONS/INTERVENTIONS	RATIONALE
Wound Care (NIC)	
Independent	
Observe wounds, noting characteristics of drainage.	Postoperative hemorrhage is most likely to occur during the first 48 hours, whereas infection may develop at any time. Depending on type of wound closure, complete healing may take 6 to 8 months.
Change dressings as needed.	Large amounts of serous drainage require that dressings be changed frequently to reduce skin irritation and potential for infection.
Encourage side-lying position with head elevated. Avoid prolonged sitting.	Promotes drainage from perineal wound/drains, reducing risk of pooling. Prolonged sitting increases perineal pressure, reducing circulation to wound, and may delay healing.
Collaborative	
Irrigate wound as indicated, using normal saline (NS) or specified antimicrobial solution.	May be required to treat preoperative inflammation, infection, or intraoperative contamination.
Provide sitz baths, if indicated, based on surgical procedure.	Promotes perineal cleanliness and facilitates healing, especially after packing is removed—usually day 3 to 5.

NURSING DIAGNOSIS: risk for deficient Fluid Volume

Risk Factors May Include

Excessive losses through normal routes—preoperative emesis and diarrhea; high-volume ileostomy output
Loss of fluid through abnormal routes—nasogastric (NG) or intestinal tube, perineal wound drainage tubes
Deviations affecting intake—medically restricted intake, absorption of fluid—loss of colon function
Factors influencing fluid needs—hypermetabolic states (inflammation, healing process)

Possibly Evidenced By

(Not applicable; presence of signs and symptoms establishes an *actual* diagnosis)

Desired Outcomes/Evaluation Criteria—Client Will

Hydration (NOC)

Maintain adequate hydration as evidenced by moist mucous membranes, good skin turgor and capillary refill, stable vital signs, and individually appropriate urinary output.

ACTIONS/INTERVENTIONS	RATIONALE
Fluid/Electrolyte Management (NIC)	
Independent	
Monitor intake and output (I&O) carefully and measure ostomy effluent. Weigh regularly.	Provides direct indicators of fluid balance. *Note:* Maintaining an appropriate fluid intake and electrolyte balance is significant for the ileostomist due to loss of the colon and its water absorbing properties. Postoperatively, daily output can be up to 1500 mL, gradually decreasing to around 350 to 800 mL (Black, 2000).
Monitor vital signs, noting postural hypotension and tachycardia. Evaluate skin turgor, capillary refill, and mucous membranes.	Reflects hydration status and possible need for fluid replacement.
Limit intake of ice chips during period of gastric intubation.	Ice chips can stimulate gastric secretions and wash out electrolytes.
Collaborative	
Monitor laboratory results, such as Hct and electrolytes.	Detects homeostasis or imbalance and aids in determining replacement needs.
Administer intravenous (IV) fluid and electrolytes as indicated.	May be necessary to maintain adequate tissue perfusion and organ function.

NURSING DIAGNOSIS: risk for imbalanced Nutrition: less than body requirements

Risk Factors May Include

Inability to ingest food (prolonged anorexia, altered intake preoperatively)
Inability to digest food/absorb nutrients (diarrhea)
[Hypermetabolic state—preoperative inflammatory disease; healing process]

Possibly Evidenced By

(Not applicable; presence of signs and symptoms establishes an *actual* diagnosis)

Desired Outcomes/Evaluation Criteria—Client Will

Nutritional Status (NOC)

Maintain weight or demonstrate progressive weight gain toward goal with normalization of laboratory values and be free of signs of malnutrition.
Plan diet to meet nutritional needs and limit gastrointestinal (GI) disturbances.

ACTIONS/INTERVENTIONS	RATIONALE
Nutrition Therapy (NIC)	
Independent	
Obtain a thorough nutritional assessment.	Identifies deficiencies and needs to aid in choice of interventions.
Auscultate bowel sounds.	Return of intestinal function indicates readiness to resume oral intake.
Resume solid foods slowly.	Reduces incidence of abdominal cramps and nausea.
Identify odor-causing foods, for instance, cabbage, fish, and beans, and temporarily restrict from diet. Gradually reintroduce one food at a time.	Sensitivity to certain foods is not uncommon following intestinal surgery. Client can experiment with food several times before determining whether it is creating a problem.
Recommend client increase use of yogurt, buttermilk, and acidophilus preparations, if needed.	May help prevent gas and decrease odor formation.
Suggest client with ileostomy limit prunes, dates, stewed apricots, strawberries, grapes, bananas, cabbage family, and beans, and avoid foods high in cellulose, such as peanuts.	These products increase ileal effluent. Digestion of cellulose requires colonic bacteria that are no longer present.
Discuss mechanics of swallowed air as a factor in the formation of flatus and some ways client can exercise control. Discuss use of a pouch with a filter to help with the management of gas.	Drinking through a straw, snoring, anxiety, smoking, ill-fitting dentures, and gulping down food increase the production of flatus. Too much flatus not only necessitates frequent emptying but also can cause leakage from too much pressure within the pouch.
Collaborative	
Consult with dietitian and nutrition specialist.	Helpful in assessing client's nutritional needs in light of changes in digestion and intestinal function, including absorption of vitamins and minerals.
Advance diet from liquids to low-residue food when oral intake is resumed.	Low-residue diet may be maintained during first 6 to 8 weeks to provide adequate time for intestinal healing.

ACTIONS/INTERVENTIONS (continued)	RATIONALE (continued)
Administer enteral or parenteral feedings when indicated.	In the presence of severe debilitation or intolerance of oral intake, parenteral or enteral feedings may be given to supply needed nutrients for healing and prevention of catabolic state. (Refer to CP: Total Nutritional Support: Parenteral/Enteral Feeding.)

NURSING DIAGNOSIS: Insomnia

May Be Related To

Interrupted sleep—necessity of ostomy care, excessive flatus or ostomy effluent
Physical discomfort/pain
Stress, anxiety

Possibly Evidenced By

Reports difficulty staying asleep, dissatisfaction with sleep, nonrestorative sleep
Observed lack of energy

Desired Outcomes/Evaluation Criteria—Client Will

Sleep (NOC)

Sleep or rest between disturbances.
Report increased sense of well-being and feeling rested.

ACTIONS/INTERVENTIONS	RATIONALE
Sleep Enhancement (NIC)	
Independent	
Explain necessity to monitor intestinal function in early postoperative period.	Client is more apt to be tolerant of disturbances by staff if he or she understands the reasons for, and importance of, ostomy care.
Provide adequate pouching system. Empty pouch before retiring and, if necessary, on an agreed-upon schedule, or when half full.	Excessive gas or effluent can occur despite interventions. Emptying on a regular schedule, or when half full, minimizes threat of leakage.
Let client know that stoma will not be injured when sleeping.	Client will be able to rest better if feeling secure about stoma and ostomy function.
Restrict intake of caffeine-containing foods and fluids.	Caffeine may delay client's falling asleep and interfere with REM (rapid eye movement) sleep, resulting in client not feeling well rested.
Support continuation of usual bedtime rituals.	Promotes relaxation and readiness for sleep.
Collaborative	
Determine cause of excessive flatus or effluent and possible actions, such as conferring with dietitian regarding restriction of foods if diet-related.	Identification of cause enables institution of corrective measures that may promote sleep or rest.
Administer analgesics or sedatives at bedtime, as indicated.	Pain can interfere with client's ability to fall, or remain, asleep. Timely medication can enhance rest or sleep during initial postoperative period. *Note:* Pain pathways in the brain lie near the sleep center and may contribute to wakefulness.

NURSING DIAGNOSIS: risk for Constipation/Diarrhea

Risk Factors May Include

Placement of ostomy in descending or sigmoid colon
Insufficient fiber or fluid intake
Stress, anxiety

Possibly Evidenced By

(Not applicable; presence of signs and symptoms establishes an *actual* diagnosis)

Desired Outcomes/Evaluation Criteria—Client Will

Bowel Elimination (NOC)

Establish an elimination pattern suitable to physical needs and lifestyle with effluent of appropriate amount and consistency.

ACTIONS/INTERVENTIONS	RATIONALE
Bowel Management (NIC)	
Independent	
Investigate delayed onset or absence of effluent. Auscultate bowel sounds.	Postoperative paralytic or adynamic ileus usually resolves within 48 to 72 hours, and ileostomy should begin draining within 12 to 24 hours. Delay may indicate persistent ileus or stomal obstruction, which may occur postoperatively because of edema, improperly fitting pouch (too tight), prolapse or stenosis of the stoma.
Inform client with an ileostomy that initially the effluent is liquid. If constipation occurs, it should be reported to ostomy nurse or physician immediately.	Although the small intestine eventually begins to take on water-absorbing functions to permit a more semisolid consistency, pasty discharge or absence of output may indicate an obstruction. Absence of stool requires emergency medical attention.
Review dietary pattern and amount and type of fluid intake.	Adequate intake of fiber and roughage provides bulk, and fluid is an important factor in determining the consistency of the stool.
Emphasize importance of chewing food well, adequate intake of fluids with and following meals, only moderate use of high-fiber foods, and avoidance of cellulose.	Reduces risk of bowel obstruction in client with ileostomy.
Review foods that are, or may be, a source of flatus, such as carbonated drinks, beer, beans, cabbage, onions, fish, and highly seasoned foods; or odor, such as onions, cabbage, eggs, fish, and beans.	These foods may be restricted or eliminated, based on individual reaction, for better ostomy control, or it may be necessary to empty the pouch more frequently if these foods are ingested.
Review physiology of the colon and discuss irrigation if indicated.	This knowledge helps client understand individual care needs. The client with a permanent colostomy and whose stoma is in the descending or sigmoid portion may choose to irrigate the large intestine, thereby stimulating the colon to flush out waste and allowing the client to regain control over elimination. This is because stools tend to be more formed. A client with irritable bowel syndrome, stomal problems, or stomas in the ascending or transverse colons is less likely to have success with irrigation and is, therefore, not a good candidate for colostomy irrigation. *Note:* It may take 6 to 8 weeks to achieve a predictable bowel pattern with routine irrigation. Once mastered, the irrigation procedure may eliminate the need for some clients to wear standard appliances (Wax, 2012; Rooney, 2007).
Ascertain client's previous bowel habits and lifestyle.	Assists in formulation of a timely and effective irrigation schedule for client with a colostomy. Irrigation may be done once a day or once every other day depending on client preference and ability to regulate bowel movements. It is helpful to establish a routine and irrigate at the same time of day.
Discuss and/or demonstrate use of irrigation equipment, if appropriate. Refer client/SO to physician or ostomy nurse for guidance.	If the client is in immediate postop period, irrigations will not be initiated. Once completely healed, the client with a permanent colostomy may benefit from instruction about irrigation and demonstration of equipment.
Inform client about the use of a patch, stoma cap, dressing, or adhesive strip once successful bowel control is achieved.	May enable client to participate in more desired lifestyle activities (e.g., sports, dating), to dress more in keeping with usual style, and to feel more comfortable socially.

NURSING DIAGNOSIS: risk for Sexual Dysfunction

Risk Factors May Include

Altered body structure and function
Vulnerability, [psychological concern about response of significant other]
Disruption of sexual response pattern, such as erectile difficulty

Possibly Evidenced By

(Not applicable; presence of signs and symptoms establishes an *actual* diagnosis)

Desired Outcomes/Evaluation Criteria—Client Will

Sexual Functioning (NOC)

Verbalize understanding of relationship of physical condition to sexual problems.
Identify satisfying and acceptable sexual practices and explore alternative methods.
Resume sexual relationship as appropriate.

ACTIONS/INTERVENTIONS	RATIONALE
Sexual Counseling (NIC)	
Independent	
Determine client's and SO's sexual relationship before the disease or surgery and whether they anticipate problems related to presence of ostomy.	Identifies future expectations and desires. Mutilation and loss of privacy and control of a bodily function can affect client's view of personal sexuality. When coupled with the fear of rejection by SO, the desired level of intimacy can be greatly impaired. Sexual needs are very basic, and client will be rehabilitated more successfully when a satisfying sexual relationship is continued or developed as desired.
Review with client and SO sexual functioning in relation to own situation.	Understanding if nerve damage has occurred and how it will alter sexual functioning (e.g., erection) helps client and SO to understand the need for exploring alternative methods of satisfaction.
Reinforce information given by the physician. Encourage questions. Provide additional information as needed.	Reiteration of data previously given assists client and SO to hear and process the knowledge again, moving toward acceptance of individual limitations or restrictions and prognosis, such as that it may take up to 2 years to regain potency after a radical procedure or that a penile prosthesis may be necessary.
Discuss likelihood of resumption of sexual activity in approximately 6 weeks after discharge, beginning slowly and progressing, such as cuddling and caressing until both partners are comfortable with body image and function changes. Include alternative methods of stimulation, as appropriate.	Knowing what to expect in progress of recovery helps client avoid performance anxiety and reduce risk of "failure." If the couple is willing to try new ideas, this can assist with adjustment and may help to achieve sexual fulfillment.
Encourage dialogue between partners, acknowledging that the situation is difficult but that restoration of sexual intimacy is most likely possible over time.	An ostomy can certainly impact feelings about desirability and cause worries about ability to function sexually (e.g., ability to have an erection or experience orgasm). The emotional issues can be hard for both the client and the healthy partner. In some instances where a client has had surgery for debilitating health problems, the healthy partner helps to take care of the ostomate and "certain" bodily functions. Working through these hard times without sex can take a toll on the sex life, and it can take time for these couples to adjust and regain confidence to resume a healthy sexual lifestyle again (Ostomyguide, 2010).
Suggest wearing a mini-pouch, or pouch cover, T-shirt, short nightgown, or special underwear designed for sexual contact.	Disguising ostomy appliance may aid in reducing feelings of self-consciousness and embarrassment during sexual activity.
Emphasize awareness of factors that might be distracting—fear of hurting the stoma, or unpleasant odors and pouch leakage.	Promotes resolution of solvable problems (e.g., assuring partner that stoma cannot be injured, emptying pouch before sex, use of pouch deodorizer).
Encourage use of sense of humor.	Laughter can help individuals deal more effectively with difficult situation and promote positive sexual experience.
Problem-solve alternative positions for coitus.	Minimizing awkwardness of appliance and physical discomfort can enhance satisfaction.
Discuss and role play possible interactions or approaches when dealing with new sexual partners.	Rehearsal is helpful in dealing with actual situations when they arise, reducing self-consciousness about "different" body image.
Offer reading lists and other resources (e.g., healthcare professional, local and national ostomy organizations, websites/blogs, ostomy support groups), as indicated.	There is a wealth of available information and support available to provide client and partner with answers, solutions to problems, and hope that they can look forward to a healthy sex life.
Provide birth control information as appropriate and stress that impotence does not necessarily mean client is sterile.	Most women can still conceive after ostomy surgery without any problem, so birth control may still be needed/desired. Most men remain fertile, even if they cannot achieve an erection for a period after surgery.
Collaborative	
Arrange meeting with an ostomy visitor, if appropriate.	Sharing of how these problems have been resolved by others can be helpful and reduce sense of isolation.
Refer to counseling or sex therapy, as indicated.	If problems persist longer than several months after surgery, a trained therapist may be required to facilitate communication between client and partner.

NURSING DIAGNOSIS: deficient Knowledge [Learning Need] regarding condition, prognosis, treatment, self-care, and discharge needs

May Be Related To

Lack of exposure, recall; information misinterpretation
Unfamiliarity with information resources

Possibly Evidenced By

Reports the problem
Inaccurate follow-through of instruction (performance of ostomy care)
Inappropriate or exaggerated behaviors—hostile, agitated, apathetic

Desired Outcomes/Evaluation Criteria—Client Will

Knowledge: Ostomy Care (NOC)

Verbalize understanding of condition, disease process, prognosis, and potential complications.
Verbalize understanding of therapeutic needs.
Correctly perform necessary procedures and explain reasons for the action.
Initiate necessary lifestyle changes.

ACTIONS/INTERVENTIONS	RATIONALE
Learning Facilitation (NIC)	
Independent	
Evaluate client's emotional, cognitive, and physical capabilities.	These factors affect client's ability to master care tasks and willingness to assume responsibility for ostomy care.
Include written and picture (photo, video, Internet) learning resources.	Provides reference for obtaining support, equipment, and additional information after discharge to support client efforts for independence in self-care.
Teaching: Disease Process (NIC)	
Review anatomy, physiology, and implications of surgical intervention. Discuss future expectations, including anticipated changes in character of effluent.	Provides knowledge base from which client can make informed choices and offers an opportunity to clarify misconceptions regarding individual situation.
Instruct client/SO in stomal care. Allot time for return demonstrations and provide positive feedback for efforts.	Promotes positive management and reduces risk of improper ostomy care and development of complications.
Recommend increased fluid intake during warm weather months, especially when client has ileostomy.	Loss of normal colon function of conserving water and electrolytes can lead to dehydration.
Discuss possible need to decrease salt intake.	Salt can increase ileal output, potentiating risk of dehydration and increasing frequency of ostomy care needs and client's inconvenience.
Identify symptoms of electrolyte depletion, such as anorexia, abdominal muscle cramps, feelings of faintness or cold in arms and legs, general fatigue or weakness, bloating, and decreased sensations in extremities.	Loss of colon function altering fluid and electrolyte absorption may result in sodium and potassium deficits requiring dietary correction with foods and fluids higher in sodium—bouillon and Gatorade—or potassium—orange juice, prunes, tomatoes, bananas, and Gatorade.
Discuss need for periodic evaluation and administration of supplemental vitamins and minerals, as appropriate.	Depending on portion and amount of bowel resected, lack of absorption may cause deficiencies.
Discuss resumption of presurgery level of activity. Suggest emptying the ostomy appliance before leaving home and carrying fresh supplies. Recommend resources for obtaining attractive appliances and decorative cummerbunds as appropriate.	With a little planning, client should be able to manage same degree of activity as previously enjoyed and in some cases increase activity level. A cummerbund can provide both physical and psychological support when client is involved in activities such as tennis and swimming.
Talk about the possibility of sleep disturbance, anorexia, and loss of interest in usual activities.	"Homecoming depression" may occur, lasting for months after surgery, requiring patience, support, and ongoing evaluation as client adjusts to living with a stoma.
Explain necessity of notifying healthcare providers and pharmacists of type of ostomy and avoidance of sustained-release medications for client with ileostomy.	Presence of ostomy may alter rate and extent of absorption of oral medications and increase risk of drug-related complications such as diarrhea, constipation, or peristomal excoriation. Liquid, chewable, or injectable forms of medication are preferred for clients with ileostomy to maximize absorption of drug.
Counsel client concerning medication use and problems associated with altered bowel function. Refer to pharmacist for teaching or advice, as appropriate.	Client with an ostomy has two key problems: altered disintegration and absorption of oral drugs and unusual or pronounced adverse effects. Some of the medications that client may respond to differently include salicylates, H_2-receptor antagonists, antibiotics, and diuretics.

ACTIONS/INTERVENTIONS (continued)	RATIONALE (continued)
Emphasize necessity of close monitoring of chronic health conditions requiring routine oral medications.	Monitoring of clinical symptoms and/or serum blood levels of routine medications is indicated because of altered drug absorption, which may require changes in dosage or use of another medication.
Identify community resources, such as United Ostomy Association of America (UOAA), the Crohn's and Colitis Foundation of America (CCFA), local ostomy support group, certified WOC nurse, visiting nurse, and pharmacy and medical supply house.	Continued support after discharge is essential to facilitate the recovery process and client's independence in care. WOC nurse can be very helpful in solving appliance problems, identifying alternatives to meet individual client needs.

POTENTIAL CONSIDERATIONS following acute hospitalization (dependent on client's age, physical condition and presence of complications, personal resources, and life responsibilities)

- ***risk for impaired Skin Integrity***—excretions (character and flow of effluent and flatus from stoma)
- ***ineffective Coping***—situational crises
- ***impaired Social Interaction***—self-concept disturbance (concern for loss of control of bodily functions)
- ***risk for ineffective Self-Health Management***—complexity of therapeutic regimen, economic difficulties, perceived barriers, powerlessness

APPENDECTOMY

I. Pathophysiology—Events occur so rapidly that process takes about 1 to 3 days.

- **a.** Appendix becomes blocked by feces, a foreign object, or tumor.
- **b.** Obstruction, along with continued secretion of mucus, causes the wall of the appendix to become distended.
- **c.** Blood supply to the wall of the appendix is reduced, causing ischemia and accumulation of toxins.
- **d.** Wall of the appendix starts to break down, and normal bacteria found in the gut attacks the decaying appendix.
- **e.** Leads to necrosis and perforation of the appendix.
- **f.** Perforation can spread infection throughout abdomen, causing peritonitis.

II. Staging—Stages are divided into early, suppurative, gangrenous, perforated, phlegmonous, spontaneous resolving, recurrent, and chronic (Craig, 2012).

- **a.** Early stage
  - **i.** Individual may experience spontaneous recovery from inflammation at this stage or it may progress.
  - **ii.** Obstruction of the opening of the appendix leads to formation of edema, distention due to accumulated fluid, bacterial migration, and increasing pressure.
  - **iii.** Patient perceives mild periumbilical or epigastric pain lasting 4 to 6 hours.
- **b.** Suppurative stage
  - **i.** Increasing pressure allows bacteria and fluid invasion of appendiceal wall.
  - **ii.** Patient experiences a shift of the pain from periumbilical area to the right lower quadrant (RLQ) of the abdomen, becoming continuous and more severe.
- **c.** Gangrenous stage
  - **i.** Spontaneous regression never occurs.
  - **ii.** Venous or arterial thromboses occur, which result in death of tissues.
  - **iii.** Peritonitis can be present.
- **d.** Perforated stage
  - **i.** Tissue ischemia and resulting tissue death cause perforation of the appendix.
  - **ii.** Localized or generalized peritonitis is present.
- **e.** Phlegmonous stage
  - **i.** Inflamed or perforated appendix can be walled off.
  - **ii.** An abscess forms, confirming the inflammation and infection.
- **f.** Spontaneously resolving appendicitis
  - **i.** Occurs when the obstruction to the appendix is relieved prior to gangrene setting in.
  - **ii.** Acute appendicitis may resolve without treatment.
- **g.** Recurrent appendicitis
  - **i.** Occurs in approximately 10% of cases (Craig, 2012)
  - **ii.** Diagnosed if client has similar RLQ pain that is shown to be resulting from an inflamed appendix after removal
- **h.** Chronic appendicitis
  - **i.** Occurs in approximately 1% of cases (Craig, 2012)
  - **ii.** Client has history of RLQ pain lasting at least 3 weeks.
  - **iii.** Pain is relieved after appendectomy.
  - **iv.** Symptoms are the result of chronic inflammation of the appendix wall or fibrosis of the appendix.

III. Etiology

- **a.** Peak incidence occurs in the 3rd quarter of the year (July–September).
- **b.** Peak incidence in individuals in their late teens and early 20s; occurs more commonly in men than in women.
- **c.** Children over 5 and young adults have a higher incidence of nonperforated appendicitis, with the highest incidence occurring in the 10 to 19 age range.
- **d.** The rate of perforation varies from with a higher frequency occurring in young children (age 5 or less) and in persons older than 50 years (Craig, 2012; Alloo, 2004; Nance, 2000).
- **e.** There is a higher incidence of occurrence among Caucasians and Hispanics (NIDDK, 2008).

IV. Procedures—Inflamed appendix may be removed using a single incision (open appendectomy [OA]), or using a laparoscopic approach (laparoscopic appendectomy [LA]), where several smaller incisions are made and special surgical tools are inserted through the incisions to remove the appendix.

- **a.** Presence of multiple adhesions, retroperitoneal positioning of the appendix, or the likelihood of rupture may necessitate an open or traditional procedure.

(continues on page 316)

b. Laparoscopic procedure, although it does involve a longer operative time, results in significantly less postoperative pain, lower wound infection rate, and faster return to normal activities (Wei et al, 2011).

c. Some clients, such as those older than 65, those with comorbidities, and those with complicated appendicitis, benefit more from the laparoscopic approach (Yeh et al, 2011).

V. Statistics

a. Morbidity: Approximately 250,000 cases are reported annually in the United States.

b. Mortality: In 2009, 426 deaths occurred related to diseases of the appendix in the United States (U.S. Department of Health and Human Services, 2011).

c. Cost: Estimated direct care costs $2.6 billion in 2010 (Pfunter, 2012).

GLOSSARY

Abscess: Collection of pus in any part of the body that is surrounded by inflammation and infection.

Appendix: A small out-pouching from the beginning of the ascending colon; formally called the vermiform appendix because it was thought to be wormlike.

Epigastric: Lying upon or above the stomach.

Erythema: Redness of tissues.

McBurney's point: Name given to the point over the right side of the abdomen that is one-third of the distance from the anterior superior iliac spine to the umbilicus.

Necrosis: Death of part of an organ.

Perforation: Rupture of the appendix caused by swelling and infection.

Peritonitis: Inflammation of the peritoneum, the tissue layer of cells lining the inner wall of the abdomen and pelvis.

Periumbilical: Situated adjacent to the umbilicus.

Phlegmonous: Purulent inflammation of the appendix.

Rebound tenderness: Pain felt when a hand pressing on the abdomen is suddenly released; a symptom of peritoneal inflammation.

Care Setting

Although many of the interventions included here are appropriate for the short-stay client, this plan of care addresses the traditional appendectomy care provided on a surgical unit, after being diagnosed in the emergency department (ED).

Related Concerns

Peritonitis, page 320
Psychosocial aspects of care, page 729
Surgical intervention, page 762

Client Assessment Database (Preoperative)

DIAGNOSTIC DIVISION MAY REPORT	MAY EXHIBIT
ACTIVITY/REST	
• Malaise	
CIRCULATION	• Tachycardia
ELIMINATION	
• Constipation of recent onset • Diarrhea (occasional)	• Abdominal distention, tenderness • Rebound tenderness, rigidity • Decreased or absent bowel sounds • Abdominal rigidity
FOOD/FLUID	
• Anorexia • Nausea, vomiting nearly always follows onset of pain.	
PAIN/DISCOMFORT	
• Abdominal pain around the umbilicus, which may have a gradual onset and become increasingly severe • Pain may localize in right lower quadrant (RLQ). • Pain aggravated by walking, sneezing, coughing, or deep breathing. • Increasingly severe, generalized pain or the sudden cessation of severe pain suggests perforation or infarction of the appendix.	• Guarding behavior; lying on side or back with knees flexed • Palpation may elicit pain in RLQ, at McBurney's point. • Increased RLQ pain with extension of right leg and upright position • Rebound tenderness on left side

DIAGNOSTIC DIVISION MAY REPORT (continued)	MAY EXHIBIT (continued)
RESPIRATION	• Tachypnea, shallow respirations
SAFETY	• Fever, usually low-grade
TEACHING/LEARNING • History of other conditions associated with abdominal pain, such as Crohn's disease, irritable bowel syndrome, peptic ulcer, painful ovulation, that may require differentiation from current pain problem • May occur at any age	
DISCHARGE PLAN CONSIDERATIONS • May need brief assistance with transportation and homemaker tasks ➧ Refer to section at end of plan for postdischarge considerations.	

Diagnostic Studies

TEST WHY IT IS DONE	WHAT IT TELLS ME
BLOOD TESTS	
• ***Complete blood count (CBC):*** Battery of screening tests that typically includes hemoglobin (Hgb); hematocrit (Hct); red blood cell (RBC) count, morphology, indices, and distribution width index; platelet count and size; and white blood cell (WBC) count and differential	WBCs are often elevated above 10,000/mm^3; neutrophil count often elevated to greater than 75%.
• ***C-reactive protein (CRP):*** Protein produced by the liver when bacterial infections occur	CRP levels greater than 1 mg/dl are commonly reported in client with appendicitis. High levels of CRP (greater than 5 mg/dL) have been shown to be a significant indicator of necrotic appendicitis and indicative of the need for surgical intervention (Yokoyama et al, 2009). However, CRP normalization occurs 12 hours after onset of symptoms, so test is not useful for chronic appendicitis or acute appendicitis when tests for it are performed late.
ASSOCIATED DIAGNOSTIC STUDIES	
• ***Abdominal computed tomography (CT) scan, also called CAT scan:*** X-ray procedure, using a contrast medium that produces a detailed picture of a cross-section of the abdomen	Preferred test for differentiation of appendicitis from other causes of abdominal pain, such as perforating ulcer, cholecystitis, and reproductive organ infections, or to localize drainable abscesses, particularly for those clients in which perforation is suspected
• ***Ultrasonography:*** Technique for imaging internal structures of the body by measuring and recording the reflection of pulsed or continuous high-frequency sound waves	Method for quickly scanning abdomen without using radiation. Is highly accurate in children suspected of having acute appendicitis (Krishnamoorthi et al, 2011).

Nursing Priorities

1. Prevent complications.
2. Promote comfort.
3. Provide information about surgical procedure, prognosis, treatment needs, and potential complications.

Discharge Goals

1. Complications prevented or minimized.
2. Pain alleviated or controlled.
3. Surgical procedure, prognosis, therapeutic regimen, and possible complications understood.
4. Plan in place to meet needs after discharge.

NURSING DIAGNOSIS: risk for Infection [spread]

Risk Factors May Include

Inadequate primary defenses, tissue destruction—perforation or rupture of the appendix, peritonitis, abscess formation
Increased environmental exposure to pathogens—invasive procedures, surgical incision

Possibly Evidenced By

(Not applicable; presence of signs and symptoms establishes an *actual* diagnosis)

Desired Outcomes/Evaluation Criteria—Client Will

Wound Healing: Primary Intention (NOC)

Achieve timely wound healing, free of signs of infection and inflammation, purulent drainage, erythema, and fever.

ACTIONS/INTERVENTIONS	RATIONALE
Infection Prevention (NIC)	
Independent	
Practice and instruct in good hand-washing and aseptic wound care.	Reduces risk of spread of bacteria.
Inspect incision and dressings. Note characteristics of drainage from wound or drains (if inserted) and presence of erythema.	Provides for early detection of developing infectious process and monitors resolution of preexisting peritonitis.
Monitor vital signs. Note onset of fever, chills, diaphoresis, changes in mentation, and reports of increasing abdominal pain.	Suggestive of presence of infection, developing sepsis, abscess, and peritonitis.
Obtain drainage specimens, if indicated.	Gram's stain, culture, and sensitivity testing is useful in identifying causative organism and most appropriate choice of therapy.
Collaborative	
Administer antibiotics, as appropriate.	Antibiotics given before appendectomy are primarily for prophylaxis of wound infection and are not usually continued postoperatively. Therapeutic antibiotics are administered if the appendix is ruptured or abscessed, or peritonitis has developed and continues based on clinical signs and symptoms.
Prepare for and assist with incision and drainage (I&D) if indicated.	May be necessary to drain contents of localized abscess. Occasionally abscesses may be drained for about 2 weeks while antibiotics are given to treat any infection. The remaining appendix is then removed 6 to 8 weeks later when infection and inflammation is under control (NIDDK, 2008).

NURSING DIAGNOSIS: risk for deficient Fluid Volume

Risk Factors May Include

Active fluid losses through normal routes—preoperative vomiting
Deviations affecting intake—postoperative restrictions (nothing by mouth [NPO])
Factors influencing fluid needs—hypermetabolic state (fever, healing process)
[Inflammation of peritoneum with sequestration of fluid]

Possibly Evidenced By

(Not applicable; presence of signs and symptoms establishes an *actual* diagnosis)

Desired Outcomes/Evaluation Criteria—Client Will

Hydration (NOC)

Maintain adequate fluid balance as evidenced by moist mucous membranes, good skin turgor, stable vital signs, and individually adequate urinary output.

ACTIONS/INTERVENTIONS	RATIONALE
Fluid Monitoring (NIC)	
Independent	
Monitor vital signs.	Variations help identify fluctuating intravascular volumes or changes in vital signs associated with immune response to inflammation.
Inspect mucous membranes; assess skin turgor and capillary refill.	Indicators of adequacy of peripheral circulation and cellular hydration.

ACTIONS/INTERVENTIONS (continued)	RATIONALE (continued)
Monitor intake and output (I&O); note urine color and concentration and specific gravity.	Decreasing output of concentrated urine with increasing specific gravity suggests dehydration and need for increased fluids.
Auscultate bowel sounds. Note passing of flatus and bowel movement.	Indicators of return of peristalsis and readiness to begin oral intake. *Note:* This may not occur in the hospital if client has had a laparoscopic procedure and been discharged in less than 24 hours.
Provide clear liquids in small amounts when oral intake is resumed, and progress diet as tolerated.	Reduces risk of gastric irritation and vomiting to minimize fluid loss.
Give frequent mouth care with special attention to protection of the lips.	Dehydration results in drying and painful cracking of the lips and mouth.
Collaborative	
Monitor lab tests (e.g., electrolytes, BUN/creatinine).	These tests provide important information about fluid balance.
Maintain nasogastric (NG) and intestinal suction, as indicated.	Although not frequently needed, an NG tube may be inserted preoperatively and maintained in immediate postoperative phase to decompress the bowel, promote intestinal rest, and prevent vomiting.
Administer intravenous (IV) fluids and electrolytes.	Needed to promote homeostasis for general well-being and postoperative healing. *Note:* If peritonitis exists, the peritoneum reacts to irritation and infection by producing large amounts of intestinal fluid, pulling fluid from the vascular space and possibly reducing the circulating blood volume, resulting in dehydration and relative electrolyte imbalances.

NURSING DIAGNOSIS: acute Pain

May Be Related To

Physical agents—presence of surgical incision, distention of intestinal tissues (inflammation)

Possibly Evidenced By

Verbal/coded reports of pain
Facial grimacing, muscle guarding
Changes in vital signs

Desired Outcomes/Evaluation Criteria—Client Will

Pain Level (NOC)

Report pain is relieved or controlled.
Appear relaxed, able to sleep and rest appropriately.

ACTIONS/INTERVENTIONS	RATIONALE
Pain Management (NIC)	
Independent	
Note client's age, developmental level, and current condition (infant/child, critically ill, ventilated, sedated, or cognitively impaired).	Impacts ability to report pain parameters.
Assess pain reports, noting location, characteristics, and severity (0 to 10 [or similar] scale). Investigate and report changes in pain, as appropriate.	Pain is a subjective experience. Ongoing assessment is needed for evaluating effectiveness of medication and progression of healing. Changes in characteristics of pain may indicate developing abscess or peritonitis, requiring prompt medical evaluation and intervention.
Observe nonverbal cues and pain behaviors (e.g., how client holds body, facial expressions such as grimacing, withdrawal, narrowed focus, crying).	Nonverbal cues may or may not support client's pain intensity, but may be the only indicator if client is unable to verbalize.
Monitor skin color and temperature, as well as vital signs (e.g., heart rate, blood pressure, respirations).	May be altered by acute pain.
Keep at rest in semi-Fowler's position.	Gravity localizes inflammatory exudate into lower abdomen or pelvis, relieving abdominal tension, which is accentuated by supine position.
Encourage early ambulation.	Promotes normalization of organ function; stimulates peristalsis and passing of flatus, reducing abdominal discomfort.
Provide comfort measures (e.g., touch, repositioning, quiet environment, focused breathing).	To promote nonpharmacological pain management.

(continues on page 320)

ACTIONS/INTERVENTIONS (continued)	RATIONALE (continued)
Provide diversional activities.	Refocuses attention, promotes relaxation, and may enhance coping abilities.
Collaborative	
Keep NPO and maintain NG suction initially.	Decreases discomfort of early intestinal peristalsis and gastric irritation or vomiting.
Administer analgesics, as indicated, to maximum dosage needed to maintain comfort.	Promotes comfort and facilitates cooperation with other therapeutic interventions, such as ambulation.
Place ice bag on abdomen periodically during initial 24 to 48 hours, as appropriate.	Soothes and relieves pain through desensitization of nerve endings. *Note:* Do not use heat because it may cause tissue congestion and increase edema formation.

NURSING DIAGNOSIS: deficient Knowledge [Learning Need] regarding condition, prognosis, treatment, self-care, and discharge needs

May Be Related To

Lack of exposure or recall; information misinterpretation

Unfamiliarity with information resources

Possibly Evidenced By

Reports the problem

Inaccurate follow-through of instruction

Desired Outcomes/Evaluation Criteria—Client Will

Knowledge: Acute Illness Management (NOC)

Verbalize understanding of disease process and potential complications.

Verbalize understanding of therapeutic needs.

Participate in treatment regimen.

ACTIONS/INTERVENTIONS	RATIONALE
Teaching: Disease Process (NIC)	
Independent	
Identify symptoms requiring medical evaluation—increasing pain, edema and erythema of wound, presence of drainage, and fever.	Prompt intervention reduces risk of serious complications, such as delayed wound healing and peritonitis.
Review postoperative activity restrictions—heavy lifting, exercise, sexual activity, sports, and driving.	Provides information for client to plan for return to usual routines without untoward incidents.
Encourage progressive activities as tolerated with periodic rest periods.	Prevents fatigue, promotes healing and feeling of well-being, and facilitates resumption of normal activities.
Recommend use of mild laxative or stool softeners as necessary and avoidance of enemas.	Assists with return to usual bowel function; prevents undue straining for defecation.
Discuss care of incision, including dressing changes, bathing restrictions, and return to physician for suture and staple removal.	Understanding promotes cooperation with therapeutic regimen, enhancing healing and recovery process.

POTENTIAL CONSIDERATIONS following acute hospitalization (dependent on client's age, physical condition, presence of complications, personal resources, and life responsibilities)

- ***risk for ineffective Self-Health Management***—perceived seriousness or susceptibility, perceived benefit, demands made on individual (family, work), economic difficulties

PERITONITIS

I. Pathophysiology

a. Inflammation of the serosal membrane that lines the abdominal cavity and its viscera

b. Intra-abdominal infection may be localized or generalized, with or without abscess formation.

II. Classification (Daley et al, 2011)

a. Categorized as primary, secondary, or tertiary

i. Primary, or bacterial peritonitis, is rare, with the peritoneum spontaneously infected via the blood and lymphatic circulation.

ii. Secondary peritonitis is related to a pathological process in a visceral organ such as perforation or trauma.
iii. Tertiary peritonitis often develops in the absence of the original visceral organ pathology and/or is a persistent or recurrent infection after adequate initial therapy.
b. Can be acute or chronic in nature

III. Etiology

a. Infectious agents
i. Most common pathogens include gram-negative organisms, such as *Escherichia coli* and *Klebsiella,* gram-positive organisms, such as *Streptococcus,* anaerobic, such as *Bacteroides.*
ii. Resistant and unusual organisms, such as *Enterococcus, Candida,* and *Enterobacter,* are found in a significant proportion of tertiary cases.
b. Other sources of inflammation
i. Primary peritonitis: Caused by acute bacterial infection of the peritoneal cavity, occurs spontaneously, and usually occurs in a person who has an accumulation of fluid in the abdomen (ascites) caused by heart failure or cirrhosis
ii. Secondary peritonitis: Rupture or perforation of internal organ or instillation of irritating substance causing chemical irritation
1. Gastrointestinal (GI) tract: Ruptured appendix; perforated gastric or duodenal ulcer; cholecystitis with stone perforation; perforated colon caused by diverticulitis or cancer; pancreatitis; ulcerative colitis; and Crohn's disease
2. Ovaries and uterus: Pelvic inflammatory disease, ovarian cyst
3. Traumatic injuries: Blunt and penetrating trauma
4. Iatrogenic trauma to GI tract, such as during endoscopic procedures; inadvertent bowel injury or anastomosis dehiscence; instrumentation such as occurs with peritoneal dialysis or percutaneous stent placement (Daley et al, 2011)

IV. Statistics

a. Morbidity: As many as 70% of survivors of primary peritonitis have a recurrent episode within 1 year; dialysis-related secondary peritonitis rate is approximately 1 in 24 patient-treatment months (Keane et al, 2000).
b. Mortality: It is difficult to isolate mortality rates because of the many and varied conditions (subgroups) that can be associated with peritonitis in death reports. Daley reports "the overall mortality rate of patients with spontaneous bacterial peritonitis (SBP) may exceed 30% if diagnosis and treatment are delayed, but the mortality rate is less than 10% in fairly well-compensated patients with early therapy. In comparison with patients with other forms of peritonitis, patients who develop tertiary peritonitis have ... higher mortality rates (50–70%)" (Daley et al, 2011).
c. Cost: Direct care costs in 2004 estimated to be $2.5 billion (Everhart, 2008).

GLOSSARY

Ascites: Accumulation of serous fluid in the peritoneal cavity.
Borborygmus: Intermittent loud, rushing bowel sounds.
Peritoneum: Serous membrane that lines the abdominal cavity and covers the visceral organs.
Peritonitis: Inflammation of the peritoneum that may be generalized throughout the peritoneum, affecting the visceral and parietal surfaces of the abdominal cavity, or localized in one area as an abscess.
Postural hypotension: A drop in blood pressure (hypotension) due to a change in body position (posture) when a person moves to a more vertical position.
Rebound tenderness (also known as Blumberg sign): Pressing a hand on the abdomen elicits less pain than releasing the hand abruptly, which will aggravate the pain, as the peritoneum snaps back into place.
Viscera: Internal organs enclosed within the abdominal cavity.

Care Setting

The client is admitted to an inpatient acute medical or surgical unit.

Related Concerns

Appendectomy, page 315
Inflammatory bowel disease (IBD): ulcerative colitis, Crohn's disease, page 291
Pancreatitis, page 426
Peritoneal dialysis (PD), page 539
Psychosocial aspects of care, page 729
Sepsis/septicemia, page 665
Surgical intervention, page 762
Total nutritional support: parenteral/enteral feeding, page 437
Upper gastrointestinal/esophageal bleeding, page 281

Client Assessment Database

DIAGNOSTIC DIVISION MAY REPORT	MAY EXHIBIT
CIRCULATION	• Tachycardia, diaphoresis, pallor, hypotension (signs of shock) • Tissue edema
ELIMINATION • Inability to pass stool or flatus • Occasional diarrhea	• Hiccups • Decreased urinary output, dark color • Decreased or absent bowel sounds (ileus) • Intermittent loud, rushing bowel sounds • Abdominal rigidity, distention, rebound tenderness; hyperresonance or tympani (ileus) • Loss of dullness over liver (free air in abdomen)
FOOD/FLUIDS • Loss of appetite • Nausea, vomiting • Thirst	• Hypoactive bowel sounds (generalized ileus) • Projectile vomiting • Dry mucous membranes, swollen tongue, poor skin turgor
PAIN/DISCOMFORT • Sudden, severe, or persistent severe abdominal pain • Pain may be generalized, localized, referred to shoulder, intensified by movement	• Abdominal distention, rigidity, rebound tenderness • Distraction behaviors, restlessness, self-focus • Muscle guarding of abdomen, flexion of knees • Lying in rigid position, almost unmoving (Movious, 2006)
RESPIRATION	• Shallow respirations • Tachypnea
SAFETY	• Fever—usually greater than 101°F (38°C), although hypothermia may be present with severe sepsis • Chills
SEXUALITY • History of pelvic organ inflammation (salpingitis), puerperal infection, septic abortion, retroperitoneal abscess	
TEACHING/LEARNING • History of recent trauma with abdominal penetration, such as gunshot or stab wound or blunt trauma to the abdomen, bladder perforation or ruptured gallbladder, perforated carcinoma of the stomach, perforated gastric or duodenal ulcer, gangrenous obstruction of the bowel, perforation of diverticulum, ulcerative colitis (UC), regional ileitis, strangulated hernia	
DISCHARGE PLAN CONSIDERATIONS • Assistance with homemaker and maintenance tasks ➧ Refer to section at end of plan for postdischarge considerations.	

Diagnostic Studies

TEST WHY IT IS DONE	WHAT IT TELLS ME
DIAGNOSTIC STUDIES	
• *Abdominal x-ray:* Identifies pathology within the abdomen.	Shows edematous and gaseous distention of the small and large bowel. With perforation of a visceral organ, the x-ray shows air in the abdominal cavity and an elevation of the diaphragm.
• *Computed tomography (CT) scan (abdominal/pelvic):* X-ray procedure that uses a computer to produce a detailed picture of a cross-section of the body.	Reveals fluid and inflammation.
• *Ultrasound scan (abdominal/pelvic):* Scan that uses sound waves to produce an electronic image of the organs of the pelvis.	Can often diagnose cause of peritonitis, such as cholecystitis, perihepatic abscess, pancreatitis, ruptured appendix, ovarian abscess, or diverticulitis. Ultrasonography can also detect increased amounts of ascites and peritoneal fluid.
• *Peritoneal tap or lavage (paracentesis):* Puncture of the wall of a cavity with a needle in order to draw off excess fluid and to obtain a sample for cell count with differential, culture analysis for antimicrobial sensitivity.	The neutrophil count is the single best predictor of infection, and one greater then 250 to 500 cells/mm^3 is indicative of infection (Tan, 2008).
ASSOCIATED TESTS	
• *Complete blood count (CBC):* Battery of screening tests that typically includes hemoglobin (Hgb); hematocrit (Hct); red blood cell (RBC) count; white blood cell (WBC) count and differential.	WBCs are elevated—sometimes more than 20,000—except in elderly or immunocompromised person, or client with certain infections, such as fungal or cytomegalovirus, who may demonstrate leukopenia. RBCs, Hgb, and Hct may be increased, indicating hemoconcentration secondary to extracellular fluid loss into the peritoneal cavity.
• *Serum protein/albumin:* Visceral proteins considered to be markers for fluid and nutrition status.	May be decreased because of fluid shifts, lack of food intake, and nothing by mouth (NPO) status.
• *Serum amylase and lipase:* Enzymes produced by the pancreas, which aid in digestion of starches and fats.	Usually elevated when pancreatitis is cause.
• *Serum electrolytes:* Substances that dissociate into ions in solution and acquire the capacity to conduct electricity. Common electrolytes include sodium, potassium, chloride, calcium, and phosphate. Provides baseline data and can be used to evaluate and monitor fluid and electrolyte balance.	Water and electrolytes are lost in vomitus and drainage from the gastrointestinal tubes, and the client cannot take anything by mouth. Large quantities of body fluids and electrolytes collect in the peritoneal cavity instead of circulating normally throughout the body, increasing the problems of water and electrolyte imbalance.
• *Cultures:* Specimens may be taken from blood, exudate, or secretions; ascites fluid; or peritoneal dialysate to evaluate source and causative organism (aerobic and anaerobic).	Causative organisms, including *E. coli* or streptococci, are often cultured. Rarely, pneumococcus is the cause. Sensitivities may also be done to identify effective antimicrobial agent. Gram's stain and aerobic and anaerobic cultures can show multiple organisms. *Note*: Blood culture results are positive for the offending agent in as many as 33% of individuals with SBP and may help guide antibiotic therapy (Daley et al, 2011).
• Stool cultures	Specific cultures (i.e, *salmonella, shigella,* cytomegalovirus [CMV]) may be done in client with diarrhea if history suggests infectious enterocolitis as cause for peritonitis.

Nursing Priorities

1. Control infection.
2. Restore and/or maintain circulating volume.
3. Promote comfort.
4. Maintain nutrition.
5. Provide information about disease process, possible complications, and treatment needs.

Discharge Goals

1. Infection resolved.
2. Complications prevented or minimized.
3. Pain relieved.
4. Disease process, potential complications, and therapeutic regimen understood.
5. Plan in place to meet needs after discharge.

NURSING DIAGNOSIS: risk for Infection [septicemia]

Risk Factors May Include

Inadequate primary defenses—broken skin, traumatized tissue, altered peristalsis
Inadequate secondary defenses—immunosuppression
Invasive procedures

Possibly Evidenced By

(Not applicable; presence of signs and symptoms establishes an *actual* diagnosis)

Desired Outcomes/Evaluation Criteria—Client Will

Infection Status (NOC)

Achieve timely healing, be free of purulent drainage or erythema, and be afebrile.

Risk Control (NOC)

Verbalize understanding of the individual causative or risk factor(s).

ACTIONS/INTERVENTIONS	RATIONALE
Infection Control (NIC)	
Independent	
Note individual risk factors: abdominal trauma, acute appendicitis, and peritoneal dialysis.	Influences choice of interventions.
Assess vital signs frequently, noting unresolved or progressing hypotension, decreased pulse pressure, tachycardia, fever, and tachypnea.	Signs of impending septic shock. Circulating endotoxins eventually produce vasodilation, shift of fluid from circulation, and a low cardiac output state. *Note:* These clients frequently are critically ill and medical or postsurgical intensive care is required. (Refer to CP: Sepsis/Septicemia.)
Note changes in mental status, such as new onset confusion and stupor.	Hypoxemia, hypotension, and acidosis can cause deteriorating mental status.
Note skin color, temperature, and moisture.	Warm, flushed, dry skin is early sign of septicemia. Later manifestations include cool, clammy, pale skin and cyanosis as shock becomes refractory.
Monitor urine output.	Oliguria develops as a result of decreased renal perfusion, circulating toxins, and effects of antibiotics.
Maintain strict aseptic technique in caring for abdominal drains, incisions or open wounds, dressings, and invasive sites. Cleanse with appropriate solution.	Prevents access or limits spread of infecting organisms and cross-contamination.
Perform and model good hand-washing technique. Monitor staff and client compliance with hand washing.	Reduces risk of cross-contamination and spread of infection.
Observe drainage from wounds or drains.	Provides information about status of infection.
Maintain sterile technique when catheterizing client, provide catheter care, and encourage perineal cleansing on a routine basis.	Prevents access and limits bacterial growth in urinary tract.
Monitor or restrict visitors and staff, as appropriate. Provide protective isolation if indicated.	Reduces risk of exposure to, or acquisition of, secondary infection in immunosuppressed client.
Collaborative	
Obtain specimens for culture and monitor results of serial blood, urine, and wound cultures.	Culture identifies causative microorganisms and helps in assessing effectiveness of antimicrobial regimen.
Assist with peritoneal aspiration, if indicated.	May be done to remove fluid and to identify infecting organisms so appropriate antibiotic therapy can be instituted.
Administer antimicrobials, for example, cephalosporins, such as cefotetan (Cefotan); extended spectrum penicillins, such as piperacillin/tazobactam (Zosyn); carbapenems, such as meropenem (Merrem); fluoroquinolones, such as norfloxacin (Noroxin); macrolides, such as clindamycin (Cleocin); antifungals, such as metronidazole (Flagyl); aminoglycosides, such as gentamicin (Garamycin).	Therapy is systemic and directed at the particular identified organism(s), such as anaerobic bacteria, fungus, and gram-negative bacilli. Optimal duration of antimicrobial therapy depends on the underlying pathology, severity of infection, and speed and effectiveness of source control. Antimicrobials may initially be selected from those that can be administered intravenously (IV) or by intraoperative lavage.
Prepare for surgical intervention, as indicated:	
Open incision, laparoscopic débridement and lavage	Surgery may be treatment of choice and curative in acute, localized peritonitis, for example, to drain localized abscess; remove peritoneal exudates, ruptured appendix or gallbladder; plicate perforated ulcer; or resect bowel. The operative approach is directed by the underlying disease process and the type and severity of the intra-abdominal infection. Intraoperative lavage may be used to remove necrotic debris and treat inflammation that is poorly localized or diffuse. Multiple

ACTIONS/INTERVENTIONS (continued)	RATIONALE (continued)
	additional operations may be needed to control source of infection, drain abscesses, or clean out necrotic material. In this instance, the abdominal closure is temporary, using various dressings and coverings or a vacuum-assisted closure device, thus providing ready access to affected area while also preventing contamination from the outside. Later surgical procedures may also be required for permanent closure or repair of abdominal wall (Peralta et al, 2011).
Ostomy procedure	Temporary fecal diversion procedure may be performed if the colon is source of infection, such as in ruptured diverticulum, to facilitate treatment of the infection and bowel healing. (Refer to CP: Fecal Diversion.)

NURSING DIAGNOSIS: deficient Fluid Volume

May Be Related To
Active fluid volume loss—vomiting; medically restricted intake; nasogastric (NG) or intestinal aspiration
Failure of regulatory mechanisms—fever, hypermetabolic state, fluid shifts from extracellular, intravascular, and interstitial compartments into intestines and/or peritoneal space

Possibly Evidenced By
Dry mucous membranes, decreased skin turgor, decreased pulse volume
Decreased urinary output; increased urine concentration
Hypotension; tachycardia

Desired Outcomes/Evaluation Criteria—Client Will
Fluid Balance (NOC)
Demonstrate improved fluid balance as evidenced by adequate urinary output with normal specific gravity, stable vital signs, moist mucous membranes, good skin turgor, prompt capillary refill, and weight within acceptable range.

ACTIONS/INTERVENTIONS	RATIONALE
Fluid/Electrolyte Management (NIC)	
Independent	
Monitor vital signs, noting presence of hypotension (including postural changes), tachycardia, tachypnea, and fever. Measure central venous pressure (CVP) if available.	Aids in evaluating degree of fluid deficit, effectiveness of fluid replacement therapy, and response to medications.
Maintain accurate intake and output (I&O) and correlate with daily weights. Include measured and estimated losses, such as with gastric suction, drains, dressings, Hemovacs, diaphoresis, and abdominal girth for third spacing of fluid.	Reflects overall hydration status. Urine output may be diminished because of hypovolemia and decreased renal perfusion, but weight may still increase, reflecting tissue edema or ascites accumulation (third spacing). Gastric suction losses may be large, and a great deal of fluid can be sequestered in the bowel and peritoneal space (ascites).
Measure urine specific gravity.	Reflects hydration status and changes in renal function, which may warn of developing acute renal failure in response to hypovolemia and effect of toxins. *Note:* Many antibiotics also have nephrotoxic effects that may further affect kidney function and urine output.
Observe skin and mucous membrane dryness and turgor. Note peripheral and sacral edema.	Hypovolemia, fluid shifts, and nutritional deficits contribute to poor skin turgor and taut edematous tissues.
Eliminate noxious sights or smells from environment. Limit intake of ice chips.	Reduces gastric stimulation and vomiting response. *Note:* Excessive use of ice chips during gastric aspiration can increase gastric washout of electrolytes.
Change position frequently, provide frequent skin care, and maintain dry, wrinkle-free bedding.	Edematous tissue with compromised circulation is prone to breakdown.
Collaborative	
Monitor laboratory studies: Hgb/Hct, electrolytes, protein, albumin, BUN, and creatinine (Cr).	Provides information about hydration and organ function. Significant consequences to systemic function are possible as a result of fluid shifts, hypovolemia, hypoxemia, circulating toxins, and necrotic tissue products.
Administer plasma, blood, fluids, electrolytes, and diuretics, as indicated.	Replenishes and maintains circulating volume and electrolyte balance. Colloids, such as plasma or blood, help move water back into intravascular compartment by increasing

(continues on page 326)

ACTIONS/INTERVENTIONS (continued) | RATIONALE (continued)

ACTIONS/INTERVENTIONS	RATIONALE
	osmotic pressure gradient. Diuretics may be used to assist in excretion of toxins and to enhance renal function.
Maintain NPO status with nasogastric (NG) or intestinal aspiration.	Reduces vomiting caused by hyperactivity of bowel and endotoxins; manages stomach and intestinal fluids.

NURSING DIAGNOSIS: acute Pain

May Be Related To

Chemical agent—irritation of the parietal peritoneum (toxins)
Physical agent—tissue trauma, accumulation of fluid in abdominal and peritoneal cavity (abdominal distention)

Possibly Evidenced By

Verbalized/coded reports of pain
Guarding behavior; expressive behavior—restlessness, irritability
Facial mask, self-focus
Changes in vital signs

Desired Outcomes/Evaluation Criteria—Client Will

Pain Control (NOC)

Report pain is relieved or controlled.
Demonstrate use of relaxation skills or other methods to promote comfort.

ACTIONS/INTERVENTIONS	RATIONALE
Pain Management (NIC)	
Independent	
Note client's age, developmental level, and current condition (infant/child, critically ill, ventilated, sedated, or cognitively impaired).	Impacts ability to report pain parameters.
Investigate pain reports, noting location, duration, intensity (0 to 10 [or similar] scale), and characteristics such as dull, sharp, or constant.	Changes in location or intensity are not uncommon but may reflect developing complications. Pain tends to become constant, more intense, and diffuse over the entire abdomen as inflammatory process accelerates; pain may localize if an abscess develops.
Observe nonverbal cues and pain behaviors (e.g., how client holds body, facial expressions such as grimacing, withdrawal, narrowed focus, crying).	Nonverbal cues may or may not support client's pain intensity, but may be the only indicator if client is unable to verbalize.
Maintain semi-Fowler's position as indicated.	Facilitates fluid and wound drainage by gravity, reducing diaphragmatic irritation and abdominal tension, thereby reducing pain.
Move client slowly and deliberately, splinting painful area.	Reduces muscle tension and guarding, which may help minimize pain of movement.
Provide comfort measures, such as massage, back rubs, and deep breathing. Instruct in relaxation and visualization exercises.	Promotes relaxation and may enhance client's coping abilities by refocusing attention.
Provide frequent oral care. Remove noxious environmental stimuli.	Reduces nausea and vomiting, which can increase intra-abdominal pressure and pain.
Collaborative	
Administer medications, as indicated, for example:	
Analgesics and opioids	Reduces metabolic rate and intestinal irritation from circulating and local toxins, which aid in pain relief and promote healing. *Note:* Pain is usually severe and may require opioid pain control.
Antiemetics, such as dolasetron (Azemet), metoclopramide (Reglan)	Reduces the nausea and vomiting that can increase abdominal pain.
Antipyretics, such as acetaminophen (Tylenol)	Reduces discomfort associated with fever.

NURSING DIAGNOSIS: risk for imbalanced Nutrition: less than body requirements

Risk Factors May Include

Inability to ingest—nausea, vomiting

Inability to digest food/absorb nutrients—intestinal dysfunction, metabolic abnormalities

[Increased metabolic needs]

Possibly Evidenced By

(Not applicable; presence of signs and symptoms establishes an *actual* diagnosis)

Desired Outcomes/Evaluation Criteria—Client Will

Nutritional Status (NOC)

Maintain usual weight and positive nitrogen balance.

ACTIONS/INTERVENTIONS	RATIONALE
Nutrition Management (NIC)	
Independent	
Auscultate bowel sounds, noting absent and hyperactive sounds.	Although bowel sounds are frequently absent, inflammation of the intestine may be accompanied by intestinal hyperactivity, diminished water absorption, and diarrhea.
Monitor NG tube output. Note presence of vomiting and diarrhea.	Large amounts of gastric aspirant, or severe vomiting and diarrhea, suggest bowel obstruction, requiring further evaluation.
Measure abdominal girth.	Provides quantitative evidence of changes in intestinal distention and accumulation of ascitic fluid.
Assess abdomen frequently for return to softness, reappearance of normal bowel sounds, and passage of flatus.	Indicates return of normal bowel function and ability to resume oral intake.
Weigh regularly.	Initial losses or gains reflect changes in hydration, but sustained losses suggest nutritional deficit.
Collaborative	
Monitor BUN, protein, prealbumin or albumin, glucose, and nitrogen balance, as indicated.	Reflects organ function and nutritional deficits and needs.
Administer enteral or parenteral feedings, as indicated.	Enteral feedings, even at low volumes, have been shown to maintain gut mucosal integrity and to reduce the incidence of infectious complications, making the choice of enteral feedings preferable over parenteral solutions whenever possible. (Refer to CP: Total Nutritional Support: Enteral/Parenteral Feedings.)
Advance diet as tolerated—clear liquids to soft food.	Client may have some degree of gut dysfunction for quite some time, making it necessary for careful progression of diet when oral intake is resumed.

NURSING DIAGNOSIS: Anxiety [specify level]

May Be Related To

Situational crisis

Threat of death; change in health status

Possibly Evidenced By

Apprehensive, uncertainty, worried

Focus on self; irritability; increased tension

Increased pulse, respirations, blood pressure; restlessness

Desired Outcomes/Evaluation Criteria—Client Will

Anxiety Self-Control (NOC)

Verbalize awareness of feelings and healthy ways to deal with them.

Report anxiety is reduced to a manageable level.

Appear relaxed.

ACTIONS/INTERVENTIONS	RATIONALE
Anxiety Reduction (NIC)	
Independent	
Evaluate anxiety level, noting client's perception of situation and verbal and nonverbal responses. Encourage free expression of emotions.	Apprehension may be escalated by severe pain, severity of illness, urgency of diagnostic procedures, and possibility of surgery.
Review physiological factors present, such as sepsis or toxins related to infection, medications, and metabolic imbalances.	These factors are present in seriously ill client and can cause or contribute to anxiety.
Provide ongoing information regarding disease process and anticipated treatment.	Knowing what to expect can reduce anxiety for both client and significant other (SO). Also, ongoing review helps to identify those factors adding to anxiety that could be changed—client getting more uninterrupted sleep or adding or deleting medications.
Provide presence. Acknowledge anxiety and fear. Do not deny or reassure client that everything will be all right. Be accurate and factual in providing information. Correct misconceptions about disease process and possible treatments.	Affirms client's value as a human being in need of assistance in dealing with a serious health threat; helps client and SO identify and deal with reality.
Schedule adequate rest and uninterrupted periods for sleep.	Limits fatigue, conserves energy, and can enhance coping ability.
Provide comfort measures: family presence, quiet environment, soft music, back rub, and Therapeutic Touch (TT).	Promotes relaxation and enhances ability to deal with situation.

Refer to CP: Psychosocial Aspects for Care, for additional interventions.

NURSING DIAGNOSIS: deficient Knowledge [Learning Need] regarding condition, prognosis, treatment, self-care, and discharge needs

May Be Related To

Lack of exposure, recall
Information misinterpretation
Unfamiliarity with information resources

Possibly Evidenced By

Reports the problem
Inaccurate follow-through of instruction

Desired Outcomes/Evaluation Criteria—Client Will

Knowledge: Acute Illness Management (NOC)

Verbalize understanding of disease process and potential complications.
Identify relationship of signs and symptoms to the disease process and correlate symptoms with causative factors.
Verbalize understanding of therapeutic needs.
Correctly perform necessary procedures and explain reasons for actions.

ACTIONS/INTERVENTIONS	RATIONALE
Teaching: Disease Process (NIC)	
Independent	
Review underlying disease process and recovery expectations.	Provides knowledge base from which client can make informed choices.
Identify signs and symptoms requiring medical evaluation, such as recurrent abdominal pain or distention, vomiting, fever, chills, or presence of purulent drainage, swelling, and erythema of surgical incision (if present).	Early recognition and treatment of developing complications may prevent more serious illness or injury.
Discuss medication regimen, schedule, and possible side effects.	Antibiotics may be continued for varying periods of time after discharge depending on extent of the infection and length of stay in acute care facility.
Recommend gradual resumption of usual activities, allowing for adequate rest.	Prevents fatigue and enhances feeling of well-being.
Review activity limitations, such as avoiding heavy lifting.	Reduces chance of undue intra-abdominal pressure and muscle tension.
Demonstrate sterile or clean dressing change as appropriate. Have client/SO demonstrate ability to manage these procedures.	Client/SO may have a long period of home management of surgical wound(s), depending on extent of infection and treatment. Slow recovery time is often associated with such a complex condition.

ACTIONS/INTERVENTIONS (continued)	RATIONALE (continued)
Emphasize importance of medical follow-up care.	Necessary to monitor resolution of infection and effectiveness of therapeutic interventions.
Refer to community resources, as needed or desired, such as visiting nurse, home healthcare, and durable medical equipment suppliers.	Supports transition to home, promotes self-care, and increases likelihood of successful outcome.

POTENTIAL CONSIDERATIONS following acute hospitalization (dependent on client's age, physical condition, presence of complications, personal resources, and life responsibilities)

- ***Fatigue***—stress; anxiety; disease state
- ***acute Pain***—chemical agent—irritation of the peritoneum

CHOLECYSTITIS WITH CHOLELITHIASIS

I. Pathophysiology—An acute or chronic inflammation of the gallbladder associated with obstruction by gallstones

- **a.** Common bile duct stones are formed in the bile duct (primary) or formed in and transported from the gallbladder (secondary).
- **b.** Cholelithiasis is usually asymptomatic.
- **c.** Cholecystitis can result if stone becomes lodged in one of the ducts.

II. Etiology

- **a.** Stones most often develop in and obstruct the common bile duct or the cystic duct; also found in the hepatic, small bile, and pancreatic ducts.
    - **i.** Ninety percent of cases involve stones in the cystic duct (calculous cholecystitis), whereas the other 10% involve cholecystitis without stones (acalculous cholecystitis) (Bloom et al, 2011; Huffman, 2010, 2009).
    - **ii.** Stones are made up of cholesterol (about 80%), calcium bilirubinate, or a mixture caused by changes in the bile composition (Heuman, 2011).
- **b.** Bile cultures are positive for bacteria in 50% to 75% of cases; however, bacterial proliferation may be a result or consequence of cholecystitis, but not the precipitating factor (Bloom et al, 2011).
- **c.** Other causes include stasis of bile or bacterial infection or ischemia of the gallbladder.
- **d.** Failure to remove impacted stone can lead to bile stasis or bacteremia and septicemia causing cholangitis—a medical emergency.

III. Statistics (Bloom et al, 2011)

- **a.** Morbidity: Gallstones are two to three times more frequent in females than in males; perforation occurs in 10% to 15% of cases, and 25% to 30% of clients either require surgery or develop complications.
- **b.** Mortality: With uncomplicated calculous cholecystitis, there was a reported 0.4% mortality rate in 2004; with acalculous cholecystitis, a 10% to 50% mortality rate (Heuman, 2011; NIDDK, 2004).

GLOSSARY

Acalculous cholecystitis: Inflammation of the gallbladder in the absence of gallstones.

Biliary colic: Typically constant and slowly progressive pain that is usually located in the epigastrium or right upper quadrant; most common presenting symptom in cholelithiasis.

Cholangitis: Inflammation of the common bile duct due to an impacted stone obstructing bile drainage, which can lead to bacteremia and septicemia.

Cholecystitis: Inflammation of the gallbladder.

Cholelithiasis: Stones in the gallbladder.

Clay-colored stool: Reflects absence of bile in stool due to infection of liver or blockage of bile flow out of the liver.

Dyspepsia: Feeling of fullness and bloating after eating; also involves belching, heartburn, nausea, and sometimes vomiting.

Eructation: Belching.

Gallstones: Generally the result of cholesterol precipitating out of bile (cholesterol stones) or of free bilirubin combining with calcium to create bile pigment stones.

Hematemesis: Bloody vomitus.

Jaundice: Yellow tinge to skin and sclera in eyes due to bile absorption into circulatory system.

Lithotripsy: Use of high-energy shock waves to fragment and disintegrate gallstones.

Melena: Black, tarry feces due to presence of digested blood in stool.

Murphy's sign: Inability to take in a breath due to pain when examiner's hand is pressing on gallbladder.

Sonographic Murphy's sign: Pain when the ultrasound probe is pushed directly on the gallbladder.

Steatorrhea: Fatty stools.

Care Setting

Severe acute attacks may require brief hospitalization on a medical unit. This plan of care deals with the acutely ill, hospitalized client. Surgery is usually performed after symptoms have subsided, but during the hospitalization, for acute illness. (Refer to CP: Cholecystectomy.)

Related Concerns

Cholecystectomy, page 335
Fluid and electrolyte imbalances, page 885
Psychosocial aspects of care, page 729
Total nutritional support: parenteral/enteral feeding, page 437

Client Assessment Database

DIAGNOSTIC DIVISION MAY REPORT	MAY EXHIBIT
ACTIVITY/REST	
• Fatigue	• Restlessness
CIRCULATION	
	• Tachycardia • Diaphoresis • Hypotension, if septic
ELIMINATION	
• Change in color of urine and stools	• Abdominal distention • Palpable mass in right upper quadrant (RUQ) • Dark, concentrated urine • Clay-colored stool, or steatorrhea
FOOD/FLUID	
• Anorexia, nausea, and vomiting • Intolerance of fatty and "gas-forming" foods, recurrent regurgitation, heartburn, indigestion, flatulence, dyspepsia • Belching	• Obesity or recent weight loss • Normal to hypoactive bowel sounds
PAIN/DISCOMFORT	
• Severe epigastric and right upper abdominal pain, may radiate to midback, right shoulder and scapula, or to front of chest • Pain increases with movement • Midepigastric colicky pain associated with eating, especially after meals rich in fats • Episodes of severe or ongoing pain starting suddenly, sometimes at night, with episodes of constant pain typically lasting 1 to 5 hours • Recurring episodes of similar pain	• Rebound tenderness, muscle guarding, or abdominal rigidity when RUQ is palpated • Positive Murphy's sign
RESPIRATION	
	• Increased respiratory rate • Splinted respiration marked by short, shallow breathing
SAFETY	
	• Low-grade fever • High fever and chills indicating septic complications • Jaundice with dry, itching skin (pruritus) • Bleeding tendencies caused by vitamin K deficiency
TEACHING/LEARNING	
• Familial tendency for gallstones • Recent pregnancy and delivery; history of diabetes mellitus (DM), inflammatory bowel disease (IBD), blood dyscrasias	
DISCHARGE PLAN CONSIDERATIONS	
• May require support with dietary changes and weight reduction ➧ Refer to section at end of plan for postdischarge considerations.	

Diagnostic Studies

TEST WHY IT IS DONE	WHAT IT TELLS ME
DIAGNOSTIC STUDIES	
• ***Abdominal/biliary system ultrasound:*** Most common screening test, also identifies abnormalities of surrounding tissues.	Right upper abdominal ultrasound is 90% to 95% sensitive for cholecystitis and 98% sensitive and specific for simple cholelithiasis (Bloom et al, 2011).
• ***Hepatoiminodiacetic acid (HIDA) scan:*** Imaging test used to examine the gallbladder and the ducts leading into and out of the gallbladder.	HIDA scan has been found to be up to 95% accurate in diagnosing acute cholecystitis, although scanning can miss stones due to loops of bowel obstructing view (Bloom et al, 2011).
• ***Abdominal radiographs (multipositional):*** X-rays of the abdomen.	An abdominal x-ray is obtained primarily to exclude other diagnoses. Disorders such as empyema of the gallbladder and gallstone ileus may be suggested by findings on plain x-rays. (Khan et al, 2011).
• ***Computed tomography (CT) scan:*** X-ray procedure that uses a computer to produce a detailed picture of a cross-section of the body. May be done with or without contrast.	In acute cholecystitis some of the CT scan findings can include: enlargement of the gallbladder (if it visualizes); stones in the gallbladder, the cystic duct, or both; thickening of the gallbladder wall; biliary sludge; and gallbladder mucosal sloughing (Khan et al, 2011).
• ***Magnetic resonance imaging (MRI) and/or cholangiopancreatography (MRCP):*** An MRI scan uses a strong magnetic field and radio waves to create pictures, on a computer, of tissues, organs, and other structures inside the body. A MRCP is an application of magnetic resonance imaging of the hepatobiliary and pancreatic system.	MRI may depict the same pathologic features as CT scanning does. The MRCP is a less invasive alternative to endoscopic retrograde cholangiopancreatography (ERCP) to evaluate the liver, bile ducts, gallbladder, and pancreas for gallstones, infection, or inflammation.
• ***Endoscopic retrograde cholangiopancreatography (ERCP):*** Endoscopic procedure that allows direct visualization of the biliary anatomy and may be used therapeutically to remove stones.	Visualizes biliary tree by cannulation of the common bile duct through the duodenum. Allows endoscopic removal of 90% of stones. Allows stenting of common bile ducts that are damaged, inflamed, or strictured. Larger stones can be reduced in size and/or removed by mechanical lithotripsy during ERCP.
ASSOCIATED TESTS	
• ***Complete blood count (CBC):*** Assesses relationship of red blood cells to fluid volume, or viscosity, and may indicate risk factors, such as anemia, blood loss, or hypercoagulability.	Moderately elevated white blood cell (WBC) count (leukocytosis) may be present in acute cholecystitis; however, a normal WBC count does not rule out cholecystitis. The hematocrit (Hct) rises when the number of red blood cells (RBCs) increases or when the plasma volume is reduced, as in dehydration from nausea and vomiting, or blood loss from any point in the digestive tract.
• ***Alkaline phosphatase (ALP):*** A liver enzyme that helps in protein metabolism.	Elevated level is observed in 25% of clients with gallbladder disease or bile duct obstruction (Bloom et al, 2011).
• ***Alanine aminotransferase (ALT) and aspartate aminotransferase (AST):*** Enzymes primarily found in the liver that assist in the making of proteins.	ALT and AST may both be elevated in cholecystitis or with common bile duct obstruction.
• ***Bilirubin:*** A yellowish pigment produced from the breakdown of hemoglobin (Hgb) and RBCs.	Serum bilirubin levels may be elevated. The two different tests of bilirubin (total and direct) are often evaluated together if a person has jaundice. Jaundice is an indication that the bile duct is blocked and bile is accumulating in the bloodstream.
• ***Amylase:*** An enzyme produced in the pancreas.	Cholecystitis can elevate this enzyme due to the close proximity of the liver to the pancreas.
• ***Prothrombin levels:*** Evaluates the ability of the blood to clot properly.	Reduced when obstruction to the flow of bile into the intestine decreases absorption of vitamin K.

Nursing Priorities

1. Relieve pain and promote rest.
2. Maintain fluid and electrolyte balance.
3. Prevent complications.
4. Provide information about disease process, prognosis, and treatment needs.

Discharge Goals

1. Pain relieved.
2. Homeostasis achieved.
3. Complications prevented and minimized.
4. Disease process, prognosis, and therapeutic regimen understood.
5. Plan in place to meet needs after discharge.

NURSING DIAGNOSIS: acute Pain

May Be Related To

Biological agents—obstruction or ductal spasm, inflammatory process, tissue ischemia

Possibly Evidenced By

Verbal/coded reports of pain
Facial mask; guarding behavior
Changes in blood pressure (BP), pulse, respirations
Self-focus; narrowed focus

Desired Outcomes/Evaluation Criteria—Client Will

Pain Control (NOC)

Report pain is relieved or controlled.
Demonstrate use of relaxation skills and diversional activities as indicated for individual situation.

ACTIONS/INTERVENTIONS	RATIONALE
Pain Management	
Independent	
Observe and document location, severity (0 to 10 [or similar] scale), and character of pain, such as steady, intermittent, or colicky.	Assists in differentiating cause of pain and provides information about disease progression or resolution, development of complications, and effectiveness of interventions.
Note response to medication, and report to physician if pain is not being relieved.	Severe pain not relieved by routine measures may indicate developing complications and the need for further intervention.
Promote bedrest, allowing client to assume position of comfort.	Bedrest in low-Fowler's position reduces intra-abdominal pressure; however, client will naturally assume least painful position.
Use soft cotton linens; calamine lotion; oil bath; and cool, moist compresses, as indicated.	Reduces irritation and dryness of the skin and itching sensation that can occur if bile salts are deposited in skin tissues.
Control environmental temperature.	Cool surroundings aid in minimizing dermal discomfort.
Encourage use of relaxation techniques such as guided imagery, visualization, and deep-breathing exercises. Provide diversional activities.	Promotes rest, redirects attention, and may enhance coping.
Make time to listen to and maintain frequent contact with client.	Helpful in alleviating anxiety and refocusing attention, which can relieve pain.
Collaborative	
Maintain nothing by mouth (NPO) status; insert and maintain nasogastric (NG) suction, as indicated.	Removes gastric secretions that stimulate release of cholecystokinin and gallbladder contractions.
Administer medications, as indicated, for example:	
Opioids, such as oral oxycodone/acetaminophen (Percocet) or oxycodone/acetaminophen (Vicodin); IV or injected analgesics such as meperidine (Demerol)	Promotes rest and relaxation of smooth muscle, relieving pain.
Antibiotics may be given IV in acute attack, and may include such drugs as piperacillin/tazobactam (Zosyn), ampicillin/sulbactam (Unasyn) meropenem (Merrem).	Given to treat infectious process, reducing inflammation and potential for systemic complications. Treatment for acute cholecystitis usually requires single-agent therapy, but for more serious infections, combination drug treatment has increased broad-spectrum coverage.
Prepare for procedures, such as the following:	
Sphincterotomy plus extraction of stones during endoscopic retrograde cholangiopancreatography (ERCP)	The procedure may be done to widen the mouth of the common bile duct where it empties into the duodenum, or to extract common bile duct stones and to facilitate endotherapy (e.g., placement of stents) (Jamidar, 2011). Once gallstones have been identified, the physician will typically either capture the stones using a basket, or push the stones down into

ACTIONS/INTERVENTIONS	RATIONALE
	the duodenum with a retrieval (or occlusion) balloon where they will pass through the intestine (Cleveland Clinic, 2009).
Laparoscopic or open surgical intervention	Cholecystectomy may be indicated because of the size of stones, degree of tissue involvement, or presence of necrosis or sepsis. (Refer to CP: Cholecystectomy.)

NURSING DIAGNOSIS: risk for deficient Fluid Volume

Risk Factors May Include

Active fluid loss—vomiting, altered clotting process
Loss of fluids through abnormal routes—gastric suction; gastric hypermotility
Deviations affecting intake—medically restricted intake

Possibly Evidenced By

(Not applicable; presence of signs and symptoms establishes an *actual* diagnosis)

Desired Outcomes/Evaluation Criteria—Client Will

Hydration (NOC)

Demonstrate adequate fluid balance evidenced by stable vital signs, moist mucous membranes, good skin turgor, capillary refill, individually appropriate urinary output, and absence of vomiting.

ACTIONS/INTERVENTIONS	RATIONALE
Fluid/Electrolyte Management (NIC)	
Independent	
Maintain accurate record of intake and output (I&O), noting output less than intake and increased urine specific gravity. Assess skin and mucous membranes, peripheral pulses, and capillary refill.	Provides information about fluid status and circulating volume and replacement needs.
Monitor for continued vomiting, possibly accompanied by abdominal cramps, weakness, twitching, seizures, irregular heart rate, paresthesias, hypoactive or absent bowel sounds, and depressed respirations.	Prolonged vomiting, gastric aspiration, and restricted oral intake can lead to deficits in sodium, potassium, and chloride. Such electrolyte imbalances can rapidly result in systemic complications.
Eliminate noxious sights and smells from environment.	Reduces stimulation of vomiting center.
Perform frequent oral hygiene with alcohol-free mouthwash; apply lubricants.	Decreases dryness of oral mucous membranes and reduces risk of oral bleeding.
Assess for unusual bleeding: oozing from injection sites, epistaxis, bleeding gums, ecchymosis, petechiae, hematemesis, and melena.	Prothrombin is reduced and coagulation time could become prolonged when bile flow is obstructed over time, increasing risk of bleeding or hemorrhage in the critically ill client.
Collaborative	
Keep client NPO as necessary.	Decreases gastrointestinal (GI) secretions and hypermotility.
Insert NG tube, connect to suction, and maintain patency, as indicated.	Provides rest for GI tract and relief of vomiting.
Administer antiemetics, such as promethazine (Phenergan), prochlorperazine (Compazine), or ondansetron (Zofran).	Helpful in reducing nausea and vomiting often associated with cholecystitis and, particularly, common bile duct obstruction.
Review laboratory studies such as Hgb/Hct, electrolytes, arterial blood gases (ABGs) (pH), and clotting times.	Aids in evaluating circulating volume, identifies deficits, and influences choice of intervention for replacement or correction.
Administer IV fluids and electrolytes, as indicated.	Maintains circulating volume and corrects imbalances.

NURSING DIAGNOSIS: risk for imbalanced Nutrition: less than body requirements

Risk Factors May Include

Inability to ingest food (e.g., self-imposed or prescribed dietary restrictions, nausea, vomiting, dyspepsia, pain)
Inability to digest foods (e.g., obstruction of bile flow)

Possibly Evidenced By

(Not applicable; presence of signs and symptoms establishes an *actual* diagnosis)

(continues on page 334)

NURSING DIAGNOSIS: risk for imbalanced Nutrition: less than body requirements (continued)

Desired Outcomes/Evaluation Criteria—Client Will

Nutritional Status (NOC)

Report relief of nausea and vomiting.

Demonstrate progression toward desired weight gain or maintain weight as individually appropriate.

ACTIONS/INTERVENTIONS	RATIONALE
Nutrition Management (NIC)	
Independent	
Assess for abdominal distention, frequent belching, guarding, and reluctance to move.	Nonverbal signs of discomfort associated with impaired digestion and pain.
Consult with client about symptoms associated with diet or foods that cause distress.	Client may restrict many foods because of experience with or fear of nausea, vomiting, or pain. Foods that are high in fat and cholesterol are often the cause of onset of a gallbladder attack; however, some clients seem to experience pain with anything they eat, rather than just select food groups. Gallstones are known to be associated with prolonged fasting, with total parenteral nutrition, and rapid weight loss associated with severe caloric and fat restriction (e.g., fasting diet, gastric bypass surgery) (Bloom et al, 2011; Heuman, 2011).
Encourage client to keep food diary during assessment period, if indicated. Estimate or calculate caloric intake. Weigh, as indicated.	Identifies food intolerances and nutritional deficiencies and needs.
Collaborative	
Consult with dietitian and nutritional support team, as indicated.	Useful in establishing individual nutritional needs and most appropriate route.
Begin low-fat liquid diet after NG tube is removed. Advance diet as tolerated, usually low-fat, nonspicy, high-fiber. Restrict foods and fluids high in fat such as butter, fried foods, and nuts.	Limiting fat content reduces stimulation of gallbladder and pain associated with incomplete fat digestion and is helpful in preventing recurrence.
Monitor laboratory studies: blood urea nitrogen (BUN), prealbumin, albumin, total protein, and transferrin levels.	Provides information about nutritional deficits and effectiveness of therapy.
Administer parenteral or enteral feedings as indicated.	Alternative feeding may be required depending on severity of gallbladder involvement, client's overall nutritional status, and need for prolonged gastric rest.

NURSING DIAGNOSIS: deficient Knowledge [Learning Need] regarding condition, prognosis, treatment, self-care, and discharge needs

May Be Related To

Lack of knowledge or recall

Information misinterpretation

Unfamiliarity with information resources

Possibly Evidenced By

Reports the problem

Inaccurate follow-through of instruction

Desired Outcomes/Evaluation Criteria—Client Will

Knowledge: Acute Illness Management (NOC)

Verbalize understanding of disease process, prognosis, and potential complications.

Verbalize understanding of therapeutic needs.

Initiate necessary lifestyle changes and participate in treatment regimen.

ACTIONS/INTERVENTIONS	RATIONALE
Teaching: Disease Process (NIC) *Independent*	
Provide explanations of and reasons for test procedures and preparation needed.	Information can decrease anxiety, thereby reducing sympathetic stimulation.
Review disease process and prognosis. Discuss hospitalization and expected treatment as indicated. Encourage questions and expression of concerns.	Provides knowledge base from which client can make informed choices. Effective communication and support at this time can diminish anxiety and promote healing.
Review drug regimen if chemical stone dissolution is chosen or drug is used for prophylaxis.	Some clients with established cholesterol gallstones may be treated with ursodeoxycholic acid (Ursodiol), which results in gradual gallstone dissolution (e.g., over 6 to 18 months). Clients remain at risk for gallstone complications until dissolution is completed. This medication may also be used to prevent gallstones in client undergoing rapid weight loss (e.g., bariatric surgery or very low calorie diet) (Heuman, 2011).
Discuss weight reduction programs, if indicated.	Obesity is a risk factor associated with cholecystitis, and weight loss is beneficial in medical management of chronic condition.
Instruct client to avoid food and fluids high in fats.	May prevent recurrence of and limit severity of gallbladder attacks.
Review signs and symptoms requiring medical intervention, such as recurrent fever; persistent nausea and vomiting; pain; jaundice of skin or eyes; itching; dark urine; clay-colored stools; blood in urine, stools, or vomitus; or bleeding from mucous membranes.	Indicative of progression of disease process and development of complications requiring further intervention.

POTENTIAL CONSIDERATIONS following acute hospitalization (dependent on client's age, physical condition and presence of complications, personal resources, and life responsibilities)

- ***acute Pain***—recurrence of obstruction or ductal spasm, inflammation, tissue ischemia

CHOLECYSTECTOMY

I. Indications—For the treatment of symptomatic gallstones, infection of the gallbladder or biliary ducts, calcified gallbladder, or cancer or trauma

II. Procedures

a. Laparoscopic cholecystectomy: for removal of gallstones; performed using video endoscopy, with instruments inserted through small abdominal incisions

b. Open cholecystectomy: for multiple or large gallstones, common bile duct stones, history of previous surgeries with scarring, or unsuccessful laparoscopic cholecystectomy

III. Statistics

a. Morbidity: In 2004 approximately 700,000 Americans developed symptoms or complications of gallstones, requiring cholecystectomy (NIDDK, 2010).

b. Mortality: No conclusive numbers were discovered, likely because it is difficult to discern when cholecystectomy was actual versus incidental cause of death, whether the procedure was performed electively or as an emergency, and what type of operation (lap versus open) was performed. Sources agree that when cholecystectomy is performed as an elective surgery, the mortality rates are very low (less than 0.5% and in 0.7% to 2% in older persons). Emergency cholecystectomy has a much higher mortality rate (as high as 19% in ill elderly patients) (Nagesh-Bandi, 2011; Simon, 2009).

c. Cost: Direct care costs estimated to be over $5.7 billion in 2004 (Everhart, 2008).

GLOSSARY

Adventitious sounds: Abnormal breath sounds heard when listening to the chest, which may include crackles (rales), rhonchi, or wheezes.

Cholecystitis: Inflammation of the gallbladder.

Cholelithiasis: Stones in the gallbladder.

Gallstones: Solid masses made of cholesterol or bilirubin that form in the gallbladder or bile ducts; majority of gallstones in clients (in United States) are composed of cholesterol, resulting from cholesterol precipitating out of bile; bile pigment stones are a result of free bilirubin combining with calcium (Sartin, 2005a).

Hematemesis: Vomiting of blood.

Jaundice: Yellow tinge to skin and sclera in eyes due to bile absorption into circulatory system.

Melena: Black, tarry feces due to digestion of blood in stool.

T-tube: Drain tube inserted into cystic duct at the point of surgical closure and exiting through stab wound in skin to allow bile to drain.

Care Setting

This procedure is usually done on a one-day or short-stay basis; however, in the presence of suspected complications such as empyema, gangrene, or perforation, an inpatient stay on a surgical unit is indicated.

Related Concerns

Cholecystitis with cholelithiasis, page 329
Pancreatitis, page 426
Peritonitis, page 320
Psychosocial aspects of care, page 729
Surgical intervention, page 762

Client Assessment Database (Preoperative)

Refer to CP: Cholecystitis with Cholelithiasis.

DIAGNOSTIC DIVISION MAY REPORT	MAY EXHIBIT
TEACHING/LEARNING	
DISCHARGE PLAN CONSIDERATIONS • May require assistance with wound care, supplies, and homemaker tasks ➧ Refer to section at end of plan for postdischarge considerations.	

Diagnostic Studies

Refer to CP: Cholecystitis with Cholelithiasis.

Nursing Priorities

1. Promote respiratory function.
2. Prevent complications.
3. Provide information about disease, procedure(s), prognosis, and treatment needs.

Discharge Goals

1. Ventilation and oxygenation adequate for individual needs.
2. Complications prevented or minimized.
3. Disease process, surgical procedure, prognosis, and therapeutic regimen understood.
4. Plan in place to meet needs after discharge.

NURSING DIAGNOSIS: ineffective Breathing Pattern

May Be Related To

Pain
Muscular impairment
Fatigue

Possibly Evidenced By

Tachypnea
Alterations in depth of breathing; decreased vital capacity
Altered chest excursion—holding breath, reluctance to cough

Desired Outcomes/Evaluation Criteria—Client Will

Respiratory Status: Ventilation (NOC)
Establish effective breathing pattern.
Experience no signs of respiratory compromise or complications.

ACTIONS/INTERVENTIONS	RATIONALE
Respiratory Monitoring	
Independent	
Observe respiratory rate and depth.	Shallow breathing, splinting with respirations, and holding breath may result in hypoventilation and atelectasis.
Auscultate breath sounds.	Areas of decreased or absent breath sounds suggest atelectasis, whereas adventitious sounds reflect congestion.

ACTIONS/INTERVENTIONS (continued)	RATIONALE (continued)
Assist client to turn, cough, and deep-breathe periodically. Demonstrate how to splint incision. Instruct in effective breathing techniques.	Promotes ventilation of all lung segments and mobilization and expectoration of secretions.
Elevate head of bed; maintain low-Fowler's position. Support abdomen when coughing or ambulating.	Facilitates lung expansion. Splinting provides incisional support and decreases muscle tension to promote cooperation with therapeutic regimen.
Collaborative	
Assist with respiratory treatments, such as incentive spirometer.	Maximizes expansion of lungs to prevent or resolve atelectasis.
Administer analgesics regularly or continuously as indicated.	Facilitates movement and effective coughing, deep breathing, and activities.

NURSING DIAGNOSIS: risk for deficient Fluid Volume

Risk Factors May Include

Losses through abnormal routes—nasogastric (NG) aspiration, vomiting; altered coagulation
Deviations affecting intake—medically restricted intake

Possibly Evidenced By

(Not applicable; presence of signs and symptoms establishes an *actual* diagnosis)

Desired Outcomes/Evaluation Criteria—Client Will

Hydration (NOC)

Display adequate fluid balance as evidenced by stable vital signs, moist mucous membranes, good skin turgor, capillary refill, and individually appropriate urinary output.

ACTIONS/INTERVENTIONS	RATIONALE
Fluid/Electrolyte Management (NIC)	
Independent	
Monitor intake and output (I&O), including drainage from NG tube, T-tube, and wound. Weigh client periodically.	Provides information about replacement needs and organ function. Initially, 200 to 1000 mL of bile drainage per 24 hours may be expected via the T-tube, decreasing as more bile enters the intestine. Continuing large amounts of bile drainage may be an indication of unresolved obstruction or, occasionally, a biliary fistula. *Note:* Sudden cessation of drainage may indicate blockage of tube.
Monitor vital signs. Assess mucous membranes, skin turgor, peripheral pulses, and capillary refill.	Indicators of adequacy of circulating volume and perfusion.
Observe for signs of bleeding, such as hematemesis, melena, petechiae, ecchymosis, epistaxis, and oozing from incision and injection sites.	Prothrombin is reduced and coagulation time prolonged when bile flow is obstructed, increasing risk of bleeding or hemorrhage.
Use small-gauge needles for injections, and apply firm pressure for longer than usual after venipuncture.	Reduces trauma and risk of bleeding or hematoma formation.
Have client use soft toothbrush or cotton or sponge swabs and alcohol-free mouthwash instead of a toothbrush, if bleeding is a problem.	Avoids trauma, mucosal drying, and bleeding of the gums.
Collaborative	
Monitor laboratory studies, such as complete blood count (CBC), electrolytes, prothrombin and clotting time, and amylase.	Provides information about circulating volume, electrolyte balance, and adequacy of clotting factors. The hematocrit (Hct) rises when plasma volume is reduced, as in dehydration from vomiting. Falling hemoglobin (Hgb) and Hct and prolonged clotting time may reflect bleeding as a complication of obstructed bile flow, surgical procedure, or preexisting bleeding disorder. Elevated white blood cells (WBCs) can indicate inflammation from surgery, peritonitis, or pancreatitis or other infection. Damage to the pancreas is indicated by elevated levels of amylase.
Administer the following, as indicated:	
Intravenous (IV) fluids, blood products, and vitamin K	Maintains adequate circulating volume and aids in replacement of clotting factors.
Electrolytes (such as potassium, sodium, and chloride)	Imbalances resulting from excessive gastric or surgical fluid losses may require replacement via oral and parenteral routes.

NURSING DIAGNOSIS: impaired Skin/Tissue Integrity

May Be Related To

Chemical substance—bile, stasis of secretions

Imbalanced nutritional state (obesity); impaired metabolic state

Possibly Evidenced By

Disruption of skin or subcutaneous tissues

Invasion of body structure—T-tube punctures or incision

Desired Outcomes/Evaluation Criteria—Client Will

Wound Healing: Primary/Secondary Intention (NOC)

Achieve timely wound healing without complications.

Demonstrate behaviors to promote healing and prevent skin breakdown.

ACTIONS/INTERVENTIONS	RATIONALE
Wound Care (NIC)	
Independent	
Observe the color and character of NG and T-tube (biliary drainage).	Initially, drainage may contain blood and blood-stained fluid, normally changing to greenish-brown (bile color) after the first several hours.
Maintain T-tube in closed collection system.	Prevents skin irritation and reduces risk of contamination.
Check the T-tube and incisional drains; make sure they are free-flowing.	T-tube may remain in common bile duct for 7 to 10 days to remove retained tiny stones and gravel. Incision site drains are used to remove any accumulated fluid and bile. Correct positioning prevents backup of the bile in the operative area.
Anchor drainage tube, allowing sufficient tubing to permit free turning and avoid kinks and twists.	Avoids dislodging tube and occlusion of the lumen.
Change dressings often initially, then as needed. Clean the skin with soap and water. Use sterile petroleum jelly gauze, zinc oxide, or other skin protectant around the incision.	Keeps the skin around the incision clean and provides a barrier to protect skin from excoriation from bile leaking outside of T-tube.
Apply Montgomery straps for client who had open cholecystectomy.	Facilitates frequent dressing changes and minimizes skin trauma.
Use a disposable ostomy bag over a stab wound drain.	Ostomy appliance may be used to collect heavy drainage for more accurate measurement of output and protection of the skin.
Place client in low- or semi-Fowler's position, and encourage early ambulation.	Facilitates drainage of bile.
Monitor abdominal puncture sites (three to five) if laparoscopic procedure is done.	These areas may bleed, or staples and Steri-Strips may loosen at puncture wound sites.
Observe for hiccups, abdominal distention, or other signs of peritonitis such as rigid abdomen, fever, and severe right upper quadrant (RUQ) abdominal pain suggesting pancreatitis.	Dislodgment of the T-tube can result in diaphragmatic irritation or more serious complications if bile drains into abdomen or pancreatic duct is obstructed.
Observe skin for itching, sclera for jaundice, and urine for change in color to dark brown.	May indicate obstruction of bile flow from retained gallstone(s).
Note color and consistency of stools.	Clay-colored stools result when bile is not present in the intestines.
Investigate reports of increased or unrelenting RUQ pain, development of fever and tachycardia, and leakage of bile drainage around tube or from wound.	Signs suggestive of abscess or fistula formation, requiring medical intervention.
Collaborative	
Administer antibiotics, as indicated.	Necessary for treatment of abscess or infection.
Clamp the T-tube per schedule.	Tests the patency of the common bile duct before tube is removed. Also, if tube is left in place for a long time, clamping may be done 1 hour before and after meals, which diverts the bile back to the duodenum to aid digestion (Antipuesto, 2010).
Prepare for surgical interventions, as indicated.	Drainage of blocked duct or fistulectomy may be required to treat abscess or repair fistula. Bile duct injury will require stenting of duct or surgical repair if stenting not successful.
Monitor laboratory studies, for instance, WBC count.	Leukocytosis reflects inflammatory process, for example, abscess formation or development of peritonitis or pancreatitis.

NURSING DIAGNOSIS: deficient Knowledge [Learning Need] regarding condition, prognosis, treatment, self-care, and discharge needs

May Be Related To

Lack of exposure, information misinterpretation
Unfamiliarity with information resources
Lack of recall

Possibly Evidenced By

Reports the problem
Inaccurate follow-through of instructions

Desired Outcomes/Evaluation Criteria—Client Will

Knowledge: Acute Illness Management (NOC)

Verbalize understanding of disease process, surgical procedure and prognosis, and potential complications.
Verbalize understanding of therapeutic needs.
Correctly perform necessary procedures and explain reasons for the actions.
Initiate necessary lifestyle changes and participate in therapeutic regimen.

ACTIONS/INTERVENTIONS	RATIONALE
Teaching: Disease Process (NIC) *Independent*	
Review disease process, surgical procedure, and prognosis.	Provides knowledge base on which client can make informed choices.
Demonstrate care of incisions and dressings and drains.	Promotes independence in care and reduces risk of complications, such as infection and biliary obstruction.
Instruct in periodic drainage of T-tube collection bag and recording of output, if indicated.	Reduces risk of reflux, strain on tube, and appliance seal. Provides information about resolution of ductal edema and return of ductal function for appropriate timing of T-tube removal.
Emphasize importance of maintaining low-fat diet, eating frequent small meals, and gradual reintroduction of foods and fluids containing fats over a 4- to 6-month period.	During initial 6 months after surgery, low-fat diet limits need for bile and reduces discomfort associated with inadequate digestion of fats.
Discuss use of medication such as dehydrocholic acid (Decholin).	Oral replacement of bile salts may be required in certain clients to facilitate digestion and treat malabsorption of fats.
Discuss avoiding or limiting use of alcoholic beverages.	Minimizes risk of pancreatic involvement.
Inform client that loose stools may occur for several months.	Intestines require time to adjust to stimulus of continuous output of bile.
Advise client to note and avoid foods that seem to aggravate the diarrhea.	Although radical dietary changes are not usually necessary, certain restrictions may be helpful, such as fats in small amounts. After a period of adjustment, client usually will not have problems with most foods.
Identify signs and symptoms requiring notification of healthcare provider, such as dark urine, jaundiced sclera and skin, clay-colored stools, excessive stools, or recurrent heartburn and bloating.	Indicators of obstruction of bile flow or altered digestion, requiring further evaluation and intervention.
Review activity limitations, depending on individual situation.	Resumption of usual activities is normally accomplished within 4 to 6 weeks.

POTENTIAL CONSIDERATIONS following acute hospitalization (dependent on client's age, physical condition, presence of complications, personal resources, and life responsibilities)

- ***Diarrhea***—inflammation, irritation, malabsorption
- ***risk for Infection***—invasive procedure, broken skin, traumatized tissues

CHAPTER 8

Metabolic and Endocrine Disorders

EATING DISORDERS: ANOREXIA NERVOSA/ BULIMIA NERVOSA

I. Pathophysiology: Eating disorders encompass a spectrum of psychological problems that involve insufficient or excessive food intake, resulting in significant health problems across the life span. The cause of eating disorders is thought to stem from a mixture of social, psychological, and biological factors. How much each factor contributes to the development of these disorders is a matter of debate.

a. Physiological factors

i. Genetic factors

1. Some studies suggest that genetics contribute to about 50% of the variance for eating disorders.
2. Clinical depression also has a genetic risk with anorexia.
3. Genes seem to influence eating regulation, personality, and emotion and may be factors in these disorders.

ii. Neurobiological factors

1. The neurotransmitter serotonin has a correlation with mood, sleep, emesis, sexuality, and appetite.
2. Anorexia may be linked to a disturbed serotonin system.
3. Cause and effect are not easily separated, as other factors, such as starvation, may be involved.
4. After recovery, personality characteristics, anxiety, and perfectionism remain, suggesting that they may be causal factors.

iii. Nutritional factors

1. Zinc deficiency is known to cause a decrease in appetite and has been recommended for the treatment of anorexia.
2. Other nutrients, such as tyrosine and tryptophan, as well as vitamin B_1 may also be deficient and contribute to malnutrition.

b. Psychological factors

i. Biases in thinking and perception are believed to maintain and contribute to developing anorexia.

ii. Feelings of fatness and unattractiveness are overestimated, perceived, and evaluated by the affected persons as being true, regardless of reality of their body, food, and eating.

iii. A "transdiagnostic model" (Fairburn et al, 2009) proposes that all major eating disorders (with the exception of obesity) share some core types of psychopathology that help maintain the eating disorder behavior. These core psychopathologies include clinical perfectionism, chronic low self-esteem, mood intolerance, and interpersonal difficulties.

c. Social and environmental factors

i. The media, which has promoted the concept of thinness as the ideal female form, is believed to contribute to the development of eating disorders.

ii. Those in professions where there is pressure to be thin—models, dancers, and sports—may develop anorexia.

iii. Child sexual abuse is noted in people with anorexia and while it is not a specific risk factor, it is for mental illness in general.

iv. The Internet has become a source of contact and communication for those with eating disorders and may or may not be helpful for them (Gibson, 2012).

II. Characteristics

a. Anorexia nervosa (AN)

i. Serious, chronic illness of starvation associated with a severe disturbance of body image and a morbid fear of obesity

ii. Constellation of factors involved include an individual's genetic makeup, personality, and psychological and emotional challenges.

iii. Divided into early, mild, or established stages

b. Bulimia nervosa (BN)

i. Chronic cycle involving binge eating and purging

ii. Characterized by binges of overeating, which may be extreme, followed by self-induced vomiting, purging, and misuse of laxatives, diuretics, or enemas; may also involve nonpurging behaviors such as excessive exercise and fasting

iii. Fear of gaining weight motivates purging or compensatory behaviors.

iv. Often seen in persons of normal weight, but may be seen in overweight clients

c. Binge eating disorder (BED)

i. Characterized by binge eating without inappropriate compensatory behaviors such as purging or fasting

ii. Ingestion of large amounts of food with a sense of loss of control; frequent dieting without weight loss

III. Etiology (Murphy, 2007)

a. The hypothalamus, which regulates appetite by signaling hunger and satiety, may not release balanced amounts of neurotransmitters, such as serotonin or pancreatic polypeptides.

b. Occurs in either sex and in people of any race, age, or social stratum

c. Both AN and BN can be present in the same individual.
d. Risk factors
  i. Personal characteristics: low self-esteem and feelings of helplessness
  ii. Social factors: popular cultural preferences, media images, peer pressure, occupational expectations, for example, model, dancer, athlete
  iii. Family structure: Theory suggests that girls who live in families that highly value perfection are at a greater risk for developing an eating disorder.
  iv. Presence of psychiatric comorbidities: anxiety, depression, addictive behavior, or impulse control disorders
  v. Genetics: Family and twin studies have suggested that genes influencing not only eating regulation but also personality and emotion may be important contributing factors (Gibson, 2012; Bernstein, 2012).

IV. Statistics

a. AN, BN, BED
  i. Morbidity: Up to 24 million people of all ages and genders suffer from an eating disorder (anorexia, bulimia, and binge eating disorder) in the United States; only 1 in 10 individuals with an eating disorder receives treatment (Anorexia Nervosa and Associated Disorders [ANAD], 2013).
  ii. Mortality: Eating disorders have the highest mortality rate of any mental illness (ANAD, 2013). Studies show recent increased mortality in bulimia nervosa and other not otherwise specified (NOS) eating disorders, e.g., crude mortality rates were 4% to 5.9% for anorexia nervosa, 1.9% to 3.9% for bulimia nervosa, and 1.9% to 5.2% for eating disorder (NOS)(Bernstein, 2012; Crow et al, 2009).
  iii. Cost: Total hospital costs were $277 million with average length of stay 8.1 days (Zhoa, 2011).
b. AN
  i. Morbidity: More common in girls and women, although approximately 10% of cases occur in males (Bernstein, 2012); only about 50% of those affected will recover, with best results occurring if treatment is begun within the first 6 months of onset and supportive parents and family are present (Speranza, 2007).
  ii. Mortality: AN has the highest mortality rate among all psychological disorders (The Alliance, 2013), with 20% of deaths attributed to suicide.
c. BN
  i. Morbidity: Most common in white (more than 95%) adolescents (more than 75%) and young adults, affecting primarily adolescent girls (6%) and college-aged women (5%); lifetime prevalence about 3% (National Institute of Mental Health, 2007).
  ii. Mortality: Up to 3% eventually die of complications from the disease; leading cause of death is suicide, which is more common in persons with BN than those with AN (Quigley & Moreno, 2011).
d. BED
  i. Morbidity: Most common eating disorder in the United States; estimated 3.5% American females and 2% males affected (The Alliance, 2013).

GLOSSARY

Abnormal involuntary movement scale (AIMS): System used to assess abnormal involuntary movements, such as hand tremors or rhythmic movements of the tongue and jaw, which may result from the long-term administration of psychotropic drugs.

Electroconvulsive therapy (ECT): Use of an electric shock to produce convulsions and thereby treat drug-resistant psychiatric disorders, such as some cases of major depression, bipolar disorder, suicidal ideation, and schizophrenia.

Family therapy: Focuses on the interdependent relationships within the family as a whole.

Margination: Adhesion of leukocytes to the walls of blood vessels during early stage of inflammatory process.

Obsessive-compulsive disorder (OCD): Chronic anxiety disorder most commonly characterized by obsessive, distressing, intrusive thoughts and related compulsions.

Osteopenia: Decrease in the amount of bone density.

Recovery environment: The individual in treatment and the supportive family members work together to create an environment in which all feel safe to express their feelings without judgment, criticism, or guilt.

Refeeding syndrome: Serious complication of electrolyte imbalance and cardiopulmonary compromise, which occurs with rapid increase of nutritional intake or total parenteral nutrition (TPN).

Total parenteral nutrition (TPN): Nutritional therapy specifically designed to prevent or correct protein-calorie malnutrition, which is administered via an enteral or parenteral route.

Care Setting

Acute care is provided through inpatient stay on a medical or behavioral unit and for correction of severe nutritional deficits and electrolyte imbalances or initial psychiatric stabilization. Long-term care is provided in an outpatient or day treatment program (partial hospitalization) or in the community.

Related Concerns

Dysrhythmias, page 87
Fluid and electrolyte imbalances, page 885
Metabolic alkalosis—primary base bicarbonate excess, page 455
Psychosocial aspects of care, page 729
Total nutritional support: parenteral/enteral feeding, page 437

Client Assessment Database

DIAGNOSTIC DIVISION MAY REPORT	MAY EXHIBIT
ACTIVITY/REST	
• Disturbed sleep patterns—early-morning insomnia, fatigue • Feeling "hyper" or anxious • Increased activity, avid exerciser, participation in high-energy sports • Employment in positions or professions that emphasize and require strict weight control, such as gymnasts, bodybuilders, and other athletes, jockeys, models, dancers, skaters, actors, wrestlers, flight attendants, and others for whom thinness is emphasized and overly rewarded (Goldfield, 2006)	• Periods of hyperactivity, constant vigorous exercising (AN)
CIRCULATION	
• Feeling cold even when room is warm	• Low blood pressure (BP), orthostatic changes in BP or heart rate • Cold hands and feet • Tachycardia, bradycardia, dysrhythmias
EGO INTEGRITY	
• Lack of control over eating, for example, cannot stop eating or cannot control what or how much is eaten (BN) • Feeling disgusted with self, depressed, or very guilty because of overeating • Distorted or unrealistic body image; reports self as fat regardless of weight (denial), and sees thin body as fat • Persistent overconcern with body shape and weight • Unrealistic pleasure in weight loss, while denying oneself pleasure in other areas • High self-expectations • Stress factors—family move, divorce, onset of puberty • Suppression of angry feelings	• Emotional states of depression, withdrawal, anger, anxiety, pessimistic outlook • Psychiatric illness, such as depression, anxiety, bipolar disorder, OCD
ELIMINATION	
• Diarrhea or constipation • Laxative and diuretic abuse	
FOOD/FLUID	
• Constant hunger or denial of hunger; normal or exaggerated appetite that rarely vanishes until late in the disorder (AN) • Intense fear of gaining weight (females); may have prior history of being overweight (particularly males) • Preoccupation with food, such as calorie counting, gourmet cooking • Recurrent episodes of binge eating, a feeling of lack of control over behavior during eating binges, a minimum average of two binge-eating episodes a week for at least 3 months (BN) • Regularly engages in self-induced vomiting either independently or as a complication of anorexia, or strict dieting or fasting	• Weight loss and maintenance of body weight 15% or more below that expected; refusal to maintain body weight over minimal norm for age and height (AN) • Weight may be normal or slightly above or below normal (BN) • No medical illness evident to account for weight loss • Cachectic appearance, skin may be dry, yellowish, pale, with poor turgor (AN) • Preoccupation with food—calorie counting, hiding food, cutting food into small pieces, rearranging food on plate • Irrational thinking about eating, food, and weight • Swollen salivary glands; sore, inflamed buccal cavity; continuous sore throat (BN) • Vomiting, bloody vomitus (may indicate esophageal tearing—Mallory-Weiss syndrome) • Excessive gum chewing
HYGIENE	
	• Increased hair growth on body (lanugo), hair loss (axillary, pubic), hair is dull, not shiny • Brittle nails • Erosion of tooth enamel, gums in poor condition, ulcerations of mucosa • Enlarged salivary glands; dry mouth; reddened, dry, cracked lips

DIAGNOSTIC DIVISION MAY REPORT (continued)	MAY EXHIBIT (continued)
NEUROSENSORY	• Appropriate affect (except in regard to body and eating) or depressive affect • *Mental changes:* Apathy, confusion, memory impairment brought on by malnutrition or starvation • Hysterical or obsessive personality style; absence of other psychiatric illness or thought disorder—although a significant number may show evidence of an affective disorder
PAIN/DISCOMFORT • Headaches • Sore throat or mouth • Generalized vague complaints • Vague abdominal pain and distress, bloating	
SAFETY	• Body temperature below normal • Recurrent infectious processes (indicative of depressed immune system) • Eczema and other skin problems, abrasions and calluses may be noted on back of hands from sticking finger down throat to induce vomiting (BN)
SEXUALITY • Absence of at least three consecutive menstrual cycles due to decreased levels of estrogen in response to malnutrition (AN) • Promiscuity or loss of sexual interest • History of sexual abuse • Homosexual or bisexual orientation—higher percentage in male clients than in general population	• Breast atrophy • Amenorrhea related to hypothalamic function
SOCIAL INTERACTION • Middle-class or upper-class family background • History of being a quiet, cooperative child • Problems of control issues in relationships, difficult communications with others, especially authority figures • Poor communication within family of origin • Engagement in power struggles • An emotional crisis of some sort, such as divorce, the onset of puberty, or an unwanted family move • Altered relationships or problems with relationships, withdrawal from friends and social contacts • Abusive family relationships • Sense of helplessness • History of legal difficulties— shoplifting, drug use	• Passive father, dominant mother • Family members closely fused • Togetherness prized • Personal boundaries not respected
TEACHING/LEARNING • Family history of higher than normal incidence of depression • Other family members with eating disorders (genetic predisposition) • Health beliefs and practice—certain foods have "too many" calories, use of "health" foods, and so forth • Substance abuse • Use of herbal or over-the-counter (OTC) preparations to control weight gain, such as bitter orange, green tea extract, guarana rhodiola, laxatives (bisacodyl, cascara, senna), high-fiber supplements • Use of prescription diet medications—Meridia, phenteramine, Xenical (often obtained without prescription via Internet)	

(continues on page 344)

Client Assessment Database (continued)

DIAGNOSTIC DIVISION MAY REPORT (continued)	MAY EXHIBIT (continued)
DISCHARGE PLAN CONSIDERATIONS • Assistance with maintenance of treatment plan ➧ Refer to section at end of plan for postdischarge considerations.	

Diagnostic Studies

TEST WHY IT IS DONE	WHAT IT TELLS ME
BLOOD TESTS	
• ***Complete blood count (CBC):*** Battery of screening tests that typically include hemoglobin (Hgb); hematocrit (Hct); red blood cell (RBC) count, morphology, indices, and distribution width index; platelet count and size; white blood cell (WBC) count and differential.	Determines presence of anemia (not due to blood loss). WBCs are reduced (leukopenia) due to margination; lymphocytes are increased (lymphocytosis). Platelets show significantly less than normal activity (thrombocytopenia). Hgb may be elevated in extreme dehydration.
• ***Basic metabolic profile (BMP):*** Provides baseline data and can be used to evaluate and monitor fluid and electrolyte balance.	Imbalances may include decreased potassium, sodium, chloride, and magnesium. Hypokalemia and hypochloremic metabolic alkalosis are observed with vomiting; acidosis is present in cases of laxative abuse (BN). Hyponatremia may be a result of excess water intake (AN). May show elevated bicarbonate levels. In AN, hypoglycemia is often present because of lack of carbohydrates in the diet or low glycogen levels in the liver. Blood urea nitrogen (BUN) and creatinine (Cr) may be normal or low. BUN may be elevated if severe dehydration is present.
• ***Erythrocyte sedimentation rate (ESR):*** Helps exclude unrecognized chronic medical conditions.	Tends to be low in presence of eating disorders
• ***Albumin or prealbumin:*** Transport proteins in plasma and assist in maintaining oncotic pressure within the vascular bed	Serum protein and albumin are often normal in AN because, although the amount of food is restricted, it often contains high-quality proteins.
• ***Amylase:*** Digestive enzyme primarily located in pancreas and salivary glands	Elevated in up to 30% of clients in presence of repeated vomiting; reflects hypersecretion of the salivary glands
• ***Aspartate aminotransferase/alanine aminotransferase (AST/ALT), aluminum phosphide (ALP), total bilirubin, and direct bilirubin:*** Liver function tests to determine associated impairment or damage and gallbladder involvement	Liver function studies may be minimally elevated (AN). In severe starvation states, AST/ALT levels are elevated. In BN, liver function tests are usually normal, although amylase may be elevated because of vomiting (Quigley & Moreno, 2012).
• ***Cholesterol, high-density lipoprotein (HDL), low-density lipoprotein (LDL), and triglycerides:*** Types of lipids	Dramatic elevations in cholesterol are observed in cases of starvation. This elevation may be secondary to (1) decrease in triiodothyronine (T_3) levels, (2) low cholesterol-binding globulin, and (3) leakage of intrahepatic cholesterol.
• ***T_3, thyroxine (T_4), and thyroid-stimulating hormone (TSH):*** Thyroid function tests	T_4 levels are usually normal; however, circulating T_3 levels may be low. TSH response to thyrotropin-releasing hormone (TRH) is abnormal in AN, reflecting euthyroid sick syndrome.
• ***Pituitary function:*** Propranolol-glucagon stimulation test studies the response of human growth hormone (hGH).	Depressed in anorexia. Gonadotropic hypofunction is noted.
• ***Cortisol:*** Hormone involved in a variety of different bodily functions, including the immune system, regulation of blood sugar, liver function, and response to stress	May be elevated.
• ***Dexamethasone suppression test (DST):*** Evaluates hypothalamic-pituitary function.	Dexamethasone resistance indicates cortisol suppression, suggesting malnutrition or depression (positive in BN).
• ***Estrogen and luteinizing hormone (LH) secretions test:*** Produced by the anterior lobe of the pituitary gland that stimulates ovulation and the development of the corpus luteum in females and the production of testosterone by the interstitial cells of the testis in males	Pattern often resembles those of prepubertal girls.

TEST WHY IT IS DONE (continued)	WHAT IT TELLS ME (continued)
Associated Studies	
• ***Urinalysis***	Ketones in the urine represent starvation.
• ***Fecal occult blood:*** Identifies associated gastrointestinal (GI) complications.	Positive result may indicate esophagitis, gastritis, or repeated colon irritation from laxative use. May reveal presence of emetine, which is a by-product of ipecac use.
• ***Electrocardiogram (ECG)*** Record of the electrical activity of the heart.	Abnormal tracing with low-voltage, T-wave inversion, prolonged QT interval, bradycardia, and dysrhythmias may be present, reflecting electrolyte imbalances.
• ***Chest x-ray or computed tomography (CT) scan:*** Determine presence of associated complications.	May reveal rib fractures associated with repeated vomiting in presence of hypocalcemia or evidence of osteopenia. Changes reflecting emphysema (AN) may resolve with refeeding and weight gain. Heart size may be decreased.
• ***Dual energy absorptiometry (DEXA) scan:*** Measures bone density and is used to assess risk for fracture.	May reveal osteoporosis.
• ***Genetic testing:*** Determines familial risk factor that may contribute to disturbance in appetite regulation.	Gene for agouti-related protein, which may affect body mass index (BMI), fat mass, and percent of body fat, has been found to be higher in anorexic clients than in the general population.

Nursing Priorities

1. Obtain client's cooperation in treatment.
2. Reestablish adequate, appropriate nutritional intake.
3. Correct fluid and electrolyte imbalance.
4. Assist client to develop realistic body image and improve self-esteem.
5. Provide support and involve significant other (SO), if available, in treatment program.
6. Coordinate total treatment program with other disciplines.
7. Provide information about disease, prognosis, and treatment to client and SO.

Discharge Goals

1. Adequate nutrition and fluid intake maintained.
2. Maladaptive coping behaviors and stressors that precipitate anxiety recognized.
3. Adaptive coping strategies and techniques for anxiety reduction and self-control implemented.
4. Self-esteem increased.
5. Disease process, prognosis, and treatment regimen understood.
6. Plan in place to meet needs after discharge.

NURSING DIAGNOSIS: imbalanced Nutrition: less than body requirements

May Be Related To

Inability to digest food—self-induced vomiting
Psychological factors—distorted view of body, fear of gaining weight

Possibly Evidenced By

Reports food intake less than recommended daily allowance
Body weight 20% or more below ideal weight range (AN)
Aversion to eating; satiety immediately after ingesting food (AN)
Capillary fragility; pale mucous membranes, poor muscle tone; excessive hair loss (AN)
Sore buccal cavity (BN)
Diarrhea (AN/BN)
Misconceptions—see's self as fat (AN/BN)

Desired Outcomes/Evaluation Criteria—Client Will

Knowledge: Healthy Diet (NOC)
Verbalize understanding of nutritional needs.
Establish a dietary pattern with caloric intake adequate to regain or maintain appropriate weight.
Demonstrate weight gain toward individually expected range.

ACTIONS/INTERVENTIONS	RATIONALE
Eating Disorders Management (NIC)	
Independent	
Establish a minimum weight goal and daily nutritional requirements.	Provides comparative baseline for effectiveness of therapy. *Note:* Malnutrition is a mood-altering condition, leading to depression and affecting cognitive function and decision making. Improved nutritional status enhances thinking ability, allowing initiation of psychological work.
Contract with client regarding commitment to therapeutic program and meeting specific dietary needs and goals.	Individual success is enhanced when client commits to a contract.
Use a consistent approach. Sit with client while eating; present and remove food without persuasion or comment. Promote pleasant environment and record intake.	Client detects urgency and may react to pressure. Any comment that might be seen as coercion provides focus on food. When staff responds in a consistent manner, client can begin to trust staff responses. The single area in which client has exercised power and control is food and eating, and she or he may experience guilt or rebellion if forced to eat. Structuring meals and decreasing discussions about food will decrease power struggles with client and avoid manipulative games.
Provide small, frequent, and nutritionally dense meals and supplemental snacks, as appropriate.	Gastric dilation may occur if refeeding is too rapid following a period of starvation dieting. Client may feel bloated for weeks while body adjusts to increased food intake. *Note:* Client at risk for developing refeeding syndrome.
Make selective menu available, and allow client to control choices as much as possible.	Client who gains confidence in self and feels in control of environment is more likely to eat preferred foods.
Be alert to choices of low-calorie foods and beverages, hoarding food, and disposing of food in various places, such as pockets or wastebaskets.	Client will try to avoid taking in what is viewed as excessive calories and may go to great lengths to avoid eating.
Maintain a regular weighing schedule, such as Monday and Friday before breakfast in same attire, and graph results.	Provides accurate ongoing record of weight loss or gain. Also diminishes obsessing about changes in weight.
Weigh with back to scale, depending on program protocols.	Although some programs prefer that client does not see the results of the weighing, this can force the issue of trust in client who usually does not trust others.
Avoid room checks and other control devices whenever possible.	External control reinforces feelings of powerlessness and therefore is usually not helpful.
Provide one-to-one supervision and have client with bulimia remain in the day room area or in sight with no bathroom privileges for a specified period, such as 2 to 3 hours, following eating if contracting is unsuccessful.	Prevents vomiting during or immediately after eating. Client may desire food and eating, but use a binge-purge syndrome to control weight. *Note:* Some clients purge for the first time in response to establishment of a weight-gain program.
Monitor exercise program and set limits on physical activities. Chart activity and level of work—pacing and so on.	Moderate exercise helps in maintaining muscle tone and combating depression; however, client may exercise excessively to burn calories.
Maintain matter-of-fact, nonjudgmental attitude if giving tube feedings, parenteral fluids, and so on.	Perception of punishment is counterproductive to client's self-confidence and faith in own ability to control destiny.
Be alert to possibility of client disconnecting feeding tube and emptying enteral or parenteral fluids if used. Check measurements and tape tubing snugly.	Sabotage behavior is common in attempt to prevent weight gain.
Monitor for signs of refeeding syndrome reflecting fluid and electrolyte disorders, increased cardiac workload, and oxygen consumption.	Refeeding syndrome and congestive heart failure can occur because of too rapid an increase in oral intake. Heart size diminishes because of malnutrition and may have a difficult time compensating for an increase in circulating volume.
Collaborative	
Provide nutritional therapy within a hospital treatment program, as indicated when condition is life-threatening.	Cure of the underlying problem cannot happen without improved nutritional status. Hospitalization provides a controlled environment in which food intake, vomiting, elimination, medications, and activities can be monitored. It also separates client from SO, who may be a contributing factor, and provides exposure to others with the same problem, creating an atmosphere for sharing.
Involve client in setting up and carrying out program of behavior modification. Provide reward for weight gain as individually determined; ignore loss.	Provides structured eating situation while allowing client some control in choices. Behavior modification may be effective in mild cases or for short-term weight gain.
Provide diet and snacks with substitutions of preferred foods when available.	Having a variety of foods available enables client to have a choice of potentially enjoyable foods.
Administer nutritional diet by prescribed means—regular food with supplements, high-calorie liquid diet, or tube feedings if needed.	When caloric intake is insufficient to sustain metabolic needs, nutritional support can be used to prevent malnutrition and death while therapy is continuing. High-calorie liquid

ACTIONS/INTERVENTIONS (continued)	RATIONALE (continued)
	feedings may be given as medication, at preset times separate from meals, or as an alternative means of increasing caloric intake.
Run through a blender anything left on the tray after a given period of time and tube-feed, if indicated.	This method of feeding may be used as part of a behavior modification program to provide total intake of needed calories.
Administer enteral or parenteral nutrition, as appropriate.	TPN, or hyperalimentation, may be required for life-threatening situations; however, enteral feedings are preferred because they preserve GI function and reduce atrophy of the gut.
Avoid giving laxatives.	Use is counterproductive because they may be used by client to rid body of food or calories.
Administer medication, as indicated, for example:	
Vitamins, minerals, electrolytes	In AN, medication is usually limited to use in managing medical complications, such as calcium and vitamin D for osteopenia (which can be severe), potassium, magnesium, and phosphorus. Restoring electrolytes before refeeding decreases the risk of refeeding syndrome.
Serotonin and histamine antagonist, such as cyproheptadine (Periactin)	May be used for client with severe anorexia and no binging and purging. A serotonin and histamine antagonist that may be used in high doses to stimulate the appetite, decrease preoccupation with food, and combat depression. Does not appear to have serious side effects, although decreased mental alertness may occur.
Selective serotonin reuptake inhibitors (SSRIs), such as fluoxetine (Prozac) and other antidepressants, such as tricyclics, for example, amitriptyline (Elavil) and imipramine (Tofranil); dopamine reuptake blocker, such as bupropion (Wellbutrin); 5-HT2 blocker, such as trazadone (Desryel)	Various antidepressants may be used to lift depression, stimulate appetite, and stabilize AN. Many of these same drugs are also found to be useful in reducing binge-purge cycles in BN. *Note:* Use must be closely monitored because of potential side effects, although side effects from SSRIs are less significant than those associated with tricyclics.
Monoamine oxidase inhibitors (MAOIs), such as phenelzine (Nardil) and tranylcypromine sulfate (Parnate)	May be used to treat depression when other drug therapy is ineffective; decreases urge to binge in BN.
Antipsychotic drugs, such as risperadone (Risperdal), olanzapine (Zyprexa), chlorpromazine (Thorazine), and lithium (Eskalith, Lithane, Lithobid)	Newer antipsychotic drugs, such as Risperdal or Zyprexa, are being used to manage eating disorders, especially in presence of dual disorder, such as with bulimia and bipolar disorder. These drugs can reduce tension, anxiety, and nervousness and increase cooperation with psychotherapeutic program. However, some antipsychotic drugs are used only when absolutely necessary for severely delusional, overactive, hospitalized client as a last resort (e.g., Thorazine). Possibility of extrapyramidal side effects is a concern.
Perform AIMS (Abnormal Involuntary Movement Scale) after initiation of, and periodically during, treatment with antipsychotic medications.	Provides baseline and monitors for the development of extrapyramidal side effects, indicating need for change in therapy.
Monitor electrolytes, as indicated.	Refeeding syndrome may develop with rapid decrease in potassium, magnesium, and phosphate levels.
Prepare for or assist with electroconvulsive therapy (ECT), if indicated. Discuss reasons for use and help client understand this is not punishment.	In rare and difficult cases in which malnutrition is severe or life-threatening, a short-term ECT series may enable client to begin eating and become accessible to psychotherapy.

NURSING DIAGNOSIS: risk for deficient Fluid Volume

Risk Factors May Include

Active fluid loss—misuse of diuretics, laxatives, enemas; diarrhea (AN/BN); induced vomiting (BN); extremes of weight (AN)

Possibly Evidenced By

(Not applicable; presence of signs and symptoms establishes an *actual* diagnosis)

Desired Outcomes/Evaluation Criteria—Client Will

Hydration (NOC)

Maintain and demonstrate appropriate fluid balance, as evidenced by adequate urine output, stable vital signs, moist mucous membranes, and good skin turgor.

Risk Control (NOC)

Verbalize understanding of causative factors and behaviors necessary to maintain or correct fluid balance.

ACTIONS/INTERVENTIONS	RATIONALE
Fluid/Electrolyte Management (NIC)	
Independent	
Monitor vital signs, capillary refill, status of mucous membranes, and skin turgor.	Indicators of adequacy of circulating volume. Orthostatic hypotension may occur with risk of falls and injury following sudden changes in position.
Monitor amount and types of fluid intake. Measure urine output accurately.	Client may abstain from all intake, with resulting dehydration, or substitute fluids for caloric intake, disturbing electrolyte balance.
Discuss strategies to stop vomiting and laxative or diuretic use.	Helping client deal with the feelings that lead to vomiting and laxative or diuretic use will prevent continued fluid loss. *Note:* Client with bulimia has learned that vomiting provides a release of anxiety.
Identify actions necessary to regain or maintain optimal fluid balance, such as specific fluid intake schedule.	Involving client in plan to correct fluid imbalances improves chances for success.
Collaborative	
Review electrolyte and renal function test results.	Fluid and electrolyte shifts or depressed renal function can adversely affect cerebral function and client's recovery, requiring correction before therapeutic interventions can begin.
Administer intravenous (IV) fluids and electrolytes, as indicated.	Used to correct fluid and electrolyte imbalances and prevent cardiac dysrhythmias.

NURSING DIAGNOSIS: disturbed Body Image

May Be Related To

Biophysical—morbid fear of obesity
Cognitive—perceived loss of control in some aspect of life; perceptual—continual negative evaluation of self

Possibly Evidenced By

Behaviors of monitoring one's body; refusal to verify actual change
Reports feelings/perceptions that reflect an altered view of one's body in appearance
Reports negative feelings about body (e.g., feelings of helplessness, hopelessness, powerlessness)
Change in social involvement; reports fear of rejection by others

Desired Outcomes/Evaluation Criteria—Client Will

Body Image (NOC)

Establish a more realistic internal picture of self.
Engage in strategies to enhance appearance.
Verbalize acceptance of positive feedback about self.

ACTIONS/INTERVENTIONS	RATIONALE
Body Image Enhancement (NIC)	
Independent	
Have client draw picture of self.	Provides opportunity to discuss client's perception of self and body image, and realities of individual situation
Listen to but avoid challenging irrational or illogical thinking. Present reality concisely and briefly.	It is difficult to respond logically when thinking ability is physiologically impaired. Client needs to hear reality, but challenging client leads to distrust and frustration. *Note:* Even though client may gain weight, she or he may continue to struggle with attitudes and behaviors typical of eating disorders, major depression, and substance dependence.
Involve in personal development program, preferably in a group setting. Provide information about proper application of makeup and grooming.	Learning about methods to enhance personal appearance may be helpful to long-range sense of self-esteem and image. Feedback from others can promote feelings of self-worth.
Recommend consultation with an image consultant.	Positive image enhances sense of self-esteem.
Suggest disposing of "thin" clothes as weight gain occurs.	Provides incentive to at least maintain and not lose weight. Not seeing "thin" clothes removes visual reminder of thinner self.
Assist client to confront changes associated with puberty and sexual fears. Provide sex education as necessary.	Major physical and psychological changes in adolescence can contribute to development of eating disorders. Feelings of powerlessness and loss of control of feelings, in particular sexual sensations, can lead to an unconscious desire to desexualize self. Client often believes that these fears can be

ACTIONS/INTERVENTIONS	RATIONALE
	overcome by taking control of bodily appearance, development, and function.
Note athletic activities, as well as excessive/compulsive exercise. Discuss menstrual problems, e.g., amenorrhea.	There is a similar risk for eating disorders in athletes as in nonathletes (Greenleaf et al, 2010; Petrie et al, 2007; Torstveit, 2005), but there is a higher level of menstrual dysfunction in athletes (Sundgot-Borgen, 2010; Coelho et al, 2010).
Note body image concerns in men such as muscle dysmorphia, drive for masculinity, low testosterone, and bone loss. Encourage client to take control of activities, avoid overtraining.	Males may be preoccupied with increased muscle mass, be dissatisfied with body, and need to learn to focus on a healthy body image.
Collaborative	
Encourage participation in directed activities such as group hiking, bicycle tours, and wilderness adventures, such as the Outward Bound Program.	Although exercise is often used negatively by these clients, participation in directed activities provides an opportunity to learn self-reliance, enhance self-concept, and realize that food is the fuel required by the body to do its work. Athletes, especially, may need to moderate their exercise in order to maintain their training levels, while avoiding overtraining.
Refer to therapist trained in dealing with sexuality, as indicated.	May need professional assistance to deal with sexuality issues and accept self as a sexual individual.

NURSING DIAGNOSIS: chronic low Self-Esteem

May Be Related To
Lack of membership in group; perceived lack of belonging
Perceived discrepancy between self and cultural norms
Repeated negative reinforcement
Psychiatric disorder; depression

Possibly Evidenced By
Dependent on others' opinions
Exaggerates negative/rejects positive feedback about self
Indecisive behavior; overly conforming; passive
Reports feelings of guilt, shame

Desired Outcomes/Evaluation Criteria—Client Will
Self-Esteem (NOC)
Acknowledge self as an individual.
Accept responsibility for own actions.
Verbalize positive feelings about own self-worth.

ACTIONS/INTERVENTIONS	RATIONALE
Self-Esteem Enhancement (NIC)	
Independent	
Establish a therapeutic nurse-client relationship.	Within a helping relationship, client can begin to trust and try out new thinking and behaviors.
Be aware of client's distorted thinking ability.	Allows care providers to have more realistic expectations of client and provide appropriate information and support.
Promote self-concept without moral judgment.	Client sees self as weak-willed even though part of person may feel sense of power and control, for example, through dieting and weight loss.
State rules clearly regarding weighing schedule, remaining in sight during medication and eating times, and consequences of not following the rules. Without undue comment, be consistent in carrying out rules.	Consistency is important in establishing trust. As part of the behavior modification program, client knows risks involved in not following established rules (e.g., decrease in privileges). Failure to follow rules is viewed as client's choice and accepted by staff in matter-of-fact manner so as not to provide reinforcement for the undesirable behavior.
Confront denial and respond with reality when client makes unrealistic statements such as "I'm gaining weight, so there's nothing really wrong with me."	Client may be denying the psychological aspects of own situation and is often expressing a sense of inadequacy and depression.
Be aware of own reaction to client's behavior. Avoid arguing.	Feelings of disgust, hostility, and infuriation are not uncommon when caring for these clients. Prognosis often remains poor even with a gain in weight because other problems

(continues on page 350)

ACTIONS/INTERVENTIONS (continued)	RATIONALE (continued)
	may remain. Many clients continue to see themselves as fat, and there is also a high incidence of affective disorders, social phobias, obsessive-compulsive symptoms, drug abuse, and psychosexual dysfunction. Nurse needs to deal with own feelings so they do not interfere with care of client.
Assist client to assume control in areas other than dieting and weight loss, such as management of own daily activities and work and leisure choices.	Feelings of personal ineffectiveness, low self-esteem, and perfectionism are often part of the problem. Client feels helpless to change and requires assistance to problem-solve methods of control in life situations.
Help client formulate goals for self not related to eating and create a manageable plan for reaching those goals, one at a time, progressing from simple to more complex.	Client needs to recognize ability to control other areas in life and may need to learn problem-solving skills to achieve this control. Setting realistic goals fosters success.
Note client's withdrawal from or discomfort in social settings.	May indicate feelings of isolation and fear of rejection and judgment by others. Avoidance of social situations and contact with others can compound feelings of worthlessness.
Encourage client to take charge of own life in a more healthful way by making own decisions and accepting self as she or he is at this moment.	Client often does not know what she or he may want for self. Parents, generally mother, often make decisions for client. Client may also believe she or he has to be the best in everything and holds self responsible for being perfect.
Let client know that it is acceptable to be different from family, particularly mother.	Developing a sense of identity separate from family and maintaining sense of control in other ways besides dieting and weight loss is a desirable goal of therapy and program.
Encourage client to express anger and acknowledge when it is verbalized.	Important to know that anger is part of self and as such is acceptable. Expressing anger may need to be taught to client because anger is generally considered unacceptable in the family, and therefore client does not express it.
Assist client to learn strategies other than eating for dealing with feelings. Have client keep a diary of feelings, particularly when thinking about food.	Feelings are the underlying issue, and client often uses food instead of dealing with feelings appropriately. Client needs to learn to recognize feelings and how to express them clearly.
Assess feelings of helplessness and hopelessness.	Lack of control is a common and underlying problem for this client and may be accompanied by more serious emotional disorders.
Be alert to suicidal ideation and behavior.	Intense anxiety and panic about weight gain, depression, and hopeless feelings may lead to suicidal attempts, particularly if client is impulsive.
Collaborative	
Use cognitive-behavioral or interpersonal psychotherapy approach rather than interpretive therapy.	Although both therapies have similar results, cognitive-behavioral seems to work more quickly. Interaction between individuals is more helpful for client to discover feelings, impulses, and needs from within own self. Client has not learned this internal control as a child and may not be able to interpret or attach meaning to behavior.
Involve in group therapy.	Provides an opportunity to talk about feelings and try out new behaviors.
Refer to occupational and recreational therapy.	Can develop interest and skills to fill time that has been occupied by obsession with eating. Involvement in recreational activities encourages social interactions with others and promotes fun and relaxation.
Refer to therapist trained in dealing with sexuality, as indicated.	May need professional assistance to deal with sexuality issues and accept self as a sexual adult.

NURSING DIAGNOSIS: impaired Parenting

May Be Related To

Deficient knowledge about parenting skills; unrealistic expectations; inability to put child's needs before own
Lack of family cohesiveness; poor communication skills
Maladaptive coping strategies; poor problem-solving skills
History of mental illness—depression, obsessive-compulsive disorder; substance abuse

Possibly Evidenced By

Inappropriate caretaking skills; inconsistent behavior management; frequently punitive
Reports frustration; negative statements about child
Parent-child interaction deficits; child abuse

NURSING DIAGNOSIS: impaired Parenting (continued)

Desired Outcomes/Evaluation Criteria—Family Will

Parenting (NOC)

Demonstrate individual involvement in problem-solving process directed at encouraging client toward independence.
Express feelings freely and appropriately.
Demonstrate more autonomous coping behaviors with individual family boundaries more clearly defined.
Recognize and resolve conflict appropriately with the individuals involved.

ACTIONS/INTERVENTIONS	RATIONALE
Family Therapy (NIC)	
Independent	
Identify patterns of interaction. Encourage each family member to speak for self. Prevent two members discussing a third without that member's participation.	Helpful information for planning interventions. The enmeshed, overinvolved family members often speak for each other and need to learn to be responsible for their own words and actions.
Discourage members from asking for approval from each other. Be alert to verbal or nonverbal checking with others for approval. Acknowledge competent actions of client.	Each individual needs to develop own internal sense of self-esteem. Individual often is living up to others' (family's) expectations rather than making own choices. Acknowledgment provides recognition of self in positive ways.
Listen with regard when client speaks.	Sets an example and provides a sense of competence and self-worth in that client has been heard and attended to.
Encourage individuals not to answer to everything.	Reinforces individualization and return to privacy.
Communicate message of separation—that it is acceptable for family members to be different from each other.	Individuation needs reinforcement. Such a message confronts rigidity and opens options for different behaviors.
Encourage and allow expression of feelings, such as crying or anger by individuals.	Often these families have not allowed free expression of feelings and need help and permission to learn and accept this.
Prevent intrusion in dyads by other members of the family.	Inappropriate interventions in family subsystems prevent individuals from working out problems successfully.
Reinforce importance of parents as a couple who have rights of their own.	The focus on the child with anorexia is very intense and often is the only area around which the couple interacts. The couple needs to explore their own relationship and restore the balance within relationship to help prevent its disintegration.
Prevent client from intervening in conflicts between parents. Assist parents in identifying and solving their marital differences.	Triangulation occurs in which a parent-child coalition exists. Sometimes the child is openly pressed to ally self with one parent against the other. The symptom (anorexia) is the regulator in the family system, and the parents deny their own conflicts.
Be aware and confront sabotage behavior on the part of family members.	Feelings of blame, shame, and helplessness may lead to unconscious behavior designed to maintain the status quo.
Collaborative	
Refer to community resources, such as:	
Parents' groups, Parent Effectiveness classes	May help reduce overprotectiveness, and support and facilitate the process of dealing with unresolved conflicts and change.
Family therapy groups	Eating disorders are not caused by families but are a family problem. Family therapy groups provide a forum for families to talk about their concerns and misconceptions, learning from others. As family members gain knowledge, they can use it to learn new skills of communication and encouragement, instead of using emotion.
Individual family therapy, as indicated	Individual family therapy focuses on developing a recovery environment in which family members work together to create a safe environment.

NURSING DIAGNOSIS: risk for impaired Skin Integrity

Risk Factors May Include

Changes in skin turgor; impaired circulation; skeletal prominences
Imbalanced nutrition state (e.g., emaciation, obesity)
Immunological factors

Possibly Evidenced By

(Not applicable; presence of signs and symptoms establishes an *actual* diagnosis)

(continues on page 352)

NURSING DIAGNOSIS: risk for impaired Skin Integrity (continued)

Desired Outcomes/Evaluation Criteria—Client Will

Risk Control (NOC)

Verbalize understanding of causative factors and absence of itching.

Identify and demonstrate behaviors to maintain soft, supple, intact skin.

ACTIONS/INTERVENTIONS	RATIONALE
Skin Surveillance (NIC)	
Independent	
Observe for reddened, blanched, and excoriated areas.	Indicators of increased risk of breakdown, requiring more intensive treatment.
Encourage bathing every other day instead of daily if this is an area of concern.	Frequent baths contribute to dryness of the skin.
Use skin cream twice a day and after bathing.	Lubricates skin and decreases itching.
Massage skin gently, especially over bony prominences.	Improves circulation to the skin and enhances skin tone.
Discuss importance of frequent position changes and need for remaining active.	Enhances circulation and perfusion to skin by preventing prolonged pressure on tissues.
Emphasize importance of adequate nutrition and fluid intake. (Refer to ND: imbalanced Nutrition: less than body requirements.)	Improved nutrition and hydration will improve skin condition.

NURSING DIAGNOSIS: ineffective Self-Health Management

May Be Related To

Decisional conflicts; powerlessness; family conflict

Complexity of therapeutic regimen

Deficient knowledge; perceived benefits

Possibly Evidenced By

Failure to include treatment regimens in daily living

Ineffective choices in daily living for meeting health goals

Failure to take action to reduce risk factors

Desired Outcomes/Evaluation Criteria—Client Will

Knowledge: Eating Disorder Management (NOC)

Verbalize plan for lifestyle changes to maintain healthy weight.

Identify relationship of signs and symptoms, such as weight loss and tooth decay, to behaviors of not eating or binging-purging.

Identify strategies to prevent relapse.

Establish realistic exercise/activity program.

Assume responsibility for own learning.

Seek out sources and resources to assist with making identified changes.

ACTIONS/INTERVENTIONS	RATIONALE
Learning Facilitation (NIC)	
Independent	
Determine level of knowledge and readiness to learn.	Learning is easier when it begins where the learner is.
Note blocks to learning, including physical, intellectual, and emotional issues.	Malnutrition, family problems, drug abuse, affective disorders, and obsessive-compulsive symptoms can be blocks to learning requiring resolution before effective learning can occur.
Teaching: Disease Process (NIC)	
Discuss familial tendencies and genetic risk for eating disorder.	Recent research supports the findings suggesting that anorexia and bulimia are disorders that occur in families; for example, this client is more likely to have an immediate family member or even a more distant relative with either disorder. The disease may be inheritable with single or multiple genes combined with environmental factors and traits such as perfectionism, maturity fears, and low self-esteem.
Provide written information for client and SOs.	Helpful as reminder of and reinforcement for learning.

ACTIONS/INTERVENTIONS (continued)	RATIONALE (continued)
Discuss consequences of behavior and potential for recovery and relapse.	Sudden death can occur because of electrolyte imbalances and suppression of the immune system. Liver damage may result from protein deficiency, or gastric rupture may follow binge eating and vomiting.
Review dietary needs, answering questions as indicated. Encourage inclusion of high-fiber foods and adequate fluid intake.	Client and family may need assistance with planning for new way of eating. Constipation may occur when laxative use is curtailed.
Encourage the use of relaxation and other stress management techniques, such as visualization, guided imagery, and biofeedback.	New ways of coping with feelings of anxiety and fear help client manage these feelings in more effective ways, assisting in giving up maladaptive behaviors of not eating or binging-purging.
Assist with establishing a sensible exercise program. Caution regarding overexercise. Modify sports workouts if necessary and use coach-athletic relationship.	Exercise can assist with developing a positive body image and combats depression—release of endorphins in the brain enhances sense of well-being. However, client may use excessive exercise as a way to control weight. *Note:* It may not be helpful to remove from sports, especially if there is a positive coach-athlete relationship. Sports might be individual's identity and can be maintained unless client is noncompliant with treatment regimen.
Discuss need for information about sex and sexuality.	Because avoidance of own sexuality is an issue for this client, realistic information can be helpful in beginning to deal with self as a sexual being.
Refer to National Association of Anorexia Nervosa and Associated Disorders, Overeaters Anonymous, and other local resources, as appropriate.	May be a helpful source of support and information for client and SO.

POTENTIAL CONSIDERATIONS following acute hospitalization (dependent on client's age, physical condition and presence of complications, personal resources, and life responsibilities)

- ***risk for imbalanced Nutrition: less than body requirements***—psychological factors (dysfunctional eating patterns)
- ***ineffective Self-Health Management***—complexity of therapeutic regimen, perceived seriousness/benefits, excessive demands made on individual, family conflict

Sample clinical pathway follows in Table 8.1.

TABLE 8.1 Sample Pathway: Eating Disorders Program. ELOS: 28 Days Behavioral Unit (Combined Hospitalization and Intensive Outpatient Program)

ND and Categories of Care	Time Dimension	Goals/Actions	Time Dimension	Goals/Actions	Time Dimension	Goals/Actions
imbalanced Nutrition: less than body requirements R/T psychological factors (inadequate intake, self-induced vomiting, laxative use)	Ongoing	Gain 3 lb/wk as indicated	Day 2–28	Consume at least 75% of food provided at each meal	Day 15–28	Demonstrate ability to select foods to meet at least 80% of nutritional needs
risk for deficient Fluid Volume R/T deviations affecting intake, active losses (self-induced vomiting, laxative use)	Ongoing	Be free of S/S of dehydration	Day 2–28	Ingest at least 1500 mL fluid/day	Day 22–28	Refrain from self-induced vomiting
	Ongoing	Display balanced I&O	Day 3	Vital signs WNL	Day 28	Be free of S/S of malnutrition, with all laboratory results WNL
Referral	Day 1 & prn	Dietitian				
Diagnostic studies	Day 1	Electrolytes, CBC, BUN/Cr, lipid profile, glucose, plasma proteins, thyroid function UA ECG, as indicated	Day 14	Repeat selected studies		
Additional assessments	Day 1–2	Vital signs/I&O q shift	Day 3–7	q a.m.	Day 8–28	As indicated
	Day 1	Weight	Day 7, 14	7:30 a.m./same clothes		
	Day 1–28	Types of amount of food/fluid intake Behavior/purging following meals Level of activity				
Medications Allergies: ______ ______	Day 1–28	Appetite stimulant Tricyclic antidepressant Vitamin supplement				
Client education	Day 1 & prn	Orient to unit and schedule	Day 7–14	Principles of nutrition; foods for maintenance of wellness	Day 21–28	Incorporating nutritional plan into lifestyle and home setting
		Behavior modification program Minimum weight goal and initial nutritional needs				

Additional nursing actions	Day 1–3	Assist client with formulation of behavioral contract and monitoring of cooperation	Day 7–28	Involve mother/SO as appropriate in nutritional counseling and planning for future		
	Day 1–7	Administer tube feeding or food that has been ground in a blender as indicated				
	Day 1–21	Bathroom locked for 1 hr following meals				
	Day 1–28	Provide social setting for meals				
ineffective Denial R/T overwhelming stress, lack of control of life events, fear of loss of autonomy, lack of emotional support from others	Ongoing	Participate in behavior modification program and adhere to unit policies	Day 8–28	Attend and contribute to group and multifamily sessions	Day 18–28	Verbalize acceptance of reality that eating behaviors are maladaptive
	Day 2–28	Cooperate with therapy to restore nutritional well-being	Day 14	Develop trusting relationship with at least one staff member on each shift	Day 28	Demonstrate ability to cope more adaptively Identify ways to gain control in life situation Refrain from use of manipulation of others to achieve control Plan in place to meet needs after discharge
Referrals	Day 5 (or when physical condition stable)	Psychologist, social worker, psychodramatist	Day 8–28	Groups: psychotherapy; psychoeducational; multifamily	Day 25	Community resource contact person(s)
Additional assessments	Day 1/ongoing	Degree and stage of denial	Day 5–7	Readiness to participate in group sessions		
	Day 1–17	Perception of situation	Day 7–28	Congruence between verbalizations and behaviors (insight)		
		Ability to trust	Day 8–28	Degree/quality of involvement in group sessions		

(continues on page 356)

TABLE 8.1 Sample Pathway: Eating Disorders Program. ELOS: 28 Days Behavioral Unit (Combined Hospitalization and Intensive Outpatient Program) (continued)

ND and Categories of Care	Time Dimension	Goals/Actions	Time Dimension	Goals/Actions	Time Dimension	Goals/Actions
		Use of manipulation to achieve control				
Client education	Day 1 and prn	Privileges and responsibilities of behavior modification	Day 3/ongoing	Eating disorder and consequences of eating behavior	Day 21	Role of support group/ community resources
		Consequences of behaviors				
Additional nursing actions	Day 1/ongoing	Encourage expression of feelings	Day 5–28	Promote involvement in unit activities	Day 21–28	Involve family as appropriate in long-range planning for meeting individual needs
		Avoid agreeing with inaccurate statements/ perceptions	Day 8–28	Support interactions with family members		
		Provide positive feedback for desired insight and behaviors		Encourage interactions in group sessions		
		Set limits on maladaptive behavior				
disturbed Body Image R/T perceptual (altered view of body), psychosocial (negative feelings about body, refusal to verify actual change)	Day 7	Acknowledge that attention will not be given to discussion of body image and food	Day 21	Acknowledge misperception of body image as fat	Day 28	Demonstrate realistic body image and self-awareness
				Verbalize positive self-attributes		Verbalize acceptance of self, including "imperfections"
						Acknowledge self as sexual being
Referrals	Day 1 (or when physical condition stable)	Therapists: occupational, recreational, music, art	Day 14	Image consultant	Day 28	Therapist to address issue of sexuality postdischarge as indicated
Additional assessments	Day 1–7	Suicidal ideation or behaviors	Day 8	Individual strengths and weaknesses		
	Day 3	Sexual history including abuse	Day 8–28	Congruency of feelings and perceptions with actions		
	Day 3–28	Perception of body image				
		Family patterns of interaction				

Client education	Day 1–28	Responsibility for self in family setting	Day 8–10	General wellness needs	Day 21–28	Sex education reflecting individual sexuality and needs
	Day 7–28	Clarify misconceptions of body image	Day 8–28	Human behavior and interactions with family and others		
			Day 14	Personal appearance and grooming		
			Day 14–28	Alternative coping strategies for dealing with feelings		
Additional nursing actions	Day 1	Develop therapeutic relationship	Day 7	Compare actual measurement of client's body with client's perceptions	Day 14–28	Have client keep diary of feelings, especially when thinking of food
	Day 1–28	Provide positive feedback for participation and independent decision making	Day 7–9	Assist with planning to meet individual goals		Role-play new behaviors for dealing with feelings and conflicts
		Confront sabotage behavior by family members	Day 8–28	Involve in physical activity/exercise program		
	Day 3–5	Encourage control in areas other than diet				
	Day 4–6	Support development of goals not related to eating				

Key: BUN/Cr, blood urea nitrogen/creatinine; CBC, complete blood count; ECG, electrocardiogram; ELOS, estimated length of stay; I&O, intake and output; ND, nursing diagnosis; prn, as needed; q, every; q a.m., every morning; R/T, related to; SO, significant other; SS, signs and symptoms; UA, urinalysis; WNL, within normal limits.

EATING DISORDERS: OBESITY

I. Pathophysiology

a. A chronic accumulation of excess body fat, at least 20% over average desired weight for age, sex, and height, or a body mass index (BMI) greater than 30 for persons of either sex

b. Negatively impacts all body systems and increases risk of multiple physical and psychological pathologies, including hypertension, heart disease, diabetes, arthritis, depression and anxiety disorders, difficulty maintaining personal relationships, prejudice and discrimination, and limited access to public conveniences

II. Etiology

a. Causes are multiple, complex, and cannot be attributed simply to a disorder of willpower or the result of insufficient exercise.
   - i. Variations in metabolism, body fat distribution, and appetite regulation can be attributed to genetic factors (Farooqi & O'Rahilly, 2007).
   - ii. Physiological factors
     1. Lesions in the hypothalamus—appetite and satiety centers
     2. Hypothyroidism—may interfere with basal metabolism
     3. Diabetes mellitus—decreased insulin production or utilization
     4. Cushing's disease—increased cortisone production
   - iii. Environmental influences, behavioral and societal issues: includes availability of high-fat, calorie-dense convenience foods, large portions, and sedentary lifestyle
   - iv. Psychosocial influences: possibility of unresolved dependency needs with individual fixed in the oral stage of psychosexual development, with food believed to be a coping mechanism for dealing with life's problems

b. Classifications: Although several classifications and definitions for degrees of obesity are accepted, the two most widely accepted classifications are those from the World Health Organization (WHO, 2013; Hamdy et al, 2013):
   - i. Grade 1 overweight (commonly and simply called overweight)—BMI of 25 to 29.9 kg/m^2
   - ii. Grade 2 overweight (commonly called obesity)—BMI of 30 to 39.9 kg/m^2
   - iii. Grade 3 overweight (commonly called severe or morbid obesity)—BMI greater than or equal to 40 kg/m^2

c. Surgical literature often uses a different classification to recognize particularly severe obesity (Hamdy et al, 2013):
   - i. Severe obesity—BMI greater than 40 kg/m^2
   - ii. Morbid obesity—BMI of 40 to 50 kg/m^2
   - iii. Super obese—BMI greater than 50 kg/m^2

d. Most likely influenced by multiple factors as demonstrated by the Transactional Model of Stress/Adaptation (Townsend, 2006)

III. Statistics

a. Morbidity: Over 78 million adults and 12.5 million young Americans were termed obese in 2009–2010 (CDC/NCHS 2012).

b. Mortality: Many methodological and conceptual difficulties arise in attempting to estimate the number of deaths in the United States that are attributable to obesity. Obesity itself may not be the only contributing factor but rather a marker for other factors such as sedentary behavior or adverse body fat distribution (Flagel et al, 2004). As a group, people who are severely obese have a 6- to 12-fold increase in the all-cause mortality rate. Although numbers may be in dispute (figures range from 112,000 to 365,000 deaths annually), overweight and obesity are indisputably linked to more deaths worldwide than underweight (WHO, 2013; Allison et al, 2004).

c. Cost: In 2008, more than $147 billion was spent to manage obesity in the United States (CDC, 2012).

GLOSSARY

Anthropometric measurements: Body measurements, including height, weight, body mass index (BMI), waist-to-hip ratio, and percentage of body fat.

Appestat: Control mechanism in the brain that signals either hunger or fullness.

Body mass index (BMI): Number calculated from an individual's weight and height, measured in kilograms divided by height in square meters, correlating to direct measures of body fat.

Circadian rhythm: Internal body clock that regulates the 24-hour cycle of biological processes, including sleep, wakefulness, and hunger.

Cushing's syndrome: Endocrine (hormonal) disorder resulting from excessive exposure to or production of the hormone cortisol.

Endomorphic body type: Descriptive of a type of body that is soft and round or pear-shaped with disposition of fat predominately in the abdomen, hips, thighs, and buttocks.

Energy balance: Weight is balanced by the amount of energy calories obtained from food equating to the energy the body uses.

Hyperlipidemia: Elevated high levels of total cholesterol and triglycerides, normal or elevated low-density lipoprotein (LDL, "bad cholesterol"), and low high-density lipoprotein (HDL, "good cholesterol").

Obesity: Having a high amount of extra body fat, with BMI greater than 30.

Overweight: Having extra body weight from muscle, bone, fat, and/or water, with BMI between 25 and 29.9.

Pickwickian syndrome: Extreme obesity along with shallow breathing, sleep apnea, excessive sleepiness, and heart failure.

Polycythemia: Excess number of red blood cells in circulating blood, which can contribute to blood clots.

Sarcopenic obesity: Process characterized by loss of lean muscle and concomitant increase in body fat as a person ages. It is often seen in sedentary individual, whether or not the person is overweight.

Transactional model of stress/adaptation: Begins with the precipitating event, leading to predisposing factors, cognitive appraisal, primary and secondary responses, and quality of individual's response, resulting in adaptive (effective) or maladaptive (refusal to eat and other ineffective behaviors).

Yo-yo dieting: Repeatedly losing weight by dieting and subsequently regaining it.

Care Setting

Community level unless morbid obesity requires brief inpatient stay.

Related Concerns

Cerebrovascular accident (CVA)/stroke, page 214
Cholecystitis with cholelithiasis, page 329
Cirrhosis of the liver, page 412
Diabetes mellitus/diabetic ketoacidosis, page 377
Heart failure: chronic, page 43
Hypertension: severe, page 33
Myocardial infarction, page 75
Obesity: bariatric surgery, page 367
Psychosocial aspects of care, page 729
Thrombophlebitis: Venous Thromboembolism (Including Pulmonary Emboli Considerations), page 109

Client Assessment Database

DIAGNOSTIC DIVISION MAY REPORT	MAY EXHIBIT
ACTIVITY/REST	
• Fatigue, constant drowsiness • Inability or lack of desire to be active or engage in regular exercise, sedentary lifestyle • Dyspnea with exertion • Relying on cars, instead of walking • Environmental problems such as lack of sidewalks, safe places to walk • Work schedules that leave little time for exercise	• Increased heart rate or respirations with activity
CIRCULATION	
	• Hypertension • Edema
EGO INTEGRITY	
• Cultural and lifestyle factors affecting food choices • Weight may or may not be perceived as a problem • Eating relieves unpleasant feelings—loneliness, frustration, boredom • Perception of body image as undesirable • Significant other's (SO's) resistance to weight loss (may sabotage client's efforts)	• Reluctant to engage in social activities
FOOD/FLUID	
• Normal and excessive ingestion of food • Experimentation with numerous types of diets (yo-yo dieting) with varied or short-lived results • History of recurrent weight loss and gain	• Weight disproportionate to height • Endomorphic body type • Failure to adjust food intake to diminishing requirements—change in lifestyle from active to sedentary, aging
PAIN/DISCOMFORT	
• Pain or discomfort on weight-bearing joints or spine	• Difficulty with movement, negotiating stairs, long walks
RESPIRATION	
• Dyspnea	• Cyanosis, respiratory distress if Pickwickian syndrome is present
SEXUALITY	
• Menstrual disturbances, amenorrhea • Problems with relationships • Menopause • Pregnancy(ies)	• Hormone regulation problems, such as polycystic ovarian syndrome

(continues on page 360)

Client Assessment Database (continued)

DIAGNOSTIC DIVISION MAY REPORT (continued)	MAY EXHIBIT (continued)
TEACHING/LEARNING • Problem may be lifelong or related to life event • Family history of obesity • Concomitant health problems may include hypertension, diabetes, gallbladder and cardiovascular disease, hypothyroidism **DISCHARGE PLAN CONSIDERATIONS** • May require support with therapeutic regimen; home modifications, assistive devices and equipment ➧ Refer to section at end of plan for postdischarge considerations.	

Diagnostic Studies

TEST WHY IT IS DONE	WHAT IT TELLS ME
BLOOD TESTS (MAY INCLUDE, NOT LIMITED TO, THE FOLLOWING)	
• ***Lipid profile:*** Total cholesterol, triglycerides, and HDL and LDL: Fats circulating in the blood.	Obesity is often associated with hyperlipidemia, which is defined as high total cholesterol, elevated triglycerides, normal or elevated LDL, and low HDL. HDL cholesterol <40 mg/dL in men or <50 mg/dL, and/or triglycerides ≥150 mg/dL has been shown to be associated with metabolic syndrome and increased risk of cardiovascular disease (AHA, 2012).
• ***Endocrine function (thyroid, pituitary, growth hormone, pancreas, etc.):*** Determines which gland(s) are involved and may determine the cause of obesity. May involve measuring hormone levels and their metabolites in the blood and urine.	The goal of testing is to identify the hormone(s) that are being under- or overproduced, which may be negatively affecting client's weight. Examples of conditions may include hypothyroidism, hypopituitarism, hypogonadism, hyperglycemia and hyperinsulinemia, and elevated cortisol.
OTHER DIAGNOSTIC TESTS	
• ***Anthropometric measurements (including and not limited to the following):***	Body mass index (BMI) calculation, waist circumference, and waist/hip ratio are the common measures of the degree of body fat used in routine clinical practice (Hamdy et al, 2013).
• ***Body mass index (BMI):*** Measures relative body fat. Typically calculated as weight (kg) ÷ height (m^2).	BMI is a weight-for-height index commonly used to classify overweight and obesity in adults. For children and teens, BMI is age- and sex-specific and is often referred to as BMI-for-age (WHO, 2013; CDC, 2011). Research reveals increased mortality with BMIs above the level of 25 (Daniels & Nicoll, 2012).
• ***Waist to hip ratio (WHR):*** Based on waist and hip measurements.	A WHR >1.0 in men and >0.85 in women indicates abdominal fat accumulation (Obesity Education Network, 2012) and is considered the strongest anthropometric measure associated with myocardial infarction risk and is a better predictor than BMI alone (Cash & Glass, 2011).
• ***Waist circumference (WC):*** Used to assess abdominal (visceral) fat.	Considered a better measure of visceral fat than the WHR (Obesity Education Network, 2012). Increased WC is associated with risk of type 2 diabetes, hypertension, dyslipidemia, and cardiovascular disease across all categories of overweight and obesity. Risk is considered extremely high in men with WC greater than 40 inches and in women with WC greater than 35 inches (AHA, 2013; National Heart Lung and Blood Institute [NHLBI], 2012).

Nursing Priorities

1. Assist client to identify a workable method of weight control, incorporating healthful foods and activity.
2. Promote improved self-concept, including body image and self-esteem.
3. Encourage healthy practices to provide for weight control throughout life.

Discharge Goals

1. Healthy patterns for eating and weight control identified.
2. Weight loss toward desired goal established.
3. Positive perception of self verbalized.
4. Plans developed for future weight control.
5. Plan in place to meet needs after discharge.

NURSING DIAGNOSIS: imbalanced Nutrition: more than body requirements

May Be Related To

Excessive intake in relation to metabolic need/physical activity (caloric expenditure)

Possibly Evidenced By

Weight 20% or more over ideal for height and frame; triceps skinfold >15 in men, >25 in women
Dysfunctional eating patterns, eating in response to external cues or internal cues other than hunger
Sedentary lifestyle

Desired Outcomes/Evaluation Criteria—Client Will

Knowledge: Diet (NOC)

Identify inappropriate behaviors and consequences associated with overeating or weight gain.
Demonstrate appropriate change in lifestyle and behaviors, including eating patterns and food quantity and quality, and involvement in individual exercise program.

Nutritional Status (NOC)

Display weight loss with optimal maintenance of health.

ACTIONS/INTERVENTIONS	RATIONALE
Weight-Reduction Assistance (NIC)	
Independent	
Review individual cause for obesity, e.g., excess intake vs. metabolic or disease condition.	Identifies and influences choice of some interventions
Ascertain previous dieting history. Determine which diets and strategies have been used, results, and individual frustrations and factors interfering with success.	Client may have tried multiple diets, with little lasting change in body weight and feel negatively about embarking on another plan.
Implement and review daily food diary, for example, total caloric intake, types and amounts of food, and eating habits and associated feelings.	Provides the opportunity for the individual to focus on a realistic picture of the amount of food ingested and corresponding eating habits and feelings. Identifies patterns requiring change and a base on which to tailor the dietary program.
Determine client's motivation for weight loss, for instance, health issues, own satisfaction, and to gain approval from others.	Helps to clarify client's motivation and potential for success in weight reduction.
Discuss client's and SO's view of self, including familial and cultural influences.	Client's family and cultural practices greatly influence client's self-view regarding food and body image.
Notice occurrence of negative feedback from SO(s).	Feedback from family may reveal control issues impacting motivation for change.
Formulate an eating plan with the overweight client, using knowledge of individual's height, body build, age, gender, and individual patterns of eating, as well as energy and nutrient requirements.	An important factor in the success of any weight-loss program is adherence to a sound nutritional plan. Although there is little basis for recommending one commercial diet plan over another, a good reducing diet should contain foods from all basic food groups, with a focus on low-fat intake and adequate protein intake to prevent loss of lean muscle mass. It is helpful to keep the plan as similar to client's usual eating pattern as possible. A plan developed with and agreed to by the client is more likely to be successful.
Emphasize the importance of avoiding fad diets.	Elimination of needed components can lead to metabolic imbalances; for example, excessive reduction of carbohydrates can lead to fatigue, headache, instability, weakness, and metabolic acidosis (ketosis), thus interfering with effectiveness of weight-loss program.
Discuss need to give self permission to include desired or craved food items in dietary plan.	Denying self by always excluding favorite foods results in a sense of deprivation and feelings of guilt and failure when

(continues on page 362)

ACTIONS/INTERVENTIONS (continued)	RATIONALE (continued)
	individual "succumbs to temptation." These feelings can sabotage weight loss.
Be alert to binge eating and develop strategies for dealing with these episodes, such as substituting other actions for eating.	The client who binges experiences guilt about it, which is also counterproductive because negative feelings may sabotage further weight-loss efforts.
Identify realistic incremental goals for weekly weight loss.	Reasonable weight loss of 1 to 2 lb/wk results in longer-lasting effects. Excessive or rapid loss may result in fatigue and irritability and ultimately lead to failure in meeting goals for weight loss. Motivation is more easily sustained by meeting "stair-step" goals.
Weigh periodically as individually indicated, and obtain appropriate body measurements.	Provides information about effectiveness of therapeutic regimen and visual evidence of success of client's efforts. During hospitalization for controlled fasting, daily weighing may be required. Weekly weighing is more appropriate after discharge.
Determine current activity level and exercise program.	Long-term exercise promotes weight loss by reducing appetite, burning fat while improving lean muscle mass and strength (Benton, 2011).
Develop an appetite reeducation plan with client (e.g., avoiding sugary snacks, increasing protein foods, drinking water throughout day, brushing teeth or using mouthwash, eating something that takes up a lot of room in stomach but has few calories, such as soup).	Appetite is both a psychological and physical phenomenon, requiring thoughtful attention and preparedness.
Emphasize the importance of avoiding tension at mealtimes and not eating too quickly.	Reducing tension provides a more relaxed eating atmosphere and encourages more leisurely eating patterns. This is important because a period of time is required for the appestat mechanism to know the stomach is full.
Encourage client to eat only at a designated eating place and to avoid standing while eating.	Techniques that modify behavior may be helpful in avoiding diet failure.
Discuss restriction of salt intake and diuretic drugs if used.	Water retention may be a problem because of increased fluid intake and fat metabolism.
Reassess caloric requirements every 2 to 4 weeks; provide additional support when plateaus occur.	Changes in weight and exercise necessitate changes in plan. As weight is lost, changes in metabolism occur, resulting in plateaus when weight remains stable for periods of time. This can create distrust and lead to accusations of "cheating" on caloric intake, which are not helpful. Client may need additional support at this time.
Collaborative	
Perform comprehensive nutritional assessment to determine calorie, nutrient, and vitamin and supplement requirements for individual.	Intake can be calculated by several different formulas, but weight reduction is based on the basal caloric requirement for 24 hours depending on client's sex, age, current or desired weight, and length of time estimated to achieve desired weight. *Note:* Standard tables are subject to error when applied to individual situations, and circadian rhythms and lifestyle patterns need to be considered.
Provide medications, as indicated.	Currently, there are three major groups of drugs used to manage obesity: (1) centrally acting medications that impair dietary intake (such as appetite suppressants); (2) medications that act peripherally to impair dietary absorption (such as lipase inhibitors); and (3) medications that increase energy expenditure (such as caffeine and other stimulants (Hamdy et al, 2013).
Appetite-suppressant drugs, such as: Diethylpropion (Tenuate), mazindol (Sanorex), and sibutramine (Meridia)	May be used with caution and supervision at the beginning of a weight-loss program to support client during stress of behavioral changes. They are effective for only a few weeks and may cause problems of dependence in some people.
Lipase inhibitors, such as orlistat (Xenical, Alli)	These drugs induce weight loss by inhibiting fat absorption. *Note:* Use of lipase inhibitors may reduce absorption of some fat-soluble vitamins (A, D, E, K) and beta carotene. Vitamin supplement should be given at least 2 hours before or after Xenical.
CNS stimulants, such as phenteramine (Adipex-P), benzphetamine (Didrex)	Adrenergic agonists that release tissue stores of epinephrine, causing subsequent alpha- and/or beta-adrenergic stimulation, have provided benefits to individuals with severe obesity who are under physician-supervised weight-loss programs. They are approved for short-term use (8 to 12 weeks) in adults.

ACTIONS/INTERVENTIONS (continued)	RATIONALE (continued)
Hospitalize for fasting regimen or stabilization of medical problems, when indicated.	Aggressive therapy and support may be necessary to initiate weight loss, although fasting is not generally a treatment of choice. Client can be monitored more effectively in a controlled setting to minimize complications such as orthostatic hypotension, anemia, and cardiac irregularities.
Prepare for bariatric surgical interventions, such as gastric banding or bypass, as indicated.	These interventions may be necessary to help the client lose weight when obesity is life-threatening. (Refer to CP: Obesity: Bariatric Surgery.)

NURSING DIAGNOSIS: sedentary Lifestyle

May Be Related To

Lack of interest, motivation, or resources
Deficient knowledge of the health benefit of physical exercise

Possibly Evidenced By

Demonstrates physical deconditioning
Chooses daily routine lacking physical exercise

Desired Outcomes/Evaluation Criteria—Client Will

Exercise Participation (NOC)

Verbalize understanding of importance of regular exercise to weight loss and general well-being.
Identify necessary precautions and safety concerns and self-monitoring techniques.
Formulate realistic exercise program with gradual increase in activity.

ACTIONS/INTERVENTIONS	RATIONALE
Exercise Promotion (NIC)	
Independent	
Review necessity for and benefits of regular exercise.	Exercise promotes weight loss by reducing appetite, increasing energy, toning muscles, and enhancing cardiac fitness and sense of well-being and accomplishment.
Determine current activity level and plan progressive exercise program tailored to the individual's physical condition, goals, and choice.	Commitment on the part of the client enables the setting of more realistic goals and adherence to the plan.
Identify perceived and actual barriers to exercise.	Lack of resources, including proper apparel such as supportive shoes and comfortable clothing, a safe place to walk, or facility membership for water aerobics, reduces the likelihood of individual adhering to specific program. In addition, fear of discrimination or ridicule by others may limit client's willingness to exercise in public.
Discuss appropriate warm-up exercises, cool-down activities, and specific techniques to avoid injury.	Preventing muscle injuries allows client to stay active. Time spent recuperating from exercise-induced injuries may result in relapse to sedentary habits.
Determine optimal exercise heart rate. Demonstrate proper technique to monitor pulse and discuss signs and symptoms requiring modification of activity.	Promotes safety as client exercises to tolerance, not peer pressure.
Identify alternatives to chosen activity program to accommodate weather, travel, and so forth.	Promotes continuation of program.
Discuss use of mechanical devices or equipment for weight reduction.	Fat loss occurs on a generalized overall basis, and there is no evidence that spot reducing or mechanical devices aid in weight loss in specific areas; however, specific types of exercise or equipment may be useful in toning specific body parts.
Recommend keeping a graph of activity as exercise program advances.	Provides visual record of progress and positive reinforcement for efforts.
Suggest client identify an exercise buddy.	Provides support and companionship, increasing likelihood of adherence to program.
Encourage involvement in social activities that are not centered on food—bike ride or nature hike, attending musical event, and group sporting activities.	Provides opportunity for pleasure and relaxation not associated with food.

(continues on page 364)

ACTIONS/INTERVENTIONS (continued)	RATIONALE (continued)
Collaborative	
Involve physical therapist or exercise physiologist in developing progressive program.	Facilitates development of an appropriate program of activities that are geared to obese individual and considers impact of client's weight on ability to perform specific activities and safety concerns.

NURSING DIAGNOSIS: disturbed Body Image

May Be Related To

Biophysical factor—changes in health status

Psychosocial factors—client's view of self; changes in body image, personal identity; control, sex, and love issues

Culture, family, or subculture encouragement of overeating

Possibly Evidenced By

Reports feelings/perceptions that reflect an altered view of one's body in appearance

Reports negative feelings about body (e.g., hopelessness, powerlessness)

Change in social involvement; fear of reaction by others

Preoccupation with change—attempts to lose weight

Desired Outcomes/Evaluation Criteria—Client Will

Body Image (NOC)

Verbalize a more realistic self-image.

Demonstrate some acceptance of self as is rather than an idealized image.

Self-Esteem (NOC)

Seek information and actively pursue appropriate weight loss.

Acknowledge self as an individual who has responsibility for self.

ACTIONS/INTERVENTIONS	RATIONALE
Body Image Enhancement (NIC)	
Independent	
Determine client's view of being fat and what it does for the individual.	Mental image includes our ideal and is usually not up-to-date. Fat and compulsive eating behaviors may have deep-rooted psychological implications, such as compensation for lack of love and nurturing or a defense against intimacy. In addition, chronically obese client may report long-term discrimination in family, social, and professional settings. She or he may experience mixed feelings of fear and shame or compensate for psychological trauma by developing a strong or "big" personality.
Determine client perception of threat to self.	Client's perception of what problem weight poses is more important than what the threat really is and needs to be dealt with before reality can be addressed.
Identify basic sense of self-worth and image client has of existential, physical, and psychological self. Determine locus of control.	Provides insight into view of self as fat and own ability to control weight. Information necessary to determine individual needs and treatment plan.
Promote open communication, avoiding criticism or judgment about client's behavior.	Supports client's own responsibility for weight loss, enhances sense of control, and promotes willingness to discuss difficulties and setbacks and to problem-solve. *Note:* Distrust and accusations of "cheating" on caloric intake are not helpful.
Assist client to identify feelings that lead to compulsive eating. Encourage journaling.	People often eat because of depression, anger, and guilt. Awareness of emotions that lead to overeating can be the first step in changing behavior.
Have client recall coping patterns related to food in family of origin and explore how these may affect current situation.	Parents act as role models for the child. Maladaptive coping patterns, such as overeating, are learned within the family system and are supported through positive reinforcement. Food may be substituted by the parent for affection and love, and eating is associated with a feeling of satisfaction, becoming the primary defense.
Develop strategies for doing something besides eating for dealing with dysfunctional eating, such as talking with a friend.	Replacing eating with other activities helps retrain old patterns and establish new ways to deal with feelings.
Identify client's motivation for weight loss and assist with goal setting.	The individual may harbor repressed feeling of hostility, which may be expressed inward on the self. Because of a poor

ACTIONS/INTERVENTIONS	RATIONALE
	self-concept, the person often has difficulty with relationships. *Note:* When losing weight for someone else, the client is less likely to be successful or maintain weight loss.
Outline and clearly state responsibilities of client and nurse.	It is helpful for each individual to understand area of own responsibility in the program so that misunderstandings do not arise.
Graph weight on a weekly basis.	Provides ongoing visual evidence of weight changes, reinforcing reality.
Encourage client to use imagery to visualize self at desired weight and to practice handling of new behaviors.	Mental rehearsal is very useful in helping the client plan for and deal with anticipated change in self-image or occasions that may arise, such as family gatherings or special dinners, where constant decisions about eating many foods will occur.
Suggest client enhance current self through the application of makeup, current hairstyles, and dressing to maximize figure assets.	Enhances feelings of self-esteem and promotes improved body image.
Encourage buying clothes instead of food treats as a reward for weight loss and life successes.	Properly fitting clothes enhance the body image as small losses are made and the individual feels more positive. Waiting until the desired weight loss is reached can become discouraging.
Suggest the client dispose of "fat clothes" as weight loss occurs.	Removes the "safety valve" of having clothes available "in case" the weight is regained. Retaining fat clothes can convey the message that the weight loss will not occur or be maintained.
Be alert to myths the client and SO may have about weight and weight loss.	Beliefs about what an ideal body looks like or unconscious motivations can sabotage efforts to lose weight. Some of these include the feminine thought of "If I become thin, men will view me as a sexual object"; the masculine counterpart, "I don't trust myself to stay in control of my sexual feelings"; as well as issues of strength, power, or the "good cook" image.
Determine relationship history and possibility of sexual abuse.	May contribute to current issues of self-esteem and patterns of coping.
Ensure availability of properly sized equipment, including gowns and other apparel; blood pressure cuff; wider and strong wheelchair, bed, commode, scales, and transfer devices, when providing inpatient care.	Healthcare providers have a moral and legal obligation to meet the client's needs for dignity, comfort, and safety (Cheung et al, 2006).
Provide privacy during care activities. Assist with personal care, as needed.	Individual knows size makes it hard to care for her or him and usually is sensitive and self-conscious about body.
Help staff be aware of and deal with own feelings when caring for client.	Judgmental attitudes, feelings of disgust, anger, and weariness can interfere with care and be transmitted to client, reinforcing negative self-concept and image.
Collaborative	
Refer to community support and/or therapy group.	Weight-loss groups can provide companionship, enhance motivation, decrease loneliness and social ostracism, and give practical solutions to common problems. Group therapy can be helpful in dealing with underlying psychological concerns.

NURSING DIAGNOSIS: impaired Social Interaction

May Be Related To
Self-concept disturbance
Limited physical mobility

Possibly Evidenced By
Discomfort in social settings
Dysfunctional interaction with others

Desired Outcomes/Evaluation Criteria—Client Will

Social Involvement (NOC)
Verbalize awareness of feelings that lead to poor social interactions.
Become involved in achieving positive changes in social behaviors and interpersonal relationships.

ACTIONS/INTERVENTIONS	RATIONALE
Socialization Enhancement (NIC)	
Independent	
Review family patterns of relating and social behaviors.	Social interaction is primarily learned within the family of origin. When inadequate patterns are identified, actions for change can be instituted.
Encourage client to express feelings and perceptions of problems.	Helps identify and clarify reasons for difficulties in interacting with others, such as feeling unloved or unlovable and insecure about sexuality.
Assess client's use of coping skills and defense mechanisms.	May have coping skills that will be useful in the process of weight loss. Defense mechanisms used to protect the individual may contribute to feelings of aloneness or isolation.
Have client list behaviors that cause discomfort.	Identifies specific concerns and suggests actions that can be taken to effect change.
Involve in role playing new ways to deal with identified behaviors or situations.	Practicing these new behaviors enables the individual to become comfortable with them in a safe situation.
Discuss negative self-concepts and self-talk, such as, "No one wants to be with a fat person," "Who would be interested in talking to me?"	May be impeding positive social interactions.
Encourage use of positive self-talk such as telling oneself "I am OK" or "I can enjoy social activities and do not need to be controlled by what others think or say."	Positive strategies enhance feelings of comfort and support efforts for change.
Collaborative	
Refer for ongoing family or individual therapy, as indicated.	Client benefits from involvement of SO to provide support and encouragement.

NURSING DIAGNOSIS: ineffective Self-Health Management

May Be Related To
Complexity of therapeutic regimen
Family pattern of healthcare
Perceived seriousness/barriers or benefits
Deficient knowledge
Social support deficit

Possibly Evidenced By
Reports difficulty with prescribed regimen
Ineffective choices in daily living for meeting health goals
Failure to include treatment regimen in daily living or to take action to reduce risk factors

Desired Outcomes/Evaluation Criteria—Client Will

Knowledge: Eating Disorder Management (NOC)
Verbalize understanding of need for lifestyle changes to maintain or control weight.
Establish individual goal and plan for attaining that goal.
Begin to look for information about nutrition and ways to control weight.

ACTIONS/INTERVENTIONS	RATIONALE
Teaching: Prescribed Diet (NIC)	
Independent	
Determine level of nutritional knowledge and what client believes is most urgent need.	Necessary to know what additional information to provide. When client's views are listened to, trust is enhanced.
Identify individual long-term goals for health, such as lowering blood pressure, controlling serum lipid and glucose levels.	A high relapse rate at 5-year follow-up suggests obesity cannot be reliably reversed. Shifting the focus from initial weight loss and percentage of body fat to overall management of wellness may enhance rehabilitation.
Provide information about ways to maintain satisfactory food intake in settings away from home.	"Smart" eating when dining out or when traveling helps individual manage weight while still enjoying social outlets.
Identify other sources of information—Internet sites, books, community classes, and groups.	Using different avenues of accessing information furthers client's learning. Involvement with others who are also losing weight can provide support.
Teaching: Individual (NIC)	
Emphasize necessity of continued follow-up care or counseling, especially when plateaus occur.	As weight is lost, changes in metabolism occur, interfering with further loss by creating a plateau as the body activates a

survival mechanism, attempting to prevent "starvation." This requires new strategies and aggressive support to continue weight loss.

Discuss use of medications; advise client to discuss with physician and pharmacist any additions to regimen such as over-the-counter (OTC) medications, antibiotics, and herbal supplements.

Obesity can alter the pharmacokinetic properties of medications. Changes in dosages may be needed based on the degree to which drugs are absorbed, resulting in subtherapeutic or toxic drug levels or dangerous side effects and interactions that might occur.

Instruct client about risk of deep vein thrombosis (DVT) and self-care including ankle exercises, walking to limit of ability, and reporting any unusual discomfort in legs.

The very obese client is at higher risk for DVT and pulmonary embolism than the general population because of immobility, stasis, and polycythemia related to chronic respiratory insufficiency.

Discuss necessity of good skin care, especially in skinfolds, such as pendulous abdomen, breasts, groin, perineal areas, during hot weather and times of immobility or following exercise.

Client is at risk for developing pressure ulcers and can be prone to yeast infections. Frequent skin care such as cleansing and drying the tissues and using antifungal creams in skinfolds, as appropriate, can prevent skin breakdown.

Identify alternative ways to "reward" self and family for accomplishments or to provide solace.

Reduces likelihood of relying on food to deal with feelings.

POTENTIAL CONSIDERATIONS following acute hospitalization (dependent on client's age, physical condition and presence of complications, personal resources, and life responsibilities in addition to above nursing diagnoses)

- ***ineffective Self-Health Management***—complexity of therapeutic regimen, perceived seriousness and benefits, excessive demands made on individual; family conflict

OBESITY: BARIATRIC SURGERY

I. Indications

a. Weight and health of extremely obese persons can be favorably changed by bariatric surgery.

b. Benefits are being reported in improvement in comorbid conditions associated with morbid obesity such as hypertension, hyperlipidemia, back pain, and sleep apnea. Studies are supporting that bariatric surgery is effective in remitting type 2 diabetes in 50% to 85% of indiviuals (Dixon, 2009; Levi et al, 2007).

II. Procedures

a. Open approaches with abdominal incisions or by laparoscopy

b. Extremely obese individuals, or those with previous abdominal surgery or complicating medical problems, may require open approach.

c. Two types of surgical procedures are offered (Gagnon, 2012).

i. Restrictive

1. Small pouch with a restricted outlet is created across the stomach just distal to the gastroesophageal junction; a small opening remains through which food passes into lower stomach.
2. Reduces the amount of food the stomach can hold and slows passage of food through the stomach, resulting in a feeling of fullness
3. Most common procedures include stapling or banding of the stomach.
   a. Adjustable gastric banding (AGB, also may be called LAP-BAND): This reversible laparoscopic procedure is the second most common bariatric procedure (Demaria et al, 2010) and is considered by some to be the safest procedure (Favoretti et al, 2009; Salemeh, 2006). The tightness of the band can be adjusted depending on client's tolerance. Digestion is slowed by allowing smaller-than-normal amounts of food through to the remainder of the gastrointestinal tract.
   b. Vertical banded gastroplasty (VBG, or "stomach stapling): This procedure is restrictive and reversible. A line of staples is placed to section off a small portion of the upper stomach, creating a small pouch anchored distally by a prosthetic band. Digestion is slowed by allowing smaller-than-normal amounts of food through to the remainder of the gastrointestinal tract.

ii. Combined restrictive and malabsorptive

1. Roux-en-Y gastric bypass (RYGB): Involves creating a small stomach pouch and attaching it directly to the small intestine using a Y-shaped limb of the small bowel; the larger stomach portion and the duodenum are bypassed. The procedure is irreversible, may be done by open abdomen or laparoscopy, works both by restricting intake and by slowing the digestion and absorption, and is the most common bariatric procedure performed (71% to 81%) (Gagnon, 2012; LABS, 2009).
2. Vertical sleeve gastrectomy (VSG, or simply sleeve gastrectomy): Performed in high-risk individuals with severe obesity (BMI of 50 kg/m^2 or greater). This restrictive, irreversible procedure, usually performed laparoscopically, removes 80% to 90% of the stomach, leaving only a gastric "sleeve." This operation is believed to be safer than the gastric bypass procedure, due to the fact that the natural anatomy of the gastrointestinal tract is not changed and therefore has no malabsorptive component (Moy et al, 2008).

(continues on page 368)

3. Biliopancreatic diversion with duodenal switch (BPD-DS): Considered for individuals with severe obesity. The surgery involves removing 65% to 70% of the stomach, leaving the pyloric valve intact. The remaining portion of the stomach is then connected to the proximal portion of the ileum. The surgery restricts intake and slows digestion and absorption. Most people lose 75% to 80% of their excess weight and stay at their new weight (Colquitt et al, 2009).

III. Complications (Gagnon, 2012; Thompson, 2011)

a. Early complications include bleeding (0.6% to 4%), anastomotic leaks (1.5% to 6%) (Adair, 2013).

b. Perioperative cardiovascular or pulmonary complications (e.g., heart failure, deep venous thrombosis, pulmonary embolism) appear to be related to comorbiditires in the morbidly obese but can sometimes be related to anastomotic leaks.

c. Late complications: Cholelithiasis (common); stomal stenosis, gastric remnant distention, ulceration at margins, hernias (all relatively uncommon)

d. Wound infections: Open abdomen procedures have been associated with higher risk of infection (10% to 15%) than laparoscopic procedures (3% to 4%).

e. Nutritional side effects: Malabsorptive effects include risk for deficiencies (e.g., iron, calcium, thiamine, folate, and vitamin B_{12}); deficiencies can occur early or late and are long-term.

IV. Statistics

a. Morbidity: Recent numbers of bariatric surgeries vary, e.g., total procedures reported by the National Association for Weight Loss Surgery as 171,000 in 2005 (NAWLS, 2005–2012); Livingston reported a plateau of 113,000/year in 2006 (Livingston, 2010); but Agaba et al reported over 200,000 procedures performed in 2007 (Agaba et al, 2008).

b. Mortality: Rates vary somewhat by procedures, but are generally low (e.g., 0.5% to 1.6%) (Demaria et al, 2010; Agaba et al, 2008).

c. Cost: Annual direct care costs of bariatric surgery estimated at least $1.5 billion (Livingston, 2010).

GLOSSARY

Bariatric surgery: Term is synonymous with "obesity surgery" or "weight-loss surgery."

Body mass index (BMI): Uses individual's weight in kilograms divided by height in meters squared to produce a unit of measure for classifying body composition.

Comorbidities: In the context of obesity, means medical conditions that a client may have that are either caused by, or exacerbated by, obesity. Examples include diabetes type 2, hypertension, cardiopulmonary disease, sleep apnea, gastroesophageal reflux disease (GERD), and musculoskeletal problems.

Dumping syndrome: A group of symptoms that result from the quick "dumping" of food into the small intestine. The most typical forms may occur after gastric bypass, although not all individuals develop dumping syndrome. Early dumping occurs shortly after a meal and consists of any combination of light-headedness, flushing, diarrhea, and extreme weakness. Delayed dumping may occur an hour or later after a meal and is believed to be a result of hypoglycemia.

Intertriginous dermatitis (ITD): An inflammatory condition of opposing skin surfaces caused by moisture. People with more skinfolds, especially the obese, often have ITD under the abdominal or pubic panniculi. Following weight-loss surgery, surplus skin remains and is also a site for the development of ITD.

Laparoscopic surgery: A way of performing various bariatric surgical procedures through multiple small holes or incisions in the abdomen.

Malabsorptive surgery: A type of bariatric surgery that causes weight loss by bypassing a portion of the small intestine, where almost all of the absorption of nutrients takes place.

Panniculus: Term used to describe an excess fold or layer (apron) of skin and tissue that hangs dependently. Abdominal panniculi can grow over and beyond the abdomen, eventually covering the genitals and potentially extending even further, passing the knees. This can cause considerable discomfort and disability. Other areas of the body that may develop panniculi include the neck, upper back, flank, upper-medial thigh, posterior legs and ankles.

Restrictive surgery: A type of bariatric surgery that induces weight loss by making only a small portion of the stomach (the pouch or, in the case of sleeve gastrectomy, a tube) available to receive food from the esophagus.

Skinfolds: Areas where one skin layer rests on or against another. These folds tend to be dark, moist, and warm, making them an ideal breeding ground for organisms like bacteria and fungi. Individuals can develop severe skin infections and may experience large ulcerations and lesions from unchecked growth of microorganisms.

Care Setting

Care is provided in an inpatient acute surgical unit.

Related Concerns

Eating disorders: obesity, page 358
Peritonitis, page 320
Psychosocial aspects of care, page 729
Surgical intervention, page 762
Thrombophlebitis: Venous Thromboembolism (Including Pulmonary Emboli Considerations), page 109

Client Assessment Database

Refer to Endocrine Disorders: Obesity Database for additional assessment information.

DIAGNOSTIC DIVISION MAY REPORT	MAY EXHIBIT
ACTIVITY/REST	
• Difficulty sleeping • Exertional discomfort, inability to participate in desired activity or sports	• Exertional dyspnea and/or chest discomfort • Slow to move, inability to participate in desired activity
EGO INTEGRITY	
• Motivated to lose weight for oneself (or for gratification of others) • Embarrassment that they've been unable to lose weight by other means • Worry that even after surgery will fail to lose weight • Hates body image, inability to be and do as others • Fear or anxiety about procedure and ability to deal with postoperative adjustments • Feels lonely, isolated, disconnected from others • History of psychiatric illness or treatment	• Anxiety, depression
ELIMINATION	
• Urinary stress incontinence	
FOOD/FLUID	
• History of yo-yo dieting, years of failed dieting; weight fluctuations; dysfunctional eating patterns	• Weight exceeding ideal body weight by 100 lb, or BMI more than 40 (morbid obesity), or BMI of 25 to 40 with comorbid conditions, such as diabetes, sleep apnea, or heart disease
HYGIENE	
• Difficulty with dressing, bathing, toileting, perineal care, or other self-care activities	• Poor general hygiene, or constant attention to hygiene practices • Body odor
PAIN/DISCOMFORT	
• Incisional pain	• Guarding behavior • Positioning to avoid pain • Facial mask, grimacing • Restlessness, moaning, irritability
RESPIRATION	
• History of chronic respiratory diseases; use of respiratory aids (including oxygen, medications) • Sleep apnea (may use CPAP) • History of/current smoking	• Shortness of breath with activity or rest • Breath sounds may be distant (chest depth and shallow respirations)
SAFETY	
• History of falls/other accidental injuries due to unstable gait, arthritis, joint problems • Use of ambulatory or other assistive devices for transportation (e.g., wheelchair) • Skin injuries, dermatitis, and other skin problems associated with skinfolds and hanging fat and tissue deposits (panniculi)	• Areas of skin breakdown including breast, abdominal, and other body skinfolds • Intertrigonous dermatitis, pressure ulcers, candidiasis, incontinence-associated dermatitis, lower leg ulcers (Blackett et al, 2011)
SEXUALITY/SOCIAL INTERACTIONS	
• Problems with menstruation, fertility, and/or childbearing • Problems with relationships that client perceives is related to condition • History of bullying, discrimination, and abuse	• May or may not have support people present

(continues on page 370)

DIAGNOSTIC DIVISION MAY REPORT (continued)	MAY EXHIBIT (continued)
TEACHING/LEARNING • Presence of chronic conditions—hypertension, diabetes, heart failure, arthritis, sleep apnea, Pickwickian syndrome, infertility • Learning about lifelong healthy eating and physical activity habits, medical follow-up, and vitamin and mineral supplementation **DISCHARGE PLAN CONSIDERATIONS** • May require support with therapeutic regimen and weight loss, assistance with self-care, homemaker and maintenance tasks ➧ Refer to section at end of plan for postdischarge considerations.	

Diagnostic Studies

Studies depend on individual situation and are used to rule out underlying disease and provide a preoperative workup, including psychiatric evaluation.

Nursing Priorities

1. Support respiratory function.
2. Prevent or minimize complications.
3. Provide appropriate nutritional intake.
4. Provide information regarding surgical procedure, postoperative expectations, and treatment needs.

Discharge Goals

1. Ventilation and oxygenation adequate for individual needs.
2. Complications prevented or controlled.
3. Nutritional intake modified for specific procedure.
4. Procedure, prognosis, and therapeutic regimen understood.
5. Plan in place to meet needs after discharge.

NURSING DIAGNOSIS: ineffective Breathing Pattern

May Be Related To
Obesity; body position
Pain, anxiety
Fatigue

Possibly Evidenced By
Feeling breathless; dyspnea
Tachypnea, alteration in depth of breathing; decreased vital capacity

Desired Outcomes/Evaluation Criteria—Client Will

Respiratory Status: Ventilation (NOC)
Maintain adequate ventilation.
Experience no cyanosis or other signs of hypoxia, with ABGs within acceptable range.

ACTIONS/INTERVENTIONS	RATIONALE
Ventilation Assistance (NIC) *Independent*	
Monitor respiratory rate and depth. Auscultate breath sounds. Investigate presence of pallor and cyanosis, increased restlessness, or confusion.	Respirations may be shallow because of incisional pain, analgesia, immobility, and obesity itself, causing hypoventilation and potentiating risk of atelectasis and hypoxia. *Note:* Many anesthetic agents are fat soluble, so risk of postoperative "resedation" and the potential for respiratory complications is increased.
Elevate head of bed 30 to 45 degrees.	Encourages optimal diaphragmatic excursion and lung expansion and minimizes pressure of abdominal contents on the

ACTIONS/INTERVENTIONS (continued)	RATIONALE (continued)
	thoracic cavity. *Note:* When kept recumbent, obese clients are at high risk for severe hypoventilation.
Encourage deep-breathing exercises. Assist with coughing and splint incision.	Promotes maximal lung expansion and aids in clearing airways, thus reducing risk of atelectasis and pneumonia. *Note:* Use of abdominal binder—properly fitted and placed at least 2 inches below the xiphoid process—can encourage deep breathing.
Turn periodically and ambulate as early as possible.	Promotes aeration of all segments of the lung, mobilizing and aiding movement of secretions. *Note:* If client was a good candidate for bariatric surgery, she or he was probably relatively healthy before operation and is usually able to turn self, walk, and transfer to chair within 8 hours of surgery.
Pad side rails and teach client to use them as armrests.	Using the side rail as an armrest allows for greater chest expansion.
Use small pillow under head, when indicated.	Many obese clients have large, thick necks, and use of large, fluffy pillows may obstruct the airway.
Collaborative	
Administer supplemental oxygen.	Maximizes available O_2 for exchange and reduces work of breathing.
Assist in use of blow bottle or incentive spirometer, as indicated.	Enhances lung expansion; reduces potential for atelectasis.
Monitor ABGs or pulse oximetry, as indicated.	Reflects ventilation, oxygenation, and acid-base status. Used as a basis for evaluating need for and effectiveness of respiratory therapies.
Monitor patient-controlled analgesia (PCA) and administer analgesics, as appropriate.	Maintenance of comfort level enhances participation in respiratory therapy and promotes increased lung expansion. *Note:* For the first 48 hours after the procedure, intravenous (IV) PCA is the method of choice.

NURSING DIAGNOSIS: risk for ineffective Tissue Perfusion [specify]

Risk Factors May Include

Deficient knowledge of disease process or aggravating factors
Hypertension; diabetes mellitus
Sedentary lifestyle

Possibly Evidenced By

(Not applicable; presence of signs and symptoms establishes an *actual* diagnosis)

Desired Outcomes/Evaluation Criteria—Client Will

Circulation Status (NOC)

Maintain perfusion as individually appropriate—skin warm and dry, peripheral pulses present and strong, and vital signs within acceptable range.

Risk Control (NOC)

Identify causative or risk factors.
Demonstrate behaviors to improve or maintain circulation.

ACTIONS/INTERVENTIONS	RATIONALE
Surveillance (NIC)	
Independent	
Monitor vital signs, palpate peripheral pulses routinely, and evaluate capillary refill and changes in mentation. Note 24-hour fluid balance.	Indicators of circulatory adequacy. (Refer to ND: risk for deficient Fluid Volume, below.)
Encourage frequent range-of-motion (ROM) exercises for legs and ankles. Maintain schedule of sequential compression devices (SCD) on lower extremities when used.	Stimulates circulation in the lower extremities, reduces high-risk complications associated with venous stasis, such as DVT and pulmonary embolus (PE).
Assess for redness, edema, and discomfort in calf.	Indicators of thrombus formation, but warning signs may not always be present in obese individuals.
Encourage early ambulation; discourage sitting and dangling legs at the bedside.	Sitting constricts venous flow, whereas walking encourages venous return.

(continues on page 372)

ACTIONS/INTERVENTIONS (continued)	RATIONALE (continued)
Evaluate for complications, such as rigid abdomen, nonincisional abdominal pain, fever, tachycardia, and low blood pressure.	Although rare, client can develop abdominal complications, such as abdominal compartment syndrome, sepsis or septic shock secondary to anastomotic leak or wound infection, requiring intensive interventions or return to surgery.
Collaborative	
Administer heparin therapy, as indicated.	May be used prophylactically to reduce risk of thrombus formation or to treat thromboemboli.
Monitor hemoglobin (Hgb), hematocrit (Hct), and coagulation studies, such as prothrombin time (PT) and International Normalized Ratio (INR).	Provides information about circulatory volume and alterations in coagulation and indicates therapy needs and effectiveness.

NURSING DIAGNOSIS: risk for deficient Fluid Volume

Risk Factors May Include

Extremes of weight
Excessive gastric losses—nasogastric suction, diarrhea
Deviations affecting intake—limited oral intake

Possibly Evidenced By

(Not applicable; presence of signs and symptoms establishes an *actual* diagnosis)

Desired Outcomes/Evaluation Criteria—Client Will

Hydration (NOC)

Maintain adequate fluid volume with balanced intake and output (I&O) and be free of signs reflecting dehydration.

ACTIONS/INTERVENTIONS	RATIONALE
Fluid/Electrolyte Management (NIC)	
Independent	
Assess vital signs, noting changes in blood pressure (BP), such as orthostatic hypotension, tachycardia, and fever. Assess skin turgor, capillary refill, and moisture of mucous membranes.	Indicators of dehydration and hypovolemia and adequacy of current fluid replacement. *Note:* Adequately sized cuff must be used to ensure factual measurement of BP. If cuff is too small, reading will be falsely elevated.
Monitor I&O, including nasogastric (NG) suction losses.	Changes in gastric capacity and intestinal motility and nausea greatly influence intake and fluid needs, increasing risk of dehydration.
Evaluate muscle strength and tone. Observe for muscle tremors.	Large gastric losses may result in decreased magnesium and calcium, leading to neuromuscular weakness and tetany.
Establish individual needs and replacement schedule.	Determined by amount of measured losses and estimated insensible losses and dependent on gastric capacity.
Encourage increased oral intake when able, beginning with clear liquids and advancing to full liquids. Encourage frequent small sips of fluids.	Intake capacity is drastically reduced (to as little as 15 to 30 mL), so client may need IV fluid support for a while, but once oral fluids are resumed, client must drink frequently in order to be hydrated. Small sips will reduce nausea.
Collaborative	
Administer IV fluids, as indicated.	Replaces fluid losses and restores fluid balance in immediate postoperative phase until client is able to take sufficient oral fluids.
Monitor electrolyte levels and replace, as indicated.	Use of NG tube, and changes in GI function can deplete electrolytes, affecting organ function.

NURSING DIAGNOSIS: risk for imbalanced Nutrition: less than body requirements

Risk Factors May Include

Inability to ingest food—restricted intake, early satiety
Inability to absorb nutrients—malabsorption of nutrients and impaired absorption of vitamins

Possibly Evidenced By

(Not applicable; presence of signs and symptoms establishes an *actual* diagnosis)

NURSING DIAGNOSIS: risk for imbalanced Nutrition: less than body requirements (continued)

Desired Outcomes/Evaluation Criteria—Client Will

Eating Disorder Self-Control (NOC)
Identify individual nutritional needs.
Display behaviors to maintain adequate nutritional intake.
Demonstrate appropriate weight loss with normalization of laboratory values.

ACTIONS/INTERVENTIONS	RATIONALE
Diet Staging: Weight-Loss Surgery (NIC)	
Independent	
Establish hourly intake schedule. Measure and provide food and fluids in amount specified.	After gastric restriction procedures, stomach capacity is reduced to approximately 30 to 50 mL, necessitating frequent, small feedings.
Instruct in how to eat slowly. Take small bites, using a baby spoon. Chew food thoroughly. Take 30 to 60 minutes to eat meal, then refrain from eating until next scheduled mealtime.	Increases satiety and reduces risk of overeating.
Avoid taking fluids with meals and for 30 minutes before or after meals. Encourage almost constant sipping of fluids between scheduled eating times.	Although fluids are a necessary part of the client's intake, the stomach is too small to hold food and fluids at the same time.
Avoid high-calorie fluids—milkshakes, sodas, and alcoholic beverages.	These can sabotage weight loss.
Emphasize importance of recognizing satiety and stopping intake.	Overeating may cause nausea and vomiting, as well as having the potential to damage surgical anastomosis.
Require that client sit up to drink and eat.	Reduces possibility of aspiration.
Determine foods that are gas forming and eliminate them from diet.	May cause nausea and bloating, interfering with digestion and causing client to restrict nutritional intake.
Discuss food preferences with client and include those foods in puréed diet when possible.	May enhance intake and promote sense of participation and control.
Weigh on regular schedule.	Monitors losses and aids in assessing nutritional needs and effectiveness of therapy.
Collaborative	
Refer to dietitian or multidisciplinary team.	Provides assistance in planning a diet that meets client's nutritional needs as well as offering individualized treatment and support. *Note:* Because quantity is strictly limited, foods should be nutrient dense, low in fat and sugars, and high in protein (Gagnon, 2012).
Administer vitamin supplements (may use chewable vitamins) and vitamin B_{12} injections, folate, and calcium, as indicated.	When absorption is impaired, supplements will be needed for life to prevent complications associated with vitamin deficiencies. Increased intestinal motility following bypass procedure lowers calcium level and increases absorption of oxalates, which can lead to urinary stone formation.

NURSING DIAGNOSIS: impaired Skin Integrity

May Be Related To
Mechanical factors (e.g., shearing forces, pressure, surgical procedure)
Impaired circulation
Imbalanced nutritional state—obesity

Possibly Evidenced By
Disruption of skin surface/skin layers

Desired Outcomes/Evaluation Criteria—Client Will

Wound Healing: Primary Intention (NOC)
Display timely wound healing without complications.
Demonstrate behaviors that reduce tension on suture line.

Tissue Integrity: Skin and Mucous Membranes (NOC)
Display intact skin free of signs of pressure or breakdown.

ACTIONS/INTERVENTIONS	RATIONALE
Incision Site Care (NIC)	
Independent	
Support and instruct client in incisional support when turning, coughing, deep breathing, and ambulating.	Reduces possibility of dehiscence and incisional hernia.
Observe incisions periodically, noting approximation of wound edges, hematoma formation and resolution, and presence of bleeding and drainage.	Verifies status of healing, provides for early detection of developing complications requiring prompt evaluation and influencing choice of interventions.
Provide routine incisional care, being careful to keep dressing dry and sterile. Assess and maintain patency of drains.	Promotes healing. Accumulation of serosanguineous drainage in subcutaneous layers increases tension on suture line, may delay wound healing, and serves as a medium for bacterial growth.
Pressure Ulcer Prevention (NIC)	
Encourage frequent positional change, inspect pressure points, and massage gently, as indicated. Apply transparent skin barrier to elbows and heels, if indicated.	Reduces pressure on skin, promoting peripheral circulation and reducing risk of skin breakdown. Skin barrier reduces risk of shearing injury.
Skinfold management (Black et al, 2011; Blackett et al, 2011):	
Inspect all skin surfaces, paying particular attention to multiple skinfolds common in the very obese client.	Client may have intertriginous dermatitis (ITD), thought to arise from skin-on-skin friction that initially leads to mild erythema and may progress to more intense inflammation with erosion, oozing, exudation, maceration, and crusting. Moisture or excoriation enhances growth of yeast and bacteria that can lead to chronic skin infections and raise the risk of postoperative wound infection from local contamination (Black et al, 2011).
Bathe/cleanse skin carefully, using a mild skin cleanser instead of ordinary soap.	Gentle mechanical actions should be used when cleansing the skin, and scrubbing should be avoided. The cleanser should be free of perfumes or potential irritants, and its pH should be similar to that of normal skin. One option is pH-balanced disposable cleansing cloths or soft baby washcloths, since regular washcloths can be abrasive. *Note*: The pH of ordinary soap is usually due to alkaline, which may increase skin irritation.
Apply skin moisturizers, as indicated.	May be needed to keep skin supple if at risk for cracking or fissuring from excessive dryness.
Use absorptive fabric/padding and loose fitting clothing, as indicated.	Obese client tends to sweat profusely. The combination of increased perspiration and larger skinfolds increases the risk for maceration and for friction damage. Use of absorptive materials in skinfolds helps keep them dry and reduces risk of skin rashes and breakdown. Client should be encouraged to wear loose-fitting, lightweight clothing made from natural fibers to absorb moisture from skinfolds. Other options include athletic clothing specifically designed to draw moisture away from the skin.
Utilize draw sheets to form sling to lift or shift large tissue areas (e.g., abdominal panniculus) when moving client in bed.	Reduces risk of friction and shear injuries and pain.
Collaborative	
Provide foam, water, or air mattress, as indicated.	Reduces skin pressure and enhances circulation.
Refer to skin/wound specialist nurse if indicated.	May be desired/needed in client with severe skin and/or tissue conditions. Management strategies must focus on elimination of skin-to-skin contact without causing harm to friable tissue, as well as education of client/SO in skin care.

NURSING DIAGNOSIS: risk for Infection

Risk Factors May Include

Inadequate primary defenses—broken skin, traumatized tissues, decreased ciliary action, stasis of body fluids

Invasive procedures

Possibly Evidenced By

(Not applicable; presence of signs and symptoms establishes an *actual* diagnosis)

Desired Outcomes/Evaluation Criteria—Client Will

Infection Severity (NOC)

Be free of healthcare-acquired infection.

Achieve timely wound healing free of signs of local or generalized infectious process.

ACTIONS/INTERVENTIONS	RATIONALE
Infection Protection (NIC)	
Independent	
Emphasize and model proper hand-washing technique.	Prevents spread of bacteria and cross-contamination.
Maintain aseptic technique in dressing changes and invasive procedures.	Reduces risk of healthcare-associated infection.
Inspect surgical incisions and invasive line sites for erythema and purulent drainage.	Early detection of developing infection provides for prevention of more serious complications.
Encourage frequent position changes, deep breathing, coughing, and use of respiratory adjuncts, such as incentive spirometer.	Promotes mobilization of secretions, reducing risk of pneumonia.
Provide routine catheter care and provide or assist with good perineal care. Remove catheter as early as possible.	Prevents ascending bladder infections.
Encourage client to drink acid-ash juices, such as cranberry.	Maintains urine acidity and prevents bacteria from adhering to the bladder wall to retard bacterial growth.
Observe for reports of abdominal pain, especially after third postoperative day, elevated temperature, and increased white blood cell (WBC) count.	Suggests possibility of developing peritonitis.
Collaborative	
Apply topical antimicrobials or antibiotics, as indicated.	Reduces bacterial or fungal colonization on skin; prevents infection in the wound.
Administer IV antibiotics, as indicated.	A prophylactic antibiotic regimen is usually standard in these clients to reduce risk of perioperative contamination and peritonitis.
Obtain specimen of purulent drainage or sputum for culture and sensitivity.	Identifies infectious agent; aids in choice of appropriate therapy.

NURSING DIAGNOSIS: Diarrhea

May Be Related To

Inflammation; irritation; malabsorption

Possibly Evidenced By

Loose, liquid stools

Hyperactive bowel sounds

Desired Outcomes/Evaluation Criteria—Client Will

Knowledge: Treatment Regimen (NOC)

Verbalize understanding of causative factors and rationale of treatment regimen.

Follow through with treatment recommendations.

Gastrointestinal Function (NOC)

Regain near-normal bowel function.

ACTIONS/INTERVENTIONS	RATIONALE
Diarrhea Management (NIC)	
Independent	
Observe and record stool frequency, characteristics, and amount.	Diarrhea often develops after resumption of diet because of shortened transit time through the GI tract and dumping syndrome. This condition is usually self-limiting but can cause discomfort and social difficulties when persistent.
Encourage diet high in fiber and bulk within dietary limitations, with moderate fluid intake as diet resumes.	Increases consistency of the effluent. Although fluid is necessary for optimal body function, excessive amounts contribute to diarrhea.
Restrict fat intake, as indicated.	Low-fat diet reduces risk of steatorrhea and limits laxative effect of decreased fat absorption.
Observe for signs of dumping syndrome such as instant diarrhea, sweating, nausea, and weakness after eating.	Rapid emptying of food from the stomach may result in gastric distress and alter bowel function.
Assist with frequent perianal care, using ointments as indicated. Provide whirlpool bath.	Anal irritation, excoriation, and pruritus occur because of diarrhea. The client often cannot reach the area for proper cleansing and may be embarrassed to ask for help.

(continues on page 376)

ACTIONS/INTERVENTIONS (continued)	RATIONALE (continued)
Collaborative	
Administer medications such as diphenoxylate with atropine (Lomotil), as indicated.	Antidiarrheals may be necessary to control frequency of stools until body adjusts to changes in function brought about by surgery.
Monitor serum electrolytes.	Large gastric losses potentiate the risk of electrolyte imbalance, which can lead to more serious or life-threatening complications.

NURSING DIAGNOSIS: deficient Knowledge [Learning Need] regarding condition, prognosis, treatment, self-care, and discharge needs

May Be Related To

Lack of exposure, unfamiliarity with information resources
Information misinterpretation
Lack of recall

Possibly Evidenced By

Reports the problem
Inaccurate follow-through of instructions

Desired Outcomes/Evaluation Criteria—Client Will

Knowledge: Disease Process (NOC)

Verbalize understanding of surgical procedure, potential complications, and postoperative expectations.

Knowledge: Treatment Regimen (NOC)

Verbalize understanding of therapeutic needs and rationale for actions.
Initiate necessary lifestyle changes and participate in treatment regimen.

ACTIONS/INTERVENTIONS	RATIONALE
Teaching: Individual (NIC)	
Independent	
Review specific surgical procedure and postoperative expectations.	Provides knowledge base from which informed choices can be made and goals formulated. Initial weight loss is rapid, with client often losing half of the total weight loss during the first 6 months. Weight loss then gradually stabilizes over a 2-year period.
Address concerns about altered body size and image.	Anticipation of problems can be helpful in dealing with situations that arise. (Refer to CP: Eating Disorders: Obesity; ND: disturbed Body Image.)
Review medication regimen, dosage, and side effects.	Knowledge may enhance client's involvement with therapeutic regimen. *Note:* As client loses weight, the dosages of many medications may need to be recalculated because body fat alters the pharmacokinetics of many medications.
Recommend avoidance of alcohol.	High caloric count contributes to slowed weight loss as well as liver and pancreatic dysfunction.
Discuss responsibility for self-care with client and significant other (SO).	Full involvement in weight-loss program is important for successful outcome after procedure.
Emphasize importance of regular medical follow-up, including laboratory studies, and discuss possible health problems.	Periodic assessment and evaluation, for example, over 3 to 12 months, promotes early recognition of such complications as liver dysfunction, malnutrition, electrolyte imbalances, and kidney stones, which may develop following bypass procedure.
Diet Staging: Weight Loss Surgery (NIC)	
Encourage progressive exercise and activity program balanced with adequate rest periods.	Promotes weight loss, enhances muscle tone, and minimizes postoperative complications while preventing undue fatigue.
Review proper eating habits; for example, eat small amounts of food slowly and chew well and sit at table in calm, relaxed environment; eat only at prescribed times, avoid between-meal snacking, and do not "make up" skipped feedings.	Focuses attention on eating, increasing awareness of intake and feelings of satiety.
Identify signs of hypokalemia, for example, diarrhea, muscle cramps, weakness of lower extremities, weak or irregular pulse, and dizziness with position changes.	Increasing dietary intake of potassium (e.g., milk, coffee, potatoes, carrots, bananas, oranges) may correct deficit, preventing serious respiratory or cardiac complications.

ACTIONS/INTERVENTIONS (continued)	RATIONALE (continued)
Discuss symptoms that may indicate dumping syndrome: weakness, profuse perspiration, nausea, vomiting, faintness, flushing, and epigastric discomfort or palpitations occurring during or immediately following meals. Problem-solve solutions.	Generally occurring in early postoperative period (1 to 3 weeks), syndrome is usually self-limiting but may become chronic and require medical intervention.
Review symptoms requiring medical evaluation, including persistent nausea or vomiting, abdominal distention or tenderness, change in pattern of bowel elimination, fever, purulent wound drainage, excessive weight loss, plateauing, or weight gain.	Early recognition of developing complications allows for prompt intervention, preventing serious outcome.
Collaborative	
Refer to bariatric postoperative program or community support groups.	Involvement with others who have dealt with same problems enhances coping; may promote cooperation with therapeutic regimen and long-term positive recovery.

POTENTIAL CONSIDERATIONS following acute hospitalization (dependent on client's age, physical condition and presence of complications, personal resources, and life responsibilities)

- ***risk for imbalanced Nutrition: more than body requirements***—dysfunctional eating patterns, observed use of food as reward or comfort measure, history of morbid obesity
- ***risk for delayed Surgical Recovery***—obesity; pain; excessive surgical procedure
- ***risk for ineffective Self-Health Management***—complexity of therapeutic regimen; family patterns of healthcare; perceived benefit/barriers; social support deficit

Refer to Potential Considerations in Surgical Intervention plan of care.

DIABETES MELLITUS/DIABETIC KETOACIDOSIS

I. Pathology

a. Diabetes mellitus (DM) is a chronic metabolic disorder characterized by high blood glucose levels, in which the body cannot metabolize carbohydrates, fats, and proteins because of a lack of, or ineffective use of, the hormone insulin.

b. Diabetic ketoacidosis (DKA) is a life-threatening emergency caused by a relative or absolute deficiency of insulin.

c. Diabetes is the leading cause of kidney failure, nontraumatic lower-limb amputations, and new cases of blindness as well as a major cause of heart disease and stroke among adults in the United States (American Diabetes Association [ADA], 2013).

II. Classification

a. Three primary types that are different disease entities but share the symptoms and complications of hyperglycemia
   - i. Type 1—formerly called *juvenile* or *insulin dependent diabetes*
   - ii. Type 2—formerly known as *adult onset* or *non-insulin dependent*
   - iii. Pre-diabetes, also sometimes known as *impaired glucose tolerance* and formerly known as *borderline diabetes*. This classification includes gestational diabetes (GD), which applies to women in whom glucose intolerance develops or is first discovered during pregnancy. GD develops in 2% to 18% of all pregnant women, but disappears after delivery (ADA, 2013).

III. Etiology

a. Conditions or situations known to exacerbate glucose and insulin imbalance
   - i. Previously undiagnosed or newly diagnosed type 1 diabetes
   - ii. Food intake in excess of available insulin
   - iii. Adolescence and puberty
   - iv. Exercise in uncontrolled diabetes
   - v. Stress associated with illness, infection, trauma, or emotional distress

b. Type 1 diabetes
   - i. An autoimmune disease possibly triggered by genetic and environmental factors, such as with virus, toxins, stress
     1. Destroys beta-cells in the pancreas
     2. When 80% to 90% of the beta cells are destroyed, overt symptoms occur.
   - ii. Totally insulin-deficient; clients require exogenous insulin to survive.
   - iii. Characteristics
     1. Usually occurs before 30 years of age, but can occur at any age
     2. Peak incidence occurs during puberty
     3. Abrupt onset of signs and symptoms of hyperglycemia
     4. Prone to ketoacidosis
     5. Five percent of people with diabetes have this type (ADA, 2013).

(continues on page 378)

c. Type 2 diabetes
  i. Involves a decreased ability to use the insulin produced in the pancreas
    1. Decreased insulin secretion in response to glucose levels
    2. Insulin resistance blocking cells from absorbing glucose
    3. Excess production of glucose because of defective insulin secretory response
  ii. Accounts for approximately 90% to 95% of all diabetes in the United States
  iii. Characteristics
    1. Usually occurs after 30 years of age, but is now occurring in children and adolescents
    2. Increased prevalence in some ethnic groups—African Americans, Hispanic/Latino, Native Americans, Asian Americans, and Pacific Islanders
    3. Strong genetic predisposition
    4. Frequently obese
    5. Not prone to ketoacidosis until late in course or with prolonged hyperglycemia

d. Prediabetes (formerly called borderline diabetes)
  i. Blood glucose levels are higher than normal but not high enough for diagnosis of diabetes. Person is at risk for developing type 2 diabetes as well as heart disease and strokes. Diagnosis of diabetes may be delayed or prevented with weight loss and increased exercise (CDC, 2011).
  ii. Accounts for 35% of 29 million Americans aged 20 years or older (CDC, 2013)
  iii. Based on fasting blood glucose or A1C levels

IV. Statistics

a. Morbidity: More than 25.8 million Americans have diabetes; affects 26% of people over the age of 65 years. Approximately 1.9 million people (age 20 and older) were newly diagnosed diabetics in 2010 (CDC, 2011).

b. Mortality: Risk of death among people with diabetes is approximately twice that of those at a similar age, but without diabetes (CDC, 2011; Molinaro, 2011). In 2007, diabetes was reported to be the seventh leading cause of death. This ranking is based on the 71,382 death certificates in 2007 in which diabetes was the underlying cause of death (CDC, 2011).

c. Cost: Direct medical care costs of $176 billion annually (ADA, 2013)

GLOSSARY

A1C: Test (also known as HbA1c, glycated hemoglobin or glycosylated hemoglobin) is a blood test that correlates with a person's average blood glucose level over a span of a few months.

Acetone: Chemical formed in the blood when the body uses fat instead of glucose for energy. Acetone passes through the body into the urine. Someone with high levels of acetone can have breath that smells fruity and is called "acetone breath."

Beta cells: Cells that make insulin found in areas of the pancreas called the Islets of Langerhans.

Blood glucose: The main sugar that the body makes from food. Glucose is carried through the bloodstream to provide energy to all of the body's living cells.

Dawn phenomenon: An abrupt increase in fasting levels of serum glucose concentrations between the hours of 5 a.m. and 9 a.m., without preceding hypoglycemia, especially in diabetic patients receiving insulin therapy.

Diabetic neuropathy: Family of nerve disorders caused by diabetes, causing numbness, pain, and weakness in the hands, arms, feet, and legs. About half of all diabetics have some form of neuropathy.

Gastroparesis: Delayed emptying of food and secretions from the stomach to the small bowel due to autonomic neuropathy.

Gestational diabetes: A pregnant woman who is not diagnosed with diabetes but develops high blood glucose levels, usually at the 24th week of pregnancy. Affects approximately 18% of pregnancies. If not controlled, it places the baby and mother at risk with an increased chance of developing type 2 diabetes later in life.

Hyperglycemia: High blood glucose.

Hypoglycemia: Low blood glucose.

Insulin: Hormone produced by the pancreas that helps the body use blood glucose for energy. A person lacking this hormone is dependent on supplemental, outside (exogenous) sources.

Insulin resistance: Body is unable to use the insulin that it makes because of cell-receptor defect resulting in inability of cells to absorb glucose.

Ketoacidosis: Condition in which very high blood sugar levels along with a very low level of insulin result in a dangerous accumulation of ketones in the blood and urine. Coma or death can result if condition is not treated.

Ketones: Chemical substances produced when the body breaks down fat for energy. When ketones build up in the body over a long period of time, serious illness or coma can result.

Kussmaul respirations: Abnormal respiratory pattern characterized by rapid, deep breathing, often seen in client with metabolic acidosis.

Lactic acidosis: The buildup of lactic acid in the body. Cells make lactic acid when they use glucose for energy. If too much lactic acid stays in the body, the balance tips and the person begins to feel ill. Lactic acidosis may be caused by diabetic ketoacidosis or liver or kidney disease.

Metabolic acidosis: A pH imbalance in which the body has accumulated too much acid and does not have enough bicarbonate to effectively neutralize the effects of the acid. It can be brought on by a lack of insulin, a starvation diet, a gastrointestinal (GI) disorder, or a major organ dysfunction. For a person with diabetes, this can lead to diabetic ketoacidosis.

Paresthesias: Sensation of numbness or tingling, indicating nerve irritation, which may be due to diabetic neuropathy.

Somogyi effect: A swing to a high level of glucose in the blood from an extremely low level; usually occurs after an untreated insulin reaction during the night. The swing is caused by the release of stress hormones to counter low glucose levels.

Care Settings

DM is managed in the community setting. Diabetic ketoacidosis (DKA) may be encountered in any setting, with mild DKA managed at the community level; however, severe metabolic imbalance requires inpatient acute care on a medical unit.

Related Concerns

Amputation, page 616
Fluid and electrolyte imbalances, page 885
Metabolic acidosis—primary base bicarbonate deficiency, page 450
Psychosocial aspects of care, page 729

Client Assessment Database

Data depend on the severity and duration of metabolic imbalance, length and stage of diabetic process, and effects on other organ function.

DIAGNOSTIC DIVISION MAY REPORT	MAY EXHIBIT
ACTIVITY/REST	
• Sleep and rest disturbances • Weakness, fatigue, difficulty walking and moving • Muscle cramps, decreased muscle strength	• Tachycardia and tachypnea at rest or with activity • Lethargy, disorientation, coma • Decreased muscle strength and tone
CIRCULATION	
• History of hypertension; acute myocardial infarction (MI), claudication, numbness, tingling of extremities (long-term effects) • Leg ulcers, slow healing	• Tachycardia • Postural blood pressure (BP) changes; hypertension • Decreased and absent pulses • Dysrhythmias • Crackles; jugular vein distention (JVD)—if heart failure present • Hot, dry, flushed skin; sunken eyeballs—if dehydration is severe
EGO INTEGRITY	
• Life stressors, including financial concerns related to condition	• Anxiety, irritability
ELIMINATION	
• Change in usual voiding pattern • Excessive urination (polyuria) • Nocturia • Pain and burning, difficulty voiding (infection neurogenic bladder) • Recent and recurrent urinary tract infections (UTIs) • Abdominal tenderness, bloating, diarrhea	• Pale, yellow, dilute urine • Polyuria may progress to oliguria and anuria if severe hypovolemia occurs • Cloudy, odorous urine (infection) • Abdomen firm, distended • Bowel sounds diminished or hyperactive (diarrhea)
FOOD/FLUID	
• Loss of appetite, nausea and vomiting • Not following prescribed diet, increased intake of glucose and carbohydrates • Weight loss over a period of days or weeks • Thirst • Use of medications exacerbating dehydration, such as diuretics	• Dry and cracked skin, poor skin turgor • Abdominal rigidity and distention • Halitosis and sweet, fruity breath odor
NEUROSENSORY	
• Fainting spells, dizziness • Headaches • Tingling, numbness, weakness in muscles • Visual disturbances	• Confusion, disorientation • Drowsiness, lethargy, stupor and coma (later stages) • Deep tendon reflexes (DTRs) may be decreased • Seizure activity (late stages of DKA or hypoglycemia)
PAIN/DISCOMFORT	
• Abdominal bloating and pain	• Facial grimacing with abdominal palpation, guarding

(continues on page 380)

Client Assessment Database (continued)

DIAGNOSTIC DIVISION MAY REPORT (continued)	MAY EXHIBIT (continued)
RESPIRATION • Air hunger (late stages of DKA) • Cough, with and without purulent sputum (infection)	• Tachypnea • Kussmaul's respiration (metabolic acidosis) • Rhonchi, wheezes • Yellow or green sputum (infection)
SAFETY • Dry, itching skin, skin ulcerations • Paresthesia (diabetic neuropathy)	• Fever, diaphoresis • Skin breakdown, lesions and ulcerations • Decreased general strength and range of motion (ROM) • Weakness and paralysis of muscles, including respiratory musculature—if potassium levels are markedly decreased
SEXUALITY • Vaginal discharge (prone to infection) • Problems with impotence (men), orgasmic difficulty (women)	
TEACHING/LEARNING • Familial risk factors, such as diabetes mellitus, heart disease, stroke, hypertension • Slow and delayed healing • Use of drugs, such as steroids, thiazide diuretics, phenytoin (Dilantin), and phenobarbital (can increase glucose levels) • May or may not be taking diabetic medications as ordered	
DISCHARGE PLAN CONSIDERATIONS • May need assistance with dietary regimen, glucose monitoring, medication administration, supplies, and self-care ➧ Refer to section at end of plan for postdischarge considerations.	

Diagnostic Studies

TEST WHY IT IS DONE	WHAT IT TELLS ME
BLOOD TESTS • ***Serum glucose:*** The gold standard for diagnosing diabetes is an elevated blood sugar level after an overnight fast. A value above 140 mg/dL on at least two occasions typically means a person has diabetes. Normal fasting sugar levels run between 70 and 110 mg/dL.	DKA is defined as glucose greater than 250 mg/dL in association with an arterial pH of less than 7.30 or serum bicarbonate of less than 15 mEq/L and ketonemia (serum ketones).
• ***Total serum ketones:*** Types of naturally occurring and synthetic lipid compounds.	When insulin levels are too low or there is not enough glucose to use for energy, the body burns fatty acids for energy. The body then makes ketone bodies, waste products that cause the acid level in the blood to become too high. This in turn may lead to ketoacidosis. Ketones are positive at 1:2 dilution and may also be present in the urine as levels reach threshold and "spill" over into the urine.
• ***Serum osmolality:*** Measures the concentration of particles found in the fluid part of blood to help evaluate the body's water balance. Normal calculated values range from 280 to 303 mOsm/K.	Osmolality increases with dehydration and decreases with overhydration. In DKA, osmolality is elevated.

TEST WHY IT IS DONE (continued)	WHAT IT TELLS ME (continued)
• *Glucogon:* Hormone that raises the blood glucose level.	Elevated level is associated with conditions that produce (1) actual hypoglycemia; (2) relative lack of glucose, such as trauma or infection; or (3) lack of insulin. Therefore, glucagon may be elevated with severe DKA despite hyperglycemia.
• *Hemoglobin A_{1C} ($HgbA_{1C}$):* Test that determines how much glucose has been sticking to part of the Hgb during the past 3 to 4 months, with the previous 2 weeks most heavily weighted. Target level is <7%.	Currently, the gold standard for measuring glycemic control. Useful in differentiating inadequate control versus incident-related DKA. A result greater than 8% represents average blood glucose of 200 mg/dL or greater and signals a need for changes in treatment.
• *Serum insulin:* Peptide hormone that enables the body to metabolize and use glucose.	May be decreased or absent (type 1) or normal to high (type 2), indicating insulin insufficiency or improper use (endogenous and exogenous). Insulin resistance may develop secondary to formation of antibodies.
• *Electrolytes:* Substances that dissociate into ions in solution and acquire the capacity to conduct electricity. Common electrolytes include sodium, potassium, chloride, calcium, and phosphate.	Sodium may be low, normal, or high (total body depletion). Initial potassium level may be high, normal, or low (total body depletion). Potassium may be falsely elevated, reflecting cellular shifts, then markedly decrease with treatment of the DKA. Phosphate may be normal or low; chloride may be high. Levels are determined by amount of solute and water loss, which is not always equal.
• *Arterial blood gases (ABGs):* Assessment of ABG levels of oxygen (PaO_2), carbon dioxide ($PaCO_2$), bicarbonate (HCO_3^-), and pH.	Usually reflect low pH and decreased HCO_3– (metabolic acidosis) with compensatory respiratory alkalosis.
• *Complete blood count (CBC):* Battery of screening tests, which typically includes Hgb; hematocrit (Hct); red blood cell (RBC) count, morphology, indices, and distribution width index; platelet count and size; white blood cell (WBC) count and differential.	Hct may be elevated reflecting dehydration; increased WBCs or leukocytosis suggests hemoconcentration, response to stress or infection.
OTHER DIAGNOSTIC STUDIES	
• *Urine:* Urine glucose correlates poorly with blood glucose, being dependent on renal glucose threshold (150 to 300 mg/dL) and should be used only if measuring of blood glucose is not possible or as a confirmatory test. Ketones should be self-monitored during febrile illness or when DKA symptoms are present.	In DKA, urine tests are positive for glucose and ketones. Specific gravity and osmolality may be elevated if dehydration is present.
• *Cultures and sensitivities:* Specimens may include urine, sputum, or wound drainage.	May reveal source of infection and identify effective antimicrobial agent.

Nursing Priorities

1. Restore fluid, electrolyte, and acid-base balance.
2. Correct or reverse metabolic abnormalities.
3. Identify and assist with management of underlying cause or disease process.
4. Prevent complications.
5. Provide information about disease process, prognosis, self-care, and treatment needs.

Discharge Goals

1. Homeostasis achieved.
2. Causative and precipitating factors corrected or controlled.
3. Complications prevented or minimized.
4. Disease process, prognosis, self-care needs, and therapeutic regimen understood.
5. Plan in place to meet needs after discharge.

NURSING DIAGNOSIS: deficient Fluid Volume [specify]

May Be Related To

Active fluid losses—diarrhea, vomiting, osmotic diuresis

Possibly Evidenced By

Increased urine output (hyperglycemia); decreased urine output, increased urine concentration (dehydration)
Weakness, thirst, sudden weight loss

(continues on page 382)

NURSING DIAGNOSIS: deficient Fluid Volume [specify] (continued)

Dry skin and mucous membranes, poor skin turgor
Decreased blood pressure, increased pulse rate, decreased pulse pressure
Change in mental state

Desired Outcomes/Evaluation Criteria—Client Will

Fluid Balance (NOC)

Demonstrate adequate hydration as evidenced by stable vital signs, palpable peripheral pulses, good skin turgor and capillary refill, individually appropriate urinary output, and electrolyte levels within normal range.

ACTIONS/INTERVENTIONS	RATIONALE
Fluid/Electrolyte Management (NIC)	
Independent	
Obtain history from client and significant other (SO) related to duration and intensity of symptoms, such as vomiting and excessive urination.	Helps estimate total volume depletion. Symptoms may have been present for varying amounts of time—hours to days. Presence of infectious process results in fever and hypermetabolic state, increasing insensible fluid losses.
Monitor vital signs:	
Note orthostatic BP changes.	Hypovolemia may be manifested by hypotension and tachycardia. Estimates of severity of hypovolemia may be made when client's systolic BP drops more than 10 mm Hg from a recumbent to a sitting or standing position. *Note:* Cardiac neuropathy may block reflexes that normally increase heart rate.
Respiratory pattern, such as Kussmaul's respirations, acetone breath	Lungs remove carbonic acid through respirations, producing a compensatory respiratory alkalosis or ketoacidosis. Acetone breath is due to breakdown of acetoacetic acid and should diminish as ketosis is corrected.
Respiratory rate and quality; use of accessory muscles, periods of apnea, and appearance of cyanosis	Correction of hyperglycemia and acidosis will cause the respiratory rate and pattern to approach normal. In contrast, increased work of breathing—shallow, rapid respirations—and presence of cyanosis may indicate respiratory fatigue and that client is losing ability to compensate for acidosis.
Temperature, skin color, and moisture	Although fever, chills, and diaphoresis are common with infectious process, fever with flushed, dry skin may reflect dehydration. *Note:* Although fever is a common precipitating factor for DKA, clients may be normothermic or hypothermic because of peripheral vasodilation.
Assess peripheral pulses, capillary refill, skin turgor, and mucous membranes.	Indicators of level of hydration and adequacy of circulating volume.
Monitor intake and output (I&O); note urine specific gravity.	Provides ongoing estimate of volume replacement needs, kidney function, and effectiveness of therapy.
Weigh daily.	Provides the best assessment of current fluid status and adequacy of fluid replacement.
Maintain fluid intake of at least 2500 mL/day within cardiac tolerance when oral intake is resumed.	Maintains hydration and circulating volume.
Promote comfortable environment. Cover client with light sheets.	Avoids overheating, which could promote further fluid loss.
Investigate changes in mentation and sensorium.	Changes in mentation can be due to abnormally high or low glucose, electrolyte abnormalities, acidosis, decreased cerebral perfusion, or developing hypoxia. Regardless of the cause, impaired consciousness can predispose client to aspiration.
Collaborative	
Administer fluids, as indicated:	
Isotonic (0.9%) or lactated Ringer's solution without additives	Type and amount of fluid depends on degree of deficit and individual client response. *Note:* Client with DKA is often severely dehydrated and commonly needs 5 to 10 L of isotonic saline, 2 to 3 L within first 2 hours of treatment.
Albumin, plasma, dextran	Plasma expanders may occasionally be needed if the deficit is life-threatening and BP does not normalize with rehydration efforts.
Insert and maintain indwelling urinary catheter.	Provides for accurate and ongoing measurement of urinary output, especially if autonomic neuropathies result in neurogenic

ACTIONS/INTERVENTIONS (continued)	RATIONALE (continued)
	bladder with urinary retention and overflow incontinence. May be removed when client is stable to reduce risk of infection.
Monitor laboratory studies, such as the following:	
Hct	Assesses level of hydration; Hct is often elevated because of hemoconcentration associated with osmotic diuresis.
Blood urea nitrogen (BUN)/creatinine (Cr)	Elevated values may reflect cellular breakdown from dehydration or signal the onset of renal failure.
Serum osmolality	Elevated because of hyperglycemia and dehydration.
Sodium	May be decreased, reflecting shift of fluids from the intracellular compartment as with osmotic diuresis. High sodium values reflect severe fluid loss and dehydration or sodium reabsorption in response to aldosterone secretion.
Potassium	Initially, hyperkalemia occurs in response to metabolic acidosis, but as this potassium is lost in the urine, the absolute potassium level in the body is depleted. As insulin is replaced and acidosis is corrected, serum potassium deficit becomes apparent.
Administer potassium and other electrolytes intravenously (IV) or by oral route, as indicated.	Potassium should be added to the IV as soon as urinary flow is adequate, to prevent hypokalemia. *Note:* Potassium phosphate may be drug of choice when IV fluids contain sodium chloride in order to prevent chloride overload. Phosphate concentrations tend to decrease with insulin therapy.
Administer bicarbonate, if indicated, for example, if pH is less than 7.1.	Not routinely necessary and given with caution to help correct acidosis in the presence of hypotension or shock, lactic acidosis, or severe hyperkalemia.
Insert nasogastric (NG) tube and attach to suction, as indicated.	Decompresses stomach and may relieve vomiting.

NURSING DIAGNOSIS: unstable Blood Glucose Level

May Be Related To

Lack of diabetes management or adherence to diabetes management plan; inadequate blood glucose monitoring or medication management

Weight gain or loss

Rapid growth periods; pregnancy

Physical health status; stress; [infectious process]

Possibly Evidenced By

Increased urinary output, dilute urine

Reported inadequate food intake, lack of interest in food

Weakness, fatigue, poor muscle tone

Altered level of consciousness (LOC)

Increased ketones

Desired Outcomes/Evaluation Criteria—Client Will

Blood Glucose Level (NOC)

Maintain glucose in satisfactory range.

Self-Management: Diabetes (NOC)

Acknowledge factors that lead to unstable glucose and DKA.

Verbalize understanding of body and energy needs.

Verbalize plan for modifying factors to prevent or minimize complications.

ACTIONS/INTERVENTIONS	RATIONALE
Hyperglycemia Management (NIC)	
Independent	
Determine individual factors that may have contributed to current situation. Note client's age, developmental level, and awareness of needs.	Occasionally, client with unknown diabetes will present with DKA, especially a young person with some type of precipitating infection. However, many times DKA is precipitated by failure of diabetes management, possibly related to dietary factors, activity, or medications. Because DKA presents more frequently in the young client with type 1 diabetes, there may be a failure to account for developmental changes, such as an adolescent growth spurt or pregnancy.

(continues on page 384)

ACTIONS/INTERVENTIONS (continued)	RATIONALE (continued)
Perform fingerstick glucose testing. Ascertain whether client and SO(s) are adept at blood glucose monitoring and are testing according to plan.	All available glucose monitors will provide satisfactory readings if properly used and maintained and routinely calibrated. *Note:* Unstable blood glucose is often associated with failure to perform testing on a regular schedule.
For client on oral diabetes medications: Determine class of drug (e.g., sulfonylureas such as chlorpropamide [Diabinese]; biguonides such as metformin [Glucophage]; meglitinides such as repaglinide [Prandin]); and note client's compliance with therapy.	Client may or may not have been on medications. Various oral preparations have been found to manage most diabetes symptoms and diabetes-related complications. Sometimes client has not followed prescribed therapeutic regimen, which can contribute to treatment failure. *Note:* A client presenting in ketoacidosis may not have been on either oral drugs or insulin, or glucose may not be well controlled on current meds (Nazario, 2011).
For client receiving insulin: Review type(s) of insulin used, such as rapid, short-acting, intermediate, long-acting, premixed. Note delivery method—subcutaneous injections, insulin jet injector, insulin infuser, or pump. Note times when short-acting, intermediate-acting, and long-acting insulins are administered, duration, and when they peak.	These factors affect timing of effects and provide clues to potential timing of glucose instability (National Diabetes Information Clearinghouse [NDIC], 2011).
Check injection sites.	Insulin absorption can vary from day to day in healthy sites and is less absorbable in lypohypertrophic (lumpy) tissues.
Review client's dietary program and usual pattern; compare with recent intake.	Identifies deficits and deviations from therapeutic plan, which may precipitate unstable glucose and uncontrolled hyperglycemia.
Weigh daily or as indicated.	Assesses adequacy of nutritional intake—both absorption and utilization. *Note:* Eating disorders are a contributing factor in 20% of recurrent DKA in young clients (Polin, 2012).
Auscultate bowel sounds. Note reports of abdominal pain and bloating, nausea, or vomiting. Maintain nothing by mouth (NPO) status, as indicated.	Hyperglycemia and fluid and electrolyte disturbances decrease gastric motility and function resulting in gastroparesis, affecting choice of interventions. *Note:* Long-term difficulties with gastroparesis and poor intestinal motility suggest autonomic neuropathies affecting the GI tract and requiring symptomatic treatment.
Provide liquids containing nutrients and electrolytes as soon as client can tolerate oral fluids; progress to more solid food as tolerated.	Oral route is preferred when client is alert and bowel function is restored.
Identify food preferences, including ethnic and cultural needs.	Incorporating as many of the client's food preferences into the meal plan as possible increases cooperation with dietary guidelines after discharge.
Include SO in meal planning, as indicated.	Promotes sense of involvement; provides information for SO to understand nutritional needs of client. *Note:* Various methods available for dietary planning include carbohydrate counting, exchange list, point system, or preselected menus.
Observe for signs of hypoglycemia—changes in LOC, cool and clammy skin, rapid pulse, hunger, irritability, anxiety, headache, light-headedness, and shakiness.	Once carbohydrate metabolism resumes, blood glucose level will fall, and as insulin is being adjusted, hypoglycemia may occur. If client is comatose, hypoglycemia may occur without notable change in LOC. This potentially life-threatening emergency should be assessed and treated quickly per protocol. *Note:* Type 1 diabetics of long standing may not display usual signs of hypoglycemia because normal response to low blood sugar may be diminished.
Collaborative	
Monitor laboratory studies, such as serum glucose, acetone, pH, and HCO_3^-.	Blood glucose will decrease slowly with controlled fluid replacement and insulin therapy. With the administration of optimal insulin dosages, glucose can then enter the cells and be used for energy. When this happens, acetone levels decrease and acidosis is corrected.
Collaborate in treatment of hyperglycemia complication, e.g., DKA.	Treatment is focused on correction of metabolic imbalances and includes (1) correction of fluid loss with intravenous fluids; (2) correction of hyperglycemia with insulin; (3) correction of electrolyte disturbances, particularly potassium loss; (4) correction of acid-base balance; and (5) treatment of concurrent infection, if present (Raghavan et al, 2013).

ACTIONS/INTERVENTIONS (continued)	RATIONALE (continued)
Administer rapid-acting insulin, such as regular (Humulin R), lispro (Humalog), or aspart (Novalog) by intermittent or continuous IV method, for example, IV bolus followed by a continuous drip via pump of approximately 5 to 10 units/hr so that glucose is reduced by 50 to 75 mg/dL/hr.	Rapid-acting insulin is used in hyperglycemic crisis. The IV route is the initial route of choice because absorption from subcutaneous tissues may be erratic. Many believe the continuous method is the optimal way to facilitate transition to carbohydrate metabolism and reduce incidence of hypoglycemia. *Note:* Intermediate insulin, such as NPH, Humulin N, Lente, and long-acting insulin, such as Ultralente, protamine zinc insulin (PZI), and glargine (Lantus), may be part of the client's usual or added insulins, but are not part of crisis hyperglycemic treatment.
Administer glucose solutions, for example, 5% dextrose and half-normal saline.	Glucose solutions may be added after insulin and fluids have brought the blood glucose to approximately 180 mg/dL (Raghavan et al, 2013). As carbohydrate metabolism approaches normal, care must be taken to avoid hypoglycemia.
Consult with nutritionist or dietitian for resumption of oral intake.	Useful in calculating and adjusting diet to meet client's specific needs; answer questions and assist client and SO in developing meal plans.
Provide diet of approximately 60% carbohydrates, 20% proteins, and 20% fats in designated number of meals and snacks.	Complex carbohydrates help to maintain more stable glucose levels, reduce serum cholesterol levels, and promote satiation. Food intake is scheduled according to specific insulin characteristics, such as peak effect, and individual client response. *Note:* A snack of complex carbohydrates at bedtime is especially important if insulin is given in divided doses to prevent hypoglycemia during sleep and potential Somogyi response.

NURSING DIAGNOSIS: risk for Infection

Risk Factors May Include

Chronic disease—diabetes mellitus; leucopenia; invasive procedure
[Preexisting respiratory infection or UTI]

Possibly Evidenced By

(Not applicable; presence of signs and symptoms establishes an *actual* diagnosis)

Desired Outcomes/Evaluation Criteria—Client Will

Risk Control: Infectious Process (NOC)

Identify interventions to prevent or reduce risk of infection.
Demonstrate techniques and lifestyle changes to prevent development of infection.

ACTIONS/INTERVENTIONS	RATIONALE
Infection Prevention (NIC)	
Independent	
Observe for signs of infection and inflammation—fever, flushed appearance, wound drainage, purulent sputum, and cloudy urine.	Client may be admitted with infection, which could have precipitated the ketoacidotic state, or may develop a nosocomial infection.
Promote good hand washing by staff and client.	Reduces risk of cross-contamination.
Maintain aseptic technique for IV insertion procedure, administration of medications, and providing site care. Rotate IV sites, as indicated.	High glucose in the blood creates an excellent medium for bacterial growth.
Provide catheter and perineal care. Teach the female client to clean from front to back after elimination.	Minimizes risk of UTI. Comatose client may be at particular risk if urinary retention occurred before hospitalization. *Note:* Elderly female diabetic clients are especially prone to UTIs and vaginal yeast infections. Many UTIs are asymptomatic, possibly related to neurogenic bladder.
Provide conscientious skin care, gently massage bony areas, keep the skin dry, and keep linens dry and wrinkle-free.	Peripheral circulation may be impaired, placing client at increased risk for skin irritation and breakdown and infection.
Inspect client's feet, noting presence of ulcers or infected ingrown toenails, or other problems requiring medical or nursing intervention.	Foot injuries and impaired circulation are associated with many complications in diabetics, including cellulitis and amputations. *Note:* Cellulitis can precipitate episode of DKA.
Auscultate breath sounds.	Rhonchi indicate accumulation of secretions possibly related to pneumonia or bronchitis that may have precipitated the DKA.

(continues on page 386)

ACTIONS/INTERVENTIONS (continued)	RATIONALE (continued)
Place in semi-Fowler's position.	Facilitates lung expansion and reduces risk of aspiration.
Reposition and encourage coughing and deep breathing if client is alert and cooperative. Otherwise, suction airway, using sterile technique, as needed.	Aids in ventilating all lung areas and mobilizing secretions. Prevents stasis of secretions with increased risk of infection.
Provide tissues and trash bag in a convenient location for sputum and other secretions. Instruct client in proper handling of secretions.	Minimizes spread of infection.
Encourage and assist with oral hygiene.	Reduces risk of oral and gum disease.
Encourage adequate dietary and fluid intake (at least 2500 mL/day if not contraindicated by cardiac or renal dysfunction), including 8 oz of cranberry juice per day, as appropriate.	Decreases susceptibility to infection. Increased urinary flow prevents stasis and aids in maintaining urine acidity, reducing bacteria growth and flushing organisms out of system. *Note:* Use of cranberry juice can help prevent bacteria from adhering to the bladder wall, reducing the risk of recurrent UTI.
Collaborative	
Obtain specimens for culture and sensitivities, as indicated.	Identifies organism(s) so that most appropriate drug therapy can be instituted.
Administer antibiotics, as appropriate.	Early treatment may help prevent sepsis.

NURSING DIAGNOSIS: [risk for disturbed Sensory Perception, (specify)]

Risk Factors May Include

Biochemical imbalance (e.g., glucose, insulin, electrolyte)

Possibly Evidenced By

(Not applicable; presence of signs and symptoms establishes an *actual* diagnosis)

Desired Outcomes/Evaluation Criteria—Client Will

Neurological Status (NOC)

Maintain usual level of mentation.

Recognize and compensate for existing sensory impairments.

ACTIONS/INTERVENTIONS	RATIONALE
Neurological Monitoring (NIC)	
Independent	
Monitor vital signs and mental status.	Provides a baseline from which to compare abnormal findings; for instance, fever may affect mentation.
Address client by name; reorient as needed to place, person, time, and situation. Give short explanations, speaking slowly and enunciating clearly.	Decreases confusion and helps maintain contact with reality.
Schedule nursing time to provide for uninterrupted rest periods.	Promotes restful sleep, reduces fatigue, and may improve cognition.
Keep client's routine as consistent as possible. Encourage participation in activities of daily living (ADLs) as able.	Helps keep client in touch with reality and maintain orientation to the environment.
Protect client from injury—avoid or limit use of restraints as able, place bed in low position—when cognition is impaired. Pad bed rails if client is prone to seizures.	Disoriented client is prone to injury, especially at night, and precautions need to be taken as indicated. Seizure precautions reduce risk of physical injury.
Evaluate visual acuity, as indicated.	Retinal edema or detachment, hemorrhage, presence of cataracts, or temporary paralysis of extraocular muscles may impair vision, requiring corrective therapy or supportive care. *Note:* Retinopathy is a very common microvascular complication associated with diabetes and is the cause of 10,000 new cases of blindness annually (Deshpande et al, 2008).
Investigate reports of hyperesthesia, pain, or sensory loss in the feet and legs. Look for ulcers, reddened areas, pressure points, and loss of pedal pulses.	Peripheral neuropathies may result in severe discomfort and absent or distorted tactile sensation, potentiating risk of dermal injury and impaired balance.
Provide bed cradle. Keep hands and feet warm, avoiding exposure to cool drafts, hot water, or heating pad.	Reduces discomfort and potential for dermal injury. *Note:* Sudden development of cold hands and feet may reflect hypoglycemia, suggesting need to evaluate serum glucose level.
Assist with ambulation or position changes.	Promotes client safety, especially when sense of balance is affected.
Collaborative	
Carry out prescribed regimen for correcting DKA, as indicated.	Alteration in thought processes and potential for seizure activity is usually alleviated once hyperosmolar state is corrected.

ACTIONS/INTERVENTIONS (continued)	RATIONALE (continued)
Monitor laboratory values, such as blood glucose, serum osmolality, Hgb/Hct, and BUN/Cr.	Imbalances can impair mentation. *Note:* If fluid is replaced too quickly, water intoxication can occur—sodium concentration falls, water enters brain cells, and confusion, disorientation, or coma may develop.

NURSING DIAGNOSIS: Fatigue

May Be Related To
Disease states; poor physical condition; stress
Altered body chemistry—insufficient insulin
Increased energy demands—hypermetabolic state, infection

Possibly Evidenced By
Reports an overwhelming lack of energy, inability to maintain usual routines, decreased performance
Compromised concentration; listless; disinterest in surroundings

Desired Outcomes/Evaluation Criteria—Client Will

Fatigue Level (NOC)
Verbalize increase in energy level.
Display improved ability to participate in desired activities.

ACTIONS/INTERVENTIONS	RATIONALE
Energy Management (NIC)	
Independent	
Discuss with client the need for activity. Plan schedule with client and identify activities that lead to fatigue.	Education may provide motivation to increase activity level even though client may feel too weak initially.
Alternate activity with periods of rest and uninterrupted sleep.	Prevents excessive fatigue.
Monitor pulse, respiratory rate, and BP before and after activity.	Indicates physiological levels of tolerance.
Discuss ways of conserving energy while bathing, transferring, and so on.	Client will be able to accomplish more with a decreased expenditure of energy.
Increase client participation in ADLs, as tolerated.	Increases confidence level, self-esteem, and tolerance level. *Note:* Elder clients may experience a "lag effect" in which exercise may precipitate hypoglycemia as late as 24 hours after exercising, leading to extensive fatigue and muscle tremors.

NURSING DIAGNOSIS: ineffective Coping

May Be Related To
Situational crisis (long-term, progressive illness that is not curable)
Inadequate level of perception of control

Possibly Evidenced By
Reports inability to ask for help
Inadequate problem-solving
Lack of goal-directed behavior

Desired Outcomes/Evaluation Criteria—Client Will

Health Beliefs: Perceived Control (NOC)
Verbalize sense of control.
Adapt to life changes.
Use effective coping strategies.

ACTIONS/INTERVENTIONS	RATIONALE
Coping Enhancement (NIC)	
Independent	
Encourage client and SO to express feelings about hospitalization and disease in general.	Identifies concerns and facilitates problem-solving.
Acknowledge normality of feelings.	Recognition that these reactions are normal can help client problem-solve and seek help as needed. Diabetic control is a full-time job that serves as a constant reminder of both presence of condition and threat to client's health and life.
Assess how client has handled problems in the past; identify locus of control.	Knowledge of individual's style helps determine needs for treatment goals. Client whose locus of control is internal usually looks at ways to gain control over own treatment program. Client who operates with an external locus of control wants to be cared for by others and may project blame for circumstances onto external factors.
Provide opportunity for SO to express concerns and discuss ways in which he or she can be helpful to client.	Enhances sense of being involved and gives SO a chance to problem-solve solutions to help client prevent recurrence.
Ascertain expectations and goals of client and SO.	Unrealistic expectations and pressure from others or self may result in feelings of frustration or loss of control and may impair coping abilities. *Note:* Even with rigid adherence to medical regimen, complications and setbacks may occur.
Determine whether a change in relationship with SO has occurred.	Constant energy and thought required for diabetic control often shifts the focus of a relationship. Development of psychological concerns and visceral neuropathies affecting self-concept, especially sexual role function, may add further stress.
Encourage client to make decisions related to care, such as ambulation, time for activities, and so forth.	Communicates to client that some control can be exercised over care.
Support participation in self-care and give positive feedback for efforts.	Promotes feeling of control over situation.

NURSING DIAGNOSIS: ineffective Self-Health Management

May Be Related To
Complexity of healthcare regimen
Deficient knowledge
Perceived susceptibility/barriers
Economic difficulties
Family patterns of healthcare

Possibly Evidenced By
Reports difficulty with prescribed regimen
Ineffective choices in daily living for meeting health goals
Failure to take actions to reduce risk factors
Unexpected acceleration of illness symptoms

Desired Outcomes/Evaluation Criteria—Client Will

Knowledge: Diabetes Management (NOC)
Verbalize understanding of disease process and potential complications.
Identify relationship of signs and symptoms to the disease process and correlate symptoms with causative factors.

Self-Management: Diabetes (NOC)
Correctly perform necessary procedures and explain reasons for the actions.
Initiate necessary lifestyle changes and participate in treatment regimen.

ACTIONS/INTERVENTIONS	RATIONALE
Learning Facilitation (NIC)	
Independent	
Create an environment of trust by listening to concerns and being available.	Rapport and respect need to be established before client will be willing to take part in the learning process.
Work with client in setting mutual goals for learning.	Participation in the planning promotes enthusiasm and cooperation with the principles learned.

ACTIONS/INTERVENTIONS (continued)	RATIONALE (continued)
Select a variety of teaching strategies, such as demonstrating needed skills and having client do return demonstration, incorporating new skills into the hospital routine.	Use of different means of accessing information promotes information retention.
Teaching: Disease Process (NIC)	
Discuss essential elements, such as the following:	
Explain the normal blood glucose range and how it compares with client's level, the type of diabetes the client has, and the relationship between insulin deficiency and a high glucose level.	Provides knowledge base from which client can make informed lifestyle choices.
Reasons for the ketoacidotic episode	Knowledge of the precipitating factors may help avoid recurrences.
Acute and chronic complications of the disease, including visual disturbances, neurosensory and cardiovascular changes, renal impairment, and hypertension	Awareness helps client be more consistent with care and may prevent or delay onset of complications.
Demonstrate fingerstick testing, or similar procedure, such as palm or armstick, or continuous glucose monitoring system (GlucoWatch). Have client and SO return demonstration of obtaining sample and operating blood glucose until proficient.	Frequent (up to 6 to 8 times daily) self-monitoring of blood glucose (SMBG) is the foundation of intensive diabetes management. Desired blood glucose ranges are based on each individual's needs, but frequent testing promotes tighter control of serum levels. The American Diabetes Association suggests general targets for nonpregnant adults to be 60 to 130 mg/dL before meals, and after meal peak level of less than 180 mg/dL (ADA, 2013). There are many different blood glucose monitors available. The client/SO may desire recommendations for a meter that best meets the client's needs, e.g., large numbers on the screen because of poor eyesight; or client needs a simple meter rather than one that is complex.
Review client's particular dietary plan. In general, plan should include avoiding sugar and limiting intake of fat, salt, and alcohol; eating complex carbohydrates, especially those high in fiber such as fruits, vegetables, whole grains.	Medical nutrition therapy for diabetes encourages client to make meal choices based on individual unique needs and preferences. Awareness of importance of dietary control aids client in planning meals and sticking to regimen. Fiber can slow glucose absorption, decreasing fluctuations in serum levels but may cause GI discomfort, increase flatus, and affect vitamin and mineral absorption.
Review medication regimen, including onset, peak, and duration of prescribed insulin, as applicable, with client and SO.	Understanding all aspects of drug usage promotes proper use. Dose algorithms are created, taking into account drug dosages established during inpatient evaluation, usual amount and schedule of physical activity, and meal plan. Including SO provides additional support and resource for client.
Review client's type of basal insulin—lente, NPH, ultralente, glargine (Lantus)—and bolus insulin—regular, lispro, aspart (Novolog)—as indicated.	Verifies understanding and correctness of procedure. Identifies potential problems, (e.g., impaired vision or cognition) so that alternative solutions can be found for insulin administration. *Note:* If multiple daily injections are required, combinations of types (e.g., rapid-acting plus short-acting, intermediate, and long-acting insulin) are used. If the pump method is used, only rapid-acting insulin (e.g., lispro, aspart, glulisine) is used, and client programs own basal and bolus settings. *Note:* DKA is rare among pump users who perform SMBG adequately but can develop quickly because of the short half-life of rapid-acting insulin analogues commonly used in pumps (American Association of Diabetes Educators [AADE], 2009).
Review self-administration of insulin, either injection or pump, and care of equipment. Have client demonstrate procedure: drawing up and injecting insulin, insulin pen technique, or use of continuous pump.	Confirms that client is proficient in skills or will require assistance or full care in managing procedures and equipment.
Discuss timing of insulin injection and mealtime.	One of the many inconveniences people with diabetes cope with is having to decide at least 30 to 60 minutes in advance when they are going to have a meal for the timely administration of regular human injections. Insulin lispro (Humalog) or aspart (Novolog) may be helpful because it works best when taken within 15 minutes of eating. With the onset twice as fast as regular human insulin and a duration approximately half as long, Humalog and Novolog closely mimic pancreatic activity. However, hypoglycemia may develop more rapidly and be more severe than with use of

(continues on page 390)

ACTIONS/INTERVENTIONS (continued)	RATIONALE (continued)
	regular insulin. A blood glucose level below 80 mg/dL indicates that insulin should be injected after eating rather than before the meal.
Emphasize importance and necessity of maintaining diary of glucose testing, medication dose and time, dietary intake, activity, feelings, sensations, and life events.	Aids in creating overall picture of client situation to achieve better disease control and promotes self-care and independence.
Discuss factors that play a part in diabetic control such as aerobic versus isometric exercise, stress, surgery, and illness. Review "sick day" rules.	This information promotes diabetic control and can greatly reduce the occurrence of ketoacidosis. *Note:* Aerobic exercise such as walking and swimming promotes effective use of insulin, lowering glucose levels, and strengthens the cardiovascular system. A "sick day" management plan helps maintain equilibrium during illness, minor surgery, severe emotional stress, exogenous steroids (as with spinal or joint injections or any oral treatment for asthma and arthritis), or any condition that might send glucose spiraling upward.
Review effects of smoking. Encourage cessation of smoking.	Nicotine constricts the small blood vessels, and insulin absorption is delayed for as long as these vessels remain constricted.
Establish regular exercise or activity schedule and identify corresponding insulin concerns.	Exercise times should not coincide with the peak action of insulin. A snack should be ingested before or during exercise as needed, and rotation of injection sites should avoid the muscle group that will be used in the activity (for instance, abdominal site is preferred over thigh or arm before jogging or swimming) to prevent accelerated uptake of insulin.
Identify the symptoms of hypoglycemia—weakness, dizziness, lethargy, hunger, irritability, diaphoresis, pallor, tachycardia, tremors, headache, and changes in mentation—and explain causes.	May promote early detection and treatment, preventing or limiting occurrence. However, approximately 30% of insulin-dependent clients are asymptomatic when hypoglycemic. *Note:* Early-morning hyperglycemia may reflect the "dawn phenomenon," indicating need for additional insulin, or the Somogyi effect, requiring a decrease in medication dosage and/or change in diet such as bedtime or hour of sleep (HS) snack. Testing serum levels at 3 a.m. aids in identifying the specific problem.
Instruct SO in emergency use of glucagon.	Given for treatment of severe hypoglycemia when client is unable to take oral carbohydrates. Prompt intervention may prevent more serious complications.
Instruct in importance of routine daily examination of the feet and proper foot care. Demonstrate ways to examine feet, inspect shoes for fit, and care for toenails, calluses, and corns. Encourage use of natural-fiber stockings.	Prevents or delays complications associated with peripheral neuropathies and circulatory impairment, especially cellulitis, gangrene, and amputation. *Note:* Studies show that approximately 15% of all clients with diabetes will develop a foot or leg ulcer during the course of the disease. Also, 50% of all nontraumatic lower extremity amputations occur in people with diabetes (Reiber, 1998). Prevention is therefore critical.
Emphasize importance of regular eye examinations, especially for clients who have had type 1 diabetes for 5 years or more.	Changes in vision may be gradual and are more pronounced in persons with poorly controlled DM and BP. Problems include changes in visual acuity and may progress to retinopathy and blindness. *Note:* Retinopathy is the most frequent cause of new blindness among adults 20 to 74 years of age.
Arrange for vision aids when needed, such as magnifying sleeve for insulin syringe, prefilled insulin pens, large-print instructions, and one-touch or talking glucose meters.	Adaptive aids have been developed in recent years to help the visually impaired manage their own DM more effectively.
Discuss sexual functioning and answer questions client and SO may have.	Impotence may be first symptom of onset of DM. *Note:* Counseling and use of penile prosthesis may be of benefit.
Emphasize importance of using medical alert ID bracelet or necklace.	Can promote quick entry into the health system and appropriate care with fewer resultant complications in the event of an emergency.
Recommend reading product labels and avoidance of over-the-counter (OTC) drugs without prior discussion with healthcare provider.	These products may contain sugars and interact with prescribed medications.
Discuss importance of follow-up care.	Helps maintain tighter control of disease process and may prevent exacerbations of DM, retarding development of systemic complications.
Review signs and symptoms requiring medical evaluation—fever, cold, or flu symptoms; cloudy, odorous urine; painful urination; delayed healing of cuts or sores; sensory changes with pain or tingling of lower extremities; changes in blood sugar level; and presence of ketones in urine.	Prompt intervention may prevent development of more serious or life-threatening complications.

ACTIONS/INTERVENTIONS (continued)	RATIONALE (continued)
Identify community resources such as the American Diabetic Association, Internet resources and online diabetes bulletin boards, visiting nurse, weight-loss or smoking cessation clinics, contact person, or diabetic instructor.	Continued support is usually necessary to sustain lifestyle changes and promote well-being.

POTENTIAL CONSIDERATIONS following acute hospitalization (dependent on client's age, physical condition and presence of complications, personal resources, and life responsibilities)

- *risk for unstable Blood Glucose Level*—lack of acceptance of diagnosis, inadequate blood glucose monitoring, activity level, stress
- *ineffective Self-Health Management*—complexity of therapeutic regimen, economic difficulties, perceived susceptibility (recurrence of problem)
- *risk for Trauma*—reduced sensation; poor vision
- *risk for Sexual Dysfunction*—altered body function (disease process)

HYPERTHYROIDISM (GRAVES' DISEASE, THYROTOXICOSIS)

I. Pathophysiology: Failure of a complex feedback mechanism resulting in excessive secretion or release of thyroid hormone

II. Etiology

a. Metabolic imbalance resulting from overproduction of the thyroid hormones triiodothyronine (T_3) and thyroxine (T_4)

b. Thyrotoxic crisis or thyroid storm—untreated or inadequately treated severe hyperthyroidism creating a life-threatening emergency

c. Varied causation

i. Autoimmune

1. Toxic diffuse goiter or Graves' disease: most common cause, accounting for 80% of hyperthyroidism diagnoses (Ogunyem, 2012; Bahn et al, 2011)
2. Subacute and "silent" thyroiditis

ii. Toxic multinodular goiter (TMNG): second most common cause of hyperthyroidism (Fisher, 2002; Schraga, 2012)

iii. Thyroid or pituitary tumors

iv. Drug-induced: iodine, excessive thyroid hormone replacement, certain other drugs, such as amiodarone

v. Bacterial or viral infections

vi. Pregnancy: hyperthyroidism affects 0.1% to 0.4% of pregnancies (Ogunyem, 2012).

vii. Iatrogenic: manipulation of thyroid gland during surgery

III. Statistics (Schraga, 2012)

a. Morbidity: The overall incidence of hyperthyroidism in the United States is estimated between 0.05% and 1.3%. Approximately 1% to 2% of patients with hyperthyroidism progress to thyroid storm.

b. Mortality: Adult mortality rate from thyroid storm is approximately 10% to 20%, but may be as high as 75% in hospitalized individuals due to comorbidities.

GLOSSARY

Ablation: Removal or excision, usually carried out surgically, but may be done chemically with radioactive iodine.

Autoimmune disease: Illness that occurs when the body tissues are attacked by its own immune system.

Diaphoresis: Excessive sweating; may be associated with exercise or with emotional, physical, and mental stress.

Endocrine gland: Gland that releases a chemical messenger, known as a hormone, directly into the bloodstream, which will affect other parts of the body. The thyroid is an endocrine gland.

Euthyroid: Situation where thyroid-stimulating hormone (TSH) test values are in the normal range and the thyroid is neither hyperthyroid nor hypothyroid.

Exophthalmos: Abnormal bulging of the eye, with resulting inability to close lid.

Extraocular muscles: The six muscles that control the movements of the eye. The actions of the extraocular muscles depend on the position of the eye at the time of muscle contraction.

Goiter: Enlargement of the thyroid gland.

Graves' disease: A condition caused by excessive production of thyroid hormone and characterized by an enlarged thyroid gland, protrusion of the eyeballs, a rapid heartbeat, and nervous excitability. Also called exophthalmic goiter.

Inotropic support: Substance that influences the contractility of heart cells.

Nodule: A small, solid collection of tissue that is palpable.

Plasmapheresis: The process of separating certain cells, such as excess antibodies, from the plasma in the blood by a machine; only the cells are returned to the person.

Pretibial myxedema: A skin condition associated with Graves' disease characterized by swollen, itchy patches of skin on the front of the lower legs or shins.

Radioactive iodine (RAI): An isotope of the chemical element iodine that is radioactive. Used in diagnostic tests as well as in radiotherapy of a hyperactive thyroid gland, most often due to Graves' disease.

(continues on page 392)

GLOSSARY (continued)

Subclinical hyperthyroiism: Mild form of hyperthyroidism, characterized by low TSH and normal T_3 and T_4. The client may have no symptoms at all, or mild symptoms (e.g., weight loss, anxiety) and possibly experience heart and bone problems (Franklyn, 2013).

Subtotal thyroidectomy: Surgical removal a portion of the gland (amount varies), leaving a small amount of thyroid tissue to produce thyroid hormone.

Thyroid storm (thyrotoxicosis): Most commonly associated with Graves' disease, thyrotoxic crisis is caused by a heightened response in the catecholamine receptor sites that intensifies sympathetic nervous system effects on the body. Clinical manifestations include fever, cardiovascular changes, and neurological issues. Without prompt treatment, patients can die from heart failure (Crawford, 2012).

Tremor: Abnormal repetitive shaking movement of the body due to varied causes, including thyroid disease.

Care Setting

Most people with classic hyperthyroidism rarely need hospitalization. Critically ill clients and those with extreme manifestations of thyrotoxicosis, plus a significant concurrent illness, require inpatient acute care on a medical unit.

Related Concerns

Heart failure: chronic, page 43
Psychosocial aspects of care, page 729
Thyroidectomy, on Davis*Plus*

Client Assessment Database

Data depend on the severity and duration of hormone imbalance and involvement of other organs.

DIAGNOSTIC DIVISION MAY REPORT	MAY EXHIBIT
ACTIVITY/REST	
• Nervousness, irritability • Insomnia • Muscle weakness • Incoordination • Extreme fatigue	• Muscle atrophy
CIRCULATION	
• Palpitations • Chest pain (angina)	• Dysrhythmias—atrial fibrillation, gallop rhythm • Tachycardia at rest • Murmurs • Elevated blood pressure (BP) with widened pulse pressure • Circulatory collapse, shock (thyrotoxic crisis)
ELIMINATION	
• Urinating in large amounts • Stool changes; diarrhea	
EGO INTEGRITY	
• Recent stressful experience—emotional and physical	• Emotional lability—mild euphoria to delirium • Anxiety and depression
FOOD/FLUID	
• Recent and sudden weight loss • Increased appetite, large meals, frequent meals, thirst • Nausea and vomiting	• Enlarged thyroid, goiter • Diaphoresis (may be profuse with thyrotoxicosis) • Nonpitting edema, especially in front of the shinbone
NEUROSENSORY	
	• Rapid and hoarse speech • Mental status and behavior alterations—confusion, disorientation, nervousness, irritability, delirium, frank psychosis, stupor, coma

DIAGNOSTIC DIVISION MAY REPORT (continued)	MAY EXHIBIT (continued)
	• Fine tremor in hands; purposeless, quick, jerky movements of body parts • Hyperactive deep tendon reflexes (DTRs) • Paralysis (thyrotoxic hypokalemia)
PAIN/DISCOMFORT • Eye pain, sensitivity to light	
RESPIRATION • Difficulty breathing	• Increased respiratory rate, tachypnea • *Breath sounds:* crackles, wheezes (pulmonary edema associated with thyrotoxic crisis)
SAFETY • Heat intolerance, excessive sweating • Itching skin • Allergy to iodine (may be used in testing)	• Elevated temperature • Skin smooth, warm, and flushed • Exophthalmos, lid retraction, conjunctival irritation, tearing • Pruritic, erythematous lesions—often in pretibial area—that become brawny
SEXUALITY • Decreased libido • Hypomenorrhea, amenorrhea • Impotence	
TEACHING/LEARNING • Family history of thyroid problems • History of hypothyroidism, thyroid hormone replacement therapy or antithyroid therapy, premature withdrawal of antithyroid drugs, recent partial thyroidectomy • History of insulin-induced hypoglycemia, cardiac disorders or surgery, recent illness (pneumonia), trauma, x-ray contrast studies	
DISCHARGE PLAN CONSIDERATIONS • May require assistance with treatment regimen, self-care activities, homemaker and maintenance tasks ➧ Refer to section at end of plan for postdischarge considerations.	

Diagnostic Studies

TEST WHY IT IS DONE	WHAT IT TELLS ME
BLOOD TESTS • *Thyroid function tests:*	
• *TSH:* Measures the amount of TSH in the blood; it is done first to evaluate thyroid function.	TSH is suppressed in hyperthyroidism and suppressed to unmeasurable levels in thyrotoxicosis (except when etiology is a TSH-secreting pituitary tumor or pituitary resistant to thyroid hormone).
• *Tyyroxine (T_4):* Produced by the thyroid gland when the pituitary gland releases TSH. Free T_4 can be measured directly (FT_4) or calculated by index (FTI). Total T_4 measures both bound and free T_4. Free T_4 affects tissue function, whereas bound T_4 does not.	Total T_4, FT_4, and FTI are elevated in hyperthyroidism.

(continues on page 394)

TEST WHY IT IS DONE (continued)	WHAT IT TELLS ME (continued)
• *Triiodothyronine (T_3):* Small amount produced directly by thyroid gland. Most T_3 is made by other tissues that convert T_4 into T_3. T_4 has a greater effect on metabolism than T_3 even though T_3 is normally present in lower amounts than T_4. Total T_3 measures both bound and free T_3 (FT_3).	Both T_3 and T_4 are increased in hyperthyroidism; however, T_3 appears to be the more accurate diagnostic indicator of hyperthyroidism than T_4. T_3 becomes abnormal earlier than T_4 and returns to normal later than T_4 in hyperthyroidism.
• *Triiodothyronine uptake (T_3U):* An indirect measurement of the amount of the protein thyroxine-binding globulin (TBG) that can bind T_3 and T_4.	A high T_4 value combined with a high T_3U value usually confirms the presence of hyperthyroidism.
• *Thyroid antibodies* (the most specific being antithyroid peroxidase [anti-TPO] antibody)	In almost all clients with autoimmune hypothyroidism and up to 80% of those with Graves' disease, anti-TPO levels are elevated (Simmons, 2010).
OTHER DIAGNOSTIC STUDIES	
• *Radioactive iodine uptake (RAIU) thyroid scan:* Measures both thyroid function and thyroid size. During this procedure, the amount of iodine "taken up" by the thyroid is measured and images are taken. A gamma camera scan operating in a fixed position views the entire thyroid gland at once. A computerized rectilinear thyroid (CRT) scan uses computer technology to enhance thyroid nodules.	Shows increased uptake of radioactive iodine in Graves' disease and, usually, in toxic multinodular goiter and toxic adenoma.
• *Thyroid ultrasound:* Uses high-frequency sound waves to obtain an image of the thyroid gland, obtain accurate measurements, and identify nodules. Also aids in performing thyroid needle biopsy by improving accuracy if the nodule cannot be felt easily on examination.	Differentiates a "solid" nodule from a fluid-filled cyst; however, it does not differentiate as to whether a nodule is benign or malignant. Determines if a nodule is getting smaller or is growing larger during treatment.
• *Needle or open biopsy:* May be done to determine cause of thyroid nodules.	Differentiates malignant from benign nodules.

Nursing Priorities

1. Reduce metabolic demands and support cardiovascular function.
2. Provide psychological support.
3. Prevent complications.
4. Provide information about disease process, prognosis, and therapy needs.

Discharge Goals

1. Homeostasis achieved.
2. Current situation being dealt with effectively.
3. Complications prevented and minimized.
4. Disease process, prognosis, and therapeutic regimen understood.
5. Plan in place to meet needs after discharge.

NURSING DIAGNOSIS: risk for decreased Cardiac Output

Risk Factors May Include

Altered preload (changes in venous return)
Altered afterload (systemic vascular resistance)
Alterations in rate, rhythm
(Hypermetabolic state)

Possibly Evidenced By

(Not applicable; presence of signs and symptoms establishes an *actual* diagnosis)

Desired Outcomes/Evaluation Criteria—Client Will

Circulation Status (NOC)

Maintain adequate cardiac output for tissue needs as evidenced by stable vital signs, palpable peripheral pulses, good capillary refill, usual mentation, and absence of dysrhythmias.

ACTIONS/INTERVENTIONS	RATIONALE
Hemodynamic Regulation (NIC)	
Independent	
Monitor BP lying, sitting, and standing, if able. Note widened pulse pressure.	General and orthostatic hypotension may occur as a result of excessive peripheral vasodilation and decreased circulating volume. Widened pulse pressure reflects compensatory increase in stroke volume and decreased SVR.
Monitor central venous pressure (CVP), if available.	Provides more direct measure of circulating volume and cardiac function.
Investigate reports of chest pain and angina.	May reflect increased myocardial oxygen demands and ischemia.
Assess pulse and heart rate while client is sleeping.	Provides a more accurate assessment of tachycardia.
Auscultate heart sounds, noting extra heart sounds and development of gallops and systolic murmurs.	Prominent S_1 and murmurs are associated with forceful cardiac output of hypermetabolic state. Development of S_3 may warn of impending cardiac failure.
Monitor ECG, noting rate and rhythm. Document dysrhythmias.	Tachycardia greater than normally expected, with fever and increased circulatory demand, may reflect direct myocardial stimulation by thyroid hormone. Dysrhythmias often occur and may compromise cardiac function and output.
Auscultate breath sounds, noting adventitious sounds such as crackles.	Early sign of pulmonary congestion, reflecting developing cardiac failure.
Monitor temperature, provide cool environment, limit bed linens and clothes, and administer tepid sponge baths.	Fever, which may exceed 104°F (40.0°C), can occur as a result of excessive hormone levels increasing diuresis and dehydration, causing increased peripheral vasodilation, venous pooling, and hypotension.
Observe for signs and symptoms of severe thirst, dry mucous membranes, weak and thready pulse, poor capillary refill, decreased urinary output, and hypotension.	Rapid dehydration can occur, which reduces circulating volume and compromises cardiac output.
Record intake and output (I&O). Note urine specific gravity.	Significant fluid losses through vomiting, diarrhea, diuresis, or diaphoresis can lead to profound dehydration, concentrated urine, and weight loss.
Weigh daily. Encourage chair rest and bedrest; limit nonessential activity.	Activity increases metabolic and circulatory demands, which may potentiate cardiac failure.
Note history of asthma and bronchoconstrictive disease, sinus bradycardia and heart blocks, advanced heart failure (HF), or current pregnancy.	Presence and potential recurrence of these conditions affects choice of therapy; for example, use of beta-adrenergic blocking agents is contraindicated.
Observe for adverse side effects of adrenergic antagonists, such as severe decrease in pulse and BP, signs of vascular congestion and HF, and cardiac arrest.	Indicates need for reduction and discontinuation of therapy.
Collaborative	
Administer intravenous (IV) fluids, as indicated.	Rapid fluid replacement may be necessary to improve circulating volume, but must be balanced against signs of cardiac failure and need for inotropic support.
Administer medications, as indicated, such as:	
Beta blockers, for example, propranolol (Inderal), atenolol (Tenormin), nadolol (Corgard), and pindolol (Visken)	Beta blockers are the mainstay of symptomatic therapy for thyrotoxicosis, such as tachycardia, tremors, and nervousness. However, their onset is slow and benefit is limited in reducing T_3, so they are typically given along with a thionimide (Ross, 2012).
Thionimides (also called thyroid hormone antagonists), for example, propylthiouracil (PTU) and methimazole (Tapazole)	Antithyroid drugs block thyroid hormone synthesis and inhibit conversion of T_4 to T_3. May be definitive long-term treatment or used to prepare client for surgery, but effect is slow and will not relieve thyroid storm. *Note:* Once PTU therapy is begun, abrupt withdrawal may precipitate thyroid crisis.
Oral iodide-iodine solution (Lugol's solution) or supersaturated potassium iodide (SSKI,PIMA)	May be used in short term (1 to 2 weeks) in preop preparation for thyroidectomy for Graves' disease, or in severe hyperthyroidism, or as an adjunct to antithyroid drugs. *Note:* Should be started 1 to 3 hours after initiation of antithyroid drug therapy to minimize hormone formation from the iodine (Ross, 2012; Schraga, 2012).
Corticosteroids, for example, dexamethasone (Decadron)	Provides glucocorticol support, decreases hyperthermia, relieves relative adrenal insufficiency, inhibits calcium absorption, and reduces peripheral conversion of T_4 to T_3. *Note:* May be given before thyroidectomy and discontinued after surgery.
Digoxin (Lanoxin)	May be required in clients with HF before beta-adrenergic blocking therapy can be considered and safely initiated.

(continues on page 396)

ACTIONS/INTERVENTIONS (continued)	RATIONALE (continued)
Furosemide (Lasix)	Diuresis may be necessary if HF occurs. *Note:* It also may be effective in reducing calcium level if neuromuscular function is impaired.
Potassium (KCl, K-Lyte)	Increased losses of K^+ through intestinal and renal routes may result in dysrhythmias if not corrected.
Acetaminophen (Tylenol)	Drug of choice to reduce temperature and associated metabolic demands. Aspirin is contraindicated because it actually increases level of circulating thyroid hormones by blocking binding of T_3 and T_4 with thyroid-binding proteins.
Sedatives and barbiturates	Promote rest, thereby reducing metabolic demands and cardiac workload.
Muscle relaxants	Reduce shivering associated with hyperthermia, which can further increase metabolic demands.
Monitor laboratory and diagnostic studies, as indicated:	
Serum potassium	Hypokalemia resulting from intestinal losses, altered intake, or diuretic therapy may cause dysrhythmias and compromise cardiac function and output.
Serum calcium	Elevation may alter cardiac contractility.
Sputum culture	Pulmonary infection is most frequent precipitating factor of crisis.
Obtain serial ECGs and other cardiac diagnostic studies (e.g., echocardiogram, myocardial perfusion studies), if indicated.	May demonstrate effects of electrolyte imbalance and/or ischemic changes reflecting inadequate myocardial oxygen supply in presence of increased metabolic demands or dysrhythmias. *Note:* Studies have associated subclinical hyperthyroidism with a higher prevalence of atrial fibrillation (AF) in older clients, confirmed by ECG than those with normal serum TSH (Bahn et al, 2011; Gammage et al, 2007).
Chest x-rays	Cardiac enlargement may occur in response to increased circulatory demands. Pulmonary congestion may be noted with cardiac decompensation.
Provide supplemental oxygen (O_2), as indicated.	May be necessary to support increased metabolic demands and O_2 consumption.
Provide hypothermia blanket, as indicated.	Occasionally used to lower uncontrolled hyperthermia (104°F [40.0°C] and higher) to reduce metabolic demands, O_2 consumption, and cardiac workload.
Prepare for radioactive iodine ablation (RAI) or surgical intervention.	RAI is often the treatment of choice for hyperthyroidism, with the purpose of reversing the overactivity This is referred to as radioactive iodine ablation, or chemical ablation. Peak results take 6 to 12 weeks, and occasionally a second treatment may be necessary; however, a single dose controls hyperthyroidism in about 90% of clients. *Note:* This therapy is contraindicated during pregnancy and breastfeeding (Ross, 2012). Thyroidectomy may be performed once euthyroid state is achieved in individuals who are intolerant of antithyroid medications or who refuse RAI therapy (Schraga, 2012; American Association of Clinical Endocrinologists [AACE], 2006).

NURSING DIAGNOSIS: Fatigue

May Be Related To
Altered body chemistry—hypermetabolic state

Possibly Evidenced By
Reports overwhelming lack of energy, inability to maintain usual routine, decreased performance
Compromised concentration

Desired Outcomes/Evaluation Criteria—Client Will

Fatigue Level (NOC)
Verbalize increase in level of energy.
Display improved ability to participate in desired activities.

ACTIONS/INTERVENTIONS	RATIONALE
Energy Management (NIC)	
Independent	
Monitor vital signs, noting pulse rate at rest and when active.	Pulse is typically elevated, and even at rest tachycardia may be noted.
Note development of tachypnea, dyspnea, pallor, and cyanosis.	O_2 demand and consumption are increased in hypermetabolic state, potentiating risk of hypoxia with activity.
Provide quiet environment, cool room, decreased sensory stimuli, soothing colors, and quiet music.	Reduces stimuli that may aggravate agitation, hyperactivity, and insomnia.
Encourage client to restrict activity and rest in bed as much as possible.	Helps counteract effects of increased metabolism.
Provide comfort measures—judicious touch and massage and cool showers.	May decrease nervous energy, promoting relaxation.
Provide for calming diversional activities—e.g., reading, computer games, television.	Allows for use of nervous energy in a constructive manner, serves as a distraction, and may reduce anxiety.
Avoid topics that irritate or upset client. Discuss ways to respond to these feelings.	Increased irritability of the CNS may cause client to be easily excited, agitated, and prone to emotional outbursts.
Discuss with SO reasons for fatigue and emotional lability.	Understanding that the behavior is physically based may enhance coping with current situation and encourage SO to respond positively and provide support for client.
Collaborative	
Administer medications, as indicated, such as sedatives and anti-anxiety agents.	May be prescribed to help combat nervousness, hyperactivity, and insomnia.

NURSING DIAGNOSIS: risk for imbalanced Nutrition: less than body requirements

Risk Factors May Include

Biological factors—metabolic demands, relative insulin insufficiency, hyperglycemia
Inability to ingest food or absorb nutrients (nausea, vomiting, diarrhea)

Possibly Evidenced By

(Not applicable; presence of signs and symptoms establishes an *actual* diagnosis)

Desired Outcomes/Evaluation Criteria—Client Will

Nutritional Status (NOC)

Demonstrate stable weight with normal laboratory values and be free of signs of malnutrition.

ACTIONS/INTERVENTIONS	RATIONALE
Nutrition Therapy (NIC)	
Independent	
Monitor daily food intake. Weigh daily and report losses.	Continued weight loss in face of adequate caloric intake may indicate failure of antithyroid therapy.
Encourage client to eat and increase number of meals and snacks, using high-calorie foods that are easily digested.	Aids in keeping caloric intake high enough to keep up with rapid expenditure of calories caused by hypermetabolic state.
Avoid foods that increase peristalsis, such as tea, coffee, fibrous and highly seasoned foods, and fluids that cause diarrhea—apple and prune juice.	Increased motility of gastrointestinal (GI) tract may result in diarrhea and impair absorption of needed nutrients.
Collaborative	
Consult with dietitian to provide diet high in calories, protein, carbohydrates, and vitamins.	May need assistance to ensure adequate intake of nutrients, identify appropriate supplements.
Administer medications, as indicated, such as glucose and vitamin B complex.	Given to meet energy requirements and prevent or correct hypoglycemia.

NURSING DIAGNOSIS: Anxiety [specify level]

May Be Related To

Stress; situational crisis (CNS stimulation, pseudocatecholamine effect of thyroid hormones); change in health status

Possibly Evidenced By

Apprehensive; jittery; shakiness; distressed
Difficulty concentrating
Focus on self; restlessness; tremors
Sleep disturbance

Desired Outcomes/Evaluation Criteria—Client Will

Anxiety Level (NOC)

Appear relaxed.
Report anxiety reduced to a manageable level.

Anxiety Self-Control (NOC)

Identify healthy ways to deal with feelings.
Recognize changes in thinking and behavior and causative factors.

ACTIONS/INTERVENTIONS	RATIONALE
Anxiety Reduction (NIC)	
Independent	
Monitor changes in behavior. Note behavior indicative of level of anxiety.	May be hypervigilant, restless, extremely sensitive, or crying, or may develop frank psychosis. Mild anxiety may be displayed by irritability and insomnia. Severe anxiety progressing to panic state may produce feelings of impending doom, terror, inability to speak or move, shouting, and swearing. *Note*: Anxiety may alter thought processes and ability to think clearly.
Assess thinking processes, such as memory; attention span; and orientation to person, place, time, and situation.	Determines extent of interference with sensory processing.
Monitor physical responses, noting palpitations, repetitive movements, hyperventilation, and insomnia.	Increased number of beta-adrenergic receptor sites, coupled with effects of excess thyroid hormones, produces clinical manifestations of catecholamine excess even when normal levels of norepinephrine and epinephrine exist.
Stay with client, maintaining calm manner. Acknowledge feelings and allow client's behavior to belong to client.	Affirms to client and SO that although client feels out of control, environment is safe. Avoiding personal responses to inappropriate remarks or actions prevents conflicts and overreaction to stressful situation and client behavior.
Describe and explain procedures, surrounding environment, or sounds that may be heard by client. Present reality concisely and briefly without challenging illogical thinking.	Provides accurate information, which reduces distortions and misinterpretations that can contribute to anxiety and fear reactions. Avoiding challenging of distorted thinking limits defensive reaction.
Speak in brief statements, using simple words.	Attention span may be shortened and concentration reduced, limiting ability to assimilate information.
Reduce external stimuli. Place in quiet, cool room; provide soft, soothing music; reduce bright lights; limit procedures and reduce number of persons interacting with client.	Creates a therapeutic environment, shows recognition that unit activity and personnel may increase client's anxiety. May decrease hyperactivity and CNS irritability.
Provide safety measures, such as padded side rails, close supervision, or use of soft restraints as last resort, as necessary.	Prevents injury to client who may be hallucinating and disoriented.
Discuss with client and SO reasons for emotional lability or psychotic reaction.	Understanding that behavior is physically based enhances acceptance of situation and encourages different responses and approaches.
Reinforce expectation that emotional control should return as drug therapy progresses.	Provides information and reassures client that the situation is temporary and will improve with treatment.
Collaborative	
Administer medications as indicated, e.g., anti-anxiety agents or sedatives, and monitor effects.	May be used in conjunction with medical regimen to reduce effects of hyperthyroid secretion. Promotes relaxation and reduces CNS hyperactivity and agitation, enhancing thinking ability and sense of control. *Note:* Antithyroid drugs combined with beta-adrenoreceptor antagonists are the treatment of choice for hyperthyroidism, as well as the psychiatric disorders and mental symptoms caused by the disorder (Bunevicius, 2006).

ACTIONS/INTERVENTIONS (continued)	RATIONALE (continued)
Refer to support systems, as needed, including counseling, social services, and pastoral care.	Ongoing therapy support may be desired and required by client and SO if crisis precipitates lifestyle alterations. *Note:* When psychiatric symptoms remain after restoration of euthyroidism, specific treatment with psychotropic drugs may be indicated (Bunevicius, 2006).

NURSING DIAGNOSIS: risk for Dry Eye

Risk Factors May Include

Altered protective mechanisms of eye—reduced ability to blink, eye dryness
Periorbital edema

Possibly Evidenced By

(Not applicable; presence of signs and symptoms establishes an *actual* diagnosis)

Desired Outcomes/Evaluation Criteria—Client Will

Dry Eye Severity (NOC)

Maintain moist eye membranes, free of ulcerations.

Risk Control: Dry Eye (NOC)

Identify measures to provide protection for eyes and prevent complications.

ACTIONS/INTERVENTIONS	RATIONALE
Surveillance (NIC)	
Independent	
Encourage use of dark glasses when awake and taping the eyelids shut during sleep, as needed.	Protects exposed cornea if client is unable to close eyelids completely because of edema and fibrosis of fat pads.
Elevate the head of the bed and restrict salt intake, if indicated.	Decreases tissue edema when appropriate.
Instruct client in extraocular muscle exercises, if appropriate.	Improves circulation and maintains mobility of the eyelids.
Provide opportunity for client to discuss feelings about altered appearance and measures to enhance self-image.	Protruding eyes may be viewed as unattractive. Appearance can be enhanced with proper use of makeup, overall grooming, and use of shaded glasses.
Collaborative	
Administer medications, as indicated, for example:	In severe Graves' disease the eyes may be protruding, the eyelids may not close all of the way during sleep or normal blinking, causing irritation of the eyeballs and increased pressure (glaucoma).
Eye drops, ointments, and artificial tears, corticosteroids, and antithyroid drugs	To minimize eye irritation, artificial tears may be used several times per day and ointments may be applied at night to prevent the eyes from drying out. Steroids may be given to reduce swelling behind the eyes (Bahn, 2011; Bedinghaus, 2008).
Prepare for surgery, as indicated.	Although these procedures are rare, an orbital decompression surgery may be performed if the eyes are markedly protruding. The removal of the thin bones that make up the orbit of the eye allows the eyes to move back to a more normal position. Eye muscle surgery may be performed, and eyeglass prisms may be prescribed if the eye muscles are so swollen that the eyes can no longer be aligned properly (Bedinghaus, 2008).

NURSING DIAGNOSIS: deficient Knowledge [Learning Need] regarding condition, prognosis, treatment, self-care, and discharge needs

May Be Related To

Lack of exposure or recall
Information misinterpretation
Unfamiliarity with information resources

(continues on page 400)

NURSING DIAGNOSIS: deficient Knowledge [Learning Need] regarding condition, prognosis, treatment, self-care, and discharge needs (continued)

Possibly Evidenced By

Reports the problem
Inaccurate follow-through of instructions

Desired Outcomes/Evaluation Criteria—Client Will

Knowledge: Acute Illness Care (NOC)

Verbalize understanding of disease process and potential complications.
Identify relationship of signs and symptoms to the disease process and correlate symptoms with causative factors.
Verbalize understanding of therapeutic needs.
Participate in treatment regimen.
Initiate necessary lifestyle changes.

ACTIONS/INTERVENTIONS	RATIONALE
Teaching: Disease Process (NIC)	
Independent	
Review disease process and future expectations.	Provides knowledge base from which client can make informed choices.
Provide information appropriate to individual situation.	Severity of condition, cause, age, and concurrent complications determine course of treatment.
Identify stressors and discuss precipitators to thyroid crises—personal, social, and job concerns; infection; and pregnancy.	Psychogenic factors are often of prime importance in the occurrence and exacerbation of this disease.
Discuss drug therapy, including need for adhering to regimen and expected therapeutic and side effects.	Antithyroid medication, either as primary therapy or in preparation for thyroidectomy, requires adherence to a medical regimen over an extended period to inhibit hormone production. Agranulocytosis (lack of enough of a specific type of white blood cells, called neutrophils or granulocytes) is the most serious side effect that can occur, and alternative drugs may be given if problems arise.
Identify signs and symptoms requiring medical evaluation, such as fever, sore throat, and skin eruptions.	Early identification of toxic reactions (thiourea therapy) and prompt intervention are important in preventing development of agranulocytosis.
Explain need to check with physician and pharmacist before taking other prescribed or over-the-counter (OTC) drugs.	Antithyroid medications can affect or be affected by numerous other medications, requiring monitoring of medication levels, side effects, and interactions.
Emphasize importance of planned rest periods.	Prevents undue fatigue and reduces metabolic demands. As euthyroid state is achieved, stamina and activity level will improve.
Review need for nutritious diet and periodic review of nutrient needs; avoid caffeine, red and yellow food dyes, and artificial preservatives.	Provides adequate nutrients to support hypermetabolic state. As hormonal imbalance is corrected, diet will need to be readjusted to prevent excessive weight gain. Irritants and stimulants should be limited to avoid cumulative systemic effects.
Emphasize necessity of continued medical follow-up.	Required to monitor effectiveness of therapy and for prevention of potentially fatal complications.

POTENTIAL CONSIDERATIONS following acute hospitalization (dependent on client's age, physical condition and presence of complications, personal resources, and life responsibilities)

- ***risk for imbalanced Nutrition: more than body requirements***—decrease in metabolic rate, excessive intake in relation to metabolic needs.

HEPATITIS

I. Pathophysiology

a. Causes widespread damage to liver cells (hepatocytes) either directly or indirectly from inflammation or autoimmune response

b. May be acute or chronic

i. Acute: Swelling of hepatocytes reduces ability to detoxify drugs; produce clotting factors, plasma proteins, bile, and glycogen; and store fat-soluble vitamins.

ii. Chronic: Inflammation and necrosis of liver of more than 6 months' duration. Approximately 20% of patients with chronic hepatitis B or hepatitis C eventually develop cirrhosis, as evidenced by the histologic changes of severe fibrosis and nodular regeneration (Buggs, 2012).

II. Etiology

a. Infectious causes: viral, bacterial, fungal, or parasitic
   i. Viruses are designated by letters A through G, with several terms used interchangeably, for example, hepatitis B is known as HBV or HepB.
   ii. HAV, HBV, HCV, and HDV are the only hepatitis viruses endemic to the United States.
   iii. HAV, HBV, and HCV are responsible for more than 90% of U.S. cases of acute viral hepatitis, with HAV the most common cause of acute hepatitis and HCV the most common cause of chronic hepatitis (Buggs, 2012; Gilroy, 2012).
   iv. Transmission frequency: The following are typical patterns by which hepatitis viruses are transmitted, with + symbols indicating the frequency of transmission (i.e., more + symbols indicate increased frequency): (1) Fecal-oral: HAV (+++), HEV (+++); (2) Parenteral: HBV (+++), HCV (+++), HDV (++), HGV (++), HAV (+); (3) Sexual: HBV (+++), HDV (++), HCV (+); and (4) Perinatal: HBV (+++), HCV (+), HDV (+) (Buggs, 2012).
   v. Other viruses: cytomegalovirus (CMV), Epstein-Barr virus (EBV), *Mycobacterium avium* complex (MAC), herpes simplex, varicella-zoster, toxoplasmosis, and histoplasmosis

b. Noninfectious causes: physical or toxic chemical agents, autoimmune
   i. Toxic agents: carbon tetrachloride, vinyl chloride; alcohol, cocaine, acetaminophen, isoniazid, anabolic steroids, methyldopa, erythromycin; poisonous mushrooms
   ii. Autoimmune: no identifiable etiology; two types, with type 1 most common form in North America

III. Statistics

a. Morbidity
   i. Between 1995 and 2006, reported hepatitis A incidence declined by 90% to the lowest rate ever recorded, 1.2 cases per 100,000 population (Wasley, 2008). The Centers for Disease Control and Prevention (CDC) reported 1,670 acute clinical cases of HAV in 2010, estimated clinical cases at 7,000; and estimated that the number of new infections in the United States would be around 17,000 (CDC, 2012).
   ii. According to the CDC, 3374 acute cases of HBV were reported in 2010, down from 3350 in 2008. However, CDC estimated that 9000 clinical cases were unreported; and it estimated 38,000 new infections for 2010, with 22,000 of those being pregnant women in the United States who could transmit the virus to their newborns.
   iii. CDC data show 853 cases of acute clinical HCV reported for 2010, with an estimated 2800 acute clinical cases and 17,000 estimated new infections (CDC, 2012).

b. Mortality: Deaths reported by CDC National Vital Statistics to be directly related to hepatitis (per mortality/death certificates) for the year 2007 were as follows: HAV: 85; HBV: 1.815; HVC: 15,106 (Xu et al, 2010).

c. Cost: Direct care costs for all forms of viral hepatitis estimated at over $1.3 billion in 2004 (Everhart, 2008).

GLOSSARY

Acute hepatitis: Often self-limiting, although approximately 5% to 10% of clients with HBV and 80% to 85% of clients with HCV progress to a chronic state (Buggs 2012).

Anorexia: Loss of appetite as result of disease.

Ascites: Buildup of fluid in the abdomen due to a number of conditions, including severe liver disease.

Asterixis: Involuntary jerking movements of hands and feet associated with hepatic encephalopathy.

Autoimmune: Persistent inflammation and necrosis with hypergammaglobulinemia and autoantibodies without other common causes of hepatitis.

Biological response modifiers (BMRs): Substances that stimulate the body's response to infection and disease.

Chronic hepatitis: Persistent inflammation and necrosis lasting more than 6 months, commonly due to hepatitis B, C, or D virus.

Ecchymosis: Skin discoloration consisting of a large, irregularly formed hemorrhagic area, with colors changing from blue-black to greenish-brown or yellow; commonly called a bruise.

Fulminant hepatitis: Occurs suddenly and with great intensity or severity, progressing to encephalopathy within 8 weeks of onset and death if liver transplant is not performed.

Hepatic encephalopathy: Brain dysfunction directly due to the liver dysfunction most often seen in advanced cirrhosis. Encephalopathy may cause disturbances of consciousness and progress to coma.

Hepatocyte: Parenchymal liver cell.

Jaundice: Yellow staining of the skin and sclerae (and sometimes other tissues and body fluids) by abnormally high blood levels of the bile pigment bilirubin.

Melena: Bloody stools.

Palmar erythema: Redness of the palms of the hands caused by dilation and congestion of capillaries.

Pruritus: Severe itching of the skin.

Right upper quadrant (RUQ): Anatomic location of the liver.

Spider angiomas: Abnormal collection of blood vessels near the surface of the skin, which can occur anywhere but are most common on the face and trunk.

Splenomegaly: Enlarged spleen.

Toxic hepatitis: Liver inflammation often due to common drugs used to treat disease or chemicals found in the workplace.

Urticaria: Vascular reaction of the skin marked by transient appearance of slightly elevated patches, which are more red or pale than the surrounding skin and often are accompanied by severe itching; may also be called hives.

Care Setting

Care is most often provided in the outpatient setting or at the community level. In states of acute hepatic inflammation, brief inpatient acute care on a medical unit may be required to monitor and treat hepatic failure or hepatic encephalopathy.

Related Concerns

Alcohol: acute withdrawal, page 800
Cirrhosis of the liver, page 412
Psychosocial aspects of care, page 729
Renal dialysis—general considerations, page 529
Substance use disorders, page 815
Total nutritional support: parenteral/enteral feeding, page 437

Client Assessment Database

Data depend on the cause (type of hepatitis) and severity of liver involvement and damage.

DIAGNOSTIC DIVISION MAY REPORT	MAY EXHIBIT
ACTIVITY/REST	
• Fatigue • Weakness, general malaise, muscle aches	
CIRCULATION	
	• Bradycardia—in severe hyperbilirubinemia • Jaundiced sclera, skin, mucous membranes
ELIMINATION	
• Dark urine, clay-colored stools • Diarrhea, constipation	
FOOD/FLUID	
• Loss of appetite, weight loss • Weight gain—edema, ascites • Nausea, vomiting	• Ascites • Abdominal distention due to liver enlargement
NEUROSENSORY	
	• Irritability, drowsiness, lethargy • Asterixis
PAIN/DISCOMFORT	
• Abdominal cramping, RUQ tenderness • Joint pain • Headache	• Muscle guarding, restlessness
SAFETY	
• Blood transfusions or organ transplant received prior to viral screening tests • Tattoos (possible equipment source) • Itching (pruritus)	• Fever—usually low grade • Urticaria, maculopapular lesions, irregular patches of erythema • Spider angiomas, palmar erythema, gynecomastia in men (sometimes present in alcoholic hepatitis) • Splenomegaly, posterior cervical node enlargement
SEXUALITY	
• Lifestyle or behaviors increasing risk of exposure—unprotected sexual intercourse with infected person	
TEACHING/LEARNING	
• History of known or possible exposure to virus, bacteria, or toxins—from contaminated food, water, needles, surgical equipment or blood; carriers (symptomatic or asymptomatic); recent surgical procedure with halothane anesthesia; exposure to toxic chemicals, such as carbon tetrachloride, vinyl chloride	

DIAGNOSTIC DIVISION MAY REPORT (continued)	MAY EXHIBIT (continued)
• History of known or possible exposure to hepatotoxic prescription, such as sulfonamides, phenothiazines, isoniazid, or over-the-counter (OTC) drug use, such as acetaminophen • Use of herbal supplements associated with hepatotoxicity, such as chaparral, Jin Bu Huan, germander, comfrey, mistletoe, skullcap, margosa oil, pennyroyal • Use of street injection drugs or alcohol • Travel to or immigration from China, Africa, Southeast Asia, Middle East (HBV and HCV are endemic in these areas) • Concurrent diabetes, heart failure (HF), malignancy, or renal disease **Discharge Plan Considerations** • May require assistance with homemaking, maintenance tasks, shopping, transportation ➧ Refer to section at end of plan for postdischarge considerations.	

Diagnostic Studies

TEST WHY IT IS DONE	WHAT IT TELLS ME
Blood Tests	
• ***Acute viral hepatitis panel:*** Used to help detect and/or diagnose an acute liver infection due to one of the three most common hepatitis viruses: hepatitis A virus (HAV), hepatitis B virus (HBV), or hepatitis C virus (HCV).	These tests are used to determine if symptoms are due to a current infection with a virus and to identify which virus in particular is causing the disease. These tests may also help determine if someone has been exposed to one of the viruses even before symptoms develop. An acute hepatitis panel typically consists of the following tests (adapted from Labtestsonline 2010): • Hepatitis A antibody, IgM—Body produces antibodies early after exposure. so positive Hepatitis A IgM test is usually considered diagnostic for acute Hepatitis A. • Hepatitis B core antibody, IgM—The first antibody produced in response to a Hepatitis B infection and, when detected, may indicate an acute infection. It may also be present in people with chronic hepatitis B when flares occur. • Hepatitis B surface Ag—Earliest indicator of acute infection but may also be present in blood of person chronically infected. • Hepatitis C antibody—Test detects antibodies produced in response to HCV infection. It cannot distinguish between an active or previous infection. If positive, it is typically followed up with other tests to determine if the infection is a current one.
• ***Liver enzymes/isoenzymes:*** Of limited value in differentiating viral from nonviral hepatitis.	Abnormal—may be 4 to 10 times normal values.
• ***Alanine aminotransferase (ALT):*** Considered best liver enzyme test for detecting hepatitis.	Elevation usually occurs before other symptoms, such as jaundice, are noted.
• ***Complete blood count (CBC):*** Battery of screening tests that typically includes hemoglobin (Hgb); hematocrit (Hct); red blood cell (RBC) count, morphology, indices, and distribution width index; platelet count and size; white blood cell (WBC) count and differential—the percentage of each of the five types of mature WBCs: neutrophils, lymphocytes (B cells and T cells), monocytes, eosinophils, and basophils.	RBCs are decreased because of shortened life span of RBCs—liver enzyme alterations or hemorrhage. WBCs may be abnormally low (leukopenia) or high (leukocytosis); monocytes may be increased (monocytosis), and lymphocytes may be increased and atypical in appearance.

(continues on page 404)

Diagnostic Studies (continued)

TEST WHY IT IS DONE (continued)	WHAT IT TELLS ME (continued)
• *Serum albumin:* Measures the main body protein manufactured by the liver.	Level is decreased.
• *Prothrombin time (PT):* One of several clotting factors that is produced by the liver. Evaluates the body's ability to produce a clot in a reasonable amount of time.	May be prolonged—liver dysfunction.
• *Serum bilirubin:* Yellow-red substance that results from the breakdown of Hgb, a normal process of the liver, then excreted via the intestines.	High level indicates the liver is incapable of adequately removing bilirubin in a timely manner due to blockage of bile ducts or liver disease, such as acute hepatitis. Accumulation of bilirubin is responsible for jaundice of the skin and mucous membranes.
Associated Tests	
• *Liver biopsy:* Considered if diagnosis is uncertain or if clinical course is atypical or unduly prolonged.	Provides initial assessment of disease severity in client with chronic HBV or chronic HVC.
• *Urinalysis:* Checks the urine for bilirubin for the nonjaundiced client with suspected viral hepatitis.	Elevated bilirubin levels and proteinuria and hematuria may occur.

Nursing Priorities

1. Reduce demands on liver while promoting physical well-being.
2. Prevent complications.
3. Enhance self-concept and acceptance of situation.
4. Provide information about disease process, prognosis, and treatment needs.

Discharge Goals

1. Basic self-care needs are met.
2. Complications prevented or minimized.
3. Dealing with reality of current situation.
4. Disease process, prognosis, transmission, and therapeutic regimen understood.
5. Plan in place to meet needs after discharge.

NURSING DIAGNOSIS: impaired Liver Function

May Be Related To

Viral infection (e.g., viruses A, B, C, D), Epstein-Barr
HIV coinfection
Hepatotoxic medications (e.g., acetaminophen, statins)
Substance abuse (e.g., alcohol, cocaine)

Possibly Evidenced By

Presence of virus or antibodies, abnormal liver function tests
Presence of jaundice, hepatic enlargement

Desired Outcomes/Evaluation Criteria—Client Will

Knowledge: Acute Illness Management (NOC)
Demonstrate behaviors or lifestyle changes to limit effects of condition.

Liver Function (NOC)
Be free of signs of liver failure as evidenced by liver function studies within normal limits (WNL) and absence of jaundice, hepatic enlargement, or altered mental status.

ACTIONS/INTERVENTIONS	RATIONALE
Infection Control/Substance Use Treatment (NIC)	
Independent	
Determine presence of condition(s), as listed above. Note whether problem is acute—viral hepatitis or acetaminophen overdose—or chronic—long-standing alcoholic or viral hepatitis.	Influences choice of interventions.
Review usual and/or occasional use medications—sulfonamides, phenothiazines, isoniazid—for hepatotoxic drugs or OTC drug use such as acetaminophen.	May require changes in usual medication regimen and client education about hepatic effects of OTC drugs.

ACTIONS/INTERVENTIONS	RATIONALE
Ascertain if client works in high-risk occupation; for example, performs tasks that involve contact with blood, blood-contaminated body fluids, other body fluids, or sharps or needles.	Helps in identifying source of infection—occupational high risk for exposure to HBV and HCV.
Assess for exposure to contaminated food or untreated drinking water or for evidence of poor sanitation practices by food-service workers, if source is known.	Helps in identifying source of infection—risk for exposure to enteric viruses, such as HAV and HEV.
Collaborative	
Review results of laboratory tests, such as hepatitis viral titers, liver function, and other diagnostic studies.	Identifies cause of hepatitis, influences choice of interventions, and monitors response to therapies.
Assist with treatment of underlying condition.	Supports organ function and minimizes liver damage and risk of organ failure. For chronic HBV and HCV infections, in particular, the goals of therapy are to reduce liver inflammation and fibrosis and to prevent progression to cirrhosis and the associated complications (Buggs, 2012).
Administer medications, as indicated, for example:	The particular or combination of medication used depends on the type of infection. Because treatment regimens for hepatitis are being actively researched, medication recommendations, indications, and dosages are all subject to change.
Antivirals, such as ribavirin (Rebetol), boceprivir (Victrelis), famciclovir (Famvir), entecavir (Baraclude)	Inhibit viral reproduction. Used in conjunction with interferon or peginterferon to improve the effectiveness of these drugs (Buggs 2012), especially in removing the higher HCV RNA loads associated with HIV coinfection (Hepbfoundation, 2012). Combination therapy has a lower relapse rate than monotherapy (National Institute of Diabetes and Digestive and Kidney Disorders [NIDDK], no date). *Note:* These treatments lead to improvement, not cure, of the disease.
Nucleoside analogues, such as lamivudine (Epivar), adefovir (Hespera), entecavir (Baraclude), tenofovir (Viread)	Help reduce viral load and treat chronic active HBV. Often used in combinations. Alternative choice for individuals unable or unwilling to use interferon, or in the presence of impaired immune function such as coinfection with HIV (Hepbfoundation, 2012).
Interferons such as IFN alpha-2a (Roferon A) and IFN alpha-2b (Intron A)	These agents are naturally produced proteins with antiviral, antitumor, and immunomodulatory actions. IFN alpha, beta, and gamma may be given topically, systemically, and intralesionally (Buggs, 2012). Reduces viral load and may lead to temporary improvement in liver function in HVB, C, and D (Hepbfoundation, 2010).
Pegylated interferons, such as pegIFN alpha-2a (Pegasys) and pegIFN alpha-2b (Peg-Intron)	These agents have largely replaced standard interferons in the treatment of HCV and may be used in combination therapy with antivirals such as ribavirin (Rebetol), boceprivir (Victrelis), and protease inhibitor such as TVR (Incivek) (Yee et al, 2012).
Steroid therapy, such as prednisone (Deltasone), alone or in combination with azathioprine (Imuran)	Steroids may be contraindicated because they can increase risk of relapse or development of chronic hepatitis in clients with viral hepatitis; however, anti-inflammatory effect may be useful in chronic active hepatitis, especially idiopathic, to reduce nausea and vomiting and to enable client to retain food and fluids. A brief course may also be useful in cholestatic HAV to shorten the illness (Buggs, 2012). Steroids may decrease serum aminotransferase and bilirubin levels, but they do not affect liver necrosis or regeneration. Combination therapy has fewer steroid-related side effects.
Administer antidote or assist with procedures as indicated, such as lavage, catharsis, or hyperventilation, depending on route of exposure.	Removal of causative agent in toxic hepatitis may limit degree of tissue involvement and damage.
Refer to specialist or liver treatment center for consideration of other treatment options, for example, transplantation, as indicated.	Currently, almost one-half of all liver transplants in the United States are performed for end-stage HCV. However, reinfection of the transplanted liver by the virus usually occurs and may require a second transplant (Verna, 2006).

NURSING DIAGNOSIS: Fatigue

May Be Related To
Disease states
Stress
Altered body chemistry (e.g., changes in liver function, effect on target organs)

Possibly Evidenced By
Reports of unremitting lack of energy, inability to maintain usual routines
Decreased performance
Increase in physical complaints

Desired Outcomes/Evaluation Criteria—Client Will

Fatigue Level (NOC)
Report improved sense of energy.
Perform activities of daily living (ADLs) and participate in desired activities at level of ability.

ACTIONS/INTERVENTIONS	RATIONALE
Energy Management (NIC)	
Independent	
Encourage bedrest and chair (recliner) rest during toxic state, and frequent rest periods during recovery. Provide quiet environment and limit visitors as needed.	Available energy can be used for healing. Activity and an upright position are believed to decrease hepatic blood flow, which prevents optimal circulation to the liver cells.
Recommend changing position frequently. Model and instruct caregiver in good skin care.	Promotes optimal respiratory function and minimizes pressure areas to reduce risk of tissue breakdown.
Do necessary tasks quickly and at one time, as tolerated.	Allows for extended periods of uninterrupted rest.
Determine and prioritize role responsibilities, alternative providers, and possible community resources available, such as Meals on Wheels and homemaker and housekeeper services.	Promotes problem-solving of most pressing needs of individual and family.
Identify energy-conserving techniques, such as sitting to shower and brush teeth, planning steps of activity so that all needed materials are at hand, and scheduling rest periods.	Helps minimize fatigue, allowing client to accomplish more and feel better about self.
Increase activity as tolerated. Demonstrate and perform range-of-motion (ROM) exercises.	Prolonged bedrest can be debilitating. This can be offset by limited activity alternating with rest periods.
Encourage and instruct in stress management techniques, such as progressive relaxation, visualization, and guided imagery, as desired. Discuss appropriate diversional activities, such as music, Internet surfing and/or games, TV, and reading.	Promotes relaxation and conserves energy, redirects attention, and may enhance coping.
Monitor for recurrence of anorexia and liver tenderness and enlargement.	Indicates lack of resolution or exacerbation of the disease, requiring further rest and change in therapeutic regimen.
Collaborative	
Administer medications, as indicated, for example, sedatives and anti-anxiety agents, such as diazepam (Valium) and lorazepam (Ativan).	Assists in managing required rest. *Note:* Use of certain medications such as prochlorperazine (Compazine) and chlorpromazine (Thorazine) is contraindicated because of hepatotoxic effects.
Monitor serial liver enzyme levels.	Aids in determining appropriate levels of activity because premature increase in activity potentiates risk of relapse.

NURSING DIAGNOSIS: imbalanced Nutrition: less than body requirements

May Be Related To
Inability to ingest food—anorexia, nausea, vomiting
Inability to digest food/absorb nutrients—reduced peristalsis, bile stasis
[Increased caloric demands]

Possibly Evidenced By
Aversion to eating, lack of interest in food; reported altered taste sensation
Abdominal pain, cramping
Loss of weight, poor muscle tone

NURSING DIAGNOSIS: imbalanced Nutrition: less than body requirements (continued)

Desired Outcomes/Evaluation Criteria—Client Will

Weight Maintenance Behavior (NOC)
Initiate behaviors and lifestyle changes to regain or maintain appropriate weight.

Nutritional Status (NOC)
Demonstrate progressive weight gain toward goal with normalization of laboratory values and no signs of malnutrition.

ACTIONS/INTERVENTIONS	RATIONALE
Weight Gain Assistance (NIC)	
Independent	
Note reports of/presence of anorexia, nausea and vomiting, diarrhea.	May be present because of the underlying disease or from side effects of certain treatments.
Monitor dietary intake and calorie count, if indicated.	May be required if client is severely anorexic, to assess deficits and needs.
Provide meals in several small feedings and offer largest meal at breakfast.	Large meals are difficult to manage when client is anorexic. Anorexia may also worsen during the day, making intake of food difficult later in the day.
Offer and make available snacks and calorie-dense fluids between meals, and whenever client feels some appetite.	Improves total daily intake of nutrients, especially if client has access to foods that do not require cooking, e.g., liquid food supplements, single-package foods, snacks that don't require refrigeration.
Encourage intake of plenty of fluids throughout the day (e.g., glass of water at beginning and end of day, ice chips or water bottle handy at all times).	Some treatments (e.g., ribavirin) cause dehydration, dry mouth, and thick saliva, which can interfere with food intake.
Limit fluids at mealtime and/or carbonated sugar containing beverages.	These can fill the stomach rapidly and interfere with appetite for food.
Provide bland foods, and foods and fluids high in soluble fiber and electrolytes, as indicated.	These may be helpful if client has diarrhea associated with disease process or treatments.
Encourage mouth care before meals and after-dinner mints, chewing gum, etc.	Rinsing mouth with saline or soda water, tea, ginger ale before eating can help clear taste buds and eliminate unpleasant taste associated with disease condition or treatments. Lemon drops, zinc lozenges, mints, or gum can help get rid of bad or "off" tastes that linger after eating.
Recommend eating in upright position.	Reduces sensation of abdominal fullness and may enhance intake.
Encourage intake of fruit juices or smoothies, milk shakes, iced tea, other noncarbonated beverages; saltines or animal crackers; hard candy throughout the day.	These supply extra calories and may be more easily digested and tolerated than other fluids and foods.
Collaborative	
Consult with dietitian or nutritional support team to provide diet according to client's needs, with fat and protein intake as tolerated.	Useful in formulating dietary program to meet individual needs. Fat metabolism varies according to bile production and excretion and may necessitate restriction of fat intake if diarrhea develops. If tolerated, a normal or increased protein intake helps with liver regeneration. Protein restriction may be indicated in severe disease, such as fulminating hepatitis, because the accumulation of the end products of protein metabolism can potentiate hepatic encephalopathy (Daniel, 2008).
Monitor serum glucose, as indicated.	Hyperglycemia or hypoglycemia may develop, necessitating dietary changes or insulin administration. Fingerstick monitoring may be done by client on a regular schedule to determine therapy needs.
Administer medications, as indicated, for example:	
Antiemetics, such as metoclopramide (Reglan) and trimethobenzamide (Tigan)	Given before meals, these drugs may reduce nausea and increase food tolerance. *Note:* Prochlorperazine (Compazine) is contraindicated in hepatic disease.
Antiulcer agents and antacids, such as lansoprazole (Prevacid), esomeprazole (Nexium), and magnesium hydroxide/aluminum hydroxide (Maalox, Mylanta), as indicated	Counteracts gastric acidity, reducing irritation and risk of bleeding.
Vitamins, such as B complex, C, and other dietary supplements, as indicated	Corrects deficiencies and aids in the healing process.
Provide supplemental feedings, enteral or parenteral nutrition if needed.	May be necessary to meet nutrient requirements if marked deficits are present and intestinal symptoms are prolonged.

NURSING DIAGNOSIS: risk for deficient Fluid Volume/Bleeding

Risk Factors May Include

Excessive losses through normal routes—vomiting, diarrhea
Failure of regulatory mechanisms—third-space shift
Active fluid loss—altered clotting process

Possibly Evidenced By

(Not applicable; presence of signs and symptoms establishes an *actual* diagnosis)

Desired Outcomes/Evaluation Criteria—Client Will

Fluid Balance (NOC)

Maintain adequate hydration, as evidenced by stable vital signs, good skin turgor, capillary refill, strong peripheral pulses, and individually appropriate urinary output.

Blood Coagulation (NOC)

Be free of signs of hemorrhage with clotting times WNL.

ACTIONS/INTERVENTIONS	RATIONALE
Fluid/Electrolyte Management (NIC)	
Independent	
Monitor intake and output (I&O) and compare periodic weights. Note enteric losses, such as vomiting and diarrhea.	Provides information about replacement needs and effects of therapy. *Note:* Diarrhea may be due to transient flulike response to viral infection or may represent a more serious problem of obstructed portal blood flow with vascular congestion in the gastrointestinal (GI) tract. Or, it may be the intended result of medication use, such as neomycin or lactulose, to decrease serum ammonia levels in the presence of hepatic encephalopathy.
Assess vital signs, peripheral pulses, capillary refill, skin turgor, and mucous membranes.	Indicators of circulating volume and perfusion.
Bleeding Precautions (NIC)	
Check for ascites and edema formation. Measure abdominal girth, as indicated.	Useful in monitoring progression and resolution of fluid shifts associated with edema and ascites.
Use small-gauge needles for injections, applying pressure for longer than usual after venipuncture.	Reduces possibility of bleeding into tissues.
Have client use cotton or sponge swabs and alcohol-free mouthwash instead of toothbrush.	Avoids trauma and bleeding of the gums. *Note:* Alcohol-based mouthwash may be irritating to dry mucosa.
Observe for signs of bleeding—hematuria and melena, ecchymosis, and oozing from gums or puncture sites.	Prothrombin levels are reduced and coagulation times prolonged when vitamin K absorption is altered in GI tract, and synthesis of prothrombin is decreased in affected liver.
Fluid/Electrolyte Management (NIC)	
Collaborative	
Monitor periodic laboratory values, such as Hgb/Hct, sodium, albumin, and clotting times.	Reflects hydration status and identifies sodium retention and protein deficits, which may lead to edema formation. Deficits in clotting potentiate risk of bleeding.
Administer antidiarrheal agents, such as diphenoxylate with atropine (Lomotil).	Reduces fluid and electrolyte loss from GI tract.
Provide intravenous (IV) fluids (usually glucose) and electrolytes:	Provides fluid and electrolyte replacement in acute toxic state.
Protein hydrolysates.	Correction of albumin and protein deficits can aid in return of fluid from tissues to the circulatory system. May follow albumin administration with an IV diuretic to pull fluids from interstitial space into intravascular space to reduce ascites.
Bleeding Precautions (NIC)	
Administer medications, as indicated, for example:	
Vitamin K	Because absorption is altered, supplementation may prevent coagulation problems, which may occur if clotting factors are decreased.
Antacids or H_2-receptor antagonists, such as lansoprazole (Prevacid) and cimetidine (Tagamet)	Neutralizes or reduces gastric secretions to lower risk of gastric irritation and bleeding.
Infuse fresh-frozen plasma (FFP), as indicated.	May be required to replace clotting factors in the presence of coagulation defects.

NURSING DIAGNOSIS: risk for situational low Self-Esteem

May Be Related To
Physical illness
Disturbed body image

Possibly Evidenced By
(Not applicable; presence of signs and symptoms establishes an *actual* diagnosis)

Desired Outcomes/Evaluation Criteria—Client Will

Self-Esteem (NOC)
Verbalize feelings.
Identify methods for coping with negative perception of self.
Verbalize acceptance of self in situation, including length of recovery and need for isolation.
Acknowledge self as worthwhile; be responsible for self.

ACTIONS/INTERVENTIONS	RATIONALE
Self-Esteem Enhancement (NIC)	
Independent	
Contract with client regarding time for listening. Encourage discussion of feelings and concerns.	Establishing time enhances trusting relationship. Providing opportunity to express feelings allows client to feel more in control of the situation. Verbalization can decrease anxiety and depression and facilitate positive coping behaviors. Client may need to express feelings about being ill, length and cost of illness, possibility of infecting others, and (in severe illness) fear of death. May have concerns regarding the stigma of the disease.
Avoid making moral judgments regarding lifestyle, such as alcohol use, drug abuse, and sexual practices.	Client may already feel upset or angry and condemn self; judgments from others will further damage self-esteem.
Discuss recovery expectations.	Recovery period may be prolonged (months), potentiating family and situational stress and necessitating need for planning, support, and follow-up.
Assess effect of illness on economic factors of client and significant other (SO).	Financial problems may exist because of loss of client's role functioning in the family and prolonged recovery.
Offer diversional activities based on energy level.	Enables client to use time and energy in constructive ways that enhance self-esteem and minimize anxiety and depression.
Suggest client wear bright reds or blues and blacks instead of yellows or greens.	Enhances appearance because yellow skin tones are intensified by yellow and green colors. *Note:* Jaundice usually peaks within 1 to 2 weeks, then gradually resolves over 2 to 4 weeks.
Collaborative	
Make appropriate referrals for help as needed, such as community case manager, social services, and other community agencies.	Can facilitate problem-solving and help involved individuals cope more effectively with situation.

NURSING DIAGNOSIS: risk for Infection [secondary/spread]

Risk Factors May Include
Inadequate secondary defenses—leukopenia, suppressed inflammatory response, immunosuppression
Malnutrition

Possibly Evidenced By
(Not applicable; presence of signs and symptoms establishes an *actual* diagnosis)

Desired Outcomes/Evaluation Criteria—Client Will

Risk Control: Infectious Process (NOC)
Verbalize understanding of individual causative and risk factor(s).
Demonstrate techniques and initiate lifestyle changes to avoid reinfection and transmission to others.

ACTIONS/INTERVENTIONS	RATIONALE
Infection Control (NIC)	
Independent	
Establish isolation techniques for enteric and respiratory infections according to infection guidelines and policy. Model and emphasize need for effective hand washing.	Prevents transmission of viral disease to others. Thorough hand washing is effective in preventing virus transmission. HAV and HEV are transmitted by oral-fecal route and contaminated water, milk, and food, especially inadequately cooked shellfish. Types A, B, C, and D are transmitted by contaminated blood or blood products; needle punctures; open wounds; and contact with saliva, urine, stool, and semen. Incidence of both HBV and HCV has increased among healthcare providers and high-risk clients. *Note:* Toxic and alcoholic types of hepatitis are not communicable and do not require special measures or isolation.
Emphasize need to monitor and restrict visitors, as indicated.	Client exposure to infectious processes, especially respiratory, potentiates risk of secondary complications.
Explain isolation procedures to client and SO.	Understanding reasons for safeguarding themselves and others can lessen feelings of isolation and stigmatization. Isolation may last 2 to 3 weeks from onset of illness, depending on type and duration of symptoms.
Collaborative	
Administer anti-infective medications, as appropriate.	Used to treat or limit secondary infections.

NURSING DIAGNOSIS: risk for impaired Tissue Integrity

Risk Factors May Include

Chemical irritants—bile salt accumulation in the tissues
Mechanical factors (e.g., scratching)

Possibly Evidenced By

(Not applicable; presence of signs and symptoms establishes an *actual* diagnosis)

Desired Outcomes/Evaluation Criteria—Client Will

Tissue Integrity: Skin and Mucous Membranes (NOC)
Display intact skin and tissues free of excoriation.
Report absence or decrease of pruritus and scratching.

ACTIONS/INTERVENTIONS	RATIONALE
Skin Surveillance (NIC)	
Independent	
Encourage use of cool showers and baking soda or starch baths. Avoid use of alkaline soaps. Apply calamine lotion, as indicated.	Prevents excessive dryness of skin. Provides relief from itching associated with accumulation of bile salts in jaundiced skin.
Provide diversional activities.	Aids in refocusing attention and reducing tendency to scratch.
Suggest use of knuckles if desire to scratch is uncontrollable. Keep fingernails cut short and apply gloves on comatose client or during hours of sleep. Recommend wearing loose-fitting clothing. Provide soft cotton linens.	Reduces potential for dermal injury.
Provide a soothing massage at bedtime.	May be helpful in promoting sleep by reducing skin irritation.
Observe skin for areas of redness and breakdown.	Early detection of problem areas allows for additional intervention to prevent complications and promote healing.
Avoid comments regarding client's appearance.	Minimizes psychological stress associated with skin changes.
Collaborative	
Administer medications, as indicated, for example:	
Antihistamines, such as diphenhydramine (Benadryl) and azatadine (Optimine)	Relieves itching. *Note:* Use cautiously in severe hepatic disease.
Antilipemic, such as cholestyramine (Questran)	May be used to bind bile acids in the intestine and prevent their absorption. Note side effects of nausea and constipation.

NURSING DIAGNOSIS: deficient Knowledge [Learning Need] regarding condition, prognosis, treatment, self-care, and discharge needs

May Be Related To
Lack of exposure or recall, information misinterpretation
Unfamiliarity with resources

Possibly Evidenced By
Reports the problem
Inaccurate follow-through of instructions

Desired Outcomes/Evaluation Criteria—Client Will

Knowledge: Chronic Illness Care (NOC)
Verbalize understanding of disease process, prognosis, and potential complications.
Identify relationship of signs and symptoms to the disease and correlate symptoms with causative factors.
Verbalize understanding of therapeutic needs.
Initiate necessary lifestyle changes and participate in treatment regimen.

ACTIONS/INTERVENTIONS	RATIONALE
Teaching: Disease Process (NIC)	
Independent	
Assess level of understanding of the disease process, prognosis, and possible treatment options.	Identifies areas of lack of knowledge or misinformation and provides opportunity to give additional information as necessary. *Note:* Liver transplantation may be needed in the presence of fulminating disease with liver failure.
Provide specific information regarding prevention and transmission of disease: for example, contacts may require gamma globulin; personal items should not be shared; and observe strict hand washing and sanitizing of clothes, dishes, and toilet facilities while liver enzymes are elevated. Avoid intimate contact, such as kissing and sexual contact, and exposure to infections, especially respiratory infections.	Needs vary with type of hepatitis, causative agent, and individual situation.
Plan resumption of activity, as tolerated, with adequate periods of rest. Discuss restriction of heavy lifting, strenuous exercise, and contact sports.	It is not necessary to wait until serum bilirubin levels return to normal, which may take as long as 2 months, to resume activity. Strenuous activity needs to be limited until the liver returns to normal size. When client begins to feel better, he or she needs to understand the importance of continued adequate rest in preventing relapse or recurrence.
Help client identify appropriate diversional activities.	Enjoyable activities promote rest and help client avoid focusing on prolonged convalescence.
Encourage continuation of balanced diet.	Promotes general well-being and enhances energy for healing process and tissue regeneration.
Identify ways to maintain usual bowel function, such as adequate intake of fluids and dietary roughage and moderate exercise to tolerance.	Decreased level of activity, changes in food and fluid intake, and slowed bowel motility may result in constipation.
Discuss the side effects and dangers of taking OTC and certain prescribed drugs that are known to have adverse effects on the liver. Advise client to notify pharmacists and all future healthcare providers of diagnosis.	Some drugs are toxic to the liver; many others are metabolized by the liver and should be avoided in severe liver diseases because they may cause cumulative toxic effects or chronic hepatitis.
Discuss restrictions on donating blood.	Most state laws prevent accepting as donors those who have a history of any type of hepatitis.
Emphasize importance of follow-up physical examination and laboratory evaluation.	Disease process may take several months to resolve. If symptoms persist longer than 6 months, liver biopsy may be required to verify presence of chronic hepatitis.
Discuss need for immunizations.	Recovery from hepatitis A and B results in protective antibodies in the client, so he or she will not get those strains again. There is currently no vaccine available against HCV. However, people should be vaccinated against HAV and HBV. Guidelines include immunizing everyone under the age of 18 years, individuals exposed to blood and body fluids or sharing a household with an infected person, screening all pregnant women for HBsAg and providing immunoprophylaxis to infants of HBV-infected women, people traveling to areas where infection rates are known to be high, men who have sex with men, illicit injection drug users, and persons

(continues on page 412)

ACTIONS/INTERVENTIONS	RATIONALE
	receiving hemodialysis or who have clotting disorders or liver disease.
Give information regarding availability of gamma globulin, immune serum globulin (ISG), hepatitis immune globulin (H-BIG), HBV vaccine (Recombivax HB, Engerix-B) through health department or family physician.	Immune globulins may be effective in preventing viral hepatitis in those who have been exposed, depending on type of hepatitis and period of incubation.
Review necessity of avoidance of alcohol, illicit drugs, and tobacco.	These substances increase hepatic irritation and interfere with recovery.
Collaborative	
Refer to community resources and drug and alcohol treatment program, as indicated.	May need additional assistance to withdraw from substance and maintain abstinence to avoid further liver damage.

POTENTIAL CONSIDERATIONS following acute hospitalization (dependent on client's age, physical condition and presence of complications, personal resources, and life responsibilities)

- ***Fatigue***—altered body chemistry, malnutrition, stress, depression
- ***impaired Home Maintenance***—illness, insufficient finances, inadequate support systems, unfamiliarity with neighborhood resources
- ***imbalanced Nutrition: less than body requirements***—inability to ingest/digest food (anorexia, nausea, vomiting); inability to absorb nutrients; [increased metabolic demands]
- ***risk for Infection***—inadequate secondary defenses; malnutrition
- ***risk for impaired Liver Function***—viral infection, co-infections, substance abuse
- ***risk for ineffective Self-Health Management***—complexity of therapeutic regimen, economic difficulties, family patterns of healthcare, perceived barriers, social support deficit

CIRRHOSIS OF THE LIVER

I. Pathophysiology (Garcia-Tsao, 2009; Murphy, 2006)

a. Alteration in structure and degenerative changes resulting from buildup of diffuse bands of fibrotic connective tissue causing widespread destruction of hepatic cells, impairing liver function, and impeding blood flow through the liver

b. Compensated cirrhosis: Liver function may continue for some time, even with significant scarring, but metabolic abnormalities can occur, such as coagulation defects and malnutrition.

c. Decompensated cirrhosis: progression of failure with significant complications, such as portal hypertension with bleeding varices (~50%), spontaneous bacterial infections (SPBs) (10% to 20%), ascites (~30%), hepatorenal syndrome, and encephalopathy

II. Etiology

a. Rate of progression of fibrosis to cirrhosis varies for unknown reasons.

b. Multiple causation (Wolf, 2012)

  i. Hepatitis C (26%); combined B, and D (15%)

  ii. Alcoholic liver disease (21%); Hep C plus alcoholic liver disease (15%). Note: Some sources place alcoholic liver disease as high as 60% to 70% (Heidelbaugh, 2006).

  iii. Cholestatic diseases: biliary atresia, primary biliary cirrhosis, cystic fibrosis, primary sclerosing cholangitis

  iv. Miscellaneous liver disorders, including autoimmune, Wilson's disease, alpha$_1$-antitrypsin deficiency, hemochromatosis

  v. Injury from trauma, drugs (e.g., isoniazid, herbal supplements such as germander), toxins such as arsenic, or environmental toxins

III. Treatment

a. Goals are to slow the progression of the disease and alleviate the symptoms.

b. Liver transplantation is currently the only life-saving procedure for end-stage disease.

IV. Statistics

a. Morbidity: In 2009, chronic liver disease or cirrhosis was the first listed diagnosis in 101,000 hospitalizations. In 2010, approximately 16,000 individuals were listed on the waiting list for liver transplant (American Liver Foundation [ALA], 2012; Scientific Registry of Transplant Recipients [SRTR], 2011; CDC, 2009).

b. Mortality: In 2011, cirrhosis and other liver disorders were listed as the 12th leading cause of death in the United States (approximately 34,000/year) (Hoyart et al, 2011).

c. Cost: Direct care costs for acute and chronic liver diseases (excluding viral hepatitis and cancer) estimated to be more than $2.5 billion in 2004 (Everhart, 2008).

GLOSSARY

Ascites: Buildup of fluid in the abdomen due to a number of conditions including severe liver disease.

Asterixis: Involuntary jerking movements of hands and feet associated with hepatic encephalopathy.

Ecchymosis: Skin discoloration consisting of a large, irregularly formed hemorrhagic area with colors changing from blue-black to greenish-brown or yellow; commonly referred to as a bruise.

Fetor hepaticus: Particularly foul-smelling breath, which frequently precedes hepatic coma.

Hematemesis: Bloody vomitus.

Hepatic encephalopathy: Brain dysfunction directly due to liver dysfunction seen in advanced cirrhosis, resulting in disturbances of consciousness and progressing to coma.

Hepatomegaly: Enlarged liver.

Hepatorenal syndrome: Represents a continuum of kidney dysfunction observed in individuals with cirrhosis caused by the vasoconstriction of large and small renal arteries.

Jaundice: Yellow staining of the skin and sclerae (and sometimes other tissues and body fluids) because of abnormally high blood levels of bilirubin.

Melena: Bloody stools.

Oliguria: Urinary output less than 400 mL/day.

Palmar erythema: Redness of the palms of the hands caused by dilation and congestion of capillaries.

Peritoneovenous shunt: Surgically implanted device for continuous draining of ascitic fluid into the venous system. Fluid is removed via a pressure-sensitive one-way valve. It is connected to a tube under the subcutaneous tissue of the chest wall to the neck, where it enters the internal jugular vein and terminates in the superior vena cava.

Petechiae: Tiny red dots on the skin caused by minute hemorrhage, indicating low platelet count or other blood disorder.

Spider angiomas: Abnormal collection of blood vessels near the surface of the skin; can occur anywhere, but are most common on the face and trunk.

Splenomegaly: Enlarged spleen.

Telangiectasis: Visibly dilated blood vessel on the skin or mucosal surface.

Care Setting

Client may be hospitalized on a medical unit during initial or recurrent acute episodes with potentially life-threatening complications. Otherwise, this condition is managed at the community, outpatient level.

Related Concerns

Acute renal injury (acute renal failure), page 505
Alcohol: acute withdrawal, page 800
Fluid and electrolyte imbalances, page 885
Psychosocial aspects of care, page 729
Renal dialysis—general considerations, page 529
Substance use disorders, page 815
Total nutritional support: parenteral/enteral feeding, page 437
Upper gastrointestinal/esophageal bleeding, page 281

Client Assessment Database

Data depend on underlying cause of the condition.

DIAGNOSTIC DIVISION MAY REPORT	MAY EXHIBIT
ACTIVITY/REST	
• Weakness • Fatigue, exhaustion	• Lethargy • Decreased muscle mass and tone
CIRCULATION	
• History of or recent onset of heart failure (HF), pericarditis, rheumatic heart disease, or cancer, causing liver impairment leading to failure • Easy bruising, nosebleeds, bleeding gums	• Hypertension or hypotension (fluid shifts) • Dysrhythmias, extra heart sounds—S_3, S_4 • Jugular vein distention (JVD), distended abdominal veins, spider angiomas, collateral circulation • Ecchymosis, petechiae • Anemia, leukopenia, thrombctyopenia, coagulation disorders, splenomegaly

(continues on page 414)

DIAGNOSTIC DIVISION MAY REPORT (continued)	MAY EXHIBIT (continued)
ELIMINATION • Flatulence • Diarrhea or constipation • Gradual abdominal enlargement	• Abdominal distention (hepatomegaly, splenomegaly, ascites) • Decreased or absent bowel sounds • Clay-colored stools, melena • Hemorrhoidal varices • Dark, concentrated urine; oliguria (hepatorenal syndrome, failure)
FOOD/FLUID • Anorexia • Food intolerance, ingestion • Nausea, vomiting • Hematemesis	• Weight loss or gain (fluid) • Tissue wasting, delayed wound healing • Edema generalized in tissues • Dry skin, poor turgor • Halitosis or fetor hepaticus, bleeding gums • Hypoalbuminemia
NEUROSENSORY • Significant other (SO)/family may report personality changes, depressed mentation	• Changes in mentation, confusion, hallucinations, coma • Slowed, slurred speech • Asterixis
PAIN/DISCOMFORT • Abdominal tenderness and right upper quadrant (RUQ) pain • Severe itching • Pins-and-needles sensation, burning pain in extremities (peripheral neuropathy)	• Guarding or distraction behaviors • Self-focus
RESPIRATION • Dyspnea	• Tachypnea, shallow respiration, adventitious breath sounds • Limited thoracic expansion because of ascites • Hypoxia
SAFETY • Itching, dryness of the skin (pruritus)	• Fever—more common in alcoholic cirrhosis • Jaundiced skin and sclera • Spider angiomas, telangiectasis • Palmar erythema • Confusion progressing to delirium and coma (hepatic encephalopathy) • Unsteady or shaky, jerking movements
SEXUALITY • Menstrual disorders (women) • Impotence (men)	• Testicular atrophy, gynecomastia, loss of hair—chest, underarm, pubic
TEACHING/LEARNING • History of long-term alcohol or injection drug use or abuse, alcoholic liver disease, use of drugs affecting liver function • History of biliary system disease, hepatitis, exposure to toxins, liver trauma	
DISCHARGE PLAN CONSIDERATIONS • May need assistance with self-care and other activities of daily living (ADLs), homemaking and maintenance tasks ➧ Refer to section at end of plan for postdischarge considerations.	

Diagnostic Studies

TEST WHY IT IS DONE	WHAT IT TELLS ME
BLOOD TESTS	
• *Liver enzymes: such as alanine aminotransferase (ALT), aspartate aminotransferase (AST), lactate dehydrogenase (LDH), alkaline phosphatase (ALP):* Assess liver functioning and detect liver damage.	Liver enzyme levels are elevated because of cellular damage and release of enzymes. Which enzymes are elevated and how much they are elevated varies depending on the cause(s) for liver disease (Heidelbaugh, 2006).
• *Serum bilirubin (total and indirect unconjugated):* Bilirubin results from the breakdown of hemoglobin.	Elevated because of cellular disruption, or biliary obstruction, causing jaundice.
• *Serum albumin:* Protein of the highest concentration in plasma. Transports substances, such as bilirubin, calcium, progesterone, and drugs, and regulates osmotic pressure of blood, keeping fluid from leaking out into the tissues.	Because albumin is made by the liver, decreased serum albumin may result from liver disease and affect bleeding/clotting and nutrition.
• *Immunoglobulin (Ig) A, G, and M:* Proteins found in blood or other bodily fluids used by the immune system to identify and neutralize foreign objects, such as bacteria and viruses.	Levels are increased.
• *Complete blood count (CBC):* Battery of screening tests, which typically includes hemoglobin (Hgb); hematocrit (Hct); red blood cell (RBC) count, morphology, indices, and distribution width index; platelet count and size; white blood cell (WBC) count and differential.	Hb, Hct, and RBCs may be decreased because of bleeding and RBC destruction. Anemia is seen with hypersplenism and iron deficiency. Leukopenia may be present as a result of hypersplenism.
• *Bleeding/Clotting:*	
• *Prothrombin time (PT):* Measures length of time required for blood sample to clot.	Prolonged because of decreased production of clotting proteins and fat-soluble vitamin K deficiency, leading to easy bleeding.
• *Fibrinogen and other clotting factors:* Used to monitor the progression of liver disease over time.	Decreased; chronically low levels seen in end-stage liver disease.
• *Blood urea nitrogen (BUN):* Urea is the end product of protein metabolism formed in the liver from amino acids and from ammonia compounds.	Elevation indicates breakdown of blood proteins and possible kidney dysfunction because of diuretic use in treatment of ascites.
• *Serum ammonia:* Product of breakdown of protein, which is normally converted to urea and excreted.	Elevated because of inability to convert ammonia to urea. Elevated levels will cause hepatic encephalopathy.
• *Serum glucose:* One of the simple sugars in the blood, which serves as primary energy source for cells.	Low blood glucose (hypoglycemia) suggests impaired synthesis of glycogen from glucose (glycogenesis).
• *Electrolytes:* Substances that dissociate into ions in solution and acquire the capacity to conduct electricity. Common electrolytes include sodium, potassium, chloride, calcium, and phosphate.	Low potassium (hypokalemia) may reflect increased aldosterone, although various imbalances may occur. Low calcium (hypocalcemia) may occur because of impaired absorption of vitamin D.
OTHER DIAGNOSTIC STUDIES	
• *Abdominal ultrasonography with Doppler:* Diagnostic technique that uses sound waves to produce an image of internal body structures.	May be first assessment performed in individual with suspected liver disease to detect ascites and enlarged liver and spleen. It can also identify biliary duct obstruction or bile stones. Nodularity, irregularity, and atrophy are ultrasonographic hallmarks of cirrhosis. In advanced disease, the gross liver appears small and multinodular, ascites may be detected, and Doppler flow can be significantly decreased in the portal circulation.
• *Liver biopsy:* Biopsy can be performed via percutaneous, transjugular, laparoscopic, open operative, or computed tomography (CT)-guided fine-needle approaches. Samples are obtained for microscopic evaluation.	Definitive test for cirrhosis, revealing hepatic tissue destruction and fibrosis.
• *Urine and stool urobilinogen:* Serves as guide for differentiating liver disease, hemolytic disease, and biliary obstruction.	May or may not be present.

Nursing Priorities

1. Maintain adequate nutrition.
2. Prevent complications.
3. Enhance self-concept and acceptance of situation.
4. Provide information about disease process, prognosis, potential complications, and treatment needs.

Discharge Goals

1. Nutritional intake adequate for individual needs.
2. Complications prevented or minimized.
3. Deals effectively with current reality.
4. Disease process, prognosis, potential complications, and therapeutic regimen understood.
5. Plan in place to meet needs after discharge.

NURSING DIAGNOSIS: imbalanced Nutrition: less than body requirements

May Be Related To

Inability to ingest food (e.g., anorexia, nausea, vomiting, indigestion)
Inability to digest food

Possibly Evidenced By

Weight loss
Lack of interest in food; satiety immediately after ingesting food
Hyperactive bowel sounds
Poor muscle tone
Abnormal laboratory studies (e.g., decreased albumin)

Desired Outcomes/Evaluation Criteria—Client Will

Nutritional Status (NOC)
Demonstrate progressive weight gain toward goal.
Experience no further signs of malnutrition.

Nutritional Status: Biochemical Measures (NOC)
Display appropriate normalization of laboratory values.

ACTIONS/INTERVENTIONS	RATIONALE
Nutrition Therapy (NIC) *Independent*	
Note client reports of inability to eat. Assess for presence of conditions that can interfere with food intake.	Client with cirrhosis may have been sick for quite a while and have no appetite; presence of nausea and/or vomiting; or abdominal ascites which causes early satiety.
Evaluate client's risk for malnutrition, noting such things as emaciated appearance, muscle wasting, obvious lack of interest in food, expressed aversion to eating, etc.	The presence of malnutrition is estimated to be as high as 80% in patients with cirrhosis and is related to the degree of liver disease. Client may have malabsorption syndrome due to inability to process or digest nutrients, anorexia, nausea or vomiting, indigestion, or early satiety associated with ascites. Deficiencies in water-soluble vitamins are common in alcoholic cirrhosis, while deficiencies in fat-soluble vitamins are more common in cholestatic liver disease. In more advanced stages, both fat-soluble and water-soluble vitamin deficiencies occur (Nardi et al, 2009).
Determine ability to chew, swallow, and taste. Discuss usual eating habits, including food preferences, intolerances, or aversions.	Factors that affect ingestion and digestion of nutrients.
Evaluate total daily food intake, using food diary if needed.	Provides information about intake, needs, and deficiencies. Client with cirrhosis requires a balanced protein diet providing 2000 to 3000 calories per day to permit liver cell regeneration.
Weigh, as indicated. Consider fluid status and recent weight history.	It may be difficult to use weight as a direct indicator of nutritional status in view of edema and ascites.
Assist or encourage client to eat; explain reasons for the types of diet. Feed client if tiring easily, or have SO assist client. Consider preferences in food choices.	Improved nutrition is vital to recovery. Client may eat better if family is involved and preferred foods are included as much as possible. Client and family must understand protein intake limitations and how best to meet needs and desires within limitations.
Recommend or provide small, frequent meals.	Poor tolerance to larger meals may be due to increased intra-abdominal pressure or ascites.

ACTIONS/INTERVENTIONS (continued)	RATIONALE (continued)
Limit such high-salt foods as canned soups and vegetables, processed meats, and condiments. Provide salt substitutes if allowed, avoiding those containing ammonia.	Salt limitations can help manage fluid complications in cirrhosis, including ascites or tissue edema. Salt substitutes enhance the flavor of food and aid in increasing appetite; ammonia potentiates risk of encephalopathy.
Restrict intake of caffeine and gas-producing or spicy and excessively hot or cold foods.	Aids in reducing gastric irritation, diarrhea, and abdominal discomfort that may impair oral intake and digestion.
Encourage or provide frequent mouth care, especially before meals.	Client is prone to sore and bleeding gums and bad taste in mouth, which contributes to anorexia.
Provide assistance with activities as needed. Promote undisturbed rest periods, especially before meals.	Conserving energy reduces metabolic demands on the liver and promotes cellular regeneration.
Recommend cessation of smoking.	Reduces excessive gastric stimulation and risk of irritation and bleeding.
Collaborative	
Monitor laboratory studies, e.g., glucose, prealbumin or albumin, total proteins, and ammonia.	Glucose may be decreased because of impaired glycogenesis, depleted glycogen stores, or inadequate intake. Protein may be low because of impaired metabolism, decreased hepatic synthesis, or loss into peritoneal cavity (ascites). Protein-calorie malnutrition contributes to further development of fatty liver and deterioration of function. Elevation of ammonia level may require restriction of protein intake to prevent serious complications.
Maintain nothing by mouth (NPO) status, when indicated.	Gastrointestinal (GI) rest may be required in acutely ill clients to reduce demands on the liver and production of ammonia and urea in the GI tract. When this is the case, nutrition must be supplied by another method—enteral or parenteral feedings.
Determine nutritional and caloric needs using appropriate methods, such as total energy expenditure (TEE), body mass index (BMI), Harris-Benedict equation, or indirect calorimetry test, as indicated.	Useful in assessing changes in muscle mass, energy expenditure, and subcutaneous fat reserves. May be used in stable client to help quantify nutritional status and determine needs for long-term nutritional plan.
Collaborate with nutritional team to provide diet that is individualized to client's needs.	Because client's intake is usually limited, calorie-dense foods are desired. Carbohydrates supply readily available energy. Fats are poorly absorbed because of liver dysfunction and may contribute to abdominal discomfort. Proteins are needed to improve serum protein levels, reducing edema and promoting liver cell regeneration. However, protein can also elevate ammonia levels and must be restricted if ammonia level is elevated or if client has clinical signs of hepatic encephalopathy.
Provide enteral tube feedings or total parenteral nutrition (TPN), if indicated.	May be required to supplement diet or to provide nutrients when client is too nauseated or anorexic to eat or when esophageal varices interfere with oral intake. (Refer to CP: Total Nutritional Support: Parenteral/Enteral Feedings.)
Administer medications, as indicated, for example:	
Vitamin supplements (especially fat-soluble vitamins A, D, E, K) and B vitamins (thiamine, iron, folic acid)	Replacement required because of the inability of the liver to process or store vitamins.
Antiemetics, such as trimethobenzamide (Tigan)	Used with caution to reduce nausea and vomiting and enhance oral intake.

NURSING DIAGNOSIS: risk for excess Fluid Volume

May Be Related To

Compromised regulatory mechanism—syndrome of inappropriate antidiuretic hormone (SIADH), decreased plasma proteins

Excess sodium and fluid intake

Possibly Evidenced By

(Not applicable; presence of signs and symptoms establishes an *actual* diagnosis)

Desired Outcomes/Evaluation Criteria—Client Will

Fluid Balance (NOC)

Demonstrate stabilized fluid volume, with balanced intake and output (I&O), stable weight, vital signs within client's normal range, and absence of edema.

ACTIONS/INTERVENTIONS	RATIONALE
Fluid/Electrolyte Management (NIC)	
Independent	
Measure I&O, noting positive balance—intake in excess of output. Weigh daily, and note.	Reflects circulating volume status, developing or resolving fluid shifts, and response to therapy. Positive fluid balance and weight gain often reflects continuing fluid retention. *Note:* Decreased circulating volume and fluid shifts can directly affect renal function and urine output, resulting in hepatorenal syndrome.
Weigh daily or as prescribed and document changes, noting both gains and losses.	Monitoring is needed to help direct therapy, as weight may increase, decrease, or fluctuate. For example, steady weight gain may reflect continuing fluid retention (renal impairment) or development of ascites. Or adjustments in dosage may be required in client on diuretic therapy for ascites who is losing more than a pound a day (Garcia-Tsao, 2009).
Monitor BP and CVP, if available. Note JVD and abdominal vein distention.	BP elevations are usually associated with fluid volume excess but may not occur because of fluid shifts out of the vascular space. JVD and presence of distended abdominal veins are associated with vascular congestion.
Assess respiratory status, noting increased respiratory rate and dyspnea.	Indicative of pulmonary congestion or edema.
Auscultate lungs, noting diminished or absent breath sounds and developing adventitious sounds—crackles.	Increasing pulmonary congestion may result in consolidation, impaired gas exchange, and complications, such as pulmonary edema.
Monitor for cardiac dysrhythmias. Auscultate heart sounds, noting development of S_3/S_4 gallop rhythm.	May be caused by HF, decreased coronary arterial perfusion, or electrolyte imbalance.
Assess degree of peripheral and dependent edema.	Fluids shift into tissues as a result of sodium and water retention, decreased albumin, and increased antidiuretic hormone (ADH).
Measure abdominal girth.	Reflects accumulation of fluid or ascites resulting from loss of plasma proteins and fluid into peritoneal space. *Note:* Ascites is one of the most frequent complications of late-stage cirrhosis (~30%) (Garcia-Tsao et al, 2009).
Provide frequent mouth care and occasional ice chips, particularly if NPO; schedule fluid intake around the clock.	Decreases sensation of thirst, especially when fluid intake is restricted.
Collaborative	
Monitor serum albumin and electrolytes, particularly potassium and sodium.	Decreased serum albumin affects plasma colloid osmotic pressure, resulting in edema formation. Reduced renal blood flow, accompanied by elevated ADH and aldosterone levels and the use of diuretics to reduce total body water, may cause various electrolyte shifts and imbalances.
Monitor serial chest x-rays.	Vascular congestion, pulmonary edema, and pleural effusions frequently occur.
Restrict sodium and fluids, as indicated.	Sodium may be restricted to minimize fluid retention in extravascular spaces. Fluid restriction may be necessary to correct dilutional hyponatremia.
Administer salt-free albumin and plasma expanders, as indicated.	Albumin may be given to increase the colloid osmotic pressure in the vascular compartment, thereby increasing effective circulating volume and decreasing formation of ascites. *Note:* In client with tense ascites in whom other complications are absent or have been resolved, a total paracentesis (i.e., removal of the maximal amount of ascites) may be an initial treatment for ascites with concomitant albumin infusion followed by the administration of diuretics (Garcia-Tsao, 2009).
Administer medications, as indicated, for example:	
Diuretics, such as spironolactone (Aldactone) given alone or in combination with furosemide (Lasix)	Spironolactone is the diuretic of choice to control edema and ascites, block effect of aldosterone, and increase water excretion while sparing potassium. Diuretics given in coordination with albumin administration may enhance fluid removal.
Potassium	Serum and cellular potassium are usually depleted because of liver disease and urinary losses.
Positive inotropic drugs and arterial vasodilators	Given to increase cardiac output and improve renal blood flow and function, thereby reducing excess fluid.
Prepare for/assist with procedures as indicated in client with ascites unresponsive to medical therapies, e.g.:	
Paracentesis, either single or serial	Therapeutic paracentesis may be performed in client who requires rapid symptomatic relief for refractory or tense

ascites. The removal of 5 L of fluid or more is considered large-volume paracentesis (LVP) (Runyon, 2009).

Peritoneovenous shunting (PVS)
This surgically placed shunt creates a passage between the peritoneum and the jugular vein to return ascitic fluid to the central venous system. The procedure is an alternative to LVP and may be used in client with refractory ascites who is not a candidate for transplant or other shunting procedures (Shah, 2012).

Transjugular intrahepatic portosystemic shunt (TIPS)
This procedure places a stent between the right jugular vein and the hepatic vein, creating a connection between the portal and systemic circulations. TIPS is gradually becoming the standard of care in patients with diuretic-refractory ascites (Shah, 2012; Runyon, 2009).

NURSING DIAGNOSIS: risk for Infection

Risk Factors May Include

Inadequate primary defenses—stasis of body fluids
Inadequate secondary defenses—immunosupression
Malnutrition

Possibly Evidenced By

(Not applicable; presence of signs and symptoms establishes an *actual* diagnosis)

Desired Outcomes/Evaluation Criteria—Client Will

Infection Severity (NOC)

Be free of fever and abdominal pain.

Risk Control: Infectious Process (NOC)

Acknowledge individual risk factors for infection.
Engage in actions to reduce risk of infection.
Be free of preventable complications.

ACTIONS/INTERVENTIONS / RATIONALE

Infection Protection (NIC)

Independent

Identify client at risk, i.e., presence of cirrhosis and ascites; immunocompromised state; malnutrition; invasive lines and procedures.
This client is at risk for any healthcare-related infection (e.g., pneumonia, urinary tract infection, skin/wound infections) (Bonnel, 2011) and especially blood-borne infections resulting in sepsis. Client with cirrhosis who has recently undergone surgery/other procedural instrumentation of the abdomen, variceal hemorrhage, or who is suspected of having some type of abscess is at risk for secondary bacterial peritonitis. Hospitalized client with cirrhosis plus ascites is at significant risk (10% and 30%) for spontaneous bacterial peritonitis (SBP) (Bonnel, 2011; Garcia-Tsao, 2001). Studies have found that ascitic fluid infection is sufficiently common (12%) at the time of admission to justify a diagnostic paracentesis as a matter of course (Borzio et al, 2001).

Note client reports of new onset abdominal pain or change in usual level of abdominal discomfort. Determine intensity using 0 to 10 or similar coded scale.
Client with chronic cirrhosis does not always have abdominal pain and may characterize it as discomfort, depending on presence/degree of ascites. Thus if client is reporting new onset or unusual abdominal pain, interventions should be geared toward finding the cause, not just relieving pain.

Monitor vital signs, noting onset of fever.
Fever usually accompanies bacterial infections but is not always present in immunocompromised client.

Evaluate body systems, e.g., respiratory, skin, urinary tract for signs of infection.
Infection may be anywhere in the body. If not found in most likely places, client must be evaluated for more unusual infectious causes.

Promote safe healthcare environment:
First-line defense against healthcare-associated infections.

- Emphasize and practice proper hand washing before and after direct contact. Wear gloves when appropriate.
This is important for staff, clients, and visitors to reduce the cross-contamination especially for immunocompromised clients.

(continues on page 420)

ACTIONS/INTERVENTIONS (continued)	RATIONALE (continued)
Maintain sterile technique for all invasive procedures (e.g., IV, urinary catheter, pulmonary suctioning).	Reduces risk of device-related infections.
Change surgical or other wound dressings, as indicated, using proper technique for changing/disposing of contaminated materials.	Dressing changes maintain dry, clean wound area to promote healing. Proper disposal of contaminated material reduces risk of spread of infection to others.
Encourage deep breathing and coughing, position changes, and early ambulation.	To limit complications associated with stasis of respiratory secretions and shallow breathing.
Maintain adequate hydration; encourage regular voiding or maintain urinary catheter as indicated. Provide/assist with pericare.	Prevents infections associated with urinary stasis and/or presence of catheter, which can be associated with ascending urinary tract infections.
Collaborative	
Prepare for/assist with medical procedures (e.g., paracentesis).	May be performed to obtain specimen of ascitic fluid for analysis.
Review laboratory test results (e.g., WBCs with differential, urinalysis, ascitic fluid and/or blood cultures).	Helps reveal source of infection. Additional tests may be done on ascites fluid (e.g., total protein, LDH, glucose) to help differentiate secondary bacterial peritonitis from spontaneous bacterial peritonitis when other sources of infection (e.g., pneumonia, perforated gut, or abdominal abscess) have been ruled out.
Administer antibiotics, as indicated.	Therapy will be determined by the site and type of infection found. Broad-spectrum therapy is used in client with suspected ascitic fluid infection until the results of susceptibility testing are available. Cefotaxime or a similar third-generation cephalosporin appears to be the treatment of choice for suspected SBP; it covers 95% of the flora, including the three most common isolates: *Escherichia coli*, *Klebsiella pneumoniae*, and pneumococci (Runyon, 2009).

NURSING DIAGNOSIS: risk for impaired Skin Integrity

Risk Factors May Include

Impaired circulation
Imbalanced nutritional state; impaired metabolic state
Chemical substance—accumulation of bile salts in skin
Changes in skin turgor, skeletal prominence, changes in fluid status (e.g., edema, ascites)

Possibly Evidenced By

(Not applicable; presence of signs and symptoms establishes an *actual* diagnosis)

Desired Outcomes/Evaluation Criteria—Client Will

Risk Control (NOC)

Maintain skin integrity.
Identify individual risk factors and demonstrate behaviors or techniques to prevent skin breakdown.

ACTIONS/INTERVENTIONS	RATIONALE
Skin Surveillance (NIC)	
Independent	
Discuss itching with client, addressing areas involved and time of day when client is most uncomfortable.	Pruritus affects about two-thirds of clients with primary biliary cirrhosis; the cause is unknown. The itching often worsens during the evening and improves during the day. It typically begins in the palms and soles, and then spreads to the rest of the body. Prolonged, repeated scratching can result in excoriations and thickening and darkening of the skin (Heathcote, 2000).
Inspect skin surfaces and pressure points routinely. Gently massage bony prominences or areas of continued stress. Use emollient lotions and limit use of soap for bathing.	Edematous tissues are more prone to breakdown and to the formation of decubitus ulcers. Ascites may stretch the skin to the point of tearing in severe cirrhosis.
Encourage and assist with repositioning on a regular schedule, while in bed or chair, and active or passive range-of-motion (ROM) exercises, as appropriate.	Repositioning reduces pressure on edematous tissues to improve circulation. Exercises enhance circulation and improve or maintain joint mobility.
Recommend elevating lower extremities.	Enhances venous return and reduces edema formation in extremities, which increases risk of skin irritation and breakdown.

ACTIONS/INTERVENTIONS (continued)	RATIONALE (continued)
Keep linens dry and free of wrinkles.	Moisture aggravates pruritus and increases risk of skin breakdown.
Suggest clipping fingernails short and provide mittens or gloves, if indicated.	Prevents client from inadvertently injuring the skin, especially while sleeping.
Encourage, or provide, perineal care following urination and bowel movement.	Prevents skin excoriation breakdown from gastrointestional or urinary excretions or bile salts.
Collaborative	
Use alternating pressure mattress, egg-crate or foam mattress, waterbed, or sheepskins, as indicated.	Reduces dermal pressure, increases circulation, and diminishes risk of tissue ischemia and breakdown.
Apply calamine lotion and provide baking soda baths.	May be soothing and provide relief of itching.
Administer medications, such as cholestyramine (Questran), colestipol (Colestid), hydroxyzine (Atarax), and dronabinol (Marinol), if indicated.	Although the cause of pruritus is unknown, it may respond to these treatments (Pyrsopoulos, 2012).

NURSING DIAGNOSIS: risk for ineffective Breathing Pattern

Risk Factors May Include

Hypoventilation (ascites with decreased lung expansion)
Fatigue

Possibly Evidenced By

(Not applicable; presence of signs and symptoms establishes an *actual* diagnosis)

Desired Outcomes/Evaluation Criteria—Client Will

Respiratory Status: Ventilation (NOC)

Maintain effective respiratory pattern and be free of dyspnea and cyanosis, with arterial blood gases (ABGs) and vital capacity within acceptable range.

ACTIONS/INTERVENTIONS	RATIONALE
Respiratory Monitoring (NIC)	
Independent	
Monitor respiratory rate, depth, and effort.	Rapid, shallow respirations or dyspnea may be present because of hypoxia or fluid accumulation in abdomen.
Auscultate breath sounds, noting crackles, wheezes, and rhonchi.	Indicates developing complications—presence of adventitious sounds reflects accumulation of fluid while diminished sounds suggest atelectasis—increasing risk of pulmonary infection.
Investigate changes in level of consciousness (LOC).	Changes in mentation may reflect hypoxemia and respiratory failure, which often accompany hepatic coma.
Keep head of bed elevated. Position client on side.	Facilitates breathing by reducing pressure on the diaphragm and minimizes risk of aspiration of secretions.
Encourage frequent repositioning, deep-breathing exercises, and coughing, as appropriate.	Aids in lung expansion and mobilizing secretions.
Monitor temperature. Note presence of chills, increased coughing, and changes in color or character of sputum.	Indicative of onset of infection, such as pneumonia. *Note:* Severely ill client is immunocompromised and may not be able to mount a febrile response to infection.
Collaborative	
Monitor serial ABGs, pulse oximetry, vital capacity measurements, and chest x-rays.	Reveals changes in respiratory status and developing pulmonary complications.
Ventilation Assistance (NIC)	
Provide supplemental oxygen (O_2) as indicated.	May be necessary to treat or prevent hypoxia. If respirations or oxygenation are inadequate, mechanical ventilation may be required.
Demonstrate and assist with respiratory adjuncts, such as incentive spirometer.	Reduces incidence of atelectasis and enhances mobilization of secretions.
Prepare for/assist with acute care procedures, such as paracentesis.	Occasionally may be done to remove ascites fluid to relieve abdominal pressure when respiratory embarrassment is not corrected by other measures.

NURSING DIAGNOSIS: risk for Bleeding

Risk Factors May Include

Impaired liver function

Gastrointestinal disorders (e.g., varices)

Possibly Evidenced By

(Not applicable; presence of signs and symptoms establishes an *actual* diagnosis)

Desired Outcomes/Evaluation Criteria—Client Will

Blood Coagulation (NOC)

Maintain homeostasis with absence of bleeding.

Risk Control (NOC)

Demonstrate behaviors to reduce risk of bleeding.

ACTIONS/INTERVENTIONS	RATIONALE
Bleeding Precautions (NIC)	
Independent	
Assess for signs and symptoms of GI bleeding; for instance, check all secretions for frank or occult blood. Observe color and consistency of stools, nasogastric (NG) drainage, or vomitus.	The GI tract—especially esophagus and rectum—is the most usual source of bleeding because of its mucosal fragility and alterations in homeostasis associated with cirrhosis.
Observe for presence of petechiae, ecchymosis, and bleeding from one or more sites.	Subacute disseminated intravascular coagulation (DIC) may develop secondary to altered clotting factors.
Monitor pulse, BP, and CVP, if available.	An increased pulse with decreased BP and CVP may indicate loss of circulating blood volume, requiring further evaluation.
Note changes in mentation and LOC.	Changes may indicate decreased cerebral perfusion secondary to hypovolemia or hypoxemia.
Avoid rectal temperature; be gentle with GI tube insertions.	Rectal and esophageal vessels are most vulnerable to rupture.
Encourage use of soft toothbrush and electric razor, avoiding straining for stool, forceful nose blowing, and so forth.	In the presence of clotting factor disturbances, minimal trauma can cause mucosal bleeding.
Use small needles for injections. Apply pressure to small bleeding or venipuncture sites for longer than usual.	Minimizes damage to tissues, reducing risk of bleeding and hematoma.
Recommend avoidance of aspirin-containing products.	Prolongs coagulation, potentiating risk of hemorrhage.
Collaborative	
Monitor Hgb and Hct, platelets, and clotting factors.	Indicators of anemia, active bleeding, or impending complications, such as DIC.
Administer medications, as indicated, for example:	
Supplemental vitamins, such as vitamins K, D, and C	Promotes prothrombin synthesis and coagulation, if liver is functional. Vitamin C deficiencies increase susceptibility of GI system to irritation and bleeding.
Stool softeners	Prevents straining for stool with resultant increase in intra-abdominal pressure and risk of bleeding hemorrhoidal varices, especially when client has portal hypertension.
Provide gastric lavage with cool saline solution or water, as indicated.	In presence of acute bleeding, evacuation of blood from GI tract may reduce ammonia production and risk of hepatic encephalopathy. (Refer to CP: Upper Gastrointestinal/Esophageal Bleeding.)
Assist with insertion and maintenance of intestinal or esophageal tube, such as Sengstaken-Blakemore tube.	Temporarily controls bleeding of esophageal varices by balloon tamponade when control by other means, such as lavage, and hemodynamic stability cannot be achieved.
Prepare for procedures, such as direct ligation or banding of varices, esophagogastric resection, transjugular intrahepatic portosystemic shunt (TIPS), and splenorenal-portacaval anastomosis.	May be needed to control active hemorrhage or to decrease portal and collateral blood vessel pressure to minimize risk of recurrence of bleeding. TIPS is an interventional radiological procedure involving stent placement from the right jugular vein to the hepatic vein, thereby creating a connection between the portal and systemic circulations to relieve portal hypertension and decompress varices.

NURSING DIAGNOSIS: risk for acute Confusion

Risk Factors May Include

Substance abuse (alcohol)

Liver impairment [inability to detoxify certain enzymes and drugs]

Possibly Evidenced By

(Not applicable; presence of signs and symptoms establishes an *actual* diagnosis)

Desired Outcomes/Evaluation Criteria—Client Will

Cognition (NOC)

Maintain usual level of mentation and reality orientation.

Alcohol/Drug Abuse Cessation Behavior (NOC)

Initiate behaviors or lifestyle changes to prevent or minimize recurrence of problem.

ACTIONS/INTERVENTIONS	RATIONALE
Substance Use Treatment: Alcohol Drug Withdrawal (NIC)	
Independent	
Observe for changes in behavior and mentation: lethargy, confusion, drowsiness, slowing or slurring of speech, and irritability. Arouse client at intervals, as indicated.	Ongoing assessment of behavior and mental status is important because of fluctuating nature of hepatic encephalopathy or impending hepatic coma.
Review current medication regimen.	Adverse drug reactions or interactions may potentiate or exacerbate confusion.
Evaluate sleep and rest schedule.	Difficulty falling asleep or staying asleep leads to sleep deprivation, exacerbating cognition problems and fatigue.
Note development or presence of asterixis, fetor hepaticus, and seizure activity.	Suggests elevating serum ammonia levels and increased risk of progression to encephalopathy.
Consult with SO about client's usual behavior and mentation.	Provides baseline for comparison of current status.
Have client write name periodically and keep this record for comparison. Report deterioration of ability. Have client do simple arithmetic computations.	Easy test of neurological status and muscle coordination.
Reorient to time, place, person, and situation, as needed.	Assists in maintaining reality orientation, reducing confusion and anxiety.
Maintain a pleasant, quiet environment and approach in a slow, calm manner. Encourage uninterrupted rest periods.	Reduces excessive stimulation and sensory overload, promotes relaxation, and may enhance coping.
Provide continuity of care. If possible, assign same nurse over a period of time.	Familiarity provides reassurance, aids in reducing anxiety, and provides a more accurate documentation of subtle changes.
Reduce provocative stimuli and confrontation. Refrain from forcing activities. Assess potential for violent behavior.	Avoids triggering agitated, violent responses; promotes client safety.
Discuss current situation and future expectations.	Client and SO may be reassured that intellectual as well as emotional function may improve as liver involvement resolves.
Maintain bedrest and assist with self-care activities.	Reduces metabolic demands on liver, prevents fatigue, and promotes healing, lowering risk of ammonia buildup.
Identify and provide for safety needs, such as supervision during smoking, bed in low position, side rails up, and pad, if necessary. Provide close supervision.	Reduces risk of injury when confusion, seizures, or violent behavior occurs.
Investigate temperature elevations. Monitor for signs of infection.	Clients with cirrhosis are immunocompromised and susceptible to infections. Infection may precipitate hepatic encephalopathy caused by tissue catabolism and release of nitrogen.
Recommend avoidance of narcotics or sedatives, anti-anxiety agents, and limiting or restricting use of medications metabolized by the liver.	Certain drugs are toxic to the liver, whereas other drugs may not be metabolized because of cirrhosis, causing cumulative effects that affect mentation, mask signs of developing encephalopathy, or precipitate coma.
Collaborative	
Monitor laboratory studies, such as ammonia, electrolytes, pH, blood urea nitrogen (BUN), glucose, and CBC with differential.	Elevated ammonia levels, hypokalemia, metabolic alkalosis, hypoglycemia, anemia, and infection can precipitate or potentiate development of hepatic coma.
Eliminate or restrict protein in diet. Provide glucose supplements and adequate hydration.	Ammonia is responsible for mental changes in hepatic encephalopathy. Dietary changes may result in constipation, which also increases bacterial action and formation of ammonia. Glucose provides a source of energy, reducing need for protein catabolism.

(continues on page 424)

ACTIONS/INTERVENTIONS (continued) / RATIONALE (continued)

Administer medications, as indicated, for example:

Ursodeoxycholic acid (urosodiol, UDCA, Actigall) — Major medication used to slow the progression of the disease; may delay need for transplantation.

Immunosuppressive agents, such as corticosteroids (Prednisolone, DeltaCortef), methotrexate (Rheumatrex/Folex), and cyclosporine (Sandimmune/Neoral); anti-inflammatory agents, such as colchicines — These agents may inhibit immune reactions that mediate inflammatory processes and progression of the disease.

Electrolytes — Corrects imbalances and may improve cerebral function and metabolism of ammonia.

Stool softeners, colonic purges such as magnesium sulfate, enemas, and lactulose — Removes protein and blood from intestines. Acidifying the intestine produces diarrhea and decreases production of nitrogenous substances, reducing risk or severity of encephalopathy. *Note:* Long-term use of lactulose may be required for clients with hepatic encephalopathy to reduce ammonia on a daily or regular basis.

Bactericidal agents, such as neomycin (Mycifradin) and kanamycin (Kantrex) — Destroys intestinal bacteria, reducing production of ammonia, to prevent encephalopathy.

Administer supplemental O_2. — Mentation is affected by O_2 concentration and utilization in the brain.

Assist with procedures as indicated, such as dialysis, plasmapheresis, or extracorporeal liver perfusion. — May be used to reduce serum ammonia levels if encephalopathy develops or other measures are not successful.

NURSING DIAGNOSIS: disturbed Body Image

May Be Related To
Biophysical changes, altered physical appearance

Possibly Evidenced By
Reports perceptions that reflect an altered view of one's body in appearance
Reports fear of reaction by others
Reports negative feelings about body (e.g., helplessness, powerlessness)

Desired Outcomes/Evaluation Criteria—Client Will

Body Image (NOC)

Verbalize understanding of changes and acceptance of self in the present situation.
Identify feelings and methods for coping with negative perception of self.

ACTIONS/INTERVENTIONS / RATIONALE

Body Image Enhancement (NIC)

Independent

Discuss situation and encourage verbalization of fears and concerns. Explain relationship between nature of disease and symptoms. — Client is very sensitive to body changes and may also experience feelings of guilt when cause is related to alcohol or other drug use.

Support and encourage client; provide care with a positive, friendly attitude. — Caregivers sometimes allow judgmental feelings to affect the care of client and need to make every effort to help client feel valued as a person.

Encourage family/SO to verbalize feelings, visit freely, and participate in care. — Family/SO may feel guilty about client's condition and may be fearful of impending death. They need nonjudgmental emotional support and free access to client. Participation in care helps them feel useful and promotes trust between staff, client, and family/SO.

Assist client/SO to cope with change in appearance; suggest clothing that does not emphasize altered appearance, such as use of red, blue, or black clothing. — Client may present unattractive appearance as a result of jaundice, ascites, and ecchymotic areas. Providing support can enhance self-esteem and promote client's sense of control.

Collaborative

Refer to support services, such as counselors, psychiatric resources, social service, clergy, and alcohol treatment program. — Increased vulnerability and concerns associated with this illness may require services of additional professional resources.

NURSING DIAGNOSIS: ineffective Self-Health Management

May Be Related To

Complexity of therapeutic regimen
Perceived benefits/barriers
Economic difficulties
Social support deficit

Possibly Evidenced By

Reports difficulty with prescribed regimen
Ineffective choices in daily living for meeting health goals
Failure to take action to reduce risk factors
Unexpected acceleration of illness symptoms

Desired Outcomes/Evaluation Criteria—Client Will

Self-Management: Chronic Disease (NOC)

Verbalize understanding of disease process, prognosis, and potential complications.
Correlate symptoms with causative factors.
Identify and initiate necessary lifestyle changes.
Actively participate in care.

ACTIONS/INTERVENTIONS	RATIONALE
Teaching: Disease Process (NIC)	
Independent	
Review disease process and future expectations.	Provides knowledge base from which client can make informed choices.
Emphasize importance of avoiding alcohol. Give information about medical and community services available to aid in alcohol rehabilitation, if indicated.	Alcohol is one of the leading causes for the development of cirrhosis.
Inform client of altered effects of medications with cirrhosis and the importance of using only drugs prescribed or cleared by a healthcare provider who is familiar with client's history.	Some drugs are hepatotoxic, especially opioids, sedatives, and hypnotics. In addition, the damaged liver has a reduced ability to metabolize all drugs, potentiating cumulative effect and aggravation of bleeding tendencies.
Instruct client with ascites to avoid using NSAIDs.	NSAIDs have been shown to blunt the effect of diuretics, which can negatively effect treatment of ascites (Garcia-Tsao, 2009).
Review procedure for maintaining function of peritoneovenous shunt when present.	Several types of shunts are available, so it is important that client and SO understand care needed for client's shunt. For example, Denver shunt requires client to periodically pump the chamber to maintain patency of the device, and client with a LeVeen shunt may wear an abdominal binder or engage in a Valsalva's maneuver to maintain shunt function.
Assist client with identifying support person(s).	Because of length of recovery, potential for relapses, and slow convalescence, support systems are extremely important in maintaining behavior modifications.
Emphasize the importance of good nutrition. Recommend avoidance of high-protein and salty foods, onions, and strong cheeses. Provide written dietary instructions.	Proper dietary maintenance and avoidance of foods high in sodium and protein aid in remission of symptoms and help prevent ammonia buildup and further liver damage. Written instructions are helpful for client to refer to at home.
Stress necessity of follow-up care and adherence to therapeutic regimen.	Chronic nature of disease has potential for life-threatening complications. Provides opportunity for evaluation of effectiveness of regimen, including patency of shunt if used.
Discuss sodium and salt substitute restrictions and necessity of reading labels on food, OTC drugs, and herbal agents.	Minimizes ascites and edema formation. Overuse of substitutes may result in other electrolyte imbalances. Food, OTC medications, and personal care products, including antacids and some mouthwashes, may contain sodium or alcohol and may be toxic to the liver or be primarily metabolized by the liver.
Encourage scheduling activities with adequate rest periods.	Adequate rest decreases metabolic demands on the body and increases energy available for tissue regeneration.
Promote diversional activities that are enjoyable to client.	Prevents boredom, facilitates rest, and minimizes anxiety and depression.
Recommend avoidance of persons with infections, especially upper respiratory infections.	Decreased resistance, altered nutritional status, and impaired immune responses potentiate risk of infection.
Instruct client and SO of signs and symptoms that warrant notification of healthcare provider, such as increased abdominal	Prompt reporting of symptoms provides opportunity to treat complications before they become life-threatening.

(continues on page 426)

ACTIONS/INTERVENTIONS (continued)	RATIONALE (continued)
girth, rapid weight loss or gain, increased peripheral edema, increased dyspnea, fever, blood in stool or urine, excess bleeding of any kind, and jaundice.	*Note:* Client may be evaluated for additional medical or surgical interventions, including liver transplantation.
Instruct SO to notify healthcare providers of any confusion, untidiness, night wandering, tremors, or personality change.	Changes reflecting deterioration in mental status may be apparent to SO, although insidious changes may be noted by others with less frequent contact with client.

POTENTIAL CONSIDERATIONS following acute hospitalization (dependent on client's age, physical condition and presence of complications, personal resources, and life responsibilities)

- ***Fatigue***—disease state, malnutrition, poor physical condition, negative life events, altered body chemistry (e.g., alcohol withdrawal, changes in liver function, effect on target organs)
- ***imbalanced Nutrition: less than body requirements***—inability to ingest food (anorexia, nausea and vomiting, indigestion), inability to digest food/absorb nutrients
- ***risk for ineffective Self-Health Management***—perceived benefit, social support deficit, complexity of therapeutic regimen, economic difficulties
- ***dysfunctional Family Processes***—substance abuse, resistance to treatment, inadequate coping and/or lack of problem-solving skills
- ***risk for Caregiver Role Strain***—illness severity of care receiver, substance abuse codependency; family dysfunction before caregiving situation; presence of situational stressors that normally affect families (e.g., economic vulnerability)

PANCREATITIS

I. Pathophysiology

a. Inflammation of pancreas with premature activation of pancreatic enzymes resulting in localized damage to the pancreas, autodigestion, and fibrosis of the pancreas

b. Leads to wide range of metabolic consequences and life-threatening complications, such as hypovolemia, shock, acute renal failure, diabetes, acute respiratory distress syndrome (ARDS), and multiorgan failure

II. Types

a. Acute
- i. Sudden inflammation occurs over a short period of time.
- ii. Severity ranges from mild abdominal discomfort to a life-threatening illness.
- iii. Can result in bleeding into the gland, serious tissue damage, infection, and cyst formation
- iv. Release of enzymes and toxins into bloodstream can damage other vital organs, including the heart, lungs, and kidneys.

b. Chronic
- i. Commonly follows acute episode when inflammation is ongoing
- ii. Development may be delayed, as in alcohol abuse.

III. Etiology

a. Acute
- i. Biliary tract disease, such as obstruction by gallstones, is most common cause—about 40% (Gardner, 2013).
- ii. Long-standing alcohol abuse, particularly binge drinking—approximately 35% (Whitcomb et al, 2008)
- iii. Trauma: blunt or penetrating
- iv. Procedures: endoscopic or surgical
- v. Viral infections: mumps, mononucleosis, varicella
- vi. Bacterial infections: *Mycoplasma pneumoniae,* salmonellosis, tuberculosis
- vii. Drugs: many are implicated, including sulfonamides, glucocorticoids, thiazide diuretics, combination cancer chemotherapy drugs (especially asparaginase, 5-aminosalicylic acid compounds, nonsteroidal anti-inflammatory drugs (NSAIDs)
- viii. Unknown cause—about 10% to 15% of cases

b. Chronic (Huffman, 2012)
- i. Intraductal obstruction: alcohol abuse, stones, or tumors
- ii. Alcohol abuse—about 60% of cases
- iii. Direct toxins and toxic metabolites
- iv. Recurrent acute pancreatitis that heals with fibrosis
- v. Ischemia from obstruction and fibrosis exacerbates or perpetuates disease, rather than initiates disease.
- vi. Autoimmune disorders: primary biliary cirrhosis, renal tubular acidosis

IV. Statistics

a. Morbidity: More than 220,000 were estimated to be hospitalized for acute pancreatitis in 2007 (Gardner et al, 2008). In 2010, it was reported that chronic pancreatitis resulted in more more than 56,000 hospitalizations per year (Stevens, 2010).

b. Mortality: Mortality is substantially increased in necrotizing pancreatitis (less than 1% for interstitial pancreatitis, 10% for sterile necrosis, 30% for infected necrosis) (Stevens, 2010).

c. Cost: Direct care cost for acute and chronic pancreatitis combined estimated at over $2.5 billon in 2004 (Everhart, 2008).

GLOSSARY

Atelectasis: Collapse of lung tissue affecting all or part of the lung.

Chyme: Thick liquid made of partially digested food and stomach juices that is made in the stomach and moves into the small intestine for further digestion.

Coagulopathy: Defect in the blood-clotting mechanisms.

Cullen's sign: Blue-black bruising around the umbilicus area, indicative of intraperitoneal hemorrhage.

Disseminated intravascular coagulopathy: Pathological process where the blood starts to coagulate throughout the whole body. This depletes the body of platelets and coagulation factors, which results in a paradoxical situation in which there is a high risk for simultaneous catastrophic thromboembolism and massive hemorrhage.

Endocrine function: Pertains to hormones and the glands that make and secrete them into the bloodstream where they travel to distant organs. The Islets of Langerhans produce and secrete insulin.

Exocrine function: Refers to glands that secrete their products into ducts. Pancreatic enzymes are produced in the pancreas, accumulate in the intralobular ducts, and empty into the main pancreatic duct, which drains into the duodenum when needed for digestion.

Hemorrhagic pancreatitis: Hemorrhage caused by digestion of vessel walls by pancreatic enzymes.

Ileus: Partial or complete blockage of the small and/or large intestine.

Interstitial edema: Abnormally large fluid volume in tissues between the body's cells (interstitial spaces).

Pancreas: Gland located in the upper, posterior abdomen responsible for insulin production and the manufacture and secretion of digestive enzymes leading to carbohydrate, fat, and protein metabolism.

Pancreatic pseudocyst: Collection of tissue, fluid, debris, pancreatic enzymes, and blood. The fluid is usually pancreatic juice that has leaked out of a damaged pancreatic duct.

Peristalsis: Pattern of smooth muscle contractions that propels food and fluid through the esophagus and intestines.

Pleural effusion: An abnormal accumulation of fluid in the pleural space around the lungs.

Steatorrhea: Symptom in which fecal matter is frothy or foul-smelling and floats because of a high fat content.

Systemic inflammatory response syndrome (SIRS): Inflammation of the whole body (the "system") without a proven source of infection. It is a medical emergency.

Care Setting

The client is treated in an inpatient acute medical unit or intensive care unit (ICU) for initial incident or exacerbations with serious complications; otherwise, condition is managed at the community level.

Related Concerns

Acute renal injury (acute renal failure), page 505
Alcohol: acute withdrawal, page 800
Diabetes mellitus/diabetic ketoacidosis, page 377
Peritonitis, page 320
Psychosocial aspects of care, page 729
Sepsis/septicemia, page 665
Substance use disorders, page 815
Total nutritional support: parenteral/enteral feeding, page 437
Upper gastrointestinal/esophageal bleeding, page 281

Client Assessment Database

DIAGNOSTIC DIVISION MAY REPORT	MAY EXHIBIT
ACTIVITY/REST • Malaise, fatigue	• Agitation, restlessness, apprehension
CIRCULATION	• Hypertension (acute pain) • Hypotension and tachycardia accompany hypovolemic shock or sepsis or SIRS • Generalized edema • Ascites • Skin pale, mottled areas; flushing may be present in acute stage from systemic inflammation; jaundiced (inflammation or obstruction of common duct); Cullen's sign from accumulation of blood (hemorrhagic pancreatitis)

(continues on page 428)

Client Assessment Database (continued)

DIAGNOSTIC DIVISION MAY REPORT (continued)	MAY EXHIBIT (continued)
ELIMINATION • Diarrhea • Absence of bowel movements • Abdominal bloating • Dark and decreased urine	• ***Bowel sounds:*** May be decreased or absent—reduced peristalsis or ileus • Dark amber or brown, foamy urine (bile) • Steatorrhea • Scanty urine (oliguria) progressing to absence of urine (anuria), which may be a compensatory response to hypovolemia
FOOD/FLUID • Food intolerance, loss of appetite • Frequent or persistent vomiting, retching, dry heaves • Weight loss	• Diffuse abdominal tenderness to palpation • Abdominal rigidity, distention • Hypoactive bowel sounds
NEUROSENSORY	• Confusion, agitation • Coarse tremors of extremities from hypocalcemia
PAIN/DISCOMFORT • Unrelenting, severe, deep abdominal pain, usually located in the epigastrium and periumbilical regions, but may radiate to the back (acute pancreatitis) • Onset may be sudden and may follow an episode of heavy drinking or a large meal • Poorly localized, dull, cramping, burning, deep, or aching abdominal pain may be reported with long-term or chronic pancreatitis • Radiation to chest and back • May increase in supine position	• Abdominal tenderness and guarding (68% in acute pancreatitis) (Gardner, 2013) • May curl up on left side with both arms over abdomen and knees and hips flexed • Abdominal rigidity
RESPIRATION	• Tachypnea with or without dyspnea • Decreased depth of respiration with splinting or guarding actions • Bibasilar crackles—associated with pleural effusion
SAFETY	• Fever (76% in acute pancreatitis) (Gardner, 2013)
SEXUALITY • Current pregnancy (third trimester) with shifting of abdominal contents and compression of biliary tract	• Agitation, confusion
TEACHING/LEARNING • Family history of pancreatitis • Signs and symptoms of hyperglycemic crisis • History of cholelithiasis with partial or complete common bile duct obstruction, gastritis, duodenal ulcer, duodenitis, diverticulitis, Crohn's disease, recent abdominal surgery (such as procedures on the pancreas, biliary tract, stomach, or duodenum), external abdominal trauma • Excessive alcohol intake (90% of cases) • Use of medications—salicylates, pentamidine, antihypertensives, opiates, thiazides, steroids, some antibiotics, estrogens • Infectious diseases—mumps, hepatitis B, Coxsackie viral infection	

DIAGNOSTIC DIVISION MAY REPORT (continued)	MAY EXHIBIT (continued)
DISCHARGE PLAN CONSIDERATIONS • May require assistance with dietary program and activities of daily living (ADLs) at home ➧ Refer to section at end of plan for postdischarge considerations.	

Diagnostic Studies

TEST WHY IT IS DONE	WHAT IT TELLS ME
BLOOD TESTS	
• ***Serum amylase:*** Common biochemical marker for acute pancreatitis.	Increased because of obstruction of normal outflow of pancreatic enzymes. May be five or more times the normal level in acute pancreatitis, and then fall back within normal ranges because serum half-life is short. Levels are elevated in chronic pancreatitis, but not as high as in acute phase, and may return to near normal levels in late stage of chronic disease.
• ***Serum lipase:*** More specific to the pancreas than amylase and has a longer half-life.	Elevates along with amylase, but stays elevated longer. Levels are elevated to a lesser degree in chronic pancreatitis, and return to normal levels in late stage of chronic disease.
• ***Alanine aminotransferase (ALT):*** An enzyme found mainly in the liver, but also in smaller amounts in the kidneys, heart, and pancreas.	An increased ALT can be indicative of gallstones, which is commonly associated with pancreatitis.
• ***Serum bilirubin:*** Substance formed when red blood cells (RBCs) break down and are excreted by the liver.	Elevation is common (may be caused by alcoholic liver disease or compression of common bile duct). Excessive bilirubin causes jaundice and may be excreted in urine and stools.
• ***Alkaline phosphatase:*** Enzyme concentrated in liver and biliary tract.	Usually elevated if pancreatitis is accompanied by biliary disease.
• ***Creactive protein (CRP):*** An acute-phase reactant protein produced in the liver.	Level greater than 10 mg/dL strongly indicates severe pancreatitis. Higher levels have been shown to correlate with a propensity toward organ failure (Gardner et al, 2013).
• ***Serum albumin:*** Most abundant plasma protein transports substances such as bilirubin, calcium, progesterone, and drugs, and creates oncotic pressure to keep fluid from leaking out into the tissues.	May be decreased because of increased capillary permeability and movement of fluid into extracellular space.
• ***Serum calcium:*** Chemical element necessary for the normal function of the heart, nerves, and bones.	Hypocalcemia occurs early on because of the release of fatty acids combining with calcium, rendering it unusable to the body. May be decreased because of increased capillary permeability and movement of fluid into extracellular space. Hypoalbuminemia and marked elevations of LDH (lactic dehydrogenase) are associated with an increased mortality rate (Fauci, 2009).
• ***Potassium:*** Electrolyte needed to regulate water balance, levels of acidity, and blood pressure.	Hypokalemia may occur because of gastric losses; hyperkalemia may develop secondary to tissue necrosis, acidosis, and renal insufficiency.
• ***Magnesium:*** Essential mineral needed for protein, bone, and fatty acid formation, making new cells, activating B vitamins, relaxing muscles, clotting of blood, and producing and using insulin.	Diuretic therapy, chronic alcoholism, cirrhosis, and pancreatitis can all cause excessive magnesium loss, as can losses from the gastrointestinal (GI) tract through nasogastric suctioning, fistula drainage, and diarrhea (Astle, 2005).
• ***Triglycerides:*** One of the many fats formed by the union of glycerol and fatty acids and may indicate cause of condition.	High triglyceride levels are often indicative of high levels of insulin. Levels may exceed 1700 mg/dL and may be causative agent in acute pancreatitis.
• ***Complete blood count (CBC):*** Battery of screening tests that typically includes hemoglobin (Hgb); hematocrit (Hct); RBC count, morphology, indices, and distribution width index;	WBC count of 10,000 to 25,000 is present in 80% of clients with acute pancreatitis. Hgb may be lower because of bleeding. Hct may be elevated because of hemoconcentration associated

(continues on page 430)

Diagnostic Studies (continued)

TEST WHY IT IS DONE (continued)	WHAT IT TELLS ME (continued)
platelet count and size; white blood cell (WBC) count and differential.	with vomiting, hypovolemia, or from effusion of fluid into pancreas or retroperitoneal area.
• *Serum glucose:* One of the simple sugars in the blood.	Transient elevations of more than 200 mg/dL are common, especially during initial or acute attacks. Sustained hyperglycemia reflects widespread pancreatic cell damage and necrosis and is a poor prognostic sign.
OTHER DIAGNOSTIC TESTS	
• *Ultrasound of abdomen:* Technique that uses sound waves to produce an image of internal body structures.	Most useful initial test to determine etiology of pancreatitis and to identify pancreatic inflammation, abscesses, pseudocysts, or obstruction of biliary tract by gallstones.
• *Computed tomography (CT) scan:* X-ray procedure that uses a computer to produce a detailed picture of a cross section of the body to look for complications of pancreatitis and determine treatment options.	Indicated in client with severe acute pancreatitis and is the imaging study of choice for assessing complications, such as fluid around the pancreas, abscess, or pancreatic pseudocyst.
• *Endoscopic retrograde cholangiopancreatography (ERCP):* Test that combines endoscopy with x-rays to provide an accurate view of the pancreatic and bile ducts.	Enables accurate visualization of the pancreatic ductal system and is regarded as the criterion standard for diagnosing chronic pancreatitis (Huffman et al, 2012).
ASSOCIATED TESTS	
• *Fecal tests*	Because maldigestion and malabsorption do not occur until more than 90% of the pancreas has been destroyed, steatorrhea is a manifestation of advanced chronic pancreatitis (Huffman et al, 2012).

Nursing Priorities

1. Control pain and promote comfort.
2. Prevent and treat fluid and electrolyte imbalance.
3. Reduce pancreatic stimulation while maintaining adequate nutrition.
4. Prevent complications.
5. Provide information about disease process, prognosis, and treatment needs.

Discharge Goals

1. Pain relieved or controlled.
2. Hemodynamically stable.
3. Complications prevented or minimized.
4. Disease process, prognosis, potential complications, and therapeutic regimen understood.
5. Plan in place to meet needs after discharge.

NURSING DIAGNOSIS: acute Pain

May Be Related To

Physical agent—obstruction of pancreatic/biliary ducts
Chemical agent—contamination of peritoneal surfaces by pancreatic exudate, autodigestion of pancreas, extension of inflammation to the retroperitoneal nerve plexus

Possibly Evidenced By

Verbalized/coded report of pain
Guarding behavior—positioning to avoid pain
Expressive behavior (e.g., grimacing)
Self-focus
Changes in vital signs

Desired Outcomes/Evaluation Criteria—Client Will

Pain Level (NOC)
Report pain is relieved or controlled.

Pain Control (NOC)
Follow prescribed therapeutic regimen.
Demonstrate use of methods that provide relief.

ACTIONS/INTERVENTIONS	RATIONALE
Pain Management (NIC)	
Independent	
Investigate verbal reports of pain, noting specific location and intensity (0 to 10 scale). Note factors that aggravate and relieve pain.	Pain is often diffuse, severe, and unrelenting in acute or hemorrhagic pancreatitis. Severe pain is often the major symptom in client with chronic pancreatitis. Isolated pain in the right upper quadrant (RUQ) reflects involvement of the head of the pancreas. Pain in the left upper quadrant (LUQ) suggests involvement of the pancreatic tail. Localized pain may indicate development of pseudocysts or abscesses.
Maintain bedrest during acute attack and provide quiet, restful environment.	Decreases stimulation of pancreatic secretions, thereby reducing pain.
Promote position of comfort, such as on one side with knees flexed or sitting up and leaning forward.	Reduces abdominal pressure and tension, providing some measure of comfort and pain relief. *Note:* Supine position often increases pain.
Provide alternative comfort measures, including repositioning and back rub, and quiet diversional activities such as TV or radio. Encourage relaxation techniques, such as guided imagery and visualization.	Promotes relaxation and enables client to refocus attention; may enhance coping.
Keep environment free of food odors.	Sensory stimulation can activate pancreatic enzymes, increasing pain.
Administer intravenous (IV) analgesics in timely manner and in smaller, more frequent doses, during acute episode. Consider use of patient-controlled analgesia (PCA), if appropriate.	Severe or prolonged pain can aggravate shock and is more difficult to relieve, requiring larger doses of medication, which can mask underlying problems and complications and may contribute to respiratory depression.
Maintain meticulous skin care, especially in presence of draining abdominal wall fistulas.	Pancreatic enzymes can digest the skin and tissues of the abdominal wall, creating abscesses and ulceration.
Collaborative	
Administer medication, as indicated, for example:	
Opioid analgesics, such as meperidine (Demerol), morphine sulfate, hydrocodone (Vicodin), tramadol (Ultram)	Meperidine is usually effective in relieving pain and may be preferred over morphine, which may have a side effect of biliary-pancreatic spasms. *Note:* Pain in clients who have recurrent or chronic pancreatitis may be more difficult to manage because they can develop tolerance to normal doses of the opioids given for pain control. Tricyclic antidepressants (e.g., clomaparmamine [Anafranil]) may be introduced in these clients to ameliorate pain and potentiate the effects of opiates (Huffman et al, 2012).
Histamine blockers, such as lansoprazole (Prevacid), cimetidine (Tagamet), ranitidine (Zantac), and famotidine (Pepcid)	Decreasing production of hydrochloric acid inhibits pancreatic enzyme activity and associated pain.
Withhold food and fluid, as indicated.	Client should be kept on nothing by mouth (NPO) status until pain and nausea subside to limit or reduce release of pancreatic enzymes and resultant pain.
Maintain gastric suction when used.	Nasogastric (NG) tube may be used for client with ileus or protracted vomiting to prevent accumulation of gastric secretions and pancreatic enzyme activity.
Prepare for surgical intervention, if indicated.	Surgical exploration may be required in presence of intractable pain or complications involving the biliary tract, such as pancreatic abscess or pseudocyst. *Note:* Surgery is not performed during acute stage, unless it would actually cure the problem, such as removing stone causing biliary tract obstruction.

NURSING DIAGNOSIS: risk for deficient Fluid Volume

Risk Factors May Include

Excessive losses through normal routes—vomiting, gastric suctioning

Failure of regulatory mechanisms (e.g., third-space fluid transudation, ascites formation, vasodilatation, alteration of clotting process)

Possibly Evidenced By

(Not applicable; presence of signs and symptoms establishes an *actual* diagnosis)

Desired Outcomes/Evaluation Criteria—Client Will

Fluid Balance (NOC)

Maintain adequate hydration as evidenced by stable vital signs, good skin turgor, prompt capillary refill, strong peripheral pulses, and individually appropriate urinary output.

ACTIONS/INTERVENTIONS	RATIONALE
Fluid/Electrolyte Management (NIC)	
Independent	
Auscultate heart sounds; note rate and rhythm. Monitor and document rhythm and changes.	Cardiac changes and dysrhythmias may reflect hypovolemia or electrolyte imbalance, commonly hypokalemia and hypocalcemia. Hyperkalemia may occur related to tissue necrosis, acidosis, and renal insufficiency and may precipitate lethal dysrhythmias if uncorrected. *Note:* Cardiovascular complications are common in severe pancreatitis and include myocardial infarction (MI), pericarditis, and pericardial effusion with or without tamponade.
Monitor blood pressure (BP), noting trends. Measure central venous pressure (CVP), if available.	Fluid sequestration with shifts into third space, bleeding, and release of vasodilators (kinins) and cardiac depressant factor triggered by pancreatic ischemia may result in profound hypotension. Reduced cardiac output and poor organ perfusion can precipitate widespread systemic complications. Systemic infection (septic shock) is also possible, exacerbating hypovolemic status.
Investigate changes in sensorium: confusion and slowed responses.	Changes may be related to hypovolemia, hypoxia, electrolyte imbalance, or impending delirium tremens (in client with acute pancreatitis secondary to excessive alcohol intake). Severe pancreatic disease may cause toxic psychosis.
Measure intake and output (I&O), including vomiting or gastric aspirate, and diarrhea. Calculate 24-hour fluid balance.	Indicators of replacement needs and effectiveness of therapy.
Note decrease in urine output (less than 400 mL/24 hr).	Oliguria may occur, signaling renal impairment or acute tubular necrosis (ATN), related to increase in renal vascular resistance or altered renal blood flow.
Record color and character of gastric drainage, measure pH, and note presence of occult blood.	Risk of gastric hemorrhage is high because of esophageal varices or erosion of other large vessels (Gardner et al, 2013). Refer to CP: Upper Gastrointestinal/Esophageal Bleeding, if indicated.
Weigh, as indicated; correlate with calculated fluid balance.	Weight loss may suggest hypovolemia; however, edema, fluid retention, and ascites, or hemorrhage into the peritoneal cavity may be reflected by increased weight, or stable weight in the presence of muscle wasting.
Note poor skin turgor, dry skin and mucous membranes, or reports of thirst.	Further physiological indicators of dehydration.
Observe and record peripheral and dependent edema. Measure abdominal girth if ascites present.	Edema and fluid shifts occur as a result of increased vascular permeability, sodium retention, and decreased colloid osmotic pressure in the intravascular compartment.
Inspect skin for petechiae, hematomas, and unusual wound or venipuncture bleeding. Note hematuria, mucous membrane bleeding, and bloody gastric contents.	Disseminated intravascular coagulation (DIC) may be initiated by release of active pancreatic proteases into the circulation. The most frequently affected organs are the kidneys, skin, and lungs.
Observe and report coarse muscle tremors, twitching, and positive Chvostek's sign.	These are symptoms of calcium imbalance. Calcium binds with free fats in the intestine and is lost by excretion in the stool. *Note:* Chvostek's sign is evaluated by tapping the cheek over the facial nerve and then observing for the development of a lip twitch or facial spasm, which is indicative of muscular irritability. Trousseau sign was previously used as an evaluation for hypocalcemia (carpal spasm development when a BP cuff is applied and the circulation transiently occluded) but may be painful and is not preferred (Elisha et al, 2010).
Collaborative	
Administer fluid replacement, as indicated, such as saline solutions, albumin, blood and blood products, and dextran.	Choice of replacement solution may be less important than rapidity and adequacy of volume restoration. Saline solutions and albumin may be used to promote mobilization of fluid back into vascular space. Low-molecular-weight dextran is sometimes used to reduce risk of renal dysfunction and pulmonary edema associated with pancreatitis.
Monitor laboratory studies—Hgb/Hct, protein, albumin, electrolytes, blood urea nitrogen (BUN), creatinine, urine osmolality, sodium and potassium, and coagulation studies.	Identifies deficits, replacement needs, and developing complications.
Replace electrolytes—sodium, potassium, chloride, and calcium, as indicated.	Decreased oral intake and excessive losses greatly affect electrolyte and acid-base balance, which is necessary to maintain optimal cellular and organ function.
Prepare for and assist with peritoneal lavage or hemoperitoneal dialysis.	Removes toxins and pancreatic enzymes and may allow for more rapid correction of metabolic abnormalities in severe acute pancreatitis.

NURSING DIAGNOSIS: imbalanced Nutrition: less than body requirements

May Be Related To

Inability to ingest food (e.g., vomiting, prescribed dietary restrictions)
Inability to digest food/absorb nutrients (e.g., loss of digestive enzymes)

Possibly Evidenced By

Reported inadequate food intake
Aversion to eating, reported altered taste sensation, lack of interest in food
Weight loss
Poor muscle tone

Desired Outcomes/Evaluation Criteria—Client Will

Nutritional Status (NOC)

Demonstrate progressive weight gain toward goal with normalization of laboratory values.
Experience no signs of malnutrition.

Knowledge: Prescribed Diet (NOC)

Demonstrate behaviors or lifestyle changes to regain and maintain appropriate weight.

ACTIONS/INTERVENTIONS	RATIONALE
Nutrition Management (NIC)	
Independent	
Assess abdomen, noting presence and character of bowel sounds, abdominal distention, and reports of nausea.	Gastric distention and intestinal atony are frequently present, resulting in reduced or absent bowel sounds. Return of bowel sounds and relief of symptoms signal readiness for discontinuation of NG.
Provide frequent oral care.	Decreases vomiting stimulus and soothes inflamed, dry mucous membranes associated with dehydration and mouth breathing when NG tube is in place.
Assist client in selecting food and fluids that meet nutritional needs and restrictions when diet is resumed.	Previous dietary habits may be unsatisfactory in meeting current needs for tissue regeneration and healing. Use of gastric stimulants, such as caffeine, alcohol, cigarettes, or gas-producing foods, or ingestion of large meals, may result in excessive stimulation of the pancreas and recurrence of symptoms.
Observe color, consistency, and amount of stools. Note frothy consistency and foul odor.	Steatorrhea may develop in chronic pancreatitis from incomplete digestion of fats.
Maintain NPO status and gastric suctioning during acute phase.	Prevents stimulation and release of pancreatic enzymes (secretin) when chyme and hydrochloric acid enter the duodenum.
Resume oral intake with liquids and advance diet slowly to provide high-protein, high-carbohydrate diet, when indicated.	Oral feedings given too early in the course of illness may exacerbate symptoms.
Collaborative	
Administer enteral or parenteral feedings, as indicated.	Enteral feedings may be preferred via nasogastric or jejunostomy tube to prevent gut atrophy in early or uncomplicated pancreatitis or when surgery is performed; however, parenteral feedings (TPN) should be instituted early when oral or enteral feedings are not possible. (Refer to CP: Total Nutritional Support: Parenteral/Enteral Feedings.)
Administer medications, as indicated, for example:	
Vitamins, such as A, D, E, and K	Replacement required because fat metabolism is altered, reducing absorption and storage of fat-soluble vitamins.
Replacement enzymes, such as pancreatin (Dizymes) and pancrelipase (Protilase, Cotazym)	Used in chronic pancreatitis to correct deficiencies to promote digestion and absorption of nutrients.

NURSING DIAGNOSIS: risk for unstable Blood Glucose Level

Risk Factors May Include

Dietary intake; [decreased insulin production, increased glucagon release]
Physical health status, stress

Possibly Evidenced By

(Not applicable; presence of signs and symptoms establishes an *actual* diagnosis)

Desired Outcomes/Evaluation Criteria—Client Will

Blood Glucose Level (NOC)

Maintain glucose in satisfactory range.

ACTIONS/INTERVENTIONS	RATIONALE
Hyperglycemia Management (NIC)	
Independent	
Note signs of increased thirst and urination or changes in mentation and visual acuity.	May warn of developing hyperglycemia associated with increased release of glucagon (damage to alpha cells) or decreased release of insulin (damage to beta cells).
Perform and monitor results of bedside fingerstick glucose testing and dipstick testing of urine for sugar and acetone (ketones).	Early detection of inadequate glucose utilization may prevent development of hyperglycemic crisis. IV insulin may be required to control serum glucose within normal ranges.
Collaborative	
Monitor serum glucose, as indicated.	Indicator of insulin needs because hyperglycemia is frequently present, although not usually in levels high enough to produce ketoacidosis.
Provide insulin, as appropriate.	Corrects persistent hyperglycemia caused by injury to cells and increased release of glucocorticoids. Insulin therapy is usually short-term unless permanent damage to pancreas occurs.
Advance diet as tolerated and based on specific nutritional needs.	Loss of pancreatic function or reduced insulin production may require initiation of a diabetic diet.

NURSING DIAGNOSIS: risk for Infection [sepsis]

Risk Factors May Include

Inadequate primary defenses: stasis of body fluids, altered peristalsis, change in pH of secretions, tissue destruction
Inadequate secondary defenses: immunosuppression
Malnutrition
Chronic disease

Possibly Evidenced By

(Not applicable; presence of signs and symptoms establishes an *actual* diagnosis)

Desired Outcomes/Evaluation Criteria—Client Will

Infection Status (NOC)
Achieve timely healing; be free of signs of infection.
Be afebrile.

Risk Control: Infectious Process (NOC)
Participate in activities to reduce risk of infection.

ACTIONS/INTERVENTIONS	RATIONALE
Infection Protection (NIC)	
Independent	
Use strict aseptic technique when changing surgical dressings or working with IV lines, indwelling catheters, tubes, or drains. Change soiled dressings promptly.	Limits sources of infection, which can lead to sepsis in a compromised client.
Model and emphasize importance of good hand washing.	Reduces risk of cross-contamination.
Observe rate and characteristics of respirations and breath sounds. Note occurrence of cough and sputum production.	Pulmonary complications of pancreatitis include atelectasis, pleural effusion, pneumonia, and ARDS. Fluid accumulation and limited mobility predisposes client to respiratory infections and atelectasis. Accumulation of ascites fluid may cause elevated diaphragm and shallow abdominal breathing.
Encourage frequent position changes, deep breathing, and coughing. Assist with ambulation as soon as stable.	Enhances ventilation of all lung segments and promotes mobilization of secretions.
Observe for signs of infection, such as the following:	
Fever and respiratory distress in conjunction with jaundice	Cholestatic jaundice and decreased pulmonary function may be first sign of sepsis or ARDS.
Increased abdominal pain, rigidity and rebound tenderness, diminished or absent bowel sounds	Suggestive of peritonitis.
Increased abdominal pain and tenderness, recurrent fever (higher than 101°F [38.3°C]), leukocytosis, hypotension, tachycardia, and chills	Abscesses can occur 2 weeks or more after the onset of pancreatitis and should be suspected whenever client is deteriorating despite supportive measures.
Collaborative	
Obtain culture specimens, such as blood, wound, urine, sputum, or pancreatic aspirate.	Identifies presence of infection and causative organism.

ACTIONS/INTERVENTIONS (continued)	RATIONALE (continued)
Administer anti-infective therapies as indicated, such as imipenem/cilastatin (Primaxin), metronidazole (Flagyl), and levofloxacin (Levaquin); cephalosporins, such as ceftriaxone (Rocephin); and aminoglycosides, such as gentamicin (Garamycin) and tobramycin (Nebcin).	Antibiotics are not given routinely for fever, especially early in the disease course, because this symptom is almost universally secondary to the inflammatory response and typically does not reflect an infectious process. However, broad-spectrum anti-infectives are generally recommended for acute pancreatitis sepsis; however, long-term therapy will be based on the specific organisms cultured (Gardner et al, 2013).
Prepare for surgical intervention, as necessary.	Abscesses may be surgically drained with resection of necrotic tissue. Sump tubes may be inserted for antibiotic irrigation and drainage of pancreatic debris. Pseudocysts (persisting for several weeks) may be drained because of the risk and incidence of infection and rupture.

NURSING DIAGNOSIS: impaired Gas Exchange

May Be Related To
Alveolar-capillary membrane changes—interstitial edema, pulmonary congestion

Possibly Evidenced By
(Not applicable; presence of signs and symptoms establishes an *actual* diagnosis)

Desired Outcomes/Evaluation Criteria—Client Will

Respiratory Status (NOC)
Maintain adequate ventilation with respiratory rate and rhythm normal for client, breath sounds clear, and free of dyspnea or shortness of breath.
Display arterial blood gases (ABGs) within client's normal range.

ACTIONS/INTERVENTIONS	RATIONALE
Respiratory Monitoring (NIC)	
Independent	
Evaluate respiratory rate and depth. Note respiratory effort, for example, presence of dyspnea, use of accessory muscles, and nasal flaring.	Client responses are variable. Rate and effort may be increased by pain, accumulation of secretions, or abdominal distention. Respiratory depression can occur with use of opioid analgesics. Early recognition and treatment of abnormal ventilation may prevent complications.
Auscultate breath sounds. Note areas of diminished or absent breath sounds and presence of adventitious sounds, such as rhonchi or crackles.	Loss of active breath sounds in an area of previous ventilation may reflect atelectasis. Crackles or rhonchi may be indicative of fluid accumulation due to interstitial edema, pulmonary congestion, or infection.
Encourage client participation and responsibility for deep-breathing exercises, use of adjuncts, and coughing, as indicated. Reposition frequently.	Stimulates respiratory function and lung expansion. Effective in preventing and resolving pulmonary congestion.
Reinforce splinting of abdomen with pillows during deep breathing or coughing.	May enhance effectiveness of cough effort.
Note increasing restlessness, confusion, and lethargy.	May indicate impaired gas exchange and possible ARDS, requiring prompt evaluation and intervention.
Collaborative	
Monitor and graph serial ABGs and pulse oximetry, and review chest x-ray reports.	Decreasing oxygen level or saturation and increasing $PaCO_2$ and changes in chest x-rays suggest developing complications requiring further evaluation and treatment.
Administer supplemental oxygen O_2, if indicated.	Increases available O_2 for tissue and organ function. *Note:* Inability to maintain adequate oxygenation indicates need for more aggressive therapy or mechanical ventilation. (Refer to CP: Ventilation Assistance [Mechanical].)

NURSING DIAGNOSIS: ineffective Self-Health Management

May Be Related To

Complexity of therapeutic regimen; deficient knowledge
Perceived barriers
Economic difficulties
Social support deficit

Possibly Evidenced By

Reports difficulty with prescribed regimen
Ineffective choices in daily living for meeting health goals
Unexpected acceleration of illness symptoms

Desired Outcomes/Evaluation Criteria—Client Will

Knowledge: Acute Illness or Chronic Disease Management (NOC)

Verbalize understanding of condition, disease process, and potential complications.
Verbalize understanding of therapeutic needs.
Correctly perform necessary procedures and explain reasons for the actions.
Initiate necessary lifestyle changes and participate in treatment regimen.

ACTIONS/INTERVENTIONS	RATIONALE
Teaching: Disease Process (NIC)	
Independent	
Review specific cause of current episode and prognosis.	Provides knowledge base on which client can make informed choices.
Discuss other causative and associated factors such as excessive alcohol intake, gallbladder disease, duodenal ulcer, and some drugs—oral contraceptives, thiazide diuretics, glucocorticoids, and sulfonamides.	Client may or may not be able to impact risk, but avoidance of certain substances and drugs may help limit damage and prevent development of a chronic condition.
Explore availability of treatment programs for chemical dependency, if indicated.	Alcohol abuse is currently the most common cause of recurrence of chronic pancreatitis. Usage of other drugs, whether prescribed or illicit, is increasing as a factor. *Note:* Pain of pancreatitis can be severe and prolonged and may lead to narcotic dependence. It may benefit from referral to a pain clinic.
Emphasize the importance of follow-up care, and review symptoms that need to be reported immediately to physician, such as recurrence of pain, persistent fever, nausea and vomiting, abdominal distention, frothy or foul-smelling stools, and general intolerance of food.	Prolonged recovery period requires close monitoring to prevent or limit recurrence and complications, such as infection and pancreatic pseudocysts.
Review importance of initially continuing bland, low-fat diet with frequent small feedings and restricted caffeine and gradual resumption of a normal diet within individual tolerance.	Understanding the purpose of the diet in maximizing the use of available enzymes while avoiding overstimulation of the pancreas may enhance client involvement in self-monitoring of dietary needs and responses to foods.
Instruct in use of pancreatic enzyme replacements and bile salt therapy as indicated, avoiding concomitant ingestion of hot foods or fluids.	If permanent damage to the pancreas has occurred, exocrine deficiencies will occur, requiring long-term replacement. Hot foods or fluids can inactivate enzymes.
Recommend cessation of smoking. Refer for medical and support interventions, if client desires.	Nicotine stimulates gastric secretions and unnecessary pancreatic activity.
Discuss signs and symptoms of diabetes mellitus: polydipsia, polyuria, weakness, and weight loss.	Damage to the beta cells may result in a temporary or permanent alteration of insulin production.

POTENTIAL CONSIDERATIONS following acute hospitalization (dependent on client's age, physical condition and presence of complications, personal resources, and life responsibilities)

- ***imbalanced Nutrition: less than body requirements***—inability to ingest food (prescribed dietary restrictions, persistent nausea and vomiting), inability to digest food/absorb nutrients (imbalances in digestive enzymes)
- ***risk for unstable Blood Glucose Level***—lack of acceptance of diagnosis; deficient knowledge of diabetes management; medication management
- ***acute/chronic Pain***—chemical agents (e.g., irritation of peritoneal surfaces by pancreatic enzymes, general inflammatory process), physical agent (e.g., spasms of biliary ducts)
- ***dysfunctional Family Processes***—alcohol abuse, family history of resistance to treatment, inadequate coping, lack of problem-solving skills
- ***ineffective Self-Health Management***—complexity of therapeutic regimen, economic difficulties, perceived benefit, social support deficits

TOTAL NUTRITIONAL SUPPORT: PARENTERAL/ENTERAL FEEDING

I. Pathophysiology: Malnutrition is a disorder of body composition in which nutritional intake is less than required and results in reduced organ function, abnormalities in blood chemistry, reduced body mass, and worsened clinical outcomes.

a. Nutritional status is affected by multiple factors, including eating behaviors, disease states, economics, and environment.

b. In the acutely or chronically ill client, the impact of malnutrition includes muscle mass loss, progressive weakness, potential for infection, poor healing, and a higher rate of systemic complications.

c. When oral intake is inadequate or not possible, specifically designed nutritional therapy can be administered via an enteral or parenteral route to prevent or correct protein-calorie malnutrition.

II. Clinical Indication for Feeding

a. Preexisting nutritional deprivation; unplanned or unexplained loss of 10% in body weight

b. Anticipated or actual inadequate energy intake by mouth, such as inability to consume food or drink orally for 7 days or more, based on individual nutritional status

c. Critically ill individuals, because of their increased metabolic demands and limited nutritional reserve, commonly require nutritional support.

d. The Joint Commission for Accreditation of Healthcare Organizations (JCAHO) recognizes the negative impact of malnutrition in hospitals and long-term care institutions and has, in turn, made nutritional assessment, support, and ongoing reassessment an essential part of accreditation requirements (JCAHO, 2002).

III. Etiology of Malnutrition

a. Can exist in persons who are underfed or overfed, occurring in both extremely thin and obese individuals

b. May result from an inadequate or unbalanced diet, digestive difficulties, absorption problems, or other medical conditions

   i. Acute conditions, such as surgery, severe burns, infections, and trauma, that drastically increase short-term nutritional requirements

   ii. Chronic diseases associated with nutrient loss, nutrient demand, and with malabsorption, such as celiac disease, cystic fibrosis, pancreatic insufficiency, pernicious anemia

   iii. Conditions and treatments associated with malnutrition through decreased intake, such as depressed appetite, difficulty swallowing, and nausea associated with both cancer and chemotherapy, as well as with HIV/AIDS and its drug therapies

c. Certain age groups, such as elderly clients, require fewer calories but continue to require adequate nutritional support because they are often less able to absorb nutrients, due in part to decreased stomach acid production, and are more likely to have one or more chronic ailments that may affect their nutritional status.

IV. Routes for Feeding

a. Enteral nutrition

   i. Gastrointestinal (GI) intubation is preferred for clients with functional GI tract but who are unable to consume an adequate nutritional intake or for whom oral intake is contraindicated or impossible.

   ii. Feeding may be done via flexible catheter (such as nasogastric [NG], orogastric tube) or enterostomy (such as gastrostomy, duodenostomy, or jejunostomy tube).

   iii. Feeding may be short-term for supplementation of oral intake or long-term to provide for all of client's nutrition.

   iv. Formulas can be manufactured to meet certain needs for the body, e.g., *polymeric* is a standard formula, and *elemental* is for those with malabsorptive guts, but also there are special formulas for diabetes, for acute and chronic renal failure, for immune system enhancement, and for hepatic encephalopathy (Diaz et al, 2004).

b. Parenteral nutrition

   i. May be chosen because of altered metabolic states or when mechanical or functional abnormalities of the GI tract prevent enteral feeding

   ii. Goals are to improve the client's nutritional status; establish and maintain a positive nitrogen balance; improve or maintain muscle strength and mass; promote weight gain; and encourage the healing process through infusion of amino acids, fat, carbohydrates, trace elements, vitamins, and electrolytes, as indicated.

   iii. The average adult requires approximately 1500 calories per day in order to maintain energy stores before illness is factored in.

   iv. Nutritional support is provided via an intravenous (IV) route, either centrally or peripherally.

      1. Central: Formula is concentrated hyperosmolar and must be infused via a central vein (subclavian or jugular) into the superior vena cava or peripherally inserted central catheter (PICC), inserted into the arm and passed into a major blood vessel.

      2. Peripheral: Formula is similar, but less concentrated than central formula and is infused via a peripheral vein.

GLOSSARY

Basal metabolic rate (BMR): Number of calories the body burns at rest to maintain normal body functions.

Bitot's spots: Triangular, shiny, gray spots on the conjunctiva seen in vitamin A deficiency.

Cachexia: Profound and marked state of general ill health and malnutrition.

Catabolism: Metabolic breakdown of complex molecules into simpler ones, often resulting in a release of energy.

Harris-Benedict equation: Formula that uses BMR and then applies an activity factor to determine total daily energy expenditure (calories).

(continues on page 438)

GLOSSARY (continued)

Ideal body weight (IBW): Calculation for men: 106 lbs for first 5 feet plus 6 lbs for each additional inch of height. Women: 100 lbs for first 5 feet plus 5 lbs for each additional inch of height.

Indirect caliometry: Estimation of energy expenditure via the measurement of oxygen consumption and carbon dioxide production.

Lipids: Lipids are fat emulsion of 10% to 20%. It contains triglycerides, egg phospholipids, glycerol, and water. If lipids are needed with TPN, they are given intermittently or mixed in with the TPN solution (Tortorice, 2007).

Malabsorption: Inability of the body to use one or more available nutrients.

Partial parenteral nutrition (PPN): Normally prescribed for clients who can tolerate some oral feedings but cannot ingest adequate amounts of food to meet their nutritional needs. It is usually administered through a peripheral intravenous catheter. Two types of solutions are commonly used in a number of combinations for PPN: lipid emulsions and amino acid-dextrose solutions.

Protein calorie malnutrition (PCM), also called protein energy malnutrition (PEM): Severe deficiency of protein plus inadequate caloric intake to meet energy needs.

Total energy expenditure (TEE): Amount of energy spent, on average, in a typical day measured in calories (k/day).

Total parenteral nutrition (TPN): IV nutrition support using a formulation of amino acids, carbohydrates, lipids, electrolytes, multiple vitamins, minerals, and supplemental medications (e.g., insulin or H2 blockers).

TPN IV access: Central access lines for TPN may include a triple lumen catheter (TLC), a peripherally inserted central line (PICC), tunneled central venous catheters (e.g., Broviac, or Hickman), and implanted central venous catheter (e.g., Port-A-Cath). The first two categories are likely to be used in shorter-term parenteral therapy, while the latter two categories may be reserved for long-term and permanent therapy.

Care Setting

Client may be treated in any setting, including community or home care.

Related Concerns

Acquired immunodeficiency syndrome (AIDS), page 689
Anemias, page 459
Burns: thermal, chemical, and electrical—acute and convalescent phases, page 638
Cancer, page 827
Chronic obstructive pulmonary disease (COPD) and asthma, page 118
Cirrhosis of the liver, page 412
Diabetes mellitus/diabetic ketoacidosis, page 377
Eating disorders: anorexia nervosa/bulimia nervosa, page 340
Eating disorders: obesity, page 358
Fluid and electrolyte imbalances, page 885
Fractures, page 601
Inflammatory bowel disease (IBD): ulcerative colitis, Crohn's disease, page 291
Obesity: bariatric surgery, page 367
Pancreatitis, page 426
Psychosocial aspects of care, page 729
Renal failure: chronic, page 517
Surgical intervention, page 762

Client Assessment Database

Clinical signs listed here depend on the degree and duration of malnutrition and include observations indicative of vitamin, mineral, protein, and calorie deficiencies.

DIAGNOSTIC DIVISION MAY REPORT	MAY EXHIBIT
ACTIVITY/REST	• Muscle wasting—temporal, intercostal, gastrocnemius, dorsum of hand • Thin extremities • Flaccid muscles • Decreased activity tolerance

DIAGNOSTIC DIVISION MAY REPORT (continued) / MAY EXHIBIT (continued)

Circulation

May Exhibit

- Tachycardia, bradycardia
- Diaphoresis
- Pallor, cyanosis

Elimination

May Report

- Diarrhea or constipation, flatulence associated with food intake

May Exhibit

- Abdominal distention, increased girth, ascites
- Abdominal tenderness on palpation
- Stools may be loose, hard-formed, fatty, or clay-colored

Food/Fluid

May Report

- Recent weight loss or weight loss of 10% or more of body weight within previous 6 months
- Unplanned weight loss of more than 20 lb in the last 3 months
- Problems with chewing, swallowing, choking, or saliva production
- Changes in the taste of food
- Anorexia
- Nausea, vomiting
- Inadequate oral intake (nothing by mouth [NPO]) status for 7 to 10 days

May Exhibit

- Actual measured weight as compared with usual, or weight is less than 90% of IBW for height, sex, and age
- Actual weight equal to or greater than 120% of IBW
- A distorted actual body mass weight may occur because of the presence of edema, ascites, organomegaly, tumor bulk
- Bowel sounds diminished, hyperactive, or absent
- Thyroid, parotid enlargement
- Lips and mucous membranes dry, cracked, red, swollen
- Tongue may be smooth, pale, slick, coated; color often magenta, beefy red; lingual papillae atrophy or swelling
- Gums swollen, bleeding
- Dentition may be poor, such as lack of teeth, multiple cavities, denture problems

Neurosensory

May Exhibit

- Lethargy, apathy, listlessness, irritability, disorientation
- Gag and swallow reflex may be decreased or absent
- Loss of balance and coordination

Respiration

May Exhibit

- Increased respiratory rate; respiratory distress
- Dyspnea, increased sputum production
- Breath sounds, crackles (protein deficiency-related fluid shifts)

Safety

May Report

- Recent course of radiation therapy (radiation enteritis)

Sexuality

May Report

- Loss of libido
- Amenorrhea

May Exhibit

- Hair may be fragile, coarse, lackluster, falling out (alopecia); decreased pigmentation may be present
- Skin dry, scaly, tented; "flaky paint" dermatosis; edematous
- Draining or unhealed wounds; pressure sores
- Ecchymosis; perifollicular petechiae
- Subcutaneous fat loss
- Eyes sunken, dull, dry, with pale conjunctiva; Bitot's spots or scleral icterus
- Nails may be brittle, thin, flattened, ridged, spoon-shaped

Teaching/Learning

May Report

- History or presence of conditions causing protracted protein and caloric losses—malabsorption or short-gut syndrome, diarrhea, acute pancreatitis, renal dialysis, fistulas, draining wounds, thermal injuries, problems with chewing or swallowing (such as due to stroke or Parkinson's disease)
- Presence of factors known to alter nutritional requirements and increase energy demands—single or multiorgan failure, sepsis, fever, AIDS, cancer, trauma, extensive burns, use of steroids, antitumor agents, immunosuppressants

(continues on page 440)

Client Assessment Database (continued)

DIAGNOSTIC DIVISION MAY REPORT (continued)	MAY EXHIBIT (continued)
• Use of treatments that greatly alter intake and medications that cause untoward drug and nutrient interactions—laxatives, anticonvulsants, diuretics, antacids, opioids, immunosuppressants, radiation, high-dose chemotherapy • Illness of psychiatric origin—anorexia nervosa or bulimia • Educational and social factors—lack of nutrition knowledge or kitchen facilities, reduced or limited financial resources **DISCHARGE PLAN CONSIDERATIONS** • May require assistance with solution preparation, therapy supplies, and maintenance of feeding device for home nutritional care ➧ Refer to section at end of plan for postdischarge considerations.	

Diagnostic Studies

TEST WHY IT IS DONE	WHAT IT TELLS ME
ANTHROPOMETRICS	
• Techniques that deal with the measurement of the size, weight, and proportions of the human body.	
• ***Weight:*** What people are expected to weigh based on age, sex, and height.	A malnourished person could weigh less or more than their IBW. Weight may be inaccurate because of factors such as edema or ascites.
• ***Body mass index (BMI):*** Calculates body composition.	Measures ratios of lean-to-fat body weight. Classifications include underweight (less than 18.5), normal weight (18.5 to 24.9), overweight (25 to 29.9), and obese (greater than 30).
• ***Skinfold measurement:*** Estimates subcutaneous body fat by measuring skinfold thickness using calipers. Measurements can use from three to nine different standard anatomical sites around the body.	Fat reserves less than in the 10th percentile suggest advanced depletion; levels less than the 30th percentile suggest mild-to-moderate depletion.
BLOOD TESTS	
• ***Visceral proteins:*** Nonmuscular proteins useful in monitoring nutritional status.	Deficits suggest malnutrition.
• ***Glucose:*** Carbohydrates provide energy and spare body protein.	During the critical phase of illness or injury, or in states of malnutrition, carbohydrate metabolism is radically altered. Hyperglycemia is a hallmark of stress and is frequently a side effect of nutritional support. Blood sugars are usually checked every 6 hours during therapy and treated, as needed, using a sliding-scale insulin regimen.
• ***Serum albumin:*** Protein deficiency results in decreased synthesis of albumin. Protein, which is available in varying concentrations in TPN and enteral feeding formulas, is an essential nutrient that functions to promote tissue growth, repair, and wound healing.	An albumin level of less than 3 g/day often indicates malnutrition. However, overhydration and dehydration affect its concentration, and its long half-life makes it unreliable as a nutrition marker, especially in acute depletion or repletion. It is more accurate in chronic protein deficiency states (Mears, 2005).
• ***Serum transferrin:*** An iron-transport protein more sensitive to changes in visceral protein stores than albumin; also, its shorter half-life and smaller blood pool makes it a more accurate early marker for protein depletion.	Level of less than 150 mg/dL is considered severe depletion.
• ***Prealbumin (PAB), also called transthyretin and thyroxine transport protein:*** Excellent sensitivity to nutritional status. PAB has a shorter half-life than albumin, and levels respond quickly to nutritional therapy, making it a more sensitive indicator of improvement and change in protein status.	Levels of less than 17 mg/dL are noted with end-stage liver disease; it is affected by inflammation, infection, and trauma (Mears, 2005).

TEST WHY IT IS DONE (continued)	WHAT IT TELLS ME (continued)
• *Retinol-binding protein (RBP):* Carrier protein of vitamin A.	Concentration falls during protein and calorie deprivation and rises rapidly with supplementation (Mears, 2005).
• *C-reactive protein (CRP):* Acute inflammation phase protein.	Increases dramatically during systemic inflammation and catabolism, while visceral proteins fall. CRP values return to normal once the body starts to synthesize proteins, such as PAB.
• *Total lymphocyte count:* Indicator of the status of the immune system.	Less than 1500 cells/mm^3 indicates leukopenia and results from decreased generation of T cells, which are very sensitive to malnutrition. Less than 800 cells/mm^3 indicates severe depletion. Levels are also altered by severe stress, renal failure, cancer, infection, and administration of corticosteroids.
• *Tests of micronutrients:* Trace elements and electrolytes required for body to produce enzymes, hormones, and substances required for growth and development, as well as numerous body regulations, functions, and balance.	Deficiency occurs with inadequate intake and with loss of electrolyte-containing fluids—urine, diarrhea, vomiting, fistula drainage, and continuous NG suctioning. Imbalances occur also when excessive or deficient amounts of electrolytes and other micronutrients are supplied in TPN for the daily allowance for nutrition. Protocols should be in place for laboratory studies.
• *Nitrogen balance studies:* Nitrogen excretion via urine, stool, and insensible losses often exceeds nitrogen intake in the acutely ill, reflecting catabolic response to stress and use of endogenous protein stores for energy production (gluconeogenesis).	Blood urea nitrogen (BUN) may be severely decreased because of chronic malnutrition and depletion of skeletal protein stores.
OTHER DIAGNOSTIC STUDIES	
• *24-hour creatinine (Cr) excretion:* Because Cr is concentrated in muscle mass, there is a correlation between lean body mass and 24-hour Cr excretion. Actual values are compared with ideal values based on height and weight times 100.	Cr height index of 60% to 80% indicates moderate depletion; less than 60% indicates severe depletion.
• *Chest x-ray:* Procedure used to evaluate organs and structures within the chest for symptoms of disease.	May be normal or show evidence of pleural effusion; small heart silhouette in severely malnourished individual. *Note:* Chest x-ray will also be done after central line is inserted prior to beginning TPN to determine it is a location safe for infusion of hyperosmolar solutions.
• *Electrocardiogram (ECG):* A record of the electrical activity of the heart that provides important information concerning the spread of electricity to the different parts of the heart.	May be normal or demonstrate low voltage, dysrhythmias, and patterns reflective of electrolyte imbalances.
• *Monitoring tests once client is on TPN:*	Guides changes in TPN formula (Diaz et al, 2004).
• Basic metabolic panel, C-Reactive Protein (CRP), magnesium (Mg), and phosphorus (Phos)	May be done on days 1 and 2 and prn. *Note:* Blood glucose may be checked every 6 hours for first 72 hours.
• Liver function studies, pre-albumin, and triglycerides	May be checked weekly and prn.
• Resting Energy Expenditure (REE): Measures body's energy at rest using a heat process called calorimetry (via a portable cart available at point-of-care)	May be done every 2 weeks.

Nursing Priorities

1. Promote consistent intake of adequate calorie and protein requirements.
2. Prevent complications.
3. Minimize energy losses and needs.
4. Provide information about condition, prognosis, and treatment needs.

Discharge Goals

1. Nutritional intake adequate for individual needs.
2. Complications prevented or minimized.
3. Fatigue alleviated.
4. Condition, prognosis, and therapeutic regimen understood.
5. Plan in place to meet needs after discharge.

NURSING DIAGNOSIS: imbalanced Nutrition: less than body requirements

May Be Related To

Inability to ingest/digest food and/or absorb nutrients (e.g., cancer and associated treatments, anorexia, surgical procedures, dysphagia, decreased level of consciousness, hypermetabolic states)

Possibly Evidenced By

Body weight 20% or more under ideal; loss of weight with adequate food intake
Lack of interest in food; aversion to eating
Abdominal pain, cramping
Poor muscle tone
Hyperactive bowel sounds; diarrhea; steatorrhea
[Abnormal laboratory studies]

Desired Outcomes/Evaluation Criteria—Client Will

Nutritional Status (NOC)

Demonstrate stable weight or progressive weight gain toward goal, with normalization of laboratory values and no signs of malnutrition.

ACTIONS/INTERVENTIONS	RATIONALE
Nutrition Therapy (NIC) *Independent* **General**	
Assess nutritional status continually during daily nursing care, noting energy level; condition of skin, nails, hair, oral cavity; and desire to eat.	Provides the opportunity to observe deviations from normal client baseline and influences choice of interventions.
Weigh daily and compare with admission weight.	Establishes baseline, aids in monitoring effectiveness of therapeutic regimen, and alerts nurse to inappropriate trends in weight loss or gain.
Document oral intake by use of 24-hour recall, food history, and calorie counts, as appropriate.	Identifies imbalance between estimated nutritional requirements and actual intake.
Ensure accurate collection of specimens (urine and stool) for nitrogen balance studies.	Inaccurate collection can alter test results, leading to improper interpretation of client's current status and needs.
When client is receiving nutrition solutions:	
Administer nutritional solutions at prescribed rate via infusion control device, as needed. Adjust rate to deliver prescribed hourly intake. Do not increase rate to "catch up" if infusion slows.	Nutritional support prescriptions are based on individually estimated caloric and protein requirements. A consistent rate of nutrient administration ensures proper utilization with fewer side effects, such as hyperglycemia or dumping syndrome. *Note:* Continuous and cyclic infusions of enteral formulas are generally better tolerated than bolus feedings and result in improved absorption.
Be familiar with electrolyte content of nutritional solutions.	Metabolic complications of nutritional support often result from a lack of appreciation of changes that can occur because of refeeding—hyperglycemia, hyperosmolar nonketotic coma (HHNC), and electrolyte imbalances.
Total Parenteral Nutrition (TPN) Administration (NIC)	
Observe appropriate "hang" time of parenteral solutions per protocol.	Effectiveness of IV vitamins diminishes and solution degrades after 24 hours.
Monitor fingerstick glucose per protocol, such as every 6 hours (Diaz et al. 2004) during initiation of therapy.	High glucose content of solutions may lead to pancreatic fatigue, requiring use of supplemental insulin to prevent hyperglycemic complications. *Note:* Fingerstick determination of glucose level is more accurate than urine testing because of variations in renal glucose threshold.
Enteral Tube Feeding (NIC)	
Assess GI function and tolerance to enteral feedings, knowing type of tube used, such as NG or small bowel. Note bowel sounds, reports of nausea and abdominal discomfort, presence of diarrhea or constipation, development of weakness, light-headedness, diaphoresis, tachycardia, and abdominal cramping.	Because protein turnover of the GI mucosa occurs approximately every 3 days, the GI tract is at great risk for early dysfunction and atrophy from disease and malnutrition. Intolerance of formula or presence of dumping syndrome may require alteration of rate of administration, concentration or type of formula, or possibly change to parenteral administration. *Note:* Use of postpyloric feeding tube eliminates need for active bowel sounds as a criterion for tolerance.
Check gastric residuals if bolus feedings are done and as otherwise indicated. Hold feeding and return aspirate per protocol	Delayed gastric emptying can be caused by a specific disease process, such as paralytic ileus, surgery, shock; by drug

ACTIONS/INTERVENTIONS (continued)	RATIONALE (continued)
for type and rate of feeding used if residual is greater than predetermined level.	therapy, especially opioids; or the protein and fat content of the individual formula. *Note:* Replacement of gastric aspirate reduces loss of gastric acid and electrolytes.
Maintain patency of enteral feeding tubes by flushing with 20 mL warm water before and after feeding and as indicated, such as between multiple doses of medications or when checking gastric residuals.	Enteral formulas contain protein that can clog feeding tubes (more likely with small-bore or silicone than with polyurethane tubes), necessitating removal or replacement of tube. *Note:* Cranberry juice or colas are not recommended because they may actually cause an obstruction by promoting formula coagulation. Pancrelipase, a pancreatic enzyme, may be effective in clearing tubing of persistent clog.
Transitional	
Emphasize importance of transition to oral feedings as appropriate.	Although client may have little interest in food or desire to eat, transition to oral feedings is preferred in view of potential side effects and complications of nutritional support therapy.
Assess gag reflex, ability to chew or swallow, and motor skills when progressing to transitional feedings.	May require additional interventions, such as retraining by dysphagia expert or speech therapist, or long-term nutritional support.
Provide self-help utensils as indicated, such as plate guard, utensils with built-up handles, and lidded cups.	Clients with neuromuscular deficits, such as those due to stroke or brain injury, may require use of special aids developed to facilitate feeding.
Create optimal environment, such as removing noxious stimuli, bedpans, and soiled linens. Provide cheerful, attractive tray or table, soft music, and companionship.	Encourages client's attempts to eat, reduces anorexia, and introduces some of the social pleasures usually associated with mealtime.
Allow adequate time for chewing, swallowing, and savoring food; provide socialization and feeding assistance, as indicated.	Clients need encouragement and assistance to overcome underlying problems such as anorexia, fatigue, and muscular weakness.
Offer small, frequent feedings; incorporate client's likes and dislikes in meal planning as much as possible, and include "home foods," as appropriate.	May enhance client's desire for food and amount of intake.
Provide calorie-containing beverages when oral intake is possible, such as juices, Jell-O, water, and dietary supplements (Boost, Sustacal, Ensure); add Polycase to beverages or water.	Maximizes calorie intake when oral intake is limited or restricted.
Collaborative	
Refer to nutritional team and registered dietitian.	Aids in identification of nutrient deficits and specific need for parenteral or enteral nutritional intervention.
Determine nutritional and caloric needs, using appropriate method, such as TEE, BMI, Harris-Benedict equation, and indirect calorimetry test, as indicated.	Several methods are available to provide an estimation of calorie and protein needs. TEE is based on resting and activity energy expenditure and thermic effect of food. BMI estimates caloric needs according to energy requirements per kilogram of body weight. Harris-Benedict provides a reasonable estimate of resting energy expenditure in kilocalories per day. Indirect calorimetry test measures oxygen (O_2) consumption at basal or resting metabolic rate to aid in estimating calorie and protein requirements. *Note:* Although any of these tests may accurately determine individual needs, a standard formula for projecting energy requirements in the ill client is to provide 30 kcal/kg for weight maintenance, 25 kcal/kg for weight loss, or 35 kcal/kg for weight gain.
Enteral Tube Feeding/TPN Administration (NIC)	
Assist with insertion and confirm proper placement of feeding tube as appropriate, such as using chest x-ray for central venous catheter or aspiration of green gastric fluid or golden small bowel contents from feeding tube, before administration of solutions. Check pH (0 to 5) of aspirated stomach contents.	Reduces risk of feeding-induced complications, including pneumothorax or hemothorax, hydrothorax, air embolus, arterial puncture with central venous line, or aspiration from NG tube.
Administer dextrose-electrolyte or dextrose–amino acid and lipid emulsions (3-in-1) solutions, as indicated.	Solutions provide calories, essential amino acids, and micronutrients, usually combined with lipids for complete nutrition known as total nutrient admixtures (TNA). Solutions are modified to meet specific needs, such as lower protein in renal and liver failure or higher fat in respiratory failure. *Note:* 3-in-1 solution bags are larger (2 to 3 L) and

(continues on page 444)

ACTIONS/INTERVENTIONS (continued)	RATIONALE (continued)
	can infuse over a 24-hour period, eliminating the need for frequent bag changes and reducing line manipulation and risk of contamination.
Co-infuse lipid emulsions if 3-in-1 solutions are not used.	Useful in meeting excessive caloric requirements (e.g., due to burns) or as a source of essential fatty acids during long-term hyperalimentation. *Note:* Lipid solutions may be contraindicated in clients with alterations in fat metabolism or in the presence of pancreatitis, liver damage, anemia, coagulation disorders, or pulmonary disease.
Administer medications, as indicated, for example:	
Multivitamin preparations	Water-soluble vitamins are added to parenteral solutions. Other vitamins may be given for identified deficiencies.
Insulin	High glucose content of solutions may require exogenous insulin for metabolism, especially in presence of pancreatic insufficiency or disease. *Note:* Now insulin is usually added directly to parenteral solution.
Diphenoxylate with atropine (Lomotil), camphorated tincture of opium (paregoric), and metoclopramide (Reglan)	GI side effects of enteral feeding may need to be controlled with antidiarrheal agents (Lomotil/paregoric) or peristaltic stimulants (Reglan) if more conservative measures such as alteration of rate or strength or type of formula are not successful.
Monitor laboratory studies: serum glucose, electrolytes, transferrin, prealbumin, albumin, total protein, phosphate, BUN/Cr, liver enzymes, complete blood count (CBC), and arterial blood gases (ABGs).	Serum chemistries, blood counts, and lipid profiles are performed before initiation of therapy, providing a baseline for comparison with repeat studies to determine therapy needs and monitor for complications. Untoward metabolic effects of TPN include hypokalemia, hyponatremia and fluid retention, hyperglycemia, hypophosphatemia, increased CO_2 production resulting in respiratory compromise, elevation of liver function tests, and renal dysfunction.

NURSING DIAGNOSIS: risk for Infection

Risk Factors May Include

Invasive procedures—insertion of venous catheter, surgically placed gastrostomy or jejunostomy feeding tube, access devices in place for extended periods

Malnutrition, chronic disease

Environmental exposure—improper preparation and handling or contamination of the feeding solution

Possibly Evidenced By

(Not applicable; presence of signs and symptoms establishes an *actual* diagnosis)

Desired Outcomes/Evaluation Criteria—Client Will

Infection Severity (NOC)

Experience no fever or chills.

Demonstrate clean catheter insertion sites, free of drainage and erythema or edema.

ACTIONS/INTERVENTIONS	RATIONALE
Infection Protection (NIC)	
Independent	
Emphasize and model proper hand-washing technique.	Reduces risk of cross-contamination.
Maintain sterile technique for invasive procedures. Provide routine site care, as appropriate.	Prevents entry of bacteria, reducing risk of nosocomial infections.
Encourage frequent position changes and being out of bed or ambulation, as tolerated.	Limits stasis of body fluids, promotes optimal functioning of organ systems and GI tract.
Screen visitors and care providers for infectious processes, especially upper respiratory infection (URI).	Reduces risk of transmission of viruses that are difficult to treat.
Monitor and assist with respiratory exercises and use of adjuncts, such as incentive spirometer. Auscultate lungs for adventitious sounds.	Promotes deep breathing to clear airways and reduce risk of pneumonia. Presence of wheezes suggests retained secretions and potential complications requiring intervention.
Assess vital signs, including temperature, per protocol.	A rise in pulse and temperature may provide warning of infectious process unless client's immune system is too compromised to respond.

ACTIONS/INTERVENTIONS (continued)	RATIONALE (continued)
Total Parenteral Nutrition (TPN) Administration (NIC)	
Maintain an optimal aseptic environment during bedside insertion of central venous catheters and during changes of TPN bottles and administration tubing.	Catheter-related sepsis may result from entry of pathogenic microorganisms through skin insertion tract or from touch contamination during manipulations of TPN system.
Secure external portion of catheter and administration tubing to dressing with tape. Note intactness of skin suture.	Manipulation of catheter in and out of insertion site can result in tissue trauma or coring and potentiate entry of skin organisms into catheter tract.
Maintain a sterile occlusive dressing over catheter insertion site. Perform central or peripheral venous catheter dressing care per protocol.	Protects catheter insertion sites from potential sources of contamination. *Note:* Central venous catheter sites can easily become contaminated from tracheotomy or endotracheal secretions, or from wounds of the head, neck, and chest.
Inspect insertion site of catheter for erythema, induration, drainage, and tenderness.	The catheter is a potential irritant to the surrounding skin and subcutaneous skin tract, and extended use may result in insertion site irritation and infection.
Refrigerate premixed solutions before use; observe a 24-hour hang time for amino acid or total nutrient admixtures solutions and a 12-hour hang time for IV fat emulsions.	TPN solutions and fat emulsions have been shown to support the growth of a variety of pathogenic organisms once contaminated.
Monitor urinary output and serum glucose levels.	A rise in temperature or loss of glucose tolerance (glycosuria, hyperglycemia) is an early indication of possible catheter-related sepsis.
Enteral Tube Feeding (NIC)	
Keep manipulations of enteral feeding system to a minimum and wash hands before opening system. Handle the system as little as possible.	Touch contamination of formula is caused by caregiver administration technique.
Alternate nares for tube placement in long-term NG feedings.	Reduces risk of trauma and infection of paranasal tissue, especially important in facial trauma or burns.
Provide daily and as needed site care to abdominally placed feeding tubes.	GI secretions leaking through or around gastrostomy or jejunostomy tube tracts can cause skin breakdown severe enough to require removal of the feeding tube.
Refrigerate reconstituted enteral formulas before use; observe a hang time of 4 to 8 hours; discard unused formula after 24 hours.	Enteral formulas easily support bacterial growth due to high concentration of glucose and lipids and can be contaminated from several sources, including when preparation is mixed or poured or via frequent aspiration of gastric or small bowel contents, use of open system, and use of blue dye.
Infection Protection (NIC)	
Collaborative	
Aseptically prepare parenteral solutions or enteral formulas for administration. When possible, use prepackaged sterile enteral feeding formula.	TPN solutions should be prepared under a laminar flow hood in the pharmacy. Enteral formulas should be mixed in a clean environment in the dietary or pharmacy department. *Note:* Additives to TPN solutions, as a rule, should not be made on the unit because of the potential for contamination and drug incompatibilities.
Notify physician if signs of infection are present. Follow protocol for obtaining appropriate culture specimens of blood and solutions, and change bottle and tubing, as indicated.	Necessary to identify source of infection and initiate appropriate therapy. May require removal of TPN line and culture of catheter tip.
Administer antibiotics, as indicated.	May be given prophylactically or for specifically identified organism.

NURSING DIAGNOSIS: risk for Injury

Risk Factors May Include

Physical (e.g., catheter-related complications such as air emboli and septic thrombophlebitis)
Malnutrition
Effects of therapy, drug interactions

Possibly Evidenced By

(Not applicable; presence of signs and symptoms establishes an *actual* diagnosis)

Desired Outcomes/Evaluation Criteria—Client Will

Risk Control (NOC)

Be free of complications associated with nutritional support.
Modify environment and correct hazards to enhance safety for in-home therapy.

ACTIONS/INTERVENTIONS — RATIONALE

Surveillance (NIC)

Independent

Parenteral

Maintain a closed central IV system using Luer-Lock (or similar) connections.

Inadvertent disconnection of central IV system can result in lethal air emboli.

Administer appropriate TPN solution via peripheral or central venous route, including peripherally inserted central catheter (PICC) lines and tunneled catheters.

Solutions containing high concentrations of dextrose more than 10% must be delivered via a central vein because they result in chemical phlebitis when delivered through small peripheral veins.

Monitor for potential drug and nutrient interactions.

Various interactions are possible, such as digoxin in conjunction with diuretic therapy, which can cause hypomagnesemia; hypokalemia may result from chronic use of laxatives, mineralocorticoid steroids, diuretics, or amphotericin.

Assess catheter for signs of displacement out of central venous position: extended length of catheter on skin surface, leaking of IV solution onto dressing, client complaints of neck/arm pain, tenderness at catheter site, or swelling of extremity on side of catheter insertion.

Assess catheter for signs of displacement out of central venous position: extended length of catheter on skin surface, leaking of IV solution onto dressing, client complaints of neck/arm pain, tenderness at catheter site, or swelling of extremity on side of catheter insertion.

Inspect peripheral TPN catheter site routinely and change sites at least every other day or per protocol.

Peripheral TPN solutions, although less hyperosmolar, can still irritate small veins and cause phlebitis. Peripheral venous access is often limited in malnourished clients, but site should still be changed if signs of irritation develop.

Investigate reports of severe chest pain or coughing in clients with central line. Turn client to left side in Trendelenburg position, if indicated, and notify physician.

Suggests presence of air embolus requiring immediate intervention to displace air into apex of heart away from the pulmonary artery.

Maintain an occlusive dressing on catheter insertion sites for 24 hours after subclavian catheter is removed.

Extended catheter use may result in development of catheter skin tract. Once the catheter is removed, air embolus is still a potential risk until skin tract has sealed.

Enteral

Assess gastrostomy or jejunostomy tube sites for evidence of malposition.

Indwelling and mushroom catheters are still used for feeding tubes inserted via the abdomen. Migration of the catheter balloon can result in duodenal or jejunal obstruction. Improperly sutured gastrostomy tubes may easily fall out.

Collaborative

Review chest x-ray, as indicated.

Central parenteral line placement is routinely confirmed by x-ray.

Consult with pharmacist in regard to site and time of delivery of drugs that might have action adversely affected by enteral formula.

Absorption of vitamin D is impaired by administration of mineral oil, which inhibits micelle formation of bile salts, and by neomycin, which inactivates bile salts. Aluminum-containing antacids bind with the phosphorus in the feeding solution, potentiating hypophosphatemia.

NURSING DIAGNOSIS: risk for Aspiration

Risk Factors May Include

Presence of gastrointestinal tube, tube feedings

Increased intragastric pressure, delayed gastric emptying

Possibly Evidenced By

(Not applicable; presence of signs and symptoms establishes an *actual* diagnosis)

Desired Outcomes/Evaluation Criteria—Client Will

Respiratory Status: Airway Patency (NOC)

Maintain clear airway, free of signs of aspiration.

ACTIONS/INTERVENTIONS — RATIONALE

Aspiration Precautions (NIC)

Independent

Confirm placement of nasoenteral feeding tubes. Determine feeding tube position in stomach by x-ray, confirm pH of 0 to 5 for the gastric fluid withdrawn through tube, or auscultate injected air before intermittent feedings. Observe for ability to speak and cough.

Malplacement of nasoenteral feeding tubes may result in aspiration of enteral formula. Clients at particular risk include those who are intubated or obtunded and those who have had a cerebrovascular accident (CVA) or surgery of the head, neck, and upper GI system. *Note:* The reliability of the pH

ACTIONS/INTERVENTIONS (continued)	RATIONALE (continued)
	method is reduced if antacids or certain other medications have been given orally or via NG in the past 4 hours. In addition, when using auscultatory method to assess tube placement, air sounds can be transmitted to the epigastrium even if the tube is malpositioned in lung or proximal jejunum.
Maintain aspiration precautions during enteral feedings, such as the following:	
Keep head of bed elevated at 30 to 45 degrees during feeding and for at least 1 hour after feeding.	Reduces risk of regurgitation or gastric reflux.
Inflate tracheostomy cuff during and for 1 hour after intermittent feeding.	Aspiration of enteral formulas is highly irritating to the lung parenchyma and may result in pneumonia and respiratory compromise.
Interrupt continuous feeding when client is in prone position.	
Monitor gastric residuals between or before bolus feedings (as previously noted in ND: imbalanced Nutrition: less than body requirements).	Presence of large gastric residuals may potentiate an incompetent esophageal sphincter, leading to vomiting and aspiration.
Note characteristics of sputum and tracheal aspirate. Investigate development of dyspnea, cough, tachypnea, and cyanosis. Auscultate breath sounds.	Presence of formula in tracheal secretions or signs and symptoms reflecting respiratory distress suggest aspiration.
Note indicators of NG tube intolerance, such as absence of gag reflex, high risk of aspiration, and frequent removal of NG feeding tubes.	May require consideration of surgically placed feeding tube, percutaneous endoscopic gastrostomy (PEG), or jejunostomy (J tube) for client safety and consistency of enteral formula delivery.
Collaborative	
Review abdominal x-ray if performed.	Confirmation of placement of gastric feeding tube should be obtained by x-ray.

NURSING DIAGNOSIS: risk for deficient Fluid Volume

Risk Factors May Include

Active fluid loss or failure of regulatory mechanisms specific to underlying disease process or trauma; complications of nutrition therapy—high-glucose solutions, hyperglycemia (hyperosmolar nonketotic coma and severe dehydration)

Inability to obtain or ingest fluids

Possibly Evidenced By

(Not applicable; presence of signs and symptoms establishes an *actual* diagnosis)

Desired Outcomes/Evaluation Criteria—Client Will

Fluid Balance (NOC)

Display moist skin, moist mucous membranes, stable vital signs, and individually adequate urinary output; be free of edema and excessive weight loss or inappropriate gain.

ACTIONS/INTERVENTIONS	RATIONALE
Fluid Management (NIC)	
Independent	
Assess for clinical signs of dehydration such as thirst, dry skin and mucous membranes, hypotension, or fluid excess, including peripheral edema, tachycardia, and adventitious breath sounds.	Early detection and intervention may prevent occurrence of excessive fluctuation in fluid balance. *Note:* Severely malnourished clients have an increased risk of developing refeeding syndrome, such as life-threatening fluid overload, intracellular electrolyte shifts, and cardiac strain occurring during initial 3 to 5 days of therapy. This potentially catastrophic complication can usually be prevented by starting feedings at low rates and advancing them slowly over several days (Mehler et al, 2010).
Incorporate knowledge of caloric density of enteral formulas into assessment of fluid balance.	Enteric solutions are usually concentrated and do not meet free water needs.
Provide additional water and flush tubing, as indicated.	With higher calorie formula, additional water is needed to prevent dehydration or hyperglycemic complications.
Record intake and output (I&O), calculate fluid balance, and measure urine specific gravity.	Excessive urinary losses may reflect developing HHNC. Specific gravity is an indicator of hydration and renal function.
Weigh daily, or as indicated; evaluate changes.	Rapid weight gain reflecting fluid retention can predispose or potentiate heart failure (HF) or pulmonary edema. Gain of more than 0.5 lb/day indicates fluid retention and not deposition of lean body mass.

(continues on page 448)

ACTIONS/INTERVENTIONS (continued)	RATIONALE (continued)
Collaborative	
Monitor laboratory studies, such as the following:	
Serum potassium and phosphorus	Hypokalemia and phosphatemia can occur because of intracellular shifts during initial refeeding and may compromise cardiac function if not corrected.
Hematocrit (Hct)	Reflects hydration and circulating volume.
Serum albumin	Hypoalbuminemia and decreased colloidal osmotic pressure leads to third spacing of fluid and edema.
Serum transferrin	Reacts quickly to changes in protein status.
Prealbumin	Sensitive to low levels of protein.
Dilute formula or change from hypertonic to isotonic formula, as indicated.	May decrease gastric intolerance, reducing occurrence of diarrhea and associated fluid losses.

NURSING DIAGNOSIS: Fatigue

May Be Related To

Disease states; malnutrition; stress

Poor physical condition

Altered body chemistry (e.g., medications, chemotherapy)

Possibly Evidenced By

Reports an overwhelming lack of energy, inability to maintain usual routines or usual level of physical activity

Lethargy; compromised concentration

Desired Outcomes/Evaluation Criteria—Client Will

Fatigue Level (NOC)

Report increased sense of well-being and energy level.

Demonstrate measurable increase in physical activity.

ACTIONS/INTERVENTIONS	RATIONALE
Energy Management (NIC)	
Independent	
Monitor physiological response to activity, including changes in blood pressure (BP) or heart and respiratory rates.	Tolerance varies greatly, depending on the stage of the disease process, nutritional state, and fluid balance.
Establish realistic activity goals with client.	Provides for a sense of control and feelings of accomplishment.
Plan care to allow for rest periods. Schedule activities for periods when client has most energy. Involve client and caregiver in planning schedule.	Frequent rest periods are needed to restore or conserve energy. Planning allows client to be active during times when energy level is higher, which may restore a feeling of well-being and a sense of control.
Encourage client to do self-care when appropriate, such as sitting up in chair and walking. Increase activity level, as indicated.	Increases strength and stamina and enables client to become more active without undue fatigue.
Provide passive and active range-of-motion (ROM) exercises to bedridden clients.	The development of healthy lean muscle mass depends on the provision of both isotonic and isometric exercises. Prevents muscle wasting.
Keep bed in low position and walkways clear of furniture; assist with ambulation.	Protects client from injury during activities.
Assist with self-care needs, as necessary.	Generalized weakness may make activities of daily living (ADLs) almost impossible for client to complete.
Collaborative	
Provide supplemental O_2, as indicated.	Presence of anemia or hypoxemia reduces O_2 available for cellular uptake and contributes to fatigue and decreased immune response.
Refer to physical or occupational therapy.	Programmed daily exercises and activities help client maintain or increase strength and muscle tone and enhance sense of well-being.

NURSING DIAGNOSIS: deficient Knowledge [Learning Need] regarding condition, prognosis, treatment, self-care, and discharge needs

May Be Related To

Lack of exposure or recall, information misinterpretation

Cognitive limitation

Possibly Evidenced By

Reports the problem

Inaccurate follow-through of instructions

Desired Outcomes/Evaluation Criteria—Client/Caregiver Will

Knowledge: Disease Process (NOC)

Verbalize understanding of condition or the disease process and individual nutritional needs.

Knowledge: Treatment Procedure (NOC)

Correctly perform necessary procedures and explain reasons for the actions.

ACTIONS/INTERVENTIONS	RATIONALE
Enteral Tube Feeding/Total Parenteral Nutrition (TPN) Administration (NIC)	
Independent	
Assess client's and significant other's (SO's) knowledge of nutritional state.	Determines content matter to be presented.
Review individual situation, signs and symptoms of malnutrition, future expectations, and transitional feeding needs.	Provides information from which client and SO can make informed choices. Knowledge of the interaction between malnutrition and illness is helpful in understanding need for special therapy.
Discuss reasons for use of parenteral or enteral nutrition support.	May experience anxiety regarding inability to eat and may not comprehend the nutritional value of the prescribed TPN or tube feedings.
Provide adequate time for teaching client and SO when client is going home on enteral or parenteral feedings. Document client's and SO's understanding, ability, and competence to deliver safe home therapy.	Generally, 3 to 4 days is sufficient for client and SO to become proficient with tube feedings. Parenteral therapy is more complex, and client and SO may require a week or longer to feel ready for home management; follow-up in the home is required.
Discuss proper handling, storage, and preparation of nutritional solutions or food prepared by a blender; also discuss aseptic or clean techniques for care of insertion sites and use of dressings.	Reduces risk of formula or solution-related problems, metabolic complications, and infection.
Review use and proper care of nutritional support devices.	Client understanding and cooperation are key to the safe insertion and maintenance of nutritional support access devices and prevention of complications.
Review specific precautions, depending on type of feeding, such as checking placement of tube, sitting upright for enteral feeding, maintaining patency of tube, anchoring of tubing, and adequate length of tubing for nighttime feeding.	Promotes safe self-care and reduces risk of complications.
Discuss and demonstrate reinsertion of enterostomal feeding tube, if appropriate.	Tube may be changed routinely or inserted only for feedings. Intermittent feedings enhance client mobility and aid in transition to regular feeding pattern.
Identify signs and symptoms requiring medical evaluation—nausea and vomiting, abdominal cramping or bloating, diarrhea, rapid weight changes, erythema, drainage, foul odor at tube insertion site, fever and chills, coughing and choking, or difficulty breathing during enteral feeding.	Early evaluation and treatment of problems such as feeding intolerance, infection, and aspiration may prevent progression to complications that are more serious.
Instruct client and SO in glucose monitoring, if indicated.	Timely recognition of changes in blood glucose levels reduces risk of hyperglycemic or hypoglycemic reactions in client on hyperalimentation.
Discuss signs, symptoms, and treatment of hyperglycemia and hypoglycemia.	Hyperglycemia is more common for clients receiving parenteral feedings and those who have pancreas or liver disease or are taking large doses of corticosteroids. Rebound hypoglycemia can occur when feedings are intentionally or accidentally discontinued.

(continues on page 450)

ACTIONS/INTERVENTIONS (continued)	RATIONALE (continued)
Encourage use of diary for recording test results, physical feelings and any reactions, activity level, oral intake if any, I&O, and weekly weight.	Provides resource for review by healthcare providers for optimal management of individual situation.
Recommend daily exercise and activity to tolerance, scheduling of adequate rest periods.	Enhances gastric motility for enteral transition feedings, promotes feelings of general well-being, and prevents undue fatigue.
Ascertain that all supplies are in place in the home before discharge; make arrangements as needed with suppliers, such as hospital, pharmacy, medical equipment company, and laboratory.	Provides for successful, smooth transition from acute care setting to home and competent home therapy.
Refer to nutritional support team, home healthcare agency, and counseling resources. Provide with immediate-access phone numbers.	Client and SO need readily available support persons to assist with nutrition therapy, equipment problems, and emotional adjustments in long-term or home-based therapy.

POTENTIAL CONSIDERATIONS following acute hospitalization (dependent on client's age, physical condition and presence of complications, personal resources, and life responsibilities)

- ***Fatigue***—disease states; malnutrition; stress; altered body chemistry (e.g., medications, chemotherapy)
- ***risk for Injury***—physical (e.g., catheter-related complications—catheter breaks, dislodgement, occlusion air emboli, septic thrombophlebitis); malnutrition; effects of therapy, drug interactions
- ***risk for Infection***—invasive tubes, environmental exposure, malnutrition, chronic disease
- ***interrupted Family Processes***—situational crises; shift of health status of a family member; shift in family roles

METABOLIC ACID-BASE IMBALANCES

I. Pathophysiology

a. The body has the remarkable ability to maintain plasma pH within the narrow range of 7.35 to 7.45; this is accomplished by means of chemical buffering mechanisms involving the kidneys and the lungs.

b. Although single acid-base (such as metabolic acidosis) imbalances do occur, mixed acid-base imbalances are more common—metabolic acidosis and respiratory acidosis as occur with cardiac arrest.

METABOLIC ACIDOSIS—PRIMARY BASE BICARBONATE (HCO_3^-) DEFICIENCY

I. Pathophysiology

a. Reflects a relative excess of acid or hydrogen (H^+) and a deficit of base or bicarbonate (HCO_3^-)

b. Gain of strong acid may be *endogenous* (for example, ketoacids from lipid metabolism) or *exogenous* (for example, NH_4Cl infusion).

c. Bicarbonate loss may occur via the bowel or kidneys.

II. Etiology: Characterized by normal or high anion gap situations (Thomas, 2013; Brandis, update 2008)

a. *Normal anion gap* (or hyperchloremic) acidosis is associated with loss of bicarbonate from the body, gain of chloride, or decreased ammonia production.

- **i.** Gastrointestinal (GI) losses: vomiting, diarrhea, small-bowel and pancreatic or biliary fistulas, ileal loop bladder
- **ii.** Early renal failure
- **iii.** Obstructed ileostomy
- **iv.** Infusion of ammonium chloride, hyperalimentation; intravenous (IV) sodium chloride in presence of preexisting kidney dysfunction; acidifying drugs

b. *High anion gap* acidosis reflects accumulation of organic anions.

- **i.** Diabetic ketoacidosis
- **ii.** Severe malnutrition or starvation; high-fat, low-carbohydrate diets; parenteral lipid administration
- **iii.** Alcoholic lactic acidosis
- **iv.** Renal tubular necrosis
- **v.** Poisoning: salicylate intoxication (after initial stage); drug therapy including acetazolamide (Diamox), isoniazid (INH); or NH_4Cl

c. Compensatory mechanisms

- **i.** Hyperventilation to reduce $PaCO_2$
- **ii.** Decreased renal secretion of H^+, less production of ammonia, and excretion of HCO_3^-
- **iii.** Treatment of underlying condition

III. Statistics: Morbidity and mortality are primarily related to the underlying disease; therefore, separate statistics are not collected.

GLOSSARY

Acidemia: Blood disorder characterized by an increased concentration of H^+ ions in the blood.

Acidosis: An increased acidity or increased H^+ ion concentration. If not further qualified, it refers to acidity of the blood plasma. Acidosis is said to occur when arterial pH falls below 7.35.

Base excess/deficit: A calculated number that represents a sum total of the metabolic buffering agents (anions) in the blood; these anions include hemoglobin, proteins, phosphates, and HCO_3^- (the dominant anion); these anions try to compensate for imbalances in the pH caused by diseases or conditions that affect the lungs (respiratory acidosis and alkalosis) or kidneys (metabolic acidosis and alkalosis).

Carbonic acid (H_2CO_3): If too much acid is present, the HCO_3^- ions take up the H^+ ions, creating H_2CO_3, which is then excreted through the lungs in the form of carbon dioxide (CO_2) and water (H_2O). Conversely, if too little acid is present in extracellular fluid, the H_2CO_3 portion of the HCO_3^- buffer system releases H^+ ions. For the pH to remain within normal range (7.35 to 7.45), the ratio of HCO_3^- ions to H_2CO_3 must be 20:1 (Felver, 2005).

CO_2: Respiratory acid—the only acid that can be exhaled via the lungs.

Endogenous: Produced or originating from within the body.

Exogenous: Originating outside the body.

H^+: The ion that is left when the hydrogen atom loses its electron, forming a proton.

HCO_3^-: A measurement of the metabolic component of the acid-base balance. HCO_3^- is excreted and reabsorbed or conserved by the kidneys in response to pH imbalances and is directly related to the pH level; as the amount of HCO_3^- rises, so does the pH.

Kussmaul's respiration: An abnormal respiratory pattern characterized by rapid, deep breathing; often seen in metabolic acidosis.

Partial pressure of carbon dioxide ($PaCO_2$): Reflects the balance between the production of CO_2 and its elimination. Unless the metabolic rate changes, the amount of CO_2 produced is roughly constant and determines the amount of ventilation required and the level of PCO_2. The normal value in arterial blood is 40 mm Hg. In the healthy, awake individual, the end-exhaled value is usually similar.

pH: A measure of the level of H^+ ion, which indicates the acid-base status of blood; the pH decreases (becomes more acidic) with increased amounts of PCO_2 and other acids, and the pH increases (blood becomes more alkaline) with decreased PCO_2 or increased amounts of bases like HCO_3^-.

Care Setting

This condition does not occur in isolation but rather is a complication of a broader problem that may require inpatient care in a medical-surgical or subacute unit.

Related Concerns

Plans of care are specific to predisposing factors.

Diabetes mellitus/diabetic ketoacidosis, page 377
Fluid and electrolyte imbalances, page 885
Renal dialysis—general considerations, page 529
Renal failure, chronic (end-stage renal failure), page 517
Respiratory acidosis (primary carbonic acid excess), page 179
Respiratory alkalosis (primary carbonic acid deficit), page 184

Client Assessment Database

Data depend on the underlying cause.

DIAGNOSTIC DIVISION MAY REPORT	MAY EXHIBIT
ACTIVITY/REST	
• Lethargy, fatigue • Muscle weakness	
CIRCULATION	
	• Hypotension, wide pulse pressure • Pulse may be weak, irregular. • Jaundiced sclera, skin, mucous membranes (liver failure)
ELIMINATION	
• Diarrhea	• Dark/concentrated urine

(continues on page 452)

Client Assessment Database (continued)

DIAGNOSTIC DIVISION MAY REPORT (continued)	MAY EXHIBIT (continued)
FOOD/FLUID • Anorexia • Nausea, vomiting	• Poor skin turgor, dry mucous membranes
NEUROSENSORY • Drowsiness, changes in thinking ability	• Changes in sensorium—stupor, confusion, lethargy, depression, delirium, coma • Decreased deep-tendon reflexes, muscle weakness
PAIN/DISCOMFORT • Headache • Abdominal pain	
RESPIRATION • Dyspnea on exertion	• Hyperventilation, Kussmaul's respiration
SAFETY • Transfusion of blood and blood products • Exposure to hepatitis virus	• Fever, signs of sepsis
TEACHING/LEARNING • History of diabetes, alcohol abuse, or prolonged starvation • Use of carbonic anhydrase inhibitors or anion-exchange resins—cholestyramine (Questran) • Ingestion of drugs or toxins, such as salicylates, acetazolamide, cyclosporine, ethylene glycol, methanol	
DISCHARGE PLAN CONSIDERATIONS • May require change in therapies for underlying disease process, condition ➧ Refer to section at end of plan for postdischarge considerations.	

Diagnostic Studies

TEST WHY IT IS DONE	WHAT IT TELLS ME
BLOOD TESTS • ***Arterial blood gases (ABGs):***	Measure how much O_2, CO_2 and bicarbonate (HCO_3^-) is in arterial blood. They also look at the acidity (pH) of the blood.
• ***Arterial pH:*** Adult normal range is 7.35 to 7.45.	Decreased in uncompensated metabolic acidosis (below 7.35) because of excess metabolic acids.
• ***HCO_3^-:*** Adult normal range is 22 to 26 mEq/L.	Decreased, less than 22 mEq/L
• ***$PaCO_2$:*** Adult normal range is 36 to 44 mm Hg.	Level is below 35 mm Hg.
• ***Base excess:*** Adult normal base values are between (2.3 and +2.3 mmol/L^{-1}.	Value of more than +3 mmol/L^{-1} indicates metabolic acidosis.
• ***Anion gap:*** The anion gap (AG) is the difference between the cations and anions found in the extracellular space (i.e., AG = [sodium + potassium] − [chloride + bicarbonate]). Normal values of AG vary according to different normal values for electrolytes, depending on laboratory methods or measurement and whether or not potassium is used in the formula (Pagana, 2011).	This calculation is most often helpful in identifying the cause of metabolic acidosis. As acids accumulate in the bloodstream, bicarbonate neutralizes them to maintain a normal pH. Mathematically, when bicarbonate decreases, the AG increases. In general, most metabolic acidotic states are associated with an increased AG. A decreased AG is very rare but can occur (Pagana, 2011).

TEST WHY IT IS DONE (continued)	WHAT IT TELLS ME (continued)
• *Electrolytes:* The electrolyte panel is composed of the individual tests for sodium, potassium, chloride, and total carbon dioxide.	Potassium level may be low due to excessive body losses or may be high secondary to renal insufficiency, tissue breakdown, or shift of potassium from the intracellular space to the extracellular space as a result of acidemia. Serum chloride levels may be increased.
ASSOCIATED TESTS	
• *Serum glucose:* Simple sugar in the blood.	Hypoglycemia associated with a metabolic acidosis can be caused by adrenal insufficiency or liver failure. Hyperglycemia will be present in metabolic acidosis in the presence of diabetic ketoacidosis.
• *Serum and urine ketones:* Acidic substances produced when the body uses fat instead of sugar for energy.	Increased in ketoacidosis, starvation, and alcohol intoxication.
• *Plasma lactic acid:* Acid produced by glucose-burning cells when these cells have an insufficient supply of oxygen.	Elevated in lactic acidosis.

Nursing Priorities

1. Achieve homeostasis.
2. Prevent or minimize complications.
3. Provide information about condition, prognosis, and treatment needs, as appropriate.

Discharge Goals

1. Physiological balance restored.
2. Free of complications.
3. Condition, prognosis, and treatment needs understood.
4. Plan in place to meet needs after discharge.

Because no current nursing diagnosis speaks clearly to metabolic imbalances, the following interventions are presented in a general format for inclusion in the primary plan of care.

NURSING DIAGNOSIS:

Desired Outcomes/Evaluation Criteria—Client Will

Electrolyte & Acid/Base Balance (NOC)

Display serum HCO_3- and electrolytes within normal limits (WNL).

Be free of symptoms of imbalance—absence of neurological impairment and vital signs WNL.

ACTIONS/INTERVENTIONS	RATIONALE
Acid-Base Management: Metabolic Acidosis (NIC)	
Independent	
Monitor BP.	Arteriolar dilation or decreased cardiac contractility (such as occurs with sepsis) and hypovolemia occur, resulting in systemic shock, evidenced by hypotension and tissue hypoxia.
Assess level of consciousness (LOC) and note progressive changes in neuromuscular status—strength, tone, and movement.	Decreased mental function, confusion, seizures, weakness, and flaccid paralysis can occur because of hypoxia, hyperkalemia, and decreased pH of cerebrospinal and interstitial fluids (Felver, 2005).
Provide seizure and coma precautions—bed in low position, use of padded side rails, and frequent observation.	Protects client from injury resulting from decreased mentation and convulsions.
Monitor heart rate and rhythm.	Acidemia may be manifested by changes in ECG configuration and presence of bradydysrhythmias as well as increased ventricular irritability such as fibrillation—signs of hyperkalemia. Life-threatening cardiovascular collapse may also occur because of vasodilation and decreased cardiac contractility. *Note:* Hypokalemia can occur as acidosis is corrected, resulting in premature ventricular contractions (PVCs) or ventricular tachycardia.

(continues on page 454)

ACTIONS/INTERVENTIONS (continued)	RATIONALE (continued)
Observe for altered respiratory excursion, rate, and depth.	Hyperventilation, or Kussmaul's respiration, may be noted as a compensatory mechanism to eliminate excess acid; however, as potassium shifts out of cells in an attempt to correct acidosis, respiration may become depressed. Transient respiratory depression may be the result of overcorrection of metabolic acidosis with sodium bicarbonate.
Assess skin temperature, color, and capillary refill.	Evaluates circulatory status, tissue perfusion, and effects of hypotension.
Auscultate bowel sounds; measure abdominal girth, as indicated.	In the presence of coexisting hyperkalemia, GI distress, including abdominal distention, diarrhea, and colicky pain, may be present.
Monitor intake and output (I&O) closely and weigh regularly.	Marked dehydration may be present because of GI losses. Therapy needs are based on underlying cause and fluid balance.
Monitor urine pH.	Kidneys attempt to compensate for acidosis by excreting excess hydrogen in the form of weak acids and ammonia. Maximum urine acidity is pH of 4.
Provide oral hygiene with sodium bicarbonate washes and lemon and glycerin swabs.	Neutralizes mouth acids and provides protective lubrication.
Collaborative	
Assist with identification and treatment of underlying cause.	Addressing the primary condition, such as diabetic ketoacidosis (DKA), liver or renal failure, drug poisoning (e.g., salicylates or alcohol), and sepsis, promotes correction of the acid-base disorder.
Monitor and graph serial arterial blood gases (ABGs).	Evaluates therapy needs and effectiveness. Blood bicarbonate and pH should slowly move toward normal levels.
Monitor serum electrolytes, such as potassium.	As acidosis is corrected, serum hypokalemia may occur as potassium shifts back into the cells.
Replace fluids, as indicated, depending on underlying etiology.	Choice of solution varies with cause of acidosis. *Note:* Lactate-containing solutions may be contraindicated in the presence of lactic acidosis.
Administer medications, as indicated, such as:	
Alkalizing agents, e.g., sodium bicarbonate, tromethamine (THAM) IV	Sodium bicarbonate is a systemic alkalinizer and primary treatment used to increase serum or urinary HCO_3– concentration and raise pH. THAM combines with hydrogen ions to form a bicarbonate buffer and is used to prevent and correct systemic acidosis. These agents are given in life-threatening hypokalemia and severe acidosis but are used with caution to correct pH to no greater than 7.20 because rebound metabolic alkalosis can occur (Thomas, 2013). *Note:* Clinicians are not entirely in agreement about the use of sodium bicarbonate, with some believing that it may do more harm than good, and that treatment of the underlying condition is much more beneficial (Brandis, update 2008).
Potassium	Potassium citrate is useful when acidosis is accompanied by hypokalemia but should be used cautiously in persons with renal impairment and must be avoided in those with hyperkalemia.
Phosphate	May be administered to enhance acid excretion in presence of chronic acidosis with hypophosphatemia.
Calcium	May be given to improve neuromuscular conduction and function.
Modify diet as indicated, such as low-protein, high-carbohydrate diet in presence of renal failure, or adjust medical nutritional therapy for the person with diabetes.	Restriction of protein may be necessary to decrease production of acid waste products, whereas addition of complex carbohydrates will correct acid production from the metabolism of fats.
Administer exchange resins and assist with dialysis, as indicated.	May be desired to reduce acidosis by decreasing excess potassium and acid waste products if pH less than 7.1 and other therapies are ineffective or heart failure (HF) develops.

POTENTIAL CONSIDERATIONS:
Refer to Potential Considerations relative to underlying cause of acid-base disorder.

METABOLIC ALKALOSIS—PRIMARY BASE BICARBONATE EXCESS

I. Pathophysiology

a. Increase in base or bicarbonate (HCO_3^-) concentration, generally reflecting a relative loss or shift of hydrogen (H^+) and/or gain in HCO_3^-

b. Organ systems most often involved are the kidneys and the gastrointestinal (GI) tract.

c. Consequences of the condition on organ systems dependent on degree of alkalemia and underlying pathology.

d. Loss of gastric acid (e.g., vomiting, NG drainage) and diuretic use account for about 90% of metabolic alkalosis (Brandis, 2008).

II. Etiology (Yaseen, 2011; Brandis, 2008): Processes responsible for maintenance of metabolic alkalosis are chloride depletion or potassium depletion. Chloride depletion primarily occurs through the GI system, while potassium depletion occurs primarily through the renal system and the clinical result is most often mixed.

a. Chloride-responsive: Urine chloride is less than 20 mEq/L and decreased extracellular fluid (ECF) volume.

i. GI acid losses: vomiting, nasogastric suction, diarrhea associated with villous adenoma

ii. Diuretics: Thiazides and loop diuretics interfere with reabsorption of sodium and chloride in the renal tubules, causing loss of chloride.

iii. HCO_3^- excess: correction of respiratory acidosis, chronic ingestion of large doses of antacids

iv. Laxative abuse

b. Chloride-resistant: Urine chloride is greater than 20 mEq/L and increased ECF volume.

i. Renal acid loss: primary or secondary hyperaldosteronism, thiazides or loop diuretics, hypokalemia and hypomagnesemia; genetic deficiency of 11-B-HSD2 or inhibition by licorice, chewing tobacco

ii. Renal artery stenosis

c. Other causes

i. Carbohydrate feeding after starvation

ii. Hypercalcemia

iii. Multiple blood transfusions

d. Compensatory mechanisms

i. Rapid excretion of HCO_3^- by the kidneys whenever plasma level exceeds 24 mmol/L—requires normal kidney function, with the ability to filter HCO_3^- and to excrete excess H^+.

ii. Hypoventilation: slow, shallow respirations to increase retention of carbonic acid

GLOSSARY

Base: Chemical opposite of acid.

Base excess/deficit: A calculated number that represents a sum total of the metabolic buffering agents or anions in the blood, including hemoglobin, proteins, phosphates, and HCO_3^- (dominant anion). These anions try to compensate for imbalances in the pH caused by diseases or conditions that affect the lungs (respiratory acidosis/alkalosis) or kidneys (metabolic acidosis/alkalosis).

Chvostek's sign: In tetany, tapping the muscles of the face causes them to go into spasm, reflecting severe hypocalcemia.

Electroneutrality: The principle that in an electrolytic solution, the concentrations of all the ions are such that the solution as a whole is neutral.

Extracellular fluid (ECF): All body fluid located outside of cells, including fluid inside blood vessels and between cells.

H^+: The ion that is left when the hydrogen atom loses its electron, forming a proton.

HCO_3^-: Measurement of the metabolic component of the acid-base balance. HCO_3^- is excreted and reabsorbed (conserved) by the kidneys in response to pH imbalances and is directly related to the pH level; as the amount of HCO_3^- rises, so does the pH.

Intracellular fluid: Fluid located inside the cell.

Kussmaul's respiration: An abnormal respiratory pattern characterized by rapid, deep breathing; often seen in metabolic acidosis.

Partial pressure of carbon dioxide ($PaCO_2$): Reflects the balance between the production of carbon dioxide and its elimination.

pH: Measure of the level of H^+ ion, which indicates the acid-base status of blood. The pH decreases or becomes more acidic with increased amounts of $PaCO_2$ and other acids, and the pH increases or blood becomes more alkaline with decreased $PaCO_2$ or increased amounts of bases such as HCO_3^-.

Tetany: Hyperexcitability of nerves and muscles because of decreased extracellular calcium.

Care Setting

This condition does not occur in isolation but rather is a complication of a broader problem that may require inpatient care in a medical-surgical or subacute unit.

Related Concerns

Plans of care are specific to predisposing factors.

Fluid and electrolyte imbalances, page 885

Renal dialysis—general considerations, page 529

Respiratory acidosis (primary carbonic acid excess), page 179

Respiratory alkalosis (primary carbonic acid deficit), page 184

Client Assessment Database

DIAGNOSTIC DIVISION MAY REPORT	MAY EXHIBIT
CIRCULATION	• Tachycardia, irregularities, or dysrhythmias • Hypotension • Cyanosis
ELIMINATION • Diarrhea—with high chloride content • Use of potassium-wasting drugs, including diuretics (e.g., Diuril, Hygroton, Lasix); some corticosteroids, large doses of insulin; epinephrine, etc. • Laxative abuse	
FOOD/FLUID • Anorexia, nausea, prolonged vomiting • High salt intake, excessive ingestion of licorice • Recurrent indigestion or heartburn with frequent use of antacids or baking soda	
NEUROSENSORY • Tingling of fingers and toes, circumoral paresthesia • Muscle twitching, weakness • Dizziness	• Hypertonicity of muscles, tetany, tremors, convulsions, loss of reflexes • Confusion, irritability, restlessness, belligerence, apathy, coma • Picking at bedclothes
SAFETY • Recent blood transfusions with citrated blood	
RESPIRATION	• Hypoventilation—increases $PaCO_2$ and conserves carbonic acid; periods of apnea
TEACHING/LEARNING • History of primary aldosteronism, Cushing's syndrome, primary reninism, Bartter's syndrome, milk-alkali syndrome, corticosteroid therapy, pyloric stenosis or ulcers, self-induced vomiting (bulimia), long-term use of diuretics	
DISCHARGE PLAN CONSIDERATIONS • May require change in therapy for underlying disease process, condition ➧ Refer to section at end of plan for postdischarge considerations.	

Diagnostic Studies

TEST WHY IT IS DONE	WHAT IT TELLS ME
BLOOD TESTS	
• ***Arterial pH:*** Adult normal range is 7.35 to 7.45.	Increased, higher than 7.45.
• ***HCO_3^-:*** Adult normal range is 22 to 26 mEq/L.	Increased, higher than 26 mEq/L (primary).
• ***$PaCO_2$:*** Adult normal range is 36 to 44 mm Hg.	Slightly increased, above 45 mm Hg (compensatory).
• ***Base excess:*** Adult normal base values are between –2.3 and +2.3 mmol/L^{-1}.	Level is increased.

TEST WHY IT IS DONE (continued)	WHAT IT TELLS ME (continued)
• *Electrolytes:* The electrolyte panel is composed of individual tests for sodium, potassium, chloride, and total carbon dioxide.	All values are usually decreased from normal range.
• *Plasma renin activity and aldosterone*	May help in finding the reason for metabolic alkalosis, especially in clients with hypertension, hypokalemic metabolic alkalosis, or renal potassium wasting without diuretic use. Low renin activity and high plasma aldosterone levels are found in primary hyperaldosteronism (Yaseen, 2011).

Nursing Priorities

1. Achieve homeostasis.
2. Prevent or minimize complications.
3. Provide information about condition, prognosis, and treatment needs, as appropriate.

Discharge Goals

1. Physiological balance restored.
2. Free of complications.
3. Condition, prognosis, and treatment needs understood.
4. Plan in place to meet needs after discharge.

Because no current nursing diagnosis speaks clearly to metabolic imbalances, the following interventions are presented in a general format for inclusion in the primary plan of care.

NURSING DIAGNOSIS:

Desired Outcomes/Evaluation Criteria—Client Will

Electrolyte & Acid/Base Balance (NOC)
Display serum HCO_3^- and electrolytes within normal limits (WNL).
Be free of symptoms of imbalance—absence of neurological impairment and irritability.

ACTIONS/INTERVENTIONS	RATIONALE
Metabolic Alkalosis Management (NIC)	
Independent	
Monitor respiratory rate, rhythm, and depth.	Hypoventilation is a compensatory mechanism to conserve carbonic acid and represents definite risks to the individual, such as hypoxemia and respiratory failure.
Assess level of consciousness and neuromuscular status—strength, tone, and movement; note presence of Chvostek's sign.	The central nervous system (CNS) may be hyperirritable related to increased pH of CNS fluid, resulting in tingling, numbness, dizziness, restlessness, or apathy and confusion. Hypocalcemia may contribute to tetany, although occurrence is rare. *Note:* Chvostek's sign is evaluated by tapping the cheek over the facial nerve and then observing for the development of a lip twitch or facial spasm, which is indicative of muscular irritability. Trousseau sign was previously used as an evaluation for hypocalcemia (carpal spasm development when a BP cuff is applied and the circulation transiently occluded) but may be painful and is not preferred (Elisha, 2010).
Monitor heart rate and rhythm.	Atrial or ventricular ectopic beats and tachydysrhythmias may develop.
Record amount and source of output.	Helpful in identifying source of acid loss—potassium and hydrochloric (HCl) acid are lost in vomiting and GI suctioning.
Monitor intake and daily weight.	Useful in monitoring fluid status.
Restrict oral intake and reduce noxious environmental stimuli, use intermittent or low suction during nasogastric (NG) suctioning, and irrigate gastric tube with isotonic solutions rather than water.	Limits gastric losses of HCl, potassium, and calcium.
Provide seizure safety precautions, as indicated—padded side rails, airway protection, bed in low position, and frequent observation.	Changes in mentation and neuromuscular hyperirritability may result in client harm, especially if tetany or convulsions occur.

(continues on page 458)

ACTIONS/INTERVENTIONS (continued)	RATIONALE (continued)
Encourage intake of foods and fluids high in potassium and possibly calcium, dependent on blood level—canned grapefruit and apple juices, bananas, cauliflower, dried peaches, figs, and wheat germ.	Useful in replacing potassium losses when oral intake permitted.
Review medication regimen for use of diuretics, such as thiazides (Diuril, Hygroton), furosemide (Lasix), and ethacrynic acid (Edecrin).	Discontinuation of these potassium-wasting drugs may prevent recurrence of imbalance.
Instruct client to avoid use of excessive amounts of sodium HCO_3^- antacids, such as Alka-Seltzer or baking soda.	Ulcer clients can cause alkalosis by taking over-the-counter (OTC) products containing sodium HCO_3^-, especially when taken in addition to prescribed alkaline antacids.
Collaborative	
Assist with identification and treatment of underlying disorder.	Addressing the primary condition, such as prolonged vomiting and diarrhea, hyperaldosteronism, and Cushing's syndrome, promotes correction of the acid-base disorder.
Monitor laboratory studies as indicated, such as arterial blood gases (ABGs)/pH, serum electrolytes, especially potassium, and blood urea nitrogen (BUN).	Evaluates therapy needs and effectiveness and monitors renal function.
Administer medications, as indicated, for example:	
Chloride solutions, such as sodium chloride by mouth (PO) or Lactated Ringer's solution intravenously (IV), unless contraindicated	Correcting sodium, water, and chloride defects may be all that is needed to permit kidneys to excrete HCO_3^- and correct alkalosis but must be used with caution in clients with heart failure (HF) or renal insufficiency.
Potassium chloride	Hypokalemia is frequently present. Chloride is needed so kidneys can absorb sodium with chloride, enhancing excretion of HCO_3^-.
Ammonium chloride or arginine hydrochloride	Although used only in severe cases, ammonium chloride may be given to increase amount of circulating H^+ ions. Monitor administration closely to prevent too rapid a decrease in pH and hemolysis of red blood cells. *Note:* May cause rebound metabolic acidosis and is usually contraindicated in clients with renal or hepatic failure.
Carbonic anhydrase inhibitor, such as acetazolamide (Diamox), or a potassium-sparing diuretic, such as spironolactone (Aldactone)	Blocks HCO_3^- reabsorption in the proximal convoluted renal tubules, promoting renal excretion of HCO_3^-. Effective in treating chloride-resistant alkalosis and its excess fluid volume effects.
Avoid or limit use of sedatives or hypnotics.	If respirations are depressed, may cause hypoxia or respiratory failure.
Encourage fluids IV and PO.	Replaces ECF losses, and adequate hydration facilitates removal of pulmonary secretions to improve ventilation.
Administer supplemental oxygen (O_2), as indicated, and respiratory treatments to improve ventilation.	Respiratory compensation for metabolic alkalosis is hypoventilation, which may cause decreased PaO_2 levels and hypoxemia.
Prepare client for and assist with dialysis, as needed.	Useful when renal dysfunction prevents clearance of HCO_3^-.

POTENTIAL CONSIDERATIONS:
Refer to Potential Considerations relative to underlying cause of acid-base disorder.

CHAPTER 9

Diseases of the Blood/Blood-Forming Organs

ANEMIAS—IRON DEFICIENCY, ANEMIA OF CHRONIC DISEASE, PERNICIOUS, APLASTIC, HEMOLYTIC

I. Pathophysiology: Decreased number of circulating red blood cells (RBCs), reduction in the amount of hemoglobin (Hgb) in the RBCs, or a combination of both, resulting in diminished oxygen-carrying capacity of the blood (Maakaron, 2011)

- **a.** Iron deficiency anemia (ID): inadequate iron stores, which results in insufficient Hgb (key molecule in RBCs), causing cells to appear abnormal, unusually small (microcytic), and pale (hypochromic)
- **b.** Anemia of chronic disease (ACD): accompanies chronic inflammatory, infectious, or neoplastic disorders. Studies have shown that anemia is prevalent in 30% to 90% of persons with cancers (Knight, 2004).
- **c.** Pernicious anemia (PA): lack of intrinsic factor in the stomach results in inability to absorb vitamin B_{12}, causing abnormal RBC formation.
- **d.** Aplastic anemia: failure of bone marrow to produce cells, including RBCs and white blood cells (WBCs) and platelets
- **e.** Hemolytic anemia: premature destruction of RBCs

II. Etiology (National Institutes of Health [NIH], 2012; Maakaron, 2011)

- **a.** Three main causes of anemia exist. They are blood loss, increased RBC destruction, and decreased RBC production. Within these causes there are a number of specific etiologies. Some examples of these specifics include genetic (e.g., thalassemia); nutritional (e.g., iron deficiency); physical (e.g., trauma, enlarged or injured spleen); chronic disease (e.g., kidney disease); malignant (e.g., neoplasms); infectious (e.g., viral, bacterial, and protozoal).
- **b.** Adult anemia is usually defined as a Hgb level lower than 11 g/dL, with severe anemia defined as Hgb lower than 8 g/dL. Not all sources agree with these numbers. For example, Maakaron opines that anemia is defined by the lower limits set for the Hgb range and that "the World Health Organization (WHO) chose 12.5 g/dL for both adult males and females. In the United States, limits of 13.5 g/dL for men and 12.5 g/dL for women are probably more realistic" (Maakaron, 2011).
- **c.** Anemia is a common condition, occurring in all age groups, both male and female, and in all races and ethnic groups.
- **d.** Anemias are associated with many physiological complications, including dyspnea, fatigue, dizziness, decreased cognition, impaired sleep, sexual dysfunction, and significant debilitation.
- **e.** ID
  - **i.** Lack of iron in the body due to a variety of causes (Nabili, 2012)
    1. Blood loss due to disease, such as gastric or duodenal ulcers, diverticula, hemorrhoids, ulcerative colitis; injury or trauma; or certain medications, including aspirin or nonsteroidal anti-inflammatory drugs (NSAIDs)
    2. Inadequate nutrition, such as not eating enough foods that contain iron
    3. Malabsorption syndromes, such as not utilizing iron from food that is eaten
    4. Lead exposure
  - **ii.** Most frequently occurring form of anemia
- **f.** ACD
  - **i.** Primarily due to slowed production of RBCs as a result of low reticulocyte production
  - **ii.** Develops slowly and is only evident after time
  - **iii.** Symptoms are usually associated with the disease causing the anemia rather than the anemia itself. Examples are the anemias associated with chronic kidney disease, chronic malnutrition, or cancers (Nabili, 2012).
  - **iv.** Second most prevalent form of anemia (Hebbar, 2006; Corwin, 2001)
- **g.** PA—an autoimmune disorder
  - **i.** Characterized by the production of autoantibodies to gastric parietal cells and their secretory product—intrinsic factor—which is needed for vitamin B_{12} absorption
  - **ii.** Conditions that interfere with the body's absorption and use of B_{12} include Crohn's and Whipple's diseases, gastrectomy or gastric bypass, and the use of chemotherapeutic medications.
- **h.** Aplastic anemia—bone marrow failure
  - **i.** May be associated with conditions that affect erythropoietin production and secretion, such as certain cancers and cancer treatments and renal, hepatic, or endocrine disorders
  - **ii.** Other known causes include exposure to chemicals, such as benzene, insecticides, solvents; certain drugs, such as chemotherapy, gold, seizure medications, some antibiotics; viruses, such as HIV, Epstein-Barr; immune conditions, such as systemic lupus erythematosus, rheumatoid arthritis; radiation; and certain inherited disorders, such as Fanconi's anemia.

(text continues on page 460)

i. Hemolytic anemia—marked by an accelerated destruction of RBCs
   i. Several types of hemolytic anemias, including sickle cell anemia (Nabili, 2012). (See CP: Sickle Cell Crisis.)
   ii. Causes include hereditary factors, such as sickle cell trait or disease; blood transfusion reactions; immune disorders, acute viral or infectious agents; certain drugs, such as quinidine, penicillin, and methyldopa; and toxins, such as chemicals and venoms.

III. Statistics

a. Morbidity: Approximately 4.5 million Americans have anemia, with 429,000 hospitalized with some type of anemia as the first-listed diagnosis (National Hospital Discharge Survey, 2009).
b. Mortality: 4,956 people died from anemia in the United States in preliminary reports for 2011 (Hoyert et al, 2012).
c. Cost: Direct care costs estimated at $4.7 billion in 2009 (NHLBI, 2012).

GLOSSARY

Aquired anemia: Client is not born with anemia, but develops it. Includes conditions and factors that can lead to anemia, such as poor diet, abnormal hormone (erythropoetin) levels, bone marrow suppression due to cancer treatment, certain medications and toxins, and pregnancy. Some anemias are mixed acquired and inherited (e.g., aplastic).

Cheilitis: Inflammation of the lips with cracking at the corners of the mouth.

Ecchymosis: Superficial bleeding (bruising) under the skin or mucous membrane.

Erythropoiesis: Red blood cell (RBC) production in the bone marrow.

Glossitis: Inflammation of tongue.

Hematemesis: Bloody vomitus.

Inherited anemia: Gene for certain anemia is passed on by parents. Anemias of this type include sickle cell, thalassemia, Fanconi, and others. Some anemias are mixed acquired and inherited (e.g., aplastic).

Koilonychia: Dystrophy of the nails, resulting in thinning and concave or spoon shape.

Lymphadenopathy: Enlargement of the lymph nodes.

Melena: Black, tarry stools due to digested blood in the gastrointestinal (GI) tract.

Petechiae: Small, purplish, hemorrhagic spots on the skin.

Pica: Insatiable craving to eat nonfood items, such as starch, clay, crayons, and paper.

Red blood cell characterization of anemias: Based on the mean corpuscular volume (MCV), or average RBC size, reported in the CBC test: (1) *microcytic:* most commonly caused by iron deficiency; other causes include thalassemia, anemia of chronic disease, and sideroblastic anemia; (2) *normocytic:* may be caused by hemorrhage, hemolysis, bone marrow failure, anemia of chronic inflammation, or renal insufficiency; and (3) *macrocytic*: the larger red cells are always associated with insufficient *numbers* of cells and often also insufficient hemoglobin content per cell. Most is megaloblastic (cells are larger because they cannot produce DNA quickly enough to divide at the right time) and include vitamin B_{12} or folate deficiencies caused by insufficient uptake or inadequate absorption through lack of intrinsic factor (pernicious anemia) (Rogers et al, 2012).

Romberg's sign: Inability to maintain body balance when eyes are shut and feet are close together, sometimes noted with movement disorders accompanying pernicious anemia.

Stomatitis: Inflammation, ulceration of mucosal lining of any structures in the mouth.

Care Setting

Clients are treated at the community level except in the presence of severe cardiovascular or immune compromise. Although the medical treatments vary widely due to the many variations in anemia presentation, nursing care for the anemic client has a common theme: managing physical symptoms and maximizing quality-of-life issues.

Related Concerns

Acquired immunodeficiency syndrome (AIDS), page 689
Burns: thermal, chemical, and electrical—acute and convalescent phases, page 689
Cancer, page 827
Cirrhosis of the liver, page 412
Heart failure: chronic, page 43
Psychosocial aspects of care, page 729
Pulmonary tuberculosis (TB), page 170
Renal failure: chronic (end-stage renal disease), page 517
Rheumatoid arthritis (RA), page 709
Upper gastrointestinal/esophageal bleeding, page 281

DIAGNOSTIC DIVISION MAY REPORT	MAY EXHIBIT
ACTIVITY/REST • Fatigue, weakness, general malaise • Loss of productivity, diminished enthusiasm for work • Low exercise tolerance • Greater need for rest and sleep	• Tachycardia and tachypnea, dyspnea on exertion or at rest (severe or aplastic anemia) • Lethargy, withdrawal, apathy, lassitude, and lack of interest in surroundings • Muscle weakness and decreased strength • Ataxia, unsteady gait • Slumping of shoulders, drooping posture, slow walk, and other cues indicative of fatigue
CIRCULATION • History of chronic blood loss, such as chronic GI bleeding, heavy menses (ID) • Angina (particularly in elderly) • History of chronic infective endocarditis • Palpitations (compensatory tachycardia) • Cold hands and feet • Brittle nails	• Tachycardia • Blood pressure (BP)—increased systolic with stable diastolic and a widened pulse pressure, postural hypotension • Bounding pulse and throbbing carotid pulsations reflect increased cardiac output as a compensatory mechanism to provide oxygen and nutrients to cells. • Dysrhythmias, electrocardiogram abnormalities—ST-segment depression and flattening or depression of the T wave, tachycardia • Systolic murmur (ID) • *Extremities:* color—pallor of the skin, palms, and nailbeds, or grayish cast in black client; waxy, pale skin (aplastic, PA) or bright lemon-yellow (PA) • Sclera blue or pearl white (ID), jaundice (PA), pale mucous membranes—conjunctiva, mouth, pharynx, lips • Capillary refill delayed due to diminished blood flow to the periphery, resulting in vasoconstriction • Nails brittle, spoon-shaped or koilonychia (ID)
EGO INTEGRITY • Negative feelings about self, ability to handle situation, events	• Depression
ELIMINATION • History of pyelonephritis, renal failure (ACD) • Flatulence, malabsorption syndrome (ID) • Hematemesis, fresh blood in stool, melena • Diarrhea or constipation • Diminished urine output	• Abdominal distention
FOOD/FLUID • Low food intake, low intake of animal protein, high intake of cereal products (ID) • Mouth or tongue soreness, difficulty swallowing, ulcerations in pharynx (PA) • Nausea, vomiting, dyspepsia, anorexia • Recent weight loss • Pica	• Beefy red, smooth appearance of tongue (PA, folic acid and vitamin B_{12} deficiencies) • Dry, pale mucous membranes • Skin turgor poor with dry, shriveled appearance and loss of elasticity (ID) • Stomatitis and glossitis (deficiency states) • Cheilitis (ID)
HYGIENE • Difficulty maintaining activities of daily living (ADLs)	• Unkempt appearance, poor personal hygiene • Hair dry, brittle, thinning; premature graying (PA)
NEUROSENSORY • Headaches, fainting, dizziness, vertigo, tinnitus, inability to concentrate • Insomnia, diminished vision, and spots before eyes • Weakness, poor balance, wobbly legs, paresthesias of hands or feet (PA)	• Irritability, restlessness, depression, drowsiness, apathy • Mentation—notable slowing and dullness in response • Retinal hemorrhages (aplastic, PA) • Epistaxis, bleeding from other orifices (aplastic)

(continues on page 462)

Client Assessment Database (continued)

DIAGNOSTIC DIVISION MAY REPORT (continued)	MAY EXHIBIT (continued)
• Sensation of being cold	• Disturbed coordination, ataxia, decreased vibratory and position sense, positive Romberg's sign, paralysis (PA)
PAIN/DISCOMFORT • Vague abdominal pains, headache (ID) • Oral pain	
RESPIRATION • Shortness of breath at rest and with activity	• Tachypnea • Dyspnea, particularly during and after exercise • Orthopnea
SAFETY • History of occupational exposure to chemicals—benzene, lead, insecticides, phenylbutazone, naphthalene (aplastic, hemolytic) • History of exposure to radiation, either as a treatment modality or by accident (aplastic, hemolytic) • History of cancer, cancer therapies (aplastic, hemolytic) • Cold and heat intolerance • Previous blood transfusions • Impaired vision • Poor wound healing, frequent infections • Skin problems, including cracks in side of mouth (PA)	• Low-grade fever • Generalized lymphadenopathy • Petechiae and ecchymosis (aplastic)
SEXUALITY • Changes in menstrual flow—menorrhagia or amenorrhea in women (ID) • Loss of libido—both men and women • Impotence	• Pale cervix and vaginal walls • Impotence
TEACHING/LEARNING • Family tendency for anemia (ID, PA) • Past or present use of anticonvulsants, antibiotics, chemotherapeutic agents (bone marrow failure), aspirin, anti-inflammatory drugs, or anticoagulants • Chronic use of alcohol • Religious or cultural beliefs affecting treatment choices—refusal of blood transfusions • Recent or current episode of active bleeding (ID) • Prior surgeries—splenectomy, tumor excision, prosthetic valve replacement, surgical excision of duodenum or gastric resection, partial or total gastrectomy for weight loss or diseases (ID, PA) • Problems with wound healing or bleeding, chronic infections	
DISCHARGE PLAN CONSIDERATIONS • May require assistance with treatment, such as injections, self-care activities, homemaker and maintenance tasks; changes in dietary plan ➧ Refer to section at end of plan for postdischarge considerations.	

Diagnostic Studies

TEST WHY IT IS DONE	WHAT IT TELLS ME
BLOOD TESTS	
• ***Complete blood count (CBC):*** Battery of screening tests, which typically includes hemoglobin, hematocrit; RBC count, morphology, indices, and distribution width index; platelet count and size; and WBC count and differential.	Evaluates for known or suspected anemia. Types of anemias may be differentiated by the number of red blood cells as well as their color and shape.
• ***Hemoglobin (Hgb):*** The oxygen-carrying pigment and predominant protein in the RBCs. • ***Hematocrit (Hct):*** The proportion of packed RBCs to serum.	Usual Hgb varies somewhat among healthy individuals, making a universal "normal" value elusive. For client with a known baseline level, a decrease of 2 g/dL or more is cause for concern and assessment. Both Hgb and Hct are decreased with blood loss, and bone marrow suppression (Rogers et al, 2012).
• ***Hgb electrophoresis:*** Identifies type of Hgb structure.	Aids in determining source of hemolytic anemia or anemias related to deficiencies in dietary intake or malabsorption. Sometimes used when a person has a family history of anemia; this test provides information on sickle cell anemia or thalassemia (Nabili, 2012).
• ***RBC (also called erythrocyte) count:*** Number of RBCs per unit volume.	Decreased in ID and PA; severely decreased in aplastic anemia.
• ***Reticulocyte count:*** Immature RBCs. Helps assess bone marrow function.	Decreased in PA and aplastic anemia. Elevated in blood loss and hemolytic and compensated anemias.
• ***RBC survival time:*** Evaluates age of RBCs.	Useful in the differential diagnosis of anemias because RBCs have shortened life spans in pernicious and hemolytic anemias.
• ***Erythrocyte fragility test:*** Evaluates susceptibility of RBCs to break down (hemolysis) under certain conditions.	Decreased in ID. Increased fragility confirms hemolytic and autoimmune anemias.
• ***Erythrocyte sedimentation rate (ESR):*** Measures rate at which RBCs settle.	While not specific to a certain anemia, higher ESR indicates presence of inflammatory reaction, such as increased RBC destruction or malignant disease.
• ***WBCs:*** Total cell count and specific WBCs, called differential.	May be increased as in hemolytic anemia or decreased in aplastic anemia.
• ***Platelet count:*** Platelets have essential function in coagulation.	Decreased in blood loss and aplastic anemias. Increased in ID, posthemorrhagic, and hemolytic anemias.
• ***Erythropoietin:*** Hormone that stimulates bone marrow to produce red blood cells.	Determines whether the amount of erythropoietin being produced is appropriate for the level of anemia present. It may be ordered to distinguish between a condition that is suppressing bone marrow function and an insufficiency of erythropoietin.
• ***Serum iron:*** Measures the level of iron in the liquid part of blood.	Iron is needed to help form adequate numbers of normal RBCs. Iron may be decreased or absent (ID) or elevated (hemolytic and aplastic anemias).
• ***Total iron-binding capacity (TIBC):*** Measures the amount of iron that can be carried through blood by transferrin.	Increased in ID; normal or slightly reduced in PA.
• ***Serum ferritin:*** Reflects the amount of stored iron in body.	Decreased in ID.
• ***Vitamin B_{12} (cobalamin) and folate (folic acid, RBC folate):*** Measures the concentration of vitamin B_{12} and folate in the serum. The amount of folate inside RBCs may also be measured; it will normally be at a higher concentration inside the cell than in the serum.	Anemia caused by folic acid deficiency is common. Helps diagnose the cause of anemia or neuropathy (nerve damage) or to evaluate nutritional status in some clients.
• ***Serum bilirubin:*** Product that results from the breakdown of Hgb.	Direct or total bilirubin is elevated in PA and hemolytic anemia.
• ***Serum lactate dehydrogenase (LDH):*** Serum LDH levels may occasionally be ordered to monitor damage caused by muscle trauma or injury and to help identify hemolytic anemia.	May be elevated in PA and hemolytic anemia.
OTHER ASSOCIATED STUDIES	
• ***Schilling's test:*** Evaluates vitamin B_{12} excretion by measuring urinary excretion.	The Schilling's test and a therapeutic trial of vitamin B_{12} injections help distinguish folic acid deficiency anemia from pernicious anemia.

(continues on page 464)

Diagnostic Studies (continued)

TEST WHY IT IS DONE (continued)	WHAT IT TELLS ME (continued)
• *Guaiac:* Tests for hidden or occult blood.	May be positive in urine, stools, and gastric contents, reflecting acute or chronic bleeding (ID).
• *Bone marrow aspiration/biopsy examination:* May be done by needle aspirate or biopsy to identify changes in number, size, and shape of blood cells, helping to differentiate type of anemia.	Megaloblasts increased in PA; fatty marrow, with diminished or absence of blood cells at several sites, found in aplastic anemia.
• *Upper endoscopy—also called esophagogastroduodenoscopy (EGD):* Visualizes esophagus, stomach, and duodenum, using a thin flexible tube that can be looked through or seen on a TV monitor.	Checks for bleeding sites—acute or chronic GI bleeding—causing blood loss anemia.
• *Lower endoscopy—also called colonoscopy:* Visualizes rectum and colon using a thin flexible tube that can be looked through or seen on a TV monitor.	

Nursing Priorities

1. Enhance tissue perfusion.
2. Provide nutritional and fluid needs.
3. Prevent complications.
4. Provide information about disease process, prognosis, and treatment regimen.

Discharge Goals

1. ADLs met by self or with assistance of others.
2. Complications prevented or minimized.
3. Disease process, prognosis, and therapeutic regimen understood.
4. Plan in place to meet needs after discharge.

NURSING DIAGNOSIS: Activity Intolerance

May Be Related To

Imbalance between oxygen supply and demand (anemia)

Possibly Evidenced By

Reports fatigue, feeling weak
Abnormal heart rate or blood pressure response to activity
Exertional dyspnea

Desired Outcomes/Evaluation Criteria—Client Will

Endurance (NOC)

Report an increase in activity tolerance, including ADLs.
Demonstrate a decrease in physiological signs of intolerance—pulse, respirations, and BP remain within client's normal range.
Display laboratory values (Hgb/Hct) within acceptable range.

ACTIONS/INTERVENTIONS	RATIONALE
Energy Management (NIC)	
Independent	
Assess client's ability to perform normal tasks and ADLs, noting reports of weakness, fatigue, and difficulty accomplishing tasks.	Influences choice of interventions and needed assistance.
Note changes in balance, gait disturbance, and muscle weakness.	May indicate neurological changes associated with vitamin B_{12} deficiency, affecting client safety and increasing risk of injury.
Monitor BP, pulse, and respirations during and after activity. Note adverse responses to increased levels of activity—increased heart rate and BP, dysrhythmias, dizziness, dyspnea, tachypnea, and cyanosis of mucous membranes and nailbeds.	Cardiopulmonary manifestations result from attempts by the heart and lungs to supply adequate amounts of oxygen to the tissues.
Recommend frequent rest periods or bedrest (rare), as indicated.	Activity may need to be curtailed until severe anemia is at least partially corrected to lower body's oxygen requirements and reduce strain on the heart and lungs.

ACTIONS/INTERVENTIONS (continued)	RATIONALE (continued)
Elevate head of bed, as tolerated.	Enhances lung expansion to maximize oxygenation for cellular uptake. *Note:* May be contraindicated if hypotension is present.
Suggest client change position slowly; monitor for dizziness.	Postural hypotension or cerebral hypoxia may cause dizziness, fainting, and increased risk of injury.
Assist client to prioritize ADLs and desired activities. Alternate rest periods with activity periods.	Promotes adequate rest, maintains energy level, and alleviates strain on the cardiac and respiratory systems.
Provide or recommend assistance with activities and ambulation as necessary, allowing client to be an active participant as much as possible.	Although help may be necessary, self-esteem is enhanced when client does some things for self.
Plan activity progression with client, including activities that client views as essential. Increase activity levels, as tolerated.	Promotes gradual return to a more normal activity level and improved muscle tone and stamina. Increases self-esteem and sense of control.
Identify and implement energy-saving techniques: shower chair and sitting to perform tasks.	Encourages client to do as much as possible, while conserving limited energy and preventing fatigue.
Instruct client to stop current activity if palpitations, chest pain, shortness of breath, weakness, or dizziness occur.	Cellular ischemia potentiates risk of infarction, and excessive cardiopulmonary strain and stress may lead to decompensation and failure.
Discuss importance of maintaining environmental temperature and body warmth, as indicated.	Vasoconstriction with shunting of blood to vital organs decreases peripheral circulation, impairing tissue perfusion. Client's comfort and need for warmth must be balanced with need to avoid excessive heat with resultant vasodilation, which reduces organ perfusion.
Collaborative	
Monitor laboratory studies, such as Hgb/Hct, RBC count, and arterial blood gases (ABGs).	Identifies deficiencies in RBC components affecting oxygen transport, treatment needs, and response to therapy.
Provide supplemental oxygen as indicated.	Maximizing oxygen transport to tissues improves ability to function.
Administer the following, as indicated:	
Whole blood, packed RBCs (PRCs); blood products as indicated. Monitor closely for transfusion reactions.	Increases number of oxygen-carrying cells; corrects deficiencies to reduce risk of hemorrhage in acutely compromised individuals. *Note:* Transfusions are reserved for severe blood loss anemias with cardiovascular compromise and are used after other therapies have failed to restore homeostasis.
Erythropoiesis-stimulating agents (ESAs), such as epoetin-Alpha (Procrit, Epogen[EPO]; darbepoetin [Aranesp])	EPO has been shown to be effective in increasing erythrocyte and Hgb levels and reducing need for RBC transfusions in many clients with ACD. Concerns have been raised about ESAs and other health risks (e.g., thromboembolic phenomena, tumor progress in cancer, and increased mortality), and research continues (Schrier, 2013; RxList, 2012).
Prepare for surgical intervention, if indicated.	Surgery is useful to control bleeding in clients who are anemic because of bleeding, such as in ulcers and uterine bleeding; or to remove spleen as treatment of autoimmune hemolytic anemia. Bone marrow and stem cell transplantation may be done in presence of bone marrow failure—aplastic anemia.

NURSING DIAGNOSIS: imbalanced Nutrition: less than body requirements

May Be Related To

Failure to ingest or inability to digest food or absorb nutrients

Possibly Evidenced By

Reports food intake less than recommended daily allowances
Weight loss or weight below ideal range
Pale mucous membranes
Abnormal laboratory studies

Desired Outcomes/Evaluation Criteria—Client Will

Nutritional Status (NOC)

Demonstrate progressive weight gain or stable weight, with normalization of laboratory values.
Experience no signs of malnutrition.
Demonstrate behaviors or lifestyle changes to regain and maintain appropriate weight.

ACTIONS/INTERVENTIONS	RATIONALE
Nutrition Therapy (NIC)	
Independent	
Review nutritional history, including food preferences.	Identifies deficiencies and suggests possible interventions. *Note:* Daily meal diary over period of time may be necessary to identify anemia related to nutrient deficiencies such as no meat in diet—iron and vitamin B_{12} deficiency, or few leafy vegetables in diet—folic acid deficiency.
Observe and record client's food intake.	Monitors caloric intake or insufficient quality of food consumption.
Weigh periodically as appropriate, such as weekly.	Monitors weight loss and effectiveness of nutritional interventions.
Recommend small, frequent meals and between-meal nourishment.	May enhance intake while preventing gastric distention. Use of liquid supplements such as Ensure, Boost, or similar product provides additional protein and calories.
Suggest bland diet, low in roughage, avoiding hot, spicy, or very acidic foods, as indicated.	When oral lesions are present, pain may restrict type of foods client can tolerate.
Have client record and report occurrence of nausea or vomiting, flatus, and other related symptoms, such as irritability or impaired memory.	May reflect the effects of anemias (e.g., hypoxia or vitamin B_{12} deficiency) on body organs and systems.
Encourage or assist with good oral hygiene before and after meals; use soft-bristled toothbrush for gentle brushing. Provide dilute, alcohol-free mouthwash if oral mucosa is ulcerated.	Enhances appetite and oral intake. Diminishes bacterial growth, minimizing possibility of infection. Special mouth-care techniques may be needed if tissue is fragile, ulcerated, or bleeding and pain is severe.
Collaborative	
Consult with nutritionist/dietitian.	Aids in establishing dietary plan to meet individual needs.
Monitor laboratory studies, such as Hgb/Hct, blood urea nitrogen (BUN), prealbumin and albumin, protein, transferrin, serum iron, vitamin B_{12}, folic acid, TIBC, and serum electrolytes.	Evaluates effectiveness of treatment regimen, including dietary sources of needed nutrients.
Administer medications, as indicated, for example:	
Vitamin and mineral supplements, such as cyanocobalamin (vitamin B_{12}), folic acid (Folvite), and ascorbic acid (vitamin C)	Replacements needed depend on type of anemia and presence of poor oral intake and identified deficiencies.
Oral iron supplements, such as ferrous sulfate (Feosol, Mol-Iron, Fer-In-Sol), ferrous gluconate (Fergon), and ferrous fumarate (Ircon, Femiron)	May be useful in some types of iron deficiency anemias. Oral preparations are taken between meals to enhance absorption and usually correct anemia and replace iron stores over a period of several months.
Iron dextran (InFeD) intramuscularly/intravenously (IM/IV)	Administered until estimated deficit is corrected. Reserved for those who cannot absorb or comply with oral iron therapy or when blood loss is too rapid for oral replacement to be effective.
Antifungal or anesthetic mouthwash, if indicated	May be needed in the presence of stomatitis or glossitis to promote oral tissue healing and facilitate intake.

NURSING DIAGNOSIS: Constipation/Diarrhea

May Be Related To

Poor eating habits, changes in gastrointestinal motility
Medication side effects

Possibly Evidenced By

Changes in frequency, characteristics, and amount of stool
Reports of abdominal pain, urgency, cramping
Altered bowel sounds

Desired Outcomes/Evaluation Criteria—Client Will

Bowel Elimination (NOC)

Establish return to normal patterns of bowel functioning.
Demonstrate changes in behaviors or lifestyle, as necessitated by causative or contributing factors.

ACTIONS/INTERVENTIONS	RATIONALE
Bowel Management (NIC)	
Independent	
Determine stool color, consistency, frequency, and amount.	Assists in identifying causative or contributing factors and appropriate interventions.
Auscultate bowel sounds.	Bowel sounds are generally increased in diarrhea and decreased in constipation.
Monitor intake and output (I&O) with specific attention to food and fluid intake.	May identify dehydration and excessive loss of fluids or aid in identifying dietary deficiencies.
Encourage fluid intake of 2500 to 3000 mL/day within cardiac tolerance.	Assists in improving stool consistency if constipated. Helps maintain hydration status if diarrhea is present.
Recommend avoiding gas-forming foods.	Decreases gastric distress and abdominal distention.
Assess perianal skin condition frequently, noting changes or beginning breakdown. Encourage and assist with perineal care after each bowel movement (BM) if diarrhea is present.	Prevents skin excoriation and breakdown.
Discuss use of stool softeners, mild stimulants, bulk-forming laxatives, or enemas, as indicated. Monitor effectiveness.	Facilitates defecation when constipation is present.
Collaborative	
Consult with dietitian to provide well-balanced diet high in fiber and bulk.	Fiber resists enzymatic digestion and absorbs liquids in its passage along the intestinal tract and thereby produces bulk, which acts as a stimulant to defecation.
Administer antidiarrheal medications, such as diphenoxylate hydrochloride with atropine (Lomotil), and water-absorbing drugs, such as Metamucil.	Decreases intestinal motility when diarrhea is present.

NURSING DIAGNOSIS: risk for Infection

Risk Factors May Include

Inadequate secondary defenses—decreased hemoglobin, leukopenia, or decreased granulocytes; suppressed inflammatory response

Inadequate primary defenses—broken skin, stasis of body fluids, invasive procedures, chronic disease, malnutrition

Possibly Evidenced By

(Not applicable; presence of signs and symptoms establishes an *actual* diagnosis)

Desired Outcomes/Evaluation Criteria—Client Will

Risk Control (NOC)

Identify behaviors to prevent and reduce risk of infection.

Infection Severity (NOC)

Be free of signs of infection; achieve timely wound healing if present.

ACTIONS/INTERVENTIONS	RATIONALE
Infection Protection (NIC)	
Independent	
Perform and promote meticulous hand washing by caregivers and client.	Prevents cross-contamination or bacterial colonization. *Note:* Client with severe or aplastic anemia may be at risk from normal skin flora.
Maintain strict aseptic techniques with procedures and wound care.	Reduces risk of bacterial colonization and infection.
Provide meticulous skin, oral, and perianal care.	Reduces risk of skin or tissue breakdown and infection.
Encourage frequent position changes and ambulation, coughing, and deep-breathing exercises.	Promotes ventilation of all lung segments and aids in mobilizing secretions to prevent pneumonia.
Promote adequate fluid intake.	Assists in liquefying respiratory secretions to facilitate expectoration and prevent stasis of body fluids in lungs and bladder.
Emphasize need to monitor and limit visitors, as indicated. Provide protective isolation, if appropriate. Restrict live plants and cut flowers.	Limits exposure to infectious agents. Protective isolation may be required in aplastic anemia, when immune response is most compromised.
Monitor temperature. Note presence of chills and tachycardia with or without fever.	Reflective of inflammatory process or infection, requiring evaluation and treatment. *Note:* With bone marrow suppression, leukocytic failure may lead to fulminating infections.
Observe for wound erythema and drainage.	Indicators of local infection. *Note:* Pus formation may be absent if granulocytes are depressed.

(continues on page 468)

ACTIONS/INTERVENTIONS (continued)	RATIONALE (continued)
Collaborative	
Obtain specimens for culture and sensitivity, as indicated.	Verifies presence of infection, identifies specific pathogen, and influences choice of treatment.
Administer topical antiseptics and systemic antibiotics.	May be used prophylactically to reduce colonization or used to treat specific infectious process.

NURSING DIAGNOSIS: **deficient Knowledge [Learning Need] regarding condition, prognosis, treatment, self-care, prevention of crisis, and discharge needs**

May Be Related To

Lack of exposure, recall
Information misinterpretation
Unfamiliarity with information resources

Possibly Evidenced By

Reports the problem
Inaccurate follow-through of instructions

Desired Outcomes/Evaluation Criteria—Client Will

Knowledge: Chronic Disease Management (NOC)

Verbalize understanding of the nature of the disease process, diagnostic procedures, and potential complications.
Identify causative factors.
Verbalize understanding of therapeutic needs.
Initiate necessary behaviors or lifestyle changes.

ACTIONS/INTERVENTIONS	RATIONALE
Teaching: Disease Process (NIC)	
Independent	
Provide information about specific anemia and explain that therapy depends on the type and severity of the anemia.	Provides knowledge base from which client can make informed choices. Allays anxiety and may promote cooperation with therapeutic regimen to manage a condition that may be long-lasting.
Discuss effects of anemias on preexisting conditions.	Anemia aggravates many underlying conditions, and resolution of anemia is impacted by aging and developmental issues, nutritional and socioeconomic issues, and acute and chronic conditions.
Review purpose and preparations for diagnostic studies.	Knowledge of what to expect can diminish anxiety.
Explain that blood taken for laboratory studies will not worsen anemia.	This is often an unspoken concern that can potentiate client's anxiety.
Review required diet alterations to meet specific dietary needs, as determined by type of anemia and deficiency.	Red meat, liver, seafood, green leafy vegetables, whole wheat bread, and dried fruits are sources of iron. Green vegetables, whole grains, liver, and citrus fruits are sources of folic acid and vitamin C, which enhances absorption of iron.
Discuss foods to avoid, such as coffee, tea, egg yolks, milk, fiber, and soy protein, at the time when client is eating high-iron foods.	These foods block absorption of iron and should be taken at a different meal. For example, red meat and milk taken at the same time can block absorption of the iron from the meat.
Assess resources, including financial, and ability to obtain and prepare food.	Inadequate resources may affect ability to purchase and prepare appropriate food items.
Encourage cessation of smoking.	Smoking decreases available oxygen and causes vasoconstriction.
Provide information about purpose, dosage, schedule, precautions, and potential side effects, interactions, and adverse reactions to all prescribed medications.	Information enhances cooperation with regimen. Recovery from anemias can be slow, requiring lengthy treatment and prevention of secondary complications.
Emphasize importance of reporting signs of fatigue, weakness, paresthesias, irritability, and impaired memory.	Indicates that anemia is progressing or failing to resolve, necessitating further evaluation and treatment changes.
For the client on iron preparations:	
Discuss importance of taking only prescribed dosages.	Overdose of iron medication can be toxic.
Advise taking with meals or immediately after meals.	Iron is best absorbed on an empty stomach. However, iron salts are gastric irritants and may cause dyspepsia, diarrhea, and abdominal discomfort if taken on an empty stomach.

ACTIONS/INTERVENTIONS (continued)	RATIONALE (continued)
Dilute liquid preparations, preferably with orange juice, and administer through a straw.	Undiluted liquid iron preparations may stain the teeth. Ascorbic acid promotes iron absorption.
Discuss possibility of iron infusions and refer to healthcare provider.	Depressed iron stores may be best treated in this manner, if client is not responding or is intolerant of oral or injected iron preparations.
Suggest use of protective devices, such as sheepskin, egg-crate, alternating air pressure, or water mattress; heel and elbow protectors; and pillows, as indicated.	Avoids skin breakdown by preventing or reducing pressure against skin surfaces.
Review good oral hygiene and necessity for regular dental care.	Effects of anemia such as oral lesions and use of iron supplements increase risk of infection and bacteremia.
Instruct to avoid use of aspirin products.	Increases bleeding tendencies.
Refer to appropriate community resources when indicated, such as social services for food stamps and Meals on Wheels.	May need assistance with groceries and meal preparation.

POTENTIAL CONSIDERATIONS following acute hospitalization (dependent on client's age, physical condition and presence of complications, personal resources, and life responsibilities)

- ***Activity Intolerance***—imbalance between oxygen supply and demand
- ***imbalanced Nutrition: less than body requirements***—failure to ingest or inability to digest food or absorb nutrients
- ***risk for Infection***—inadequate secondary defenses (e.g., decreased hemoglobin, leukopenia, or decreased granulocytes, suppressed inflammatory response); inadequate primary defenses (e.g., broken skin, stasis of body fluids; invasive procedures); chronic disease; malnutrition
- ***ineffective Self-Health Management***—economic difficulties, perceived benefits/susceptibility

SICKLE CELL CRISIS

I. Pathophysiology

a. Formation of abnormal hemoglobin chains containing hemoglobin S. When red blood cells (RBCs) are exposed to low oxygen saturation states, hemoglobin S causes the beta globin chain of hemoglobin to polymerize and contract and clump together inside the cell, leading to the formation of distorted RBCs, causing hemolysis and obstruction of blood flow.

b. These sickled cells clump together and obstruct blood flow, rendering the individual vulnerable to repeated painful crises, which can progressively destroy vital organs. Sickle cell disease (SCD) is associated with the following:

   i. Vaso-occlusive crisis (also called sickle cell crisis), responsible for a wide variety of clinical complications of SCD, including pain syndromes, stroke, leg ulcers, spontaneous abortion, and renal insufficiency (Yale, 2000). Triggers for crisis include hypoxemia (as might occur with acute chest syndrome/other respiratory complications); concomitant medical conditions (e.g., diabetes, herpes); dehydration; physical or psychological stress; changes in body and/or environmental temperatures; pregnancy and alcohol.

   ii. Anemia usually present, chronic and hemolytic in nature (Maakaron et al, 2013)

   iii. Cerebrovascular accidents (24% of people with sickle cell disease [SCD] have a stroke by the age of 45 years) (Verduzco, 2009).

   iv. Splenic crisis: rapid enlargement of spleen and life-threatening anemia

   v. Acute chest syndrome: a sudden onset pulmonary condition (see Glossary) that affects about 12% of adults and is more common in children (about 25%) (Meier 2012; Bernard, 2007). Some common causes include pulmonary infections, fat emboli, and rib infarction.

   vi. Pulmonary hypertension: emerging as a relatively common complication and is one of the leading causes of morbidity and mortality in adults with SCD (Dahoui et al, 2010).

   vii. P Cholelithiasis: common in children (Maakaron et al, 2013)

   viii. Priapism: Frequency in adults has been reported to range from 30% to 45% and P 5% to 10% in boys between 5 and 20 years of age (Maples, 2004).

   ix. P Dactylitis (hand-foot syndrome): often first symptom noted in children (Pack-Mabien, 2009)

c. Plasma clotting factors likely participate in the microthrombi in the prearterioles.

d. After recurrent episodes of sickling, membrane damage occurs and the cells are no longer capable of resuming their normal shape upon reoxygenation.

II. Etiology

a. Sickle hemoglobinopathies compose a group of genetic diseases, consisting of four genotypes: sickle cell anemia (HbSS), sickle hemoglobin C disease (HbSC), and the sickle cell thalassemias (Sβ+- and Sβ°-thalassemia) (Ellison, 2012).

b. Primarily affects black populations of African descent as well as people of South and Central American, Caribbean, Mediterranean, Arabian, and East Indian descent (Raj, n.d.; Creary, 2007)

(continues on page 470)

c. Vaso-occlusive crisis is often triggered by infection, dehydration, fever, or local trauma.

d. As of January 2006, all states in the United States as well as the District of Columbia, Puerto Rico, the Virgin Islands, and Guam have utilized universal screening for SCD in all newborns (Pack-Mabian, 2009; Yusuf et al, 2011).

III. Statistics

a. Morbidity: Sickle cell anemia is the most common inherited blood disorder in the United States, affecting 1 in 625, seen more commonly in African Americans. There are approximately 89,000 cases of HbSS in the United States annually (Maakaron et al, 2013; Yusuf et al, 2011; Brousseau et al, 2009).

b. Mortality: Median survival rate for individuals with SCD is 48 years for women and 42 years for men (Maakaron et al, 2013). In 2008, there were 501 adult deaths (National Heart, Lung and Blood Institute [NHLBI], 2012).

c. Cost: In 2009, approximately $1.1 billion for treatment of sickle cell anemia with roughly 80% of that amount spent for hospital costs (Reuters Health, 2009). For an average patient with SCD reaching age 45, total lifetime healthcare costs were estimated to be $953,640 (Kauf et al, 2009).

GLOSSARY

Acute chest syndrome: A life-threatening complication defined as an infiltrate on a chest x-ray, accompanied by two or more other symptoms, which can include fever, cough, wheezing, tachypnea, or chest pain (reflects the unique nature of acute pulmonary illness in client with SCD), with a peak incidence in early childhood (Meier 2012; Bernard, 2007).

Bruit: Abnormal sound heard over an artery or vascular channel, reflecting turbulence of blood flow.

Dactylitis: Swollen, tender digits of the hands and feet, causing severe pain. Often first sign of sickle cell disease in babies.

Genetic disease: The ultimate unit of inheritance, carried by the chromosome. Genes determine various characteristics, such as hair texture, skin color, height, shape of nose, lips, and so on, including the kind of hemoglobin in red blood cells (RBCs).

Hemoglobin (Hgb): An iron-containing protein of the RBC, which carries oxygen to the tissues and gives the cell its red color.

Hemolysis: Destruction of RBCs and subsequent release of hemoglobin.

Hyperhemolytic crisis: A rapid, higher-than-normal rate of hemolysis; reticulocytes are increased in peripheral blood, and bone marrow is hyperplastic, leading to anemia and jaundice due to effects of hemolysis. Often associated with vaso-occlusive crisis.

Hypoplastic/aplastic crisis: May be secondary to severe (usually viral) infection or folic acid deficiency, resulting in cessation of production of RBCs and bone marrow.

Icterus (jaundice): Yellowing of the skin and the whites of the eyes caused by an accumulation of bile pigment in the blood.

Kyphosis: Exaggerated outward curvature of the spine.

Lordosis: Curvature of spinal column characterized by an abnormal hollow at the small of the back; also known as swayback.

Priapism: Abnormal, painful, sustained erection of the penis, usually occurring without sexual desire. Can last for hours or days.

Pulmonary hypertension: Increased pressure in the pulmonary arteries that carry blood from the heart to the lungs to pick up oxygen.

Reticulocytes: Immature RBCs, typically composing about 1% of the red cells in the human body. Reticulocytes develop and mature in the red bone marrow and then circulate for about a day in the bloodstream before developing into mature RBCs.

Sickle cell disease (SCD): An inherited disorder of the RBCs where the individual inherits two genes for hemoglobin S, or a single S gene is combined with a second variant gene such as C or Thal.

Sickle cell trait: The inheritance of one gene for the usual hemoglobin (A) and one gene for sickle hemoglobin (S). A person who has sickle cell trait (AS) is a carrier of the sickle gene but does not have the disease or incur painful episodes and is generally not affected by the sickle hemoglobin.

Splenic sequestration crisis: Occurs when the spleen suddenly traps large numbers of RBCs, causing splenomegaly, a drop in hemogloblin greater than or equal to 20%, hypovolemia, shock, and possible death.

Thalassemia (Thal): An inherited disorder of the gene in the RBCs, which results in the impaired ability to produce hemoglobin.

Vaso-occlusive/sickle cell crisis: Related to infection, dehydration, fever, hypoxia, and characterized by multiple infarcts of bones, joints, and target organs, with tissue pain and necrosis caused by plugs of sickled cells in the microcirculation.

Care Setting

Sickle cell disease is generally managed at the community level, with many of the interventions included here being appropriate for this focus; however, this plan of care addresses sickle cell crisis, which usually requires hospitalization during the acute phase to address oxygenation and severe pain.

Related Concerns

Cerebrovascular accident (CVA)/stroke, page 214
Cholecystitis with cholelithiasis, page 329
Heart failure: chronic, page 43
Pediatric considerations, page 872
Pneumonia, page 129
Psychosocial aspects of care, page 729
Seizure disorders, page 188
Sepsis/septicemia, page 665
Transplantation considerations—postoperative and lifelong, page 719

Client Assessment Database

Depends on severity of condition and presence of complications.

DIAGNOSTIC DIVISION MAY REPORT	MAY EXHIBIT
ACTIVITY/REST • Lethargy, fatigue, weakness, general malaise • Loss of productivity • Decreased exercise tolerance, impaired mobility • Greater need for sleep and rest	• Listlessness, severe weakness, and increasing pallor (aplastic crisis) • Gait disturbances (pain, kyphosis, lordosis), inability to walk (pain) • Poor body posture • Decreased range of motion (ROM) • Joint, bone deformities • Generalized retarded growth, tower-shaped skull with frontal bossing, disproportionately long arms and legs, short trunk, narrowed shoulders and hips, and long, tapered fingers
CIRCULATION • Palpitations or anginal chest pain due to concomitant coronary artery disease (CAD), myocardial ischemia, or acute chest syndrome • Intermittent pain in legs when walking • Swelling of hands and feet (often initial symptom in infants)	• Apical pulse—point of maximal impulse (PMI) may be displaced to the left • Tachycardia, S-T elevation • Systolic heart murmurs may be heard over entire precordium • Blood pressure (BP)—widened pulse pressure • P Hypertension or abnormal blood pressure patterns (elevations and dips) in children (Maakaron et al, 2013) • Generalized symptoms of shock—hypotension; rapid, thready pulse; and shallow respirations during sequestration crisis • Peripheral pulses throbbing on palpation • Bruits—reflects compensatory mechanisms of anemia; may also be auscultated over the spleen because of multiple splenic infarcts • Capillary refill delayed (anemia or hypovolemia) • ***Skin color:*** Pallor or cyanosis of skin, mucous membranes, and conjunctiva (*Note:* Pallor may appear as yellowish-brown color in brown-skinned clients and as ashen gray in black-skinned clients.) • Scleral icterus, generalized icteric coloring due to excessive RBC hemolysis • Dry skin and mucous membranes • P Puffy, tender hands and feet, refusal to bear weight, irritability in children less than 2 years of age (Pack-Mabien, 2009)
ELIMINATION • Frequent voiding, voiding in large amounts • Nocturia	• Right upper quadrant (RUQ) abdominal tenderness, enlargement due to hepatomegaly or ascites • Left upper quadrant (LUQ) abdominal fullness; spleen may be enlarged and nonfunctional and may eventually become fibrotic and shrunken. • Dilute, pale, straw-colored urine; hematuria or smoky appearance from multiple renal infarcts • Asymptomatic proteinuria
EGO INTEGRITY • Resentment and frustration with disease, fear of rejection from others • Negative feelings about self, ability to deal with life or situation • Concern regarding being a burden to significant others (SOs), financial concerns, possible loss of insurance benefits, lost time at work or school, fear of genetic transmission of disease	• Anxiety, restlessness, irritability, apprehension, withdrawal, narrowed focus, self-focusing, unresponsiveness to questions, regression, depression, decreased self-concept • Dependent relationship with whomever can offer security and protection

(continues on page 472)

Client Assessment Database (continued)

DIAGNOSTIC DIVISION MAY REPORT (continued)	MAY EXHIBIT (continued)
FOOD/FLUID • Thirst • Anorexia • Nausea, vomiting	• (P) Child's height and weight usually in the lower percentiles (Maakaron et al, 2013) • Poor skin turgor with visible tenting during sequestration crisis, infection, and dehydration • Dry skin and mucous membranes • Jugular vein distention (JVD) and general peripheral edema (concomitant heart failure [HF])
HYGIENE • Difficulty maintaining activities of daily living (ADLs) (pain or severe anemia)	• Unkempt appearance, poor personal hygiene
NEUROSENSORY • Headaches or dizziness • Visual disturbances due to retinal vascular changes • Tingling in the extremities • Disturbances in pain and position sense	• Mental status usually unaffected except in cases of severe sickling (cerebral infarction and intracranial hemorrhage) • Weakness of the mouth, tongue, and facial muscles; aphasia (in cerebral infarction of dominant hemisphere) • Abnormal reflexes, decreased muscle strength and tone, abnormal involuntary movements, hemiplegia or sudden hemiparesis, quadriplegia • Ataxia, seizures • Meningeal irritation (intracranial hemorrhage)—decreasing level of consciousness (LOC), nuchal rigidity, focal neurological deficits, vomiting, severe headache
PAIN/DISCOMFORT • Pain may be acute and severe, throbbing, of varied locations (two or more sites). • Pain may be localized or migratory and most commonly involves the back, legs, knees, arms, chest, and abdomen. Recurrent, sharp, transient headaches • Joint or bone pain may be low-level and chronic or acute and accompanied by warmth, tenderness, erythema, and occasional effusions (vaso-occlusive crisis). • Abdominal tenderness and pain	• Sensitivity to palpation over affected areas • Guarding or holding joints in position of comfort, decreased ROM, resulting from joint pain and swelling • Maladaptive pain behaviors—guilt for being ill, denial of any aspect of disease, indulgence in precipitating factors such as overwork, strenuous exercise
RESPIRATION • Dyspnea on exertion or at rest • History of repeated pulmonary infections, infarctions, pulmonary fibrosis, pulmonary hypertension or cor pulmonale	• Acute respiratory distress—dyspnea, chest pain, and cyanosis (especially in crisis) • (P) Cough with fever (children with acute chest syndrome) (Bernard, 2007) • Bronchial or bronchovesicular sounds in lung periphery, diminished breath sounds (pulmonary fibrosis) • Crackles, rhonchi, wheezes, diminished breath sounds (HF) • Increased anteroposterior (AP) diameter of the chest (barrel chest)
SAFETY • History of repeated, frequent blood transfusions • Jaundice with skin itching • Leg ulcers • Impaired vision (sickle retinopathy), decreased visual acuity (temporary or permanent blindness)	• Fever with chills (adult with acute chest syndrome) (Bernard, 2007) • Leg ulcers—especially common on the internal and external malleoli and the medial aspect of the tibia

DIAGNOSTIC DIVISION MAY REPORT (continued)	MAY EXHIBIT (continued)
SEXUALITY • Loss of libido • Amenorrhea • Complications of pregnancy, including placenta previa and abruption; premature birth or fetal death • Priapism, impotence	• Delayed sexual maturity • Pale cervix and vaginal walls (anemia)
TEACHING/LEARNING • Chronic anemic state • Pulmonary hypertension or cor pulmonale (multiple pulmonary infections and infarctions) • Chronic leg ulcers, delayed healing	
DISCHARGE PLAN CONSIDERATIONS • May need assistance with shopping, transportation, self-care, homemaker and maintenance tasks ➧ Refer to section at end of plan for postdischarge considerations.	

Diagnostic Studies

TEST WHY IT IS DONE	WHAT IT TELLS ME
BLOOD TESTS	
• ***Complete blood count (CBC):*** Battery of screening tests, which typically includes Hgb; hematocrit (Hct); RBC count, morphology, indices, and distribution width index; platelet count and size; and white blood cell (WBC) count and differential.	Hgb and total RBCs are decreased.. Young WBCs (leukocytes) are elevated, especially in vaso-occlusive crisis. Platelets are often increased. *Note:* Anemia is often well tolerated by the client; however, a major drop in Hgb from previously recorded values indicates a hematologic crisis. If the reticulocyte count is normal, splenic sequestration is the probable cause. If the reticulocyte count is low, an aplastic crisis is the probable cause.
• ***Red blood cells***	
• ***Reticulocyte count:*** Measures how fast red blood cells are made by the bone marrow and released into the blood.	Young RBCs (reticulocytes) can be low or elevated if anemia is long-standing. If the reticulocyte count is normal, splenic sequestration is the probable cause. If the reticulocyte count is low, an aplastic crisis is the probable cause.
• ***Stained RBC (erythrocyte) examination:*** Evaluates changes in morphology of RBCs.	Demonstrates partially or completely sickled, crescent-shaped cells, Howell-Jolly bodies, basophilic stippling, and occasional nucleated RBCs (normoblasts).
• ***Hemoglobin electrophoresis:*** Determines type of hemoglobin the individual has. When an electric charge is passed through a solution of hemoglobin, distinct hemoglobins move different distances, depending on their composition. This technique differentiates between usual hemoglobin (A), sickle hemoglobin (S), and many other different kinds of hemoglobin.	Identifies any abnormal hemoglobin types and differentiates between sickle cell trait and sickle cell anemia. Results may be inaccurate if client has received a blood transfusion within 3 to 4 months before testing.
• ***Sickle-turbidity tube test (Sickledex):*** Detects the presence of hemoglobin S in blood.	Positive if 10% of hemoglobin S is present but does not differentiate between sickle cell anemia and sickle cell trait.
• ***Alkaline phosphatase (ALP):*** Enzyme found primarily in the liver.	Elevated during vaso-occlusive crisis, reflecting bone and liver damage.
• ***Lactate dehydrogenase (LDH):*** Indicator of the existence and severity of acute or chronic tissue damage.	Elevated because of RBC hemolysis.

(continues on page 474)

Diagnostic Studies (continued)

TEST WHY IT IS DONE (continued)	WHAT IT TELLS ME (continued)
• *Serum iron:* Iron balance is not easily achieved in sickle cell disease.	Deficiency is associated with premature destruction of young RBCs. However, the iron stores released by hemolysis may be available for reuse; therefore, serum iron deficiency is not always present. (P) A very high iron level is associated with frequent blood transfusions for sickle cell anemia—a condition more common in children than adults. A single transfusion can contain approximately 250 mg of iron. Excess iron cannot be excreted without additional medication being given (Mohanty et al, 2008; Iron Disorders Institute, 2006).
Other Diagnostic Studies	
• *Urine/fecal urobilinogen:* Substance formed in the intestine from the breakdown of bilirubin; some is excreted in feces and some is reabsorbed and excreted in bile or urine.	These sensitive indicators of RBC destruction are increased.
• *Abdominal/pelvic ultrasound:* Performed to evaluate condition of organs.	Documents spleen size and presence of biliary or kidney stones.
• *Bone x-rays:* Evaluate skeletal changes.	May demonstrate bone infarction, osteomyelitis, avascular necrosis of hip, and so forth.
• *Chest x-ray:* Performed to check for pulmonary infiltrate.	May confirm presence of acute chest syndrome if infiltrate accompanied by other symptoms such as chest pain, elevated temperature, or hypoxemia (Ellison, 2012). A lateral chest x-ray detects the characteristic "Lincoln log" deformity. This spinal abnormality develops in many adults and some adolescents with sickle cell anemia, leaving the vertebrae resembling logs that form the corner of a cabin (*Nurse's 3-minute Clinical Reference*, 2008).
• *Magnetic Resonance Imaging (MRI):* An imaging test that uses magnets and radio waves to create pictures of the body.	The definitive test to rule out cerebral infarct (Ellison, 2012). Also identifies bone marrow changes due to acute and chronic bone marrow infarction, marrow hyperplasia, osteomyelitis, and osteonecrosis (Maakaron et al, 2013).
• *Transcranial Doppler studies:* a noninvasive ultrasound technology for imaging blood flow in the cerebral arteries and veins.	Detects large vessel disease that is often involved in overt cerebral vascular accidents in patients with SCD (Meier, 2012).
• *Echocardiography*	Can identify pulmonary hypertension

Nursing Priorities

1. Promote adequate cellular oxygenation and perfusion.
2. Alleviate pain.
3. Prevent complications.
4. Provide information about disease process, prognosis, and treatment needs.

Discharge Goals

1. Oxygenation and perfusion are adequate to meet cellular needs.
2. Pain relieved or controlled.
3. Complications prevented or minimized.
4. Disease process, future expectations, potential complications, and therapeutic regimen understood.
5. Plan in place to meet needs after discharge.

NURSING DIAGNOSIS: impaired Gas Exchange

May Be Related To

Decreased oxygen-carrying capacity of the blood, reduced RBC life span or premature destruction, abnormal RBC structure, sensitivity to low oxygen tension due to strenuous exercise, increase in altitude

Increased blood viscosity—occlusions created by sickled cells packing together within the capillaries

Pulmonary congestion—impairment of surface phagocytosis

Predisposition to bacterial pneumonia, pulmonary infarcts

Possibly Evidenced By

Dyspnea, use of accessory muscles

Restlessness, confusion

Tachycardia

Cyanosis (hypoxia)

Desired Outcomes/Evaluation Criteria—Client Will

Respiratory Status: Gas Exchange (NOC)

Demonstrate improved ventilation and oxygenation as evidenced by respiratory rate within normal limits, absence of cyanosis, use of accessory muscles, and clear breath sounds.

Participate in ADLs without weakness and fatigue.

Display improved or normal pulmonary function tests.

ACTIONS/INTERVENTIONS	RATIONALE
Respiratory Monitoring (NIC)	
Independent	
Monitor respiratory rate and depth, use of accessory muscles, and areas of cyanosis.	Indicators of adequacy of respiratory function or degree of compromise and therapy needs and effectiveness.
Auscultate breath sounds, noting presence or absence, and adventitious sounds.	Development of atelectasis and stasis of secretions can impair gas exchange.
Monitor vital signs; note changes in cardiac rhythm.	Changes in vital signs and development of dysrhythmias reflect effects of hypoxia on cardiovascular system.
Investigate reports of chest pain and increasing fatigue. Observe for signs of increased fever, cough, and adventitious breath sounds.	Reflective of developing acute chest syndrome, which increases the workload of the heart and oxygen demand.
Assess LOC and mentation regularly.	Brain tissue is very sensitive to decreases in oxygen, and changes in mentation may be an early indicator of developing hypoxia.
Ventilation Assistance	
Assist in turning, coughing, and deep-breathing exercises.	Promotes optimal chest expansion, mobilization of secretions, and aeration of all lung fields; reduces risk of stasis of secretions and pneumonia.
Evaluate activity tolerance; limit activities to those within client's tolerance or place client on bedrest. Assist with ADLs and mobility, as needed.	Reduction of the metabolic requirements of the body reduces the oxygen requirements and degree of hypoxia.
Encourage client to alternate periods of rest and activity. Schedule rest periods, as indicated.	Protects from excessive fatigue and reduces oxygen demands and degree of hypoxia.
Demonstrate and encourage use of relaxation techniques, such as guided imagery and visualization.	Relaxation decreases muscle tension and anxiety and, hence, the metabolic demand for oxygen.
Promote adequate fluid intake, such as 2 to 3 L/day within cardiac tolerance.	Sufficient hydration is necessary to provide for mobilization of secretions and to prevent hyperviscosity of blood with associated capillary occlusion.
Screen health status of visitors and staff.	Protects client from potential sources of respiratory infection.
Collaborative	
Administer supplemental humidified oxygen, as indicated.	Maximizes oxygen transport to tissues, particularly in presence of pulmonary insults or pneumonia. *Note:* Oxygen should be given only in the presence of confirmed hypoxemia because oxygen can suppress erythropoietin levels, further reducing the production of RBCs.
Monitor laboratory studies—CBC (especially noting Hgb and WBCs), blood cultures, arterial blood gases (ABGs) and pulse oximetry, chest x-ray, and pulmonary function tests (when available).	Client is particularly prone to acute chest syndrome and pneumonia (which is potentially fatal because of its hypoxemic effect of increased sickling). *Note:* Most individuals with sickle cell anemia have hemoglobin (Hgb) values of 6 to 10 g per dL. The hemoglobin S molecule has a low affinity for oxygen (which allows for adequate tissue oxygenation). During a vaso-occlusive crisis, a client's Hgb level often declines by at least 1 g per dL.

(continues on page 476)

ACTIONS/INTERVENTIONS (continued)	RATIONALE (continued)
Perform or assist with chest physiotherapy, intermittent positive-pressure breathing (IPPB), and incentive spirometry.	Mobilizes secretions and increases aeration of lung fields.
Administer packed RBCs (PRCs) or exchange transfusions, as indicated.	Simple blood transfusion increases the number of oxygen-carrying cells, dilutes the percentage of hemoglobin S, and improves circulation. PRCs are used because they are less likely to create circulatory overload. Exchange blood transfusions are indicated when the client's condition is deteriorating and may be done for cases of stroke and acute chest syndrome. Exchange transfusion consists of replacing the client's RBCs by normal donor RBCs, thereby decreasing hemoglobin S (Bernard, 2007). *Note:* Partial transfusions are sometimes used prophylactically in high-risk situations, such as chronic, severe leg ulcers, preparation for general anesthesia, and third trimester of pregnancy.
Administer medications, as indicated, for example:	
Antipyretic, such as acetaminophen (Tylenol)	Maintains normothermia to reduce metabolic oxygen demands without affecting serum pH, which may occur with aspirin.
Antibiotics, such as amoxicillin plus clavulanic acid (Augmentin), third-generation cephalosporins (e.g., ceftriaxone [Rocephin]) among others	Broad-spectrum antibiotics are started immediately pending culture results of suspected infections, then may be changed when the specific pathogen is identified. *Note:* Studies have shown that *Chlamydia pneumonia* and *Mycoplasma pneumoniae* are now the most common documented infectious causes of ACS (Vichinsky et al, 2000).

NURSING DIAGNOSIS: acute/chronic Pain

May Be Related To

Physical agent (e.g., intravascular sickling with localized stasis, occlusion, infarction, and necrosis; activation of pain fibers due to deprivation of oxygen and nutrients, accumulation of noxious metabolites)

Possibly Evidenced By

Verbalized/coded reports of pain
Guarding behaviors
Facial grimacing, narrowed or self-focus

Desired Outcomes/Evaluation Criteria—Client Will

Pain Level (NOC)

Verbalize relief or control of pain.

Pain Control (NOC)

Demonstrate relaxed body posture, freedom of movement, and ability to sleep and rest appropriately.

ACTIONS/INTERVENTIONS	RATIONALE
Pain Management (NIC) *Independent*	
Assess reports of pain, including location, duration, and intensity (0 to 10 or similar coded scale). Have client help differentiate current pain from typical or usual pain problems.	Acute pain in patients with sickle cell disease can be localized, migratory, or more generalized and described as throbbing, gnawing, or severe and incapacitating. Pain is caused by ischemic tissue injury resulting from the occlusion of microvascular beds by sickled erythrocytes during an acute crisis. Chronic pain occurs because of the destruction of bones, joints, and visceral organs as a result of recurrent crises. The effect of unpredictable recurrences of acute crises on chronic pain creates a unique pain syndrome (Yale, 2000). Typically, acute pain occurs deep in the bones and muscles of back, ribs, and limbs and lasts 5 to 7 days. However, client may also have chronic pain from sickle cell damage (usually bone pain that is present daily) and chronic nerve pain caused by damage from sickle cell blockage or other conditions, such as diabetes.
Observe nonverbal pain cues, such as gait disturbances, body positioning, reluctance to move, facial expressions; and	Nonverbal cues may aid in evaluation of pain and effectiveness of therapy. Pain is unique to each client; therefore, one may

ACTIONS/INTERVENTIONS (continued)	RATIONALE (continued)
physiological manifestations of acute pain—elevated BP, tachycardia, and increased respiratory rate. Explore discrepancies between verbal and nonverbal cues.	encounter varying descriptions because of individualized perceptions.
Discuss with the client/SO what pain relief measures were effective in the past.	Involves client/SO in care and allows for identification of remedies that have already been found to relieve pain. Helpful in establishing individualized treatment needs.
Explore alternative pain relief measures, such as relaxation techniques, biofeedback, yoga, meditation, and distraction—visual, auditory, tactile, kinesthetic, guided imagery, and breathing techniques.	Cognitive-behavioral interventions may reduce reliance on pharmacological therapy and enhance client's sense of control.
Provide support for and carefully position affected extremities.	Reduces edema, discomfort, and risk of injury, especially if osteomyelitis is present.
Apply local massage gently to affected areas.	Helps reduce muscle tension.
Encourage ROM exercises.	May reduce joint stiffness and possible contracture formation.
Plan activities during peak analgesic effect.	Maximizes movement of joints, enhancing mobility.
Maintain adequate fluid intake.	Dehydration increases sickling vaso-occlusion and corresponding pain.
Collaborative	
Apply warm, moist compresses to affected joints or other painful areas. Avoid use of ice or cold compresses.	Warmth causes vasodilation and increases circulation to hypoxic areas. Cold causes vasoconstriction and compounds the crisis.
Administer medications by appropriate route (such as continuous infusion or around-the-clock intermittent IV or oral, as indicated), for example:	Various types of analgesics are needed to manage different types of pain.
Opioids morphine (Astramorph, Duramorph), hydromorphone (Dilaudid), and nalbuphine (Nubain); long-acting opiate combinations, such as morphine (MS Contin) and oxycodone (Oxycontin), hydrocodone (Vicodin); oxycodone and acetaminophen (Percocet)	Opioids are the mainstay of pain control during crisis and are usually administered via patient-controlled analgesia (PCA). Oral preparations are preferred for longer-term treatment and can be initiated while client is still on IV analgesia. *Note:* Meperidine (Demerol) should not be used because its metabolite, normeperidine, can cause central nervous system (CNS) excitation—anxiety, tremors, and seizures.
Nonopioid analgesics, such as acetaminophen (Tylenol); nonsteroidal anti-inflammatory drugs (NSAIDs), such as ibuprofen (Advil, Motrin); Ketrolac	Acetaminophen and NSAIDs add to the effects of opioids during painful crisis. Acetaminophen can be used for control of headache, pain, and fever. *Note:* Aspirin should be avoided because it alters blood pH and can make cells sickle more easily.
Consult with or refer to physical therapy.	Determines and provides appropriate therapies, such as massage, heat therapies, and guided exercise.
Administer and monitor RBC transfusion.	Although transfusion does not halt the pain in an acute crisis, frequency of painful crises may be reduced by regular partial exchange transfusions to maintain population of normal RBCs.

NURSING DIAGNOSIS: risk for ineffective Tissue Perfusion [specify: cardiac, cerebral, gastrointestinal, peripheral]

May Be Related To
Coagulopathy (e.g., vaso-occlusive nature of sickling, inflammatory response)
Deficient knowledge of aggravating factors

Possibly Evidenced By
Extremity pain, bone pain, claudication, angina
Altered skin characteristics (e.g., pallor)
Changes in vital signs, diminished or absent pulses
Skin ulcerations, delayed peripheral wound healing
Decreased mentation, restlessness
Transient visual disturbances

Desired Outcomes/Evaluation Criteria—Client Will

Tissue Perfusion (NOC)
Demonstrate improved tissue perfusion as evidenced by stabilized vital signs, strong and palpable peripheral pulses, adequate urine output, absence of pain; usual mentation; normal capillary refill; skin warm and dry; nailbeds and lips of natural pale, pink color; and absence of paresthesias.

ACTIONS/INTERVENTIONS	RATIONALE
Circulatory Care: Arterial [or] Venous Insufficiency (NIC)	
Independent	
Impaired systemic and cardiovascular perfusion	
Monitor vital signs carefully. Assess pulses for rate, rhythm, and volume. Note changes in blood pressure.	Sludging and sickling in peripheral vessels may lead to complete or partial obliteration of a vessel with diminished perfusion to surrounding tissues.
Assess heart sounds and pulses for dysrhythmias.	May reflect problems with cardiac output (systemic dehydration and/or hypoxemia), electrolyte imbalances, or local or systemic sickling causing inadequate myocardial perfusion.
Assess for restlessness, changes in level of consciousness, increased capillary refill time, diminished peripheral pulses, and pale, cool skin.	Indicative of inadequate systemic perfusion.
Note onset of hypotension with rapid, weak, thready pulse and tachypnea with shallow respirations.	Sudden massive splenic sequestration of cells can lead to systemic shock.
Investigate reports of chest pain.	To evaluate for potential myocardial ischemia, inadequate systemic oxygenation or perfusion of organs.
Impaired general and peripheral perfusion	
Assess lower extremities for skin texture, edema, and ulcerations, especially of internal and external ankles.	Edema may reflect both systemic and peripheral effects of sickle cell disease. Reduced peripheral circulation often results in skin and underlying tissue changes (e.g., ulcerations) and delayed healing.
Investigate reports of eye pain or vision disturbances.	Changes may reflect occlusion of vasculature of the eye.
Evaluate for developing edema—including genitals in boys and men.	Vaso-occlusion or circulatory stasis may lead to edema of extremities and priapism, potentiating risk of tissue ischemia and necrosis.
Maintain environmental temperature and body warmth without overheating. Avoid hypothermia.	Prevents vasoconstriction, aids in maintaining circulation and perfusion. Excessive body heat may cause diaphoresis, adding to insensible fluid losses and risk of dehydration. Hypothermia may exacerbate cardiovascular compromise with severe anemia.
Monitor urine output.	Decreased output may be indicative of dehydration, impaired cardiac output or impaired renal perfusion because of vascular occlusions. (Refer to ND: risk for deficient Fluid Volume, following; and CP: Renal Failure/Acute/Chronic).
Risk for impaired respiratory system perfusion	
Monitor respirations, noting rate outside of acceptable parameters and drop in pulse oximetry. Note client reports of/demonstration of difficult breathing.	May indicate presence of oxygen exchange problems, presence of respiratory infection or acute chest syndrome.
Assess skin for coolness, pallor, cyanosis, and diaphoresis.	Changes reflect diminished circulation and hypoxia potentiating capillary occlusion. (Refer to ND: impaired Gas Exchange.)
Risk for ineffective cerebral perfusion	
Note changes in level of consciousness and menation; reports of headaches, dizziness; development of sensory or motor deficits, such as hemiparesis or paralysis; and seizure activity.	Changes may reflect diminished perfusion to the brain and central nervous system (CNS) due to ischemia or infarction (stroke). Studies reported that 24% of adults with SCD have suffered a stroke by age 45 and approximately 11% of those occur before the age of 20 (Cushman et al, 2008). (P) *Note:* Researchers have demonstrated that the scenario of high blood pressure and anemia together put children with SCD at serious danger for symptomless or so-called "silent" strokes, which cause subclinical brain damage (DeBaun et al, 2012). (Refer to CP: Cerebral Vascular Accident/Stroke).
Ineffective Gastrointestinal Perfusion	
Asculate abdomen to evaluate for peristaltic activity, especially in the presence of vomiting and abdominal pain.	May indicate presence of bowel ischemia or obstruction or other abdominal pathology, such as cholecystitis (especially common in children) (Maakaron et al, 2013).
Note increasing abdominal girth, especially when accompanied by general deterioration in clinical status (i.e., sudden weakness, pale lips, rapid breathing, excessive thirst, belly pain, and rapid heartbeat) and severe anemia.	May indicate presence of splenic sequestration (occurs when large numbers of sickled red blood cells become trapped in the spleen, causing it to suddenly enlarge). (P) This condition is more common in infants and young children. Without emergency medical care, splenic sequestration can cause death in a matter of hours (Thompson, 2010).
Collaborative	
Monitor laboratory studies, such as the following:	
Arterial blood gases (ABGs), liver and kidney function tests	Decreased tissue perfusion may lead to gradual infarction of organ tissues, such as the brain, liver, spleen, kidney, and skeletal muscle, with consequent release of intracellular enzymes.

ACTIONS/INTERVENTIONS (continued)	RATIONALE (continued)
Serum electrolytes; provide replacements as indicated.	Electrolyte losses, especially sodium and potassium, are increased during crisis because of fever, diarrhea, vomiting, and diaphoresis, and presence of acidosis.
Administer oxygen by appropriate route and assist with respiratory treatment measures, such as coughing, deep breathing exercises, and incentive spirometer.	Improves oxygenation and reduces risk of pulmonary complications. (Refer to ND: impaired Gas Exchange, above.)
Administer intravenous (IV) solutions, such as 0.45 normal saline, via an infusion pump.	Hydration lowers the hemoglobin S concentration, which decreases the sickling tendency and also reduces blood viscosity, which helps to maintain perfusion. Infusion pump may prevent circulatory overload. *Note:* Lactated Ringer's solution or D_5W may cause RBC hemolysis and potentiate thrombus formation.
Administer hydroxyurea (Droxia) and observe for possible side effects.	Hydroxyurea, a cytotoxic agent, dramatically decreases the number of sickle cell episodes and is given to prevent crises. Use of this medication has been associated with fewer episodes of pain crises and acute chest syndrome, decreased need for transfusion, and lower mortality (Steinberg et al, 2003).
Administer deferoxamine (Desferal) and vitamin C.	Chelation therapy may be indicated to correct iron overload associated with regular, frequent transfusions. Vitamin C may enhance excretion, especially in clients who are vitamin deficient. *Note:* Phlebotomy and exchange transfusions may be used in conjunction with chelation therapy.
Prepare for and assist with needle aspiration of blood from corpora cavernosa.	Sickling within the penis can cause priapism and edema. Removal of sludged sickled cells can improve circulation, decreasing psychological trauma and risk of necrosis and infection.
Prepare for surgical intervention.	Direct incision and ligation of the dorsal arteries of the penis and saphenous-cavernous shunting may be necessary in severe cases of priapism to prevent tissue necrosis.

NURSING DIAGNOSIS: risk for deficient Fluid Volume

Risk Factors May Include

Increased fluid needs (hypermetabolic state or fever, inflammatory processes)
Active fluid loss (renal parenchymal damage or infarctions limiting the kidney's ability to concentrate urine [hyposthenuria])

Possibly Evidenced By

(Not applicable; presence of signs and symptoms establishes an *actual* diagnosis)

Desired Outcomes/Evaluation Criteria—Client Will

Hydration (NOC)

Maintain adequate fluid balance as evidenced by individually appropriate urine output with a near-normal specific gravity, stable vital signs, moist mucous membranes, good skin turgor, and prompt capillary refill.

ACTIONS/INTERVENTIONS	RATIONALE
Fluid Monitoring (NIC)	
Independent	
Maintain accurate intake and output (I&O). Weigh daily.	Client may reduce fluid intake during periods of crisis because of malaise and anorexia. Dehydration from vomiting, diarrhea, and fever may reduce urine output and precipitate a vaso-occlusive crisis.
Note urine characteristics and specific gravity.	The kidney can lose its ability to concentrate urine, resulting in excessive losses of dilute urine and fixation of the specific gravity.
Monitor vital signs, comparing with client's usual or previous readings. Take BP in lying, sitting, and standing positions, if possible.	Reduction of circulating blood volume can occur from increased fluid loss, resulting in hypotension and tachycardia.
Observe for fever, changes in level of consciousness, poor skin turgor, dryness of skin and mucous membranes, and pain.	Symptoms are reflective of dehydration and hemoconcentration with consequent vaso-occlusive state.
Monitor vital signs closely during blood transfusions and note presence of dyspnea, crackles, rhonchi, wheezes, diminished breath sounds, cough, frothy sputum, and cyanosis.	Client's heart may already be weakened and prone to failure because of chronic demands placed on it by the anemic

(continues on page 480)

state. Heart may be unable to tolerate the added fluid volume from transfusions or rapid IV fluid administered to treat crisis or shock.

Collaborative

ACTIONS/INTERVENTIONS	RATIONALE
Administer IV fluids, as indicated.	Replaces fluid deficits; may reverse renal concentration of RBCs and reduce potential for kidney failure.
Monitor laboratory studies, for example: Hgb/Hct	Elevations may indicate hemoconcentration. Post-transfusion Hgb level of 8 to 9 g/dL is generally recommended to avoid the risk of hyperviscosity that may occur several days after transfusion when RBCs sequestered in the spleen may return to the circulation and increase the Hgb levels.
Serum and urine electrolytes	Kidneys' loss of ability to concentrate urine may result in serum depletions of NA^+, K^-, and CL^-, necessitating replacement.

NURSING DIAGNOSIS: impaired physical Mobility

May Be Related To

Joint stiffness; loss of integrity of bone structures (osteoporosis, osteomyelitis)
Decreased endurance
Pain/discomfort; reluctance to initiate movement
Prescribed movement restrictions (bedrest)

Possibly Evidenced By

Limited joint ROM, slowed movement, gait changes
Generalized weakness

Desired Outcomes/Evaluation Criteria—Client Will

Mobility (NOC)

Maintain or increase strength and function of affected body parts.
Participate in activities with absence of or improvement in gait disturbances, increased joint ROM, and absence of inflammatory signs.

Refer to CP: Extended Care; ND: impaired physical Mobility for appropriate actions and interventions.

NURSING DIAGNOSIS: risk for impaired Skin Integrity

Risk Factors May Include

Impaired circulation (venous stasis and vaso-occlusion); impaired sensation
Mechanical factors—pressure

Possibly Evidenced By

(Not applicable; presence of signs and symptoms establishes an *actual* diagnosis)

Desired Outcomes/Evaluation Criteria—Client Will

Tissue Integrity: Skin and Mucous Membranes (NOC)

Prevent dermal ischemic injury.
Display improvement in wound or lesion healing if present.

Risk Control (NOC)

Participate in behaviors to reduce risk factors and skin breakdown.

ACTIONS/INTERVENTIONS	RATIONALE
Skin Surveillance (NIC)	
Independent	
Reposition frequently, even when sitting in chair.	Prevents prolonged tissue pressure where circulation is already compromised, reducing risk of tissue trauma and ischemia.
Inspect skin pressure points regularly for pallor or redness and provide gentle massage.	Poor circulation may predispose to rapid skin breakdown.
Protect bony prominences with sheepskin, heel and elbow protectors, or pillows, as indicated.	Decreases pressure on tissues, preventing skin breakdown.
Keep skin surfaces dry and clean and linens dry and wrinkle-free.	Moist, contaminated areas provide excellent media for growth of pathogenic organisms.
Monitor ischemic areas, leg bruises, cuts, and bumps closely for ulcer formation.	Potential entry sites for pathogenic organisms. In presence of altered immune system, this increases risk of infection and delayed healing.
Elevate lower extremities when sitting.	Enhances venous return, reducing venous stasis and edema formation.
Collaborative	
Provide egg-crate, alternating air pressure, or water mattress.	Reduces tissue pressure and aids in maximizing cellular perfusion to prevent dermal injury.
Provide wound care as indicated, such as cleansing and débriding open wounds and ulcers according to protocol.	Improvement or delayed healing reflects status of tissue perfusion and effectiveness of interventions. *Note:* These clients are at increased risk of serious complications because of lowered resistance to infection and decreased nutrients for healing.
Prepare for and assist with hyperbaric oxygenation of ulcer sites.	Maximizes oxygen delivery to tissues, enhancing healing.

NURSING DIAGNOSIS: risk for Infection

Risk Factors May Include

Chronic disease

Inadequate primary defenses—broken skin, tissue destruction (e.g., infarction, fibrosis, loss of spleen [autosplenectomy]), stasis of body fluids, decreased ciliary action

Possibly Evidenced By

(Not applicable; presence of signs and symptoms establishes an *actual* diagnosis)

Desired Outcomes/Evaluation Criteria—Client Will

Risk Control: Infectious Process (NOC)

Verbalize understanding of individual causative or risk factors.

Identify interventions to prevent or reduce risk of infection.

Refer to CPs: Pneumonia, Sepsis/Septicemia, Fractures; ND: risk for Infection.

NURSING DIAGNOSIS: ineffective Self-Health Management

May Be Related To

Complexity of therapeutic regimen; deficient knowledge

Family patterns of healthcare

Perceived barriers

Possibly Evidenced By

Reports difficulty with regimen

Failure to take action to reduce risk factors

Ineffective choices in daily living for meeting health goals

Unexpected acceleration of illness symptoms

Desired Outcomes/Evaluation Criteria—Client Will

Self-Management: Chronic Disease (NOC)

Verbalize understanding of disease process, including symptoms of crisis and potential complications.

Verbalize understanding of therapeutic needs.

Initiate necessary behaviors or lifestyle changes to prevent complications.

Participate in continued medical follow-up, genetic counseling, and family planning services.

ACTIONS/INTERVENTIONS	RATIONALE
Teaching: Disease Process (NIC)	
Independent	
Review disease process and treatment needs.	Provides knowledge base from which client can make informed choices. *Note:* The median age at death is 48 years for women and 42 years for men, with death often being due to organ failure. However, a significant number of individuals are living much longer.
Review precipitating factors, such as the following:	
Cold environmental temperatures, failure to dress warmly when engaging in winter activities; wearing tight, restrictive clothing; stressful situations	Causes peripheral vasoconstriction, which may result in sludging of the circulation, increased sickling, and may precipitate a vaso-occlusive crisis.
Strenuous physical activity or contact-type sports and extremely warm temperatures	Increases metabolic demand for oxygen and increases insensible fluid losses (evaporation and perspiration), leading to dehydration, which may increase blood viscosity and tendency to sickle.
Travel to places more than 7000 ft above sea level or flying in unpressurized aircraft	Decreased oxygen tension present at higher altitudes causes hypoxia and potentiates sickling of cells. *Note:* Even though commercial airline cabins are pressurized, low cabin humidity increases risk of dehydration.
Encourage consumption of at least 3 to 4 L of fluid daily, during a steady state, increasing to 6 to 8 L during a painful crisis or while engaging in activities that might precipitate dehydration.	Prevents dehydration and consequent hyperviscosity that can potentiate sickling and crisis.
Discuss use of antimetabolites, such as hydroxyurea (Hydrea).	May reduce frequency of pain episodes in adults.
Encourage ROM exercise and regular physical activity with a balance between rest and activity.	Prevents bone demineralization and may reduce risk of fractures. Aids in maintaining level of resistance and decreases oxygen needs.
Review client's current diet, reinforcing the importance of diet including liver, green leafy vegetables, citrus fruits, and wheat germ. Provide necessary instruction regarding supplementary vitamins such as folic acid.	Nutritious foods, including vitamins folate and B_{12} in greater quantities than usual, are essential because of increased demands placed on bone marrow. Folic acid supplements are frequently ordered to prevent aplastic crisis.
Emphasize importance of avoiding smoking and alcohol consumption; identify appropriate medical assistance and community support groups for smoking cessation.	Nicotine induces peripheral vasoconstriction and decreases oxygen tension, which may contribute to cellular hypoxia and sickling. Alcohol increases the possibility of dehydration, which precipitates sickling. Maintaining these changes in behavior or lifestyle may require prolonged support.
Discuss principles of skin and extremity care and protection from injury. Encourage prompt treatment of cuts, insect bites, sores, and lesions.	Because of impaired tissue perfusion, especially in the periphery, distal extremities are especially susceptible to altered skin integrity and infection.
Include instructions on care of leg ulcers that might develop.	Fosters independence and maintenance of self-care at home.
Instruct client to avoid persons with infections such as upper respiratory infections (URIs).	Altered immune response places client at risk for infections, especially bacterial bronchitis and pneumonia.
Recommend avoiding cold remedies and decongestants containing ephedrine and large amounts of caffeine. Stress the importance of reading labels on over-the-counter (OTC) drugs and consulting healthcare provider before consuming any drugs or herbal supplements.	Those remedies containing vasoconstrictors may decrease peripheral tissue perfusion and cause sludging of sickled cells.
Discuss conditions for which medical attention should be sought, such as the following:	
Urine that appears blood tinged or smoky	Symptoms suggestive of sickling in the renal medulla.
Indigestion, persistent vomiting, diarrhea, high fever, and excessive thirst	Dehydration may trigger a vaso-occlusive crisis.
Severe joint or bone pain	May signify a vaso-occlusive crisis due to sickling in the bones or spleen, leading to ischemia or infarction or onset of osteomyelitis.
Severe chest pain, with or without cough	May reflect acute chest syndrome, with pulmonary infiltrates or pneumonia.
Abdominal pain; gastric distress following meals	Cholelithiasis, primarily with bilirubin stones, is present in more than 50% of adults.
Priapism episode persisting over 4 hours with no resolution	Suggestive of sickling in the penis.
Persistent fever greater than 100°F (38°C); increasing fatigue and pallor; dizziness, drowsiness; and nonhealing leg ulcers	Suggestive of infections that may precipitate a vaso-occlusive crisis if dehydration develops. *Note:* Severe infections are the most frequent cause of aplastic crisis.
Any neurological symptom or sign	Stroke can occur due to cerebral infarction, although it is more common in children than adults. Without long-term transfusion therapy, approximately one-third of clients will experience recurrent strokes.

ACTIONS/INTERVENTIONS (continued)	RATIONALE (continued)
Review and strengthen coping abilities, such as how to deal appropriately with anxiety, getting adequate information, and using relaxation techniques.	Promotes client's sense of control and may avert a crisis.
Recommend wearing a medical alert bracelet or carrying a wallet card.	May prevent inappropriate treatment in emergency situation.
Discuss genetic implications of the condition. Encourage SO and family members to seek testing to determine presence of hemoglobin S.	Screening may identify other family members with sickle cell trait. Hereditary nature of the disease with the possibility of transmitting the mutation may have a bearing on reproductive decisions.
Explore concerns regarding childbearing and family planning. Refer to community resources and obstetrician knowledgeable about sickle cell disease, as indicated.	Provides opportunity to correct misconceptions and present information necessary to make informed decisions. Evidence shows that pregnant client has increased risk of infections (e.g., pneumonia and genitourinary tract infections), gestational hypertension, intrauterine growth retardation, eclampsia, preterm labor, and postpartum infections (Vichinsky, 2012).
Encourage client to have routine follow-ups, such as the following:	
Periodic laboratory studies, such as CBC	Monitors changes in blood components; identifies need for changes in treatment regimen. When using hydroxyurea, frequent monitoring of CBC is required because of narrow margin between acceptable degree of bone marrow suppression and toxicity, including neutropenia, anemia, and thrombocytopenia.
Biannual dental examination	Sound oral hygiene limits opportunity for bacterial invasion and sepsis.
Annual ophthalmological examination	Detects development of sickle retinopathy with either proliferative or nonproliferative ocular changes predisposing to retinal hemorrhage and increased intraocular pressure.
Immunizations	Annual influenza vaccination is recommended for all clients with SCD. Vaccination against *S. pneumoniae* is also an important part of comprehensive care in prevention of pulmonary complications. (P) Current recommendations support the use of both Prevnar and the 23-valent pneumococcal polysaccharide vaccine in children with SCD. Other routine childhood vaccinations that should be given include the *H. influenzae* type b conjugate vaccine and the meningococcal vaccine (American Academy of Pediatrics, 2000 and 2003).
Determine need for vocational and career guidance.	Sedentary career may be necessary because of decreased oxygen-carrying capacity and diminished exercise tolerance.
Encourage participation in community support groups available to clients and SO, such as the Sickle Cell Disease Association of America, March of Dimes, public health nurse, and visiting nurse.	Helpful in adjustment to long-term situation; reduces feelings of isolation and enhances problem-solving through sharing of common experiences. *Note:* Failure to resolve concerns and deal with situation may require more intensive therapy and psychological support.

POTENTIAL CONSIDERATIONS following acute hospitalization (dependent on client's age, physical condition and presence of complications, personal resources, and life responsibilities)

- ***acute/chronic Pain***—physical agent (e.g., intravascular sickling with localized stasis, occlusion, infarction, and necrosis; activation of pain fibers due to deprivation of oxygen and nutrients, accumulation of noxious metabolites)
- ***risk for deficient Fluid Volume***—increased fluid needs (hypermetabolic state or fever, inflammatory processes), active fluid loss (renal parenchymal damage or infarctions limiting the kidney's ability to concentrate urine [hyposthenuria])
- ***risk for Infection***—chronic disease; inadequate primary defenses—broken skin, tissue destruction, stasis of body fluids, decreased ciliary action

ADULT LEUKEMIAS

I. Pathophysiology: Malignant disorder of the blood and bone marrow characterized by the uncontrolled accumulation of white blood cells (WBCs)

a. Blood cells originate primarily in the marrow of bones, such as the sternum, iliac crest, and cranium, and begin as immature cells (blasts or stem cells) that differentiate and mature into red blood cells (RBCs), platelets, and various types of WBCs.

b. Production of normal blood cells markedly decreased, leading to anemia, thrombocytopenia, neutropenia

c. Rapid growth of immature or ineffective WBCs and delayed cell death lead to their accumulation in bone marrow, blood, spleen, and liver.

II. Categories (Hu, 2012; Seiter, 2012; Swierzewski, update 2012; Klepin, 2009)

a. Leukemia is classified by how quickly it progresses. Acute leukemia is fast-growing and can overwhelm the body within weeks or months. Chronic leukemia is slow-growing and progressively worsens over years.

b. Leukemia is also classified according to the type of white blood cell that is multiplying—i.e., lymphocytes (immune system cells), granulocytes (bacteria-destroying cells), or monocytes (macrophage-forming cells).

c. The four types of leukemia that occur most frequently are acute myelogenous leukemia (AML), acute lymphocytic leukemia (ALL), chronic myelogenous leukemia (CML), and chronic lymphocytic leukemia (CLL).

i. Acute

1. Acute essentially refers to a disorder of rapid onset. In the acute myelogenous leukemias, the abnormal cells grow rapidly and do not mature. Most of these immature cells tend to die rapidly. In the acute lymphocytic leukemias, growth is not as rapid as that of the myelocytic cells, but the cells tend to accumulate.
2. These abnormalities result in loss of the body's ability to fight infections and prevent bleeding.
3. Most common form in adults is AML (especially adults over 60, and particularly older males) (Kleppin, 2009). The underlying pathophysiology in AML consists of arrested bone marrow cell maturation. AML is further classified into eight subtypes.
4. Acute leukemias in general progress rapidly without treatment but can be kept in remission in a high percentage of individuals who undergo appropriate therapy. As a group, older clients tend to have worse treatment outcomes than younger ones, i.e., they experience greater treatment-related toxicity, lower remission rates, shorter disease-free survival times, and shorter overall survival times.

ii. Chronic

1. In the chronic leukemias, the onset tends to be slow, and the cells generally mature abnormally and often accumulate in various organs, over long intervals. Their ability to fight infections and assist in repairing injured tissues is impaired.
2. The most common form of chronic leukemia in adults is CLL, which is characterized by abnormal increase in lymphocytes (called B lymphocytes, or B cells). These cells spread through the blood and bone marrow and can also affect the lymph nodes or other organs such as the liver and spleen, resulting in infections, anemia, and easy bleeding. CLL eventually causes the bone marrow to fail.
3. Chronic myelogenous leukemia (CML, and some cases of AML and ALL) has a particular genetic marker (the Philadelphia chromosome [Ph1]) in about 95% of individuals, which causes uncontrolled proliferation of all types of white blood cells and platelets. Another distinctive feature of CML is its invariable conversion, if untreated, to a more rapidly fulminating acute type, leading to rapid death (Swierzewski, 2012; Sherbenou, 2007).
4. CML tends to occur more in middle age and older-age persons.
5. Develops gradually and progresses more slowly than acute forms

III. Etiology

a. Exact cause is unknown.

b. Risk factors (Seiter, 2012)

i. Antecedent histological disorders: diseases of the bone marrow, such as myelodysplastic syndrome (MDS)

ii. Environmental exposures: radiation, benzene (found in some work areas, gasoline-related industries, and cigarette smoke) (Phillips, 2012)

iii. Prior chemotherapy for other malignancies

iv. Genetics or congenital disorders: some congenital disorders that predispose patients to AML include Down syndrome, Fanconi anemia, and neurofibromatosis. These individuals usually develop AML during childhood.

IV. Classification or Staging (National Cancer Institute, 2013; Hu, 2012)

a. In general, leukemias are classified rather than staged in order to determine the most appropriate therapy.

b. All leukemias are classified according to their genotypes, or their unique characteristics.

c. In addition, CML is classified by phase, i.e., chronic phase, accelerated phase, and blast phase (or "blast crisis") and are defined by the number of blasts (immature leukemia cells) in the blood and bone marrow. CLL is classified by two different staging systems, both based on the parts of the body affected by the leukemia.

V. Statistics

a. Morbidity: In 2011, an estimated 44,600 new cases of leukemia (all types) were diagnosed in the United States, more often in males than females. Chronic leukemias account for 7% more cases than acute; most cases occur in older adults, with more than half occurring after age 67 (The Leukemia & Lymphoma Society [LLS] Facts, 2012).

b. Mortality: Approximately 22,100 adult deaths from all leukemias were reported for 2010 (Hoyert & Xu, 2011). A majority (up to 82%) of those with CLL live 5 to 10 years; however, presence of complications may shorten survival to 2 to 3 years. The 5-year survival rate for CML increased from 31% for cases diagnosed during 1990–1992 to 56% for those diagnosed during 2002–2008 (ACS, 2013).

c. Cost: National direct cost for care was $5.44 billion in 2010 (National Cancer Institute [NCI], 2011).

GLOSSARY

Blast cell: Blood cell that is not fully developed and is still immature.

Lymphocytic or lymphoblastic: A cancerous change takes place in a type of marrow cell that forms lymphocytes.

Lymphopenia: Low number of lymphocytes in the blood.

Myelogenous or myeloid: Cancerous change takes place in a type of marrow cell that normally goes on to form red cells, some types of white cells, and platelets.

Neutropenia: Abnormal decrease in the number of neutrophils (type of white blood cell [WBC] that fights infection) in the blood.

Normocytic, normochromic anemia: Anemia associated with disturbances of red cell formation and related to endocrine deficiencies, chronic inflammation, and condition in which cancer is spread widely throughout the body or, in some cases, to a relatively large region of the body.

Progenitor stem cell transplant: Reestablishment of normal bone marrow function through the infusion of cells committed to forming a specific type of blood cell line—red blood cells (RBCs), WBCs, or platelets. The source of the cells may be from the peripheral blood, bone marrow, or umbilical cord and placenta. The donor may be the client himself or herself (autologous transplant), a genetically compatible relative or individual (allogeneic transplant), or donated cord blood. Syngeneic transplant describes the use of an identical twin as donor.

Thrombocytopenia: Disorder in which there are not enough platelets. This condition is sometimes associated with abnormal bleeding.

Tumor lysis syndrome: Metabolic derangement produced by rapid tumor breakdown as a consequence of therapy. It is characterized by hyperuricemia because of DNA breakdown; hyperkalemia because of cytosol breakdown; hyperphosphatemia because of protein breakdown; and hypocalcemia secondary to hyperphosphatemia. As phosphate level goes up, serum calcium goes down. These derangements can result in acute renal failure, cardiac dysrhythmias, and sudden death from hyperkalemia or hypocalcemia.

Care Setting

Client receives acute inpatient care on medical or oncology unit for initial evaluation and treatment, typically for 4 to 6 weeks, and then at the community level.

Related Concerns

Cancer, page 827
Psychosocial aspects of care, page 729
Transplantation considerations—postoperative and lifelong, page 719

Client Assessment Database

Data depend on degree and duration of the disease and other organ involvement.

DIAGNOSTIC DIVISION MAY REPORT	MAY EXHIBIT
ACTIVITY/REST	
• Fatigue, malaise • Weakness, inability to engage in usual activities • Flu-like symptoms	• Muscle wasting • Increased need for sleep, somnolence
CIRCULATION	
• Palpitations	• Tachycardia, heart murmurs • Pallor of skin, mucous membranes • Cranial nerve deficits and signs of cerebral hemorrhage
EGO INTEGRITY	
• Feelings of helplessness, hopelessness	• Depression, withdrawal, anxiety, fear, anger, irritability • Mood changes, confusion
ELIMINATION	
• Diarrhea, perianal tenderness, pain • Bright red blood on tissue paper, tarry stools • Blood in urine, decreased urine output	• Perianal abscess, hematuria
FOOD/FLUID	
• Loss of appetite, anorexia, vomiting • Change in taste	• Abdominal distention, decreased bowel sounds • Splenomegaly, hepatomegaly, jaundice

(continues on page 486)

DIAGNOSTIC DIVISION MAY REPORT (continued)	MAY EXHIBIT (continued)
• Weight loss • Sore throat, difficulty swallowing	• Stomatitis, oral ulcerations • Gum hypertrophy (gum infiltration may be indicative of AML)
NEUROSENSORY • Lack of or decreased coordination • Mood changes, confusion, disorientation, lack of concentration • Dizziness; numbness, tingling, paresthesias	• Muscle irritability • Seizure activity • Uncoordinated movements
PAIN/DISCOMFORT • Abdominal pain • Headaches • Bone, joint pain—knees, hips, shoulders • Sternal tenderness • Muscle cramping	• Guarding or distraction behaviors, restlessness • Self-focus
RESPIRATION • Shortness of breath with minimal exertion	• Dyspnea, tachypnea • Cough • Crackles, rhonchi • Decreased breath sounds
SAFETY • History of recent or recurrent infections • Falls • Visual disturbances or impairment • Nosebleeds or other hemorrhages, spontaneous uncontrollable bleeding with minimal trauma • Swollen gums	• Fever, infections • Bruises, purpura, retinal hemorrhages, gum or nose bleeding • Papilledema and exophthalmos • Leukemic infiltrates in the dermis
SEXUALITY • Changes in libido • Changes in menstrual flow, menorrhagia • Impotence	
TEACHING/LEARNING • History of exposure to chemicals—benzene (commercially used toxic liquid that is also present in lead-free gasoline), excessive levels of ionizing radiation, previous treatment with chemotherapy—especially alkalizing agents • Chromosomal disorder—Down syndrome or Fanconi's aplastic anemia • Exposure to virus—human T-cell leukemia or lymphoma virus-1 (HTLV-1)	
DISCHARGE PLAN CONSIDERATIONS • May need assistance with therapy and treatment needs and supplies, shopping, food preparation, self-care activities, homemaker and maintenance tasks, transportation ➧ Refer to section at end of plan for postdischarge considerations.	

Diagnostic Studies

TEST WHY IT IS DONE	WHAT IT TELLS ME
BLOOD TESTS	*Note:* Once a diagnosis of leukemia is obtained, additional tests may be performed. These tests may include (and are not limited to) immunophenotyping, fluorescence in situ hybridization [FISH], IgVH gene mutation test). These more sophisticated tests are not included in this text (National Cancer Institute, 2013).
• ***Complete blood count (CBC):*** The most common screening and diagnostic test to demonstrate leukemia. Typically includes hemoglobin (Hgb); hematocrit (Hct); RBC count, morphology, indices, and distribution width index; platelet count and size; and WBC count and differential.	There may be decreased or elevated WBCs, and in acute leukemia, systemic blasts may be present. The bloodstream normally carries less than 5% blasts, but in acute, newly diagnosed, or recurrent leukemia, the blast percentage may be as high as 50% of the total WBCs (Foster, 2012). RBC production can be decreased by the leukemic cells and suppression of normal bone marrow activity. Client may have mild to severe normocytic, normochromic anemia associated with hypersplenism.
• ***White blood cells (WBC) count and differential:*** Evaluates numbers and characteristics of each of the five types of WBCs: neutrophils, lymphocytes (B cells and T cells), monocytes, eosinophils, and basophils within the bloodstream.	Persons with ALL or AML often have too many leukocytes—count may be more than 50,000/cm—with increased numbers of immature WBCs ("shift to left"). Leukemic blast cells may be present.
• ***Platelet count:*** Platelets have essential function in coagulation.	May vary from normal to very low, less than 50,000/mm.
• ***Prothrombin time (PT)/activated partial thromboplastin time (aPTT):*** Determines bleeding and clotting time.	May be prolonged. Disseminated intravascular coagulation (DIC) may occur with AML, but it is especially common in acute promyelocytic leukemia.
• ***Blood chemistries:*** Measures the type and amount of enzymes, minerals, and other substances within the blood.	Identifies kidney or liver damage that may be caused by leukemic cell breakdown or by drugs used for chemotherapy.
• ***Alkaline phosphatase (ALP):*** Aids in differential diagnosis.	Elevated with CML.
• ***Lactic dehydrogenase (LDH):*** Substance released by tumors and found in blood.	It is considered an accurate marker for the severity of the disease and used to establish a baseline to monitor for response to treatment.
• ***Serum vitamin B_{12}:*** May aid in differential diagnosis of type of leukemia and other myeloproliferative conditions.	Can be increased with CML and some forms of acute leukemia; normal in CLL and undifferentiated stem cell leukemia.
• ***Uric acid:*** Waste product resulting from the breakdown of nitrogen-containing compounds (purines).	Commonly elevated in client with ALL or as a result of chemotherapy (tumor lysis syndrome).
OTHER DIAGNOSTIC STUDIES	
• ***Computed tomography (CT) scan:*** Computer-assisted x-ray that produces cross-sectional images of the body.	CT scans are not usually used in client with leukemia unless metastasis is suspected. In such cases, CT scan may detect changes in the lymph nodes around the heart, trachea, or abdomen. Lymph node enlargement is more common in patients with ALL or CLL with potential for compression of organs or internal structures, such as airway obstruction or obstructive uropathy. Scans of liver and spleen may reveal splenomegaly (National Cancer Institute, 2013).
• ***X-rays:*** Determine areas of involvement.	May reveal enlarged lymph nodes in the chest, a localized mass in the lungs, or evidence that leukemia has spread to bones or joints.
• ***Bone marrow aspiration and biopsy:*** May be done by needle aspirate or biopsy for microscopic examination of fluid and tissues within the marrow to determine the number, size, and shape of the various cell types as well as the proportion of mature to immature cells.	Although signs of leukemia are evident in CBC results and platelet counts, a bone marrow biopsy is necessary for a definitive diagnosis. The bone marrow examination determines the cell type, the type of erythropoiesis, and the maturity of the leukopoietic and erythropoietic cell. Abnormal WBCs usually make up 50% or more of the WBCs in the bone marrow. Often 60% to 90% of the cells are blast cells, with erythroid precursors, mature cells, and megakaryocytes reduced.

(continues on page 488)

Diagnostic Studies (continued)

TEST WHY IT IS DONE (continued)	WHAT IT TELLS ME (continued)
DEFINITIVE DIAGNOSTIC STUDIES	
• *Cytogenetic analysis:* Cells are studied to see if chromosomal abnormalities are present.	Examination of chromosome abnormalities from samples of peripheral blood, bone marrow, or lymph nodes can indicate prognostic features and direct treatment options.
• *Immunocytochemistry:* Uses antibodies to treat the bone marrow or biopsy samples; specific cells undergo a color change that can be identified under microscope.	Allows pathologist to identify specific types of leukemia.
• *Lumbar puncture:* Determines if cancer has spread to spinal column or brain.	May reveal leukemic cells in cerebrospinal fluid (CSF).

Nursing Priorities

1. Prevent infection during acute phases of disease and treatment.
2. Maintain circulating blood volume.
3. Alleviate pain.
4. Promote optimal physical functioning.
5. Provide psychological support.
6. Provide information about disease process, prognosis, and treatment needs.

Discharge Goals

1. Complications prevented or minimized.
2. Pain relieved or controlled.
3. Activities of daily living (ADLs) met by self or with assistance.
4. Dealing with disease realistically.
5. Disease process, prognosis, and therapeutic regimen understood.
6. Plan in place to meet needs after discharge.

Refer to CP: Cancer for further discussion and expansion of interventions related to cancer care and for client teaching.

NURSING DIAGNOSIS: risk for Infection

Risk Factors May Include

Inadequate secondary defenses—immature WBCs with low granulocyte and abnormal/ immature lymphocyte count; immunosuppression, bone marrow suppression; pharmaceutical agents
Inadequate primary defenses—stasis of body fluids, traumatized tissue, invasive procedures
Malnutrition; chronic disease

Possibly Evidenced By

(Not applicable; presence of signs and symptoms establishes an *actual* diagnosis)

Desired Outcomes/Evaluation Criteria—Client Will

Risk Control: Infectious Process (NOC)
Identify actions to prevent or reduce risk of infection.
Demonstrate techniques or lifestyle changes to promote safe environment and achieve timely healing.

ACTIONS/INTERVENTIONS	RATIONALE
Infection Protection (NIC)	
Independent	
Place in private room. Screen and limit visitors, as indicated. Prohibit use of live plants or cut flowers. Restrict fresh fruits and vegetables or make sure they are washed or peeled.	Protect client from potential sources of pathogens and infection. *Note:* Profound bone marrow suppression, neutropenia, and chemotherapy place client at great risk for infection.
Model and require good hand-washing protocol for all personnel and visitors.	Prevents cross-contamination and reduces risk of infection.
Monitor temperature. Note correlation between temperature elevations and chemotherapy treatments. Observe for fever associated with tachycardia, hypotension, and subtle mental changes.	Although fever may accompany some forms of chemotherapy, progressive hyperthermia occurs in some types of infections, and fever unrelated to drugs or blood products occurs in most leukemia clients. *Note:* Septicemia may occur without fever.

ACTIONS/INTERVENTIONS (continued)	RATIONALE (continued)
Prevent chilling. Force fluids and administer tepid sponge bath.	Helps reduce fever, which contributes to fluid imbalance, discomfort, and central nervous system (CNS) complications.
Encourage frequent turning and deep breathing.	Prevents stasis of respiratory secretions, reducing risk of atelectasis and pneumonia.
Auscultate breath sounds, noting crackles and rhonchi; inspect secretions for changes in characteristics, such as increased sputum production or change in sputum color. Observe urine for signs of infection: cloudy, foul-smelling, or presence of urgency or burning with voids.	Early intervention is essential to prevent sepsis or septicemia in immunosuppressed person.
Handle client gently. Keep linens dry and wrinkle-free.	Prevents sheet burns and skin excoriation.
Inspect skin for tender, erythematous areas and open wounds. Cleanse skin with antibacterial solutions.	May indicate local infection. *Note:* Open wounds may not produce pus because of insufficient number of granulocytes.
Inspect oral mucous membranes. Provide good oral hygiene. Use a soft toothbrush, sponge, or swabs for frequent mouth care.	The oral cavity is an excellent medium for growth of organisms and is susceptible to ulceration and bleeding.
Promote good perianal hygiene. Examine perianal area at least daily during acute illness. Provide sitz baths, using Betadine or Hibiclens, if indicated. Avoid rectal temperatures and use of suppositories.	Promotes cleanliness, reducing risk of perianal abscess; enhances circulation and healing. *Note:* Perianal abscess can contribute to septicemia and death in immunosuppressed clients.
Coordinate procedures and tests to allow for uninterrupted rest periods.	Conserves energy for healing and cellular regeneration.
Encourage increased intake of fluids and foods high in protein with adequate fiber.	Promotes healing and prevents dehydration. *Note:* Constipation potentiates retention of toxins and risk of rectal irritation and tissue injury.
Prepare for/assist with invasive procedures, such as venipuncture, insertion of semi-permanent central lines or ports, maintaining sterile technique for insertions and site care per protocol.	Break in skin could provide an entry for pathogenic and potentially lethal organisms. Use of central venous lines, such as tunneled catheter or implanted port, can effectively reduce need for frequent invasive procedures and risk of infection. *Note:* Myelosuppression may be cumulative in nature, especially when multiple drug therapy, including steroids, is prescribed.
Collaborative	
Monitor laboratory studies, such as the following:	
CBC, noting whether WBC count falls or sudden changes occur in neutrophils	Decreased numbers of normal or mature WBCs can result from the disease process or chemotherapy, compromising the immune response and increasing risk of infection.
Gram's stain cultures and sensitivity	Verifies presence of infections; identifies specific organisms and appropriate therapy.
Review serial chest x-rays.	Indicator of development or resolution of respiratory complications.
Prepare for and assist with leukemia-specific treatments, such as chemotherapy with neoplastic agents; biological therapy (immune modulators [such as interferons] and gene-directed agents [such as imatinib]); radiation, bone marrow and stem cell transplantation.	Leukemia treatment falls into two categories: (1) treatment to fight the cancer and (2) treatment to relieve symptoms of the disease and the side effects of therapy (supportive care). A variety of treatment options are available, depending on the type and staging of the client's disease. The most widely used antileukemic treatment is chemotherapy (of which there are many different drugs), typically given in cycles, sometimes referred to as induction, consolidation, and maintenance (Hu, 2012; Seiter, 2012; Druker et al, 2006).
Administer medications, as indicated, for example:	
Anti-infectives, such as ofloxacin (Ocuflox) and rifampin (Rifadin)	May be given prophylactically or to treat specific infection, especially in febrile client who has prolonged granulocytopenia or too few mature neutrophils (Seiter, 2012).
Colony-stimulating factors (CSFs), such as sargramostim (Leukine), filgrastim (Neupogen), and pegfilgrastim (Neulasta)	Restores WBCs destroyed by chemotherapy and reduces risk of severe infection and death in certain types of leukemia.
Avoid use of aspirin-containing antipyretics.	Aspirin can cause gastric bleeding and further decrease platelet count.
Provide nutritious diet, high in protein and calories, avoiding raw fruits, vegetables, or uncooked meats.	Proper nutrition enhances immune system. Minimizes potential sources of bacterial contamination (Seiter, 2012).

NURSING DIAGNOSIS: risk for deficient Fluid Volume

Risk Factors May Include

Excessive losses—vomiting, hemorrhage, diarrhea
Deviations affecting intake—nausea, anorexia
Factors influencing fluid needs—hypermetabolic state, fever, predisposition for kidney stone formation and tumor lysis syndrome

Possibly Evidenced By

(Not applicable; presence of signs and symptoms establishes an *actual* diagnosis)

Desired Outcomes/Evaluation Criteria—Client Will

Hydration (NOC)

Demonstrate adequate fluid volume, as evidenced by stable vital signs; palpable pulses; urine output, specific gravity, and pH within normal limits.

Risk Control (NOC)

Identify individual risk factors and appropriate interventions.
Initiate behaviors or lifestyle changes to prevent development of dehydration.

ACTIONS/INTERVENTIONS	RATIONALE
Fluid Management (NIC)	
Independent	
Monitor intake and output (I&O). Calculate insensible losses and fluid balance. Note decreased urine output in presence of adequate intake. Measure urine specific gravity and pH.	Tumor lysis syndrome occurs when destroyed cancer cells release toxic levels of potassium, phosphorus, and uric acid. Elevated phosphorus and uric acid levels can cause crystal formation in the renal tubules, impairing filtration and leading to renal failure.
Weigh daily.	Measure of adequacy of fluid replacement and kidney function. Continued intake greater than output may indicate renal insult or obstruction.
Monitor blood pressure (BP) and heart rate.	Changes may reflect effects of hypovolemia associated with bleeding or dehydration.
Evaluate skin turgor, capillary refill, and general condition of mucous membranes.	Indirect indicators of fluid status.
Note presence of nausea or fever.	Affects intake, fluid needs, and route of replacement.
Encourage liberal fluids when oral intake is resumed.	Promotes urine flow, prevents uric acid precipitation, and enhances clearance of antineoplastic drugs.
Bleeding Precautions (NIC)	
Inspect skin and mucous membranes for petechiae and ecchymotic areas; note bleeding gums, frank or occult blood in stools and urine, and oozing from invasive line sites.	Suppression of bone marrow and platelet production places client at risk for spontaneous or uncontrolled bleeding.
Implement measures to prevent tissue injury and bleeding: gentle brushing of teeth or gums with soft toothbrush, cotton swab, or sponge-tipped applicator; using electric razor instead of sharp razors when shaving; avoiding forceful nose blowing and needlesticks when possible; and using sustained pressure such as sandbags or pressure dressings on oozing puncture or intravenous (IV) sites.	Fragile tissues and altered clotting mechanisms increase the risk of hemorrhage following even minor trauma.
Limit oral care to mouth rinse, if indicated, such as a mixture of 1/4 tsp baking soda and 1/8 tsp salt in 8 oz water, or may use hydrogen peroxide in water or saline for bleeding or infected oral tissue. Avoid mouthwashes with alcohol.	When bleeding is present, even gentle brushing may cause more tissue damage. Alcohol has a drying effect and may be painful to irritated tissues.
Provide soft foods.	May help reduce risk of gum bleeding.
Fluid Management (NIC)	
Collaborative	
Administer IV and electrolyte solutions, as indicated.	Maintains fluid and electrolyte balance in the absence of oral intake. Prevents or minimizes tumor lysis syndrome and reduces risk of renal complications.
Administer medications, as indicated, for example:	
Antiemetics: such as ondansetron (Zofran) or granisetron (Kytril), aprepitant (Emend), dronabinol (Marinol)	Chemotherapy-induced nausea and vomiting (CINV) is one of the most feared side effects of chemotherapy. With the correct use of antiemetics, CINV can be prevented in almost 70% to up to 80% of patients (Jordan, 2007). Relieving nausea and vomiting can reduce fluid deficits and enhance oral intake.

ACTIONS/INTERVENTIONS (continued)	RATIONALE (continued)
rasburicase (Elitek)	Treats hyperuricemia. Improves renal excretion of toxic by-products from tumor lysis. Reduces the chances of nephropathy as a result of uric acid production (Held-Warmkessel, 2010).
Bleeding Precautions (NIC)	
Monitor laboratory studies: platelets, Hgb/Hct, and clotting.	When the platelet count is less than 20,000/mm because of proliferation of WBCs or bone marrow suppression, client is prone to spontaneous life-threatening bleeding. Decreasing Hgb/Hct is indicative of occult bleeding.
Assist with insertion/maintain central vascular access device, such as subclavian or tunneled catheter or implanted port, as indicated.	Eliminates peripheral venipuncture as source of bleeding.
Administer packed RBCs, platelets, and clotting factors.	Restores more normal RBC count and oxygen-carrying capacity to correct anemia. Platelets or fresh frozen plasma (FFP) may be used to prevent or treat hemorrhage (Seiter, 2012).

NURSING DIAGNOSIS: acute Pain

May Be Related To
Physical agents—enlarged organs and lymph nodes, bone marrow packed with leukemic cells
Chemical agents—antileukemic treatments
Psychological—anxiety, fear

Possibly Evidenced By
Verbalized/coded reports of pain
Guarding behaviors
Expressive behaviors—facial grimacing, restlessness
Changes in vital signs

Desired Outcomes/Evaluation Criteria—Client Will

Pain Level (NOC)
Report pain is relieved or controlled.
Appear relaxed and able to sleep and rest appropriately.

Pain Control (NOC)
Demonstrate behaviors to manage pain.

ACTIONS/INTERVENTIONS	RATIONALE
Pain Management (NIC)	
Independent	
Investigate reports of pain. Note changes in intensity (using 0 to 10 [or similar] scale) and location of pain.	Helpful in understanding client's situation and intervention needs and monitoring potential of developing complications.
Monitor vital signs, noting changes in blood pressure, heart rate, and breathing pattern. Note nonverbal cues, such as facial mask of pain, grimacing, crying, withdrawal, muscle tension, and restlessness.	Indicators of acute pain that can corroborate verbal reports or may be only indicators in client unable or unwilling to verbalize pain. Client with long-term condition may have acute pain superimposed on chronic pain issues and be reluctant to report new symptoms. Older client may or may not report pain, but may have more pain behaviors.
Determine client's acceptable level of pain and help client achieve pain control.	Pain is a subjective experience and needs to be fully addressed by care providers to promote the best-possible quality of life. Client may report having a level of discomfort that is manageable (e.g., can do desired activities when pain is reduced from a 10 to a 3). Another client may need to be pain-free in order to function.
Provide quiet environment and reduce stressful stimuli: noise, lighting, and constant interruptions.	Promotes rest and enhances coping abilities.
Place in position of comfort, and support joints and extremities with pillows and other padding.	May decrease associated bone and joint discomfort.
Reposition periodically and provide or assist with gentle range-of-motion (ROM) exercises.	Improves tissue circulation and joint mobility.

(continues on page 492)

ACTIONS/INTERVENTIONS (continued)	RATIONALE (continued)
Provide comfort measures, such as massage, cool packs, and psychological support, including encouragement and presence, as appropriate.	Enhances effects of medication.
Review and promote client's own comfort interventions—position and physical activity or nonactivity.	Successful management of pain requires client involvement. Use of effective techniques provides positive reinforcement, promotes sense of control, and prepares client for interventions to be used after discharge.
Evaluate and support client's coping mechanisms.	Using own learned perceptions and behaviors to manage pain can help client cope more effectively.
Encourage use of stress management techniques, such as deep-breathing exercises, guided imagery, visualization, and therapeutic touch.	Facilitates relaxation, augments pharmacological therapy, and enhances coping abilities.
Assist with or provide diversional activities and relaxation techniques.	Helps with pain management by redirecting attention.
Collaborative	
Monitor uric acid level as appropriate.	Rapid turnover and destruction of leukemic cells during chemotherapy can elevate uric acid, causing swollen painful joints in some clients. *Note:* Massive infiltration of WBCs into joints can also result in intense pain.
Administer medications, as indicated, for example:	
Analgesics, such as acetaminophen (Tylenol)	Given for mild pain not relieved by comfort measures. *Note:* Avoid aspirin-containing products because they may potentiate hemorrhage.
Opioids, such as codeine, morphine, and hydromorphone (Dilaudid)	Routinely scheduled medication administration or patient-controlled analgesia (PCA) is beneficial in preventing peaks and valleys associated with intermittent drug administration and increases client's sense of control.
Anti-anxiety agents, such as diazepam (Valium) and lorazepam (Ativan)	May be given to enhance the action of analgesics and opioids.

NURSING DIAGNOSIS: Fatigue

May Be Related To
Disease state; malnutrition; anemia
Stress; anxiety; negative life events
Altered body chemistry (e.g., medications, chemotherapy)

Possibly Evidenced By
Reports an overwhelming lack of energy; inability to maintain usual routines
Lethargic; listless
Decreased performance
Compromised concentration

Desired Outcomes/Evaluation Criteria—Client Will

Fatigue Level (NOC)
Report a measurable increase in activity tolerance.
Participate in ADLs to level of ability.
Demonstrate a decrease in physiological signs of intolerance—pulse, respiration, and BP remain within client's normal range.

ACTIONS/INTERVENTIONS	RATIONALE
Energy Management (NIC)	
Independent	
Evaluate reports of fatigue, noting inability to participate in desired activities or ADLs.	Effects of leukemia, anemia, tumor-induced hypermetabolic state, pain, depression, and malnutrition associated with chemotherapy can be cumulative, especially during acute and active treatment phase. *Note:* Cancer-related fatigue (CRF) is one of the most common side effects of cancer and its treatments. Usually, it comes on suddenly, does not result from activity or exertion, and is not relieved by rest or sleep (National Cancer Institute, 2013).
Encourage client to keep a diary of daily routines and energy levels for 1 week, noting activities that increase fatigue.	Helps client prioritize activities and arrange them around fatigue pattern.

ACTIONS/INTERVENTIONS (continued)	RATIONALE (continued)
Provide quiet environment and uninterrupted rest periods. Encourage rest periods before meals.	Restores energy needed for activity and cellular regeneration and tissue healing.
Implement energy-saving techniques, such as sitting rather than standing, or alternate; use shower chair, and furniture with good support; combine activities, reducing number of individual actions, reduce sudden or prolonged strains, etc. Assist with ambulation or other activities, as indicated.	Maximizes available energy for self-care tasks.
Recommend small, nutritious, high-protein meals and snacks throughout the day.	Smaller meals require less energy for digestion than larger meals. Increased intake provides fuel for energy. (Refer to CP: Cancer; ND: imbalanced Nutrition: less than body requirements.)
Collaborative	
Assist in management of underlying condition and alter treatment regimen as indicated.	Sometimes treating symptoms associated with the leukemia (e.g., anemia) will relieve the fatigue. But other interventions may be needed over time, such as discontinuation of certain anticancer drugs, titration of pain medications, nutritional interventions including iron-rich foods, supplemental iron or vitamins, and/or antidepressants or psychostimulants (National Cancer Institute, 2013).
Provide supplemental oxygen.	Maximizes oxygen available for cellular uptake, improving tolerance of activity.
Administer blood and blood components, as indicated.	Correcting anemia improves client's stamina and tolerance for activity.

NURSING DIAGNOSIS: deficient Knowledge [Learning Need] regarding disease, prognosis, treatment, self-care, and discharge needs

May Be Related To
Lack of exposure to resources
Information misinterpretation, lack of recall

Possibly Evidenced By
Reports the problem
Inaccurate follow-through of instructions

Desired Outcomes/Evaluation Criteria—Client Will
Knowledge: Acute Illness Care/Knowledge: Chronic Disease Management (NOC)
Verbalize understanding of condition, disease process, and potential complications.
Verbalize understanding of therapeutic needs.
Initiate necessary lifestyle changes.
Participate in treatment regimen.

ACTIONS/INTERVENTIONS	RATIONALE
Teaching: Disease Process (NIC)	
Independent	
Review client's specific form of leukemia and various treatment options:	Treatments can include various individual and combinations of therapies.
Chemotherapy, using a combination of drugs, such as daunorubicin (Cerubidine), cytarabine (Ara-C), idarubicin (Idamycin), and imatinib (Gleevec)	Kills leukemic cells.
Monoclonal antibodies and interferon (INF-α)	Biological therapy slows the reproduction of leukemic cells and promotes the immune system's antileukemic activity.
Radiation therapy	Kills cancer cells by exposure to high-energy radiation.
Stem cell transplantation (SCT), including peripheral stem cell transplant or umbilical cord blood transplant	After chemotherapy and/or radiation, the injured bone marrow is replenished by a transplant of stem cells, which can manufacture the necessary new blood cells.
Surgery	Surgery may be performed to remove an enlarged spleen or to install a venous access device to give medications and withdraw blood samples (Swierzewski, 2007).

(continues on page 494)

ACTIONS/INTERVENTIONS (continued)	RATIONALE (continued)
Discuss side effects of treatment, as indicated, and possible solutions.	Client may want opportunity to prepare for certain side effects, such as temporary hair loss. Client and significant other (SO) may benefit from knowledge that certain discomforts, such as nausea, vomiting, weakness, mouth sores, bruising, and anorexia, are treatment related, not indications of escalating disease, and will subside.
Inform client and SO of potential sexual side effects of treatment and provide opportunity to consider options. Discuss sperm banking and pregnancy issues, when appropriate, before beginning treatment.	In males, permanent sterility can occur as a result of radiation when combined with certain chemotherapeutic agents. In females, menstruation may cease during the active phase of treatment, with older women subsequently experiencing menopause. Pregnancy should be avoided during treatment and for 2 to 3 years after treatment as that is when recurrence is most common. Vaginal dryness can be a distressing side effect as well (Katz, 2007; Visovsky, 2006).

For additional interventions refer to CP: Cancer; ND: deficient Knowledge.

POTENTIAL CONSIDERATIONS following acute hospitalization (dependent on client's age, physical condition and presence of complications, personal resources, and life responsibilities)

- ***risk for Infection***—inadequate secondary defenses: alterations in mature WBCs (low granulocyte and abnormal lymphocyte count), increased number of immature lymphocytes, immunosuppression, bone marrow suppression (effects of therapy/transplant)
- ***ineffective Role Performance***—situational crisis, physical illness, fatigue, stress
- ***ineffective Self-Health Management***—complexity of therapeutic regimen, decisional conflicts, economic difficulties, excessive demands made on individual or family, perceived benefits, powerlessness
- ***interrupted Family Processes***—situational crisis (illness, disabling and expensive treatments); shift in health status of a family member, shift in family roles

LYMPHOMAS

I. Pathophysiology

a. Malignant growth involving reticuloendothelial and lymphoid system, resulting in accumulation of abnormal lymphocytes in lymph tissue forming masses; may travel to distant sites, including the lungs, liver, gastrointestinal (GI) tract, meninges, skin, and bones

b. Major sites of lymphoid tissue are lymph nodes, spleen, thymus gland, adenoids and tonsils, and digestive tract. Lymphoma is the second most common primary malignancy occurring in the head and neck (Dunleavy, 2012).

II. Classification (Leukemia and Lymphoma Society [LSS], 2013; Lymphoma Research Foundation, 2012; Dunleavy, 2012)

a. Lymphomas are divided into two major categories: Hodgkin lymphoma (HL) formerly called Hodgkin's disease, and non-Hodgkin lymphoma (NHL).

b. Staging (I–IV) provides a general idea of how far the disease has spread and how it should be treated. This is done after testing determines which parts of the body are affected. Letters of the alphabet are also used with the stage to describe the lymphoma. The most important ones are A and B. For example, if the client complains of fever, weight loss, or excessive night sweats (called "B" symptoms), a "B" is added to the stage description. If none of these symptoms exist, an "A" is added. If any organ that does not belong to the lymph system is involved, it is denoted with an "E" (extralymphatic organ involvement) after the stage. If the spleen is involved, the corresponding letter is "S."

i. Hodgkin lymphoma (Lymphoma Research Foundation, 2012)

1. Divided into two main classifications: classical HL (CHL, which accounts for most cases of HL) and nodular lymphocyte predominant HL.
2. A characteristic that distinguishes CHL is presence of a large malignant cell called the Reed-Sternberg (R-S) cell. This characteristic does not appear in nodular lymphocyte predominate HL.
3. Over 80% of individuals with HL are cured. Most treatments include some form of chemotherapy, and sometimes radiation therapy, as their first treatment.

ii. Non-Hodgkin lymphoma (LSS, 2013; Lymphoma Research Foundation, 2012)

1. Most common cancer of the lymphatic system
2. Incidence of NHL is consistently higher than HL, with NHL the seventh most common cancer in the United States.
3. Divided into two broad categories: B-cell or T-cell lymphomas. B-cell lymphomas develop from abnormal B cells and account for 85% of all NHLs. T-cell lymphomas develop from abnormal T cells and account for the remaining 15% of all NHLs.
4. NHLs may also be classified as indolent (slow-growing) or aggressive (fast-growing).
5. NHL treatments include chemotherapy, radiation, newer versions of established agents, novel targeted therapies, and stem cell transplantation.

III. Etiology

a. Exact causes are unknown.

b. Several factors have been linked to an increased risk.

   i. Age: Risk of NHL generally increases with advancing age, with the most dramatic increases being in age group 80–84 (LSS, 2013); HL in the older population is associated with a poorer prognosis than in younger clients.

   ii. Infection: HIV; human T-lymphocytic virus type 1 (HTLV-1); Epstein-Barr virus (EBV), one of the etiological factors in mononucleosis; *Helicobacter pylori*; hepatitis B or C virus

   iii. Medical conditions that compromise the immune system: HIV; autoimmune diseases; conditions requiring immunosuppressive therapy, such as following organ transplant; inherited immunodeficiency diseases; or treatment with phenytoin

   iv. Exposure to toxic chemicals: occupational exposure to pesticides, herbicides, or benzene and other solvents; woodworking

IV. Statistics (LSS, 2012)

a. Morbidity: In 2011, 75,190 people were diagnosed with lymphoma in the United States. The 5-year survival rate is 77% to 86.3% for HL and 69.5% for NHL.

b. Mortality: In 2011, there were an estimated 20,620 deaths from lymphoma with 1300 from HL and 19,320 from NHL. Mortality rate increases with age (Dunleavy et al, 2007).

c. Cost: In 2010, the national direct costs for care were $12.44 billion (National Cancer Institute [NCI], 2011).

GLOSSARY

ABVD therapy: Chemotherapy combination of Adriamycin, bleomycin, vinblastine, and decarbazine (DTIC-Dome) commonly used to treat HL.

Aggressive lymphoma: The National Cancer Institute (NCI) designation for high-grade and some intermediate-grade lymphomas. Aggressive lymphomas grow more quickly than indolent lymphomas but do respond well to chemotherapy.

Bone marrow transplant (BMT): Bone marrow is taken from a compatible donor or the client's own body, prior to high-dose chemotherapy and/or radiation treatment. After treatment, the marrow, which may or may not have been treated with chemotherapy, is reinfused into the patient to restore the immune system.

Hilar lymphadenopathy: Enlargement of the tracheobronchial and pulmonary lymph nodes.

Lymphopenia: Low number of lymphocytes in the blood.

Neuralgia: Pain in the distribution of a nerve or nerve pathway.

Normocytic, normochromic anemia: Anemia associated with disturbances of red blood cell (RBC) formation, which is related to endocrine deficiencies, chronic inflammation, and condition in which cancer is spread widely throughout the body or, in some cases, to a relatively large region of the body.

Pel-Ebstein fever: Fever pattern common in HL, in which temperature varies during each 24-hour period but never reaches normal.

Peripheral blood cell transplantation: The most common form of stem cell transplant with the source of stem cells being the circulating blood, rather than the bone marrow. Client with NHL can have either an autologous or an allogeneic peripheral blood cell transplant, depending on whether or not his or her own stem cells are suitable for use and whether a suitable donor can be found.

Stanford V: Chemotherapy combination of Mechlorethamine, Doxorubicin, Vinblastine, Vincristine, Bleomycin, Etoposide, and Prednisone may be used to treat HL.

Stem cell transplant: Reestablishment of normal bone marrow function through the infusion of cells committed to forming a specific type of blood cell line—RBCs, white blood cells (WBCs), or platelets. The source of the cells may be from the peripheral blood, bone marrow, or umbilical cord and placenta. The donor may be the client (autologous transplant), a genetically compatible relative or individual (allogeneic transplant), or donated cord blood. Syngeneic transplant describes the use of an identical twin as donor.

Superior vena cava syndrome: Obstruction of venous drainage from enlarged lymph nodes.

Tumor burden (also called tumor load): Refers to the number of cancer cells, the size of a tumor, or the amount of cancer in the body. Treatment has a better chance of working when a patient's tumor burden is low.

Tumor lysis syndrome: Metabolic derangement produced by rapid tumor breakdown as a consequence of therapy for some lymphomas (e.g., Burkitt lymphoma, lymphoblastic lymphoma, or B-cell acute lymphoblastic leukemia). It is characterized by hyperuricemia because of DNA breakdown; hyperkalemia because of cytosol breakdown; hyperphosphatemia because of protein breakdown; and hypocalcemia secondary to hyperphosphatemia. As phosphate level goes up, serum calcium goes down. These derangements can result in acute renal failure, cardiac dysrhythmias, and sudden death from hyperkalemia or hypocalcemia.

Care Setting

The client receives acute inpatient care on a medical unit for initial evaluation and treatment and then at the community level. This plan of care addresses potential complications that may be encountered in acute care or hospice settings.

Related Concerns

Adult leukemias, page 484
Anemias—iron deficiency, anemia of chronic disease, pernicious, aplastic, hemolytic, page 459
Cancer, page 827
Psychosocial aspects of care, page 729
Sepsis/septicemia, page 665
Transplantation considerations—postoperative and lifelong, page 719
Upper gastrointestinal/esophageal bleeding, page 281

Client Assessment Database

DIAGNOSTIC DIVISION MAY REPORT	MAY EXHIBIT
ACTIVITY/REST	
• Fatigue • Weakness or general malaise • Loss of productivity and decreased exercise tolerance	• Diminished strength, slumping of the shoulders, slow walk, and other cues indicative of fatigue
CIRCULATION	
• Palpitations, chest pain	• Tachycardia, dysrhythmias • Painless swelling of the lymph nodes, beginning in the neck and progressing to axillary, inguinal, mediastinal, and mesenteric regions • Cyanosis and edema of the face and neck or arms due to superior vena cava syndrome, a rare occurrence, but more common in lymphomas with large mediastinal mass • Pallor • Diaphoresis, night sweats
EGO INTEGRITY	
• Increased stress from school, job, family • Fear related to diagnosis and possibility of dying • Concerns about diagnostic testing and treatment modalities—chemotherapy, radiation therapy, surgery • Financial concerns—hospital costs, treatment expenses, fear of losing job-related benefits because of lost time from work • Relationship status—fear and anxiety related to being a burden on family and significant other (SO)	• Varied behaviors—angry, withdrawn, passive
ELIMINATION	
• Changes in characteristics of urine or stool • History of intestinal obstruction, such as intussusception or malabsorption syndrome (infiltration from retroperitoneal lymph nodes)	• Abdomen: Right upper quadrant (RUQ) tenderness and enlargement on palpation (hepatomegaly); left upper quadrant (LUQ) tenderness and enlargement on palpation (splenomegaly) • Decreased output, dark and concentrated urine, anuria • Bowel and bladder dysfunction (spinal cord compression occurs late)
FOOD/FLUID	
• Anorexia • Dysphagia (pressure on the esophagus) • Recent unexplained weight loss • Night sweats • Severe nausea and vomiting, often treatment related	• Ascites and edema of the lower extremities (inferior vena cava obstruction from intra-abdominal lymph node enlargement associated with NHL)
NEUROSENSORY	
• Nerve pain reflecting compression of nerve roots by enlarged lymph nodes in the brachial, lumbar, and sacral plexuses • Muscle weakness, paresthesia	• Lethargy, withdrawal, general lack of interest in surroundings

DIAGNOSTIC DIVISION MAY REPORT (continued)	MAY EXHIBIT (continued)
PAIN/DISCOMFORT	
• Tenderness or pain over involved lymph nodes—in or around the mediastinum (chest) • Stiff neck; generalized bone pain (bone involvement) • Abdominal pain	• Self-focusing; guarding behaviors
RESPIRATION	
• Dyspnea on exertion or at rest, chest pain	• Dyspnea, tachypnea • Dry, nonproductive cough (hilar lymphadenopathy) • Hoarseness, laryngeal paralysis (pressure from enlarged nodes on the laryngeal nerve)
SAFETY	
• History of frequent or recurrent infections (abnormalities in cellular immunity predispose client to systemic herpes virus infections, tuberculosis [TB], toxoplasmosis, or bacterial infections); history of infectious mononucleosis (higher risk of HL in client with high titers of EBV) • HIV—risk of NHL is 60 to 100 times higher in these clients compared with the general population (LSS, 2012) • Administration of immunosuppressive drugs after organ transplantation • History or presence of ulcers, *H. pylori* • Waxing and waning pattern of lymph node size • Cyclical pattern of evening temperature elevations lasting a few days to weeks (Pel-Ebstein fever) followed by alternate afebrile periods; drenching night sweats without chills • Itchy skin	• Unexplained, intermittent persistent fever without symptoms of infection • Tonsillar or other lymph node enlargement • Generalized pruritus and urticaria (HL) • Scleral icterus and a generalized jaundice related to liver damage and consequent obstruction of bile ducts by enlarged lymph nodes (may be a late sign) • Patchy areas of loss of melanin pigmentation (vitiligo)
SEXUALITY	
• Concern about sterility, fertility, and pregnancy (although disease does not affect either, treatment does) • Decreased libido	
TEACHING/LEARNING	
• Familial risk factors—higher incidence among families of HL than in general population • Occupational exposure to pesticides and herbicides or other chemicals—benzene, creosote, lead, formaldehyde, paint thinner	
DISCHARGE PLAN CONSIDERATIONS	
• May need assistance with medical therapies and supplies, self-care activities, and homemaker or home maintenance tasks, transportation, shopping	
➧ Refer to section at end of plan for postdischarge considerations.	

Diagnostic Studies

TEST WHY IT IS DONE	WHAT IT TELLS ME
BLOOD TESTS	
Blood studies may vary from completely normal to marked abnormalities.	In stage I, few clients have abnormal blood findings.
• *Complete blood count (CBC):* Battery of screening tests, which typically includes hemoglobin (Hgb); hematocrit (Hct); RBC count, morphology, indices, and distribution width index; platelet count and size; and WBC count and differential.	RBC production may be decreased due to the lymphoma and suppression of bone marrow activity. Client with HL may have mild to severe normocytic, normochromic anemia associated with hypersplenism. WBCs are variable; that is, they may be normal, decreased, or markedly elevated.
• *Differential WBCs:* Percentage of each of the five types of mature WBCs: neutrophils, lymphocytes (B cells and T cells), monocytes, eosinophils, and basophils.	Increased percentage of neutrophils, monocytes, basophils, and eosinophils may be found initially, but these lymphocytes can be profoundly decreased by suppression of marrow activity or by lymphoma treatments. A relative or absolute lymphopenia is a late sign.
• *Platelets:* Platelets have essential function in coagulation.	Decreased in bone marrow involvement or as a side effect of therapy.
• *Erythrocyte sedimentation rate (ESR):* Useful to monitor clients in remission and to detect early evidence of recurrence of disease.	Elevated during active stages and indicates inflammatory or malignant disease.
• *Serum lactate dehydrogenase (LDH):* Substance released by tumors; important prognostic indicator in NHL.	Elevated; may indicate a more aggressive form of NHL.
OTHER DIAGNOSTIC STUDIES	
• *Chest x-ray:* Determines lung involvement, status of airway, and presence of complications.	May reveal mediastinal or hilar adenopathy, nodular infiltrates, or pleural effusions.
• *X-rays or bone scans of thoracic, lumbar vertebrae, proximal extremities, pelvis, or areas of bone tenderness:* Determines areas of involvement and assists in staging.	Bone lesions often associated with acute form of adult T-cell or diffuse large B-cell lymphomas.
• *Whole lung, chest, abdomen, neck computed tomography (CT) scan:* Generally accepted as the primary staging modality for suspected lymphoma and for evaluating therapy response.	Used to assess the extent of disease and responsiveness to therapy. Detects enlarged lymph nodes as well as enlargement of liver and spleen. Most people have repeated CT scans to monitor the status of their disease or evaluate for recurrence.
• *Positron emission tomography (PET) scan:* A type of nuclear scan. Scan of the entire body; allows for a three-dimensional image of not only anatomy (physical structure) but also physiology (function).	May help identify hypermetabolic areas that suggest malignancy and assist with staging of the disease.
• *Abdominal ultrasound:* Aids in identifying additional sites and assesses organ status.	Evaluates extent of involvement of retroperitoneal lymph nodes and determines size of kidneys and patency of urinary tract in preparation for chemotherapy.
• *Biopsies:* Aid in diagnosis as well as determining prognosis.	Presence of Reed-Sternberg cells from blood and lymph cells confirms diagnosis of HL (Visovsky, 2006).
• *Lymph node biopsies:* Establishes the diagnosis of lymphoma and cell type involved.	The most definitive diagnostic tool for confirmation of Hodgkin lymphoma when biopsy shows the presence of Reed-Sternberg (Foster, 2012).
• *Bone marrow:* Sampling may be done by needle aspirate or biopsy to determine bone involvement and staging.	Detects different types of chromosome aberrations and can be used to plan treatment and measure the results of treatment.
• *Cytogenetic analysis:* Cells are studied to see if chromosomal abnormalities are present.	Often used to determine the type of lymphoma cells present. For example, each disease subtype has a specific pattern of markers on its cell surface.
• *Flow cytometry:* Method of counting types of cells with fluorescent tags on the surfaces of the cells.	For some of the more aggressive types of lymphoma, this test can sometimes detect residual disease long before it grows large enough to be detected by any other means.

Nursing Priorities

1. Provide physical and psychological support during extensive diagnostic testing and treatment regimen.
2. Prevent complications.
3. Alleviate pain.
4. Provide information about disease process, prognosis, and treatment needs.

Discharge Goals

1. Complications prevented or minimized.
2. Individual situation dealt with realistically.
3. Pain relieved or controlled.
4. Disease process, prognosis, possible complications, and therapeutic regimen understood.
5. Plan in place to meet needs after discharge.

Refer to CPs: Cancer for shared nursing diagnoses such as Anxiety, Self-Esteem, Grieving, Pain, and Nutrition to accomplish corresponding nursing priorities and discharge goals. See also other related cancer care plans for nursing interventions related to treatments such as radiation, chemotherapy, and bone marrow transplant.

NURSING DIAGNOSIS: risk for impaired Gas Exchange

Risk Factors May Include

[Altered oxygen-carrying capacity of blood]

[Tracheobronchial obstruction—enlarged mediastinal nodes and airway edema (HL and NHL), superior vena cava syndrome (NHL)]

Possibly Evidenced By

(Not applicable; presence of signs and symptoms establishes an *actual* diagnosis)

Desired Outcomes/Evaluation Criteria—Client Will

Respiratory Status: Ventilation (NOC)

Maintain a normal, effective respiratory pattern, free of dyspnea, cyanosis, or other signs of respiratory distress, and arterial blood gases (ABGs) within normal limits (WNL).

ACTIONS/INTERVENTIONS	RATIONALE
Ventilation Assistance (NIC)	
Independent	
Assess and monitor respiratory rate, depth, and rhythm. Note reports of dyspnea or use of accessory muscles, nasal flaring, and altered chest excursion.	Changes such as tachypnea, dyspnea, and use of accessory muscles, may indicate progression of respiratory involvement requiring prompt intervention.
Place client in position of comfort, usually with head of bed elevated or sitting upright, leaning forward with weight supported on arms, and feet dangling.	Maximizes lung expansion, decreases work of breathing, and reduces risk of aspiration.
Reposition and assist with turning periodically.	Promotes aeration of all lung segments and mobilizes secretions.
Instruct in and assist with deep-breathing techniques and pursed-lip or abdominal diaphragmatic breathing, if indicated.	Helps promote gas diffusion and expansion of small airways. Provides client with some control over respiration, helping to reduce anxiety.
Evaluate skin color, noting pallor or development of cyanosis, particularly in nailbeds, ear lobes, and lips.	Proliferation of WBCs and anemia can reduce oxygen-carrying capacity of the blood, leading to hypoxemia.
Assess respiratory response to activity. Note reports of dyspnea and increased fatigue. Schedule rest periods between activities.	Decreased cellular oxygenation reduces activity tolerance. Rest reduces oxygen demands and minimizes fatigue and dyspnea.
Encourage energy-saving techniques, such as rest periods before and after meals, use of shower chair, and sitting for care.	Aids in reducing fatigue and dyspnea and conserves energy for cellular regeneration and respiratory function.
Promote bedrest and provide care as indicated during acute or prolonged exacerbation.	Worsening respiratory involvement and hypoxia may necessitate cessation of activity to prevent more serious respiratory compromise.
Encourage expression of feelings. Acknowledge reality of situation and normality of feelings.	Anxiety increases oxygen demand, and hypoxemia potentiates respiratory distress or cardiac symptoms, which in turn escalates anxiety.
Provide calm, quiet environment.	Promotes relaxation, conserving energy and reducing oxygen demand.

(continues on page 500)

ACTIONS/INTERVENTIONS (continued)	RATIONALE (continued)
Observe for neck vein distention, headache, dizziness, periorbital or facial edema, dyspnea, and stridor.	NHL client is at risk for superior vena cava syndrome, which may result in tracheal deviation and airway obstruction, representing an oncological emergency.
Provide support to family and SOs. Encourage open expression of feelings.	Development of this complication is very frightening for client and family because it may indicate end-stage of disease process or approaching death, especially in the hospice setting. Keeping family informed may diminish their anxiety and minimize transmission to client.
Collaborative	
Assist with treatment of disease process and side effects of therapies.	Interventions to correct or manage anemia can improve oxygenation.
Provide supplemental oxygen.	Maximizes oxygen available for circulatory uptake, aids in reducing hypoxemia.
Monitor laboratory studies, such as ABGs and pulse oximetry.	Measures adequacy of respiratory function and effectiveness of therapy.
Administer analgesics and tranquilizers, as indicated.	Reducing physiological responses to pain and anxiety decreases oxygen demands and may limit respiratory compromise.
Assist with respiratory treatments and adjuncts, such as intermittent positive-pressure breathing (IPPB) and incentive spirometer, if appropriate.	Promotes maximal aeration of all lung segments, preventing atelectasis.
Assist with intubation and mechanical ventilation.	May be necessary to support respiratory function until airway edema is resolved in acutely ill hospitalized client.
Prepare for other procedures—thrombolysis, emergency radiation, endovascular stenting, or thoracentesis when indicated.	Superior vena cava syndrome, rarely presents as an acute emergency, but when it does, life-saving treatments must be immediately carried out. Thoracentesis may also be done if pleural effusion is present.

NURSING DIAGNOSIS: Nausea

May Be Related To
Chemotherapeutic agents; radiation therapy
Gastric irritation

Possibly Evidenced By
Reports nausea, gagging sensation
Aversion toward food

Desired Outcomes/Evaluation Criteria—Client Will

Nausea & Vomiting Severity (NOC)
Be free of nausea.

Nausea & Vomiting Disruptive Effects (NOC)
Manage nausea as evidenced by acceptable level of dietary intake.
Maintain weight, as appropriate.

ACTIONS/INTERVENTIONS	RATIONALE
Nausea Management (NIC)	
Independent	
Control environmental factors, such as strong or noxious odors or noise. Avoid overly sweet, fatty, or spicy foods.	Can trigger nausea and vomiting response.
Encourage use of relaxation techniques, such as visualization, guided imagery, and moderate exercise before meals.	May prevent onset or reduce severity of nausea, decrease anorexia, and enable client to increase oral intake.
Provide or encourage frequent oral hygiene.	Prevents drying of mucosa, promotes comfort, and reduces sour taste.
Evaluate effectiveness of anti-emetic agents.	Individuals respond differently to all medications. First-line anti-emetics may not work, requiring alteration in or use of combination drug therapy.
Identify client who experiences anticipatory nausea or vomiting and take appropriate measures.	Psychogenic nausea and vomiting occurring before chemotherapy generally does not respond to anti-emetic drugs. Change of treatment environment or client routine on treatment day may be effective.

ACTIONS/INTERVENTIONS (continued)	RATIONALE (continued)
Obtain client's height and weight. Weigh daily or as indicated.	Weight loss may indicate client's fat tissues, the chief source of stored energy, are depleted.
Monitor daily food intake and have client keep food diary, as indicated.	Identifies nutritional strengths and deficiencies.
Encourage client to eat high-calorie, nutrient-rich diet, with adequate fluid intake. Encourage use of supplements and frequent, smaller meals spaced throughout the day.	Metabolic tissue needs are increased, as well as fluids, in order to eliminate waste products. Supplements can play an important role in maintaining adequate caloric and protein intake.
Encourage open communication regarding anorexia.	Often a source of emotional distress, especially for SO who wants to feed client frequently. When client refuses, SO may feel rejected or frustrated.
Adjust diet before and immediately after treatment, providing such foods as clear, cool liquids; light or bland foods; candied ginger; dry crackers; toast; and carbonated drinks. Give liquids 1 hour before or 1 hour after meals.	The effectiveness of diet adjustment is very individualized in relief of post-therapy nausea. Clients must experiment to find best solution or combination. Avoiding fluids during meals minimizes becoming "full" too quickly.
Collaborative	
Administer medications, as indicated, for example:	
5-HT3 receptor antagonists, such as ondansetron (Zofran), granisetron (Kytril), and palonosetron (Aloxi); NK-1 receptor antagonist aprepitant (Emend); phenothiazines, such as prochlorperazine (Compazine) and thiethylperazine (Torecan); and antidopaminergics, such as metoclopramide (Reglan)	Most anti-emetics act to interfere with stimulation of true vomiting center, and chemoreceptor trigger zone agents also act peripherally to inhibit reverse peristalsis. These medications are often prescribed routinely before, during, and after chemotherapy to prevent nausea and vomiting.
Antacids and proton pump inhibitors, such as esomeprazole (Nexium), lansoprazole (Prevacid), and pantoprazole (Protonix)	Minimizes gastric irritation, decreases nausea, and reduces risk of mucosal ulceration. *Note:* Client with *H. pylori* gastritis is at increased risk for lymphoma; therefore it is conceivable that client with lymphoma may have gastritis or ulcers associated with *H. pylori* (Ballentine, 2011).
Administer anti-emetic on a regular schedule before, during, and after administration of antineoplastic agent, as appropriate.	Nausea and vomiting are frequently the most disabling and psychologically stressful side effects of chemotherapy.

NURSING DIAGNOSIS: Sexual Dysfunction

May Be Related To

Altered body structure or function (e.g., drugs, surgery, disease process, radiation)

Possibly Evidenced By

Verbalization of problem
Actual or perceived limitations imposed by disease or therapy
[Change in relationship with SO]

Desired Outcomes/Evaluation Criteria—Client Will

Sexual Functioning (NOC)

Verbalize understanding of individual reasons for sexual problems.
Identify stressors in lifestyle that may contribute to the dysfunction.
Discuss concerns about body image, sex role, and desirability as a sexual partner with partner or SO.

ACTIONS/INTERVENTIONS	RATIONALE
Sexual Counseling (NIC)	
Independent	
Assess knowledge of client and SO regarding sexual function and effects of current situation.	Because lymphomas often affect the relatively young who are in their reproductive years, these clients are affected more by these problems and may be less knowledgeable about the possibilities of change.
Collaborate with other healthcare team members in informing client and partner of potential sexual side effects of treatment plans and provide opportunity to consider options. Discuss sperm banking and pregnancy issues, when appropriate, before beginning treatment.	Various cancers, including some lymphomas and the treatments used for them can affect male and female sexual development, libido, fertility, and the success of pregnancy. In males, impotence and permanent sterility can occur as a result of radiation when combined with certain chemotherapeutic agents. In females, menstruation may cease during

(continues on page 502)

the active phase of treatment, and infertility may occur. The woman's age during treatment and certain chemotherapy regimens (e.g., type and dose of alkylating agent) are more likely than others to impact fertility. In addition, side effects of treatment can impact sexual enjoyment (e.g., vaginal dryness and atrophy of vaginal tissues) but can be managed when client and partner are given information and resources (Harel, 2011; Katz, 2007; Johnston, 1999).

Identify preexisting and current stress factors that may be affecting the relationship.
Client may be concerned about other issues, such as job, financial, and illness-related problems.

Determine specific pathophysiology involved and impact on, or perception of, individual.
Client's perception of the individual effects of this illness is crucial to planning interventions that will be appropriate to those affected.

Assist with treatment of underlying condition.
As illness is treated and client can see improvement, hope is restored and client can begin to look to the future.

Provide factual information.
Promotes trust in caregivers.

Encourage and accept expressions of concern, anger, grief, and fear.
Helps client identify feelings and begin to deal with them.

Encourage client to share thoughts and concerns with partner and to clarify values and impact of condition on relationship.
Helps couple begin to deal with issues that can strengthen or weaken relationship.

Collaborative

Refer to appropriate community resources or support groups for sexual dysfunction, such as the American Cancer Society.
Provides information about resources that are available to help with individual needs. Meeting with others who are dealing with the effects of devastating illness can help client and family.

Provide written material, informational Web sites such as Fertile Hope, and other resources appropriate to age and situation.
Reinforces information client has received regarding sexual and fertility issues.

Refer to psychiatric clinical nurse specialist or professional sexual therapist, as indicated.
May need additional in-depth assistance to resolve existing problems.

NURSING DIAGNOSIS: deficient Knowledge [Learning Need] regarding disease process, prognosis, treatment regimen, self-care, and discharge needs

May Be Related To

Lack of exposure, recall
Information misinterpretation
Unfamiliarity with information resources
Cognitive limitations

Possibly Evidenced By

Reports the problem
Inaccurate follow-through of instruction

Desired Outcomes/Evaluation Criteria—Client Will

Knowledge: Cancer Managementl (NOC)

Verbalize understanding of condition, prognosis, and potential complications.
Identify relationship of signs and symptoms to disease process.
Initiate necessary lifestyle changes.

ACTIONS/INTERVENTIONS — RATIONALE

Teaching: Disease Process (NIC)

Independent

Review with client and SO their understanding of client's diagnosis and outlook.
Although lymphomas are complex and have intensive treatment regimens, the outlook has improved in recent years. The 5-year survival rate after treatment in both categories of lymphomas has improved significantly, and many people live with lymphoma in remission.

Review potential treatments client may be considering:
May assist client and SO in making informed choices. In general, the goal of therapy is remission of the lymphoma, and treatments vary according to the disease process and stage.

ACTIONS/INTERVENTIONS	RATIONALE
Various combinations of chemotherapy agents, and/or radiation therapy	Chemotherapy and radiation therapy are the most commonly used treatments and may be used alone or combined. Chemotherapy is a systemic treatment that uses a combination of several drugs, given by IV injection or by mouth, typically given in cycles, based on the duration of the drug's effect and other factors. Radiation therapy targets and kills cancer cells in a specific area, using an external beam (EBRT) or radioisotope targeted therapy (see below). Since lymphoma cells are likely to be present in widespread areas, radiation therapy is not commonly used alone (Cancer Treatment Centers of America [CTCA], 2012; Ballentine, 2011).
Interferon-alpha (INF-α) and monoclonal antibodies, such as rituximab (Rituxan) and alemtuzumab (Campath)	Biological therapies may be used to treat HL or NHL.
Targeted therapies such as:	
Monoclonal antibodies (MAbs or MoAbs)	Common type of immunotherapy for NHL. *Note:* The body's immune system naturally produces antibodies. When produced in the laboratory, these substances can be programmed to make tumor cells more visible to the immune system and to block their growth signals. These agents may be attached to certain chemotherapy agents to deliver high concentrations of drugs directly to the tumor cells (CTCA, 2012).
Radioimmunotherapy (RIT) such as ibritumomab tiuxetan (Zevalin)	This therapy may be an option for NHL individuals with B-cell lymphoma, specifically those with relapsed or refractory NHL. In this therapy, radioisotopes are attached to monoclonal antibodies and delivered intravenously to target and destroy specific cancer cells. By delivering radiation directly to the tumor cells, this treatment helps limit toxic effects on normal tissues (CTCA, 2012).
Peripheral progenitor (stem) cell transplant	Stem cell transplant from bone marrow is now standard therapy for selected clients with NHL. May be combined with high-dose chemotherapy for clients with HL who have relapsed or who have experienced a failed primary chemotherapy regimen.
Discuss potential complications relative to specific therapeutic regimen.	Receiving radiation or chemotherapy increases the risk of contracting another type of lymphoma or another type of cancer, so client will continue to need monitoring after treatment. After 5 disease-free years, however, risk becomes close to normal. Radiation therapy also increases the risk of developing a solid malignancy, such as a breast or lung tumor or thyroid disease if the radiation field during treatment included these regions (Rogers, 2005).
Emphasize need for ongoing medical follow-up, post-treatment surveillance, and testing.	After completion of primary therapy, appropriate tests will be repeated to determine efficacy of therapy. Also, certain monitoring tests are continued; for example, thyroid-stimulating hormone (TSH) levels should be monitored yearly starting 8 to 10 years after radiation therapy. Yearly Pap smears are recommended for female clients because Hodgkin's cells may be found on the cervix. Women receiving radiation therapy are at higher risk of developing breast cancer and should receive yearly mammograms starting 8 years after the completion of treatment, or yearly beginning at age 40, depending on age at time of diagnosis (American Cancer Society [ACS], 2012).
Identify signs and symptoms requiring further evaluation, such as cough, fever, chills, malaise, dyspnea, weight gain, slow pulse, decreased energy level, intolerance to cold; or moderate fever, chest pain, dry cough, dyspnea, rapid pulse (pericarditis [rare]); or dyspnea, fatigue, chest pain, dizziness, or syncope (cardiomyopathy [rare]).	Prompt intervention can identify recurrence, or perhaps limit, progression of complications, thereby reducing further debilitating effects.
Recommend regular exercise in moderation, with adequate rest. Discuss energy conservation techniques. Refer for physical therapy or cancer exercise program, as indicated.	Promotes general well-being. *Note:* Fatigue is associated with disease process and treatment regimen as well as developing complications. Therefore, balancing activity with rest enhances client's ability to perform activities of daily living (ADLs).

(continues on page 504)

ACTIONS/INTERVENTIONS (continued)	RATIONALE (continued)
Determine financial needs or concerns. Identify community resources and vocational services.	Although survival rates are relatively good, clients often have limitations in physical activities and employment because of dyspnea, chronic fatigue, and difficulties in concentration or memory. Presence of the disease can also impact client's ability to work or qualify for loans or obtain health insurance.
Recommend or refer to appropriate community resources—support groups, social worker, counselor, pastor; home health assistance, medical equipment and supplies; hospice; and Lymphoma Research Foundation and American Cancer Society.	Client and SO may benefit from many available resources and networks for such help as care assistance, transportation to treatments, sources of financial resources, and long-term support or counseling.

POTENTIAL CONSIDERATIONS following acute hospitalization (dependent on client's age, physical condition and presence of complications, personal resources, and life responsibilities)

- ***Fatigue***—disease states; stress; anxiety; altered body chemistry (e.g., chemotherapy)
- ***interrupted Family Processes***—situational crisis (illness, disabling and expensive treatments)

Refer to CPs: Adult Leukemias and Cancer for additional postdischarge concerns.

CHAPTER 10

Renal and Urinary Tract

ACUTE KIDNEY INJURY (ACUTE RENAL FAILURE)

I. Pathophysiology

a. Acute renal failure has been defined as a sudden decrease in kidney function, which may or may not be associated with a decrease in urine output and results in a buildup of toxic wastes, such as urea and creatinine in the blood.

b. In 2007, the Acute Kidney Injury Network (AKIN) proposed that the term "acute kidney injury" be used to describe "the entire spectrum of acute renal failure." A universal definition utilizing urine output plus serum creatinine rise (amount plus time) and staging criteria were established for standardization of care over a wider spectrum of kidney dysfunction (Lewington, 2011; Mehta et al, 2007).

c. There are four well-defined phases: onset, oliguric/anuric, diuretic, and convalescent, also called recovery (Ali, 2011; Hudson, n.d.; Choka, 2005).

i. Onset
  1. Period lasts from hours to days
  2. Renal blood flow is reduced.
  3. Urine output is reduced, possibly 30 mL/hr.

ii. Oliguric/anuric
  1. Typically lasts 8 to 14 days
  2. Filtration capability is reduced because of debris and damage to renal tubules.
  3. Output is greatly reduced—may be less than 400 mL/24 hr.
  4. Metabolic acidosis may be present along with hyperkalemia, hyperphosphatemia, and hypocalcemia.

iii. Diuretic
  1. May skip oliguric phase and begin to make large quantities (may be several liters) of urine
  2. Client with oliguria will progress through diuretic phase during recovery.
  3. Urine is dilute because of kidney's inability to concentrate. Serum creatinine and BUN may remain elevated during this phase.

iv. Convalescent/recovery
  1. Renal blood flow and filtration improves.
  2. Process of recovery is gradual, often weeks to months; in many cases, some degree of renal insufficiency persists.

II. Etiology (Workeneh, 2013; Centers for Disease Control and Prevention [CDC], 2012)

a. Multiple causes: ischemia and toxicity (most common), obstructions

i. Prerenal failure: blood volume depletion due to hemorrhage, "third-space" sequestration of fluid as in edema or ascites in advanced liver disease, or burns; dehydration due to gastrointestinal (GI) losses or overuse of diuretics; septic or anaphylactic shock; heart failure (HF) with renal insufficiency, myocardial infarction (MI), trauma; renal artery obstruction; and certain nephrotoxic drugs, such as NSAIDs, cyclooxygenase inhibitors, angiotensin-converting enzyme (ACE) inhibitors; synthetic cannabanoids (SC)

ii. Intrarenal (intrinsic) failure: resulting from direct injury to kidney from ischemia, hypoperfusion, and primary kidney disease. Can be caused by infections, blood transfusion reaction, renal artery stenosis; and direct damage from nephrotoxic substances, such as radiocontrast media, cyclosporine, heavy metals (e.g., lead, mercury), cytotoxic drugs (e.g., certain chemotherapy agents), certain antibiotics (e.g., carbenicillins, aminoglycosides).

iii. Postrenal failure: most commonly occurs with stones in the ureters, bladder, or urethra; from trauma or edema associated with infection, prostatic hypertrophy, or cancer; cervical cancer; strictures of renal artery

iv. If underlying cause is corrected, the nephrons may recover; however, in some cases, damage is permanent and renal failure becomes chronic.

b. Community- or hospital-acquired: Most community-acquired AKI is secondary to volume depletion; as many as 90% of cases are estimated to have a potentially reversible cause (Peacock, 2011). Hospital-acquired AKI often occurs in the intensive care unit (ICU) setting (about 25%) (Cheung, 2008) and is commonly the end result of multiorgan failure.

III. Risk factors:
While there are many risk factors, the older client is at particular risk. Age-related structural and functional changes in the kidney increase the risk for prerenal and postrenal etiologies. This may be due to combordid conditions (e.g., diabetes, influenza, sepsis, heart failure); polypharmacy (including a variety of nephrotoxic drugs) and an increase in hospitalizations, and high-risk medical and surgical procedures (Cartin-Ceba et al, 2012; Ali, 2011; Rosner, 2009).

IV. Statistics

a. Morbidity: Discharge coding data from a 5% sample of U.S. Medicare beneficiaries ($n = 5.4$ million) demonstrated an 11% annual increase in AKI prevalence in hospitalized adults between 1992 and 2001 (Xue et al, 2006).

b. Mortality: Kidney disease is the ninth leading cause of death in the United States (National Kidney Foundation, 2013), and in 2011, 92,110 Americans died from all types of kidney disease (Hoyert & Xu, 2012).

GLOSSARY

Acute tubular necrosis (ATN): Structural injury or tissue necrosis within the kidney, caused by ischemia or toxic injury. Necrosis is usually patchy, but injury can be widespread. ATN should be suspected in any individual presenting after a period of hypotension secondary to cardiac arrest, hemorrhage, sepsis, drug overdose, or surgery.

Anuria: Urine output less than 100 mL/day.

Azotemia: Buildup of nitrogenous waste products, specifically urea, in the blood.

Calculus: Mass of solid material or metabolic substance—kidney or bladder stone.

Catabolic: Destructive metabolism, or breakdown, of proteins for energy results in muscle wasting, loss of lean muscle mass, and negative nitrogen balance.

Glomerular filtration rate (GFR): Rate of fluid filtration through the kidney glomeruli.

Glomerulonephritis: Inflammation of the glomerular capillary walls, causing impaired filtration.

Hydronephrosis: Kidney enlargement caused by urine backing up from the bladder into the kidney or inability of urine to drain from the kidney into bladder; excessive reflux stretches the kidney, causing functional damage to it.

Myoglobin: Form of hemoglobin found in muscle tissue and released into urine when tissue damage occurs.

Nephrotoxins: Chemical substances, including medications that can cause kidney damage.

Nonoliguric AKI: Urinary output more than 400 mL/day.

Oliguria: Urinary output less than 400 mL/day.

Orthostatic hypotension: Decrease in blood pressure when person rises from seated or lying position; often associated with hypovolemia.

Parenchymal disease: Connective tissue of the kidney is damaged and scarred.

Polyuria: Excretion of large amounts (2 to 6 L/24 hr) of urine, lacking concentration and regulation of waste products; occurs during diuretic phase of AKI with head injury (diabetes insipidus [DI]), and diabetic ketoacidosis (DKA).

Porphyrins: Nitrogen-containing chemical components of hemoglobin.

Pyelonephritis: Infection of the kidney's medulla or cortex.

Renal replacement therapy (RRT): Umbrella term used for life-saving treatments for renal failure, including hemodialysis, peritoneal dialysis, hemofiltration, and renal transplantation.

Uremia: Toxic clinical syndrome associated with fluid, electrolyte, and hormone imbalances and metabolic abnormalities due to deterioration of renal function and the deleterious effects of azotemia on organ systems.

Care Setting

Client will be treated in inpatient acute medical, surgical, or intensive care unit.

Related Concerns

Fluid and electrolyte imbalances, page 885
Metabolic acidosis—primary base bicarbonate deficiency, page 450
Psychosocial aspects of care, page 729
Renal dialysis—general considerations, page 529
Renal failure: chronic, page 517
Sepsis/septicemia, page 665
Total nutritional support: parenteral/enteral feeding, page 437
Upper gastrointestinal/esophageal bleeding, page 281

Client Assessment Database

DIAGNOSTIC DIVISION MAY REPORT	MAY EXHIBIT
ACTIVITY/REST	
• Fatigue, weakness, malaise	• Muscle weakness, loss of tone
CIRCULATION	
	• Hypotension or hypertension, including accelerated (malignant) hypertension, eclampsia, or gestational hypertension • Cardiac dysrhythmias associated with hyperkalemia and hypocalcemia • Weak, thready pulses; orthostatic hypotension (hypovolemia) • Jugular vein distention (JVD), full and bounding pulses (hypervolemia) • Generalized tissue edema, including periorbital area, ankles, sacrum • Pallor (anemia); bleeding tendencies

DIAGNOSTIC DIVISION MAY REPORT (continued)	MAY EXHIBIT (continued)
ELIMINATION • History of benign prostatic hyperplasia (BPH) or kidney or bladder stones • Change in usual urination pattern—increased frequency (early failure and early recovery) or decreased frequency or oliguria (later phase) • Dysuria, hesitancy, urgency, and retention (obstruction or infection) • Abdominal bloating, diarrhea, or constipation	• Change in urinary color; for example, ranges from absence of color to deep yellow, reddish-brown, and cloudy • Oliguria: Production of a small amount of urine with no other indicators (e.g., presence of stones or prostate enlargement) generally favors AKI. A gradually diminishing urine output may indicate a urethral stricture or bladder outlet obstruction due to prostate enlargement. • Polyuria: Occurs during diuretic phase of AKI with head injury (diabetes insipidus [DI]) and diabetic ketoacidosis (DKA). • Anuria: Abrupt anuria suggests acute urinary obstruction, acute and severe glomerulonephritis, or embolic renal artery occlusion (Workeneh, 2013).
FOOD/FLUID • Weight gain (edema), weight loss (dehydration) • Nausea, anorexia, heartburn • Vomiting • Use of diuretics	• Changes in skin turgor and moisture • Edema—generalized, dependent
NEUROSENSORY • Headache, blurred vision • Muscle cramps or twitching, "restless leg" syndrome, numbness, tingling	• Altered mental state—decreased attention span, inability to concentrate, loss of memory, confusion, decreasing level of consciousness (LOC) (azotemia, electrolyte and acid-base imbalance) • Twitching, muscle fasciculation, seizure activity
PAIN/DISCOMFORT • Flank pain, headache	• Guarding or distraction behaviors, restlessness
RESPIRATION • Shortness of breath	• Tachypnea, dyspnea, increased rate and depth; Kussmaul's respiration can be compensatory mechanism because of metabolic acidosis. • Cough productive of pink-tinged sputum (pulmonary edema)
SAFETY • Recent transfusion reaction	• Fever (sepsis, dehydration) • Petechiae, ecchymotic areas on skin • Pruritus, dry skin
TEACHING/LEARNING • Family history of polycystic disease, hereditary nephritis, urinary calculus, malignancy • History of exposure to toxins, such as drugs (cyclosporine, amphotericin B, cocaine), environmental poisons (e.g., ethyl alcohol, ethylene glycol, mercury vapors, lead, cadmium or other heavy metals), substance abuse • Current or recent use of nephrotoxic drugs, such as aminoglycoside antibiotics, amphotericin B; anesthetics; ACE inhibitors and vasodilators; NSAIDs such as ibuprofen, naproxen • Recent diagnostic testing with radiographic contrast media reaction • Concurrent conditions—tumors in the urinary tract, gram-negative sepsis, trauma or crush injuries, hemorrhage, disseminated intravascular coagulation (DIC), burns, electrocution injury, autoimmune disorders (e.g., scleroderma, vasculitis), vascular occlusion or surgery, diabetes mellitus (DM), cardiac or liver failure	

(continues on page 508)

Client Assessment Database (continued)

DIAGNOSTIC DIVISION MAY REPORT (continued)	MAY EXHIBIT (continued)
DISCHARGE PLAN CONSIDERATIONS • May require alteration or assistance with medications, treatments, supplies, transportation, and homemaker or maintenance tasks ➧ Refer to section at end of plan for postdischarge considerations.	

Diagnostic Studies

TEST WHY IT IS DONE	WHAT IT TELLS ME
BLOOD TESTS	
• ***Blood urea nitrogen (BUN):*** Measures the by-product of protein metabolism in the liver, filtered by the kidneys and excreted in urine.	Elevated BUN is highly suggestive of kidney dysfunction, although BUN levels may also be affected by liver disorders, hydration, and other factors.
• ***Creatinine (Cr):*** End product of muscle and protein metabolism filtered by the kidneys and excreted in urine.	AKI presents clinically as a rapidly rising creatinine (Cr) over several hours or days.
• ***BUN/Cr ratio:*** Ratio helps determine whether factors other than kidney failure are causing changes in the levels. Normal ratio is 10:1.	In normal individuals, and in client with intrinsic renal disease, the BUN will be approximately 10 times that of Cr. Therefore, a BUN/Cr ratio considerably greater than 10 suggests a prerenal (decreased renal perfusion) or postrenal (obstruction) cause of renal failure.
• ***Complete blood count (CBC):*** Battery of screening tests, which typically includes hemoglobin (Hgb); hematocrit (Hct); red blood cell (RBC) count, morphology, indices, and distribution width index; platelet count and size; and white blood cell (WBC) count and differential.	Hgb is decreased in presence of anemia, which is the main hematologic effect of AKI. RBCs are often decreased because of increased fragility and decreased survival time. Elevated WBC count (leukocytosis) is common in AKI.
• ***Arterial blood gases (ABGs):*** Determines the pH and the percentage of oxygen, carbon dioxide, and bicarbonate in arterial blood.	Metabolic acidosis (pH less than 7.2) may develop because of decreased renal ability to excrete hydrogen and end products of metabolism. Bicarbonate is decreased.
• ***Electrolytes or renalytes:*** Electrically charged minerals found in body tissues and blood in the form of dissolved salts. They help move nutrients into and wastes out of the body's cells, maintain water balance, and stabilize the body's pH level.	Sodium—usually increased, but may vary. Potassium—elevated related to retention and cellular shifts (acidosis) or RBC hemolysis. Rapid increase in K+ is common with AKI. Chloride, phosphorus, and magnesium—usually elevated. Calcium—commonly decreased in AKI and may require replacement.
• ***Serum osmolality:*** Measures the amount of chemicals dissolved in the serum. Kidneys excrete or reabsorb water to keep osmolality in range of 280 to 300 mOsm/kg. Chemicals that affect serum osmolality include sodium, chloride, bicarbonate, protein, and glucose.	Higher-than-normal levels can indicate dehydration or renal tubular necrosis. Lower-than-normal levels are associated with fluid volume overload or syndrome of inappropriate antidiuretic hormone secretion (SIADH).
URINE TESTS	
• ***Volume:*** In AKI, volume is variable.	Often less than 400 mL/24 hr (oliguric phase), which occurs within 24 to 48 hours after renal insult. May be less than 100 mL/24 hr (anuric phase), or more than 400 mL/24 hr (nonoliguric) when renal damage is associated with nephrotoxic agents such as contrast media or antibiotics.
• ***Color:*** Determine presence of RBCs, Hgb, myoglobin, and porphyrins.	Presence of RBCs is always pathologic (Workeneh, 2013). Reddish-brown, cola- or tea-colored urine is suggestive of glomerular damage and acute tubular necrosis (ATN) or presence of myoglobin in the urine.

TEST WHY IT IS DONE (continued)	WHAT IT TELLS ME (continued)
• *Specific gravity:* Measures density of urine compared to water with normal range of 1.005 to 1.030.	Increased in poor renal perfusion. Decreased in kidney disease, such as glomerulonephritis and pyelonephritis with loss of ability to concentrate. Specific gravity that is fixed at 1.010 reflects severe renal damage.
• *pH:* Measures level of acidity.	Alkaline urine (pH greater than 7) can be found in urinary tract infections (UTIs) and renal tubular necrosis.
• *Osmolality or osmolarity:* Measures the ratio of water and solutes, such as electrolytes, acids, and other metabolic wastes, processed by the kidneys and released in urine. When body fluid is balanced, normal urine osmolarity is in the range of 300 to 900 mOsm/L.	Urine with higher osmolarity is concentrated with less water and a higher solute load, indicating a prerenal cause. Urine with decreased osmolarity is dilute with few solutes, indicating that the cause of renal failure resides in the kidney itself.
• *Cr clearance:* Calculates glomerular filtration rate (GFR) by measuring the amount of Cr cleared from the blood and filtered into urine in 24 hours.	Best indicator of overall kidney function, as reduced Cr clearance correlates with increased circulating creatinine.
• *Sodium:* Determines hydration status and ability to conserve or excrete Na.	Usually increased if ATN is cause of AKI and if kidney is not able to reabsorb sodium, although it is typically decreased in other causes of prerenal azotemia.
• *Fractional excretion sodium (FeNa):* Calculated measure of renal tubule function.	Reveals inability of tubules to reabsorb sodium. Readings of less than 1% indicate prerenal disorders; higher than 1% reflects intrarenal disorders.
• *RBCs:* Presence of RBCs is pathologic.	May be present because of infection, stones, trauma in the renal system, inflammation, tumors, or altered GFR.
• *Protein:* The protein most likely to appear in urine is albumin. The term albuminuria is sometimes used when a urine test detects albumin specifically.	High-grade proteinuria (3 to 4+) strongly indicates glomerular damage when RBCs and casts are also present. Low-grade proteinuria (1 to 2+) and WBCs may be indicative of infection or interstitial nephritis. In ATN, proteinuria is usually minimal.
• *Casts:* Tubules in the kidneys secrete proteins. Under some circumstances, these proteins precipitate out to form cylindrical impressions of the tubules called casts.	Usually signal renal disease or infection. Cellular casts with brownish pigments and numerous renal tubular epithelial cells are diagnostic of ATN. Red casts suggest acute glomerular nephritis.
Other Diagnostic Studies	
• *Kidney/abdominal ultrasound:* Imaging technique that uses high-frequency sound waves and a computer to create images of blood vessels, tissues, and organs.	Evaluates existing renal disease and obstruction of the urinary collecting system. The degree of hydronephrosis does not necessarily correlate with the degree of obstruction.
• *Kidney, ureter, bladder (KUB) x-ray:* X-ray of the abdomen, showing the kidneys, ureters, and bladder.	Demonstrates size and structure of kidneys, ureters, and bladder; reveals presence of abnormalities, such as cysts, tumors, or stones.
• *Computed tomography (CT) scan, with or without enhancement:* X-ray procedure that uses a computer to produce a detailed picture of a cross section of the body.	Ultrasound and computed tomography (CT) are modalities of first choice in renal imaging.
• *Magnetic resonance imaging (MRI):* Imaging test that uses powerful magnets and radio waves to create pictures of the body. It does not use radiation.	Can be used in case of compromised renal function, severe contrast allergy, or in case radiation exposure is a problem (e.g., in children and pregnant women) or as a problem-solving modality when CT findings are nondiagnostic (Nikken, 2007).
• *CT or MRI urography:* Examines the urinary tract before and after administration of intravenous contrast material that includes excretory phase images.	These tests provide detailed anatomic depiction of each of the major portions of the urinary tract—the kidneys, intrarenal collecting systems, ureters, and bladder—and thus allow for comprehensive evaluation of the entire urinary system at work. MR has the advantage of not using ionizing radiation and the potential to provide more functional information than CT. Clinicians have not yet reached consensus on optimal protocols and appropriate utilization in an era of cost containment and heightened concerns about radiation exposure (Silverman, 2008).
• *Intravenous pyelogram (IVP) also called intravenous urography (IVU):* X-ray examination and fluoroscopic visualization of the kidneys, ureters, and bladder using contrast material.	This test has largely been replaced by CT, CT urography, and MRI as the primary test for evaluating the urinary system (Fulgham, 2011). Shows size, shape, and location of urinary structures. Identifies filling defects such as caused by trauma, stones, or tumors.

(continues on page 510)

Diagnostic Studies (continued)

TEST WHY IT IS DONE (continued)	WHAT IT TELLS ME (continued)
• *Aortorenal angiography:* Fluoroscopic examination using contrast to examine the renal blood vessels for signs of blockage or abnormalities.	Determines if blood vessel blockage is reducing renal flow.
• *Endourology:* Diagnostic and therapeutic operative procedures performed through instruments—cystoscopic, pelviscopic, or laparoscopic.	Provides direct visualization of urethra, bladder, ureters, and kidneys to diagnose problems or to biopsy or remove small lesions or calculi.

Nursing Priorities

1. Reestablish or maintain fluid and electrolyte balance.
2. Prevent complications.
3. Provide emotional support for client and significant other (SO).
4. Provide information about disease process, prognosis, and treatment needs.

Discharge Goals

1. Homeostasis achieved.
2. Complications prevented or minimized.
3. Current situation dealt with realistically.
4. Disease process, prognosis, and therapeutic regimen understood.
5. Plan in place to meet needs after discharge.

NURSING DIAGNOSIS: excess Fluid Volume

May Be Related To

Compromised regulatory mechanism (renal failure)

Possibly Evidenced By

Intake exceeds output, oliguria; specific gravity changes
Blood pressure (BP) changes, increased central venous pressure (CVP)
Edema, weight gain over short period of time
Pulmonary congestion
Change in mental status, restlessness
Decreased Hgb/Hct, electrolyte imbalance

Desired Outcomes/Evaluation Criteria—Client Will

Fluid Overload Severity (NOC)

Display appropriate urinary output with specific gravity and other laboratory studies near normal; stable weight and vital signs within client's normal range; and absence of edema.

ACTIONS/INTERVENTIONS	RATIONALE
Hypervolemia Management (NIC)	
Independent	
Record accurate intake and output (I&O). Include "hidden" fluids, such as intravenous (IV) antibiotic additives, liquid medications, ice chips, and frozen treats. Measure GI losses and estimate insensible losses, such as diaphoresis.	Low urine output less than 400 mL/24 hr may be first indicator of acute failure, especially in a high-risk client. Accurate I&O are necessary for determining fluid replacement needs and reducing risk of fluid overload. *Note:* Hypervolemia occurs in the anuric phase of AKI.
Monitor urine specific gravity.	Measures the kidney's ability to concentrate urine. In intrarenal failure, specific gravity is usually equal to or less than 1.010, indicating loss of ability to concentrate the urine.
Weigh daily at same time of day, on same scale, with same equipment and clothing.	Daily body weight is best monitor of fluid status. A weight gain of more than 0.5 kg/day suggests fluid retention.
Assess skin, face, and dependent areas for edema. Evaluate degree of edema (on scale of +1 to +4).	Edema occurs primarily in dependent tissues of the body, such as hands, feet, and lumbosacral area. Client can gain up to 10 lb (4.5 kg) of fluid before pitting edema is detected. Periorbital edema may be a presenting sign of this fluid shift because these fragile tissues are easily distended by even minimal fluid accumulation.

ACTIONS/INTERVENTIONS (continued)	RATIONALE (continued)
Monitor heart rate, BP, and central venous pressure (CVP), if available.	Tachycardia and hypertension can occur because of (1) failure of the kidneys to excrete urine, (2) excessive fluid resuscitation during efforts to treat hypovolemia or hypotension, and (3) changes in the renin-angiotensin system, which helps regulate long-term blood pressure and blood volume. *Note:* Invasive monitoring may be needed for assessing intravascular volume, especially in clients with poor cardiac function.
Auscultate lung and heart sounds.	Fluid overload may lead to pulmonary edema and HF, as evidenced by development of adventitious breath sounds and extra heart sounds. (Refer to ND: risk for decreased Cardiac Output, below.)
Assess level of consciousness; investigate changes in mentation and presence of restlessness.	May reflect fluid shifts, accumulation of toxins, acidosis, electrolyte imbalances, or developing hypoxia.
Plan oral fluid replacement with client, within multiple restrictions. Intersperse desired beverages throughout 24 hours. Vary offerings, such as hot, cold, and frozen.	Helps avoid periods without fluids, minimizes boredom of limited choices, and reduces sense of deprivation and thirst.
Collaborative	
Correct any reversible cause of AKI, such as replacing blood losses, maximizing cardiac output, discontinuing nephrotoxic drug, and removing obstruction via surgery.	Current treatment for AKI is mainly supportive. Maintenance of circulating volume and correction of biochemical abnormalities are the primary goals of treatment. Kidneys may be able to return to normal functioning, thus preventing or limiting long-term residual effects, although recent studies are supporting the idea that AKI can still be implicated in chronic renal failure sufficient to require dialysis one to ten years after the initial event (Goldberg, 2008).
Insert and maintain indwelling catheter, as indicated.	Catheterization excludes lower tract obstruction and provides means of accurate monitoring of urine output during acute phase; however, indwelling catheterization may be contraindicated because of increased risk of infection.
Monitor laboratory and diagnostic studies, such as the following:	
BUN, Cr	Assesses progression and management of renal dysfunction, failure. *Note:* Dialysis is indicated if ratio is higher than 10:1 or if therapy fails to correct fluid overload or metabolic acidosis.
Serum sodium	Hyponatremia may result from fluid overload (dilutional) or kidney's inability to conserve sodium. Hypernatremia indicates total body water deficit.
Serum potassium	Lack of renal excretion or selective retention of potassium by the tubules leads to hyperkalemia, requiring prompt intervention.
Hgb/Hct	Decreased values may indicate hemodilution associated with hypervolemia; however, during prolonged failure, anemia frequently develops as a result of decreased RBC production. Other possible causes—active or occult hemorrhage—should also be evaluated.
Serial chest x-rays	Increased cardiac size, prominent pulmonary vascular markings, pleural effusion, and infiltrates indicate acute responses to fluid overload or chronic changes associated with renal failure and HF.
Administer and restrict fluids, as indicated.	Fluid management is usually calculated to replace output from all sources as well as estimate insensible losses due to metabolism and diaphoresis. Prerenal failure is treated with volume replacement and vasopressors. The oliguric client with adequate circulating volume or fluid overload who is unresponsive to fluid restriction and diuretics requires dialysis.
Administer medication, as indicated, for example:	
Diuretics, such as furosemide (Lasix), bumetanide (Bumex), torsemide (Demadex), and mannitol (Osmitrol)	Given early in oliguric phase of AKI in an effort to convert to diuretic phase, flush the tubular lumen of debris, reduce hyperkalemia, and promote adequate urine volume.
Vasodilators, such as fenolodopam (Corolopam)	May be given to decrease systemic vascular resistance (SVR) and increase renal blood flow. It has been noted to improve renal function in patients with severe hypertension.
Antihypertensives, such as clonidine (Catapres), methyldopa (Aldomet), and prazosin (Minipress)	May be given to treat hypertension by counteracting effects of decreased renal blood flow and/or circulating volume overload.

(continues on page 512)

ACTIONS/INTERVENTIONS (continued)

Prepare for renal replacement therapy as indicated, such as hemodialysis (HD), peritoneal dialysis (PD), or continuous renal replacement therapy (CRRT).

RATIONALE (continued)

Done to reduce volume overload, correct electrolyte and acid-base imbalances, and remove toxins. The type of dialysis chosen for AKI depends on the degree of hemodynamic compromise and client's ability to withstand the procedure. *Note:* Although it technically can be used, peritoneal dialysis is not frequently used in patients with AKI (Workeneh, 2013). (Refer to CP: Renal Dialysis.)

NURSING DIAGNOSIS: risk for decreased Cardiac Output

Risk Factors May Include

Altered afterload—fluid deficit (excessive losses)
Altered preload—fluid shifts (venous distention)
Altered rhythm (e.g., potassium, calcium imbalance; uremic effects on cardiac muscle)

Possibly Evidenced By

(Not applicable; presence of signs and symptoms establishes an *actual* diagnosis)

Desired Outcomes/Evaluation Criteria—Client Will

Cardiac Pump Effectiveness (NOC)

Maintain cardiac output as evidenced by BP and HR and rhythm within client's normal limits and peripheral pulses strong and equal, with adequate capillary refill time.

ACTIONS/INTERVENTIONS

Hemodynamic Regulation (NIC)

Independent

Monitor BP and heart rate.

Observe ECG or telemetry for changes in rhythm.

Auscultate heart sounds.

Assess color of skin, mucous membranes, and nailbeds. Note capillary refill time.

Note occurrence of slow pulse, hypotension, flushing, nausea or vomiting, and depressed LOC—central nervous system (CNS) depression.

Investigate reports of muscle cramps, numbness or tingling of fingers, with muscle twitching and hyperreflexia.

Maintain bedrest or encourage adequate rest and provide assistance with care and desired activities.

Collaborative

Monitor laboratory studies, such as the following:

Potassium

RATIONALE

Fluid volume excess, combined with hypertension, which often occurs in renal failure, and effects of uremia increase cardiac workload and can lead to cardiac failure. In AKI, cardiac failure is usually reversible.

Changes in electromechanical function may become evident in response to accumulation of toxins and electrolyte imbalance. For example, hyperkalemia is associated with a peaked T wave, wide QRS complex, prolonged PR interval, and flattened or absent P wave. Hypokalemia is associated with flattened T wave, peaked P wave, and appearance of U waves. Prolonged QT interval may reflect calcium deficit.

Development of S_3/S_4 is associated with fluid volume excess and congestive HF. Pericardial friction rub may be only manifestation of uremic pericarditis, requiring prompt intervention and, possibly, acute dialysis.

Pallor may reflect vasoconstriction or anemia—common in AKI, whether associated with actual blood loss or abnormalities in life of RBCs. Cyanosis is a late sign and is related to pulmonary congestion or cardiac failure. A long capillary refill time is associated with hypovolemic states.

Magnesium is typically decreased with AKI. If client is also using drugs (e.g., antacids) containing magnesium, the result can be significant hypomagnesemia, potentiating neuromuscular dysfunction and risk of respiratory or cardiac arrest.

These are symptoms of hypocalcemia. Calcium levels are typically somewhat decreased with AKI. If phosphorus levels are also high, hypocalcemia can become severe, which can also affect cardiac contractility and function.

Reduces oxygen consumption and cardiac workload.

During oliguric phase, hyperkalemia is present but often shifts to hypokalemia in diuretic or recovery phase. Any potassium value associated with ECG changes requires intervention. *Note:* A serum level of 6.5 mEq or higher constitutes a medical emergency.

ACTIONS/INTERVENTIONS (continued)	RATIONALE (continued)
Calcium	In addition to its own cardiac effects, calcium deficit enhances the toxic effects of potassium.
Phosphorus	May be abnormal because of reduced renal excretion or excess release of cellular phosphate.
Magnesium	Dialysis or calcium administration may be necessary to combat the CNS-depressive effects of an elevated serum magnesium level.
Administer and restrict fluids as indicated. (Refer to NDs: excess Fluid Volume and risk for deficient Fluid Volume.)	Cardiac output depends on circulating volume—affected by both fluid excess and deficit—and myocardial muscle function.
Provide supplemental oxygen, as indicated.	Maximizes available oxygen for myocardial uptake to reduce cardiac workload and cellular hypoxia.
Administer medications, as indicated:	
Inotropic agents	May be used to improve cardiac output by increasing myocardial contractility and stroke volume.
Calcium gluconate	Serum calcium is often low but usually does not require specific treatment in AKI. Calcium gluconate may be given to treat hypocalcemia and to offset the effects of hyperkalemia by modifying or reducing cardiac irritability.
Aluminum hydroxide gels (Amphojel, Basalgel)	Increased phosphate levels may occur as a result of failure of glomerular filtration and require use of phosphate-binding antacids to limit phosphate absorption from the GI tract.
Glucose and insulin solution	Temporary measure to lower serum potassium by driving potassium into cells when cardiac rhythm is endangered.
Sodium bicarbonate or sodium citrate	May be used to correct metabolic acidosis or hyperkalemia by increasing serum pH if client is severely acidotic. Used with caution as it can exacerbate fluid overload and cause tetany by decreasing the ionized calcium concentration. Acidosis that does not respond to medical therapy is an indication for dialysis.
Prepare for and assist with dialysis, as necessary.	May be indicated for persistent dysrhythmias and progressive HF unresponsive to other therapies.

NURSING DIAGNOSIS: risk for imbalanced Nutrition: less than body requirements

Risk Factors May Include

Inability to ingest/digest food—nausea/vomiting, ulcerations of oral mucosa, dietary restrictions

[Increased metabolic needs]

Possibly Evidenced By

(Not applicable; presence of signs and symptoms establishes an *actual* diagnosis)

Desired Outcomes/Evaluation Criteria—Client Will

Nutritional Status (NOC)

Maintain or regain weight as indicated by individual situation; be free of edema.

ACTIONS/INTERVENTIONS	RATIONALE
Nutrition Therapy (NIC)	
Independent	
Assess and document dietary intake.	Aids in identifying deficiencies and dietary needs. Uremic symptoms (such as, nausea, anorexia, altered taste) and multiple dietary restrictions affect food intake.
Provide frequent, small feedings.	Minimizes anorexia and nausea associated with uremic state and diminished peristalsis.
Give client and SO a list of permitted foods and fluids and encourage involvement in menu choices.	Provides client with a measure of control within dietary restrictions. Food from home may enhance appetite.
Offer frequent mouth care and rinse with dilute (0.25%) acetic acid solution; provide gum, hard candy, or breath mints between meals.	Mucous membranes may become dry and cracked. Mouth care soothes, lubricates, and helps freshen mouth taste, which is often unpleasant because of uremia and restricted oral intake. Rinsing with acetic acid helps neutralize ammonia formed by conversion of urea.

(continues on page 514)

ACTIONS/INTERVENTIONS (continued)	RATIONALE (continued)
Weigh daily, preferably in the morning before breakfast.	The fasting and catabolic client normally loses 0.2 to 0.5 kg/day. Changes in excess of 0.5 kg may reflect shifts in fluid balance.
Collaborative	
Monitor laboratory studies, such as BUN, prealbumin or albumin, transferrin, sodium, and potassium.	Indicators of nutritional needs, restrictions, and necessity for, and effectiveness of, therapy.
Consult with dietitian or nutritional support team.	Determines individual calorie and nutrient needs within the restrictions and identifies most effective route and product—oral supplements, enteral or parenteral nutrition.
Provide high-calorie, low- or moderate-protein diet. Include complex carbohydrates and fat sources to meet caloric needs (avoiding concentrated sugar sources) and to provide essential amino acids.	The amount of needed exogenous protein is less than normal unless client is on dialysis. Carbohydrates meet energy needs and limit tissue catabolism, preventing ketoacid formation from protein and fat oxidation. Carbohydrate intolerance mimicking diabetes mellitus may occur in severe renal failure. Essential amino acids improve nitrogen balance and nutritional status, stimulate repair of tubular epithelial cells, and enhance client's ability to fight systemic complications.
Restrict potassium, sodium, and phosphorus intake, as indicated.	Restriction of these electrolytes may be needed to prevent further renal damage, especially if dialysis is not part of treatment, and during recovery phase of AKI.
Administer medications as indicated, for example:	
Iron preparations	Iron deficiency may occur if protein is restricted, client is anemic, or GI function is impaired.
Calcium carbonate	Restores normal serum levels to improve cardiac and neuromuscular function, blood clotting, and bone metabolism. *Note:* Low serum calcium is often corrected as phosphate absorption is decreased in the GI system. Calcium may be substituted as a phosphate binder.
Vitamin D	Necessary to facilitate absorption of calcium from the GI tract.
B complex and C vitamins and folic acid	Vital as coenzyme in cell growth and actions. Intake is decreased because of protein restrictions.
Antiemetics, such as prochlorperazine (Compazine) and trimethobenzamide (Tigan)	Given to relieve nausea and vomiting, and may enhance oral intake.

NURSING DIAGNOSIS: risk for Infection

Risk Factors May Include
Invasive procedures/devices
Immunosuppression
Malnutrition

Possibly Evidenced By
(Not applicable; presence of signs and symptoms establishes an *actual* diagnosis)

Desired Outcomes/Evaluation Criteria—Client Will

Infection Severity (NIC)
Experience no signs or symptoms of infection.

ACTIONS/INTERVENTIONS	RATIONALE
Infection Protection (NIC)	
Independent	
Promote good hand washing by client and staff.	Reduces risk of cross-contamination.
Avoid invasive procedures, instrumentation, and manipulation of indwelling catheters whenever possible. Use aseptic technique when caring for IV and invasive lines. Change site and dressings per protocol. Note edema and purulent drainage.	Limits introduction of bacteria into body. Early detection and treatment of developing infection may prevent sepsis.
Provide routine catheter care and promote meticulous perianal care. Keep urinary drainage system closed and remove indwelling catheter as soon as possible.	Reduces bacterial colonization and risk of ascending UTI.
Encourage deep breathing, coughing, and frequent position changes.	Prevents atelectasis and mobilizes secretions to reduce risk of pulmonary infections.

ACTIONS/INTERVENTIONS (continued) | RATIONALE (continued)

Assess skin integrity. (Refer to CP: Renal Failure: Chronic; ND: risk for impaired Skin Integrity.)

Excoriations from scratching may become secondarily infected.

Monitor vital signs.

Fever higher than 100.4°F (38.0°C) with increased pulse and respirations is typical of increased metabolic rate resulting from inflammatory process, although sepsis can occur without a febrile response.

Collaborative

Monitor laboratory studies, such as WBC count with differential.

Although elevated WBCs may indicate generalized infection, leukocytosis is commonly seen in AKI and may reflect inflammation or injury within the kidney. A shifting of the differential to the left is indicative of infection.

Obtain specimen(s) for culture and sensitivity and administer appropriate antibiotics, as indicated.

Verification of infection and identification of specific organism aids in choice of the most effective treatment. *Note:* A number of anti-infective agents require adjustments of dose or time while renal clearance is impaired.

NURSING DIAGNOSIS: risk for deficient Fluid Volume

Risk Factors May Include

Excessive loss of fluid (diuretic phase of AKI)

Possibly Evidenced By

(Not applicable; presence of signs and symptoms establishes an *actual* diagnosis)

Desired Outcomes/Evaluation Criteria—Client Will

Fluid Balance (NOC)

Display I&O near balance, good skin turgor, moist mucous membranes, palpable peripheral pulses, stable weight and vital signs, and electrolytes within normal range.

ACTIONS/INTERVENTIONS | RATIONALE

Fluid Monitoring (NIC)

Independent

Measure I&O accurately. Weigh daily.

Helps estimate fluid replacement needs. *Note*: Rising urinary volume and delayed return of tubular reabsorption capabilities may lead to hypovolemia.

Calculate insensible fluid losses.

Fluid intake should approximate losses through urine, nasogastric (NG) or wound drainage, and insensible losses—diaphoresis and metabolism. *Note:* Some sources believe that fluid replacement should not exceed two-thirds of the previous day's output to prevent prolonging the diuresis.

Encourage fluid intake. Provide allowed fluids throughout 24-hour period.

Diuretic phase of AKI may revert to oliguric phase if fluid intake is not maintained or nocturnal dehydration occurs.

Monitor BP, noting postural changes, and heart rate.

Orthostatic hypotension and tachycardia suggest hypovolemia.

Note signs and symptoms of dehydration, such as dry mucous membranes, thirst, dulled sensorium, and peripheral vasoconstriction.

In diuretic or postobstructive phase of renal failure, urine output can exceed 3 L/day. Extracellular fluid (ECF) volume depletion activates the thirst center, and sodium depletion causes persistent thirst, unrelieved by drinking water. Continued fluid losses and inadequate replacement may lead to hypovolemic state.

Collaborative

Monitor laboratory studies, such as sodium.

In nonoliguric AKI or in diuretic phase of AKI, large urine losses may result in sodium wasting, while elevated urinary sodium acts osmotically to increase fluid losses. Restriction of sodium may be indicated to break the cycle.

NURSING DIAGNOSIS: deficient Knowledge [Learning Need] regarding condition, prognosis, treatment, self-care, and discharge needs

May Be Related To

Lack of exposure or recall
Information misinterpretation
Unfamiliarity with information resources

Possibly Evidenced By

Reports the problem
Inaccurate follow-through of instructions

Desired Outcomes/Evaluation Criteria—Client Will

Knowledge: Kidney Disease Management (NOC)

Verbalize understanding of condition, disease process, prognosis, and potential complications.
Identify relationship of signs and symptoms to the disease process and correlate symptoms with causative factors.
Verbalize understanding of therapeutic needs.
Initiate necessary lifestyle changes and participate in treatment regimen.

ACTIONS/INTERVENTIONS	RATIONALE
Teaching: Disease Process (NIC)	
Independent	
Review disease process, prognosis, and precipitating factors, if known.	Provides knowledge base from which client can make informed choices.
Explain level of renal function after acute episode is over.	Client may experience residual defects in kidney function, which may or may not be permanent.
Discuss renal dialysis or transplantation if these are likely options for the future.	Although these options would have been previously presented by the physician, client may now be at a point when options need to be considered and decisions made and may desire additional input.
Review dietary plan and restrictions. Include fact sheet listing food and fluid restrictions.	Adequate nutrition is necessary to promote healing and tissue regeneration; adherence to restrictions may prevent complications.
Encourage client to observe characteristics of urine and amount and frequency of output.	Changes may reflect alterations in renal function and need for dialysis.
Establish regular schedule for weighing.	Useful tool for monitoring fluid and dietary status and needs.
Review fluid intake and restriction. Remind client to spread fluids over entire day and to include all fluids (e.g., ice) in daily fluid counts.	Depending on the cause and phase of AKI, client may need to either restrict or increase intake of fluids.
Discuss activity restriction and gradual resumption of desired activity. Encourage use of energy-saving and relaxation techniques and diversional activities.	Client with severe AKI may need to restrict activity and may feel weak for an extended period during lengthy recovery phase, requiring measures to conserve energy and reduce boredom and depression.
Discuss reality of continued presence of fatigue.	Decreased metabolic energy production, presence of anemia, and states of discomfort commonly result in fatigue.
Determine and prioritize activities of daily living (ADLs) and personal responsibilities. Identify available resources and support systems.	Helps client manage lifestyle changes that may be needed to meet personal and family needs.
Recommend scheduling activities with adequate rest periods.	Prevents excessive fatigue and conserves energy for healing and tissue regeneration.
Review medication use. Encourage client to discuss all medications, including over-the-counter (OTC) drugs and herbal supplements, with healthcare provider.	Medications that are concentrated in or excreted by the kidneys can cause toxic cumulative reactions and permanent damage to kidneys. Some supplements may interact with prescribed medications and may contain electrolytes.
Stress necessity of follow-up care and laboratory studies.	Renal function can be slow to return—up to 12 months following AKI—and deficits may persist, requiring frequent monitoring to avoid complications.
Identify symptoms requiring medical intervention, such as decreased urinary output, sudden weight gain, presence of edema, lethargy, bleeding, signs of infection, and altered mental status.	Prompt evaluation and intervention may prevent serious complications and progression to chronic renal failure (CRF).

POTENTIAL CONSIDERATIONS following acute hospitalization (dependent on client's age, physical condition and presence of complications, personal resources, and life responsibilities)
- ***deficient Fluid Volume (specify)***—dependent on cause, duration, and stage of recovery
- ***Fatigue***—disease state, malnutrition, anemia
- ***risk for Infection***—immunosuppression, malnutrition, increased environmental exposure
- ***ineffective Self-Health Management***—complexity of therapeutic regimen, economic difficulties, perceived benefit/ barriers

RENAL FAILURE: CHRONIC (END-STAGE RENAL DISEASE)

I. Pathophysiology

a. Renal failure is the end result of chronic kidney disease (CKD), which is the consequence of gradual, progressive destruction of nephrons and decrease in glomerular filtration rate (GFR) over time, resulting in loss of kidney function that produces major changes in all body systems.

b. Changes in the composition of blood (e.g., BUN/Cr) plus urine (e.g., albuminuria) are indicative of kidney damage progression.

II. CKD Stages (Pradeep, 2013; Choka, 2005; The Kidney Disease Outcomes Quality Initiative [KDOQI] of the National Kidney Foundation [NKF], 2002): Correspond to the degree of nephron loss and changes in GFR. Other markers of kidney damage (e.g., abnormalities in the composition of blood or urine or abnormalities on imaging studies) should also be present in stage 1 and stage 2 because GFR may be normal or borderline.

a. Stage 1
  - i. GFR may be normal or slightly higher than normal (>90 mL/min/1.73 m^2).
  - ii. Kidney dysfunction is present; however, it may be undiagnosed due to lack of symptoms—blood urea nitrogen/creatinine (BUN/Cr) ratio is normal and nephron loss at less than 75%.

b. Stage 2
  - i. GFR is mildly decreased (60 to 89 mL/min/1.73 m^2), slight elevation in BUN/Cr
  - ii. Client may be asymptomatic or have hypertension.
  - iii. Polyuria and nocturia present—high output failure

c. Stage 3
  - i. Moderate reduction in GFR (30 to 59 mL/min/1.73 m^2)
  - ii. Fluid and electrolyte abnormalities and other complications present
  - iii. Client may be asymptomatic or have hypertension.

d. Stage 4
  - i. Severe reduction in GFR (15 to 29 mL/min/1.73 m^2) and/or very high albuminuria (>300 mg/24 hr)
  - ii. Client has endocrine/metabolic derangements or disturbances in water or electrolyte balance, protein-energy malnutrition, loss of lean body mass, muscle weakness; peripheral and pulmonary edema
  - iii. Timely referral to a nephrologist when glomerular filtration rate approaches 30 mL/min/1.73 m^2 is believed to improve ESRD outcome and appropriate selection of dialysis modality.

e. Stage 5
  - i. GRF <15 mL/min/1.73 m^2, or on dialysis
  - ii. Client has metabolic acidosis, cardiovascular complications such as pericarditis, encephalopathy, neuropathies, and many other manifestations demonstrating end-stage disease.

III. Etiology (Pradeep, 2013; Holcomb, 2005)

a. Multiple causes, including (but not limited to):
  - i. Acute tubular necrosis (ATN) from unresolved acute kidney injury (AKI)
  - ii. Diabetes (40%) and hypertension (25.2%) are responsible for most cases of ESRD resulting in dialysis (Alper, 2012).
  - iii. Chronic infections: glomerulonephritis, pyelonephritis, beta-hemolytic *streptococci* infection; hepatitis B and C; HIV; syphilis
  - iv. Vascular diseases: hypertensive nephrosclerosis, renal artery stenosis, renal vein thrombosis, vasculitis
  - v. Obstructive processes: long-standing renal calculi, benign prostatic hyperplasia (BPH)
  - vi. Cystic disorders: polycystic or medullary kidney disease
  - vii. Collagen and connective tissue diseases: rheumatoid arthritis (RA), systemic lupus erythematosus (SLE), and collagen vascular disease
  - viii. Tumors: malignant (multiple myeloma) or benign
  - ix. Nephrotoxic agents: drugs, such as aminoglycosides, tetracyclines; contrast dyes; heavy metals, NSAIDs

b. Highest incidence of ESRD occurs in individuals older than age 75 years, increasing over 90% over the last decade (Alper, 2012).

IV. Statistics

a. Morbidity: In 2011, more than 594,000 individuals were treated for ESRD in the United States; with 90,000 new cases reported annually, 415,000 were receiving dialysis, and more than 179,000 living with a functioning kidney transplant (National Kidney Foundation [NFK], 2012).

b. Mortality: In 2010, 90,000 deaths were attributed to ESRD in the United States (U.S. Renal Data System (USRDS), 2012) and associated with (1) cardiovascular disease, (2) sepsis, and (3) cerebrovascular disease (Alper, 2012).

c. Cost: In 2010, overall per person per year (PPPY) costs for patients with CKD reached $22,323 for Medicare patients age 65 and older and $13,395 for patients age 50 to 64 in the MarketScan database, including Part D cost. These figures were substantially increased by additional diagnoses such as diabetes or cardiac disease and by racial differences (2012) (USRDS, 2012). In 2010, expenditures for ESRD rose 8.0% to $32.9 billion, including the Medicare Part D prescription drug benefit. These expenditures cover 488,938 patients in the prevalent Medicare ESRD population, along with 105,436 non-Medicare patients; these latter patients cost an additional estimated $14.5 billion (2012).

GLOSSARY

Acute tubular necrosis (ATN): Structural injury or tissue necrosis within the kidney, caused by ischemia or toxic injury. Necrosis is usually patchy, but injury can be widespread.

Anuria: Urine output less than 100 mL/24 hr.

Azotemia: Buildup of nitrogenous waste products, specifically urea, in the blood (BUN).

Chronic kidney disease or chronic renal failure: Kidney damage or decreased kidney GFR of less than 60 mL/min/1.73 m^2 for 3 or more months

Ecchymosis: Superficial bleeding under the skin—purple or black-and-blue bruise.

End-stage renal disease (ESRD): GFR less than 15 mL/min or receiving dialysis.

Glomerular filtration rate (GFR): Rate of fluid filtration through the kidney glomeruli.

Nephrotoxins: Chemical substances, including medications that can cause kidney damage.

Nocturia: Frequent urination after retiring to bed.

Oliguria: Urinary output less than 400 mL/24 hr.

Osteitis fibrosa: Bones become soft and deformed due to increased metabolism or high bone turnover associated with increased levels of parathyroid hormone. Leads to bone pain, tenderness, and increased risk of fractures.

Polyuria: Excretion of large amounts (2 to 6 L/24 hr) of urine, lacking concentration and regulation of waste products. Occurs during diuretic phase of AKI.

Porphyrins: Nitrogen-containing chemical components of hemoglobin.

Purpura: Hemorrhagic state characterized by patches of purplish discoloration, resulting from extravasation of blood into the skin. Purpura does not blanch with pressure.

Pyelonephritis: Infection of the kidney medulla or cortex.

Renal osteodystrophy: Bone disease that occurs when the kidneys fail to maintain the proper levels of calcium and phosphorus in the blood.

Uremia: Toxic clinical syndrome associated with fluid, electrolyte, and hormone imbalances and metabolic abnormalities due to deterioration of renal function and the deleterious effects of azotemia on organ systems.

Care Setting

Primary focus is at the community level, although inpatient acute hospitalization may be required for life-threatening complications.

Related Concerns

Anemias—iron deficiency, anemia of chronic disease, pernicious, aplastic, hemolytic, page 459
Fluid and electrolyte imbalances, page 885
Heart failure: chronic, page 43
Hypertension: severe, page 33
Metabolic acidosis—primary base bicarbonate deficiency, page 450
Psychosocial aspects of care, page 729
Upper gastrointestinal/esophageal bleeding, page 281

Additional associated nursing diagnoses are found in:

Acute kidney injury (acute renal failure), page 505
Renal dialysis—general considerations, page 529
Seizure disorders, page 188

Client Assessment Database

Clients with chronic renal failure may not have any symptoms at all until normal kidney function declines to 20% or less. At that stage, an array of symptoms, such as the following, may appear.

DIAGNOSTIC DIVISION MAY REPORT	MAY EXHIBIT
ACTIVITY/REST • Extreme fatigue, weakness, malaise • Sleep disturbances—insomnia, restlessness, somnolence	Muscle weakness, loss of tone, decreased range of motion (ROM)
CIRCULATION • History of prolonged or severe hypertension • Palpitations, chest pain (angina)	Hypertension, jugular vein distention (JVD) Full or bounding pulses Generalized tissue and pitting edema of feet, legs, and hands Cardiac dysrhythmias, distant heart sounds Pericardial friction rub if uremic pericarditis is present

DIAGNOSTIC DIVISION MAY REPORT (continued)	MAY EXHIBIT (continued)
	Enlargement of liver, spleen, and heart Pallor, bronze-gray, yellow skin Bleeding tendencies
EGO INTEGRITY • Stress factors—financial, relationship • Feelings of helplessness, hopelessness, powerlessness	Denial, anxiety, fear, anger, irritability, personality changes
ELIMINATION • Decreased urinary frequency, oliguria, anuria (advanced failure) • Abdominal bloating, diarrhea, or constipation	Change in urine color—deep yellow, red, brown, cloudy Oliguria, may become anuric
FOOD/FLUID • Rapid weight gain (edema), weight loss (malnutrition) • Anorexia • Heartburn, nausea, vomiting, unpleasant metallic taste in mouth • Use of diuretics	Abdominal distention, ascites, liver enlargement (end-stage) Changes in skin turgor and moisture Edema—generalized, dependent Gum ulcerations; bleeding of gums, tongue Ammonia breath Muscle wasting, decreased subcutaneous fat, debilitated appearance
HYGIENE • Difficulty performing activities of daily living (ADLs)	Thin, dry, brittle nails and hair
NEUROSENSORY • Headache, blurred vision • Muscle cramps or twitching, "restless leg" syndrome, burning numbness of soles of feet • Numbness, tingling, and weakness, especially of lower extremities (peripheral neuropathy)	Altered mental state—continuum of symptoms can be present, depending on stage of disease, such as decreased attention span, inability to concentrate, loss of memory, confusion, decreasing level of consciousness, stupor, coma Gait abnormalities Twitching, muscle fasciculation, seizure activity
PAIN/DISCOMFORT • Flank pain, headache, muscle cramps, or leg pain—worse at night	Guarding, distraction behaviors, restlessness
RESPIRATION • Shortness of breath, sudden nighttime dyspnea • Cough with or without thick, tenacious sputum	Tachypnea, dyspnea, increased rate and depth (Kussmaul's respiration may be associated with metabolic acidosis) Cough productive of pink-tinged sputum (pulmonary edema)
SAFETY • Itching skin, frequent scratching • Recent or recurrent infections • Bleeding tendencies	Scratch marks, petechiae, ecchymotic areas on skin Fever (sepsis, dehydration); normothermia may actually represent an elevation in client who has developed a lower-than-normal body temperature (effect of chronic renal failure [CRF] and depressed immune response) Bone fractures; calcium phosphate deposits (metastatic calcifications) in skin, soft tissues, joints; limited joint movement
SEXUALITY • Decreased libido, amenorrhea, infertility • Erectile dysfunction	
SOCIAL INTERACTION • Difficulties imposed by condition, such as unable to work, maintain social contacts, or usual role function in family	

(continues on page 520)

Client Assessment Database (continued)

DIAGNOSTIC DIVISION MAY REPORT (continued)	MAY EXHIBIT (continued)
TEACHING/LEARNING • Family history of polycystic disease, hereditary nephritis, urinary calculus, malignancy • History of poorly controlled hypertension or diabetes (high risk for renal failure), exposure to toxins, such as nephrotoxic drugs, drug overdose, environmental poisons • Current or recent use of nephrotoxic antibiotics, angiotensin-converting enzyme (ACE) inhibitors, chemotherapy agents, heavy metals, NSAIDs, radiocontrast agents	
DISCHARGE PLAN CONSIDERATIONS • May require alteration or assistance with medications, treatments, supplies; transportation; homemaker or maintenance tasks ➧ Refer to section at end of plan for postdischarge considerations.	

Diagnostic Studies

TEST WHY IT IS DONE	WHAT IT TELLS ME
BLOOD TESTS	
• ***Blood urea nitrogen (BUN):*** Measures the by-product of protein metabolism in the liver, filtered by the kidneys and excreted in urine.	Levels are elevated in chronic kidney disease. ESRD is characterized by marked elevation of BUN.
• ***Creatinine (Cr):*** End product of muscle and protein metabolism filtered by the kidneys and excreted in urine.	Can be quite elevated before symptoms of CRF are present in unmonitored client. Markedly elevated in late stage.
• ***BUN/Cr ratio:*** Ratio helps determine whether factors other than kidney failure are causing changes in numbers. Normal ratio is 10:1.	Ratio is less than 10:1, especially in later stages of CRF. Impaired filtration causes reduced BUN reabsorption, thereby lowering BUN/Cr ratio.
• ***Glomerular filtration rate (GFR):*** Calculated from serum Cr levels and adjusted for mean normal body surface area. GFR is approximately 90 mL/min in the healthy adult.	GFR is used to stage renal failure. Symptoms are typically absent until GFR falls below 60 (stage 3). The client in severe CRF with a GFR between 15 and 29 (stages IV to V) is a candidate for dialysis or transplantation.
• ***Complete blood count (CBC):*** Battery of screening tests, which typically includes hemoglobin (Hgb); hematocrit (Hct); red blood cell (RBC) count, morphology, indices, and distribution width index; platelet count and size; and white blood cell (WBC) count and differential.	Hgb decreases because of anemia, usually less than 7 to 8 g/dL. Anemia develops from decreased renal synthesis of erythropoietin, the hormone responsible for bone marrow stimulation for RBC production. RBC survival is decreased, and bleeding tendency is increased from the uremia-induced platelet dysfunction.
• ***Arterial blood gases (ABGs):*** Determines the pH and the percentage of oxygen, carbon dioxide, and bicarbonate in arterial blood.	Decreased pH. Metabolic acidosis (less than 7.2) occurs because of loss of renal ability to excrete hydrogen and ammonia or end products of protein catabolism. Bicarbonate and PCO_2 decreased.
• ***Electrolytes (renalytes):*** Electrically charged minerals found in body tissues and blood in the form of dissolved salts that help move nutrients into and wastes out of the body's cells, maintain water balance, and stabilize the body's pH level.	
• ***Sodium:*** Helps to evaluate hydration status and progression of renal failure.	May be low if kidney "wastes sodium" or normal, reflecting dilutional state of hypernatremia.
• ***Potassium:*** Fluctuation in levels can create life-threatening situations, affecting therapeutic choices.	Elevated related to retention, with decline in GFR below 20 to 25 mL/min, cellular shifts (acidosis), or tissue release (RBC hemolysis). In ESRD, electrocardiogram (ECG) changes may not occur until potassium is 6.5 mEq or higher. The resulting hyperkalemia poses a life-threatening emergency, which requires

TEST WHY IT IS DONE (continued)	WHAT IT TELLS ME (continued)
	frequent and immediate intervention. *Note*: Potassium may also be decreased if client is on potassium-wasting diuretics or when client is receiving dialysis treatment.
• ***Phosphorus:*** Has a direct impact on parathyroid function and bone health.	As GFR declines, less phosphate is filtered and excreted; however, serum levels may remain normal initially because of increased parathyroid hormone (PTH) secretion and the associated increase in renal excretion of phosphorus. As CRF advances to stages IV and V, serum levels rise and bone complications such as osteitis fibrosa may develop.
• ***Calcium:*** Important in feedback mechanism for inhibiting PTH synthesis and skeletal bone turnover.	Hypocalcemia may become severe as a result of low plasma calcitriol levels impairing intestinal absorption or from calcium binding to elevated serum phosphate levels.
• ***Magnesium:*** Helps maintain normal muscle and nerve function, keeps heart rhythm steady, promotes normal blood pressure, and is known to be involved in energy metabolism and protein synthesis.	In end-stage renal disease, the limited ability of the kidney to excrete an increased magnesium load may result in toxic concentrations in serum. While hypermagnesemia is a hazard when magnesium-containing drugs are given, magnesium balance may be normal or even decreased in many uremic individuals. This is usually due to decreased dietary intake combined with the impaired intestinal magnesium absorption that characterizes chronic renal failure (Mountokalakis, 1990).
• ***Proteins (especially albumin):*** Evaluates nutritional status and predicts mortality in clients receiving dialysis.	Decreased serum level may reflect protein loss via urine, fluid shifts, decreased intake, or decreased synthesis because of malnutrition.
• ***Serum osmolality:*** Measures the amount of chemicals dissolved in the serum. Kidneys excrete or reabsorb water to keep osmolality in range of 285 to 295 mOsm/kg. Chemicals that affect serum osmolality include sodium, chloride, bicarbonate, proteins, and glucose.	Higher than 285 mOsm/kg; often equal to urine.
URINE TESTS	
• ***Volume:*** Reflection of declining renal function, possible development of AKI superimposed on CRF.	Usually less than 400 mL/24 hr (oliguria) or urine is absent (anuria).
• ***Color:*** Changes in color or clarity indicate developing complications.	Abnormally cloudy urine may be caused by pus, bacteria, fat, colloidal particles, phosphates, or urates. Dirty, brown sediment indicates presence of RBCs, Hgb, myoglobin, and porphyrins.
• ***Specific gravity:*** Measures density of urine compared to water, with normal range of 1.005 to 1.030.	Less than 1.015 or fixed at 1.010 reflects severe renal damage.
• ***Protein (albuminuria):*** Dipstick test used as a screening tool to detect glomerular injury (prevalent in persons with diabetes, hypertension, or glomerular disease) that has caused glomeruli to lose selective permeability and leak protein, particularly albumin, which is excreted in the urine.	High-grade persistent proteinuria (3 to 4+) strongly indicates glomerular damage, especially when RBCs and casts are also present. Low-grade proteinuria (1 to 2+) and WBCs may be indicative of infection or interstitial nephritis.
• ***Total protein-Cr (albumin-Cr) ratio:*** Spot urine collection for total protein-to-creatinine ratio allows reliable approximation (extrapolation) of total 24-hour urinary protein excretion.	A value greater than 3.0 to 3.5 g is within the nephrotic range; less than 2.0 g is characteristic of tubulointerstitial problems.
• ***Osmolality:*** Measures the ratio of water and solutes, such as electrolytes, acids, and other metabolic wastes, processed by the kidneys and released in urine. When body fluid is balanced, normal urine osmolality is in the range of 300 to 900 mOsm/kg.	Less than 350 mOsm/kg is indicative of tubular damage, and urine/serum ratio is often 1:1.
• ***Cr clearance:*** Calculates GFR by measuring the amount of Cr cleared from the blood and filtered into urine in 24 hours.	Best indicator of overall kidney function, as reduced Cr clearance correlates with increased circulating Cr. May be significantly decreased—less than 80 mL/min in early failure; less than 10 mL/min in ESRD.
• ***Sodium:*** Determines hydration status and ability to conserve or excrete Na.	More than 40 mEq/L because kidney is not able to reabsorb sodium.
• ***Fractional excretion sodium (FeNa):*** Calculated measure of renal tubule function.	Reveals inability of tubules to reabsorb sodium. Readings of less than 1% indicate prerenal problems, whereas higher than 1% reflects intrarenal disorders.

(continues on page 522)

Diagnostic Studies (continued)

TEST WHY IT IS DONE (continued)	WHAT IT TELLS ME (continued)
OTHER DIAGNOSTIC STUDIES	
• *Renal ultrasound:* Imaging technique that uses high-frequency sound waves and a computer to create images of blood vessels, tissues, and organs.	Kidney size can be correlated with certain conditions—large kidney may be present in hyperfiltration, or small, echogenic kidney may be associated with advanced kidney disease. Ultrasound can also document presence of tumors, polycystic disease, or other obstruction in upper urinary system.
• *Computed tomographic (CT) scans:* X-ray procedure that uses a computer to produce a detailed picture of a cross section of the body.	Demonstrates vessel disorders and kidney mass.
• *Kidney, ureter, bladder (KUB) x-ray:* X-ray of the abdomen, showing the kidneys, ureters, and bladder.	Demonstrates size and structure of kidneys, ureters, and bladder; reveals presence of abnormalities, such as cysts, tumors, or stones.
• *Aortorenal angiography:* Fluoroscopic examination, which uses contrast to examine the renal blood vessels for signs of blockage or abnormality.	Assesses renal circulation and identifies extravascularities and masses. *Note:* Contrast media can precipitate renal failure in damaged kidney.
• *Voiding cystourethrogram (VCUG):* Specific x-ray that examines the bladder and urethra while the bladder fills and empties.	Shows bladder size and identifies backflow (reflux) into ureters or retention caused by postrenal obstruction or failure.
• *Renal biopsy:* Percutaneous renal biopsy currently is performed most often with ultrasound guidance.	Biopsy is generally indicated when renal impairment or proteinuria approaching the nephrotic range is present and diagnosis is still unclear.

Nursing Priorities

1. Maintain homeostasis.
2. Prevent complications.
3. Provide information about disease process, prognosis, and treatment needs.
4. Support adjustment to lifestyle changes.

Discharge Goals

1. Fluid and electrolyte balance stabilized.
2. Complications prevented or minimized.
3. Disease process, prognosis, and therapeutic regimen understood.
4. Dealing realistically with situation and initiating necessary lifestyle changes.
5. Plan in place to meet needs after discharge.

NURSING DIAGNOSIS: risk for decreased Cardiac Output

Risk Factors May Include

Altered afterload—increased SVR
Altered preload—venous distention
Altered heart rate, rhythm

Possibly Evidenced By

(Not applicable; presence of signs and symptoms establishes an *actual* diagnosis)

Desired Outcomes/Evaluation Criteria—Client Will

Cardiac Pump Effectiveness (NOC)

Maintain cardiac output as evidenced by blood pressure (BP) and heart rate within client's normal range; peripheral pulses strong and equal with prompt capillary refill time.

In addition to interventions here, refer to CP: Acute Kidney Injury; ND: risk for decreased Cardiac Output.

ACTIONS/INTERVENTIONS	RATIONALE
Hemodynamic Regulation (NIC) ***Independent***	
Auscultate heart and lung sounds. Evaluate presence of peripheral edema, vascular congestion, and reports of dyspnea.	S_3/S_4 heart sounds with muffled tones, tachycardia, irregular heart rate, tachypnea, dyspnea, crackles, wheezes, and edema or jugular distention suggest heart failure (HF).

ACTIONS/INTERVENTIONS (continued)	RATIONALE (continued)
Assess presence and degree of hypertension: Monitor BP and note postural changes, such as sitting, lying, and standing.	Significant hypertension can occur because of disturbances in the renin-angiotensin-aldosterone system caused by renal dysfunction. Although hypertension is common, orthostatic hypotension may occur because of intravascular fluid deficit, response to effects of antihypertensive medications, or uremic pericardial tamponade.
Investigate reports of chest pain, noting location, radiation, severity (0 to 10 or similar scale), and whether or not it is intensified by deep inspiration and supine position.	Although myocardial infarction (MI) is common, approximately half of CRF clients on dialysis develop pericarditis, potentiating risk of pericardial effusion and tamponade.
Evaluate heart sounds for friction rub, BP, peripheral pulses, JVD, capillary refill, and mentation.	Presence of sudden hypotension (along with paradoxical pulse, narrow pulse pressure, diminished or absent peripheral pulses, marked JVD, pallor, and a rapid mental deterioration) can indicate cardiac tamponade, a medical emergency.
Assess activity level and response to activity.	Weakness can be attributed to heart failure and anemia.
Collaborative	
Monitor laboratory and diagnostic studies, such as the following:	
Electrolytes—potassium, sodium, calcium, magnesium; BUN/Cr	Imbalances can alter electrical conduction and cardiac function.
Chest x-rays	Useful in identifying developing cardiac failure and response to therapies.
Collaborate in treatment of underlying disease or conditions, where possible.	Halting progression of CRF in early stages can be aided by interventions, such as controlling BP, managing diabetes, treating hyperlipidemia, and avoiding toxins such as NSAIDs, intravenous (IV) contrast dye, aminoglycosides.
Administer medications, as indicated, for example:	Aggressive treatment of hypertension is needed to reduce SVR or renin release to decrease myocardial workload and aid in prevention of HF and MI.
ACE inhibitors, such as enalapril (Vasotec), or angiotensin receptor blockers (ARBs), such as irbesartan (Avapro) and losartan (Cozaar)	These drugs may be prescribed not only to lower the patient's BP but more importantly to protect kidneys from further damage, especially in presence of diabetic nephropathy (Polzein, 2007).
Erythropoietin-stimulating agents (ESAs) such as Epogen, EPO or erythropoietin-stimulating proteins, such as somatropin (Nutropin) or darbepoetin alpha (Aranesp).	May be given to treat anemia associated with CRF when hemoglobin falls below 10 to improve oxygen-carrying capacity of circulating hemoglobin and reduce left ventricular strain.
Administer oxygen, as indicated.	Cardiac function can be improved with use of oxygen if client is severely anemic or metabolic acidosis and electrolyte abnormalities are causing dysrhythmias.
Prepare for renal replacement therapy, such as hemodialysis.	Reduction of uremic toxins and correction of electrolyte imbalances and fluid overload may limit or prevent cardiac manifestations, including hypertension and pericardial effusion.
Assist with pericardiocentesis, as indicated.	Accumulation of fluid within pericardial sac can compromise cardiac filling and myocardial contractility, impairing cardiac output and potentiating risk of cardiac arrest.

NURSING DIAGNOSIS: Activity Intolerance

Risk Factors May Include

Generalized weakness

Imbalance between oxygen supply/demand

Possibly Evidenced By

(Not applicable; presence of signs and symptoms establishes an *actual* diagnosis)

Desired Outcomes/Evaluation Criteria—Client Will

Activity Tolerance (NOC)

Participate in necessary activities free of physiological signs of intolerance (e.g., pulse, respirations, and blood pressure remain within client's normal range).

ACTIONS/INTERVENTIONS	RATIONALE
Energy Management (NIC)	
Independent	
Note reports of increasing fatigue and weakness. Observe for tachycardia, pallor of skin and mucous membranes, dyspnea, and chest pain.	May reflect effects of anemia and cardiac response necessary to keep cells oxygenated.
Monitor level of consciousness (LOC) and behavior.	Anemia may cause cerebral hypoxia manifested by changes in mentation, orientation, and behavioral responses.
Evaluate response to activity and ability to perform tasks. Assist as needed and develop schedule for rest.	Anemia decreases tissue oxygenation and increases fatigue, which may require intervention, changes in activity, and rest.
Collaborative	
Monitor laboratory studies, such a RBCs, Hgb/Hct.	Uremia decreases production of erythropoietin and depresses RBC production and survival time. In CRF, Hgb and Hct are usually low, but tolerated, such as client may not be symptomatic until Hgb is below 7.
Administer fresh blood and packed red cells (PRCs), as indicated.	May be necessary when client is symptomatic with anemia. PRCs are usually given when client is experiencing fluid overload or receiving dialysis treatment. Washed RBCs are used to prevent hyperkalemia associated with stored blood.
Administer medications, as indicated, for example:	
Erythropoietin-stimulating agents such as preparations (Epogen, Procrit)	Stimulates the production and maintenance of RBCs, thus decreasing the need for transfusion. Due to concern about the use of ESAs and increased cardiovascular mortality, clinicians will use the lowest ESA dose possible to reduce the need for transfusion and discontinue the ESA as quickly as possible (Alper, 2012).
Iron preparations, such as folic acid (Folvite) and cyanocobalamin (Rubesol-1000)	Useful in managing symptomatic anemia related to nutritional and dialysis-induced deficits. *Note:* Iron should not be given with phosphate binders because they may decrease iron absorption.

NURSING DIAGNOSIS: risk for Bleeding

Risk Factors May Include

Abnormal blood profile—decreased RBC production and survival, altered clotting factors (suppressed erythropoietin production or secretion)

Possibly Evidenced By

(Not applicable; presence of signs and symptoms establishes an *actual* diagnosis)

Desired Outcomes/Evaluation Criteria—Client Will

Blood Loss Severity (NOC)

Experience no signs and symptoms of bleeding or hemorrhage.
Maintain or demonstrate improvement in laboratory values.

ACTIONS/INTERVENTIONS	RATIONALE
Bleeding Precautions (NIC)	
Independent	
Observe for oozing from venipuncture sites, bleeding or ecchymotic areas following slight trauma, petechiae, and joint swelling or mucous membrane involvement—bleeding gums, recurrent epistaxis, hematemesis, melena, and hazy or red urine.	Bleeding can occur easily because of capillary fragility and altered clotting functions and may worsen anemia.
Test gastrointestinal (GI) secretions and stool for occult blood.	Mucosal changes and altered platelet function due to uremia may result in gastric mucosal erosion and GI hemorrhage.
Provide soft toothbrush and electric razor. Use smallest needle possible and apply prolonged pressure following injections or vascular punctures.	Reduces risk of bleeding and hematoma formation.
Collaborative	
Monitor laboratory studies, such as the following:	
Platelet count, clotting factors	Suppression of platelet formation and inadequate levels of factors III and VIII impair clotting and potentiate risk of bleeding. *Note:* Bleeding may become intractable in ESRD.

ACTIONS/INTERVENTIONS (continued)	RATIONALE (continued)
Prothrombin time (PT) level	Abnormal prothrombin consumption lowers serum levels and impairs clotting.
Administer medications, as indicated, for example:	
Iron preparations, such as folic acid (Folvite) and cyanocobalamin (Rubesol-1000)	Useful in managing symptomatic anemia related to nutritional and dialysis-induced deficits. *Note:* Iron should not be given with phosphate binders because they may decrease iron absorption.
Cimetidine (Tagamet), ranitidine (Zantac), and antacids	May be given prophylactically to reduce or neutralize gastric acid and thereby reduce the risk of GI hemorrhage.
Hemostatics or fibrinolysis inhibitors, such as aminocaproic acid (Amicar)	Inhibits bleeding that does not subside spontaneously or respond to usual treatment.
Stool softeners, such as Colace, and bulk laxative, such as Metamucil	Straining to pass hard-formed stool increases likelihood of mucosal or rectal bleeding.

NURSING DIAGNOSIS: risk for acute Confusion

May Be Related To

Metabolic abnormalities— electrolyte imbalances, increased blood urea nitrogen (BUN)/creatinine, azotemia, decreased hemoglobin

Fluctuations in sleep-wake cycle

Possibly Evidenced By

(Not applicable; presence of signs and symptoms establishes an *actual* diagnosis)

Desired Outcomes/Evaluation Criteria—Client Will

Cognition (NOC)

Maintain or regain optimal level of mentation.

Identify ways to compensate for cognitive impairment and memory deficits.

ACTIONS/INTERVENTIONS	RATIONALE
Reality Orientation (NIC)	
Independent	
Monitor for impairment in thinking ability, memory, and orientation. Note attention span.	Uremic syndrome's effect can begin with minor confusion or irritability and progress to altered personality, inability to assimilate information or participate in care. Awareness of changes provides opportunity for evaluation and intervention.
Ascertain from significant other (SO) client's usual level of mentation.	Provides comparison to evaluate development, progression, or resolution of impairment.
Provide SO with information about client's status.	In presence of encephalopathy some improvement in mentation may be expected with restoration of more normal levels of BUN, electrolytes, and serum pH.
Provide quiet, calm environment and judicious use of TV, radio, and visitation.	Minimizes environmental stimuli to reduce sensory overload and confusion while preventing sensory deprivation.
Reorient to surroundings, person, and so forth. Provide calendars, clocks, and outside window.	Provides clues to aid in maintaining reality.
Present reality concisely and briefly, and do not challenge illogical thinking if present.	Confrontation potentiates defensive reactions and may lead to client mistrust and heightened denial of reality.
Communicate information and instructions in simple, short sentences. Ask direct, yes or no questions. Repeat explanations as necessary.	May aid in reducing confusion when present and increases possibility that communications will be understood and remembered.
Establish a regular schedule for expected activities.	Aids in maintaining reality orientation and may reduce fear and confusion.
Promote adequate rest and undisturbed periods for sleep.	Sleep deprivation may further impair cognitive abilities.
Fluid/Electrolyte Management (NIC)	
Collaborative	
Monitor laboratory studies, such as BUN/Cr, serum electrolytes, glucose level, and ABGs (PO_2, pH).	Correction of imbalances can have profound effects on cognition.
Provide supplemental oxygen (O_2) as indicated.	Correction of hypoxia alone can improve cognition.
Avoid use of barbiturates and opiates.	Drugs normally detoxified in the kidneys will have increased half-life and cumulative effects, worsening confusion.
Prepare for dialysis.	Marked deterioration of thought processes may indicate worsening of azotemia and general condition, requiring prompt intervention to regain homeostasis.

NURSING DIAGNOSIS: risk for impaired Skin Integrity

Risk Factors May Include

Accumulation of toxins in the skin
Impaired circulation (anemia with tissue ischemia), or sensation (peripheral neuropathy)
Changes in skin turgor—edema
Reduced activity, immobility

Possibly Evidenced By

(Not applicable; presence of signs and symptoms establishes an *actual* diagnosis)

Desired Outcomes/Evaluation Criteria—Client Will

Tissue Integrity: Skin and Mucous Membranes (NOC)
Maintain intact skin.

Risk Management (NOC)
Demonstrate behaviors and techniques to prevent skin breakdown or injury.

ACTIONS/INTERVENTIONS	RATIONALE
Skin Surveillance (NIC)	
Independent	
Inspect skin for changes in color, turgor, and vascularity. Note redness and excoriation. Observe for ecchymosis and purpura.	Indicates areas of poor circulation and early breakdown that may lead to decubitus formation and infection.
Monitor fluid intake and hydration of skin and mucous membranes.	Detects presence of dehydration or fluid overload that affects circulation and tissue integrity at the cellular level.
Inspect dependent areas for edema. Elevate legs, as indicated.	Edematous tissues are more prone to breakdown. Elevation promotes venous return, limiting venous stasis and edema formation.
Change position frequently, move client carefully, pad bony prominences with sheepskin, and use elbow and heel protectors.	Decreases pressure on edematous, poorly perfused tissues to reduce ischemia.
Provide soothing skin care, restrict use of soaps, and apply ointments or creams such as lanolin or Aquaphor.	Baking soda and cornstarch baths decrease itching and are less drying than soaps. Lotions and ointments may be desired to relieve dry, cracked skin.
Keep linens dry and wrinkle-free.	Reduces dermal irritation and risk of skin breakdown.
Investigate reports of itching.	Although dialysis has largely eliminated skin problems associated with uremic frost, itching can occur because the skin is an excretory route for waste products, such as phosphate crystals associated with hyperparathyroidism in ESRD.
Recommend client use cool, moist compresses to apply pressure to, rather than scratch, pruritic areas. Keep fingernails short; encourage use of gloves during sleep, add vinegar (acetic acid) to bath water, as needed.	Alleviates discomfort and reduces risk of dermal injury.
Suggest wearing loose-fitting cotton garments.	Prevents direct dermal irritation and promotes evaporation of moisture on the skin.
Collaborative	
Provide foam or flotation mattress.	Reduces prolonged pressure on tissues, which can limit cellular perfusion, potentiating ischemia and necrosis.

NURSING DIAGNOSIS: risk for impaired Oral Mucous Membrane

Risk Factors May Include

Decreased salivation, fluid restrictions
Chemical irritation (conversion of urea in saliva to ammonia)

Possibly Evidenced By

(Not applicable; presence of signs and symptoms establishes an *actual* diagnosis)

Desired Outcomes/Evaluation Criteria—Client Will

Oral Health (NOC)
Maintain integrity of mucous membranes.

Risk Control (NOC)
Identify and initiate specific interventions to promote healthy oral mucosa.

ACTIONS/INTERVENTIONS	RATIONALE
Oral Health Maintenance (NIC)	
Independent	
Inspect oral cavity: note moistness, character of saliva, presence of inflammation, ulcerations, and leukoplakia.	Provides opportunity for prompt intervention and prevention of infection.
Provide fluids throughout 24-hour period within prescribed limit.	Prevents excessive oral dryness from prolonged period without oral intake.
Offer frequent mouth care or rinse with 0.25% acetic acid solution. Provide gum, hard candy, or breath mints between meals.	Mucous membranes may become dry and cracked. Mouth care soothes, lubricates, and helps freshen mouth taste, which is often unpleasant because of uremia and restricted oral intake. Rinsing with acetic acid helps neutralize ammonia formed by conversion of urea.
Encourage good dental hygiene after meals and at bedtime. Recommend avoidance of dental floss.	Reduces bacterial growth and potential for infection. Dental floss may cut gums, potentiating bleeding.
Recommend client stop smoking and avoid lemon and glycerin products or mouthwash containing alcohol.	These substances are irritating to the mucosa and have a drying effect, potentiating discomfort.
Provide artificial saliva as needed, such as Ora-Lube.	Prevents dryness, buffers acids, and promotes comfort.

NURSING DIAGNOSIS: ineffective Self-Health Management

May Be Related To
Complexity of therapeutic regimen; complexity of healthcare system
Economic difficulties
Perceived barriers; powerlessness
Social support deficit

Possibly Evidenced By
Reports difficulty with prescribed regimen
Reports desire to manage the illness
Ineffective choices in daily living for meeting health goals
Unexpected acceleration of illness symptoms

Desired Outcomes/Evaluation Criteria—Client Will

Self-Management: Kidney Disease (NOC)
Verbalize understanding of condition, disease process, and potential complications.
Verbalize understanding of therapeutic needs.
Correctly perform necessary procedures and explain reasons for the actions.
Demonstrate and initiate necessary lifestyle changes.
Participate in treatment regimen.

In addition to interventions here, refer to interventions outlined in CP: Acute Kidney Injury, ND: deficient Knowledge.

ACTIONS/INTERVENTIONS	RATIONALE
Teaching: Disease Process (NIC)	
Independent	
Review disease process, prognosis, and future expectations. Educate regarding natural disease progression, different dialysis modalities, renal transplantation, and client's option to refuse or discontinue chronic dialysis.	Provides knowledge base from which client can make informed choices. Kidney failure choices depend on stage of disease and include doing no treatment, hemodialysis, peritoneal dialysis, and kidney transplantation. No matter which option is chosen, the client faces many lifestyle changes, including a complicated treatment plan involving several medications, diet and exercise modification, and appointments with numerous healthcare providers. *Note:* Client at stage 4 must be evaluated and prepared for renal replacement therapy—dialysis or transplantation.
Address client's and SO's feelings, concerns, and methods of dealing with situation. Offer compassionate listening and honest answers to questions. Refer to appropriate support resources.	Common reactions to diagnosis include disbelief, anxiety, anger at self and others, and mild to severe depression (including suicidal ideation). (Refer to CP: Psychosocial Aspects of Care; ND: risk for self-/other-directed Violence.)

(continues on page 528)

ACTIONS/INTERVENTIONS (continued)	RATIONALE (continued)
Review dietary modifications or restrictions, including the following:	
Phosphorus—milk, cheese, carbonated drinks, processed foods, poultry, corn, and peanuts	Dietary restrictions to control serum phosphorus, which are routinely recommended, are usually associated with a reduction in protein intake. This may lead to protein-energy wasting and poor survival. A better solution may be the use of specific nutritional supplements high in energy and protein content but low in phosphorus (González-Parra, 2012).
Fluid, potassium, and sodium restrictions, when indicated	If fluid retention is a problem, client may need to restrict intake of fluid, such as previous day's output plus 500 mL for insensible losses, and restrict dietary potassium and sodium as prescribed. If fluid overload is present, diuretic therapy or dialysis will be part of the regimen. (Refer to CP: Acute Kidney Injury, ND: excess Fluid Volume.)
Discuss other nutritional concerns such as regulating protein intake according to level of renal function—generally 0.6 to 0.7 g/kg of body weight per day of good-quality protein, such as meat, chicken, fish, and eggs.	Metabolites that accumulate in blood derive almost entirely from protein catabolism; as renal function declines, proteins may be restricted proportionately. Too little protein can result in malnutrition. *Note:* Client on dialysis may not need to be as vigilant with protein intake.
Encourage adequate calorie intake, especially from carbohydrates in the nondiabetic client.	Spares protein, prevents wasting, and provides energy. *Note:* Use of special glucose polymer powders can add calories to enhance energy level without extra food or fluid intake.
Discuss drug therapy, including use of vitamin D, calcium supplements, and phosphate binders, such as calcium acetate (PhosLo), calcitriol (Caltrate), sevelamer (Renegel), and avoidance of magnesium antacids (Mylanta, Maalox, Gelusil).	Prevents serious complications, such as reducing phosphate absorption from the GI tract and supplying calcium to maintain normal serum levels, reducing risk of bone demineralization and fractures and tetany; however, use of aluminum-containing products should be monitored because accumulation in the bones potentiates osteodystrophy. Magnesium-containing products potentiate hypermagnesemia, which is already present late in chronic kidney disease, and carries the risk of causing neurological problems (e.g., seizures). *Note:* Supplemental vitamin D may be required to facilitate calcium absorption.
Emphasize importance of reading all product labels—drugs and foods—and not taking medications (including over-the-counter products) without prior approval of healthcare provider.	It is difficult to maintain electrolyte balance when exogenous intake is not factored into dietary restrictions; for example, hypercalcemia can result from routine supplement use in combination with increased dietary intake of calcium-fortified foods and medications containing calcium.
Instruct in or review BP or glucose monitoring at home and provide information on obtaining monitoring equipment, as indicated.	Because hypertension and poor glycemic control are high risk factors in kidney disease progression, self-monitoring and management are important. Also, hypertension is worsened by CRF, often requiring management with antihypertensive drugs, necessitating close observation of treatment effects, such as vascular response to medication.
Emphasize need for smoking cessation, if client smokes. Refer for nicotine medications and support resources.	Smoking increases renal vasoconstriction and exacerbates hypertension.
Review strategies to prevent constipation, including stool softeners, such as Colace, and bulk laxatives, such as Metamucil, but avoiding magnesium products (milk of magnesia).	Reduced fluid intake, changes in dietary pattern, and use of phosphate-binding products often result in constipation that is not responsive to nonmedical interventions. Use of products containing magnesium increases risk of hypermagnesemia.
Review measures to prevent bleeding or hemorrhage, such as use of soft toothbrush, electric razor, avoidance of constipation, forceful blowing of nose, strenuous exercise, or contact sports.	Reduces risks related to alteration of clotting factors and decreased platelet count.
Caution against exposure to external temperature extremes.	Peripheral neuropathy may develop, especially in lower extremities, because of effects of uremia and electrolyte/acid-base imbalances impairing peripheral sensation and potentiating risk of tissue injury.
Discuss role of fatigue in client's daily or desired activities. Advise establishing a routine exercise program within limits of individual ability and rest periods with activities. Instruct in energy conservation techniques.	Fatigue due to anemia, sleep disturbances, malnutrition, and failure of kidneys to clear toxins can greatly reduce client's tolerance for activity. At the same time, exercise is needed to maintain muscle tone and joint flexibility; reduces risks associated with immobility including bone demineralization.
Address sexual concerns.	Physiological effects of uremia and antihypertensive therapy may impair sexual desire and performance.

ACTIONS/INTERVENTIONS (continued)	RATIONALE (continued)
Identify available resources such as nephrologist, nutritionist, and other specialists, as indicated. Stress necessity of medical and laboratory follow-up.	Close monitoring of renal function and electrolyte balance is necessary to adjust dietary prescription, treatment, and to make decisions about possible options such as dialysis or transplantation.
Discuss quality of life concerns, such as pros and cons of each treatment option, refusing or withdrawing dialysis, medical care advance directives, and durable power of attorney.	When kidney failure is chronic or end-stage, client and SO may want to discuss issues with others, such as family, social worker, religious counselor, and should have the opportunity to receive information to make informed choices.
Identify signs and symptoms requiring immediate medical evaluation, such as the following:	
Low-grade fever, chills, changes in characteristics of urine or sputum, tissue swelling or drainage, and oral ulcerations	Depressed immune system, anemia, and malnutrition all contribute to increased risk of infection.
Numbness or tingling of digits, abdominal and muscle cramps, carpopedal spasms, and pain and tenderness in extremities	Uremia and decreased absorption of calcium may lead to peripheral neuropathies. *Note:* Client is also at risk for development of thrombophlebitic complications.
Joint swelling or tenderness, decreased ROM, and reduced muscle strength	Hyperphosphatemia with corresponding calcium shifts from the bone may result in deposition of the excess calcium phosphate as calcifications in joints and soft tissues. Symptoms of skeletal involvement are often noted before impairment in organ function is evident.
Headaches, blurred vision, periorbital or sacral edema, and red eyes	Suggestive of development and poor control of hypertension and changes in eyes caused by calcium.
Provide client and family information resources, such as books, articles, and informational Web sites; the National Kidney Foundation; and the American Association of Kidney Patients.	Offers client and SO opportunity to obtain information, support, and sources of funding.

POTENTIAL CONSIDERATIONS following acute hospitalization (dependent on client's age, physical condition and presence of complications, personal resources, and life responsibilities)

- ***excess Fluid Volume***—compromised regulatory mechanism
- ***Fatigue***—disease state, malnutrition, anemia, stress, depression
- ***ineffective Self-Health Management***—complexity of therapeutic regimen, decisional conflicts (e.g., client value system, health beliefs, cultural influences), powerlessness, economic difficulties, family conflict, social support deficit
- ***Hopelessness***—deteriorating physiological condition, long-term stress, prolonged activity limitations,

RENAL DIALYSIS—GENERAL CONSIDERATIONS

I. Procedure

a. Process that substitutes for kidney function by removing excess fluid and accumulated endogenous or exogenous toxins

b. Type of fluid and solute removal depends on the client's underlying pathophysiology, current hemodynamic status, vascular access, availability of equipment and resources, and healthcare providers' training.

II. Indications

a. Treatment for acute kidney injury (AKI) or chronic end-stage renal disease (ESRD)

b. Emergency removal of toxins due to drug overdose, acute life-threatening hyperkalemia, severe acidosis, and uremia

III. Types

a. Choice of dialysis is determined by three main factors:

i. Type of renal failure (acute or chronic)

ii. Client's particular physical condition

iii. Access to dialysis resources

b. Two primary types of dialysis

i. Hemodialysis (HD)

1. Requires placement of a venous access and a machine removing the blood from the body, running it through a dialyzer, and then returning it to the body
2. Conventional HD may be done three times a week over 3 to 4 hours, either at a facility or in the home; or, daily dialysis may be done during the day or night hours (nocturnal dialysis).

ii. Peritoneal dialysis (PD)

1. Requires a surgically placed abdominal catheter for infusing dialysate fluid into the peritoneal cavity for a predetermined dwell time and then draining it out
2. Procedure may be carried out at home through gravity system or automated pump.

IV. Statistics (National Kidney and Urologic Diseases Information Clearinghouse [NKUDIC], 2012; U.S. Renal Data System [USRDS], 2012)

a. Morbidity: In 2012, 114,083 individuals with ESRD reportedly received dialysis in the United States, with 105,900 receiving HD and approximately 8,100 receiving PD. An additional 2,863 received transplants as the initial mode of therapy (USRDS, 2012).

b. Mortality: Major causes of death associated are cardiovascular disease, infection, and withdrawal of dialysis (USRDS, 2012). The death rate in 2008 for persons on

(continues on page 530)

dialysis was reportedly 20% (NKUDIC, 2012). However, the adjusted probability of survival data for 2009 of clients receiving dialysis at 1 year is 91.4%; at 2 years, 87.5%; at 5 years,71.1%; and at 10 years, 42.7% (USRDS, 2012).

c. Costs: In 2010, Medicare payments for outpatient HD and PD were approximately $4.8 billion; inpatient costs were an added $79 million. Per patient per year costs for all dialysis patients averaged $86,600 (USRDS, 2012).

GLOSSARY

Access: Point on the body where a needle or catheter is inserted to gain entry to the bloodstream. Arteriovenous (AV) access is via graft, fistula, or central vein line.

AV fistula: Vascular access is made by joining an artery to a vein under the skin to make a bigger blood vessel.

AV graft: Soft plastic tube to join an artery and a vein under the skin.

Dialysate: Fluid used in both PD and HD that cleanses the blood and replaces needed electrolytes.

Disequilibrium syndrome: Nausea, vomiting, and hypertension, occasionally with convulsions, which develops within several hours after starting HD for renal failure; it is apparently caused by too rapid removal of urea from the extracellular fluid (ECF) compartment, with movement of water into cells and cerebral edema.

Dry weight: The lowest weight a patient can tolerate without the development of symptoms or hypotension. Because physiological dry weight is that weight resulting from normal renal function, vascular permeability, serum protein concentration, and body volume regulation, dry weight in HD should, theoretically, be lower.

Intradialytic parenteral nutrition (IDPN): Involves infusing hyperalimentation fluids during the time of dialysis—through the vascular shunt or intraperitoneally—to normalize the amounts of albumin, glucose, and other nutrients in the bloodstream and to decrease the associated morbidity and mortality associated with protein-calorie malnutrition.

Ultrafiltration: Blood management method that removes noncellular water and low-molecular-weight solutes from anticoagulated blood through an extracorporeal (external from the body) filter.

Care Setting

Primary focus is at the community level at the dialysis center, although inpatient acute stay may be required during initiation of therapy.

Related Concerns

Anemias—iron deficiency, anemia of chronic disease, pernicious, aplastic, hemolytic, page 459

Heart failure: chronic, page 43

Peritonitis, page 320

Psychosocial aspects of care, page 729

Sepsis/septicemia, page 665

Total nutritional support: parenteral/enteral feeding, page 437

Transplantation considerations—postoperative and lifelong, page 719

Client Assessment Database

Refer to CPs: Acute Kidney Injury and/or Renal Failure: Chronic, for assessment information.

DIAGNOSTIC DIVISION MAY REPORT	MAY EXHIBIT
Discharge Plan Considerations • May require assistance with treatment regimen, transportation, activities of daily living (ADLs), homemaker and maintenance tasks, end-of life decisions, palliative care. ➧ Refer to section at end of plan for postdischarge considerations.	

Diagnostic Studies

Studies and results are variable, depending on reason for dialysis, for example, removal of excess fluid or toxins and drugs, degree of renal involvement, and client considerations, such as distance from treatment center, cognition, available support, and insurance options.

Nursing Priorities

1. Promote homeostasis and general well-being.
2. Maintain comfort.
3. Prevent complications.
4. Support client independence and self-care.
5. Provide information about disease process, prognosis, and treatment needs.

Discharge Goals

1. Fluid and electrolyte balance maximized.
2. Complications prevented or minimized.
3. Discomfort alleviated.
4. Dealing realistically with current situation; independent within limits of condition.
5. Disease process, prognosis, and therapeutic regimen understood.
6. Plan in place to meet needs after discharge.

This section addresses the general nursing management issues of client receiving some form of dialysis.

NURSING DIAGNOSIS: imbalanced Nutrition: less than body requirements

May Be Related To

Inability to ingest/digest food (result of uremia or medication side effects; loss of peptides and amino acids; abdominal distention during continuous ambulatory peritoneal dialysis [CAPD])

Possibly Evidenced By

Reports food intake less than recommended; satiety immediately after ingesting food
Lack of interest in food, aversion to eating, reported altered taste sensation
Poor muscle tone
Sore, buccal cavity; pale mucous membranes

Desired Outcomes/Evaluation Criteria—Client Will

Nutritional Status (NOC)

Demonstrate stable weight or gain toward goal with normalization of laboratory values and no signs of malnutrition.

ACTIONS/INTERVENTIONS	RATIONALE
Nutrition Therapy (NIC)	
Independent	
Monitor food and fluid ingested and calculate daily caloric intake.	Identifies nutritional deficits and therapy needs, which are extremely variable, depending on client's age, stage of renal disease, other coexisting conditions, and the type of dialysis being planned.
Recommend client/significant other (SO) keep a food diary, including estimation of ingested calories, protein, and electrolytes of individual concern—sodium, potassium, chloride, magnesium, and phosphorus.	Helps client realize "big picture" and allows opportunity to alter dietary choices to meet individual desires within identified restriction.
Note presence of nausea and anorexia.	Symptoms accompany accumulation of endogenous toxins that can alter or reduce intake and require intervention.
Encourage client to participate in menu planning.	May enhance oral intake and promote sense of control.
Recommend small, frequent meals. Schedule meals according to dialysis needs.	Smaller portions may enhance intake. Type of dialysis influences meal patterns; for instance, clients receiving HD might not be fed directly before or during procedure because this can alter fluid removal, and clients undergoing PD may be unable to ingest food while abdomen is distended with dialysate.
Encourage use of herbs and spices such as garlic, onion, pepper, parsley, cilantro, and lemon.	Adds zest to food to help reduce boredom with diet, while reducing potential for ingesting too much potassium and sodium.
Suggest socialization during meals.	Provides diversion and promotes social aspects of eating.
Encourage frequent mouth care.	Reduces discomfort of oral stomatitis and metallic taste in mouth associated with uremia, which can interfere with food intake.
Collaborative	
Refer to nutritionist or dietitian to develop diet appropriate to client's needs.	It will be necessary to develop a highly individual dietary program to meet cultural and lifestyle needs within specific kilocalorie and protein restrictions while controlling phosphorus, sodium, and potassium. Nutrition-related concerns include maintenance of acceptable weight and

(continues on page 532)

ACTIONS/INTERVENTIONS (continued)	RATIONALE (continued)
	serum proteins, prevention of renal osteodystrophy (defective bone development), and reduction of cardiovascular risks associated with protein energy malnutrition, electrolyte and micronutrient deficiencies (Mailloux, 2013).
Perform complete nutrition assessment, consisting of laboratory measures (e.g., albumin), comparison of initial weight with both usual body weight and percent of ideal body weight, subjective global assessment (SGA), and review of food diaries using appropriate anthropometric and nutrition studies.	Assesses need and adequacy of nutrient utilization by measuring changes that may suggest presence or absence of tissue catabolism. Malnutrition is often present to some degree in any client with severe or chronic kidney disease. *Note:* Studies have shown that the presence of malnutrition prior to initiation of dialysis is strongly predictive of increased mortality (Chung, 2000).
Provide a balanced diet of complex carbohydrates and prescribed calories and high-quality protein.	Provides sufficient nutrients to improve energy and prevent muscle wasting (catabolism); promotes tissue regeneration and healing and electrolyte balance. Although client with kidney disease is often advised to limit protein intake, that changes with the start of dialysis. The recommended dietary protein intake for a clinically stable maintenance hemodialysis client is 1.2 g/kg body weight/d, and 1.2 to 1.3 g/kg body weight/d for individuals on peritoneal dialysis, 50% of which should come from sources high in biological value (NKF, 2000). Protein-rich foods, such as fresh meats, poultry, fish and other seafood, eggs and egg whites, and small servings of dairy products are needed for building muscles, repairing tissue, and fighting infection. However, some protein-rich foods may contain a high level of phosphorus, so a dietitian's input is essential in determining the right amount to eat (Paton, 2007).
Restrict sodium (usually to 2 g or less/day) and potassium as indicated; for example, avoid bacon, ham, other processed meats and foods, orange juice, and tomato soup.	These electrolytes can quickly accumulate, causing fluid retention, weakness, and potentially lethal cardiac dysrhythmias. *Note:* PD is not as effective in lowering elevated sodium level, necessitating tighter control of sodium intake.
Administer multivitamins, including folic acid; vitamins B_6, C, and D; and iron supplements, as indicated.	Replaces vitamin and mineral deficits resulting from malnutrition, anemia, or loss during dialysis.
Administer parenteral supplements, as indicated, or interdialytic parenteral nutrition (IDPN), as necessary.	Parenteral nutrition may be given to enhance renal tubular regeneration and resolution of underlying disease process (if that is possible); or to provide nutrients if oral or enteral feeding is contraindicated. IDPN may be required when parenteral route is also unavailable or contraindicated. *Note*: Recent treatment guidelines and reimbursement schedules indicate that IDPN should be limited to those dialysis clients with weight loss more than 10% of usual body weight within the last 6 months and with a serum albumin less than 3.4 g/dL, and only after aggressive attempts at enteral feeding (Corbello, 2009).
Monitor laboratory studies, for example:	
Serum protein, prealbumin or albumin levels	Indicators of protein needs. *Note:* PD is associated with significant protein loss. Serum albumin levels consistently below 3.4 g/dL suggest need for parenteral nutrition.
Hemoglobin (Hgb), red blood cell (RBC), and iron levels	Anemia is the most pervasive complication affecting energy levels in ESRD.
Administer medications, as appropriate, for example:	
Antiemetics, such as prochlorperazine (Compazine)	Reduces stimulation of the vomiting center.
Histamine blockers, such as famotidine (Pepcid)	Gastric distress is common and may be a neuropathy-induced gastric paresis. Hypersecretion can cause persistent gastric distress and digestive dysfunction.
Hormones and supplements as indicated, such as erythropoietin (EPO, Epogen) and iron infusions or oral supplements such as iron polysaccharide (Niferex)	Although EPO is given to increase numbers of RBCs, it is not effective without iron supplementation. Niferex is preferred because it can be given once daily and has fewer side effects than many iron preparations.
Insert and maintain nasogastric (NG) or enteral feeding tube, if indicated.	May be necessary when persistent vomiting occurs or when enteral feeding is desired.

NURSING DIAGNOSIS: risk for impaired Skin Integrity

May Be Related To
Changes in skin turgor; [edema]
Imbalanced nutritional state
Impaired circulation/sensation
Physical immobilization—lengthy dialysis procedure
Chemical substance (e.g., urea)

Possibly Evidenced By
(Not applicable; presence of signs and symptoms establishes an *actual* diagnosis)

Desired Outcomes/Evaluation Criteria—Client Will

Tissue Integrity: Skin & Mucous Membranes (NOC)
Maintain structural intactness of epidermis and dermis.

Risk Control (NOC)
Engage in techniques to promote healthy skin.

ACTIONS/INTERVENTIONS	RATIONALE
Skin Surveillance (NIC)	
Independent	
Assess activity limitations, noting presence and degree of restriction or ability.	Influences choice of interventions. *Note*: Fear of or real danger of dislodging dialysis lines or catheter may cause client to be reluctant to initiate movement.
Encourage frequent change of position when on bedrest or chair rest; support affected body parts and joints with pillows, rolls, sheepskin, and elbow and heel pads, as indicated.	Decreases discomfort, maintains muscle strength and joint mobility, enhances circulation, and prevents skin breakdown.
Provide gentle massage. Keep skin clean and dry. Keep linens dry and wrinkle-free.	Stimulates circulation and reduces skin irritation. May be of special importance in client with uremic pruritus, which is generalized and especially bothersome when it affects the back (Barnard, 1994).
Instruct in and assist with active and passive range-of-motion (ROM) exercises.	Promotes circulation, maintains joint flexibility, prevents contractures, and aids in reducing muscle tension. *Note:* A high level of phosphorus may cause calcium-phosphorus crystals to build up in the joints, muscles, and other body organs, leading to bone and joint pain. To avoid these risks, client may be prescribed a phosphate binder (Leydig, 2005).
Institute a planned activity or exercise program as appropriate, with client's input.	Increases client's energy and sense of well-being. Studies have shown that regular exercise programs have benefited clients with ESRD, both physically and emotionally. *Note*: Studies indicate that stable ESRD clients have not been shown to have adverse effects from exercise (Goodman, 2004).
Collaborative	
Provide foam, water, or air flotation mattress or soft chair cushion.	Reduces tissue pressure and may enhance circulation, thereby reducing risk of dermal ischemia and breakdown.

NURSING DIAGNOSIS: Self-Care Deficit (specify)

May Be Related To
Weakness, fatigue
Pain, discomfort
Perceptual or cognitive impairment (accumulated toxins)

Possibly Evidenced By
Impaired inability to perform ADLs

Desired Outcomes/Evaluation Criteria—Client Will

Self-Care Status (NOC)
Performs ADLs within level of own ability and constraints of the illness.

ACTIONS/INTERVENTIONS	RATIONALE
Self-Care Assistance (NIC)	
Independent	
Determine client's ability to participate in self-care activities (scale of 0 to 4).	Underlying condition dictates level of deficit, affecting choice of interventions. *Note:* Psychological factors, such as depression, motivation, and degree of support, also have a major impact on the client's abilities.
Provide assistance with activities as necessary.	Meets needs while supporting client participation and independence.
Encourage use of energy-saving techniques: sitting, not standing; using shower chair; and doing tasks in small increments.	Conserves energy, reduces fatigue, and enhances client's ability to perform tasks.
Recommend scheduling activities to allow client sufficient time to accomplish tasks to fullest extent of ability.	Unhurried approach reduces frustration and promotes client participation, enhancing self-esteem.

NURSING DIAGNOSIS: risk for Constipation

Risk Factors May Include

Change in usual foods or eating pattern; insufficient food/fluid intake
Decreased motility of gastrointestinal tract
Electrolyte imbalances

Possibly Evidenced By

(Not applicable; presence of signs and symptoms establishes an *actual* diagnosis)

Desired Outcomes/Evaluation Criteria—Client Will

Bowel Elimination (NOC)

Maintain usual or improved bowel function.

ACTIONS/INTERVENTIONS	RATIONALE
Constipation/Impaction Management (NIC)	
Independent	
Auscultate bowel sounds. Note consistency and frequency of bowel movements (BMs) and presence of abdominal distention.	Decreased bowel sounds, passage of hard-formed or dry stools suggest constipation and requires ongoing intervention to manage.
Review current medication regimen.	Side effects of some drugs, such as iron products and some antacids, may compound problem.
Ascertain usual dietary pattern and food choices.	Although restrictions may be present, thoughtful consideration of menu choices can aid in controlling problem.
Suggest adding fresh fruits, vegetables, and fiber to diet within restrictions, when indicated.	Provides bulk, which improves stool consistency.
Encourage or assist with ambulation, when able.	Activity may stimulate peristalsis, promoting return to normal bowel activity.
Provide privacy at bedside commode and bathroom.	Promotes psychological comfort needed for elimination.
Collaborative	
Administer stool softeners, such as docusate sodium (Colace), or bulk-forming laxatives, such as psyllium (Metamucil), as appropriate.	Produces a softer, more easily evacuated stool.
Keep client nothing by mouth (NPO) status; insert NG tube, as indicated.	Decompresses stomach when recurrent episodes of unrelieved vomiting occur. Large gastric output suggests ileus, a common early complication of PD, with accumulation of gas and intestinal fluid that cannot be passed rectally.

NURSING DIAGNOSIS: risk for acute Confusion

Risk Factors May Include

Metabolic abnormalities—electrolyte imbalances, increased blood urea nitrogen (BUN)/creatinine, azotemia, decreased hemoglobin
Fluctuations in sleep-wake cycle

Possibly Evidenced By

(Not applicable; presence of signs and symptoms establishes an *actual* diagnosis)

Desired Outcomes/Evaluation Criteria—Client Will

Cognition (NOC)

Maintain or regain usual or improved level of mentation.
Recognize changes in thinking and behavior and demonstrate behaviors to prevent or minimize changes.

ACTIONS/INTERVENTIONS	RATIONALE
Delirium Management (NIC)	
Independent	
Assess for behavioral changes or change in level of consciousness (LOC)—disorientation, lethargy, decreased concentration, memory loss, and altered sleep patterns.	May indicate level of uremic toxicity, developing complication of dialysis such as disequilibrium syndrome, and need for further assessment and intervention.
Keep explanations simple and reorient frequently as needed. Provide "normal" day or night lighting patterns, clock, and calendar.	Improves reality orientation.
Provide a safe environment, restrain as indicated, and pad side rails during procedure, as appropriate.	Prevents client trauma and inadvertent removal of dialysis lines or catheter.
Drain peritoneal dialysate promptly at end of specified equilibration period.	Prompt outflow will decrease risk of hyperglycemia or hyperosmolar fluid shifts affecting cerebral function.
Investigate reports of headache, associated with onset of dizziness, nausea and vomiting, confusion or agitation, hypotension, tremors, or seizure activity.	May reflect development of disequilibrium syndrome, which can occur near completion of or following HD and is thought to be caused by ultrafiltration or by the too rapid removal of urea from the bloodstream not accompanied by equivalent removal from brain tissue. The hypertonic cerebrospinal fluid (CSF) causes a fluid shift into the brain, resulting in cerebral edema and increased intracranial pressure.
Monitor changes in speech pattern, development of dementia, and myoclonus activity during HD.	Occasionally, accumulation of aluminum may cause dialysis dementia, progressing to death if untreated.
Collaborative	
Monitor lab studies such as:	
BUN/Cr and serum glucose levels, determine urea reduction ratio (URR)	Follows progression or resolution of azotemia. Pre- and postdialysis BUN levels are used to determine efficacy of procedure. URR 60% to 65% is considered desirable (NKUDIC, update 2012).
Aluminum level, as indicated	Elevation may warn of impending cerebral involvement or dialysis dementia.
Alternate or change dialysate concentrations according to protocol, and add insulin, as indicated.	Hyperglycemia may develop secondary to glucose crossing peritoneal membrane and entering circulation. May require initiation of insulin therapy.
Administer normal saline intravenously (IV), as appropriate.	Volume restoration may be sufficient to reverse effects of disequilibrium syndrome.
Administer medication, as indicated, such as phenytoin (Dilantin), mannitol (Osmitrol), and barbiturates.	If disequilibrium syndrome occurs during dialysis, medication may be needed to control seizures in addition to a change in dialysis prescription or discontinuation of therapy. After the procedure, an osmotic diuresis may be required to reduce cerebral edema, along with anticonvulsant therapy and barbiturates to slow brain metabolism.

NURSING DIAGNOSIS: Anxiety [specify level]

May Be Related To
Situational crisis, threat of death
Change in health status, role functioning, or socioeconomic status

Possibly Evidenced By
Reports concerns due to change in life events
Increased tension, apprehension, uncertainty, fear
Sympathetic stimulation, focus on self

Desired Outcomes/Evaluation Criteria—Client Will

Anxiety Self-Control (NOC)
Verbalize awareness of feelings and reduction of anxiety or fear to a manageable level.
Demonstrate problem-solving skills and effective use of resources.
Appear relaxed and able to rest and sleep appropriately.

ACTIONS/INTERVENTIONS	RATIONALE
Anxiety Reduction (NIC)	
Independent	
Assess level of concern of both client and SO. Note signs of denial, depression, or narrowed focus of attention.	Helps determine the kind of interventions required.
Explain procedures and care as delivered. Repeat explanations frequently, as needed. Provide information in multiple formats, including pamphlets and films.	Fear of unknown is lessened by information and knowledge and may enhance acceptance of permanence of ESRD and necessity for dialysis. Alteration in thought processes and high levels of anxiety or fear may reduce comprehension, requiring repetition of important information. *Note:* Uremia can impair short-term memory, requiring repetition or reinforcement of information provided.
Acknowledge normalcy of feelings in this situation.	Knowing feelings are normal can allay fear that client is losing control.
Provide opportunities for client and SO to ask questions and verbalize concerns.	Creates feeling of openness and cooperation and provides information that will assist in problem identification and solving.
Encourage SO to participate in care, as able and desired.	Involvement promotes sense of sharing, strengthens feelings of usefulness, provides opportunity to acknowledge individual capabilities, and may lessen fear of the unknown.
Acknowledge concerns of client and SO.	Prognosis and possibility of need for long-term dialysis and resultant lifestyle changes are major concerns for this client and those who may be involved in future care.
Point out positive indicators of treatment—improvement in laboratory values, stable BP, and lessened fatigue.	Promotes sense of progress in an otherwise chronic process that seems endless while client still is experiencing physical deterioration and depression.
Collaborative	
Arrange for visit to dialysis center and meeting with another dialysis client, as appropriate.	Interaction with others who have encountered similar problems may assist client and SO to work toward acceptance of chronic condition and focus on problem-solving activities.
Address financial considerations. Refer to appropriate resources.	Treatment for kidney failure is expensive, although Medicare and other health insurance programs pay much of the cost.

NURSING DIAGNOSIS: disturbed Body Image

May Be Related To

Illness, treatment regimen
Cognitive

Possibly Evidenced By

Reports negative feelings about body (e.g., feelings of helplessness, powerlessness)
Focus on past function; preoccupation with change
Reports changes in lifestyle
Extension of body boundary to incorporate environmental objects (i.e., dialysis equipment)

Desired Outcomes/Evaluation Criteria—Client Will

Body Image (NOC)

Identify feelings and methods for coping with negative perception of self.
Verbalize acceptance of body function/change in health status.

Psychosocial Adjustment: Life Change (NOC)

Demonstrate adaptation to changes and events that have occurred, as evidenced by setting realistic goals and active participation in care and life in general.

ACTIONS/INTERVENTIONS	RATIONALE
Body Image Enhancement (NIC)	
Independent	
Assess level of client's knowledge about condition and treatment and anxiety related to current situation.	Identifies extent of problem or concern and necessary interventions.
Discuss meaning of loss and change to client.	Many clients and their families have difficulty dealing with changes in life and role performance as well as the client's loss of ability to control own body.
Note withdrawn behavior, ineffective use of denial, or behaviors indicative of overconcern with body and its functions. Investigate reports of feelings of depersonalization or the bestowing of humanlike qualities on machinery.	Indicators of developing difficulty handling stress of what is happening. *Note:* Client may feel tied to and controlled by the technology central to his or her survival, even to the point of extending body boundary to incorporate dialysis equipment.

ACTIONS/INTERVENTIONS (continued)	RATIONALE (continued)
Assess for use of addictive substances, primarily alcohol, other drugs, and self-destructive or suicidal behavior.	May reflect dysfunctional coping and attempt to handle problems in an ineffective manner.
Determine stage of grieving. Note signs of severe or prolonged depression.	Identification of grief stage client is experiencing provides guide to recognizing and dealing appropriately with behavior as client and SO work to come to terms with loss and limitations associated with condition. Prolonged depression may indicate need for further intervention.
Acknowledge normalcy of feelings.	Recognition that feelings are to be expected helps client accept and deal with them more effectively.
Encourage verbalization of personal and work conflicts that may arise. Actively listen to concerns.	Helps client identify problems and problem-solve solutions. *Note:* Home dialysis may provide more flexibility and enhance sense of control for clients who are appropriate candidates for this form of therapy.
Determine client's role in family constellation and client's perception of expectation of self and others.	Long-term and permanent illness or disability alters client's ability to fulfill usual role(s) in family and work setting. Unrealistic expectations can undermine self-esteem and affect outcome of illness.
Recommend SO treat client normally and not as an invalid.	Conveys expectation that client is able to manage situation and helps maintain sense of self-worth and purpose in life.
Assist client to incorporate disease management into lifestyle.	Necessities of treatment assume a more normal aspect when they are a part of the daily routine.
Identify strengths, past successes, and previous methods client has used to deal with life stressors.	Focusing on these reminders of own ability to deal with problems can help client deal with current situation.
Help client identify areas over which he or she has some measure of control. Provide opportunity to participate in decision-making process.	Provides sense of control over seemingly uncontrollable situation, fostering independence.
Collaborative	
Recommend participation in local support group.	Reduces sense of isolation as client learns that others have been where client is now. Provides role models for dealing with situation, problem-solving, and "getting on with life." Reinforces that therapeutic regimen can be beneficial.
Refer to healthcare and community resources, such as social service, vocational counselor, and psychiatric clinical nurse specialist.	Provides additional assistance for long-term management of chronic illness and change in lifestyle.

NURSING DIAGNOSIS: risk for ineffective Self-Health Management

May Be Related To
Complexity of therapeutic regimen; perceived barriers
Deficient knowledge
Complexity of healthcare system
Economic difficulties
Decisional conflicts; powerlessness

Possibly Evidenced By
(Not applicable; presence of signs and symptoms establishes an *actual* diagnosis)

Desired Outcomes/Evaluation Criteria—Client Will

Self-Management: Kidney Disease (NOC)
Verbalize understanding of condition and relationship of signs and symptoms of the disease process and potential complications.
Verbalize understanding of therapeutic needs.
Correctly perform necessary procedures and explain reasons for actions.

ACTIONS/INTERVENTIONS	RATIONALE
Teaching: Disease Process (NIC)	
Independent	
Note level of anxiety or fear and alteration of thought processes. Time teaching appropriately.	These factors directly affect ability to access and use knowledge. In addition, during the dialysis procedure, client's cognitive function may be impaired, and clients themselves state that they feel "fuzzy." Therefore, learning may not be optimal during this time.

(continues on page 538)

ACTIONS/INTERVENTIONS (continued)	RATIONALE (continued)
Review particular disease process, prognosis, and potential complications in clear concise terms, periodically repeating and updating information, as necessary.	Providing information at the level of the client's and SO's understanding will reduce anxiety and misconceptions about what client is experiencing.
Encourage and provide opportunity for questions.	Enhances learning process, promotes informed decision making, and reduces anxiety associated with the unknown.
Acknowledge that certain feelings and patterns of response are normal during course of therapy.	Client and SO may initially be hopeful and positive about the future, but as treatment continues and progress is less dramatic, they can become discouraged and depressed, and conflicts of dependence versus independence may develop.
Emphasize necessity of reading all product labels—food, beverage, and over-the-counter (OTC) drugs—and not taking medications or herbal supplements without checking with healthcare provider.	It is difficult to maintain electrolyte balance when exogenous intake is not factored into dietary restriction; for example, hypercalcemia can result from routine supplement use in combination with increased dietary intake of calcium-fortified foods and medicines.
Emphasize importance of adhering to medication schedule required for the client's specific form of renal disease, timing of dialysis, and properties of the individual medications.	This is necessary to ensure that therapeutic levels of the drugs are reached and that toxic levels are avoided.
Discuss significance of maintaining nutritious eating habits, preventing wide fluctuation of fluid and electrolyte balance, and avoidance of crowds or people with infectious processes.	Depressed immune system, presence of anemia, invasive procedures, and malnutrition potentiate risk of infection.
Instruct client about epoetin (Epogen) or darbepoetin (Aransep), when indicated. Have client or SO demonstrate ability to administer and state adverse side effects and healthcare practices associated with this therapy.	Epogen is used for the management of the anemia associated with chronic renal failure (CRF) and ESRD. The drug is given to increase and maintain RBC production, which allows client to feel better and stronger. Darbepoetin is a nonnatural recombinant protein that can stimulate RBC production, but the half-life is about three times longer than erythropoietin, resulting in less frequent dosing. Contraindications may include adverse side effects such as polycythemia, increased clotting, failure to administer correctly or have appropriate follow-up.
Identify healthcare and community resources, such as dialysis support group, social services, and mental health clinic.	Knowledge and use of these resources assist client and SO to manage care more effectively. Interaction with others in similar situation provides opportunity for discussion of options and making informed choices, including stopping dialysis or renal transplantation.
Teaching: Procedure/Treatment (NIC)	
Discuss procedures and purpose of dialysis in terms understandable to client. Repeat explanations as required.	A clear understanding of the purpose, process, and what is expected of client and SO facilitates their cooperation with regimen and may enhance outcomes.
Instruct client and SO in home dialysis, as indicated:	Home dialysis is associated with better outcomes in general and better survival rates as dialysis is usually performed 5 to 7 days/week and is more intensive. This decreases fluctuations in fluid, solute, and electrolyte balance, more closely mimicking renal function. However, specific criteria for client and SO participation and training, home resources, and professional oversight must be met in order to consider this option.
Operation and maintenance of equipment (including vascular shunt), sources of supplies	Information diminishes anxiety of the unknown and provides opportunity for client to be knowledgeable about own care.
Aseptic or clean technique	Prevents contamination and reduces risk of infection.
Self-monitoring of effectiveness of procedure	Provides information necessary to evaluate effects of therapy and need for change.
Management of potential complications.	Reduces concerns regarding personal well-being; supports efforts at self-care.
Provide contact information for dialysis support persons.	Readily available support person can answer questions, troubleshoot problems, and facilitate timely medical intervention, when indicated, reducing risk and severity of complications. *Note:* Home dialysis clients usually are monitored by conventional dialysis center or interdisciplinary team.
Identify sources for supplies at home and when away from home.	Home dialysis clients are often capable of travel, even overseas, with proper preplanning and support.

POTENTIAL CONSIDERATIONS following acute hospitalization (dependent on client's age, physical condition and presence of complications, personal resources, and life responsibilities)
- ***Fatigue***—disease state, malnutrition, altered body chemistry, stress, depression
- ***excess Fluid Volume***—compromised regulatory mechanism
- ***risk for Infection***—invasive procedures, decreased hemoglobin, chronic disease, malnutrition
- ***ineffective Self-Health Management***—complexity of therapeutic regimen, economic difficulties, decisional conflicts; excessive demands made on individual and family
- ***risk for Caregiver Role Strain***—illness severity of care receiver, caregiver is spouse, presence of situational stressors, complexity/amount/duration of caregiving required

PERITONEAL DIALYSIS (PD)

I. Procedure

a. Requires a surgically placed abdominal catheter and uses the peritoneum to filter toxins and excess fluid from the body

b. Fluid removal is controlled by adjusting the dextrose concentration in the dialysate (e.g., 1.5%, 2.5%, 4.25%) to create an osmotic gradient for water with higher dextrose concentrations and more frequent exchanges increasing the rate of fluid removal.

c. May be preferred over hemodialysis because it uses a simpler technique and provides more gradual physiological changes

d. Long-term PD typically calls for three to four exchanges a day, each with a dwell time of 4 to 6 hours, and a long (8 to 10 hour) dwell time at night.

II. Types (Advanced Renal Education Program, 2012; National Kidney and Urologic Diseases Information Clearinghouse [NKUDIC], 2010; Sexena, 2006)

a. Continuous ambulatory peritoneal dialysis (CAPD)

i. Most commonly used type of long-term PD, allowing client to manually manage the procedure at home with bag and gravity flow

ii. Some clients experience problems with the long overnight dwell time because, as dextrose in the solution crosses into body, it becomes glucose and starts to draw fluid from the peritoneal cavity back into the body, thereby reducing the efficiency of the exchange and requiring a mini-cycler machine during the night.

b. Automated peritoneal dialysis (APD)

i. Continuous cycler-assisted peritoneal dialysis (CCPD)

1. Uses a machine (cycler) to fill and empty the abdomen three to five times during the night while the person sleeps. In the morning, the last fill remains in the abdomen with a dwell time that lasts the entire day.
2. The dialysis solution used for the long daytime dwell may have a higher concentration of dextrose.
3. May be method of choice for younger individuals engaged in school or work activities

ii. Nocturnal intermittent peritoneal dialysis (NIPD)

1. Usually reserved for individuals with substantial remaining renal function
2. May improve uremia-associated sleep apnea (Perl, 2007)

III. Statistics

a. Morbidity: In 2010, more than 27,500 Americans received PD (National Kidney and Urologic Diseases Information Clearinghouse [NKUDIC], 2012).

b. Mortality: The rate of PD mortality is similar to HD in adjusted 5-year survival rates at 33.5% and 33.9%, respectively. Several recent studies seem to indicate that PD is associated with better survival during the first 1 to 2 years of dialysis, whereas HD is associated with better survival thereafter (Advanced Renal Education Program, 2011; Sexena, 2006).

c. Costs: In 2010, Medicare payments for outpatient PD were approximately $360 million. Per patient per year costs for all PD patients averaged $66,800 (U.S. Renal Data System [USRDS], 2012).

GLOSSARY

Automated peritoneal dialysis (APD): Uses a machine to control the time of exchanges; warm, infuse, and drain the used solution at preset intervals; and fill the peritoneal cavity with new solution.

Continuous ambulatory peritoneal dialysis (CAPD): Uses three to five cycles daily and one long overnight dwell time, 7 days/week.

Continuous cycler-assisted peritoneal dialysis (CCPD): Mechanical device cycles shorter dwell times during the night (three to six cycles) with one 8-hour dwell time during daylight hours, thus increasing the client's independence.

Cycle: The infusion and drainage of a specific volume of peritoneal dialysis solution. The dwell time may vary from a few minutes to several hours.

Cycler: Machine used to infuse and drain dialysate from the peritoneal cavity.

Dialysate (dialysis fluid): A mixture of water, electrolytes, and dextrose. Electrolyte levels in dialysate are proportioned to ensure that the levels in the blood remain within physiological range. Waste products, such as BUN and creatinine, are not present in the dialysate and will readily move out of the blood into the dialysis fluid.

(continues on page 540)

GLOSSARY (continued)

Nocturnal intermittent peritoneal dialysis (NIPD): Similar to CCPD, except the number of overnight exchanges is greater (six to eight) and no exchange is performed during the day.

Peritoneal dialysis (PD): Treatment for both acute kidney injury (AKI) and end-stage renal disease (ESRD) using the peritoneum as the semipermeable membrane permitting transfer of nitrogenous waste products, toxins, and fluid from the blood into a dialysate solution.

Ultrafiltrate: The net amount of fluid resulting when the original volume of the dialysate used for a certain dwell is subtracted from the volume of the drained dialysate (effluent-infused dialysate = ultrafiltrate).

NURSING DIAGNOSIS: risk for excess Fluid Volume

Risk Factors May Include

Compromised regulatory mechanism (e.g., inadequate osmotic gradient of dialysate; fluid retention—malpositioned, kinked, or clotted catheter)

Excess fluid intake—oral (PO) or intravenous (IV)

Possibly Evidenced By

(Not applicable; presence of signs and symptoms establishes an *actual* diagnosis)

Desired Outcomes/Evaluation Criteria—Client Will

Fluid Overload Severity (NOC)

Demonstrate dialysate outflow exceeding or approximating infusion.

Experience no rapid weight gain, edema, or pulmonary congestion.

ACTIONS/INTERVENTIONS	RATIONALE
Peritoneal Dialysis Therapy (NIC)	
Independent	
Maintain a record of inflow and outflow volumes and cumulative fluid balance.	In most cases, the amount drained should equal or exceed the amount instilled. A positive balance with more fluid in than out indicates need for further evaluation.
Record serial weights, compare with intake and output (I&O) balance. Weigh client when abdomen is empty of dialysate, providing a consistent reference point.	Serial body weights are an accurate indicator of fluid volume status. A positive fluid balance with an increase in weight indicates fluid retention.
Assess patency of catheter, noting difficulty in draining. Note presence of fibrin strings or plugs.	Slowing of flow rate or presence of fibrin suggests partial catheter occlusion requiring further evaluation or possible intervention.
Check tubing for kinks; note placement of bags. Anchor catheter so that adequate inflow and outflow is achieved.	Improper functioning of equipment may result in retained fluid in abdomen and insufficient clearance of toxins.
Turn from side to side, elevate the head of the bed, and apply gentle pressure to the abdomen.	May enhance outflow of fluid when catheter is malpositioned or obstructed by the omentum.
Note abdominal distention associated with decreased bowel sounds, changes in stool consistency, and reports of constipation.	Bowel distention or constipation may impede outflow of effluent. (Refer to CP: Renal Dialysis; ND: risk for Constipation.)
Monitor blood pressure (BP) and pulse, noting hypertension, bounding pulses, neck vein distention, and peripheral edema; measure central venous pressure (CVP), if available.	Elevations indicate hypervolemia. Assess heart and breath sounds, noting S_3 and crackles and rhonchi. Fluid overload may potentiate heart failure (HF) or pulmonary edema.
Evaluate development of tachypnea, dyspnea, and increased respiratory effort. Drain dialysate and notify physician.	Abdominal distention or diaphragmatic elevation may cause respiratory distress.
Assess for headache, muscle cramps, mental confusion, and disorientation.	Symptoms suggest hyponatremia or water intoxication.
Collaborative	
Alter dialysate regimen, as indicated.	Changes may be needed in the glucose or sodium concentration to facilitate efficient dialysis.
Monitor serum sodium.	Hypernatremia may be present, although serum levels may reflect dilutional effect of fluid volume overload.
Maintain fluid restriction, as indicated.	Fluid restrictions may have to be continued to decrease fluid volume overload. Between dialysis treatments, fluids accumulate in the body, particularly in the heart, lungs, and ankles. Therefore, most nephrologists recommend restricting fluid to about 1500 mL/day (Leydig, 2005).

NURSING DIAGNOSIS: risk for deficient Fluid Volume

Risk Factors May Include

Loss of fluid through abnormal routes (e.g., use of hypertonic dialysate with excessive removal of fluid)

Possibly Evidenced By

(Not applicable; presence of signs and symptoms establishes an *actual* diagnosis)

Desired Outcomes/Evaluation Criteria—Client Will

Systemic Toxin Clearance: Dialysis (NOC)

Achieve desired alteration in fluid volume and weight with BP and electrolyte levels within acceptable range.

Experience no symptoms of dehydration.

ACTIONS/INTERVENTIONS	RATIONALE
Peritoneal Dialysis Therapy (NIC)	
Independent	
Maintain record of inflow and outflow volumes and individual and cumulative fluid balance.	Provides information about the status of client's loss or gain at the end of each exchange.
Adhere to schedule for draining dialysate from abdomen.	Prolonged dwell times, especially when 4.5% glucose solution is used, may cause excessive fluid loss.
Weigh when abdomen is empty, following initial 6 to 10 runs, then as indicated.	Detects rate of fluid removal by comparison with baseline body weight.
Monitor BP lying and sitting and pulse. Note level of jugular pulsation.	Decreased BP, postural hypotension, and tachycardia are early signs of hypovolemia.
Note reports of dizziness, nausea, and increasing thirst.	May indicate hypovolemia or hyperosmolar syndrome.
Inspect mucous membranes; evaluate skin turgor, peripheral pulses, and capillary refill.	Dry mucous membranes, poor skin turgor, and diminished pulses and capillary refill are indicators of dehydration and need for increased intake or changes in strength of dialysate.
Collaborative	
Monitor laboratory studies, as indicated, such as:	
Serum sodium and glucose levels	Hypertonic solutions may cause hypernatremia by removing more water than sodium. In addition, dextrose may be absorbed from the dialysate, thereby elevating serum glucose.
Serum potassium levels	Hypokalemia may occur and can cause cardiac dysrhythmias.

NURSING DIAGNOSIS: risk for Trauma

Risk Factors May Include

Physical (e.g., catheter inserted into peritoneal cavity, site near the bowel and bladder with potential for perforation during insertion or manipulation of the catheter)

Possibly Evidenced By

(Not applicable; presence of signs and symptoms establishes an *actual* diagnosis)

Desired Outcomes/Evaluation Criteria—Client Will

Risk Control (NOC)

Experience no injury to bowel or bladder.

ACTIONS/INTERVENTIONS	RATIONALE
Peritoneal Dialysis Therapy (NIC)	
Independent	
Have client empty bladder before peritoneal catheter insertion if indwelling catheter not present.	An empty bladder is more distant from insertion site and reduces likelihood of being punctured during catheter insertion.
Anchor catheter and tubing with appropriate connectors and/or tape. Emphasize importance of client avoiding pulling or pushing on catheter.	Reduces risk of trauma by manipulation of the catheter.
Note presence of fecal material in dialysate effluent or strong urge to defecate, accompanied by severe, watery diarrhea.	Suggests bowel perforation with mixing of dialysate and bowel contents. This requires immediate medical intervention as it is a potentially lethal complication including peritonitis, sepsis, and death.

(continues on page 542)

ACTIONS/INTERVENTIONS (continued) / RATIONALE (continued)

Note reports of intense urge to void or large urine output following initiation of dialysis run. Test urine for sugar, as indicated.
— Suggests bladder perforation with dialysate leaking into bladder. Presence of glucose-containing dialysate in the bladder will elevate glucose level of urine.

Stop dialysis if there is evidence of bowel or bladder perforation, leaving peritoneal catheter in place.
— Prompt action will prevent further injury. Immediate surgical repair may be required. Leaving catheter in place facilitates diagnosing and locating the perforation.

NURSING DIAGNOSIS: acute Pain

May Be Related To

Physical agents (e.g., insertion of catheter through abdominal wall, catheter irritation, improper catheter placement; abdominal distention)

Chemical agents (e.g., infusion of cold or acidic dialysate, rapid infusion of dialysate)

Biological agents (e.g., infection within the peritoneal cavity)

Possibly Evidenced By

Verbalization/coded reports of pain

Self-focusing

Guarding behaviors, positioning to avoid pain

Expressive behavior (e.g., restlessness, irritability)

Desired Outcomes/Evaluation Criteria—Client Will

Pain Level (NOC)

Verbalize decrease of pain and discomfort.

Demonstrate relaxed posture and facial expression; be able to sleep and rest appropriately.

ACTIONS/INTERVENTIONS / RATIONALE

Pain Management (NIC)

Independent

Investigate client's reports of pain; note intensity (using 0 to 10 [or similar] scale), location, and precipitating factors.
— Assists in identification of source of pain and appropriate interventions.

Explain that initial discomfort usually subsides after the first few exchanges.
— Information may reduce anxiety and promote relaxation during procedure.

Monitor for pain that begins during inflow and continues during equilibration phase. Slow infusion rate, as indicated.
— Pain will occur if acidic dialysate causes chemical irritation of peritoneal membrane.

Note reports of discomfort that are most pronounced near the end of inflow, and instill no more than 2000 mL of solution at a single time.
— Likely the result of abdominal distention from dialysate. Amount of infusion may have to be decreased initially.

Prevent air from entering peritoneal cavity during infusion. Note report of pain in area of shoulder blade.
— Inadvertent introduction of air into the abdomen irritates the diaphragm and results in referred pain to shoulder blade. This type of discomfort may also be reported during initiation of therapy or during infusions and usually is related to stretching or irritation of the diaphragm with abdominal distention. Smaller exchange volumes may be required until client adjusts.

Elevate head of bed at intervals. Turn client from side to side. Provide back care and tissue massage.
— Position changes and gentle massage may relieve abdominal and general muscle discomfort.

Warm dialysate to body temperature before infusing.
— Warming the solution increases the rate of urea removal by dilating peritoneal vessels. Cold dialysate causes vasoconstriction, which can cause discomfort and excessively lower the core body temperature, precipitating cardiac dysrhythmias.

Monitor for severe or continuous abdominal pain and temperature elevation, especially after dialysis has been discontinued.
— May indicate developing peritonitis. (Refer to ND: risk for Infection, following.)

Encourage use of relaxation techniques, such as deep-breathing exercises, guided imagery, and visualization. Provide diversional activities.
— Redirects attention and promotes sense of control.

Collaborative

Administer analgesics, as indicated.
— Relieves pain and discomfort.

NURSING DIAGNOSIS: risk for Infection

Risk Factors May Include

Inadequate primary defenses—skin contaminants at catheter insertion site, contamination of the catheter during insertion

Increased environmental exposure—periodic changing of tubing and bags; sterile peritonitis (response to the composition of dialysate)

Possibly Evidenced By

(Not applicable; presence of signs and symptoms establishes an *actual* diagnosis)

Desired Outcomes/Evaluation Criteria—Client Will

Risk Control (NOC)

Identify interventions to prevent or reduce risk of infection.

Infection Severity (NOC)

Experience no signs or symptoms of infection.

ACTIONS/INTERVENTIONS	RATIONALE
Infection Protection (NIC)	
Independent	
Observe meticulous aseptic technique and wear masks during catheter insertion, dressing changes, and whenever the system is opened. Change tubing per protocol.	Prevents the introduction of organisms and airborne contamination that may cause infection, the most common complication of PD. Infection can be associated with problems at the exit or skin tunnel sites or multiple disconnections of the transfer tubings during dialysis procedures, as well as impaired host defenses in the peritoneal cavity.
Change dressings as indicated, being careful not to dislodge the catheter. Note character, color, odor, or drainage (if any) from insertion site.	Moist environment promotes bacterial growth. Purulent drainage at insertion site suggests presence of local infection, often involving skin organisms, which can be difficult to treat and sometimes require catheter removal and temporary HD. *Note:* Polyurethane adhesive film (e.g., blister film) dressings have been found to decrease amount of pressure on catheter and exit site as well as incidence of site infections.
Observe color and clarity of effluent fluid.	Cloudy effluent is suggestive of peritoneal infection.
Cleanse the insertion site with antibiotic solutions such as povidone-iodine (Betadine) or chlorhexadine (CHG, Hibiclens) per protocol.	Helps reduce infective agents on the skin.
Cleanse the distal, clamped portion of catheter with CHG prior to reattachment, when intermittent dialysis therapy used.	Reduces risk of bacterial entry through catheter between dialysis treatments when catheter is disconnected from closed system.
Investigate reports of nausea or vomiting, increased or severe abdominal pain, rebound tenderness, or fever.	Signs and symptoms suggesting peritonitis, requiring prompt intervention.
Collaborative	
Monitor white blood cell (WBC) count of effluent.	Presence of WBCs initially may reflect normal response to a foreign substance; however, continued or new elevation of WBCs suggests developing infection.
Obtain specimens of blood, effluent, and drainage from insertion site, as indicated, for culture and sensitivity.	Identifies types of organism(s) present and influences choice of interventions.
Monitor renal blood urea nitrogen (BUN) and creatinine (Cr) clearance.	Choice and dosage of antibiotics are influenced by level of clearance.
Administer broad-spectrum antibiotics (e.g., cephalosporins, vancomycin) in dialysate, as indicated.	Intraperitoneal antibiotics are usually preferred over intravenous, as infection is most often localized and bacteremia is rare (Kontamwar, 2011).

NURSING DIAGNOSIS: risk for ineffective Breathing Pattern

Risk Factors May Include

Body position—abdominal pressure, restricted diaphragmatic excursion, rapid infusion of dialysate

Pain

Possibly Evidenced By

(Not applicable; presence of signs and symptoms establishes an *actual* diagnosis)

(continues on page 544)

NURSING DIAGNOSIS: risk for ineffective Breathing Pattern (continued)

Desired Outcomes/Evaluation Criteria—Client Will

Respiratory Status: Ventilation (NOC)

Display an effective respiratory pattern with clear breath sounds and arterial blood gases (ABGs) within client's normal range.

Experience no signs of dyspnea or cyanosis.

ACTIONS/INTERVENTIONS	RATIONALE
Respiratory Monitoring (NIC)	
Independent	
Monitor respiratory rate and effort. Reduce infusion rate if dyspnea is present.	Tachypnea, dyspnea, shortness of breath, and shallow breathing during dialysis suggest diaphragmatic pressure from distended peritoneal cavity or may indicate developing complications.
Auscultate lungs, noting decreased, absent, or adventitious breath sounds, such as crackles, wheezes, and rhonchi.	Decreased areas of ventilation suggest presence of atelectasis, whereas adventitious sounds may suggest fluid overload, retained secretions, or infection.
Note character, amount, and color of secretions.	Client is susceptible to pulmonary infections as a result of depressed cough reflex and respiratory effort, increased viscosity of secretions, as well as altered immune response and chronic, debilitating disease.
Elevate head of bed or have client sit up in chair. Promote deep-breathing exercises and coughing.	Facilitates chest expansion and ventilation and mobilization of secretions.
Collaborative	
Review ABGs, pulse oximetry, and serial chest x-rays.	Changes in PaO_2 and $PaCO_2$ and appearance of infiltrates and congestion on chest x-ray suggest developing pulmonary problems.
Administer supplemental oxygen, as indicated.	Maximizes oxygen for vascular uptake, thus preventing or lessening hypoxia.
Administer analgesics, as indicated.	Alleviates pain and promotes comfortable breathing and maximal cough effort.

HEMODIALYSIS (HD)

I. Procedure

- **a.** Removal of urea and other toxic products from the bloodstream and correction of fluid and electrolyte imbalances
- **b.** Blood is shunted through an artificial kidney or membrane (dialyzer) for removal of toxins and excess fluid and then returned to the venous circulation.
- **c.** Requires placement of vascular access
  - **i.** Arteriovenous (AV) fistula: usually requires at least 2 to 4 months to heal before it can be used, providing sufficient time so that those involved are prepared and can perform home hemodialysis, if appropriate
  - **ii.** AV graft: may be indicated in presence of small veins, usually ready for use within 2 to 3 weeks
  - **iii.** Temporary access: provides immediate access with insertion of a catheter into a vein in the neck, chest, or groin

II. Types

- **a.** Intermittent HD procedure
  - **i.** Requires permanent AV access, such as primary AV fistula or synthetic graft
  - **ii.** Usually performed three times per week for 3 to 5 hours per procedure, or six to seven times per week for 1.5 to 2 hours
- **b.** Continuous renal replacement therapy (CRRT) (Paton, 2007)
  - **i.** Blood is usually accessed via a central venous catheter.
  - **ii.** Treatment for acute kidney injury (AKI) with fluid and toxins removed at a continuous and slower rate than intermittent HD
  - **iii.** May be indicated for clients with AKI and who are too hemodynamically unstable to tolerate conventional hemodialysis
  - **iv.** Commonly used types of CRRT
    1. Slow continuous ultrafiltration (SCUF)
    2. Continuous venovenous hemofiltration (CVVH) via ultrafiltration and convection
    3. Continuous venovenous hemofiltration (CVVJ)
    4. Continuous venovenous hemodialysis (CVVHD)
    5. Continuous venovenous hemodiafiltration (CVVHDF)

III. Statistics (U.S. Renal Data System [RSRDS], 2012; National Kidney and Urologic Diseases Information Clearinghouse [NKUDIC], 2012)

- **a.** Morbidity: In 2010, an estimated 365,566 Americans received in-center hemodialysis, and 4511 received home dialysis.
- **b.** Mortality: The USRDS reported adjusted death rates for 2010 in the dialysis population to be 294,000, stating that was a drop of 23.7% in death rates since 1995. These figures did not differentiate types of dialysis. This is similar to mortality rates for 2008 published by the NKUDIC (2012).
- **c.** Cost: In 2010, costs averaged $88,000 annually per client; in 2010, Medicare payments for outpatient hemodialysis were approximately $4.4 billion (U.S. Renal Data System [USRDS], 2012).

GLOSSARY

Arteriovenous (AV) fistula: An artery, usually in the forearm, is surgically connected to a vein.

Arteriovenous (AV) graft: A synthetic tube or graft is surgically implanted in the arm connecting an artery and vein.

Continuous renal replacement therapy (CRRT): Continuous 24-hour dialysis therapy, which provides a more normal physiological response by removing plasma water more slowly, thus compensating for the loss of intravascular volume; particularly useful in intensive care setting.

Continuous venovenous hemodiafiltration: Removes fluid and toxins via ultrafiltration and convection using a dialysate to enhance toxin removal and a replacement fluid to help titrate fluid and electrolyte balance.

Continuous venovenous hemodialysis: Removes fluid and toxins via ultrafiltration and convection. A dialysate is added to enhance the removal of toxins via diffusion.

Continuous venovenous hemofiltration: Removes both fluid and toxins via ultrafiltration and convection with a replacement fluid infused to help titrate fluid removal and maintain electrolyte balance.

Slow continuous ultrafiltration (SCUF): Uses ultrafiltration to remove fluid only.

Thrill: Palpable vibration or buzzing sensation caused by turbulence of high-pressure arterial blood flow entering low-pressure venous system, indicating AV shunt is patent.

Venous access: The point on the body where a needle or catheter is inserted to gain entry to the bloodstream. AV access is via graft, fistula, or central venous line.

This plan of care addresses the typical HD procedure usually performed three times per week and carried out in the hospital, community dialysis center, or at home.

NURSING DIAGNOSIS: risk for Injury [loss of vascular access]

Risk Factors May Include

[Clotting, hemorrhage related to accidental disconnection, infection]

Possibly Evidenced By

(Not applicable; presence of signs and symptoms establishes an *actual* diagnosis)

Desired Outcomes/Evaluation Criteria—Client Will

Hemodialysis Access (NOC)

Maintain patent vascular access.
Be free of infection.

ACTIONS/INTERVENTIONS	RATIONALE
Hemodialysis Therapy (NIC)	
Independent	
Clotting	
Assess client's pulse and tissue color distal to shunt.	Determines general circulatory status of limb.
Monitor internal AV fistula or graft patency at frequent intervals:	Clotting (thrombosis) and fistula malfunction are the most common complications (Sofocleous, 2011).
Palpate for thrill.	Should be palpable above venous exit site. If the thrill stops, or even feels different, this could indicate clotting. With early intervention, many clots can be dissolved or removed.
Auscultate for a bruit.	Bruit is the sound caused by the turbulence of arterial blood entering the venous system and should be audible by stethoscope, although may be very faint. If the bruit gets higher in pitch, it could mean narrowing of the blood vessels; if it stops, clot may have formed.
Note color of blood and obvious separation of cells and serum.	Change of color from uniform medium red to dark purplish red suggests sluggish blood flow and early clotting. Separation in tubing is indicative of clotting. Very dark reddish-black blood next to clear yellow fluid indicates full clot formation. *Note:* Prior to insertion of an AV fistula or graft, client may have a temporary or permanent central catheter, which is maintained with heparin to inhibit clot formation. Because heparin remains active in the body for 4 to 6 hours, the client is at risk for hemorrhage during and immediately after dialysis (Leydig, 2005).
Palpate skin around shunt for warmth.	Diminished blood flow results in "coolness" of shunt.

(continues on page 546)

ACTIONS/INTERVENTIONS (continued)	RATIONALE (continued)
Notify physician and initiate declotting procedure if there is evidence of loss of shunt patency.	Rapid intervention may save access; however, declotting must be done by experienced personnel.
Evaluate reports of pain, numbness, and tingling; note extremity swelling distal to access.	May indicate inadequate blood supply.
Handle tubing gently and maintain cannula alignment. Limit activity of extremity. Avoid taking blood pressure (BP) or drawing blood samples in shunt extremity. Instruct client not to sleep on side with shunt or carry packages, books, or purse on affected extremity.	Decreases risks of shunt-related complications, (e.g., clotting, dislodgement or disconnection). It is critical that the catheter be used only for dialysis as it is the client's lifeline (Leydig, 2005).
Hemorrhage	
Attach two cannula clamps to shunt dressing. Have tourniquet available. If cannulae separate, clamp the arterial cannula first, then the venous. If tubing comes out of vessel, clamp cannula that is still in place and apply direct pressure to bleeding site. Place tourniquet above site or inflate BP cuff to pressure just above client's systolic BP.	Prevents massive blood loss while awaiting medical assistance if cannula separates or shunt is dislodged.
Infection	
Assess skin around vascular access, noting redness, swelling, local warmth, exudate, and tenderness.	Signs of local infection, which can progress to sepsis if untreated.
Avoid contamination of access site. Use aseptic technique and masks when giving shunt care, applying and changing dressings, and when starting and completing dialysis process.	Prevents introduction of organisms that may cause infection.
Monitor temperature. Note presence of fever, chills, and hypotension.	Signs of infection or sepsis requiring prompt medical intervention.
Collaborative	
Culture the site and obtain blood samples, as indicated.	Determines presence of pathogens and how best to treat.
Monitor prothrombin time (PT) and activated partial thromboplastin time (aPTT), as appropriate.	Provides information about coagulation status, identifies treatment needs, and evaluates effectiveness.
Administer medications, as indicated, for example:	
Low-dose heparin	Infused on arterial side of filter to prevent clotting in the filter without systemic side effects.
Antibiotics—systemic and topical	Prompt treatment of infection may save access and prevent sepsis.
Prepare for/assist with procedures, such as balloon angioplasty, thrombolysis, and mechanical thrombectomy, as indicated.	All three types of vascular access—AV fistula, AV graft, and venous catheter—can have complications that require further treatment or surgery. The most common complications are access infection and low blood flow due to blood clotting in the access. In the last two decades, radiological interventions have improved the care of AV access devices for treatment of stenosis and fistula thrombosis without surgery. However, shunt revision can require surgical intervention and replacement of stenotic area or placement of new vascular access (Sofocleous, 2011).

NURSING DIAGNOSIS: risk for deficient Fluid Volume

Risk Factors May Include

Loss of fluid through abnormal routes (e.g., ultrafiltration, systemic heparinization, actual blood loss—disconnection of the shunt)
Fluid restrictions

Possibly Evidenced By

(Not applicable; presence of signs and symptoms establishes an *actual* diagnosis)

Desired Outcomes/Evaluation Criteria—Client Will

Fluid Balance (NOC)

Maintain fluid balance as evidenced by stable vital signs, good skin turgor, moist mucous membranes, absence of bleeding, and appropriate weight.

ACTIONS/INTERVENTIONS	RATIONALE
Monitoring (NIC) *Independent*	
Measure all sources of intake and output (I&O). Have client keep diary.	Aids in evaluating fluid status, especially when compared with weight. *Note:* Urine output is an inaccurate evaluation of renal function in dialysis clients. Some individuals have water output with little renal clearance of toxins, whereas others have oliguria or anuria.
Weigh daily as well as before and after dialysis run.	Weight loss over precisely measured time is a measure of ultrafiltration and fluid removal. Dry weight determines how much excess fluid has been removed and serves as a guide for subsequent dialysis run time and solution.
Monitor BP, pulse, and hemodynamic pressures, if available, during dialysis.	Hypotension, tachycardia, and falling hemodynamic pressures suggest volume depletion.
Hemodialysis Therapy (NIC)	
Ascertain whether diuretics and antihypertensives are to be withheld.	Dialysis potentiates hypotensive effects if these drugs have been administered.
Verify continuity of shunt or access catheter.	Disconnected shunt or open access permits exsanguination.
Apply external shunt dressing. Permit no puncture of shunt.	Minimizes stress on cannula insertion site to reduce inadvertent dislodgement and bleeding from site.
Place client in a supine or Trendelenburg position, as necessary.	Maximizes venous return if hypotension occurs.
Assess for oozing or frank bleeding at access site, mucous membranes, or incisions and wounds. Test stools or any drainage for occult blood.	Systemic heparinization during dialysis prolongs clotting times and places client at risk for bleeding, especially during the first 4 hours after procedure.
Fluid Monitoring (NIC) *Collaborative*	
Monitor laboratory studies, as indicated, such as the following:	
Hemoglobin/hematocrit (Hgb/Hct)	May be reduced because of anemia, hemodilution, or actual blood loss.
Serum electrolytes and pH	Imbalances may require changes in the dialysate solution or supplemental replacement to achieve balance.
Clotting times—PT/aPTT and platelet count.	Use of heparin to prevent clotting in blood lines and hemofilter alters coagulation and potentiates active bleeding.
Administer IV solutions during dialysis, as indicated, for example:	
Normal saline (NS)	Saline or dextrose solutions, electrolytes, and $NaHCO_3$ may be infused in the venous side of continuous arteriovenous hemofilter when high ultrafiltration rates are used for removal of extracellular fluid (ECF) and toxic solutes.
Volume expanders, such as albumin	Volume expanders may be required during or following hemodialysis if sudden or marked hypotension occurs.
Packed red blood cells (RBCs), if needed	Destruction of RBCs (hemolysis) by mechanical dialysis, hemorrhagic losses, or decreased RBC production may result in profound and progressive anemia requiring corrective action.
Reduce rate of ultrafiltration during dialysis, as indicated.	Reduces the amount of water being removed and may correct hypotension or hypovolemia.
Administer protamine sulfate, as appropriate.	May be needed to return clotting times to normal or if heparin rebound occurs within 16 hours after hemodialysis.

NURSING DIAGNOSIS: risk for excess Fluid Volume

Risk Factors May Include

Receiving hemodialysis—rapid and excessive fluid intake (e.g., IV, blood, plasma expanders, saline given to support BP during dialysis)

Possibly Evidenced By

(Not applicable; presence of signs and symptoms establishes an *actual* diagnosis)

Desired Outcomes/Evaluation Criteria—Client Will

Fluid Balance (NOC)

Maintain "dry weight" within client's normal range; be free of edema; with clear breath sounds and serum sodium levels within normal limits.

ACTIONS/INTERVENTIONS	RATIONALE
Fluid Management (NIC)	
Independent	
Measure all sources of I&O. Weigh routinely.	Aids in evaluating fluid status, especially when compared with weight. Weight gain between treatments should not exceed 0.5 kg or approximately 1 lb/day.
Monitor BP and pulse.	Hypertension and tachycardia between hemodialysis runs may result from fluid overload and heart failure (HF).
Note rate and regularity of pulse.	Rapid rate, or irregularity in heart rate, may indicate changes in volume status.
Note presence of peripheral or sacral edema, respiratory crackles, dyspnea, orthopnea, distended neck veins.	Fluid volume excess due to inefficient dialysis or repeated hypervolemia between dialysis treatments may cause or exacerbate HF, as indicated by signs and symptoms of respiratory and systemic venous congestion.
Collaborative	
Monitor serum sodium levels. Restrict sodium intake, as indicated.	High sodium levels are associated with fluid overload, edema, hypertension, and cardiac complications.
Restrict fluid intake as indicated, spacing allowed fluids throughout a 24-hour period.	The intermittent nature of hemodialysis results in fluid retention and volume overload between procedures and may require fluid restriction. Spacing fluids helps reduce thirst.

URINARY DIVERSIONS/UROSTOMY (POSTOPERATIVE CARE)

I. Procedure

a. Diversion of urine out of the body through an opening in the abdominal wall bypassing the bladder, which requires a pouch to be worn outside the body; or, a continent diversion involving the creation of a pouch or bladder inside the body, usually using part of the digestive tract

b. Types: At present, varieties of urinary diversions are performed using different types of bowel segments and based on the individual's need and desire. The ileal conduit remains the most common form of noncontinent urinary diversion practiced worldwide today, and it is the standard to which all other urinary diversions are compared (Syracusano, 2012).

   i. Incontinent urinary diversions
      1. Ileal conduit
      2. Colonic conduit
      3. Ureterostomy

   ii. Continent urinary diversions
      1. Catheterizable urinary reservoir: Kock reservoir or Indiana (ileocecal) pouch
      2. Orthotopic continent urinary diversion: known as orthotopic neobladder reconstruction (ONR), now widely accepted as a first procedure where possible, such as for urothelial cancer (Herdiman 2013)

II. Indications (Costa 2012)

a. Bladder cancer, primary or metastatic, requiring cystectomy—fourth most common cancer in the United States

b. Neurogenic bladder, such as may occur following spinal cord injury

c. Severe radiation injury to the bladder

d. Intractable incontinence

e. Chronic pelvic pain syndromes

III. Statistics (for bladder cancer only)

a. Morbidity: This year (2013) it is estimated that 72,570 adults (54,610 men and 17,960 women) will be diagnosed with bladder cancer in the United States (American Cancer Society [ACS], 2013). Male-to-female ratio is 3:1 (National Cancer Institute [NCI] Surveillance Epidemiology and End Results (SEER), 2012).

b. Mortality: It is estimated that 15,210 deaths (10,820 men and 4,390 women) from this disease will occur in 2013. Among men, bladder cancer is the fourth most common cancer, and the eighth most common cancer in women.

c. Costs: The direct national costs for treatment of bladder cancer in 2010 were $3.98 billion (NCI, 2011).

GLOSSARY

Appliance: Pouch and accessories worn over stoma to collect urine.

Clean intermittent catheterization (CIC): Placement of a catheter to remove urine from the body. This is usually done by placing the catheter through the urethra, but may also be done by inserting the catheter through the opening of the reservoir.

Colonic conduit: Similar to an ileal conduit but uses a segment of colon instead of ileum.

Continent urinary diversion: Ureters carry urine to a pouch or reservoir created inside the body from a section of stomach or small or large intestine.

Cystectomy: Surgical removal of the urinary bladder.

Enterostomal: A surgically created permanent opening into the intestine through the abdominal wall.

Ileal conduit: Ureters are anastomosed to a segment of ileum, usually 15 to 20 cm long, and resected with the blood supply

GLOSSARY (continued)

intact. The proximal section is closed, and the distal end is brought through an opening in the skin to form a stoma or a passageway, not a storage reservoir.

Incontinent or noncontinent urinary diversions: Urine flows through ureters directly anastomosed to the abdominal wall (cutaneous ureterostomy) or into a short segment of ileum or colon also attached to the abdominal wall where the urine drains into an external collecting device through a permanent stoma.

Interrupted anastomosis: Loss of the surgical connection of two hollow organs.

Intractable incontinence: Loss of bladder control that becomes impossible to manage, alleviate, or remedy.

Kegel exercises: Pelvic muscle exercises intended to improve pelvic muscle tone and prevent urine leakage for sufferers of stress urinary incontinence.

Kock reservoir or Indiana (ileocecal) pouch: A section of intestine is used to form a pouch inside the client's abdomen, creating a reservoir that the client periodically drains by inserting a catheter through the nipple valve—or a one-way valve integrated into a stoma—thus negating the need for an external collecting device.

Nocturnal enuresis: Bed wetting at night, common to all people with neobladder procedures.

Orthotopic neobladder: A urinary reservoir fashioned from a bowel segment that is in the normal anatomic position of the bladder and attached directly to the urethra, with discharge of urine through the urethra.

Peristomal: Skin around and closest to the stoma.

Stoma: An opening that, when used in reference to ostomy care, is the segment of bowel or ureter brought to the surface of the abdomen. It is formed of mucosal tissue and is red and moist in appearance.

Ureterostomy: The ureter(s) is brought directly through the abdominal wall to form its own stoma.

Urostomy: Surgically constructed method of bypassing a dysfunctional or removed bladder in order to discharge urine. Most commonly, a conduit is created from a section of the ileum and the ureters are connected to it. The open end of the conduit is brought to the abdomen to create a stoma.

Valsalva's maneuver: Performed by holding the breath and bearing down as may be done when straining with bowel movements or to force urine from continent reservoir out through urethra.

Care Setting

Client is treated in acute surgical unit.

Related Concerns

Cancer, page 827
Peritonitis, page 320
Psychosocial aspects of care, page 729
Surgical intervention, page 762

Client Assessment Database

Data depend on underlying problem, duration, and severity, for example, malignant bladder tumor, congenital malformations, trauma, chronic infections, or intractable incontinence due to injury or disease of other body systems, such as with multiple sclerosis. (Refer to appropriate CP.)

DIAGNOSTIC DIVISION MAY REPORT	MAY EXHIBIT
TEACHING/LEARNING • ***Discharge plan considerations:*** May require assistance with management of ostomy and acquisition of supplies ➧ Refer to section at end of plan for postdischarge considerations.	

Preoperative Diagnostic Studies

TEST WHY IT IS DONE	WHAT IT TELLS ME
URINE TESTS • ***Urodynamic tests (e.g., may include uroflowmetry, postvoid residual measurement, cystometric test, leak point pressure measurement, pressure flow study, electromyography, video urodynamic tests)***	Any or all of these tests may be done preoperatively to determine the presence of urinary tract obstruction, or urine storage abnormalities, and help determine which urinary diversion will be most appropriate (Costa, 2012).

(continues on page 550)

Preoperative Diagnostic Studies (continued)

TEST WHY IT IS DONE (continued)	WHAT IT TELLS ME (continued)
• *Blood tests (e.g., serum creatinine [CR] liver function tests (LFTs])*	A contraindication to any type of continent diversion is compromised renal function that results from long-standing obstruction or chronic renal failure, with serum creatinine levels >150. Individuals with cirrhosis or abnormal liver function tests are not able to metabolize ammonia properly and would experience an increased risk for liver failure following neobladder construction. Metabolic acidosis is another potential complication of neobladder construction, due to the potential for resorption of ammonium and chloride and excessive excretion of sodium and bicarbonate (Herdiman, 2013; Mills, 1999).
OTHER DIAGNOSTIC STUDIES	
• *Imaging studies (e.g., ultrasound, CT, MRI)*	Will have been done to determine the etiology for which urinary diversion is required (Costa, 2012).
• *Intravenous pyelogram (IVP) and retrograde pyelogram:* X-ray examination and fluoroscopic visualization of the kidneys, ureters, and bladder using contrast material. Retrograde pyelogram requires cystoscopy and the placement of a small tube into the lower part of the ureter to inject contrast and opacify the ureter and renal pelvis.	Shows size, shape, and location of urinary structures. Identifies filling defects caused by tumors or other obstructive disorders. Retrograde pyelogram may also be done to delineate urinary tract system anatomy in preparation for surgery.
• *Cystoscopy with biopsy:* Diagnostic procedure that uses a cystoscope (endoscope), which is specially designed to examine the bladder, lower urinary tract, and prostate gland. It can also be used to perform biopsies. Ultraviolet cystoscopy outlines bladder lesions. Bladder washings can also be done during cystoscopy for cytological evaluation.	Initially, may be done to evaluate painless hematuria. If bladder tumor is detected, biopsy will be done to stage the malignancy.
• *Pelvic magnetic resonance imaging (MRI) or computed tomography (CT) scans:* Imaging techniques that use x-rays, or magnetic energy, and computer analysis to provide a complete picture of pelvic body tissues and structures.	Defines size of tumor mass and degree of cancer spread into surrounding tissues.

Nursing Priorities

1. Prevent complications.
2. Assist client and significant other (SO) in physical and psychosocial adjustment.
3. Support independence in self-care.
4. Provide information about procedure, prognosis, treatment needs, potential complications, and resources.

Discharge Goals

1. Complications prevented or minimized.
2. Adjusting to perceived or actual changes.
3. Self-care needs met by self or with assistance, as necessary.
4. Procedure, prognosis, therapeutic regimen, and potential complications understood and sources of support identified.
5. Plan in place to meet needs after discharge.

This plan of care primarily addresses the nursing care of the client with incontinent urinary diversion with a permanent stoma and urine-collecting device.

NURSING DIAGNOSIS: risk for impaired Skin Integrity

Risk Factors May Include

Excretions (e.g., continuous flow of urine, improper fitting of appliance)
Chemical substance (e.g., reaction to skin product or chemicals)
Mechanical factors (e.g., removal of adhesive)

Possibly Evidenced By

(Not applicable; presence of signs and symptoms establishes an *actual* diagnosis)

NURSING DIAGNOSIS: risk for impaired Skin Integrity (continued)

Desired Outcomes/Evaluation Criteria—Client Will

Tissue Integrity: Skin and Mucous Membranes (NOC)
Maintain skin integrity.

Ostomy Self-Care (NOC)
Identify individual risk factors.
Demonstrate behaviors and techniques to promote healing and prevent skin breakdown.

ACTIONS/INTERVENTIONS	RATIONALE
Ostomy Care (NIC)	
Independent	
Inspect stoma and peristomal skin. Note irritation, bruises, rashes, and status of sutures.	Stoma should be pink or reddish, similar to mucous membranes. Color changes may be temporary, but persistent changes may require surgical intervention. Early identification of stomal ischemia or fungal infection provides for timely interventions to prevent skin necrosis.
Clean with water and pat dry, or use hair dryer on cool setting.	Maintaining a clean and dry peristomal area helps prevent skin breakdown.
Touch stoma gently to prevent irritation.	Mucosa has good blood supply and bleeds easily with rubbing or trauma.
Measure stoma periodically, for example, each appliance change for first 6 weeks, then monthly times six.	As postoperative edema resolves, size of appliance must be altered to ensure proper fit so that urine is collected as it flows from the stoma and contact with the skin is prevented.
Apply effective sealant barrier, such as Skin Prep or similar product, as recommended by appliance manufacturer.	Protects skin from pouch adhesive, enhances adhesiveness of pouch, and facilitates removal of pouch when necessary. *Note:* Some barriers are designed to be used without skin sealant.
Ensure proper opening for adhesive backing of pouch. Using a stoma-measuring guide or ostomy sizer, find the smallest opening that fits over the stoma and does not allow any skin exposure. Cut the barrier to size with adequate adhesive area left to apply pouch.	Prevents trauma to the stoma tissue and protects the peristomal skin. Adequate adhesive area is important to maintain a seal. *Note:* Too tight a fit may cause stomal edema or stenosis.
Use a transparent, odor-proof, drainable pouch. Keep gauze square over stoma while cleansing area, and have client cough or strain before applying skin barrier wafer.	A transparent appliance during first 4 to 6 weeks allows easy observation of stoma and stents when used, without necessity of removing appliance and irritating skin. Covering stoma prevents urine from wetting the peristomal area during pouch changes. Coughing empties distal portion of conduit, followed by a brief pause in drainage to facilitate application of appliance.
Avoid use of karaya-type appliances.	Will not protect skin because urine melts karaya.
Apply waterproof tape around pouch edges, if desired.	Reinforces anchoring to help maintain seal.
Connect collecting pouch to continuous bedside drainage system when necessary or desired.	May be needed during times when rate of urine formation is increased, such as while intravenous (IV) fluids are administered, or at night if client prefers. Weight of the urine can cause pouch to pull loose and leak when pouch becomes more than half full.
Cleanse ostomy pouch on a routine basis, using vinegar solution or commercial solution designed for this purpose.	Frequent pouch changes are irritating to the skin and should be avoided. Emptying and rinsing the pouch with vinegar or commercial solution not only removes bacteria but also deodorizes the pouch.
Change pouch every 3 to 7 days, or as needed for leakage. Remove appliance gently while supporting skin. Use adhesive removers as indicated and wash off completely.	Prevents tissue irritation or damage associated with pulling skin barrier wafer off.
Investigate reports of burning or itching around stoma.	Suggests peristomal irritation or possibly *Candida* infection, both requiring intervention. *Note:* Continuous exposure of skin to urine can cause hyperplasia around stoma, affecting pouch fit and increasing risk of infection.
Evaluate adhesive product and appliance fit on an ongoing basis.	Provides opportunity for problem-solving. Determines need for further intervention.
Monitor for distention of lower abdomen in presence of ileal conduit; assess bowel sounds.	Intestinal distention can cause tension on new suture lines with possibility of rupture.

(continues on page 552)

ACTIONS/INTERVENTIONS (continued)	RATIONALE (continued)
Collaborative	
Consult with ostomy nurse specialist.	Ostomy nurse specialist can help client and caregiver by providing support and education, helping with problem-solving and choosing products appropriate for client's stoma characteristics, evaluating physical and mental status, and seeking financial resources. The client or caregiver should be capable of changing ostomy appliance prior to discharge or receive home care until such time as the client is competent (Colwell et al, 2001).
Apply antifungal spray or powder, as indicated.	Assists in healing if peristomal irritation is caused by fungal infection. *Note:* These products can have potent side effects and should be used sparingly. Creams and ointments are to be avoided because they interfere with adhesion of the appliance.

NURSING DIAGNOSIS: disturbed Body Image

May Be Related To

Biophysical—surgery (e.g., presence of stoma, loss of control of urine elimination)
Psychosocial—altered body structure
Illness (e.g., cancer)

Possibly Evidenced By

Reports feelings/perceptions that reflect an altered or negative view of one's body (e.g., appearance, structure, function)
Reports fear of reaction by others
Actual change in structure and function (ostomy)
Not looking at/not touching body part [stoma]

Desired Outcomes/Evaluation Criteria—Client Will

Body Image (NOC)

Demonstrate beginning acceptance by viewing and touching stoma and participating in self-care.
Verbalize feelings about stoma and illness.
Verbalize acceptance of self in situation, incorporating change into self-concept without negating self-esteem.

ACTIONS/INTERVENTIONS	RATIONALE
Body Image Enhancement (NIC)	
Independent	
Review reason for surgery and future expectations.	Client may find it easier to accept and deal with an ostomy done for chronic or long-term disease, such as intractable incontinence or infections, than for traumatic injury or cancer.
Ascertain whether counseling was initiated when the possibility or necessity of urinary diversion was first discussed.	Provides information about client's and SO's levels of knowledge about individual situation and process of acceptance. Client with new ostomy is also often struggling to adjust to cancer or other devastating medical condition requiring the diversion.
Answer all questions concerning urostomy and its function.	Establishes rapport and conveys interest and concern of caregiver. Provides additional information for client to consider.
Encourage client and SO to verbalize feelings. Acknowledge normality of feelings of anger, depression, and grief over loss.	Provides opportunity to deal with issues and misconceptions. Helps client and SO to realize that feelings are not unusual and that feeling guilty for them is not helpful.
Note behaviors of withdrawal, increased dependency, manipulation, or noninvolvement in care.	Suggestive of problems in adjustment that may require further evaluation and more extensive therapy. May reflect grief response to loss of body part and function, worry over acceptance by others, and fear of further disability or loss of life from cancer.
Provide opportunities for client and SO to view and touch stoma, using the moment to point out positive signs of healing, normal appearance, and so forth.	Although integration of stoma into body image can take months or even years, looking at the stoma and hearing comments made in a normal, matter-of-fact manner can help client with this process. Touching stoma reassures client and SO that it is not fragile and that slight movements of stoma actually reflect normal peristalsis.
Provide opportunity for client to deal with ostomy through participation in self-care.	Independence in self-care helps improve self-esteem. In the case of a continent diversion, client needs the energy, ability, and time to intubate the stoma a minimum of four times a day.

ACTIONS/INTERVENTIONS (continued)	RATIONALE (continued)
Maintain positive approach during care activities, avoiding expressions of disdain or revulsion. Do not take client's angry expressions personally.	Assists client and SO to accept body changes and feel all right about self. Anger is most often directed at the situation and lack of control individual has over what has happened.
Plan stoma care activities with client.	Promotes client's sense of control and gives message that client can handle this situation, enhancing self-esteem.
Discuss contacting ostomy or urostomy visitor and make arrangements for visit if client desires.	Can provide a good support system. Shared experiences can facilitate acceptance of change as client realizes "life does go on" and can be relatively normal.
Discuss sexual functioning and potential physical changes that may occur or medications that effect sexual function, if applicable. (Refer to ND: risk for Sexual Dysfunction.)	Client may experience anticipatory anxiety and fear of failure in relation to sex after surgery, usually because of lack of knowledge. Surgery that removes the bladder and prostate (removed with the bladder) may disrupt parasympathetic nerve fibers that control erection in men, although newer techniques are available that may be used in individual cases to preserve nerve function.

NURSING DIAGNOSIS: acute Pain

May Be Related To
Physical factors—incisions, drains
Biological factors—disease process (cancer), trauma
Psychological factors—fear, anxiety

Possibly Evidenced By
Verbalization/coded reports of pain
Guarding behaviors
Expressive behaviors—restlessness
Self-focus
Changes in vital signs

Desired Outcomes/Evaluation Criteria—Client Will

Pain Level (NOC)
Verbalize relief or control of pain.
Appear relaxed and be able to sleep and rest appropriately.

Pain Control (NOC)
Perform general comfort measures.

ACTIONS/INTERVENTIONS	RATIONALE
Pain Management (NIC)	
Independent	
Assess pain, noting location, characteristics, and intensity (0 to 10 or similar coded scale).	Helps evaluate degree of discomfort and effectiveness of analgesia or may reveal developing complications. Surgical causes for abdominal pain usually subside gradually as healing begins. Continued or increasing pain may be a sign of infection or intestinal obstruction.
Auscultate bowel sounds; note passage of flatus.	Indicates reestablishment of bowel function. Lack of return of bowel sounds and function within 72 hours may indicate presence of complication, such as peritonitis, hypokalemia, or mechanical obstruction.
Note urine flow and characteristics, and evaluate need for more intensive interventions.	Decreased flow may reflect urinary retention due to edema with increased pressure in upper urinary tract organs or leakage into peritoneal cavity with failure of anastomosis. Cloudy urine may be normal because of mucus from intestinal tract or may indicate infectious process.
Encourage client to verbalize concerns. Active-listen these concerns and provide support by acceptance, remaining with client and giving appropriate information.	Reduction of anxiety and fear can promote relaxation and comfort.
Provide comfort measures, such as back rub, repositioning, and ambulating. Assure client that position change will not injure stoma.	Activity, movement, and comfort measures can reduce muscle tension, promote relaxation, and enhance coping abilities.
Encourage use of relaxation techniques, such as guided imagery, visualization, and diversional activities.	Helps client rest more effectively and refocuses attention, which may enhance coping ability, reducing pain and discomfort.

(continues on page 554)

ACTIONS/INTERVENTIONS (continued)	RATIONALE (continued)
Assist with range-of-motion (ROM) exercises and encourage early ambulation.	Reduces muscle and joint stiffness. Ambulation returns organs to normal position, promotes return of gastrointestinal (GI) peristalsis, and enhances feelings of general well-being.
Investigate and report abdominal muscle rigidity, involuntary guarding, and rebound tenderness.	Suggestive of peritoneal inflammation, requiring prompt medical intervention.
Collaborative	
Administer medications as indicated, such as opioids, analgesics, and patient-controlled analgesia (PCA).	Relieves pain, enhances comfort, and promotes rest. PCA may be more beneficial than intermittent analgesia, especially following radical resection.
Maintain patency of nasogastric (NG) tube.	Decompresses stomach and intestines; prevents abdominal distention when intestinal function is impaired.

NURSING DIAGNOSIS: risk for Infection

Risk Factors May Include

Inadequate primary defenses—break in skin, stasis of body fluids (e.g., reflux of urine into urinary tract)
Inadequate secondary defenses—immunosuppression

Possibly Evidenced By

(Not applicable; presence of signs and symptoms establishes an *actual* diagnosis)

Desired Outcomes/Evaluation Criteria—Client Will

Infection Severity (NOC)

Achieve timely wound healing, be free of purulent drainage or erythema, and be afebrile.

Risk Control: Infectious Process (NOC)

Verbalize understanding of individual causative or risk factors.
Demonstrate techniques or lifestyle changes to reduce risk.

ACTIONS/INTERVENTIONS	RATIONALE
Infection Protection (NIC)	
Independent	
Empty ostomy pouch when it becomes one-third to one-half full, once continuous pouch drainage is discontinued.	Reduces risk of urinary reflux and maintains integrity of appliance seal if pouch does not have an antireflux valve.
Document urine characteristics and note whether changes are associated with reports of flank pain.	Cloudy, odorous urine indicates infection, possibly pyelonephritis; however, urine normally contains mucus after a conduit procedure because of natural secretions of the intestine.
Report sudden cessation of urethral drainage.	Constant drainage usually subsides within 10 days; however, abrupt cessation may indicate plugging and lead to abscess formation.
Note red rash around stoma.	Rash is most commonly caused by yeast. Urine leakage or allergy to appliance or products may also cause red, irritated areas.
Inspect incision line around stoma. Observe and document wound drainage, signs of incisional inflammation, and systemic indicators of sepsis.	Provides baseline and comparative reference. Complications may include interrupted anastomosis of intestine or ureteral conduit, with leakage of bowel contents into abdomen or urine into peritoneal cavity.
Change dressings, as indicated, when used.	Moist dressings act as a wick to the wound and provide media for bacterial growth.
Assess skinfold areas in groin, perineum, and under arms and breasts.	Use of antibiotics and trapping of moisture in skinfold areas increases risk of *Candida* infections.
Monitor vital signs.	An elevated temperature suggests incisional infection, urinary tract infection (UTI), or respiratory complications. *Note*: Infection in a neobladder is most likely to occur in the early postoperative period; the infection may be afebrile and limited to the neobladder, or it may be associated with pyelonephritis or even urosepsis. Such infections of the neobladder are typically managed with antimicrobials (Thurairaja, 2008).
Auscultate breath sounds.	Client is at high risk for development of respiratory complications because of length of time under anesthesia. Often this client is older and may already have a compromised immune system. Also, painful abdominal incisions cause client to breathe more shallowly than normal and to limit coughing effort. Accumulation of secretions in respiratory tract predisposes to atelectasis and infections.

ACTIONS/INTERVENTIONS (continued)	RATIONALE (continued)
Collaborative	
Use pouch with antireflux valve, if available.	Prevents backflow of urine into stoma, reducing risk of infection.
Obtain specimens of exudates, urine, sputum, and blood, as indicated.	Identifies source of infection and most effective treatment. Infected urine may cause pyelonephritis. *Note:* Urine specimen must be obtained from the conduit because the pouch is considered contaminated.
Administer medications, as indicated, for example:	
Cephalosporins, such as cefoxitin (Mefoxin) and cefazolin (Ancef)	Given to treat identified infection or may be given prophylactically, especially with history of recurrent pyelonephritis.
Antifungal powder	Used to treat yeast infections around stoma.

NURSING DIAGNOSIS: impaired Urinary Elimination

May Be Related To

Surgical diversion, tissue trauma, postoperative edema

Possibly Evidenced By

Incontinence (loss of continence)

Changes in amount, character of urine; urinary retention

Desired Outcomes/Evaluation Criteria—Client Will

Urinary Elimination (NOC)

Display continuous flow of urine, with output adequate for individual situation.

ACTIONS/INTERVENTIONS	RATIONALE
Urinary Elimination Management (NIC)	
Independent	
Evaluate and maintain urinary catheters and drains in the immediate postoperative period.	Most clients have Foley catheter, possibly a suprapubic catheter, and pelvic drains during perioperative phase, especially when neobladder has been constructed. Although pelvic drains and ureteral stents are usually removed within 7 to 10 days, the catheters will stay in place during the healing time (Costa, 2012).
Note presence of stents or ureteral catheters. Label "right" and "left" (or they may be color-coded), and observe urine flow through each.	Stents and ureteral catheters are placed during surgery to facilitate healing of internal anastomosis by keeping it urine free. It is necessary to verify that both kidneys and ureters are functional.
Record urinary output. Investigate sudden reduction or cessation of urine flow.	Sudden decrease in urine flow may indicate obstruction or dysfunction, such as blockage by edema or mucus, or dehydration. *Note:* Reduced urinary output not related to hypovolemia, associated with abdominal distention, fever, and clear, watery discharge from the incision; suggests urinary fistula, also requiring prompt intervention.
Observe and record color of urine. Note hematuria or bleeding from stoma.	Urine may be slightly pink, which should clear up in 2 to 3 days. Rubbing or washing stoma may cause temporary oozing because of vascular nature of mucosal tissues. Continued bleeding, frank blood in the pouch, or oozing around the base of stoma requires medical evaluation and intervention.
Position tubing and drainage pouch so that it allows unimpeded flow of urine. Monitor and protect stents.	Blocked drainage allows pressure to build within urinary tract, risking anastomosis leakage and damage to renal parenchyma. *Note:* Stents inserted to maintain patency of ureters during period of postoperative edema may be inadvertently dislodged, compromising urine flow.
Demonstrate self-catheterization techniques and reservoir irrigations, as appropriate.	After a healing time of several weeks, catheters will be removed and new voiding techniques initiated. Some clients with neobladders can void spontaneously, whereas others void by sitting down and performing Valsalva's maneuver. Clients should learn clean intermittent catheterization (CIC) in the event they cannot void spontaneously. Rarely, men will be unable to urinate by pelvic floor relaxation and Valsalva maneuver. In women, the incidence of urinary retention requiring CIC may be as high as 50% (Urology Care

(continues on page 556)

ACTIONS/INTERVENTIONS (continued)	RATIONALE (continued)
	Foundation, 2011). Periodic irrigations with sterile water or saline are needed in the continent reservoir to remove accumulated mucus.
Encourage increased fluids and maintain accurate intake.	Maintains hydration and good urine flow.
Monitor vital signs. Assess peripheral pulses, skin turgor, capillary refill, and oral mucosa. Weigh daily.	Indicators of fluid balance. Reflects level of hydration and effectiveness of fluid replacement therapy.
Collaborative	
Administer fluids, as indicated.	Assists in maintaining hydration and adequate circulating volume and urinary flow.
Monitor electrolytes and arterial blood gases (ABGs).	Impaired renal function in client with intestinal conduit increases risk of severe electrolyte or acid-base problems, such as hyperchloremic acidosis.
Prepare for diagnostic testing and procedures, as indicated.	Retrograde ileogram may be done to evaluate patency of conduit; nephrostomy tube or stents may be inserted to maintain urine flow until edema or obstruction is resolved.

NURSING DIAGNOSIS: risk for Sexual Dysfunction

Risk Factors May Include

Altered body structure and function

Vulnerability (concern about response of SO)

Possibly Evidenced By

(Not applicable; presence of signs and symptoms establishes an *actual* diagnosis)

Desired Outcomes/Evaluation Criteria—Client Will

Sexual Functioning (NOC)

Verbalize understanding of relationship of physical condition to sexual difficulties.

Identify satisfying, acceptable sexual practices and explore alternative methods.

Resume sexual relationship, as appropriate.

ACTIONS/INTERVENTIONS	RATIONALE
Sexual Counseling (NIC)	
Independent	
Ascertain client and SO's sexual relationship before surgery, if possible. Identify future expectations and desires.	Mutilation and loss of control of a bodily function can affect client's view of personal sexuality. When coupled with the fear of rejection by a partner, the desired level of intimacy can be greatly impaired. Sexual needs are very basic, and client will be rehabilitated more successfully when a satisfying sexual relationship is continued or developed. *Note:* Even with nerve-sparing procedures, 15% to 50% of men will experience erectile dysfunction, and 30% to 40% of women will experience painful intercourse (Costa, 2012).
Review with client and SO anatomy and physiology of sexual functioning in relation to own situation.	Understanding normal physiology helps client and SO understand the mechanisms of nerve damage and need for exploring alternative methods of satisfaction.
Reinforce information given by the physician. Encourage questions. Provide additional information as needed.	Reiteration of previously given information assists client and SO to hear and process the knowledge again, moving toward acceptance of individual limitations or restrictions and prognosis, for example, that it may take months to regain potency after a radical procedure or that a penile prosthesis may be necessary.
Discuss resumption of sexual activities, beginning slowly and progressing, such as cuddling and caressing until both partners are comfortable with body image and function changes. Include alternative methods of stimulation, as appropriate.	Knowing what to expect in progress of recovery helps client avoid performance anxiety and reduce risk of "failure." If the couple is willing to try new ideas, this can assist with adjustment and may help achieve sexual fulfillment.
Encourage dialogue between client and SO. Suggest wearing pouch cover, T-shirt, or short nightgown.	Disguising urostomy appliance may aid in reducing feelings of self-consciousness and embarrassment during sexual activity.
Stress awareness of factors that might be distracting—unpleasant odors and pouch leakage.	Promotes resolution of solvable problems.
Encourage use of sense of humor.	Laughter can help individuals deal more effectively with difficult situation and promote a positive sexual experience.

ACTIONS/INTERVENTIONS (continued)	RATIONALE (continued)
Problem-solve alternative positions for coitus.	Minimizing awkwardness of appliance and physical discomfort can enhance satisfaction.
Discuss and role-play possible interactions or approaches when dealing with new sexual partners.	Rehearsal helps deal with actual situations when they arise, preventing self-consciousness about "different" body image.
Provide birth control information, as appropriate, and stress that impotence does not mean client is necessarily sterile.	Confusion about impotency and sterility can lead to an unwanted pregnancy.
Collaborative	
Arrange meeting with an ostomy visitor or support group, if appropriate.	Sharing of how these problems have been resolved by others can be helpful and reduce sense of isolation.
Refer for counseling or sex therapy, as indicated.	If problems persist longer than several months after surgery, a trained therapist may be required to facilitate communication between client and partner.

NURSING DIAGNOSIS: deficient Knowledge [Learning Need] regarding condition, prognosis, treatment, self-care, and discharge needs

May Be Related To
Lack of exposure or recall, information misinterpretation
Unfamiliarity with information resources

Possibly Evidenced By
Reports the problem
Inaccurate follow-through of instruction or performance of urostomy care
Inappropriate or exaggerated behaviors—hostile, agitated, apathetic, withdrawn

Desired Outcomes/Evaluation Criteria—Client Will

Knowledge: Chronic Disease Management (NOC)
Verbalize understanding of condition, disease process, prognosis, and potential complications.

Ostomy Self-Care (NOC)
Verbalize understanding of therapeutic needs.
Correctly perform necessary procedures and explain reasons for the action.
Initiate necessary lifestyle changes.

ACTIONS/INTERVENTIONS	RATIONALE
Teaching: Disease Process (NIC)	
Independent	
Evaluate client's emotional and physical capabilities.	These factors affect client's ability to master tasks and willingness to assume responsibility for ostomy care.
Review anatomy, physiology, and implications of surgical intervention. Discuss future expectations.	Provides knowledge base from which client can make informed choices and an opportunity to clarify misconceptions regarding individual situation.
Include written and picture resources.	Provides references after discharge to support client efforts for independence in self-care.
Instruct client/SO in stomal care, as appropriate. Allow time for return demonstrations and provide positive feedback for efforts.	Promotes positive management and reduces risk of improper ostomy care.
Ensure that stoma and appliance are odorless and nonleaking.	When client feels confident about urostomy, energy and attention can be focused on other tasks.
Demonstrate padding to absorb urethral drainage; ask client to report changes in amount, odor, and character.	Small amount of leakage may continue for several weeks after prostate surgery with bladder left in place—a temporary diversion procedure.
Recommend routine trimming of hair around stoma to edges of pouch adhesive.	Hair can be pulled out when the pouch is changed, causing irritation of hair follicles and increasing risk of local infection.
Encourage clients with Kock pouch to lengthen voiding interval each week unless discomfort noted.	Increases capacity of reservoir to achieve a more normal voiding pattern. Presence of discomfort suggests reservoir is full, necessitating prompt emptying.
Review signs of reservoir overdistention and need for immediate medical intervention.	Client and caregiver will need to recognize signs, such as lower abdominal pain accompanied by feelings of fullness, bloating, or nausea associated with reservoir overdistention. Severe overdistention can result in neobladder rupture, a life-threatening complication (Costa, 2012).

(continues on page 558)

ACTIONS/INTERVENTIONS (continued)	RATIONALE (continued)
Instruct client in a progressive exercise program to include Kegel exercises that stop and start urinary stream.	Improves tone of pelvic muscles and the external sphincter to enhance continence when client voids through urethra.
Encourage optimal nutrition.	Promotes wound healing and increases utilization of energy to facilitate tissue repair. Anorexia may be present for several months postoperatively, requiring conscious effort to meet nutritional needs.
Discuss use of acid-ash diet: cranberries, prunes, plums, cereals, rice, peanuts, noodles, cheese, poultry, and fish; avoidance of salt substitutes, sodium bicarbonate, and antacids; and cautious use of products containing calcium.	May be useful in acidifying urine to decrease risk of infection and crystal or stone formation. Products containing bicarbonate or calcium potentiate risk of crystal and stone formation, affecting both urinary flow and tissue integrity. *Note:* Use of sulfa drugs requires alkaline urine for optimal absorption, necessitating acid-ash diet and vitamin C supplements withheld.
Discuss importance of maintaining normal weight.	Changes in weight can affect size of stoma and appliance fit. *Note:* Weight loss of 10 to 20 lb is not uncommon because of intestinal involvement and anorexia.
Stress necessity of increased fluid intake of at least 2 to 3 L/day and cranberry juice or ascorbic acid and vitamin C tablets. Explain to client that urine should be pale yellow to almost colorless.	Maintains urinary output and promotes acidic urine to reduce risk of infection and stone formation. *Note:* Oranges and citrus fruits make urine alkaline and are therefore contraindicated. Large doses of vitamin C can inhibit vitamin B_{12} absorption, requiring periodic monitoring of vitamin B_{12} levels.
Discuss resumption of presurgery level of activity and possibility of sleep disturbance, anorexia, and loss of interest in usual activities.	Client should be able to manage same degree of activity as previously enjoyed and in some cases increase activity level, except for contact sports. "Homecoming depression" may occur, lasting for up to 3 months after surgery, requiring patience, support, and ongoing evaluation.
Encourage regular activity and exercise program.	Immobility or inactivity increases urinary stasis and calcium shift out of bones, potentiating risk of stone formation and resultant urinary obstruction or infection.
Emphasize need for smoking cessation, if indicated. Refer for medication and smoking cessation assistance, if client is cooperative.	Smoking cessation is critical to the health of the new bladder, ureters, and kidneys because of the vasoconstrictive, acidic, and carcinogenic effects of smoking.
Identify signs and symptoms requiring medical evaluation: changes in character, amount, and flow of urine; unusual drainage from wound; fatigue or muscle weakness; anorexia; abdominal distention; and confusion.	Early detection and prompt intervention of developing problems such as UTI, stricture, and intestinal fistula, may prevent more serious complications. Urinary electrolytes, especially chloride, are reabsorbed in the intestinal conduit, which leads to compensatory bicarbonate loss, lowered serum pH or metabolic acidosis, and potassium deficit.
Stress importance of follow-up appointments.	Monitors healing and disease process and provides opportunity for discussion of appliance problems, general health, and adaptation to condition. *Note:* Bowel resection of the distal ileum creating ileal conduit can lead to vitamin B_{12} malabsorption. Therefore, long-term monitoring may be necessary as deficiency can lead to anemia, neurological problems, and anorexia (Clark, 2005; Pieper et al, 2006).
Identify community resources, such as the United Ostomy Association, local ostomy support group, enterostomal therapist, visiting nurse, and pharmacy or medical supply house.	Continued support after discharge is essential to facilitate the recovery process and client's independence in care. Enterostomal nurse can be very helpful in solving appliance problems and identifying alternatives to meet individual client needs.

POTENTIAL CONSIDERATIONS following acute hospitalization (dependent on client's age, physical condition and presence of complications, personal resources, and life responsibilities)

In addition to postsurgical concerns:

- ***impaired Urinary Elimination***—anatomic diversion
- ***situational low Self-Esteem***—loss of or altered control of body function
- ***risk for ineffective Self-Health Management***—complexity of therapeutic regimen, perceived barriers

BENIGN PROSTATIC HYPERPLASIA (BPH)

I. Pathophysiology
- a. Overgrowth of normal, nonmalignant cells that cause progressive enlargement of the prostate gland, resulting in bladder outlet obstruction with urinary retention, leakage, and frequency (Deters et al, 2013; Shiller, 2007)
- b. Additional complications: bladder wall trabeculation, detrusor muscle enlargement, narrowing of urethra, incontinence, and acute or chronic renal failure (Springhouse, 2005)

II. Classification (American Urological Association [AUA], 2010)
- a. International scoring system has been adopted worldwide.
- b. Questions, and subsequent scoring, focus on degree of incomplete emptying, frequency, intermittency, urgency, weak stream, straining, nocturia, as well as impact on quality of life.
    - i. Score of 0 to 7: mildly symptomatic
    - ii. Score of 8 to 19: moderately symptomatic
    - iii. Score of 20 to 35: severely symptomatic

III. Etiology
- a. Cause is unknown, although testosterone and other hormones may affect growth.
- b. Microscopically characterized as a hyperplastic process with the number of cells in the gland increasing with age
- c. Most commonly seen in men older than age 50 years

IV. Statistics
- a. Morbidity: BPH is the most common disorder of the prostate gland and is the most common diagnosis by urologists for male patients age 45 to 74 (Prostatehealthcures.com, 2009). An estimated 14 million men in the United States have symptoms related to benign enlargement (Deters et al, 2013).
- b. Mortality: Generally related to renal failure, infection, and complications of surgery.
- c. Cost: In 2000, the direct cost of BPH treatment was estimated to be $1.1 billion exclusive of outpatient pharmaceuticals (Wei, 2008).

GLOSSARY

Bladder outlet obstruction (BOO): Blockage at the base of the bladder causing compression of the urethra, thus reducing or preventing urine flow into the urethra.

Bladder wall trabeculation: Characterized by thick wall and hypertrophied muscle bundles; typically seen in instances of long-standing obstruction.

Dysuria: Painful, difficult urination.

LUTS: Lower urinary tract symptoms associated with BPH include urinary frequency, urgency, nocturia, decreased or intermittent force of stream, or a sensation of incomplete emptying.

Prostatitis: Inflammation of the prostate gland.

Care Settings

Client is treated at the community level, with more acute care provided during outpatient procedures.

Related Concerns

Acute kidney injury, page 505
Prostatectomy, page 566
Psychosocial aspects of care, page 729

Client Assessment Database

DIAGNOSTIC DIVISION MAY REPORT	MAY EXHIBIT
CIRCULATION	• Elevated blood pressure (BP)
ELIMINATION • Feeling need to urinate urgently, sensation of imminent loss of urine without control • Hesitancy or straining in initiating voiding, having to stand at or sit on the toilet for some time prior to producing a urinary stream • Decreased force or caliber of urinary stream, intermittent flow, dribbling • Usually voiding only small amounts of urine with each episode, sensation of incomplete emptying	• Firm mass in lower abdomen (distended bladder), bladder tenderness • Inguinal hernia, hemorrhoids—result of increased abdominal pressure required to empty bladder against resistance

(continues on page 560)

Client Assessment Database (continued)

DIAGNOSTIC DIVISION MAY REPORT (continued)	MAY EXHIBIT (continued)
• Need to urinate frequently during the day or night (nocturia), resulting in interrupted sleep • Dysuria, hematuria • Chronic constipation, resulting from protrusion of prostate into rectum	
FOOD/FLUID • Anorexia, nausea, vomiting • Recent weight loss	
PAIN/DISCOMFORT • Suprapubic, flank, or back pain; sharp, intense, with acute prostatitis • Low back pain	
SAFETY • Fever	
SEXUALITY • Concerns about effects of condition or therapy on sexual abilities • Fear of incontinence or dribbling during intimacy • Decrease in force of ejaculatory contractions	• Enlarged, tender prostate
TEACHING/LEARNING • Family history of cancer, hypertension, kidney disease • Use of antihypertensive or antidepressant medications, over-the-counter (OTC) cold and allergy medications containing sympathomimetics, urinary antibiotics or antibacterial agents • Use of nutrients or herbal supplements for self-treatment of BPH and urinary flow—saw palmetto, pygeum, pumpkin seed oil, or soy products	
DISCHARGE PLAN CONSIDERATIONS • May need assistance with management of therapy—catheter ➧ Refer to section at end of plan for postdischarge considerations.	

Diagnostic Studies

TEST WHY IT IS DONE	WHAT IT TELLS ME
BLOOD TESTS • ***Prostate-specific antigen (PSA):*** Substance manufactured solely by prostate gland cells. An elevated reading indicates an abnormal condition of the prostate gland, either benign or malignant.	In men without prostate cancer, serum PSA reflects the amount of glandular epithelium, which in turn reflects prostate size. As prostate size increases with increasing age, the PSA concentration also rises; it increases at a faster rate in elderly men. As a result, different normal reference ranges may be appropriate based upon a man's age. Prostate cancer is only one of many potential causes of an elevated PSA; anything that irritates the prostate (including BPH) will cause the PSA to rise, at least temporarily (Schmidt, 2009).

TEST WHY IT IS DONE (continued)	WHAT IT TELLS ME (continued)
URINE TESTS	
• *Urinalysis:* Laboratory examination of urine for red blood cells (RBCs) and WBCs or presence of infection or excessive protein.	Yellow, dark brown, dark or bright red (bloody) in color; appearance may be cloudy, pH of 7 or greater suggests infection; and bacteria, WBCs, and RBCs may be present microscopically.
• *Postvoid residual (PVR):* Volume of urine remaining in bladder immediately after voiding.	Determines the severity of urinary retention; may be done by catheterization or by transabdominal ultrasound.
OTHER DIAGNOSTIC STUDIES	
• *Transrectal prostatic ultrasound (TRUS):* Examination where a fingerlike probe is placed in the rectum and ultrasound pictures are made of the prostate.	Measures size of prostate and amount of residual urine, locates lesions unrelated to BPH. For client with elevated PSA levels, a TRUS-guided biopsy may be indicated.
• *Digital rectal exam (DRE):* Test performed by inserting gloved finger into rectum to detect prostate abnormalities.	Prostate size and contour can be assessed, nodules evaluated, and areas of suspected malignancy detected; also helps determine pelvic floor tone and fluctuance, such as in prostate abscess, and pain and sensitivity of gland can be assessed.
• *Uroflowmetry:* Measures urine amount and flow rate via a collection device and scale. The equipment creates a graph that shows changes in flow rate from second to second, measuring peak flow rate and how long it took to get there.	Results of this test will be abnormal if the bladder muscle is weak or urine flow is obstructed. Helps distinguish poor bladder contractibility (detrusor underactivity) from BOO caused by prostate hyperplasia.
• *Urography:* Series of x-rays of the kidney, ureters, and bladder after injection of a contrast dye into a vein.	Shows any blockage in the urinary tract causing delayed emptying of bladder, urinary retention, or presence of prostatic enlargement.
• *Cystourethrography:* Allows visualization of the bladder and urethra on x-ray, using radiopaque contrast material injected through the urethra.	May be used instead of IVP to visualize bladder and urethra because it uses localized, rather than systemic, radiopaque contrast media.
• *Cystourethroscopy:* Direct visualization of the bladder and urethra by means of a flexible fiber-optic scope.	May be done in selected individuals. Shows degree of prostatic enlargement and bladder wall changes associated with bladder trabeculation.

Nursing Priorities

1. Relieve acute urinary retention.
2. Promote comfort.
3. Prevent complications.
4. Help client deal with psychosocial concerns.
5. Provide information about disease process, prognosis, and treatment needs.

Discharge Goals

1. Voiding pattern normalized.
2. Pain or discomfort relieved.
3. Complications prevented or minimized.
4. Situation being dealt with realistically.
5. Disease process, prognosis, and therapeutic regimen understood.
6. Plan in place to meet needs after discharge.

NURSING DIAGNOSIS: [acute/chronic] Urinary Retention

May Be Related To
Blockage
[Decompensation of detrusor musculature]
[Loss of bladder tone—inability of bladder to contract adequately]

Possibly Evidenced By
Sensation of bladder fullness; dribbling
Bladder distention; residual urine (150 mL or more)

Desired Outcomes/Evaluation Criteria—Client Will

Urinary Elimination (NIC)
Void in sufficient amounts with no palpable bladder distention.
Demonstrate postvoid residuals of less than 50 mL, with absence of dribbling or overflow.

ACTIONS/INTERVENTIONS	RATIONALE
Urinary Retention Care (NIC)	
Independent	
Encourage client to void every 2 to 4 hours and when urge is noted.	May minimize urinary retention and overdistention of the bladder.
Ask client about stress incontinence when moving, sneezing, coughing, laughing, or lifting objects.	High urethral pressure inhibits bladder emptying or can inhibit voiding until abdominal pressure increases enough for urine to be involuntarily lost.
Observe urinary stream, noting size and force.	Useful in evaluating degree of obstruction and choice of intervention.
Have client document time and amount of each voiding. Note diminished urinary output. Measure specific gravity, as indicated.	Urinary retention increases pressure within the ureters and kidneys, which may cause renal insufficiency. Any deficit in blood flow to the kidney impairs its ability to filter and concentrate substances.
Percuss and palpate suprapubic area.	A distended bladder can be felt in the suprapubic area.
Encourage oral fluids, if indicated.	Increased circulating fluid maintains renal perfusion and flushes kidneys, bladder, and ureters of sediment and bacteria. *Note:* Fluids may be restricted to prevent bladder distention if severe obstruction is present or until adequate urinary flow is reestablished.
Monitor vital signs closely. Observe for hypertension, peripheral or dependent edema, and changes in mentation. Weigh daily. Maintain accurate intake and output (I&O).	Loss of kidney function results in decreased fluid elimination and accumulation of toxic wastes.
Provide and encourage meticulous catheter and perineal care.	Reduces risk of ascending infection.
Recommend sitz bath, as indicated.	Promotes muscle relaxation, decreases edema, and may enhance voiding effort.
Collaborative	
Administer medications, as indicated, for example:	Medications have long been used as a first-line therapy for clients with mild to moderate symptoms.
5-α-reductase inhibitors, such as finasteride (Proscar) and dutasteride (Avodart)	Reduces the size of the prostate and decreases symptoms if taken long-term; however, side effects, such as decreased libido and ejaculatory dysfunction, may influence client's choice for long-term use. Studies indicate that combination therapy with 5-α-reductase inhibitor plus alpha blocker may be superior to taking either drug class alone for prevention of BPH progression (AUA, 2010; National Institute of Diabetes and Digestive and Kidney Diseases [NIDDK], 2003).
Alpha-adrenergic antagonists, such as alfuzosin (UroXatral), terazosin (Hytrin), doxazosin (Cardura), and tamsulosin (Flomax)	These agents block effects of postganglionic synapses that affect smooth muscle and exocrine glands. This action can decrease adverse urinary tract symptoms and increase urinary flow.
Antibiotics and antibacterials	Given to combat infection. May be used prophylactically.
Catheterize for residual urine and leave indwelling catheter, as indicated.	Relieves and prevents urinary retention and rules out presence of ureteral stricture. Coudé catheter may be required because the curved tip eases passage of the tube around the enlarged prostate. *Note:* Bladder decompression should be done with caution to observe for signs of adverse reaction, such as hematuria due to rupture of blood vessels in the mucosa of the overdistended bladder and syncope due to excessive autonomic stimulation.
Monitor laboratory studies, such as the following:	
Blood urea nitrogen (BUN), creatinine (Cr), and electrolytes	Prostatic enlargement with obstruction eventually causes dilation of upper urinary tract, ureters, and kidneys, potentially impairing kidney function and leading to uremia.
Urinalysis and culture	Urinary stasis potentiates bacterial growth, increasing risk of urinary tract infection (UTI).
Prepare for and assist with urinary drainage, such as emergency cystostomy.	May be indicated to drain bladder during acute episode with azotemia or when surgery is contraindicated because of client's health status.
Prepare for minimally invasive therapies, such as:	These therapies rely on heat to cause destruction of prostatic tissue. Treatment is often completed in a one-time procedure carried out in the physician's office. Long-term outcomes are variable in terms of adequately treating urinary tract symptoms.
Heat therapies, such as laser, transurethral microwave thermotherapy (TUMT), Cortherm, Prostatron, and transurethral needle ablation (TUNA).	

NURSING DIAGNOSIS: acute Pain

May Be Related To
Physical agents—mucosal irritation (e.g., bladder distention, renal colic, urinary infection, radiation therapy)

Possibly Evidenced By
Verbalized/coded reports of pain
Self-focus
Expressive behaviors (e.g., restlessness, irritability)
Changes in vital signs

Desired Outcomes/Evaluation Criteria—Client Will

Pain Level (NOC)
Report pain relieved or controlled.
Appear relaxed.
Be able to sleep and rest appropriately.

ACTIONS/INTERVENTIONS	RATIONALE
Pain Management (NIC)	
Independent	
Assess pain, noting location, intensity (0 to 10 or similar coded scale), characteristics, and duration.	Provides information to aid in determining choice and effectiveness of interventions.
Tape drainage tube to thigh and catheter to the abdomen, if traction not required.	Prevents accidental dislodging of catheter with attendant urethral trauma.
Provide comfort measures, such as back rub, helping client assume position of comfort. Suggest use of relaxation and deep-breathing exercises and diversional activities.	Promotes relaxation, refocuses attention, and may enhance coping abilities.
Encourage use of sitz baths and warm soaks to perineum.	Promotes muscle relaxation.
Collaborative	
Insert catheter and attach to straight drainage, as indicated.	Draining bladder reduces bladder tension and irritability.
Administer medications, as indicated, for example:	
Opioids, such as meperidine (Demerol)	Given to relieve severe pain; provide physical and mental relaxation.
Antibacterials, such as methenamine hippurate (Hiprex)	Reduces bacteria present in urinary tract and those introduced by drainage system.
Antispasmodics and bladder sedatives, such as flavoxate (Urispas) and oxybutynin (Ditropan).	Relieves bladder irritability.

NURSING DIAGNOSIS: risk for deficient Fluid Volume

Risk Factors May Include
Failure of regulatory mechanism (e.g., postobstructive diuresis from rapid drainage of a chronically overdistended bladder)

Possibly Evidenced By
(Not applicable; presence of signs and symptoms establishes an *actual* diagnosis)

Desired Outcomes/Evaluation Criteria—Client Will

Fluid Balance (NOC)
Maintain adequate hydration as evidenced by stable vital signs, palpable peripheral pulses, good capillary refill, and moist mucous membranes.

ACTIONS/INTERVENTIONS	RATIONALE
Fluid Management (NIC)	
Independent	
Monitor output carefully. Note outputs of 100 to 200 mL/hr.	Rapid or sustained diuresis could cause client's total fluid volume to become depleted and limits sodium reabsorption in renal tubules.
Encourage increased oral intake based on individual needs.	Client may have restricted oral intake in an attempt to control urinary symptoms, reducing homeostatic reserves and increasing risk of dehydration and hypovolemia.
Monitor BP and pulse. Evaluate capillary refill and oral mucous membranes.	Enables early detection of and intervention for systemic hypovolemia.

(continues on page 564)

ACTIONS/INTERVENTIONS (continued)	RATIONALE (continued)
Promote bedrest with head elevated.	Decreases cardiac workload, facilitating circulatory homeostasis.
Collaborative	
Monitor electrolyte levels, especially sodium.	As fluid is pulled from extracellular spaces, sodium may follow the shift, causing hyponatremia.
Administer intravenous (IV) fluids—hypertonic saline as needed.	Replaces fluid and sodium losses to prevent or correct hypovolemia following outpatient procedures.

NURSING DIAGNOSIS: Anxiety [specify level]

May Be Related To

Change in health status
Threat to self-concept
Threat to role function (e.g., concern about sexual ability)

Possibly Evidenced By

Increased tension, apprehensive, worried
Reports concerns due to change in life events

Desired Outcomes/Evaluation Criteria—Client Will

Anxiety Self-Control (NOC)

Appear relaxed.
Verbalize accurate knowledge of the situation.
Demonstrate appropriate range of feelings and lessened fear.
Report anxiety is reduced to a manageable level.

ACTIONS/INTERVENTIONS	RATIONALE
Anxiety Reduction (NIC)	
Independent	
Be available to client. Establish trusting relationship with client and significant other (SO).	Demonstrates concern and willingness to help. Encourages discussion of sensitive subjects.
Provide information about specific procedures and tests and what to expect afterward, such as catheter, bloody urine, and bladder irritation. Be aware of how much information client wants.	Helps client understand purpose of what is being done and reduces concerns associated with the unknown, including fear of cancer. However, overload of information is not helpful and may increase anxiety.
Maintain matter-of-fact attitude in doing procedures and dealing with client. Protect client's privacy.	Communicates acceptance and eases client's embarrassment.
Encourage client and SO to verbalize concerns and feelings.	Defines the problem, providing opportunity to answer questions, clarify misconceptions, and problem-solve solutions.
Reinforce previous information client has been given.	Allows client to deal with reality and strengthens trust in caregivers and information presented.

NURSING DIAGNOSIS: deficient Knowledge [Learning Need] regarding condition, prognosis, treatment, self-care, and discharge needs

May Be Related To

Lack of exposure or recall, information misinterpretation
Unfamiliarity with information resources

Possibly Evidenced By

Reports the problem
Inappropriate behaviors—apathetic, withdrawn
Inaccurate follow-through of instructions

Desired Outcomes/Evaluation Criteria—Client Will

Knowledge: Disease Process (NOC)

Verbalize understanding of disease process, prognosis, and potential complications.
Identify relationship of signs and symptoms to the disease process.
Initiate necessary lifestyle or behavior changes.

Knowledge: Treatment Regimen (NOC)

Verbalize understanding of therapeutic needs.
Participate in treatment regimen.

ACTIONS/INTERVENTIONS	RATIONALE
Teaching: Disease Process (NIC)	
Independent	
Review disease process and client expectations.	Provides knowledge base from which client can make informed therapy choices. *Note:* "Watchful waiting" is one of the options in client with early BPH with no symptoms of urinary retention. Client should understand that this includes ongoing periodic evaluation for change (Neal, 2009).
Encourage verbalization of fears, feelings, and concerns.	Helping client work through feelings can be vital to rehabilitation.
Give information that the condition is not sexually transmitted.	May be an unspoken fear.
Review drug therapy, use of herbal products, and diet, such as increasing intake of fruits and soybeans.	Some clients may prefer to treat with complementary therapy because of decreased occurrence and lessened severity of side effects, such as impotence. *Note:* Nutrients known to inhibit prostate enlargement include zinc, soy protein, essential fatty acids, flaxseed, and lycopene. Herbal supplements that client may use include saw palmetto, pygeum, stinging nettle, and pumpkin seed oil. However, a recent study found no difference in efficacy or side effects between saw palmetto and a placebo, indicating a need for further research as to benefit versus variability of potency or purity of botanical products (Bent, 2006).
Review usual medication regimen.	Medications known to be associated with urinary obstruction symptoms (e.g., tricyclic antidepressants, first generation antihistamines, anticholinergic agents, diuretics, narcotics, and decongestants) may require dose adjustment or change to a different drug (Neal, 2009).
Encourage reading of labels and discuss concerns with over-the-counter (OTC) drugs.	Many OTC medications for upper respiratory symptom relief can increase urinary retention. Client with BPH should avoid these medications.
Recommend avoiding spicy foods, coffee, alcohol, long automobile rides, and rapid intake of fluids.	May cause prostatic irritation with resulting congestion. Sudden increase in urinary flow can cause bladder distention and loss of bladder tone, resulting in episodes of acute urinary retention.
Address sexual concerns—during acute episodes of prostatitis, intercourse should be avoided but may be helpful in treatment of chronic condition.	Sexual activity can increase pain during acute episodes but may serve as massaging agent in presence of chronic disease. *Note:* Medications, such as finasteride (Proscar), are known to interfere with libido and erections. Alternatives include terazosin (Hytrin), doxazosin mesylate (Cardura), and tamsulosin (Flomax), which do not affect testosterone levels.
Provide information about sexual anatomy and function as it relates to prostatic enlargement. Encourage questions and promote a dialogue about concerns.	Having information about anatomy involved helps client understand the implications of proposed treatments because they might affect sexual performance.
Review signs and symptoms requiring medical evaluation—cloudy, odorous urine; diminished urinary output; inability to void; and presence of fever or chills.	Prompt interventions may prevent more serious complications.
Discuss necessity of notifying other healthcare providers of diagnosis.	Reduces risk of inappropriate therapy, such as the use of decongestants, anticholinergics, and antidepressants, which can increase urinary retention and may precipitate an acute episode.
Reinforce importance of medical follow-up for at least 6 months to 1 year, including rectal examination and urinalysis.	Recurrence of hyperplasia and infection caused by same or different organisms is not uncommon and requires changes in therapeutic regimen to prevent serious complications.
Discuss personal safety issues and potential environmental changes.	Recent research reports increased risk of falls in presence of moderate to severe BPH associated with urgency, nocturia, and straining to void, with fall risk increasing with age and symptom severity (Parsons et al, 2008).

POTENTIAL CONSIDERATIONS following acute hospitalization (dependent on client's age, physical condition and presence of complications, personal resources, and life responsibilities)

- ***[acute/chronic] Urinary Retention***—blockage, [loss of bladder tone, decompensation of detrusor musculature]
- ***risk for Infection***—urinary stasis, invasive procedure (periodic catheterization)
- ***risk for ineffective Self-Health Management***—perceived barriers

PROSTATECTOMY

I. Indications

a. Benign prostatic hyperplasia (BPH)-related complications
   - i. Urinary retention
   - ii. Frequent urinary tract infections
   - iii. Bladder stones
   - iv. Recurrent gross hematuria
   - v. Kidney damage from long-standing blockage
   - vi. Failure to respond to medical or minimally invasive treatments

b. Prostate cancer

II. Procedures (Miles et al, 2011; American Urological Association, [AUA], 2010)

a. Minimally invasive prostatectomy
   - i. Transurethral microwave thermotherapy (TUMT)
   - ii. Transurethral needle ablation (TUNA) using low-level frequency thermal energy
   - iii. Laser ablation: includes transurethral holmium laser ablation of the prostate (HoLAP); transurethral laser enucleation of the prostate (HoLEP); holmium laser resection of the prostate (HoLRP)
   - iv. Transurethral vaporization of the prostate (TUVP)
   - v. Transurethral resection of the prostate (TURP)
     1. Most common procedure for the long-term treatment of BPH, in client with moderate to severe lower urinary tract symptoms (LUTS) and/or where significantly bothered by these symptoms
     2. Obstructive prostatic tissue of the medial lobe surrounding the urethra is removed by means of a cystoscope introduced through the urethra.

b. Open surgical approaches performed when the prostate is overly enlarged (greater than 75 g), the bladder has been damaged, or when there are complicating factors, such as cancer
   - i. Robot assisted—nerve sparing, uses a laparoscope, and several incisions are made in the abdomen
   - ii. Suprapubic prostatectomy
     1. Obstructing prostatic tissue is removed through a low midline incision made through the bladder.
     2. Preferred approach if bladder stones are present
   - iii. Retropubic prostatectomy
     1. Hypertrophied prostatic tissue mass located high in the pelvic region is removed through a low abdominal incision without opening the bladder.
   - iv. Perineal prostatectomy
     1. Laparoscopy removal of larger tumors or in presence of cancerous lymph nodes or nerve invasion
     2. Large prostatic masses low in the pelvic area are removed through an incision between the scrotum and the rectum.

III. Statistics

a. Morbidity: In 2009, 158,000 prostatectomy procedures were performed in short-stay hospitals in the United States (Centers for Disease Control and Prevention [CDC], 2009); in 2011, 4 of 5 radical prostatectomies were robotic assisted (NCI National Cancer Bulletin, 2011).

b. Mortality: Prostatectomy is a relatively low-risk procedure (generally stated as 0 or less than 1% and usually associated with cardiovascular disease) (AUA, 2010; Guilli et al, n.d.).

c. Cost: In 2010, the direct costs for treatment of prostate cancer totaled $11.85 billion (NCI, 2011); most commonly performed procedures are prostatectomy and TURP (Milenkovic et al, 2007).

GLOSSARY

Blood dyscrasias: General term used to describe any abnormality in the blood, such as low white blood cell (WBC) count, low red blood cell (RBC) count, or low platelet count.

Continuous bladder irrigation (CBI): Constant flow of normal saline or another bladder irrigant through a three-way urinary catheter to keep the catheter patent.

Hematuria: Blood in the urine.

Kegel exercises: Pelvic muscle exercises intended to improve pelvic muscle tone and prevent urine leakage for sufferers of stress urinary incontinence.

Prostatic fossa: Cavity or depression where the prostate gland lies.

Retropubic: Behind the pubic bone.

Suprapubic: Above the pubic bone.

Transurethral resection of the prostate (TURP) syndrome: Rare complication directly related to this procedure. During the surgery, excess fluid collects in the body, reducing the concentration of sodium in the bloodstream. Common symptoms include nausea, vomiting, and confusion.

Urinary retention: Inability to empty bladder.

Care Setting

Client is treated in inpatient acute surgical unit.

Related Concerns

Benign prostatic hyperplasia (BPH), page 559
Cancer, page 827
Psychosocial aspects of care, page 729
Surgical intervention, page 762

Client Assessment Database

Refer to CP: Benign Prostatic Hyperplasia (BPH) for assessment data.

DIAGNOSTIC DIVISION MAY REPORT	MAY EXHIBIT
DISCHARGE PLAN CONSIDERATIONS • Dependent upon type of procedure, needs may be minimal or client may require assistance with self-care needs, transportation, medical supplies, and home maintenance ➧ Refer to section at end of plan for postdischarge.	

Nursing Priorities

1. Maintain homeostasis and hemodynamic stability.
2. Promote comfort.
3. Prevent complications.
4. Provide information about surgical procedure, prognosis, treatment, and rehabilitation needs.

Discharge Goals

1. Urinary flow restored or enhanced.
2. Pain relieved or controlled.
3. Complications prevented or minimized.
4. Procedure, prognosis, therapeutic regimen, and rehabilitation needs understood.
5. Plan in place to meet needs after discharge.

NURSING DIAGNOSIS: impaired Urinary Elimination

May Be Related To

Anatomic obstruction (e.g., blood clots, edema, trauma, surgical procedure)
[Loss of bladder tone—preoperative overdistention or continued decompression]

Possibly Evidenced By

Frequency, urgency, hesitancy, dysuria
Incontinence; retention

Desired Outcomes/Evaluation Criteria—Client Will

Urinary Elimination (NOC)

Void normal amounts without retention.
Demonstrate behaviors to regain bladder and urinary control.

ACTIONS/INTERVENTIONS	RATIONALE
Urinary Elimination Management (NIC)	
Independent	
Assess urine output and catheter drainage system, especially during bladder irrigation.	Retention can occur because of edema of the surgical area, blood clots, and bladder spasms.
Assist client to assume normal position to void; for example, stand and walk to bathroom at frequent intervals after catheter is removed.	Encourages passage of urine and promotes sense of normality.
Record time, amount of voiding, and size of stream after catheter is removed. Note reports of bladder fullness, inability to void, and urgency.	The catheter is usually removed 2 to 5 days after surgery, but voiding may continue to be a problem for some time because of urethral edema and loss of bladder tone.
Encourage client to void when urge is noted but not more than every 2 to 4 hours per protocol.	Voiding with urge prevents urinary retention. Limiting voids to every 4 hours, if tolerated, increases bladder tone and aids in bladder retraining.
Encourage fluid intake to 2000 to 2500 mL as tolerated. Limit fluids in the evening once catheter is removed.	Maintains adequate hydration and renal perfusion for urinary flow. "Scheduling" fluid intake reduces need to void during the night.
Instruct client in perineal exercises, such as tightening buttocks and stopping and starting urine stream.	Helps regain bladder sphincter control, minimizing incontinence.
Advise client that "dribbling" is to be expected after catheter is removed and should resolve as recuperation progresses. Provide and instruct in use of continence pads when indicated.	Information helps client deal with the problem. Postoperative incontinence is usually temporary, but stress incontinence—leaking urine when coughing, laughing, and lifting—can persist indefinitely.

(continues on page 568)

ACTIONS/INTERVENTIONS (continued)	RATIONALE (continued)
Collaborative	
Maintain continuous bladder irrigation (CBI), as indicated, in early postoperative period.	Flushes bladder of blood clots and debris to maintain patency of the catheter and urinary flow.
Measure residual volumes via suprapubic catheter, if present, or with Doppler ultrasound.	Monitors effectiveness of bladder emptying. Residuals of more than 50 mL suggest need for continuation of catheter until bladder tone improves.

NURSING DIAGNOSIS: risk for Bleeding

Risk Factors May Include

Treatment-related side effects (e.g., surgery—vascular nature of surgical area)

Possibly Evidenced By

(Not applicable; presence of signs and symptoms establishes an *actual* diagnosis)

Desired Outcomes/Evaluation Criteria—Client Will

Blood Loss Severity (NOC)

Display no signs of active bleeding.

ACTIONS/INTERVENTIONS	RATIONALE
Bleeding Precautions (NIC)	
Independent	
Monitor intake and output (I&O).	Indicator of fluid balance and replacement needs. With bladder irrigations, monitoring is essential for estimating blood loss and accurately assessing urine output. *Note:* Following release of urinary tract obstruction, marked diuresis may occur during initial recovery period.
Monitor vital signs, noting increased pulse and respiration, decreased blood pressure (BP), diaphoresis, pallor, delayed capillary refill, and dry mucous membranes.	Hypovolemia requires prompt intervention to prevent impending shock. *Note:* Hypertension, bradycardia, and nausea or vomiting suggest TURP syndrome, requiring immediate medical intervention.
Investigate restlessness, confusion, and changes in behavior.	May reflect decreased cerebral perfusion (hypovolemia) or indicate cerebral edema from excessive solution absorbed into the venous sinusoids during TUR procedure (TURP syndrome).
Inspect dressings and wound drains. Weigh dressings, if indicated. Note hematoma formation.	Signs of persistent bleeding may be evident or sequestered within tissues of the perineum.
Encourage increased fluid intake, preferably water, to 2000 to 2500 mL/day unless contraindicated by medical condition.	Helps maintain fluid volume while flushing bladder of blood clots, debris, and bacteria (Wojcik & Dennison, 2006).
Bleeding Reduction (NIC)	
Anchor urethral catheter and avoid excessive manipulation.	After TURP, the client will have special catheter in place that allows traction on the prostatic fossa to minimize bleeding. The catheter also allows irrigation of the bladder. Displacement of the catheter may cause bleeding. With bladder distention, clot formation may cause plugging of the catheter.
Observe urethral and suprapubic catheter drainage, noting excessive or continued bleeding.	Bleeding is not unusual during first 24 hours for all but the perineal approach. Continued or heavy bleeding or recurrence of active bleeding requires medical evaluation and intervention.
Evaluate color, consistency of urine, for example:	
Bright red with bright red clots	Usually indicates arterial bleeding and requires aggressive therapy.
Dark burgundy with dark clots and increased viscosity	Suggests venous source, which is the most common type of bleeding and usually subsides on its own.
Bleeding with absence of clots.	May indicate blood dyscrasias or systemic clotting problems.
Avoid taking rectal temperatures and use of rectal tubes or enemas.	May result in referred irritation to prostatic bed and increased pressure on prostatic capsule with risk of bleeding.
Collaborative	
Monitor laboratory studies, as indicated, such as:	
Hemoglobin/hematocrit (Hgb/Hct) and RBCs	Useful in evaluating blood losses and replacement needs.
Coagulation studies and platelet count	May indicate developing complications that can potentiate bleeding or clotting.

ACTIONS/INTERVENTIONS (continued)	RATIONALE (continued)
Administer intravenous (IV) therapy or blood products, as indicated.	May need additional fluids, if oral intake inadequate, or blood products, if losses are excessive.
Maintain traction on indwelling catheter; tape catheter to inner thigh.	Traction on the 30-mL balloon positioned in the prostatic urethral fossa creates pressure on the arterial supply of the prostatic capsule to help prevent or control bleeding.
Release traction within 4 to 5 hours. Document period of application and release of traction, if used.	Prolonged traction may cause permanent trauma and problems with urinary control.
Administer stool softeners or laxatives, as indicated.	Prevention of constipation and straining for stool reduces risk of rectal-perineal bleeding.

NURSING DIAGNOSIS: risk for Infection

Risk Factors May Include

Inadequate primary defenses—traumatized tissue, surgical incision, invasive procedures (e.g., instrumentation during surgery, indwelling catheter, frequent bladder irrigation)

Possibly Evidenced By

(Not applicable; presence of signs and symptoms establishes an *actual* diagnosis)

Desired Outcomes/Evaluation Criteria—Client Will

Wound Healing: Primary Intention (NOC)

Experience no signs of infection.
Achieve timely healing.

ACTIONS/INTERVENTIONS	RATIONALE
Infection Protection (NIC)	
Independent	
Maintain sterile catheter system; provide regular catheter and urinary meatus care with soap and water, applying antibiotic ointment around catheter site per protocol.	Prevents introduction of bacteria and resultant infection.
Ambulate with drainage bag dependent.	Avoids backward reflux of urine, which may introduce bacteria into the bladder.
Monitor vital signs, noting low-grade fever, chills, rapid pulse and respiration, restlessness, irritability, and disorientation.	Client who has had cystoscopy or TURP is at increased risk for surgical and septic shock related to instrumentation.
Observe drainage from wounds around suprapubic catheter.	Presence of drains and suprapubic incision increases risk of infection, as indicated by erythema or purulent drainage.
Change suprapubic/retropubic and perineal incision dressings frequently, cleaning and drying skin thoroughly each time.	Wet dressings cause skin irritation and provide medium for bacterial growth, increasing risk of wound infection.
Use ostomy-type skin barriers.	Provides protection for surrounding skin, preventing excoriation and reducing risk of infection.
Collaborative	
Administer antibiotics, as indicated.	May be given prophylactically because of increased risk of infection with prostatectomy.

NURSING DIAGNOSIS: acute Pain

May Be Related To

Physical agents (e.g., irritation of bladder mucosa; reflex muscle spasm)

Possibly Evidenced By

Verbalized/coded reports of pain
Guarding behaviors
Expressive behaviors—restlessness, irritability
Self-focus
Changes in vital signs

Desired Outcomes/Evaluation Criteria—Client Will

Pain Level (NOC)

Report pain is relieved or controlled.
Appear relaxed and sleep and rest appropriately.

Pain Control (NOC)

Demonstrate use of relaxation skills and diversional activities, as indicated, for individual situation.

ACTIONS/INTERVENTIONS	RATIONALE
Pain Management (NIC)	
Independent	
Assess pain, noting location, intensity (0 to 10 or similar coded scale), and characteristics.	Changes in pain reports may indicate developing complications requiring further evaluation and intervention. *Note:* Sharp, intermittent pain with urge to void and passage of urine around catheter suggests bladder spasms, which tend to be more severe with suprapubic or TUR approaches and usually decrease within 48 hours.
Maintain patency of catheter and drainage system. Keep tubing free of kinks and clots.	Maintaining a properly functioning catheter and drainage system decreases risk of bladder distention and spasm.
Promote intake of up to 3000 mL/day, as tolerated.	Decreases irritation by maintaining a constant flow of fluid over the bladder mucosa.
Give client accurate information about catheter, drainage, bladder spasms, and potential for voiding difficulties.	Allays anxiety and promotes cooperation with necessary procedures. *Note:* Depending on the degree of preoperative urge incontinence, postoperative urge incontinence may be present for weeks or months (Mills, 2011).
Provide comfort measures, such as position changes, back rub, Therapeutic Touch, and diversional activities. Encourage use of relaxation techniques, including deep-breathing exercises, visualization, and guided imagery.	Reduces muscle tension, refocuses attention, and may enhance coping abilities.
Collaborative	
Provide sitz baths or heat lamp, if indicated.	Promotes tissue perfusion and resolution of edema and enhances healing in perineal approach.
Administer antispasmodics, such as:	
Oxybutynin (Ditropan), flavoxate (Urispas), B & O suppositories	Relaxes smooth muscle to provide relief of spasms and associated pain.
Propantheline bromide (Pro-Banthine)	Relieves bladder spasms by anticholinergic action. Usually discontinued 24 to 48 hours before anticipated removal of catheter to promote normal bladder contraction.

NURSING DIAGNOSIS: risk for Sexual Dysfunction

Risk Factors May Include

Situational crisis—incontinence/leakage of urine, involvement of genital area
Vulnerability (e.g., change in health status, threat to self-concept)

Possibly Evidenced By

(Not applicable; presence of signs and symptoms establishes an *actual* diagnosis)

Desired Outcomes/Evaluation Criteria—Client Will

Sexual Functioning (NOC)

Report understanding of sexual function and alterations that may occur following surgery.
Discuss concerns about possible changes in body image and sexual functioning with partner/significant other (SO).
Demonstrate problem-solving skills regarding solutions to difficulties that occur.

ACTIONS/INTERVENTIONS	RATIONALE
Sexual Counseling (NIC)	
Independent	
Provide openings for client and SO to talk about concerns of incontinence and sexual functioning.	May have anxieties about the effects of surgery and may be hesitant about asking necessary questions. Anxiety may have affected ability to access information given previously.
Discuss basic anatomy. Be honest in answers to client's questions.	The nerve plexus that controls erection runs posteriorly to the prostate through the capsule. In procedures that do not involve the prostatic capsule, impotence and sterility are usually not consequences. Surgical procedure may not provide a permanent cure, and hypertrophy may recur.
Give accurate information about expectation of return of sexual function.	Physiological impotence occurs when the perineal nerves are cut during radical procedures; with other approaches, sexual activity can usually be resumed within weeks. If erectile dysfunction persists after healing is complete, client may want to pursue options to restore function—use of medications such as sildenafil citrate (Viagra). *Note:* Coincident erectile dysfunction and bladder neck contracture have been

ACTIONS/INTERVENTIONS (continued)	RATIONALE (continued)
	reported postoperatively in approximately 2% to 3% of patients following suprapubic prostatectomy (Miles, 2011).
Discuss retrograde ejaculation if transurethral or suprapubic approach is used.	Seminal fluid goes into the bladder and is excreted with the urine. This does not interfere with sexual functioning, but will decrease fertility and cause urine to be cloudy. *Note*: Retrograde ejaculation has been reported in up to 80% to 90% of patients after surgery (Miles et al, 2011).
Instruct in perineal and pelvic floor exercises and interruption of urinary stream exercises.	Tightening pelvic floor muscles prior to standing, coughing, and sneezing promotes regaining bladder and, perhaps, erectile function.
Collaborative	
Refer to sexual counselor as indicated.	Persistent or unresolved problems may require professional intervention.

NURSING DIAGNOSIS: deficient Knowledge [Learning Need] regarding condition, prognosis, treatment, self-care, and discharge needs

May Be Related To

Lack of exposure or recall, information misinterpretation
Unfamiliarity with information resources

Possibly Evidenced By

Reports the problem
Inaccurate follow-through of instruction

Desired Outcomes/Evaluation Criteria—Client Will

Knowledge: Disease Process (NOC)

Verbalize understanding of surgical procedure and potential complications.
Initiate necessary lifestyle changes.

Knowledge: Treatment Regimen (NOC)

Verbalize understanding of therapeutic needs.
Correctly perform necessary procedures and explain reasons for actions.
Participate in therapeutic regimen.

ACTIONS/INTERVENTIONS	RATIONALE
Teaching: Disease Process (NIC)	
Independent	
Review implications of procedure and future expectations.	Provides knowledge base from which client can make informed choices.
Stress necessity of good nutrition; encourage inclusion of fruits and increased fiber in diet.	Promotes healing and prevents constipation, reducing risk of postoperative bleeding.
Advise client to avoid or limit intake of caffeine, citrus juices, carbonated beverages, and spicy foods for first few weeks after surgery.	Acidic substances can lower urine pH, thereby aggravating dysuria (Shiller, 2007).
Discuss initial activity restrictions, such as avoidance of heavy lifting, strenuous exercise, prolonged sitting, long car trips, and climbing more than two flights of stairs at a time.	Increased abdominal pressure and straining places stress on the bladder and prostate, potentiating risk of bleeding.
Encourage continuation of perineal exercises.	Facilitates urinary control and alleviation of incontinence.
Instruct in urinary catheter care if present. Identify source for supplies and support.	Promotes independence and competent self-care. Catheter may be in place only on day of surgery when laser procedure is done or for days to weeks with other procedures.
Instruct client to avoid tub baths after discharge.	Decreases the possibility of introduction of bacteria or undue tension on incision.
Review signs and symptoms requiring medical evaluation: erythema, purulent drainage from wound sites; inability to urinate, changes in character or amount of urine, presence of urgency or frequency; and heavy clots or bright red bleeding, fever, or chills.	Prompt intervention may prevent serious complications. *Note:* Urine may appear cloudy for several weeks until postoperative healing occurs and may appear cloudy after intercourse because of retrograde ejaculation.
Provide written information to client and SO regarding recovery expectations and home management, as indicated, regarding pain, incision care, and catheter-related problems and care.	Anxiety related to hospitalization; procedure performed; and associated diagnosis, fatigue, and postoperative pain often makes it difficult for client to absorb necessary self-care information.

(continues on page 572)

ACTIONS/INTERVENTIONS (continued)	RATIONALE (continued)
Stress importance of follow-up care—evaluation by primary healthcare provider, urologist or oncologist, and laboratory studies.	Monitoring and follow-up can reduce incidence of unaddressed complications. Persistent incontinence and other postoperative issues will require additional evaluation and treatment.
Provide information on available community resources, such as home-health services, medical equipment supply company, housekeeping, and support persons.	Can be helpful in assisting client and SO in coping with challenges they are faced with following prostatectomy, whatever the reason for procedure—BPH, cancer, incontinence, and so forth.

POTENTIAL CONSIDERATIONS following acute hospitalization (dependent on client's age, physical condition, presence of complications, personal resources, and life responsibilities)

In addition to surgical and cancer concerns:

- ***impaired Urinary Elimination***—loss of bladder tone, possible discharge with catheter in place
- ***Sexual Dysfunction***—situational crises (e.g., leakage of urine), altered body function (e.g., erectile dysfunction)

Sample clinical pathway follows in Table 10.1.

TABLE 10.1 TURP, Hospital. ELOS: 3 Days Urology or Surgical Unit

ND and Categories	Day 1 Day of Surgery_____	Day 2 POD 1 _____	Day 3 POD 2 Discharge _____
impaired Urinary Elimination R/T mechanical obstruction, loss of bladder tone, therapeutic intervention	Display urine output individually appropriate, few clots and catheter free-flowing	Verbalize understanding of home-care needs, S/S to report to healthcare provider	Void normal amounts w/o retention Demonstrate behaviors to regain bladder/urinary control Plan in place to meet postdischarge needs
Referrals		Home care	
Additional assessments	Characteristics of urinary drainage	→	Voiding frequency, character of urine
	Urinary output q8h	→	Amount per void
	Presence of spontaneous voiding	→	→
Patient education	Foley catheter function, hygiene	Perineal exercises	
		Home-care needs, activity/dietary restrictions, sexual concerns	Provide written instructions, schedule for follow-up visits
		S/S to report to healthcare provider	
Additional nursing actions	Foley catheter to straight drain, irrigate/CBI per protocol	→ D/C	
		Stand to void q2–4h	→ Per self q4h
	Bedrest if CBI	Ambulate as tolerated	→ Ad lib
	Bed flat × 8 h if epidural anesthesia	Encourage fluids to 3 L/day as indicated	→
acute Pain R/T physical agents: ureteral contractions, tissue trauma, edema	Report pain relieved/ controlled	→	→ Verbalize understanding of pain management postdischarge
Additional assessments	Pain characteristics/ changes, presence of bladder spasms	→	→
	Response to interventions	→	→
		Return of bowel function	→
Medications	Analgesic of choice IM/PO q4h	→ PO analgesic	→
Allergies: ______	Antispasmotic prn	→ D/C	
		Stool softener/laxative	→
Patient education	Reporting of pain/effects of intervention		
	Relaxation techniques		
Additional nursing actions	Routine comfort measures	→	→
	Anchor catheter, avoid manipulation	→	→
	Maintain potency of catheter	Sitz bath as indicated	→

TABLE 10.1 TURP, Hospital. ELOS: 3 Days Urology or Surgical Unit (continued)

ND and Categories	Day 1 Day of Surgery____	Day 2 POD 1 ____	Day 3 POD 2 Discharge ____
risk for deficient Fluid Volume, R/T nausea and vomiting, post-obstructive diuresis	Maintain adequate hydration with VS stable, palpable pulses, good capillary refill, adequate urinary output	→	→
	Free of active bleeding	→	→
Diagnostic studies		Hb/Hct, RBC	
Additional assessments	Characteristics of catheter drainage	→ Characteristics of urine	→ D/C
	VS per postoperative protocol	→ q8h	→
	Peripheral pulses, capillary refill, status of skin q8h	→	→ D/C
	I&O q8h	→	→ D/C
	Mental status/restlessness q4h	→ q8h	→ D/C
	Temperature q8h	→	→
Medications	IV therapy/blood products as indicated	→ D/C	
Patient education	Fluid needs/restrictions	→ D/C	
Additional nursing actions	Maintain catheter traction as indicated, release q4h per protocol	→ D/C	
	Begin PO fluids as tolerated	→ Advance diet/fluids as tolerated	→

Key: ad lib, as desired; CBI, continuous bladder irrigation; D/C, discontinue; Hb/Hct, hemoglobin/hematocrit; IM, intramuscular; I&O, intake & output; PO, by mouth; prn, as needed; q2–4h, every 2 to 4 hours; q4h, every 4 hours; q8h, every 8 hours; RBC, red blood cell; R/T, related to; S/S, signs and symptoms; VS, vital signs.

UROLITHIASIS (RENAL CALCULI)

I. Pathophysiology

a. Presence of stones anywhere in the urinary tract
- **i.** Most commonly found in the renal pelvis and calyces
  1. Stones forming in the kidney—nephrolithiasis
  2. Stones formed in the ureters—ureterolithiasis
- **ii.** May be single or multiple calculi, ranging in size from a grain of salt to the size of a pebble or staghorn calculus

b. Composition of calculi (Wolf, 2013; Miller, 2007)
- **i.** Formed of mineral deposits—predominantly calcium oxalate and calcium phosphate. Note: About 70% to 80% of renal calculi are calcium stones
- **ii.** Uric acid (5% to 10%), struvite (5% to 15%), and cystine (1%) are also calculus formers

II. Etiology

a. Slow urine flow allows accumulation of crystals—damaging the lining of the urinary tract and decreasing the number of inhibitor substances that would prevent crystal accumulation (Winkleman, 2006).

b. May remain asymptomatic until passed into a ureter or urine flow is obstructed, at which time the potential for renal damage is acute and the level of pain is at its highest

c. Causes: dehydration; heredity; excessive intake of vitamins A and D, grapefruit juice, and purines (gout); congenital renal abnormalities; and some medications, such as acetazolamide (Diamox), indinavir (Crixivan), dilantin, some antibiotics (e.g., ceftriazone [Rocephin], ciprofloxacin [Cipro]) (Wedro, 2010)

d. Risk factors: men aged 30 to 50, postmenopausal women; gender: male-to-female ratio 3:1; heredity may play a part in hypercalcuria; recurrent urinary tract infections; certain chronic conditions (e.g., cystic fibrosis, inflammatory bowel disease, hyperparathyroidism, hypertension); insulin resistance; prolonged bedrest; spinal cord injury; some geographic locations—southeastern United States; use of antacids or aspirin (Wedro, 2010)

III. Statistics (Centers for Disease Control and Prevention [CDC], 2006)

a. Morbidity: Each year in the United States more than 300,000 people go to emergency rooms for kidney stone problems (National Kidney and Urologic Diseases Information Clearinghouse [NKUDIC], 2012). Kidney stones affect approximately 1 in 11 people in the United States. These data represent a marked increase in stone disease compared with the National Health and Nutrition Examination Survey (NHANES) III cohort study of 2002 (Scales, 2012).

b. Mortality: Rare and related to development of acute kidney injury or comorbidities. Note: Mortality and morbidity are not increased with uric acid stones compared with other stones; however, the process that leads to excess uric acid production (e.g., malignancy, Lesch-Nyhan syndrome) may cause death (Fathallah-Shaykh, 2013).

c. Cost: In 2007, $10.3 billion expended for treatment of upper urinary tract stones, and almost $200 million for lower urinary tract stones (Litwin, 2012).

GLOSSARY

Calcium oxalate stones: Kidney stones formed by calcium and oxalate crystals, which usually develop in acidic urine.

Calcium phosphate stones: Kidney stones formed by calcium and phosphate crystals, which usually develop in alkaline urine.

Cystine stones: Kidney stones made of cystine crystals.

Extracorporeal shock wave lithotripsy (ESWL): Procedure whereby a shock wave is transmitted through the body to target a stone, thus fragmenting it.

Hematuria: Blood in the urine.

Hypercalciuria: High calcium in the urine—an inherited condition.

Hyperoxaluria: Excretion of excessive amounts of oxalate in the urine.

Polycythemia: Too many red blood cells (RBCs) in the circulation.

Pyuria: Pus in the urine.

Renal calyces: The perimeter of the renal pelvis is interrupted by cuplike projections called calyces. A minor calyx surrounds the renal papillae of each pyramid and collects urine from that pyramid. Several minor calyces converge to form a major calyx. From the major calyces the urine flows into the renal pelvis and from there into the ureter.

Renal colic: Flank (side) pain caused by obstruction to the flow of urine caused by kidney or ureteral stones.

Renal pelvis: The area at the center of the kidney where urine collects and is funneled into the ureter.

Renal tubular acidosis: Condition associated with dehydration, metabolic acidosis, low potassium, and high chloride. Often associated with renal stones due to hypercalciuria (high calcium in urine).

Staghorn calculi: Develops in the center of the kidney or pelvis, filling the entire pelvis and extending out into the calyces.

Stent: Tube inserted into the ureter to bypass a stone or to keep the ureter open so urine flows freely from the kidney to the bladder.

Struvite stone: Also known as magnesium ammonium phosphate—stones that are often present with infection.

Ureterovesical junction: Joining of the ureters and bladder.

Uric acid stones: Kidney stones made of pure uric acid crystals. These stones develop in acidic urine.

Care Setting

Treatment is often handled at the community level or as an outpatient; acute episodes occasionally require inpatient treatment on a medical or surgical unit. On occasion, surgery is necessary to remove the stone(s).

Related Concerns

Acute kidney injury (acute renal failure), 505
Fluid and electrolyte imbalances, page 885
Metabolic acidosis—primary base bicarbonate deficiency, page 450
Metabolic alkalosis—primary base bicarbonate excess, page 455
Psychosocial aspects of care, page 729

Client Assessment Database

Dependent on size, location, and etiology of calculi.

DIAGNOSTIC DIVISION MAY REPORT	MAY EXHIBIT
ACTIVITY/REST	
• Sedentary occupation or occupation in which client is exposed to high environmental temperatures • Activity restrictions or immobility due to a preexisting condition—debilitating disease, spinal cord injury—causing bones to release more calcium	
CIRCULATION	
	• Elevated blood pressure (BP) and pulse associated with pain, anxiety, or kidney failure • Warm, flushed skin, pallor
ELIMINATION	
• History of recent or chronic urinary tract infection (UTI) • Previous kidney stones • Decreased urinary output, bladder fullness • Burning, urgency with urination • Diarrhea	• Oliguria (retention, scant urine), hematuria, pyuria • Alterations in voiding pattern

DIAGNOSTIC DIVISION MAY REPORT (continued)	MAY EXHIBIT (continued)
FOOD/FLUID • Nausea and vomiting (common) • A high-protein, high-sodium, low-calcium diet, which may increase risk of some types of stones • Insufficient fluid intake, does not drink fluids well (common)	• Abdominal distention, decreased or absent bowel sounds
PAIN/DISCOMFORT • Acute episode of excruciating, colicky pain, with location depending on stone location; in the flank in the region of the costovertebral angle, may radiate to back, abdomen, and down to the groin and genitalia; constant dull pain suggests calculi located in the renal pelvis or calyces • May be described as acute, severe, and not relieved by positioning or any other measures	• Guarding, distraction behaviors, self-focusing • Tenderness in renal areas on palpation
SAFETY • Use of alcohol can contribute to dehydration and to uric acid stone formation. • Fever (uncommon)	
TEACHING/LEARNING • Family history of kidney stones, kidney disease, hypertension, gout, chronic UTI, or hereditary disease, such as renal tubular acidosis, cystinuria, hyperoxaluria • History of small bowel disease, previous abdominal surgery, hyperparathyroidism • Use of antibiotics, antihypertensives, sodium bicarbonate, allopurinol, phosphates, thiazides, excessive intake of calcium or vitamin D • Use of herbal remedies for kidney stones, such as valerian, skullcap, wild yam, khella, marshmallow, slippery elm	
DISCHARGE PLAN CONSIDERATIONS • May require dietary modifications, exercise program, pain management plan ➧ Refer to section at end of plan for postdischarge considerations.	

Diagnostic Studies

TEST WHY IT IS DONE	WHAT IT TELLS ME
BLOOD TESTS • ***Serum and urine blood urea nitrogen/creatinine (BUN/Cr):*** Helpful in delineating obstructive uropathy due to urolithiasis.	Blockage of urine flow below the kidneys causes postrenal azotemia (ratio greater than 15:1) without intrinsic renal disease. Abnormal levels—high in serum and low in urine—are secondary to high obstructive stones with reduced urine output.
• ***Complete blood count (CBC):*** Battery of screening tests, which typically includes hemoglobin (Hb); hematocrit (Hct); RBC count, morphology; and white blood cell (WBC) count and differential.	Hgb/Hct—abnormal if client is severely dehydrated or client is anemic (hemorrhage, kidney dysfunction or failure) RBCs—usually normal WBCs—may be increased, indicating infection
• ***Blood chemistry:*** Measures levels of calcium, phosphate, uric acid, sodium, potassium, chloride, bicarbonate, and albumin. If serum calcium levels are elevated, then testing for hyperparathyroidism is performed.	These tests are done if complications associated with kidney stones are suspected or present.

(continues on page 576)

TEST WHY IT IS DONE (continued)	WHAT IT TELLS ME (continued)
URINE TESTS	
• ***Urinalysis:*** Simple screening test may suggest type of stone and presence of infection.	Color may be yellow, dark brown, or bloody. Commonly shows RBCs, WBCs, crystals (cystine, uric acid, calcium oxalate), casts, minerals, bacteria, and pus. pH may be less than 5.0, which promotes cystine and uric acid stones, or higher than 7.5, which promotes magnesium, struvite, phosphate, or calcium phosphate stones.
• ***Urine (24-hour):*** Measures urine volume, pH, and levels of calcium, sodium, uric acid, oxalate, citrate, and creatinine.	Helps identify degree of obstruction and type of stone—especially important for long-term management in client who is prone to stone formation.
• ***Urine culture:*** Identifies presence of infection and causative agent.	May reveal UTI and identify organism (e.g., *Staphylococcus aureus, Proteus, Klebsiella, Pseudomonas*) as cause for stone development—struvite or infection stone.
OTHER DIAGNOSTIC STUDIES	
• ***Renal helical or spiral computerized tomography (CT) scan:*** Continuous motion image providing detailed views of the kidneys, ureters, and bladder in a shorter period of time.	Identifies and delineates calculi and other masses, as well as kidney, ureteral, and bladder distention. Contrast is not used because it masks the stones. *Note*: This test has largely replaced IVP as the definitive diagnostic test for stones (Wolf et al, 2013).
• ***Abdominal x-ray of kidneys-ureters-bladder (KUB):*** Usually ordered to evaluate hematuria flank pain.	Shows presence of calculi and anatomic changes in the area of the kidneys or along the course of the ureter. May show small stones that can pass unnoticed.
• ***Kidney ultrasound and intrarenal Doppler ultrasound:*** Determines obstructive changes and location of stone without the risk of kidney failure that can be induced by contrast medium.	Ultrasound is used to show obstruction to the kidney. However, small kidney stones that are not obstructing may be missed. Renal Doppler ultrasound improves the detection of early obstruction by evaluating for elevated resistive index (RI) in kidney with nondilated collecting system.
• ***Intravenous urogram (IVU; also known as intravenous pyelogram [IVP]):*** Kidney x-ray performed by injecting radiopaque contrast into a vein. Multiple pictures of the kidneys are taken to follow the uptake and excretion of the contrast by the kidneys.	Provides rapid confirmation of urolithiasis as a cause of abdominal or flank pain. Shows abnormalities in anatomical structures, such as distended ureter, and outline of calculi.

Nursing Priorities

1. Alleviate pain.
2. Maintain adequate renal functioning.
3. Prevent complications.
4. Provide information about disease process, prognosis, and treatment needs.

Discharge Goals

1. Pain relieved or controlled.
2. Fluid and electrolyte balance maintained.
3. Complications prevented or minimized.
4. Disease process, prognosis, and therapeutic regimen understood.
5. Plan in place to meet needs after discharge.

NURSING DIAGNOSIS: acute Pain

May Be Related To

Physical agents (e.g., tissue trauma, ureteral contractions, edema formation, cellular ischemia)

Possibly Evidenced By

Verbalized/coded reports of pain
Expressive behaviors (e.g., restlessness, moaning)
Self-focus; facial mask of pain (e.g., grimacing)
Guarding behaviors

Desired Outcomes/Evaluation Criteria—Client Will

Pain Level (NOC)

Report pain is relieved, with spasms controlled.
Appear relaxed and able to sleep/rest appropriately.

ACTIONS/INTERVENTIONS	RATIONALE
Pain Management (NIC)	
Independent	
Document location, duration, intensity (0 to 10 or similar coded scale), and radiation. Note nonverbal signs—elevated BP, pulse and respirations, moaning and thrashing about.	Helps evaluate site of obstruction and progress of calculi movement. Flank pain suggests that stones are in the kidney area, upper ureter. Flank pain radiates to back, abdomen, groin, and genitalia because of proximity of nerve plexus and blood vessels supplying these areas. Sudden, severe pain may precipitate apprehension, restlessness, and severe anxiety.
Explain cause of pain and importance of notifying care providers of changes in pain occurrence or characteristics.	Provides opportunity for timely administration of analgesia and alerts care providers to possibility of passing of stone or developing complications. Sudden cessation of pain usually indicates stone passage.
Provide such comfort measures as back rub and restful environment.	Promotes relaxation, reduces muscle tension, and enhances coping.
Apply warm compresses to back.	Reduces muscle tension and may reduce reflex spasms.
Assist with and encourage use of focused breathing, guided imagery, and diversional activities.	Redirects attention and aids in muscle relaxation.
Encourage frequent ambulation as indicated; increase fluid intake to at least 3 to 4 L/day within cardiac tolerance.	Renal colic can be worse in the supine position. Vigorous hydration promotes passing of stone, prevents urinary stasis, and aids in prevention of further stone formation.
Note reports of increased or persistent abdominal pain.	Complete obstruction of ureter can cause perforation and extravasation of urine into perirenal space. This represents an acuter surgical emergency.
Collaborative	
Administer medications, as indicated, for example:	
Analgesics, including narcotics (e.g., morphine sulfate [Astramorph], butorphenol [Stadol]; combination opiods such as oxycodone and acetaminophen [Percocet]; and NSAIDs such as ketorolac [Toradol], diclofenac [Voltaren], and ibuprophen	Acute renal colic may be the most painful event a person can endure. Striking without warning, the pain is often described as excruciating, and the client is unable to find a position of comfort. Parenteral narcotics have traditionally been prescribed for acute renal colic and are often required in the early phases of treatment, but NSAIDs are also effective for moderate to severe pain. *Note*: NSAIDs should be avoided in client with poor renal function or a history of gastrointestinal bleeding (Wolf, 2013; Miller, 2007).
Antispasmodics, such as flavoxate (Urispas) and oxybutynin (Ditropan); calcium channel blockers, such as nifedipine (Adalat); and alpha-adrenergic blockers, such as tamsulosin (Flomax)	Decreases reflex spasm and relaxes ureteral smooth muscle, which facilitates stone passage. *Note*: Oral analgesics, NSAIDs, and alpha-adrenergic blockers help facilitate stone passage after acute attack.
Maintain patency of catheters when used.	Prevents urinary stasis or retention, reduces risk of increased renal pressure and infection.

NURSING DIAGNOSIS: impaired Urinary Elimination

May Be Related To

Anatomic obstruction

Possibly Evidenced By

Dysuria

Urgency; frequency

Retention

Desired Outcomes/Evaluation Criteria—Client Will

Urinary Elimination (NOC)

Void in normal amounts of greater than or equal to 30 mL/hr and usual pattern.

Experience no signs of retention

ACTIONS/INTERVENTIONS	RATIONALE
Urinary Elimination Enhancement (NIC)	
Independent	
Note urine output and characteristics of urine.	Provides information about kidney function and presence of complications (such as infection and dehydration). Bleeding may also indicate increased obstruction or irritation of ureter.
Determine client's normal voiding pattern and note variations.	Calculi may cause urinary tract nerve excitability, which causes sensations of urgent need to void. Frequency and urgency usually increase as calculus nears the ureterovesical junction.
Encourage increased fluid intake, if nausea is not present.	Increased hydration dilutes urine and flushes bacteria, blood, and debris and may facilitate stone passage—especially small stones.
Strain all urine. Document any stones expelled and send to laboratory for analysis.	Retrieval of calculi allows identification of type of stone and influences choice of therapy.
Investigate reports of bladder fullness; palpate for suprapubic distention. Note decreased urine output and presence of periorbital or dependent edema.	Urinary retention may develop, causing bladder, ureteral, and kidney distention, exacerbating pain and potentiating risk of infection and renal failure.
Observe for changes in mental status, behavior, or level of consciousness (LOC).	Accumulation of uremic wastes and electrolyte imbalances can be toxic to the central nervous system (CNS).
Collaborative	
Maintain patency of indwelling catheters—ureteral, urethral, or nephrostomy—when used.	May be required to facilitate urine flow, preventing retention and corresponding complications. Catheters are positioned above the stone to promote urethral dilation and stone passage. Continuous or intermittent irrigation can be carried out to flush kidneys and ureters and adjust pH of urine to permit dissolution of stone fragments following lithotripsy.
Administer medications, as indicated, for example:	
Acetazolamide (Diamox) and allopurinol (Zyloprim)	Increases urine pH (alkalinity) to reduce formation of acid stones. Antigout agents such as allopurinol also lower uric acid production and potential of uric acid stone formation.
Alpha-adrenergic blockers, e.g., tamsulosin (Flomax), terazosin (Hytrin)	Although these drugs are designed specifically for prostatic hypertrophy, they have off-label use in treatment of kidney stones as smooth muscle relaxants, which facilitate passage of ureteral stones.
Corticosteroids, such as prednisone (Deltasone)	May be used short-term to reduce tissue edema to facilitate movement of stones.
Penicillamine (Cuprimine), tiopronin (Thiola), and potassium citrate (Polycitra-K)	Drugs may be prescribed to make urine more alkaline or bind cystine in the urine, when cystine stones cannot be controlled.
Ammonium chloride and potassium or sodium phosphate	Reduces phosphate stone formation.
Antibiotics	Antibiotics may be needed in presence of UTI or to keep urine bacteria-free to prevent struvite stone formation.
Monitor laboratory studies, for example:	
Electrolytes, BUN, and Cr	Elevated BUN, Cr, and certain electrolytes indicate presence and degree of kidney dysfunction.
Urine culture and sensitivities	Determines presence of UTI, which may be causing or complicating kidney stone symptoms; determines appropriate antibiotic therapy.
Prepare client for and assist with endoscopic procedures, such as the following:	For treatment of most kidney stones, shock wave lithotripsy, ureteroscopy, and percutaneous nephrolithotomy have largely replaced open surgery (Miller, 2007).
Basket procedure, percutaneous ultrasonic lithotripsy, and stent placement	Calculi in the distal and midureter may be removed by fiberoptic ureteroscope, which shatters the stone with a shock wave and captures it in a basket catheter.
Extracorporeal shock wave lithotripsy (ESWL)	ESWL is the most frequently used outpatient procedure for treatment of stones that are not responsive to medical therapy, and has been found effective 80% to 85% of the time (Miller, 2007). Kidney stones are pulverized by shock waves delivered from outside the body while client reclines in water bath or on soft cushion. *Note:* ESWL is not ideal for large stones.
Percutaneous nephrolithotomy or open incision stone removal	Surgery may be necessary in about 15% to 20% of clients (Wolf, 2013) to remove a stone that is (1) too large to pass through ureters (e.g., >7 mm in diameter), (2) is caught in a difficult place, (3) blocks flow of urine, (4) causes or exacerbates ongoing urinary tract infection (UTI), (5) causes constant bleeding, or (6) is potentially damaging to kidney tissue. One advantage to the open procedure is that stone fragments are removed at surgery rather than relying on natural passage from the kidneys or urinary tract. Client may have a small drainage tube left in kidney or ureters during the healing process.

NURSING DIAGNOSIS: risk for deficient Fluid Volume

Risk Factors May Include

Active fluid loss (e.g., nausea, vomiting)
Failure of regulatory mechanisms (e.g., postobstructive diuresis)

Possibly Evidenced By

(Not applicable; presence of signs or symptoms establishes an *actual* diagnosis)

Desired Outcomes/Evaluation Criteria—Client Will

Fluid Volume (NOC)

Maintain adequate fluid balance as evidenced by vital signs and weight within client's normal range, palpable peripheral pulses, moist mucous membranes, and good skin turgor.

ACTIONS/INTERVENTIONS	RATIONALE
Fluid/Electrolyte Management (NIC)	
Independent	
Monitor I&O.	Comparing actual and anticipated output may aid in evaluating presence and degree of renal stasis or impairment. *Note:* Impaired kidney functioning and decreased urinary output can result in higher circulating volumes with signs and symptoms of heart failure (HF).
Document incidence and note characteristics and frequency of vomiting and diarrhea, as well as accompanying or precipitating events.	Nausea or vomiting and diarrhea are commonly associated with renal colic because celiac ganglion serves both kidneys and stomach. Documentation may help rule out other abdominal occurrences as a cause for pain or pinpoint calculi.
Increase fluid intake to 3 to 4 L/day within cardiac tolerance.	Maintains fluid balance for homeostasis and "washing" action that may flush the stone(s) out. *Note:* Patients with recurrent kidney stones traditionally have been instructed to drink 8 glasses of fluid daily to maintain adequate hydration and decrease chance of urinary supersaturation with stone-forming salts. The goal is a total urine volume in 24 hours in excess of 2 liters (Wolf, 2013).
Monitor vital signs. Evaluate pulses, capillary refill, skin turgor, and mucous membranes.	Indicators of hydration and circulating volume and need for intervention.
Weigh daily.	Rapid weight changes suggest water loss or retention.
Collaborative	
Monitor Hgb/Hct and electrolytes.	Assesses hydration and effectiveness of, or need for, interventions.
Administer IV fluids.	Maintains circulating volume if oral intake is insufficient, promoting renal function.
Provide appropriate diet, clear liquids, and bland foods, as tolerated.	Easily digested foods decrease gastrointestinal (GI) activity or irritation and help maintain fluid and nutritional balance.
Administer medications, as indicated, for example, antiemetics, such as metoclopramide (Reglan), ondansetron (Zofran), promethazine (Phenergan), or droperidol (Inapsine).	Reduces nausea and vomiting.

NURSING DIAGNOSIS: deficient Knowledge [Learning Need] regarding condition, prognosis, treatment, self-care, and discharge needs

May Be Related To

Lack of exposure or recall; information misinterpretation
Unfamiliarity with information resources

Possibly Evidenced By

Reports the problem
Inaccurate follow-through of instructions

Desired Outcomes/Evaluation Criteria—Client Will

Knowledge: Acute Illness Management (NOC)

Verbalize understanding of disease process and potential complications.
Correlate symptoms with causative factors.
Verbalize understanding of therapeutic needs.
Initiate necessary lifestyle changes and participate in treatment regimen.

ACTIONS/INTERVENTIONS	RATIONALE
Teaching: Disease Process (NIC)	
Independent	
Review disease process and future expectations.	Provides knowledge base from which client can make informed choices.
Stress importance of increased fluid intake, such as 3 to 4 L/day if not contraindicated. Encourage client to notice dry mouth and excessive diuresis or diaphoresis and to increase fluid intake whether or not feeling thirsty.	Flushes renal system, decreasing opportunity for urinary stasis and stone formation. Increased fluid losses or dehydration require additional intake beyond usual daily needs.
Review dietary regimen, as individually appropriate, for example:	Diet depends on the type of stone. Understanding reason for modifications provides opportunity for client to make informed choices, increases cooperation with regimen, and may prevent recurrence.
Low-purine diet, such as limited lean meat, turkey, legumes, whole grains, and alcohol	Decreases oral intake of uric acid precursors.
Low-oxalate diet, such as limited chocolate, caffeine-containing beverages, beets, nuts, rhubarb, strawberries, spinach, and wheat bran	Reduces calcium-oxalate stone formation. *Note:* Research suggests that daily inclusion of coffee, tea, beer, or wine decreases the risk of stone formation, whereas regular intake of apple or grapefruit juice increases the risk (Finkielstein & Goldfarb, 2006).
Limit calcium intake to about 800 mg/day when appropriate. Use calcium citrate when supplements are required.	Although not advocating high-calcium diets, researchers are urging that calcium limitation be reexamined. Research suggests that restricting dietary calcium is not helpful in reducing calcium stone formation and may actually increase oxalate formation. Use of citrate is helpful in binding oxalate and improving calcium absorption.
Shorr regimen: low-calcium and phosphorus diet with aluminum carbonate gel 30 to 40 mL 30 minutes after meals and at bedtime	Prevents phosphoric calculi by forming an insoluble precipitate in the GI tract, reducing the load to the kidney nephrons. Also effective against other forms of calcium calculi. *Note:* May cause constipation.
Encourage foods rich in magnesium and vitamins B and K	These nutrients reduce stone formation.
Discuss medication and herbal supplement regimen; avoidance of over-the-counter (OTC) drugs, and reading all product and food ingredient labels.	Drugs will be given to acidify or alkalize urine, depending on underlying cause of stone formation. Ingestion of products containing individually contraindicated ingredients, such as calcium and phosphorus, potentiates recurrence of stones. *Note:* Some herbal supplements—valerian, skullcap, wild yam, khella, and marshmallow—are known to have antispasmodic properties or are soothing to irritated urinary tissues.
Encourage client to reveal all medications and herbals to physician or pharmacist.	To reduce risk of dangerous interactions and side effects.
Emphasize need for smoking cessation, when indicated.	Cigarette smoking may contribute to kidney stones because it increases urine levels of cadmium, a heavy metal.
Encourage regular activity and exercise program.	Inactivity contributes to stone formation through calcium shifts and urinary stasis.
Active-listen concerns about therapeutic regimen and lifestyle changes.	Helps client work through feelings and gain a sense of control over what is happening.
Identify signs and symptoms requiring medical evaluation, such as recurrent pain, hematuria, and oliguria.	With increased probability of stone recurrence, prompt interventions may prevent serious complications. *Note:* Rate of recurrence at 1 year is 14%; at 2 years, 35%; and at 10 years, 52% (Wolf, 2013).
Demonstrate proper care of incisions or catheters if present.	Promotes competent self-care and independence.

POTENTIAL CONSIDERATIONS following acute hospitalizations (dependent on client's age, physical condition and presence of complications, personal resources, and life responsibilities)

- ***impaired Urinary Elimination***—recurrence of calculi

CHAPTER 11

Women's Reproductive

HYSTERECTOMY

I. Indications—surgical removal of the uterus

- **a.** Malignancies: Cancer of the uterus, or endometrial cancer, is the most common gynecological cancer in the United States, and in 2000, 11% of hysterectomies were due to cancer (Greenlee, 2000; Encyclopedia of Surgery, n.d.).
- **b.** Nonmalignant conditions, such as endometriosis, fibroid tumors; pelvic relaxation with uterine prolapse that leads to disabling levels of pain, discomfort, uterine bleeding, emotional stress
- **c.** Life-threatening bleeding or hemorrhaging, such as obstetric or traumatic complication; irreparable rupture of the uterus
- **d.** Treatment of intractable pelvic infection

II. Procedures

- **a.** Abdominal hysterectomy
  - **i.** Subtotal or partial: removal of body of uterus; cervical stump remains
  - **ii.** Total: removal of the uterus and cervix
  - **iii.** Total with bilateral salpingo-oophorectomy: removal of uterus, cervix, fallopian tubes, and ovaries
  - **iv.** Total pelvic exenteration (TPE): Complex, aggressive surgical procedure involving radical hysterectomy with dissection of pelvic lymph nodes, bilateral salpingo-oophorectomy, total cystectomy, and abdominoperineal resection of the rectum; colostomy and/or urinary conduit are created, and vaginal reconstruction may or may not be performed. (Refer to additional care plans regarding fecal or urinary diversions, as appropriate.)
- **b.** Vaginal hysterectomy or laparoscopically assisted vaginal hysterectomy (LAVH)
  - **i.** Limited to certain conditions, such as uterine prolapse, cystocele or rectocele, carcinoma in situ, and high-risk obesity
  - **ii.** Requires removal of cervix
  - **iii.** Advantages: less pain, no visible (or much smaller) scars, shorter hospital stay, and shorter recovery period of about 3 to 4 weeks (vaginal) and 2 weeks (LAVH) versus approximately 6 weeks (abdominal)
- **c.** Laparoscopic-assisted abdominal supracervical hysterectomy (LASH)
  - **i.** Can be performed in presence of mild to moderate adhesions or large uterus
  - **ii.** A single abdominal incision is used instead of three
  - **iii.** Removal of cervix not required
  - **iv.** Usually done on outpatient basis, with a recovery period of about 1 week

III. Statistics (Centers for Disease Control and Prevention [CDC], 2008)

- **a.** Morbidity: For 2000–2004 it was reported that 600,000 hysterectomies were performed annually, and during that four-year period an estimated 3.1 million women had a hysterectomy. The three conditions most often associated with hysterectomy during that four-year period were fibroid tumors, endometriosis, and uterine prolapse.
- **b.** Mortality: Death rate is reported as 1 per thousand (Encyclopedia of Surgery, n.d.; National Women's Health Network [NWHN], 2005; Surgery.com, 2009).
- **c.** Cost: Direct care costs $3.7 billion for both abdominal and vaginal hysterectomy in 2009 (Pfunter, 2012).

GLOSSARY

Cervix: Lower end or neck of the uterus, which protrudes into the vagina.

DUB: Dysfunctional uterine bleeding (a common symptom in women undergoing hysterectomy when bleeding does not respond to other treatments).

Endometriosis: Ectopic endometrial tissue found outside the uterine cavity, usually in the ovaries, fallopian tubes, and other pelvic structures. Endometriosis is the cause for about 20% of hysterectomies (Gor, 2012).

Fibroids: Benign tumors that form in the uterine muscle; also called leiomyomas. Fibroids are the cause for about 33% of hysterectomies (Gor, 2012).

Laparoscopy: Use of a slender, light-transmitting tube to view abdominal organs or perform surgery.

Leiomyoma: Benign soft tissue tumors that arise from smooth muscle, increase in size and frequency as a woman ages, but revert to size postmenopause; also called fibroids.

Menopause: Permanent cessation of menstrual activity.

Uterine prolapse: Displacement or sagging of the uterus into the vagina. Prolapse accounts for about 5% of hysterectomies (Gor, 2012).

Care Setting

Procedure is performed in inpatient acute surgical unit or short-stay unit or outpatient, depending on type performed.

Related Concerns

Cancer, page 827
Psychosocial aspects of care, page 729
Surgical intervention, page 762
Thrombophlebitis: venous thromboembolism, page 109

Client Assessment Database

Data depend on the underlying disease process and the need for surgical intervention—cancer, prolapse, dysfunctional uterine bleeding, severe endometriosis, or pelvic infections unresponsive to medical management—and associated complications, such as anemia.

TEACHING/LEARNING

Discharge Plan Considerations

- May need temporary help with transportation and homemaker and maintenance tasks

➧ Refer to section at end of plan for postdischarge considerations.

Diagnostic Studies

WHY IT IS DONE	WHAT IT TELLS ME
• ***Pelvic examination:*** Identifies uterine and/or other pelvic organ irregularities.	May reveal masses, tender nodules, visual changes of cervix, requiring further diagnostic evaluation.
• ***Pap smear:*** Screening test for cervical cancer and certain vaginal or uterine infections.	Cellular dysplasia reflects possibility of or actual presence of cancer, which may affect choice of procedure.
• ***Pelvic ultrasound or computed tomography (CT) scan:*** Creates an electronic picture of the organs and structures within the pelvis.	Aids in identifying size and location of pelvic mass.
• ***Sonohysterogram:*** A saline-enhanced sonogram or ultrasound.	Evaluates abnormal growths inside the uterus, lining of the uterus, and deeper tissue layers. Delineates polyps and submucosal fibroids.
• ***Hysteroscopy:*** Uses fiberoptic viewing scope and a distending medium, such as carbon dioxide, to directly view the uterine cavity and/or biopsy growths.	Viewed by some to be the "gold standard." Determines cause of abnormal bleeding.
• ***Laparoscopy:*** Visualizes pathology, obtains biopsies, or performs laser treatment for endometriosis.	May reveal source of bleeding, presence of tumors, and superficial peritoneal implants of endometriosis; determines cancer staging and assesses effects of chemotherapy.
• ***Endometrial sampling:*** Dilation and curettage (D&C) with biopsy of endometrial or cervical tissue for histopathological study of cells.	Determines presence and location of cancer.
• ***Schiller's test (staining of cervix with iodine):*** Useful in identifying abnormal cells.	Cervix turns dark brown in noncancerous areas and white or yellow in possible cancerous areas.
• ***Complete blood count (CBC):*** Useful in determining general health status.	Decreased hemoglobin (Hgb) may reflect chronic anemia; decreased hematocrit (Hct) suggests active blood loss; and elevated white blood cell (WBC) count may indicate inflammation and infectious process.
• ***Sexually transmitted disease (STD) screen:*** Determines presence of infection.	Human papillomavirus (HPV) is present in 80% of clients with cervical cancer.

Nursing Priorities

1. Support adaptation to change.
2. Prevent complications.
3. Provide information about procedure, prognosis, and treatment needs.

Discharge Goals

1. Situation being dealt with realistically.
3. Complications prevented or minimized.
4. Procedure, prognosis, and therapeutic regimen understood.
5. Plan in place to meet needs after discharge.

In addition to these NDs, see nursing actions and interventions listed in CP: Surgical Intervention.

NURSING DIAGNOSIS: risk for [acute] Urinary Retention

Risk Factors May Include

Blockage (e.g., mechanical trauma, surgical manipulation, perineal swelling, hematoma)
[Sensory and motor impairment—nerve paralysis]

Possibly Evidenced By

(Not applicable; presence of signs and symptoms establishes an *actual* diagnosis)

Desired Outcomes/Evaluation Criteria—Client Will

Urinary Elimination (NOC)

Empty bladder regularly and completely.

ACTIONS/INTERVENTIONS	RATIONALE
Urinary Elimination Management (NIC)	
Independent	
Note voiding pattern and monitor urinary output, once surgical catheter is removed.	May indicate urinary retention if voiding frequently in small or insufficient amounts less than 100 mL.
Palpate bladder. Investigate reports of discomfort, fullness, and inability to void.	Perception of bladder fullness and distention of bladder above symphysis pubis indicates urinary retention.
Provide routine voiding measures, such as privacy, normal position, running water in sink, and pouring warm water over perineum.	Promotes relaxation of perineal muscles and may facilitate voiding efforts.
Provide and/or encourage good perineal cleansing and catheter care when present.	Promotes cleanliness, reducing risk of ascending urinary tract infection (UTI).
Assess urine characteristics, noting color, clarity, and odor.	Urinary retention, vaginal drainage, and possible presence of intermittent or indwelling catheter increase risk of infection, especially if client has perineal sutures.
Collaborative	
Catheterize when indicated per protocol if client is unable to void or is uncomfortable.	Edema or interference with nerve supply may cause bladder atony or urinary retention requiring decompression of the bladder. *Note:* Indwelling urethral or suprapubic catheter may be inserted intraoperatively if complications are anticipated.
Maintain patency of indwelling catheter; keep drainage tubing free of kinks.	Promotes free drainage of urine, reducing risk of urinary stasis or retention and infection.
Check residual urine volume after voiding, as indicated.	May not be emptying bladder completely; retention of urine increases possibility for infection and is uncomfortable, even painful.

NURSING DIAGNOSIS: risk for Constipation

Risk Factors May Include

Functional—abdominal muscle weakness
Mechanical—pain or discomfort in abdomen or perineal area
Physiological—decreased gastrointestinal motility, changes in dietary intake
Pharmacological—use of opiates

Possibly Evidenced By

(Not applicable; presence of signs and symptoms establishes an *actual* diagnosis)

(continues on page 584)

NURSING DIAGNOSIS: risk for Constipation (continued)

Desired Outcomes/Evaluation Criteria—Client Will

Bowel Elimination (NOC)

Display active bowel sounds and peristaltic activity.

Maintain usual pattern of elimination.

ACTIONS/INTERVENTIONS	RATIONALE
Bowel Management (NIC)	
Independent	
Auscultate bowel sounds. Note abdominal distention and presence of nausea or vomiting.	Indicators of presence or resolution of ileus, affecting choice of interventions.
Assist client with sitting on edge of bed and walking.	Early ambulation helps stimulate intestinal function and return of peristalsis.
Encourage adequate fluid intake, including fruit juices, when oral intake is resumed.	Promotes softer stool; may aid in stimulating peristalsis.
Provide sitz baths.	Promotes muscle relaxation and minimizes discomfort.
Collaborative	
Restrict oral intake as indicated.	Prevents nausea and vomiting until peristalsis returns in 1 to 2 days.
Maintain nasogastric (NG) tube, if present.	May be inserted in surgery to decompress stomach.
Provide clear or full liquids and advance to solid foods as tolerated.	When peristalsis begins, food and fluid intake promote resumption of normal bowel elimination.
Administer medications, such as stool softeners, mineral oil, and laxatives, as indicated.	Promotes formation and passage of softer stool.

NURSING DIAGNOSIS: risk for ineffective Tissue Perfusion (specify)

Risk Factors May Include

Deficient knowledge of aggravating factors (e.g., dehydration, immobility, smoking)

[Intraoperative pressure on pelvic or calf vessels; pelvic congestion, postoperative tissue inflammation, venous stasis]

Possibly Evidenced By

(Not applicable; presence of signs and symptoms establishes an *actual* diagnosis)

Desired Outcomes/Evaluation Criteria—Client Will

Tissue Perfusion: (Specify) (NOC)

Demonstrate adequate perfusion, as evidenced by stable vital signs, palpable pulses, good capillary refill, usual mentation, and individually adequate urinary output.

Be free of edema and signs of thrombus formation.

ACTIONS/INTERVENTIONS	RATIONALE
Postanesthesia Care (NIC)	
Independent	
Monitor vital signs, palpate peripheral pulses and note capillary refill, assess urinary output and characteristics, and evaluate changes in mentation.	Indicators of adequacy of systemic perfusion, fluid or blood needs, and developing complications.
Inspect dressings and perineal pads, noting color, amount, and odor of drainage. Weigh pads and compare with dry weight if client is bleeding heavily.	Proximity of large blood vessels to operative site and/or potential for alteration of clotting mechanism (e.g., cancer) increases risk of postoperative hemorrhage.
Turn client and encourage frequent coughing and deep-breathing exercises.	Prevents stasis of secretions and respiratory complications.
Assist with and/or encourage use of incentive spirometer.	Promotes lung expansion and minimizes atelectasis.
Embolus Prevention (NIC)	
Avoid high Fowler's position and pressure under the knees or crossing of legs.	Creates vascular stasis by increasing pelvic congestion and pooling of blood in the extremities, potentiating risk of thrombus formation.
Assist with and instruct in foot and leg exercises and ambulate as soon as able.	Movement enhances circulation and prevents stasis complications.
Note erythema, swelling of extremity, or reports of sudden chest pain with dyspnea.	May be indicative of development of thrombophlebitis and pulmonary embolus.

ACTIONS/INTERVENTIONS (continued)	RATIONALE (continued)
Collaborative	
Apply sequential compression devices (SCDs): antiembolism stockings or pneumatic compression stocking and boots.	Aids in venous return; reduces stasis and risk of thrombosis.
Postanesthesia Care (NIC)	
Administer intravenous (IV) fluids and blood products, as indicated.	Replacement of blood losses maintains circulating volume and tissue perfusion.

NURSING DIAGNOSIS: risk for Sexual Dysfunction

Risk Factors May Include

Altered body structure (e.g., shortening of vaginal canal)

Altered body function (e.g., changes in hormone levels, possible change in sexual response pattern—absence of rhythmic uterine contractions during orgasm, vaginal discomfort or pain)

Biopsychosocial alteration of sexuality (e.g., decreased libido; sense of femininity)

Possibly Evidenced By

(Not applicable; presence of signs and symptoms establishes an *actual* diagnosis)

Desired Outcomes/Evaluation Criteria—Client Will

Sexual Functioning (NOC)

Verbalize understanding of changes in sexual anatomy or function.

Discuss concerns about body image, sex role, and desirability as a sexual partner with SO.

Identify satisfying and acceptable sexual practices and alternative ways of dealing with sexual expression.

ACTIONS/INTERVENTIONS	RATIONALE
Sexual Counseling (NIC)	
Independent	
Listen to comments of client and SO. Provide open environment for client to discuss concerns about sexuality.	Sexual concerns are often disguised as humor and/or offhand remarks. An open environment promotes sharing of beliefs or values about sensitive subject and identifies misconceptions or myths that may interfere with adjustment to situation.
Assess client's and SO's information regarding sexual anatomy, function, and effects of surgical procedure.	May have misinformation or misconceptions that can affect adjustment. Negative expectations are associated with poor overall outcome. Changes in hormone levels can affect libido and decrease suppleness of the vagina. Although a shortened vagina can eventually stretch, intercourse initially may be uncomfortable or painful.
Identify cultural or value factors and conflicts present.	May affect return to satisfying sexual relationship.
Assist client to be aware of and deal with stage of grieving.	Acknowledging normal process of grieving for actual or perceived changes may enhance coping and facilitate resolution.
Encourage client to share thoughts or concerns with partner.	Open communication can identify areas of agreement and problems and promote discussion and resolution.
Problem-solve solutions to potential problems, such as postponing sexual intercourse when fatigued, substituting alternative means of expression, using positions that avoid pressure on abdominal incision, and using vaginal lubricant or vaginal estrogen product.	Helps client return to desired and satisfying sexual activity. It may be of help to the client/partner to learn that there is abundant evidence in the medical literature supporting favorable sexual outcomes from hysterectomy (Katz, 2003) given time for recovery.
Discuss expected physical sensations or discomforts and changes in response, as appropriate to the individual.	Vaginal pain may be significant following vaginal procedure, or sensory loss may occur because of surgical trauma. Research data show a trend toward more problems with lubrication, arousal, and altered genital sensation after total hysterectomy as compared to vaginal hysterectomy. Altered hormone levels and loss of sensation of rhythmic contractions of the uterus during orgasm can impair sexual satisfaction for some women (American College of Obstetricians and Gynecologists [ACOG], 2011). *Note:* Many women experience few negative effects because fear of pregnancy is gone, and relief from symptoms often improves sexual pleasure.
Collaborative	
Refer to counselor or sex therapist as needed.	May need additional assistance to promote a satisfactory outcome.

NURSING DIAGNOSIS: Grieving

May Be Related To
Loss of significant object (e.g., parts and processes of body/perceived sexual role or identity)

Possibly Evidenced By
Making meaning of loss
Experiencing relief

Desired Outcomes/Evaluation Criteria—Client Will

Grief Resolution (NOC)
Verbalize reality of perceived loss.
Report sense of acceptance and hope for future.

ACTIONS/INTERVENTIONS	RATIONALE
Grief Work Facilitation (NIC)	
Independent	
Provide open environment in which client feels free to discuss realistic feelings and concerns without confrontation.	Therapeutic communication skills, such as active-listening, silence, being available, and acceptance, provide opportunity and encouragement for the client to talk freely and deal with the perceived loss. Provides opportunity for reflection aiding resolution and acceptance.
Discuss client's perceptions of self, related to anticipated changes and her specific lifestyle.	Research supports the idea that hysterectomy is physiologically and psychologically stressful for a woman, even when she desires the procedure. The prospect of hysterectomy is said to engender more stress than other comparable surgeries. Cultural beliefs may result in delaying needed surgery, increasing risk of complications and negatively impacting recovery (Augustus, 2002). Although preoperative instruction and interaction are often performed at the community level, the postoperative care providers can convey interest and concern and make opportunities for support, teaching, and correction of misconceptions, such as loss of femininity and sexuality, weight gain, and menopausal body changes.
Determine client's perception and meaning of current and past losses. Note cultural factors and expectations.	Affects client's response and needs to be acknowledged in planning care. Perceptions and way of expressing self may be result of cultural expectations.
Assess emotional stress client is experiencing.	Being aware of what this operation means to client helps avoid inadvertent casualness or oversolicitude by care providers. *Note:* Women in their thirties who have hysterectomies are at risk for some degree of depression. Some of the feelings are part of the grieving process associated with never being able to bear children again. The degree of depression can be compounded by a trauma response and the significance attached to not being able to conceive. For others, depression can be the result of the abrupt hormonal changes that can accompany a hysterectomy in a woman who is not yet premenopausal (Bauers, 2010).
Encourage client to vent feelings appropriately, identifying meaning of loss.	Depending on the reason for the surgery (e.g., cancer or long-term, heavy bleeding), the client may be frightened or relieved. She may mourn the loss of ability to fulfill her reproductive role whether or not she has borne children. She may also worry about her wholeness as a woman or have heard stories about problems others have had with the procedure.
Assist family/SO to cope with client's responses.	Family may not share client's perspective and be intolerant, not recognizing needs of client.
Identify and problem-solve solutions to existing physical responses—eating, sleeping, activity levels, and sexual desire.	May need additional assistance to deal with the physical aspects of the potential for grieving.
Note withdrawn behavior, negative self-talk, and overconcern with actual or perceived changes.	May indicate difficulty in working through the grief process and need for additional interventions or support.
Discuss healthy ways of dealing with difficult situation.	Provides opportunity to look toward the future and incorporate perceived loss into lifestyle.
Collaborative	
Refer to other resources for counseling, spiritual or pastoral care, and psychotherapy, as indicated.	May need additional help to prevent development of dysfunctional grieving and help client move toward a positive future.

NURSING DIAGNOSIS: deficient Knowledge [Learning Need] regarding condition, prognosis, treatment, self-care, and discharge needs

May Be Related To
Lack of exposure or recall
Information misinterpretation
Unfamiliarity with information resources

Possibly Evidenced By
Reports the problem
Inaccurate follow-through of instructions

Desired Outcomes/Evaluation Criteria—Client Will

Knowledge: Disease Process (NOC)
Verbalize understanding of condition and potential complications.
Identify relationship of signs and symptoms related to surgical procedure and actions to deal with them.

Knowledge: Treatment Regimen (NOC)
Verbalize understanding of therapeutic needs.

ACTIONS/INTERVENTIONS — RATIONALE

Teaching: Disease Process (NIC)
Independent

Review effects of surgical procedure and future expectations; for example, the client needs to know that she will no longer menstruate or bear children, whether surgical menopause will occur, and whether hormonal replacement will be necessary.
— Provides knowledge base from which client can make informed choices.

Discuss complexity of problems anticipated during recovery, including emotional lability and expectation of feelings of depression or sadness, excessive fatigue, sleep disturbances, and urinary problems.
— Physical, emotional, and social factors can have a cumulative effect, which may delay recovery, especially if hysterectomy was performed because of cancer. Providing an opportunity for problem-solving may facilitate the process. Client and SO may benefit from the knowledge that a period of emotional lability is normal and expected during recovery.

Discuss resumption of activity. Encourage light activities initially, with frequent rest periods, increasing activities and exercise as tolerated. Stress importance of individual response in recuperation.
— Client can expect to feel tired when she goes home and needs to plan a gradual resumption of activities, with return to work an individual matter. Prevents excessive fatigue; conserves energy for healing and tissue regeneration.

Identify individual restrictions, such as avoiding heavy lifting and strenuous activities (such as vacuuming, straining at stool) and prolonged sitting or driving. Avoid tub baths and douching until physician authorizes.
— Strenuous activity intensifies fatigue and may delay healing. Activities that increase intra-abdominal pressure can strain surgical repairs, and prolonged sitting potentiates risk of thrombus formation. Showers are permitted, but tub baths and douching may cause vaginal or incisional infections and are a safety hazard.

Encourage client to report bowel dysfunction—constipation, loss of urge to defecate, severe straining, incomplete evacuation, and digital evacuation—to healthcare providers if it occurs.
— Constipation is a frequent symptom after hysterectomy and may be related to undiagnosed irritable bowel syndrome, which is often present preoperatively and/or associated with the particular procedure performed—vaginal hysterectomy with posterior repair.

Discuss dietary modifications, medicinal bulk agents, and stimulation by suppository, as indicated.
— Postsurgical bowel dysfunction may be short-term or long-term and may require simple home management measures or referral for medical intervention.

Review recommendations of resumption of sexual intercourse. (Refer to ND: risk for Sexual Dysfunction.)
— When sexual activity is cleared by the physician, it is best to resume activity easily and gently, expressing sexual feelings in other ways or using alternative coital positions.

Identify dietary needs, such as high-quality protein, complex carbohydrates, and additional iron. Provide information about foods to include and avoid in managing menopausal symptoms.
— Facilitates healing and tissue regeneration, helps correct anemia when present. *Note:* Certain vegetables, such as broccoli, cabbage, cauliflower, brussels sprouts, and turnips, may have protective action against excessive estrogen effects. Some foods and substances to avoid or limit include rich dairy products, sugar, fried foods, caffeine, alcohol, and nicotine.

Review hormone replacement therapy (HRT) and route (oral, injection, patch) when used. Clarify distinction between long-term HRT use for preventive therapy and short-term use for symptom relief.
— Total hysterectomy with bilateral salpingo-oophorectomy results in surgically induced menopause requiring replacement hormones. Benefits of HRT, particularly estrogen, include protection against osteoporosis and the

(continues on page 588)

amelioration of certain postmenopausal discomforts such as sleep disturbance, hot flashes, mood disorders, problems with memory and concentration, reduced libido, and urinary symptoms. *Note:* Regarding the media attention given in recent years to the risks of taking HRT, one author writes: "The risks of HRT—while real—are quite small for an individual person. For example, the 2002 Women's Health Initiative study found that estrogen replacement therapy (ERT) increased the risk of strokes by 39%. That sounds frighteningly high. But the actual number of people affected is very small. Out of 10,000 women who are not taking ERT, 32 have strokes each year. Out of 10,000 who *are* taking ERT, 44 have strokes each year. That's an increase of just 12 people out of 10,000" (Todd, 2012). This would seem to support the reason that most physicians continue to support the use of hormone replacement therapy, especially in younger women who have surgically induced menopause.

Encourage taking prescribed drug(s) routinely, for example, with meals or at bedtime. Determine when patch should be changed, wearing time altered.

Establishes routine for taking drug and reduces potential for discontinuing drug because of nausea that is often an early side effect.

Discuss potential side effects, such as weight gain, increased skin pigmentation or acne, breast tenderness, headaches, and photosensitivity.

Development of some side effects is expected but may require problem-solving for the client to continue the hormones, such as change in dosage; change of delivery method; and use of analgesics, sunscreen, and sunglasses.

Recommend cessation of smoking, especially when receiving estrogen therapy.

Some studies suggest an increased risk of thrombophlebitis, myocardial infarction (MI), stroke, and pulmonary emboli associated with smoking and concurrent estrogen therapy.

Inquire if client is taking or planning to take vitamins and/or herbal supplements for menopause, such as vitamin C with bioflavonoids, calcium, magnesium, selenium, evening primrose oil, black cohosh, angelica, and wild yam.

Client may express desire to use "natural hormones" and feel confused over choices. These substances are numerous and available and have been the object of media attention. They should be reviewed in terms of expected action, potential interaction, or adverse effects, depending on client's particular situation and reason for the hysterectomy.

Review incisional care, when appropriate.

Facilitates competent self-care, promoting independence.

Emphasize importance of follow-up care.

Provides opportunity to ask questions, clear up misunderstandings, and detect developing complications. *Note:* Client needs to discuss with the physician her particular requirements for follow-up pelvic exams with Pap smear, once surgical healing has occurred. The need and rationale for these exams depends upon the client's reason for hysterectomy—benign fibroids versus cervical neoplasm.

Identify signs and symptoms requiring medical evaluation, such as fever or chills, change in character of vaginal or wound drainage, and bright red bleeding.

Early recognition and treatment of developing complications, such as infection or hemorrhage, may prevent life-threatening situations.

Identify support group and appropriate Web sites, as indicated.

May desire additional information or opportunity to discuss feelings or concerns with women with similar experiences. However, instruct client to exercise caution when choosing Internet resources and sharing personal information online (Bunde et al, 2007).

POTENTIAL CONSIDERATIONS following acute hospitalization (dependent on client's age, physical condition, and presence of complications, personal resources, and life responsibilities)

In addition to surgical and cancer concerns (if appropriate):

- ***Sexual Dysfunction***—altered body structure and function, changes in hormone levels, decreased libido, possible change in sexual response pattern, vaginal discomfort or pain (dyspareunia)
- ***risk for situational low Self-Esteem***—disturbed body image; loss (e.g., perceived changes in femininity, effect on sexual relationship, inability to have children); functional impairment (e.g., changes in sexual response pattern, decreased libido)

MASTECTOMY

I. Purpose

a. Removal of breast tissue due to presence of malignant or cancerous tumor changes

b. Surgical procedures: dependent on tumor type, size, and location as well as clinical characteristics or staging

   i. Breast-conserving therapy

   ii. Lumpectomy

   iii. Partial or segmental mastectomy

   iv. Lymph node surgery

   v. Mastectomy (Mayo Clinic, 2011)

      1. Simple or total
      2. Modified radical
      3. Radical
      4. Skin-sparing mastectomy

II. Pathology—Tumor growth originates in cells of the breast tissue occurring primarily in women, although men may also be affected.

a. Types (National Comprehensive Cancer Network [NCCN], 2011)

   i. Ductal

      1. Occurs in the ducts that connect the lobes and the nipple
      2. May be in situ or invasive
      3. Represents 83% of all breast cancers (invasive ductal carcinoma [IDC]) (American Cancer Society [ACS], 2011).
      4. Note: Invasive ductal carcinoma (IDC) and invasive lobular carcinoma (ILC) are the two most common types of invasive breast cancer (Downs-Holmes, 2011).

   ii. Lobular

      1. Occurs in the lobes where milk is produced
      2. May be in situ or invasive
      3. Represents 10% to 15% of all cancers
      4. Note: Invasive ductal carcinoma (IDC) and invasive lobular carcinoma (ILC) are the two most common types of invasive breast cancer.

   iii. Inflammatory breast cancer (IBC) (Cancer Treatment Centers of America [CTCA], 2012)

      1. A rare (1% to 5%) and aggressive type of breast cancer
      2. Starts within soft tissues of the breast and causes blocking of lymph vessels in the skin of the breast
      3. Affects younger women more than other breast cancer types

b. Clinical staging (National Comprehensive Cancer Network [NCCN], 2013)

   i. Classification: noninvasive, invasive (infiltrating)

   ii. Size and spread of tumor: T stage

   iii. Number of lymph nodes involved: N stage

   iv. Metastasis: M stage

   v. Grade measured from 0 to IV, with zero resembling normal breast tissue

   vi. Some stages further divided by letters of the alphabet (A, B, C, etc.)

III. Statistics (National Cancer Institute [NCI], 2013; ACS, 2011)

a. Morbidity: As of January 2012, approximately 2,477,847 American women had a history of breast cancer; in 2013, an estimated 232,340 new cases of breast cancer were diagnosed in women and 2,240 in men.

b. Mortality: In 2009, breast cancer was the second leading cause of death in women in the United States; an estimated 39,520 women and 450 men died of breast cancer in 2011.

c. Cost: $16.5 billion spent in United States in direct costs in 2010 (NCI, 2011), averaging $11,000 per Medicare client in first year following diagnosis and rising to just under $30,000 in the last year of life (Brown et al, 2002; Cancer Action Network, 2009).

GLOSSARY

Adenocarcinoma: A carcinoma that originates in glandular tissue, or tissue responsible for the production and secretion of a substance. Breast ducts and lobules are examples of glandular tissues where adenocarcinomas may sometimes develop.

Aromatase inhibitors (AIs): Newer drugs sometimes used in women who have already gone through menopause to treat breast cancer or reduce cancer recurrence after surgery. Instead of blocking estrogen receptors, they stop a key enzyme (called aromatase) from changing other hormones into estrogen, taking away the fuel that estrogen receptor-positive breast cancers need to grow.

Breast-conserving therapy: Treatment of choice for most women with stage I or stage II breast cancer and usually followed with radiation therapy.

Carcinoma: Cancer that originates in epithelial tissue cells, which are present both in the skin (epidermis) and in the lining of internal organs. The most common type of cancer.

Grade: Determined by cellular differentiation; the lower the grade, the more it resembles normal breast tissue and the least likely it is to spread.

Infiltrating (invasive) breast cancer: Breast cancer that extends into the surrounding breast tissue and may metastasize.

In situ (noninvasive) breast cancer: Breast cancer that is contained within a structure of the breast, such as a duct or lobe.

Lumpectomy: Removes only the breast lump and a rim of normal surrounding breast tissue.

Lymph node surgery: Removal of lymph node(s) to determine if breast cancer has spread to the lymph ducts or lymph nodes in the axilla. In tumors 2 cm or smaller in size, a *sentinel* procedure may be performed to remove only the node(s) deemed most likely to contain cancerous cells. In larger tumors, or if sentinel biopsy is positive, a traditional axillary lymph node dissection is performed.

Metastasis: Cancer that has spread to other parts of the body.

Modified radical mastectomy: Removal of entire breast and some axillary (underarm) lymph nodes.

Partial or segmental mastectomy: Removes more breast tissue than a lumpectomy—up to one-quarter of the breast—which is then called a quadrantectomy.

Radical mastectomy: All the muscle under the breast is removed; however, it is rarely used today because it is no more effective than the more limited forms of mastectomy.

(continues on page 590)

GLOSSARY (continued)

Simple or total mastectomy: Entire breast is removed, but no lymph nodes from under the arm or muscle tissue from beneath the breast are removed.

Skin-sparing mastectomy: Removal of the entire breast, nipple, and areola, without removal of the breast skin for immediate or delayed breast reconstruction.

Staging: Method to classify progression of cancer in order to select treatment options and predict a prognosis.

Care Setting

Client is treated at inpatient acute surgical unit.

Related Concerns

Cancer, page 827
Psychosocial aspects of care, page 729
Surgical intervention, page 762

Client Assessment Database

DIAGNOSTIC DIVISION MAY REPORT	MAY EXHIBIT
CIRCULATION	• Unilateral engorgement in affected arm as a result of lymph node involvement
EGO INTEGRITY • Constant stressors in work or home life • Stress and fear involving diagnosis, prognosis, and future expectations	
FOOD/FLUID • Loss of appetite, recent weight loss	
PAIN/DISCOMFORT • Pain may be reported in advanced metastatic disease but rarely occurs in early malignancy • Discomfort or "funny feeling" in breast tissue occurs in some clients	
SAFETY	• Nodular axillary masses • Edema, erythema of involved skin
SEXUALITY • Changes in breast symmetry or size, pitting or dimpling of breast skin, color changes such as erythema or temperature, unusual nipple discharge, itching, burning, retracted nipple • History of early menarche younger than age 12, late menopause after age 50, late first pregnancy, such as after age 30 • Concerns about sexuality and intimacy	• Change in breast contour or symmetry • Retraction of nipple, discharge from nipple
TEACHING/LEARNING • Family history of genetically transmitted breast cancer. *Note:* BRCA1 and BRCA2 genes that have mutated account for 80% to 90% of hereditary cancers and present a lifetime risk factor 10 times that of the population (NCI, 2008); however, most breast cancer clients have no relatives with the disease, with only 5% to 10% attributable to hereditary factors.	

Client Assessment Database (continued)

DIAGNOSTIC DIVISION MAY REPORT (continued)	MAY EXHIBIT (continued)
• Previous unilateral breast cancer, endometrial cancer, or ovarian cancer • History of prolonged hormone replacement therapy, radiation, or multiple breast biopsies or procedures **Discharge Plan Considerations** • May need assistance with treatments and rehabilitation, decisions, self-care activities, and homemaker or maintenance tasks. ➧ Refer to section at end of plan for postdischarge considerations.	

Diagnostic Studies

TEST WHY IT IS DONE	WHAT IT TELLS ME
Blood tests	
• ***Hormone receptor assay:*** Test to determine whether a breast cancer's growth is influenced by hormones or if it can be treated with hormones.	Reveals whether cells of excised tumor or biopsy specimens contain hormone receptors (estrogen and progesterone). In malignant cells, the estrogen-plus receptor complex stimulates cell growth and division. About two-thirds of all women with breast cancer are estrogen-receptor positive and tend to respond favorably to the addition of hormone blocking therapy, which extends the disease-free period and increases survival time.
• ***Human epidermal growth factor receptor 2 (HER2) tumor test:*** A growth-promoting protein.	Cancer cells with too many copies of this gene tend to grow and spread more aggressively than do other breast cancers. Approximately 15% to 20% of women with breast cancer have HER2-positive tumors (NCCN, 2011).
• ***Breast cancer genes—BRCA1 and BRCA2:*** Normal genes that are associated with familial breast cancer when inherited in mutated state.	Associated with a high risk of female breast cancer and ovarian cancer, as well as male breast cancer (BRCA2), and other cancers. The tests may be performed on young women with more than one family member who has developed breast cancer at an early age. *Note:* Known BRCA1 or BRCA2 genetic mutations place women at 60% to 80% risk of breast cancer (Bland, 2009).
• ***Ploidy:*** Chromosome test that refers to the amount of DNA that cancer cells contain.	Helps predict how aggressive a cancer is likely to be. If the amount is abnormal, the cells are aneuploid. Aneuploid breast cancers tend to be faster growing and more likely to recur than other forms of breast cancers.
Other diagnostic studies	
• ***Mammography:*** Visualizes internal structure of the breast; capable of detecting nonpalpable cancers or tumors that are in early stages of development.	Women with dense breasts may benefit from digital, rather than a film, mammography.
• ***Digital mammography:*** Creates computer images, rather than images on film, which can be manipulated and transmitted for further review.	Complements findings of mammograms. Distinguishes fluid-filled cysts from solid tumors.
• ***Ultrasound:*** Uses sound waves to produce images for both screening and diagnostic staging.	Ongoing studies are evaluating whether whole-breast ultrasound should be used in conjunction with mammography to screen high-risk women with dense breast tissue (Mayo Clinic, 2011).
• ***Magnetic resonance imaging (MRI):*** Creates images that capture multiple cross-sectional pictures using a computer to generate detailed two- and three-dimensional images.	Performed when more information is needed than a mammogram, ultrasound, or clinical breast exam can provide. Ductal cancer in situ is usually better detected with an MRI than with a mammography.

(continues on page 592)

Diagnostic Studies (continued)

TEST WHY IT IS DONE (continued)	WHAT IT TELLS ME (continued)
• *Biopsy:* Removal of a sample of suspicious tissue for examination by a pathologist.	Biopsy may be done if a mammography, surgery, or other screening method reveals a mass or lesion to determine whether it is benign or cancerous.
• *Fine-needle aspiration biopsy:* A fine, hollow needle is inserted into a lump or lesion and cells are withdrawn for evaluation.	This is usually performed when a fluid-filled mass is seen on an ultrasound image or a lesion is detected during a clinical breast exam.
• *Core-needle biopsy:* A hollow needle is used to take several rice- or grain-sized cores of tissue.	With this type of biopsy, tissue structure and cells can be evaluated. When a solid mass has been detected, ultrasound may be used to guide the placement of the needle.
• *Stereotactic biopsy:* Computer-guided procedure that uses a core needle to obtain a larger tissue sample (than the fine-needle procedure), or a vacuum-assisted device (VAD) that allows collection of multiple tissue samples during one needle insertion.	When a suspicious area cannot be palpated or located by ultrasound—but is visible through mammography—the physician uses digital x-rays to guide the needle to the abnormality and perform the biopsy.
• *Ultrasound-guided core-needle biopsy:* Core-needle biopsy that uses ultrasound to produce precise images of structures within the body.	May be used in place of fine-needle biopsy or surgical biopsy to verify diagnosis.
• *Surgical biopsy:* All or part of the suspicious tissues may be removed by surgery for cytological examination.	Total removal of the tissue is called an excisional biopsy, whereas partial removal is called an incisional biopsy.
• *Sentinel node biopsy:* The lymph ducts of the breast usually drain to one lymph node first before draining to the remaining axillary lymph nodes. Lymph node mapping helps to identify that specific lymph node to determine presence of cancerous cells.	If the first node is benign, it is likely that all other nodes are the same, thereby limiting removal of additional nodes, preventing damage to the ducts and the increased potential for lymphedema and avoiding an axillary node dissection (Mayo Clinic, 2011).
• *21 gene RT-PCR (reverse transcriptase-polymerase chain reaction) assay*	May be done on excised breast tissue to help determine the risk of recurrence and the benefit of chemotherapy, assuming that 5 years of hormonal treatment is planned in early stage I or II, ER positive, HER-2 negative, and node-negative breast cancer of greater than 0.5 cm (a recent breakthrough in breast oncology care) (Lo et al, 2010; Mamounas et al, 2010).

Nursing Priorities

1. Assist client and significant other (SO) in dealing with stress of situation and prognosis.
2. Prevent complications.
3. Establish individualized rehabilitation program.
4. Provide information about disease process, procedure, prognosis, and treatment needs.

Discharge Goals

1. Situation being dealt with realistically.
2. Complications prevented or minimized.
3. Exercise regimen implemented.
4. Disease process, surgical procedure, prognosis, and therapeutic regimen understood.
5. Plan in place to meet needs after discharge.

Preoperative

NURSING DIAGNOSIS: Anxiety

May Be Related To

Situational crisis; threat to/change in health status
Threat to self-concept (e.g., change of body image; scarring/loss of body part, change in sexual attractiveness)
Threat of death (e.g., extent of disease, uncertainty of prognosis; denial of own mortality)

Possibly Evidenced By

Behavioral—reports concerns due to change in life events, restlessness
Affective—apprehensive; feelings of helplessness, inadequacy; focus on self
Physiological—increased tension
Sympathetic—changes in vital signs

NURSING DIAGNOSIS: Anxiety (continued)

Desired Outcomes/Evaluation Criteria—Client Will

Anxiety Level (NOC)
Demonstrate appropriate range of feelings regarding possibility of death or increasing hope related to prognosis.
Acknowledge acceptance of health status.

Anxiety Self-Control (NOC)
Communicate thoughts and feelings utilizing available support systems such as family, spiritual leaders, and other resources.
Demonstrate coping behaviors that reduce anxiety.

ACTIONS/INTERVENTIONS	RATIONALE
Anxiety Reduction (NIC)	
Independent	
Ascertain what information client has about diagnosis, expected surgical intervention, and future therapies. Note presence of denial or extreme anxiety.	Provides knowledge base for the nurse to enable reinforcement of needed information, helps identify client with high anxiety or a low capacity for information processing, and need for special attention. *Note:* Denial may be useful as a coping method initially; however, extreme anxiety needs to be dealt with immediately.
Explain purpose and preparation for diagnostic tests or procedures.	Promotes clear understanding of procedures and what is happening, increases feelings of control, and lessens anxiety and fear of the unknown.
Provide an atmosphere of concern and anticipatory guidance and privacy for client and family.	Facilitates therapeutic communication, active-listening, and expression of underlying unresolved issues. Privacy is needed to encourage open discussion related to feelings of anticipated loss and other concerns.
Encourage questions and provide time for expression of fears.	Provides opportunity to identify and clarify misconceptions and offer emotional support.
Offer relaxation techniques such as back massage, guided imagery, and use of touch, if culturally acceptable.	Relaxation may help in reducing anxiety and fear.
Explore previously used coping mechanisms as perceived by the client.	Reinforces effective coping mechanisms previously used for coping in a new situation.
Explore spiritual support as a resource.	Provides calmness and peace in times of uncertainty.
Discuss role of rehabilitation after surgery and use of community resources.	Promotes support systems in place in the rehabilitation process as an essential component of therapy intended to meet physical, social, emotional, and vocational needs so that client can achieve the best possible level of physical and emotional functioning.

Postoperative

NURSING DIAGNOSIS: impaired Tissue Integrity

May Be Related To
Altered circulation, sensation
Mechanical factors (e.g., surgical removal of skin and tissue)
Excess fluid volume (edema, changes in skin elasticity)
Chemical irritants (e.g., drainage); radiation

Possibly Evidenced By
Damaged/destroyed tissues

Desired Outcomes/Evaluation Criteria—Client Will

Wound Healing: Primary Intention (NOC)
Achieve timely wound healing free of purulent drainage or erythema.

Knowledge: Treatment Procedures (NOC)
Verbalize understanding of treatment plan to promote wound healing.
Demonstrate wound care techniques that facilitate increased tissue granulation at incision site.
Demonstrate behaviors that prevent complications.

ACTIONS/INTERVENTIONS	RATIONALE
Incision Site Care (NIC)	
Independent	
Assess dressings and wound for amount and characteristics of drainage.	Use of dressings depends on the extent of surgery and the type of wound closure. Pressure dressings are usually applied initially and are reinforced, not changed. Drainage occurs because of the trauma of the procedure and manipulation of the numerous blood vessels and lymphatics in the area.
Provide drain care, instructing client/family in the process, as indicated.	The Jackson-Pratt drain is most commonly used for mastectomies to maintain negative pressure in the wound and is easily managed. Simple mastectomies use one drain, whereas more complex procedures, such as those involving removal of lymph nodes, may require several drains. Drains are usually removed around the third day or when drainage ceases, possibly after client is discharged. Teaching facilitates self-care, reducing a major concern of client.
Monitor temperature.	Early recognition of developing infection enables rapid institution of treatment.
Place in semi-Fowler's position on back or unaffected side; avoid letting the affected arm dangle.	Assists with drainage of fluid through use of gravity.
Prevent or minimize edema of involved arm.	Reduces the discomfort and associated complications.
Elevate hand and arm with shoulder positioned at appropriate angles at no more than 65 degrees of flexion, 45 to 65 degrees of abduction, 45 to 60 degrees of internal rotation, and forearm resting on wedge or pillow, as indicated.	Elevation of affected arm facilitates drainage and resolution of edema. Lymphedema is present in approximately 24% to 49% postmastectomy, depending on the malignancy and the surgical procedure performed (Warren et al, 2007). This may develop immediately after surgery or years later.
Avoid measuring blood pressure (BP), injecting medications, or inserting intravenous (IV) lines in affected arm, where possible.	Increases potential of constriction, infection, and lymphedema on affected side.
Encourage wearing of loose-fitting, nonconstrictive clothing. Inform the client not to wear wristwatch or other jewelry on affected arm.	Reduces pressure on compromised tissues, which may improve circulation and healing and minimize lymphedema.
Collaborative	
Administer antibiotics, as indicated.	Provides prophylaxis to treat specific infection and enhance healing.

NURSING DIAGNOSIS: acute Pain

May Be Related To

Physical agents (e.g., surgical procedure; tissue trauma, interruption of nerves, dissection of muscles)

Possibly Evidenced By

Verbalized/coded reports of pain
Guarding behavior
Self-focus

Desired Outcomes/Evaluation Criteria—Client Will

Pain Level (NOC)

Express reduction in pain or discomfort.
Appear relaxed and able to sleep or rest appropriately.

Pain Control (NOC)

Identify factors that aggravate or relieve pain.

ACTIONS/INTERVENTIONS	RATIONALE
Pain Management (NIC)	
Independent	
Assess reports of pain and sensory alterations, noting location, duration, and intensity (0 to 10 [or similar] scale). Note reports of stiffness, swelling, and numbness or burning in chest, shoulder, and affected arm. Identify verbal and nonverbal cues.	Examines the degree of discomfort and verifies the need for analgesia and evaluates its effectiveness. The amount of tissue, muscle, and lymphatic system removed can affect the amount of pain experienced. The need to elevate arm, the size of dressings, and the presence of drains all affect client's ability to relax and rest or sleep effectively.

ACTIONS/INTERVENTIONS (continued)	RATIONALE (continued)
Explain the causes of pain to the client.	Provides understanding of sensory alterations. Destruction of nerves in axillary region causes numbness in upper arm and scapular region, which may be more intolerable than surgical pain. Pain in chest wall can occur from muscle tension, be affected by extremes in heat and cold, and continue for several months.
Acknowledge the presence of phantom breast sensations.	Provides reassurance that sensations are not imaginary and that relief can be obtained.
Provide basic comfort and diversional activities. Encourage early ambulation and use of relaxation techniques, guided imagery, and Therapeutic Touch.	Promotes relaxation, refocuses attention away from the discomfort, and may enhance coping abilities.
Provide opportunities for uninterrupted sleep.	Relieves fatigue, increasing coping ability.
Splint or support chest during coughing and deep-breathing exercises.	Facilitates participation in activity without undue discomfort.
Provide appropriate pain medication on a regular schedule before pain is severe and before activities are scheduled.	Maintains comfort level and permits client to exercise arm and to ambulate without pain hindering efforts.
Provide accurate information related to patient-controlled analgesia (PCA) or opioids to reduce fear of addiction.	Reduces fear, augmenting appropriate pain relief, to enhance mobility and coping abilities.
Describe the adverse effects of unrelieved pain.	Explains complications resulting from poor pain management both physiologically and emotionally (NCI, 2012).
Discuss previous successful methods of coping with pain.	Provides pain-relieving methods to employ based on past experiences.
Collaborative	
Administer PCA, opioids, or nonopioids, as indicated.	Provides relief from discomfort or pain and facilitates rest and participation in postoperative therapy.

NURSING DIAGNOSIS: situational low Self-Esteem

May Be Related To
Physical illness; loss
Disturbed body image (e.g., surgical change in structure or body contour)
Behaviors inconsistent with values
[Fear of rejection or reaction by others]

Possibly Evidenced By
Reports current situational challenge to self-worth
Self-negating verbalizations

Desired Outcomes/Evaluation Criteria—Client Will

Self-Esteem (NOC)
Distinguish between self-perceptions and societal stigmas.
Identify strategies to cope with self-acceptance in present situation.
Verbalize progress toward acceptance of self.
Participate in setting realistic goals involving the postoperative therapy program.

ACTIONS/INTERVENTIONS	RATIONALE
Self-Esteem Enhancement (NIC)	
Independent	
Provide active-listening when surgical dressings are removed.	Provides emotional support and client safety.
Assess for grief, depression, and ineffective coping.	Common reactions that need to be recognized immediately for timely intervention, as indicated. Grief may resurface when subsequent procedures are done, such as fitting for prosthesis or reconstructive procedure if postponed.
Validate client's feelings and address any misinformation that is revealed.	Encourages client to express feelings and provides opportunity to give or reinforce information.
Encourage questions about current situation and future expectations.	Loss of the breast causes many reactions, including feeling disfigured, fear of viewing scar, and fear of partner's reaction to change in body. Loss of body part, disfigurement, and perceived loss of sexual desirability engender grieving process that needs to be dealt with so that client can make plans for the future.
Identify role concerns as woman, wife, mother, career woman, and so forth.	Explores possible alteration in client's self-perception.

(continues on page 596)

ACTIONS/INTERVENTIONS (continued) / RATIONALE (continued)

Provide positive reinforcement for gains and improvement and participation in self-care and treatment program.
: Encourages continuation of healthy behaviors.

Review possibilities for reconstructive surgery and/or prosthetic augmentation.
: If feasible, reconstruction may be performed to provide a less disfiguring or "near-normal" cosmetic result. Variations in skin flap may be done for facilitation of reconstructive procedure, which may be performed at the same time as mastectomy. The associated emotional boost may help the client through the more complex surgical recovery process and adjunctive therapies. *Note:* Sometimes, reconstruction is not done for 3 to 6 months.

Identify concerns of client and SO regarding sexual dysfunction in order to provide acceptable practices for self and SO. Encourage communication of needs and fears of both partners.
: Negative responses actually reflect SO's concern about hurting client, fear of cancer or death, or inability to look at operative area.

Discuss and refer to support groups, as appropriate.
: Provides a place to exchange concerns and feelings with others who have had a similar experience and identifies ways SO can facilitate client's recovery.

Collaborative

Provide temporary soft prosthesis, if indicated.
: Prosthesis of nylon and Dacron fluff may be worn in bra indefinitely or until incision heals if reconstructive surgery is not performed at the time of mastectomy. This may promote social acceptance and allow client to feel more comfortable about body image at the time of discharge.

NURSING DIAGNOSIS: impaired physical Mobility

May Be Related To

Neuromuscular impairment
Pain, discomfort; reluctance to attempt movement
Decreased muscle mass/strength; joint stiffness
Difficulty turning

Possibly Evidenced By

Limited range of motion (ROM); limited ability to perform gross motor skills

Desired Outcomes/Evaluation Criteria—Client Will

Motivation (NOC)

Display willingness to participate in therapy.
Demonstrate techniques that enable resumption of activities.

Coordinated Movement (NOC)

Demonstrate increased muscle strength of affected body parts.

ACTIONS/INTERVENTIONS / RATIONALE

Exercise Therapy: Muscle Control (NIC)

Independent

Elevate affected arm, as indicated.
: Promotes venous return, lessening possibility of lymphedema.

Perform passive ROM, such as flexion and extension of elbow, pronation and supination of wrist, and clenching and extending fingers, as soon as possible.
: Early postoperative exercises are usually started in the first 24 hours to prevent joint stiffness that can further limit movement and mobility.

Encourage client to move fingers, noting sensations and color of hand on affected side.
: Lack of movement may reflect problems with the intercostal brachial nerve. Discoloration can indicate impaired circulation.

Encourage client to use affected arm for personal hygiene: feeding, combing hair, and washing face.
: Increases circulation, minimizes edema, and maintains strength and function of the arm and hand. These activities use the arm without abduction, eliminating stress on the suture line in the early postoperative period.

Assist with self-care activities, as necessary.
: Conserves client's energy and prevents undue fatigue.

Assist with ambulation and encourage correct posture.
: Client may feel unbalanced and need assistance until accustomed to change. Keeping back straight prevents shoulder from moving forward, avoiding permanent limitation in movement and posture.

Advance exercise, as indicated, for example, active extension of arm and rotation of shoulder while lying in bed, pendulum swings, rope turning, and elevating arms to touch fingertips behind head.
: Prevents joint stiffness, increases circulation, and maintains muscle tone of the shoulders and arm.

ACTIONS/INTERVENTIONS (continued)	RATIONALE (continued)
Progress to hand climbing or walking fingers up wall, clasping hands behind head, and full abduction exercises as soon as client can manage.	Because this group of exercises can cause excessive tension on the incision, they are usually delayed until healing process is well established.
Evaluate degree of exercise-related pain and changes in joint mobility. Measure upper arm and forearm if edema develops.	Monitors progression and resolution of complications. May need to postpone increasing exercises and wait until further healing occurs.
Discuss types of exercises to be done at home to regain strength and enhance circulation in the affected arm.	Exercise program needs to be continued to regain optimal function of the affected side.
Coordinate early exercise program into self-care and homemaker activities such as dressing self, washing, dusting, and mopping; and leisure activities, such as swimming.	Client is usually more willing to participate or finds it easier to maintain an exercise program that fits into her lifestyle and accomplishes tasks as well.
Assist client to identify signs/symptoms of shoulder tension, such as an inability to maintain posture or a burning sensation in the postscapular region. Instruct client to avoid sitting or holding arm in dependent position for extended periods.	Altered weight and support put tension on surrounding structures.
Collaborative	
Administer medications, as indicated, for example:	
Analgesics	Pain needs to be controlled before exercise or client may not participate optimally and incentive to exercise may be lost.
Diuretics	May be useful in treating and preventing fluid accumulation or lymphedema.
Maintain integrity of elastic bandages or custom-fitted, pressure-gradient elastic sleeve.	Promotes venous return and decreases risk or effects of edema formation.
Refer to physical and occupational therapist and lymphedema clinic or specialist.	Provides an individualized exercise program. Assesses limitations or restrictions regarding employment requirements.

NURSING DIAGNOSIS: deficient Knowledge [Learning Need] regarding condition, prognosis, treatment, self-care, and discharge needs

May Be Related To
Lack of exposure or recall
Information misinterpretation
Unfamiliarity with information resources

Possibly Evidenced By
Reports the problems
Inaccurate follow-through of instructions

Desired Outcomes/Evaluation Criteria—Client Will

Knowledge: Acute Illness Care (NOC)
Verbalize understanding of disease process and potential complications.
Perform necessary procedures correctly and explain reasons for actions.
Initiate necessary lifestyle changes and participate in treatment regimen.

ACTIONS/INTERVENTIONS	RATIONALE
Teaching: Disease Process (NIC)	
Independent	
Review disease process, surgical procedure, and future expectations.	Provides knowledge base from which client can make informed choices, including participation in radiation and/or chemotherapy programs. (Refer to CP: Cancer.)
Review and have client demonstrate care of drains and wound sites.	Shorter hospital stays may result in discharge with drains in place, requiring more complex care by client and caregivers. Drains may be removed 7 to 10 days after surgery.
Encourage continuation of exercises, increasing program as healing progresses, for at least 1 year.	Good muscle tone enhances development of collateral lymphatic channels, reduces the tightening of scar tissue, and maintains muscle strength and function. Moderation is important because strenuous activity or exercise increases heart rate and body temperature, which can potentially increase edema. Some evidence suggests that exercise lowers the risk of recurrence of breast cancer (Ligibel, 2008).
Discuss necessity for well-balanced, nutritious meals and adequate fluid intake.	Provides optimal nutrition and maintains circulating volume to enhance tissue regeneration and the healing process.

(continues on page 598)

ACTIONS/INTERVENTIONS (continued)	RATIONALE (continued)
Suggest alternating schedule of frequent rest and activity periods, especially in situations when sitting or standing is prolonged.	Prevents or limits fatigue, promotes healing, and enhances feelings of general well-being. Positions in which arm is dangling or extended intensify stress on suture lines, creating muscle tension and stiffness, and may interfere with healing.
Discuss potential for lymphedema in affected arm and signs to watch for (e.g., feeling of fullness or tightness, aching or pain, weakness, swollen fingers)	Lymphedema may or may not occur in the immediate postop period. An acute, temporary, and mild type of lymphedema occurs within a few days after surgery and usually lasts a short period of time. An acute and more painful type of lymphedema can occur about 4 to 6 weeks following surgery. However, the most common type of lymphedema is slow and painless and may occur 18 to 24 months after surgery (New York Presbyterian, 2008).
Instruct client to protect hands and arms, for example:	
Wear long sleeves and gloves when gardening, use thimble when sewing, and do not carry purse or wear jewelry or wristwatch on affected side.	Compromised lymphatic system causes tissues to be more susceptible to infection and/or injury, which may lead to lymphedema.
Use potholders when handling hot items; use plastic gloves when doing dishes.	Sensory alterations place client at risk for burns and infections.
Avoid lifting, moving heavy objects, or prolonged repetitive motions.	Prevents strain on tissues with potential for edema.
Demonstrate holding affected arm appropriately, for example, not dangling the arm, swinging arms with elbows bent when walking, and placing arm above heart level when sitting or lying down.	Helps prevent or minimize lymphedema and "frozen shoulder."
Warn against having blood withdrawn or receiving IV fluids and medications or BP measurements on the affected side.	May restrict the circulation and increase risk of infection when the lymphatic system is compromised. *Note:* Following this guideline is not always possible (e.g., bilateral mastectomy, or loss of good sites for venipuncture in nonaffected arm), but should be adhered to as much as possible, especially in early postop period.
Demonstrate use of intermittent sequential pumping or low-stretch, compression custom-made garments, as appropriate.	Used in managing lymphedema by promoting circulation and venous return.
Suggest gentle massage of healed incision with emollients.	Stimulates circulation, promotes elasticity of skin, and reduces discomfort associated with phantom breast sensations.
Recommend use of sexual positions that avoid pressure on chest wall. Encourage alternative forms of sexual expression such as cuddling or touching during initial healing process and while operative area is still tender.	Promotes feelings of femininity and sense of ability to resume sexual contact.
Encourage regular self-examination of remaining breast when mastectomy is unilateral. Determine recommended schedule for mammography.	Identifies changes in breast tissue indicative of recurrent or new tumor development.
Emphasize importance of regular medical follow-up.	Other treatment may be required as adjunctive therapy, such as radiation. Recurrence of breast cancer can be identified early and managed by an oncologist.
Identify signs and symptoms requiring medical evaluation: breast or arm red, warm, and swollen; edema and purulent wound drainage; and fever or chills.	Lymphangitis can occur as a result of infection, causing lymphedema.
Address additional concerns as indicated—ongoing therapies and expected and/or adverse side effects.	Depending on the type of cancer that required the mastectomy, the client may have ongoing cancer therapies (e.g., chemotherapy, radiotherapy), selective estrogen modulators (e.g., tamoxifen [Soltamox] and raloxifene [Evista]), or aromatase inhibitors (e.g., letrozole [Femara], anastrozole [Arimidex]) to treat cancer or prevent recurrence.

POTENTIAL CONSIDERATIONS following acute hospitalization (dependent on client's age, physical condition and presence of complications, personal resources, and life responsibilities)

In addition to surgical and cancer concerns:

- ***impaired Tissue Integrity***—altered circulation, sensation; tissue removal/destruction, radiation; drainage
- ***situational low Self-Esteem***—physical illness, loss, disturbed body image (e.g., disfiguring surgical procedure, concern about sexual attractiveness)
- ***Self-Care Deficit (specify)***—weakness, fatigue, neuromuscular impairment, pain, muscular impairment

Sample clinical pathway follows in Table 11.1.

TABLE 11.1 Sample CP: Mastectomy—Modified Radical, Hospital. ELOS: 2 Days

ND and Categories of Care	Day of Surgery ____	Postop Day 1 ____	Postop Day 2 ____ (Discharge)
impaired Tissue Integrity R/T tissue removal/destruction; altered circulation, sensation; drainage, radiation	Display wound drainage w/in established limits	Participate in self-care activities/beginning exercise program	Display minimal erythema, absence of purulent drainage, edema resolving
	Maintain usual color, sensation and motion in affected fingers/hand	Identify ways to maximize healing/minimize risk of injury to arm	Report plan in place to meet postdischarge needs
Referrals	Physical Therapist Occupational Therapist Home Care		
Additional assessments	Dressing/drainage q4h	→ q8h Wound characteristics	→
	Presence/degree of edema q8h	→ qd & Measure upper arm/forearm if edema present	→
	Donor/graft site if used q4h	→ q8h	→ D/C
	VS q1h × 4 → q4h	→ q8h	→ q12h
	I&O and wound drainage system q8h	→	→ Discharge with drain in place/ remove when less than 30 mL/24 h
	Neurovascular check—UE q1h × 4 → q4h × 2	→ q8h	→
Medications	Diuretic if edema present	→	→ D/C
Client teaching	Protection of affected arm: shaving, use of deodorant/creams, activity limitations, avoidance of heat/cold, proper posture/positioning of arm, sexual positions to prevent pressure on chest wall, wearing loose-fitting clothing	Wound care	Management of wound drain if not removed
	Graduated exercise program incorporating ADLs/homemaking activities	Gentle massage of healed incision	S/S to report to healthcare provider
		General healthcare needs to promote healing, dietary intake, fluids, rest/pacing self	Use of medical alert device
		Breast self-examination	Provide written instructions, schedule for follow-up visits/additional treatment modalities
Additional nursing actions	Position per protocol; HOB elevated 30° or more	→	→
	BRP/chair w/assist	→ Ambulate/up ad lib	→
	Elevate affected arm	→	→
	Turn, cough, deep breath or incentive spirometry q2h	→ DB/IS q2h WA	→
	Maintain elastic bandages/custom-fitted, pressure-gradient sleeve if used	→	→
	Reinforce dressing PRN	→ Assist w/dressing chg	→ D/C dressing
	Encourage progressive exercises & ambulate as tolerated	→	→
	Advance diet as tolerated	→	→
acute Pain R/T physical agents (e.g., tissue trauma, muscle dissection, interruption of nerves)	Report pain reduced to manageable level	→	Verbalize understanding of therapeutic regimen

(continues on page 600)

TABLE 11.1 Sample CP: Mastectomy—Modified Radical, Hospital. ELOS: 2 Days (continued)

ND and Categories of Care	Day of Surgery ____	Postop Day 1 ____	Postop Day 2 ____ (Discharge)
	Participate in activities to manage pain	→	→
	Pain characteristics/any changes	→	→
Additional assessments	Response to interventions	→	→
Medications	Analgesic of choice	→ PO analgesic	→
Allergies:____________	IV/PO		
Client education	Orient to unit/room	S/S of shoulder tension; possibility of phantom breast pain	Medication: dose, time/frequency, purpose, side effects
	Reporting of pain/effects of interventions	Progression of exercises as tolerated	
	Initial exercises of fingers/wrist of affected arm; ROM exercises of unaffected limbs	Home exercise program	
	Relaxation techniques		
	Splinting of chest w/coughing, exercise		
	Routine comfort measures	→	→
Additional nursing actions	Passive ROM/exercises per protocol	→ Advance exercises as tolerated	→
	Assist w/self-care	→	→
situational low Self-Esteem R/T perceived disfigurement, psychosocial concerns	Verbalize feelings, verbal/nonverbal communication congruents	→	→ Verbalize acceptance of self
		Participate in care/planning for future	→ Plan in place to meet postdischarge needs
		View incision	
Referrals	Social services		
	Reach to Recovery		
Additional assessments	Response to surgical procedure by client and SO	Future expectations, role concerns, usual coping strategies, past coping successes	
	Availability/effectiveness of support systems	Understanding of diagnosis	
Client education	Postoperative routines	Community resources for client and SO	S/S to report to healthcare provider (depression)
	Extent/outcome of surgical procedure		Written information regarding diagnosis/treatment options
	Future treatment needs		
	Use of/sources for temporary prosthesis		
	Possibilities for reconstructive surgery/prosthetic augmentation		
Additional nursing actions	Discuss normalcy of feelings	Role-play ways of handling responses of others	Identify options for managing home/work responsibilities; importance of taking time for self
	Encourage participation in self-care at level of ability	Provide support/answer questions when dressing removed	
	Provide positive reinforcement for participation in therapeutic regimen		

Key: ADLs, activities of daily living; BRP, bathroom privileges; DB/IS, deep breath/incentive spirometry; D/C, discontinue; HOB, head of bed; I&O, intake and output; IV, intravenous; PO, per mouth; PRN, as needed; q1h × 4, every hour 4 times a day; q4h, every 4 hours; q8h, every 8 hours; q12h, every 12 hours; qd, every day; ROM, range of motion; R/T, related to; SO, significant other; S/S, signs and symptoms; UE, upper extremity; VS, vital signs; WA, while awake.

CHAPTER 12

Orthopedic

FRACTURES

I. Pathophysiology
 a. Discontinuity or break in a bone
 b. May be associated with serious injury to nerves, blood vessels, muscles, and/or organs

II. Etiology (Buckley, 2012; Smeltzer, 2010)
 a. Common causes: Trauma, such as falls, blunt force, and penetrating force. (P) Note: 30% to 50% of children seen by orthopedic surgeons are the victims of nonaccidental injury (Budd, 2012).
 b. Osteoporosis, which leaves bones thinned and weakened
 c. Repetitive stress, which is associated with athletics
 d. Bone tumors
 e. Infections, such as osteomyelitis; may be acute or chronic

III. Classifications (American Academy of Orthopedic Surgeons [AAOS], 2012; Walsh, 2011)
 a. Location in the bone (e.g., proximal, midshaft, distal, through a joint)
 b. Complete (through the entire bone); incomplete (the bone is not broken into two parts); comminuted (broken into three or more parts)
 c. Other fracture patterns: Stable (bone ends may touch and are in line); transverse (horizontal fracture line); oblique (angled fracture line); (P) spiral (created by rotational force common in toddlers from relatively minor trauma, and in older children from skiing, contact sports); greenstick (common in children who fall onto arm while running); dislocated (fracture causes dislocation of part of joint, e.g., elbow, cervical vertebrae); impacted.
 d. Closed (also called simple) or open (also called compound). Open fractures are further classified as Type I (low-energy, simple fracture with wound opening less than 1 cm; Type II (higher energy with comminution and wound size greater than 1 cm; Type III (fractures are high-energy with moderate to large tissue loss and possible vascular injury).
 e. Velocity: Low-velocity injuries include falls from a standing height, athletic injuries, stab wounds, and shotgun injuries. High-velocity injuries are associated with motor vehicle crashes, pedestrian versus automobile injuries (most frequent fracture sites are tibia-fibula, and pelvis, followed by femur [Bradley, 1992]); falls from a height, and handgun injuries.
 f. (P) Salter-Harris classification: Used for children and identifies where fracture is located relative to the growth plate: S = straight across; A = above growth plate; L = lower or below; T = through; ER = erasure of growth plate (crushed)

IV. Phases of healing (Buckley, 2012; Cho et al, 2002; Frost, 1989)
 a. Reactive phase
  i. Fracture and inflammatory phase: Bone fracture is an injury, and thus incites an inflammatory response, which peaks 24 hr following the injury and is complete by the first week. Soon after fracture (3 to 5 days), the blood vessels constrict, stopping any further bleeding. During this stage cellular signaling mechanisms work through chemotaxis and an inflammatory mechanism to attract the cells necessary to initiate the healing response.
  ii. Granulation tissue formation: Within 7 days, the body forms granulation tissue between the fracture fragments. This phase lasts about 2 weeks.
 b. Reparative phase
  i. Callus formation: Cell proliferation and differentiation begin to produce osteoblasts and chondroblasts in the granulation tissue, synthesizing the extracellular organic matrices of woven bone and cartilage. Then the newly formed bone is mineralized. This stage requires 4 to 16 weeks, depending on the type and location of the fracture.
  ii. Lamellar bone deposition: The mesh-like callus of woven bone is replaced by a hard, rigid form of connective tissue (lamellar bone). Eventually, the woven bone and cartilage is replaced by trabecular bone (dense, hard, and slightly elastic connective tissue in which the fibers are impregnated with a form of calcium phosphate), restoring most of the bone's original strength. (P) Note: Pediatric fractures heal more quickly than adult fractures due to children's growth potential and a thicker, more active periosteum.
 c. Remodeling phase
  i. Trabecular bone is replaced by compact bone, remodeling to original bone contour.
  ii. The final two stages can take several years in adults. (P) Younger children have greater and more rapid remodeling potential.

V. Statistics
 a. Morbidity: In 2010, 671,000 Americans had open reduction for fractures listed on hospital discharge. (P) 94,000 of those were under the age of 15 (Centers for Disease Control and Prevention [CDC], 2010). In 2007, discharge data from U.S. nonfederal hospitals listed 1.0 million with fractures as first diagnosis. (P) About 12% of those were children (Mahar, 2011). More than one-half (531,000) were

(text continues on page 602)

aged 65 years and over. Almost one-half of the fracture hospitalizations for this age group were for hip fractures (fractures of neck of femur) (National Health Statistics Report, 2007).

b. Mortality: Dependent upon multiple factors, including the specific bone affected, severity of fracture, associated soft tissue and organ involvement, age of individual, and presence of comorbidities. Note: Most currently available mortality studies are associated with hip fractures (estimated mortality rate within one year of a hip fracture ranges from 12% to 33 % (not the focus of this care plan) (Goel, 2013).

c. Cost: In 2012, osteoporosis-related fractures were responsible for an estimated $18 billion in medical treatment expenses while the cost of care and of lost work adds billions more (National Institute of Arthritis, and Musculoskeletal and Skin Diseases [NIAMSD], 2012). For the years 2004–2006, the sum of the direct expenditures in healthcare costs and the indirect expenditures in lost wages (for bone and joint health) has been estimated to be $950 billion dollars annually (The Burden of Musculoskeletal Diseases in the United States Project, 2011).

GLOSSARY

Buckle fracture: Compression failure of bone that usually occurs at the junction of the metaphysis and the diaphysis. Commonly seen in distal radius

Closed fracture: Fracture does not extend through the skin.

Closed reduction: Nonsurgical method for reduction and stabilization of fracture through a wide range of interventions, such as simple braces or aluminum splints, plaster or fiberglass casts, metal braces, and/or traction devices.

Comminuted fracture: Bone fragments into three or more pieces.

Compartment syndrome: Excessive swelling in the tissues associated with a fracture or crush injury to a limb, which elevates tissue pressure, resulting in decreased arteriovascular pressure and impaired tissue perfusion.

Complete fracture: Fracture line involves entire cross section of the bone, and bone fragments are usually displaced.

Compression fracture: Collapsing of bone usually involves vertebra of the thoracic or lumbar spine and is often seen in elderly people as a result of osteoporosis, but may also occur traumatically.

Crepitation: Grating sound heard with movement of ends of fractured bones.

Fragility fracture: Fractures secondary to osteoporosis.

Growth plate: Softer parts of child's bones, where growth occurs. Located at each end of a bone, growth plates are the weakest sections of the skeleton.

Incomplete or greenstick fracture: Involves only a portion of the cross section of the bone; one side breaks and the other usually just bends.

Oblique fracture: Break occurs diagonally.

Open fracture: Bone fragments extend through the muscle and skin and are potentially infected.

Open reduction: Surgical method for stabilization of a fracture using rods, pins, screws, and plates.

Pathological fracture: Fracture occurs in diseased bone—such as in cancer and osteoporosis—with no (spontaneous) or only minimal trauma.

Pediatric long bones: Three main regions: epiphysis (each end of a long bone with associated joint cartilage); physis ([growth plate]: cartilage cells that create solid bone with growth); and metaphysis (wide area below the physis, closest to the diaphysis/shaft).

Periosteum: Membrane that lines the outer surface of all bones, except at the joints of long bones, and serves as the attachment mechanism for muscles and tendons.

Physeal fractures: Fractures of the growth plate. May result in progressive angular deformity, limb-length discrepancy, or joint incongruity. The distal radial physis is the most frequently injured physis.

P **Plastic deformation:** The bone is angulated beyond its elastic limit, but the energy is insufficient to produce a fracture. No fracture line is visible radiographically. Unique to children. Most commonly seen in the ulna, occasionally in the fibula.

Simple fracture: Bone breaks into two pieces.

Spiral fracture: Break follows a helical line along and around the bone; commonly associated with a twisting motion.

Stress fracture: Hairline fracture due to overuse or repeated microtrauma, such as those seen in gymnasts, runners, and tennis or basketball players, as well as those who participate in marching bands or drill teams.

Transverse fracture: Break occurs in a straight line across the bone.

Care Setting

Many fractures are managed at the community level. Although many of the interventions listed here are appropriate for this population, this plan of care addresses more complicated injuries encountered on an inpatient acute medical-surgical unit. Note: Definitive treatment of fractures may be delayed until life-threatening injuries, such as lung contusions, brain injury, or hemodynamic instability, have been stabilized (Weinstein, 2005).

Related Concerns

Craniocerebral trauma—acute rehabilitative phase, page 197
Pneumonia, page 129
Psychosocial aspects of care, page 729
Renal failure: acute, page 505
Spinal cord injury (acute rehabilitative phase), page 248
Surgical intervention, page 762
Thrombophlebitis: venous thromboembolism, page 109

Client Assessment Database

Symptoms of fracture depend on the site, severity, type, and amount of damage to other structures.

DIAGNOSTIC DIVISION MAY REPORT	MAY EXHIBIT
ACTIVITY/REST • Weakness • Fatigue • Gait and/or mobility problems • Generalized weakness	• Restriction or loss of function of affected part—may be immediate, because of the fracture, or develop secondarily from tissue swelling, pain • Weakness of affected extremity • Range-of-motion (ROM) deficits
CIRCULATION	• Hypertension—occasionally seen as a response to acute pain or anxiety, or hypotension from severe blood loss • Tachycardia—stress response, hypovolemia • Pulse diminished or absent distal to injury in extremity • Delayed capillary refill • Pallor of affected part • Tissue swelling • Bruising or hematoma mass at site of injury
ELIMINATION	• Hematuria • Sediment in urine • Changes in output—acute renal failure (ARF) with major skeletal muscle damage
NEUROSENSORY • Loss of or impaired motion or sensation • Muscle spasms worsening over time • Numbness or tingling (paresthesias)	• Local musculoskeletal deformities—abnormal angulation, posture changes, shortening of limbs, rotation, or crepitation • Muscle spasms • Visible weakness or loss of function • Giving way or collapse, locking of joints, dislocations • Agitation—may be related to pain, anxiety, or other trauma
PAIN/DISCOMFORT • Sudden severe pain at time of injury—may be localized to the area of tissue or skeletal damage and then become more diffuse; however, can diminish on immobilization • Absence of pain—suggests nerve damage • Muscle-aching pain • Muscle spasms or cramping following immobilization	• Guarding or distraction behaviors • Restlessness • Self-focus
SAFETY • Circumstances of incident may not support type of injury incurred—may be suggestive of abuse • Use of alcohol or other drugs	• Skin lacerations • Tissue avulsion • Bleeding • Color changes of skin • Localized swelling—may increase gradually or suddenly • Discrepancy in limb length • Presence of risk factors for falling—age, osteoporosis, dementia, arthritis, other chronic conditions; preexisting unrecognized fracture

(continues on page 604)

Client Assessment Database (continued)

DIAGNOSTIC DIVISION MAY REPORT (continued)	MAY EXHIBIT (continued)
TEACHING/LEARNING • Use of multiple medications—prescribed and/or over-the-counter (OTC) with interactive effects **DISCHARGE PLAN CONSIDERATIONS** • May require temporary assistance with transportation, self-care activities, and homemaker or maintenance tasks • May require additional therapy or rehabilitation postdischarge • Possible placement in assisted living or extended care facility for a period of time ➧ Refer to section at end of plan for postdischarge considerations.	

Diagnostic Studies

TEST WHY IT IS DONE	WHAT IT TELLS ME
• *Radiographic examinations:* First-line tool to determine location and extent of fractures/trauma and bone alignment.	May reveal preexisting and yet undiagnosed fracture(s).
• *Bone scans, tomograms, computed tomography (CT), and magnetic resonance imaging (MRI) scans:* Used to visualize changes of structure within the body and bone alignment. May be preferred diagnostic tool because of superior ability to image some types of injuries.	These are used to visualize fractures, bleeding, and soft tissue damage; they differentiate between stress or trauma fractures and bone neoplasms.
• *Bone densitometry:* Photons from a single- or dual-emitting source are used to measure comparative density of the spine, femur, or distal radius. These are then compared with normal values for a large patient population based on sex and age.	Procedure may be done if fracture is suspected or known to be associated with osteoporosis. *Note:* Osteoporosis is often underrecognized and undertreated, and clients with fragility fractures secondary to osteoporosis are at risk of recurrent fracture (Inderjeeth, 2006).
• *Arteriograms:* X-rays that use contrast media to evaluate arterial blood flow.	May reveal vascular damage.
• *Complete blood count (CBC):* Battery of screening tests, which typically includes hemoglobin (Hgb); hematocrit (Hct); red blood cell (RBC) count, morphology, indices, and distribution width index; platelet count and size; white blood cell (WBC) count and differential.	Hct may be increased, reflecting hemoconcentration or dehydration; or Hct may be decreased, signifying hemorrhage at the fracture site or at distant organs in multiple trauma. Increased WBC count is a normal stress response after trauma.
• *Urine creatinine (Cr) clearance:* Measures filtering ability of the kidneys.	Muscle trauma increases Cr load for renal clearance; decreased renal perfusion or impaired renal function also elevates Cr.
• *Coagulation profile:* Tests that measure blood coagulation. There are many types of coagulation tests, some of which are general and tell only whether a person's blood is clotting normally. Other tests can identify which element within the blood is causing abnormal clotting.	Alterations may occur because of blood loss, multiple transfusions, or liver injury.

Nursing Priorities

1. Prevent further bone/tissue injury.
2. Alleviate pain.
3. Prevent complications.
4. Provide information about condition, prognosis, and treatment needs.

Discharge Goals

1. Fracture stabilized.
2. Pain controlled.
3. Complications prevented or minimized.
4. Condition, prognosis, and therapeutic regimen understood.
5. Plan in place to meet needs after discharge.

NURSING DIAGNOSIS: risk for Injury

Risk Factors May Include

Physical (e.g., loss of skeletal integrity [fractures]; movement of bone fragments)

Possibly Evidenced By

(Not applicable; presence of signs and symptoms establishes an *actual* diagnosis)

Desired Outcomes/Evaluation Criteria—Client Will

Bone Healing (NOC)

Maintain stabilization and alignment of fracture(s).
Display callus formation/beginning union at fracture site as appropriate.

Risk Control (NOC)

Demonstrate body mechanics that promote stability at fracture site.

ACTIONS/INTERVENTIONS	RATIONALE
Positioning (NIC) *Independent*	
Ascertain type of fracture injury and medical treatment planned if surgery is not indicated.	Nonoperative (closed) therapy consists of casting and traction (skin and skeletal traction). Closed reduction is performed initially for any fracture that is displaced, shortened, or angulated. This is achieved by applying force (traction) to the long axis of the injured bone (usually femur) and then reversing the mechanism of injury/fracture. This is followed by subsequent immobilization through casting/splinting or traction apparatus. *Note*: With the advancement of orthopedic implant technology and operative techniques, traction is rarely used for definitive fracture/dislocation management (Buckley, 2012).
Maintain bedrest or limb rest as indicated. Provide support of joints above and below fracture site, especially when moving and turning.	Provides stability, reducing possibility of disturbing alignment and aggravating muscle spasms, which enhances healing.
Cast Care: Wet (if cast is made of plaster of Paris) (NIC)	
Support fracture site with pillows or folded blankets. Maintain neutral position of affected part with sandbags, splints, trochanter roll, or footboard.	Prevents unnecessary movement and disruption of alignment. Proper placement of pillows also can prevent pressure deformities in the drying cast.
Use the palms of the hands, not the fingertips, when touching the wet cast.	Fingertips can dent the cast before it is dry.
Obtain sufficient personnel for turning. Avoid using abduction bar for turning client with spica cast.	Hip, body, or multiple casts can be extremely heavy and cumbersome. Failure to properly support limbs in casts may cause damage to cast or injury to client and staff.
Traction/Immobilization Care (NIC)	
Evaluate splinted extremity for edema resolution.	Coaptation splint (e.g., Jones-Sugar tong) may be used to provide immobilization of fracture while excessive tissue swelling is present. As edema subsides, readjustment of splint or application of fiberglass or plaster cast may be required for continued alignment of stable fracture.
Maintain position and integrity of traction apparatus, when used.	Traction is a less frequently used modality than in times past. But it may still be used in some instances of (P) femur fracture in children and older adults or client's with multitrauma who are not current candidates for surgery. Traction permits pull on the long axis of the fractured bone and overcomes muscle tension and shortening to facilitate alignment and union. Skeletal traction using pins, wires, or tongs permits use of greater weight for traction pull than can be applied to skin tissues.
Assess integrity of external fixator device.	(P) External fixation has evolved from being used primarily as a last-resort fixation method to becoming a mainstream technique used to treat a great many bone and soft tissue pathologies in both adults and children. This device provides stabilization and rigid support for fractured bone without use of ropes, pulleys,

(continues on page 606)

ACTIONS/INTERVENTIONS (continued) / RATIONALE (continued)

or weights, thus allowing for greater client mobility and comfort and facilitating wound care (Kidsfractures.com, 2011; Fragomen, 2007).

Collaborative

Review follow-up or serial x-rays. — Provides visual evidence of proper alignment or beginning callus formation and healing process to determine level of activity and need for changes in, or additions to, the therapy plan.

Prepare client for surgery where indicated. — Surgical procedures may include open reduction and internal fixation (ORIF); flexible or rigid intramedullary nailing; insertion of plates, screws, and pins. Treatments are variable and dependent on the type, location, and severity of fracture and other internal injuries.

Initiate and maintain bone rehabilitation—early ambulation, weight-bearing activities, soft tissue massage, or electrical stimulation if used. — Promotes bone growth and healing.

NURSING DIAGNOSIS: acute Pain

May Be Related To
Physical agents (e.g., muscle spasms, movement of bone fragments, edema, soft tissue injury, traction/immobility device)
Psychological (e.g., stress, anxiety)

Possibly Evidenced By
Verbalized/coded reports of pain
Self-focusing/narrowed focus; facial mask of pain
Guarding behavior, protective gestures
Changes in vital signs

Desired Outcomes/Evaluation Criteria—Client Will

Pain Level (NOC)
Verbalize relief of pain.
Display relaxed manner, able to participate in activities, and sleep and rest appropriately.

Pain Control (NOC)
Demonstrate use of relaxation skills and diversional activities, as indicated for individual situation.

ACTIONS/INTERVENTIONS / RATIONALE

Pain Management (NIC)

Independent

Maintain immobilization of affected part by means of bedrest, cast, splint, and traction. (Refer to ND: risk for Injury.) — Relieves pain and prevents bone displacement/extension of tissue injury.

Elevate and support injured extremity. — Promotes venous return, decreases edema, and may reduce pain.

Avoid use of plastic sheets/pillows under limbs in cast. — Can increase discomfort by enhancing heat production in the drying cast.

Elevate bed covers and keep linens off toes. — Maintains body warmth without discomfort due to pressure of bedclothes on affected parts.

Evaluate and document reports of pain or discomfort, noting location and characteristics, including intensity (0 to 10, or similar coded scale), relieving, and aggravating factors. Note nonverbal pain cues, such as changes in vital signs and emotions or behavior. Listen to reports of family member/significant other (SO) regarding client's pain. — Influences choice of, and monitors effectiveness of, interventions. Many factors, including level of anxiety, may affect perception of and reaction to pain. *Note:* Absence of pain expression does not necessarily mean lack of pain.

Encourage client to discuss problems related to injury. — Helps alleviate anxiety. Client may feel need to relive the accident experience.

Explain procedures before beginning them. — Allows client to prepare mentally for activity and to participate in controlling level of discomfort.

Medicate before care activities. Let client know it is important to request medication before pain becomes severe. — Promotes muscle relaxation and enhances participation.

Perform and supervise passive or active ROM exercises. — Maintains strength and mobility of unaffected muscles and facilitates resolution of inflammation in injured tissues.

Provide alternative comfort measures, for example, massage, back rub, or position changes. — Improves general circulation; reduces areas of local pressure and muscle fatigue.

ACTIONS/INTERVENTIONS (continued)	RATIONALE (continued)
Provide emotional support and encourage use of stress management techniques—progressive relaxation, deep-breathing exercises, and visualization or guided imagery; provide Therapeutic Touch.	Refocuses attention, promotes sense of control, and may enhance coping abilities in the management of the stress of traumatic injury and pain, which is likely to persist for an extended period.
Identify diversional activities appropriate for client's age, physical abilities, and personal preferences.	Prevents boredom, reduces muscle tension, and can increase muscle strength; may also enhance coping abilities.
Investigate any reports of unusual or sudden pain or deep, progressive, and poorly localized pain unrelieved by analgesics.	May signal developing complications, such as infection, tissue ischemia, or compartment syndrome. (Refer to ND: risk for Peripheral Neurovascular Dysfunction, following.)
Collaborative	
Apply cold or ice pack first 24 to 72 hours and as necessary per facility policy or protocol.	Reduces edema and hematoma formation; decreases pain sensation. *Note:* Length of application depends on degree of client comfort and whether the skin is carefully protected.
Administer medications, as indicated: opioid and nonopioid analgesics, such as morphine, meperidine (Demerol), or hydrocodone (Vicodin); injectable and oral NSAIDs, such as ketorolac (Toradol) or ibuprofen (Motrin); and/or muscle relaxants, such as cyclobenzaprine (Flexeril) or carisoprodol (Soma).	Given to reduce pain and/or muscle spasms. Studies of Toradol have shown it to be effective in alleviating bone pain, with longer action and fewer side effects than opioid agents.
Maintain continuous intravenous (IV) or patient-controlled analgesia (PCA) using peripheral, epidural, or intrathecal routes of administration. Maintain safe and effective infusions and equipment.	Optimal pain management is essential to permit early mobilization and physical therapy and to maintain adequate blood level of analgesia, preventing fluctuations in pain relief with associated muscle tension or spasms.

NURSING DIAGNOSIS: risk for Peripheral Neurovascular Dysfunction

Risk Factors May Include

Fractures; trauma; orthopedic surgery; immobilization
Vascular obstruction
Mechanical compression (e.g., cast, dressing)

Possibly Evidenced By

(Not applicable; presence of signs and symptoms establishes an *actual* diagnosis)

Desired Outcomes/Evaluation Criteria—Client Will

Tissue Perfusion: Peripheral (NOC)

Maintain tissue perfusion as evidenced by palpable pulses; warm, dry skin; normal sensation; usual sensorium; stable vital signs; and adequate urinary output for individual situation.

ACTIONS/INTERVENTIONS	RATIONALE
Circulatory Precautions (NIC)	
Independent	
Assess client's risk for development of venous thromboembolism (VTE) and acute compartment syndrome (ACS).	Any client with severe fractures or multiple fractures, especially of long bones (femur) is at risk for VTE (including deep vein thrombosis (DVT) and pulmonary embolus (PE) particularly if long-term bedrest is required. Clients with fractures of tibia or femur can be at risk for ACS if they have sustained severe tissue injury that resulted in significant bleeding into a closed compartment, compressed blood vessels such as might occur with a crush injury, or surgery to repair blood vessels with subsequent reperfusion to a compartment. ACS can also be a complication of circumferential dressings, splints, or casts that are applied too tightly (Walsh, 2011; Wedro, 2010).
Remove jewelry from affected limb immediately.	May restrict circulation when edema occurs.
Evaluate presence and quality of peripheral pulse distal to injury via palpation or Doppler. Compare with uninjured limb.	Decreased or absent pulse may reflect vascular injury and necessitates immediate medical evaluation of circulatory status. Be aware that occasionally a pulse may be palpated even though circulation is blocked by a soft clot through which pulsations may be felt. In addition, perfusion through larger arteries may continue after increased compartment pressure has collapsed the arteriole and venule circulation in the muscle.

(continues on page 608)

ACTIONS/INTERVENTIONS (continued)	RATIONALE (continued)
Assess capillary return, skin color, and warmth distal to the fracture.	Return of color should be rapid (3–5 seconds). White, cool skin indicates arterial impairment. Cyanosis suggests venous impairment. *Note:* Peripheral pulses, capillary refill, skin color, and sensation may be normal even in the presence of compartment syndrome because superficial circulation is usually not compromised.
Circulatory Care: Arterial [or] Venous Insufficiency (NIC)	
Maintain elevation of injured extremity(ies) unless contraindicated by confirmed presence of compartment syndrome.	Promotes venous drainage and decreases edema. *Note:* In presence of increased compartment pressure, elevation of the extremity actually impedes arterial flow, decreasing perfusion. Casts or circumferential dressings can also cause arterial venous insufficiency.
Assess entire length of injured extremity for swelling and edema formation. Measure injured extremity and compare with uninjured extremity. Note appearance and spread of hematoma.	Increasing circumference of injured extremity may suggest general tissue swelling or edema but may also reflect hemorrhage. *Note:* A 1-inch increase in an adult thigh can equal approximately 1 unit of sequestered blood.
Note reports of pain extreme for type of injury or increasing pain on passive movement of extremity, development of paresthesia, muscle tension or tenderness with erythema, and change in pulse quality distal to injury. Do not elevate extremity. Report symptoms to physician at once.	Continued bleeding or edema formation within a muscle enclosed by tight fascia can result in impaired blood flow and ischemic myositis or compartment syndrome, necessitating emergency interventions to relieve pressure and restore circulation (Smeltzer, 2011). *Note:* This condition constitutes a medical emergency and requires immediate intervention.
Investigate sudden signs of limb ischemia, such as decreased skin temperature, pallor, and increased pain.	Fracture dislocations of joints, especially the knee, may cause damage to adjacent arteries, with resulting loss of distal blood flow.
Encourage client to routinely exercise digits or joints distal to injury. Ambulate as soon as possible.	Enhances circulation and reduces pooling of blood, especially in the lower extremities.
Investigate tenderness, swelling, redness, or tissue pain on dorsiflexion of foot (positive Homans' sign).	There is an increased potential for thrombophlebitis and pulmonary emboli in clients who have been immobile for several days. *Note:* The absence of a positive Homans' sign is not a reliable indicator in many people. Refer to CP: Thrombophlebitis: Venous Thromboembolism—(Including Pulmonary Emboli Considerations), as indicated.
Monitor vital signs. Note signs of general pallor or cyanosis, cool skin, and changes in mentation.	Inadequate circulating volume compromises systemic tissue perfusion.
Test stools and gastric aspirant for occult blood. Note continued bleeding at trauma or injection site(s) and oozing from mucous membranes.	Increased incidence of gastric bleeding accompanies fractures and trauma and may be related to stress or occasionally reflects a clotting disorder requiring further evaluation.
Pressure Management (NIC)	
Perform neurovascular assessments, noting changes in motor and sensory function. Ask client to localize pain or discomfort.	Impaired feeling, numbness, tingling, and increased or diffuse pain occur when circulation to nerves is inadequate or nerves are damaged.
Test sensation of peroneal nerve by pinch or pinprick in the dorsal web between the first and second toe, and assess ability to dorsiflex toes, if indicated.	Length and position of peroneal nerve increase risk of its injury in the presence of leg fracture, edema, or compartment syndrome, or because of malposition of traction apparatus.
Assess tissues around cast edges for rough places and pressure points. Investigate reports of "burning sensation" under cast.	These factors may be the cause of or be indicative of tissue pressure or ischemia, leading to breakdown and necrosis.
Monitor position and location of supporting ring of splints or sling.	Traction apparatus can cause pressure on vessels and nerves, particularly in the axilla and groin, resulting in ischemia and possible permanent nerve damage.
Circulatory Care: Arterial [or] Venous Insufficiency (NIC) *Collaborative*	
Apply ice bags around fracture site for short periods of time on an intermittent basis for 24 to 72 hours.	Reduces edema and hematoma formation, which could impair circulation. *Note:* Length of application of cold therapy is usually 20 to 30 minutes at a time.
Monitor Hgb/Hct and coagulation studies, such as prothrombin time (PT).	Assists in calculation of blood loss and needs and effectiveness of replacement therapy. Coagulation deficits may occur secondary to major trauma, in presence of fat emboli, or during anticoagulant therapy.
Administer IV fluids and blood products as needed.	Maintains circulating volume, enhancing tissue perfusion.
Administer medications, as indicated: Low-molecular-weight heparin or heparinoids, such as enoxaparin (Lovenox), dalteparin (Fragmin), or fondaparinux (Arixtra), if indicated.	Anticoagulants may be given prophylactically to reduce threat of deep venous thrombus.
Apply antiembolic hose or sequential pressure hose or compression boots, as indicated.	Decreases venous pooling and may enhance venous return, thereby reducing risk of thrombus formation.

ACTIONS/INTERVENTIONS (continued)	RATIONALE (continued)
Pressure Management (NIC)	
Split or bivalve cast as needed. Be sure to cut through wadding down to the skin.	May be done on an emergency basis to relieve restriction and improve impaired circulation resulting from compression and edema formation in injured extremity. The wadding under the cast may also be restrictive.
Refer for and monitor intracompartmental pressures as appropriate.	Diagnosis of compartment syndrome is typically performed with client under light or local anesthesia and measured by means of slit catheter or side-ported catheter. Values of 30 mm Hg or greater indicate a probable compartment problem, requiring prompt medical attention (Jagminas, 2011).
Prepare for surgical intervention, such as fasciotomy, as indicated.	Failure to relieve pressure or correct compartment syndrome within 4 to 6 hours of onset can result in severe contractures, loss of function, and disfigurement of extremity distal to injury, possibly necessitating amputation.

NURSING DIAGNOSIS: risk for impaired Gas Exchange

Risk Factors May Include

Ventilation-perfusion imbalance (e.g., altered blood flow, blood or fat emboli)
Alveolar and capillary membrane changes (e.g., interstitial congestion, pulmonary edema)

Possibly Evidenced By

(Not applicable; presence of signs and symptoms establishes an *actual* diagnosis)

Desired Outcomes/Evaluation Criteria—Client Will

Respiratory Status: Gas Exchange (NOC)

Maintain adequate respiratory function, as evidenced by absence of dyspnea or cyanosis; respiratory rate and arterial blood gases (ABGs) are within client's normal range.

ACTIONS/INTERVENTIONS	RATIONALE
Respiratory Monitoring (NIC)	
Independent	
Monitor respiratory rate and effort. Note stridor, use of accessory muscles, retractions, and development of central cyanosis.	Tachypnea, dyspnea, and changes in mentation are early signs of respiratory insufficiency and may be the only indicator of developing pulmonary emboli in the early stage. Remaining signs and symptoms reflect advanced respiratory distress and impending failure.
Auscultate breath sounds, noting development of unequal, hyperresonant sounds; also note presence of crackles, rhonchi, or wheezes and inspiratory crowing or croupy sounds.	Changes in or presence of adventitious breath sounds reflects developing respiratory complications—atelectasis, pneumonia, emboli, or acute respiratory distress syndrome (ARDS). *Note:* Early fixation of long-bone fractures (within 24 hours of injury) can reduce client's risk of developing ARDS (Kirkland, 2013; Walsh, 2011). Inspiratory crowing reflects upper airway edema and is suggestive of fat emboli as a reason for ARDS. *Note*: Fat embolus syndrome (FES) should be suspected in client with long-bone fractures who develops hypoxia, fever, bilateral pulmonary infiltrates, and a rash (Kirkland, 2013; Smeltzer, 2011).
Instruct and assist with deep-breathing and coughing exercises. Reposition frequently.	Promotes alveolar ventilation and perfusion. Repositioning promotes drainage of secretions and decreases congestion in dependent lung areas.
Note increasing restlessness, confusion, lethargy, or stupor.	Impaired gas exchange or presence of pulmonary emboli can cause deterioration in client's level of consciousness as hypoxemia and acidosis develop.
Observe sputum for signs of blood.	Hemoptysis may occur with pulmonary emboli.
Inspect skin for petechiae above nipple line, in axilla, spreading to abdomen or trunk, buccal mucosa and hard palate, and conjunctival sacs and retina.	This is the most characteristic sign of fat emboli, which may appear within 2 to 3 days after injury.
Collaborative	
Instruct in, and encourage regular use of, incentive spirometry.	Maximizes ventilation and minimizes atelectasis.
Administer supplemental oxygen, if indicated.	Increases available O_2 for optimal tissue oxygenation.

(continues on page 610)

ACTIONS/INTERVENTIONS (continued)	RATIONALE (continued)
Monitor laboratory studies, such as the following:	
Pulse oximetry or serial ABGs	Identifies situations in which oxygen desaturation is occurring and reveals complications such as impaired gas exchange and developing respiratory failure.
Hgb, calcium, erythrocyte sedimentation rate (ESR), serum lipase, fat screen, and platelets, as appropriate	Anemia, hypocalcemia, elevated ESR and lipase levels; fat globules in blood, urine, or sputum; and decreased platelet count (thrombocytopenia) are often associated with fat emboli.
Administer medications, as indicated, for example:	
Low-molecular-weight heparin or heparinoids, such as enoxaparin (Lovenox), dalteparin (Fragmin), or fondaparinux (Arixtra)	Used for prevention of thromboembolic phenomena, including deep vein thrombosis and pulmonary emboli.
Corticosteroids	Steroids have been used with some success to prevent and treat fat embolus.

NURSING DIAGNOSIS: impaired physical Mobility

May Be Related To

Loss of integrity of bone structures; decreased muscle strength or control
Pain or discomfort; reluctance to initiate movement
Prescribed movement restrictions—limb immobilization

Possibly Evidenced By

Limited range of motion; slowed movement
Difficulty turning

Desired Outcomes/Evaluation Criteria—Client Will

Skeletal Function (NOC)

Maintain position of function.
Increase strength and function of affected and compensatory body parts.

Mobility (NOC)

Regain and maintain mobility at the highest possible level.
Demonstrate techniques that enable resumption of activities, especially activities of daily living (ADLs).

ACTIONS/INTERVENTIONS	RATIONALE
Bedrest Care (NIC)	
Independent	
Assess degree of immobility produced by injury and/or treatment and note client's perception of immobility.	Client may be restricted by self-view or self-perception out of proportion with actual physical limitations, requiring information and interventions to promote progress toward wellness.
Encourage participation in diversional or recreational activities. Maintain stimulating environment—radio, TV, newspapers, personal possessions, pictures, clock, calendar, and visits from family and friends.	Provides opportunity for release of energy, refocuses attention, enhances client's sense of self-control and self-worth, and aids in reducing social isolation.
Instruct client in active, or assist with passive, ROM exercises of affected and unaffected extremities.	Increases blood flow to muscles and bone to improve muscle tone; maintain joint mobility; and prevent contractures, atrophy, and calcium resorption from disuse.
Encourage use of isometric exercises, starting with the unaffected limb.	Isometrics contract muscles without bending joints or moving limbs and help maintain muscle strength and mass. *Note:* These exercises are contraindicated while acute bleeding or edema is present.
Provide footboard, wrist splints, and trochanter or hand rolls, as appropriate.	Useful in maintaining functional position of extremities, hands or feet, and preventing complications such as contractures or footdrop.
Instruct in, and encourage use of, trapeze and "post position" for lower limb fractures.	Facilitates movement during hygiene, skin care, and linen changes; reduces discomfort of remaining flat in bed. "Post position" involves placing the uninjured foot flat on the bed with the knee bent while grasping the trapeze and lifting the body off the bed.
Assist with and encourage self-care activities such as bathing, shaving, and oral hygiene.	Improves muscle strength and circulation, enhances client control in situation, and promotes self-directed wellness.
Assist with mobility by means of wheelchair, walker, crutches, and/or canes as soon as possible. Instruct in safe use of mobility aids.	Early mobility reduces complications of bedrest, such as phlebitis, and promotes healing and normalization of organ function. Learning the correct way to use aids is important to maintain optimal mobility and client safety.

ACTIONS/INTERVENTIONS (continued)	RATIONALE (continued)
Monitor blood pressure (BP) with resumption of activity. Note reports of dizziness.	Postural hypotension is a common problem following prolonged bedrest and may require specific interventions, such as tilt table with gradual elevation to upright position.
Reposition periodically and encourage coughing and deep-breathing exercises.	Prevents or reduces incidence of skin and respiratory complications—decubitus ulcer, atelectasis, or pneumonia.
Auscultate bowel sounds. Monitor elimination habits and provide for regular bowel routine. Place on bedside commode, if feasible. Provide privacy.	Bedrest, use of analgesics, and changes in dietary habits can slow peristalsis and produce constipation. Nursing measures that facilitate elimination may prevent or limit complications.
Evaluate client's prior bowel habits.	Provides baseline for comparison with postsurgical concerns. The long-term use of opioids for pain and limited mobility causes constipation in orthopedic clients. Constipation is a major issue and needs immediate and ongoing attention.
Encourage increased fluid intake of 2000 to 3000 mL/day within cardiac tolerance, including acid ash juices such as cranberry.	Keeps the body well hydrated, decreasing risk of urinary infection and stone formation, and helps to prevent constipation.
Provide diet high in proteins, carbohydrates, vitamins, and minerals, limiting protein content until after first bowel movement.	In the presence of musculoskeletal injuries, early good feeding is needed as nutrients required for healing are rapidly depleted. This can have a profound effect on muscle mass, tone, and strength. *Note:* Protein foods increase contents in small bowel, resulting in gas formation and constipation. Therefore, gastrointestinal (GI) function should be fully restored before protein foods are increased.
Increase the amount of roughage and fiber in the diet. Limit gas-forming foods.	Adding bulk to stool helps prevent constipation. Gas-forming foods may cause abdominal distention, especially in presence of decreased intestinal motility.
Collaborative	
Consult with physical or occupational therapist and/or rehabilitation specialist.	Useful in creating aggressive individualized activity or exercise program. Client may require long-term assistance with movement, strengthening, and weight-bearing activities as well as use of adjuncts, for example, walkers, crutches, canes; elevated toilet seats; pickup sticks or reachers; special eating utensils; and help for women with actions such as hooking a brassiere.
Refer to dietitian or nutrition team, as indicated.	The client with fractures, especially when associated with trauma, may have special nutritional considerations; for example, he or she may need enteral or parenteral feedings to maximize healing of tissues and bones.
Initiate bowel program—stool softeners, enemas, or laxatives, as indicated.	Important to promote regular bowel evacuation and prevent constipation.
Refer to psychiatric clinical nurse specialist or therapist, as indicated.	Client/SO may require more intensive treatment to deal with reality of current condition, prognosis, prolonged immobility, and perceived loss of control.

NURSING DIAGNOSIS: impaired Tissue Integrity

May Be Related To

Mechanical factors (e.g., compound fracture; surgical repair; insertion of traction pins, wires, screws)
Altered sensation, circulation
Chemical irritants (e.g., accumulation of excretions or secretions)
Impaired physical mobility

Possibly Evidenced By (actual)

Damaged/destroyed tissue (e.g., abrasions, lacerations, puncture wounds, surgical incisions)

Desired Outcomes/Evaluation Criteria—Client Will

Tissue Integrity: Skin & Mucous Membranes (NOC)

Verbalize relief of discomfort.
Demonstrate behaviors or techniques to prevent skin breakdown and facilitate healing, as indicated.
Achieve timely wound or lesion healing, if present.

ACTIONS/INTERVENTIONS	RATIONALE
Skin Surveillance (NIC)	
Independent	
Examine the skin for open wounds, foreign bodies, rashes, bleeding, discoloration, duskiness, and/or blanching.	Provides information regarding skin circulation and problems that may be caused by application and/or restriction of cast, splint, or traction apparatus, or edema formation that may require further medical intervention.
Provide specialty beds and Geomatts as indicated.	Used for clients with a high risk of skin breakdown or in whom long-term immobility is expected.
Massage skin and bony prominences. Keep bed linens dry and free of wrinkles. Place water pads or other padding under elbows and heels, as indicated.	Reduces pressure on susceptible areas and risk of abrasions or skin breakdown.
Reposition frequently. Encourage use of trapeze, if possible. If not able to turn independently, a turning schedule must be maintained by the nurse.	Lessens constant pressure on same areas and minimizes risk of skin breakdown. Use of trapeze may reduce risk of abrasions to elbows and heels.
Cast Care: Wet (NIC)	
Plaster cast application and skin care:	
Cleanse skin with soap and water, rubbing gently with alcohol and/or dust with small amount of a zinc or stearate powder.	Provides a dry, clean area for cast application. *Note:* Excess powder may cake when it comes in contact with water or perspiration.
Cut a length of stockinette to cover the area and extend several inches beyond the cast.	Useful for padding bony prominences, finishing cast edges, and protecting the skin.
Use palm of hand to apply, hold, or move cast and support on pillows after application; avoid using fingertips to hold cast.	Prevents indentations or flattening over bony prominences, such as back of heels, and weight-bearing areas, which would cause abrasions or tissue trauma. An improperly shaped or dried cast is irritating to the underlying skin and may lead to circulatory impairment. Fingertips may dent the cast when it is wet.
Trim excess plaster from edges of cast as soon as casting is completed.	Uneven plaster is irritating to the skin and may result in abrasions.
Promote cast drying by removing bed linen, exposing to circulating air.	Prevents skin breakdown caused by prolonged moisture trapped under cast.
Observe for potential pressure areas, especially at the edges of and under the splint/cast.	Pressure can cause ulcerations, necrosis, and/or nerve palsies. These problems may be painless when nerve damage is present.
Pad or petal tape the edges of the cast with waterproof tape or moleskin.	Provides an effective barrier to cast flaking and moisture. Helps prevent breakdown of cast material at edges and reduces skin irritation and excoriation.
Cleanse excess plaster from skin while still wet, if possible.	Dry plaster may flake into completed cast and cause skin damage.
Protect cast and skin in perineal area, providing frequent perineal care.	Prevents tissue breakdown and infection by fecal contamination.
Instruct client/SO to avoid inserting objects inside casts.	"Scratching an itch" may cause tissue injury.
Massage the skin around the cast edges with alcohol.	Has a drying effect, which toughens the skin. Creams and lotions are not recommended because excessive oils can seal cast perimeter, not allowing the cast to "breathe." Powders are not recommended because of potential for excessive accumulation inside the cast.
Pressure Management (NIC)	
Collaborative	
Provide foam mattress, sheepskins, flotation pads, or air mattress, as indicated.	Because of immobilization of body parts, bony prominences other than those affected by the casting may suffer from decreased circulation.
Monovalve, bivalve, or cut a window in the cast, per protocol.	Cutting or hinging the cast allows the release of pressure and provides access for wound and skin care.

NURSING DIAGNOSIS: risk for Infection

Risk Factors May Include

Inadequate primary defenses—broken skin, traumatized tissues, invasive procedures, skeletal traction
Increased environmental exposure

Possibly Evidenced By

(Not applicable; presence of signs and symptoms establishes an *actual* diagnosis)

Desired Outcomes/Evaluation Criteria—Client Will

Infection Severity (NOC)
Achieve timely wound healing, be free of purulent drainage or erythema, and be afebrile.

ACTIONS/INTERVENTIONS	RATIONALE
Infection Protection (NIC)	
Independent	
Inspect the skin for preexisting irritation or breaks in continuity.	Pins or wires should not be inserted through skin infections, rashes, or abrasions—may lead to bone infection.
Assess pin sites and skin areas, noting reports of increased pain or burning sensation, or presence of edema, erythema, foul odor, or drainage.	May indicate onset of local infection or tissue necrosis, which can lead to osteomyelitis.
Provide sterile pin and wound care according to protocol, and exercise meticulous hand washing.	May prevent cross-contamination and possibility of infection.
Instruct client not to touch the insertion sites.	Minimizes risk of contamination.
Line perineal cast edges with plastic wrap.	Damp, soiled casts can promote growth of bacteria.
Observe wounds for formation of bullae, crepitation, bronze discoloration of skin, and frothy or fruity-smelling drainage.	Signs suggestive of gas gangrene infection.
Assess muscle tone, reflexes, and ability to speak.	Muscle rigidity, tonic spasms of jaw muscles, and dysphagia reflect development of tetanus.
Monitor vital signs. Note presence of chills, fever, and malaise and any changes in mentation.	Hypotension and confusion may be seen with gas gangrene; tachycardia, chills, and fever reflect developing sepsis.
Investigate abrupt onset of pain or limitation of movement with localized edema and erythema in injured extremity.	May indicate development of osteomyelitis.
Institute prescribed isolation procedures.	Presence of purulent drainage requires wound and linen precautions to prevent cross-contamination.
Collaborative	
Monitor laboratory/diagnostic studies, for example:	
CBC	Anemia may be noted with osteomyelitis; leukocytosis is usually present with infective processes.
ESR	Elevated in osteomyelitis.
Cultures and sensitivity of wound, serum, and/or bone	Identifies infective organism and effective antimicrobial agent(s).
Radioisotope scans	Hot spots signify increased areas of vascularity, indicative of osteomyelitis.
Administer medications, as indicated, for example:	
IV/topical antibiotics	Wide-spectrum antibiotics may be used prophylactically or may be geared toward a specific microorganism.
Tetanus toxoid	Given prophylactically because the possibility of tetanus exists with any open wound. *Note:* Risk increases when injury or wound(s) occur in "field conditions"—outdoors, rural areas, or the work environment.
Provide wound or bone irrigations, and apply warm, moist soaks, as indicated.	Local debridement and cleansing of wounds reduces microorganisms and incidence of systemic infection. Continuous antimicrobial drip into bone may be necessary to treat osteomyelitis, especially if blood supply to bone is compromised.
Assist with procedures such as incision and drainage, placement of drains, and hyperbaric oxygen therapy.	Numerous procedures may be carried out in treatment of local infections, osteomyelitis, and gas gangrene.
Prepare for surgery, as indicated.	Sequestrectomy, removal of necrotic bone, is necessary to facilitate healing and prevent extension of infectious process.

NURSING DIAGNOSIS: **deficient Knowledge [Learning Need] regarding condition, prognosis, treatment, self-care, and discharge needs**

May Be Related To

Lack of exposure or recall
Misinterpretation of information
Unfamiliarity with information resources

Possibly Evidenced By

Reports the problem
Inaccurate follow-through of instructions

Desired Outcomes/Evaluation Criteria—Client Will

Knowledge: Treatment Regimen (NOC)

Verbalize understanding of condition, prognosis, and potential complications.
Correctly perform necessary procedures and explain reasons for actions.

ACTIONS/INTERVENTIONS	RATIONALE
Teaching: Disease Process (NIC)	
Independent	
Review pathology, prognosis, and future expectations.	Provides knowledge base from which client can make informed choices. *Note:* Internal fixation devices can ultimately compromise the bone's strength, and intramedullary nails or rods, and plates may be removed at a future date.
Discuss prophylactic antibiotic use.	When hardware, such as pins, screws, and plates, is implanted, it provides a place for infection to develop. If there are procedures that open the GI tract to the bloodstream, such as dental procedures or a colonoscopy, antibiotics should be given.
Discuss dietary needs.	A low-fat diet adequate in quality protein and rich in calcium promotes healing and general well-being.
Discuss individual drug regimen, as appropriate.	Proper use of pain medication and antiplatelet agents can reduce risk of complications.
Reinforce methods of mobility and ambulation as instructed by physical therapist when indicated.	Most fractures require casts, splints, or braces during the healing process. Further damage and delay in healing could occur secondary to improper use of ambulatory devices.
Suggest use of a backpack.	Provides place to carry necessary articles and leaves hands free to manipulate crutches; may prevent undue muscle fatigue when one arm is casted.
List activities that the client can perform independently and those that require assistance.	Organizes activities around need and who is available to provide help.
Identify available community services, such as a rehabilitation team, home nursing care, or homemaker services.	Provides assistance to facilitate self-care and support independence. Promotes optimal self-care and recovery.
Encourage client to continue active exercises for the joints above and below the fracture.	Prevents joint stiffness, contractures, and muscle wasting, promoting earlier return to independence in ADLs.
Discuss importance of clinical and therapy follow-up appointments.	Fracture healing may take as long as a year for completion, and client cooperation with the medical regimen facilitates proper union of bone. Physical therapy and occupational therapy may be indicated for exercises to maintain or strengthen muscles and improve function. Additional modalities such as low-intensity ultrasound may be used to stimulate healing of lower-forearm or lower-leg fractures.
Review proper pin or wound care.	Reduces risk of bone and tissue trauma and infection, which can progress to osteomyelitis.
Recommend cleaning external fixator device regularly.	Keeping device free of dust or contaminants reduces risk of infection.
Identify signs and symptoms requiring medical evaluation, for example, severe pain, fever or chills, or foul odors; changes in sensation, swelling, burning, numbness, tingling, skin discoloration, paralysis, or white/cool toes or fingertips; and warm spots, soft areas, or cracks in the cast.	Prompt intervention may reduce severity of complications such as infection or impaired circulation. *Note:* Some darkening of the skin reflecting vascular congestion may occur normally when walking on the casted extremity or using casted arm; however, this should resolve with rest and elevation.
Discuss care of "green" or wet cast.	Promotes proper curing to prevent cast deformities and associated misalignment or skin irritation. *Note:* Placing a "cooling" cast directly on rubber or plastic pillows traps heat and increases drying time.

ACTIONS/INTERVENTIONS (continued)	RATIONALE (continued)
Suggest the use of a blow-dryer to dry small areas of dampened cast.	Cautious use can hasten drying.
Demonstrate use of plastic bags to cover plaster cast during wet weather or while bathing. Clean soiled cast with a slightly dampened cloth and some scouring powder.	Protects from moisture, which softens the plaster and weakens the cast. *Note:* Fiberglass casts are being used more frequently. They also need to be thoroughly dried if they get wet to avoid developing mold.
Emphasize the importance of not adjusting clamps or nuts of an external fixator device.	Tampering may alter compression and misalign fracture.
Recommend use of loose-fitting or adaptive clothing.	Facilitates dressing and grooming activities.
Suggest ways to cover toes if appropriate, for example, using stockinette or soft socks.	Helps maintain warmth and protect from injury.
Discuss postcast removal instructions:	
Instruct client to continue exercises as permitted.	Reduces stiffness and improves strength and function of affected extremity.
Inform client that the skin under the cast is commonly mottled and covered with scales or crusts of dead skin.	It will be several weeks before normal appearance returns.
Wash the skin gently with soap and water and lubricate with a protective emollient.	New skin is extremely tender because it has been protected beneath a cast.
Inform client that muscles may appear flabby and atrophied (less muscle mass); recommend supporting the joint above and below the affected part and the use of mobility aids—elastic bandages, splints, braces, crutches, walkers, or canes.	Muscle strength will be reduced and new or different aches and pains may occur secondary to loss of support.
Elevate the extremity, as needed.	Swelling and edema tend to occur after cast removal.

NURSING DIAGNOSIS: readiness for enhanced Self-Care

May Be Related To

(Not applicable; readiness diagnoses do not have related factors)

Possibly Evidenced By

Expression of desire to enhance self-care, knowledge for strategies for self-care, or responsibility for self-care

Desired Outcomes/Evaluation Criteria—Client Will

Discharge Readiness: Independent Living (NOC)

Demonstrate proactive management of chronic condition, potential complications.
Identify and use resources appropriately.
Remain free of preventable complications.

ACTIONS/INTERVENTIONS	RATIONALE
Self-Efficacy Enhancement (NIC)	
Independent	
Note age, developmental level, and presence of comorbidities.	These factors impact ability of client to meet own needs.
Discuss client's understanding of current situation.	Helps determine areas that can be clarified or strengthened.
Determine individual strengths and skills of the client, using functional status instrument if indicated.	Establishes comparative baseline for potential for growth or modifications in current strategies.
Review coping skills (e.g., assertiveness, interpersonal relations, decision making, problem-solving).	Useful for managing a wide range of stressful conditions.
Provide accurate and relevant information regarding current and future needs.	Client can incorporate information into self-care plans, while minimizing difficulties associated with change.
Active-listen client's/SO's concerns.	Exhibits regard for their values and beliefs and encourages open discussion about concerns.
Note availability and use of resources, and supportive persons and assistive devices.	Makes sure that client has means for sharing concerns, needs, and wishes, as well as has access to support and approval (family members, professionals).
Identify reliable reference sources and strategies for self-care.	Reinforces learning and promotes self-paced review.
Review safety concerns and potential for modification of therapies, activities, or environment.	May be needed to prevent complications or enhance successful functioning.
Refer to home-care provider, social services, physical or occupational therapy, durable medical equipment, rehabilitation and counseling resources as indicated or requested. Identify additional community resources (e.g., handicap transportation van for appointments, accessible and safe locations for social or sports activities).	May be helpful for education, assistance, adaptive devices, and modifications that may be desired.

POTENTIAL CONSIDERATIONS following acute hospitalization (dependent on client's age, physical condition and presence of complications, personal resources, and life responsibilities)

In addition to surgical considerations:

- *risk for Trauma*—balancing difficulties, weakness, reduced muscle coordination, history of previous trauma
- *impaired physical Mobility* —neuromuscular skeletal impairment, pain/discomfort, prescribed movement restrictions (limb immobilization)
- *Self-Care Deficit*—musculoskeletal impairment, decreased strength/endurance, pain
- *risk for Infection*—inadequate primary defenses: broken skin, traumatized tissues, environmental exposure, invasive procedures, skeletal traction

AMPUTATION

I. Pathophysiology—Partial or complete detachment of body part with residual extremity covered with well-vascularized muscle and skin, although reattachment surgery may be possible for fingers, hands, and arms

a. Primarily two types of amputations
   i. Open or provisional: Requires subsequent revisions
   ii. Closed or flap: All surgical revision is performed and the wound closed in one procedure.

b. Amputation levels (Amputation Coalition, 2012):
   i. Lower-extremity: Partial foot or toe, below knee (BKA), above knee (AKA), hip disarticulation or hemipelvectomy, and bilateral lower-limb loss
   ii. Upper-extremity amputation: Partial hand or finger, below elbow, above elbow, shoulder disarticulation or forequarter, and bilateral upper-limb loss

c. Two basic types of prosthetic designs are used: exoskeletal and endoskeletal.

II. Etiology

a. Varied causes (Ertl, 2012; Kalapatapu, 2012; Kirshner, 2011)
   i. Peripheral vascular disease (causing critical limb ischemia, often associated with diabetes (45% to 50%), usually involves lower extremity; most common in the United States, accounting for 65% of cases
   ii. Trauma: Examples include direct limb transection or a severe open fracture with an associated unreconstructable neurovascular injury (often associated with motor vehicle crashes or industrial accidents), battlefield wounds. Note: U.S. wounded in current war theaters include more than 1500 amputations to date (Huffington Post, October 2012).
   iii. Malignant bone tumors
   iv. Infections: osteomyelitis, gangrene
   v. Congenital disorders: approximately 5% of cases

b. Lower-extremity amputations are performed much more frequently than upper-extremity amputations.

c. Upper-extremity amputations generally result from trauma caused by industrial accidents.

III. Statistics

a. Morbidity: In the year 2005, 1.6 million persons were living with the loss of a limb (Ziegler-Graham, 2008). In 2008, the incidence of amputation for those with a previous incident amputation was 17.1% (Margolis et al, 2011).

b. Mortality: One review of a series of studies showed 30-day mortality rates for major amputation range from 3% to 18% (Kalapatapu, 2012). A higher level of amputation correlates with increased mortality and may reflect the severity of systemic cardiovascular disease or differences in the incidence of thromboembolism rather than the magnitude of the procedure (Dillingham, 2005). One study indicated that while there is a high prevalence of preexisting neurological disorders among lower-extremity amputees affecting the risk of mortality, age is a stronger predictor of mortality (Prvu-Bettger, 2009).

c. Costs: The average total charge equals $32,129 per amputation and cumulative inpatient hospitalization equaled $56.5 million in 2008 (Peacock, 2011).

GLOSSARY

Complete amputation: Total detachment of appendage or limb from the body.

Endoskeletal prosthetic: Aluminum, titanium, and other tubular materials form the inner structure, providing strength; external shape is removable, usually composed of foam or skin-simulating material.

Exoskeletal prosthetic: Outer plastic laminated skin with wood or urethane foam interiors where the strength is provided by the outer layer.

Neuromas: Painful proliferation of nerve fibers at the proximal end of a severed nerve.

Partial amputation: Some soft tissue remains attached to the body.

Residual limb: Remaining portion of the amputated limb (once referred to as the stump).

Care Setting

Client is treated in inpatient acute surgical unit and subacute or rehabilitation unit.

Related Concerns

Cancer, page 827
Diabetes mellitus/diabetic ketoacidosis, page 377
Psychosocial aspects of care, page 729
Surgical intervention, page 762

Client Assessment Database

Data depend on underlying reason for surgical procedure, for example, severe trauma, peripheral vascular/arterial occlusive disease, diabetic neuropathy, osteomyelitis, and cancer.

DIAGNOSTIC DIVISION MAY REPORT	MAY EXHIBIT
ACTIVITY/REST	
• Actual or anticipated limitations imposed by condition or amputation	
CIRCULATION	
	• Presence of edema • Absent or diminished pulses in affected limb or digits
EGO INTEGRITY	
• Concern about negative effects or anticipated changes in lifestyle, financial situation, reactions of others • Feelings of helplessness, powerlessness	• Anxiety, apprehension • Irritability • Anger, frustration • Withdrawal, grief • False cheerfulness
NEUROSENSORY	
• Loss of sensation in affected area • Phantom pain	
SAFETY	
• History of falls, traumatic injuries, risky behavior, or work environment resulting in injury • Loss of ability to walk; altered gait	• Necrotic or gangrenous area • Nonhealing wound • Local infection • Altered gait; increased risk for falls
SEXUALITY	
• Concern about intimate relationships	
SOCIAL INTERACTION	
• Problems related to illness or condition • Concern about role function • Concern about reaction of others	
TEACHING/LEARNING	
DISCHARGE PLAN CONSIDERATIONS	
• May require assistance with wound care and supplies, adaptation to prosthesis or other ambulatory devices, transportation, homemaker or maintenance tasks, and possibly self-care activities and vocational retraining	
➧ Refer to section at end of plan for postdischarge considerations.	

Diagnostic Studies

Studies depend on the underlying condition necessitating amputation and are used to determine the appropriate level for amputation.

TEST WHY IT IS DONE	WHAT IT TELLS ME
• *X-rays:* Used to visualize pathology and the extent of involvement.	Identify skeletal abnormalities, trauma, or mass or tumor.
• *Computed tomography (CT) scan:* Used to visualize changes of structure within the body and bone alignment.	Identifies soft tissue and bone destruction, neoplastic lesions, osteomyelitis, and hematoma formation.
• *Angiography and blood flow studies:* Evaluates circulation and tissue perfusion.	Helps predict potential for tissue healing after amputation.
• *Doppler ultrasound, laser Doppler flowmetry:* Performed to assess and measure blood flow.	Determines adequacy of skin microcirculation and helps predict tissue or muscle viability and primary wound healing.
• *Transcutaneous oxygen pressure:* Maps out areas of greater and lesser perfusion in the involved extremity.	Helps determine lowest level at which to perform amputation for maximum preservation of limb length and successful healing.
• *Thermography:* Measures temperature differences in an ischemic limb at two sites—the skin and the center of the bone.	The lower that the difference is between the two readings, the greater the chances will be for healing.
• *C-reactive protein (CPR):* Inflammatory marker as indicator of infection.	Important if osteomyelitis or sepsis is a suspected or known factor in considering amputation. A level greater than 8 mg/L indicates significant infection.
• *White blood cell (WBC) count/differential:* Assess body's ability to respond to and eliminate infection.	Elevation and "shift to left" suggest infectious process.
• *Biopsy:* Determines presence of pathology and treatment needs or options.	Confirms diagnosis of benign or malignant mass.

Nursing Priorities

1. Alleviate pain.
2. Prevent complications.
3. Promote mobility and functional abilities.
4. Support psychological and physiological adjustment.
5. Provide information about surgical procedure, prognosis, and treatment needs.

Discharge Goals

1. Pain relieved or controlled.
2. Complications prevented or minimized.
3. Mobility and function regained or compensated for.
4. Dealing with current situation realistically.
5. Surgical procedure, prognosis, and therapeutic regimen understood.
6. Plan in place to meet needs after discharge.

NURSING DIAGNOSIS: acute Pain

May Be Related To

Physical injury (e.g., tissue and nerve trauma)
Psychological (e.g., impact of loss of body part, stress, anxiety)

Possibly Evidenced By

Verbalized/coded reports of pain
Guarding behavior, protective gestures
Narrowed focus
Changes in vital signs

Desired Outcomes/Evaluation Criteria—Client Will

Pain Level (NOC)

Report pain is relieved or controlled.
Appear relaxed and able to rest and sleep appropriately.
Verbalize understanding of phantom pain and methods to provide relief.

ACTIONS/INTERVENTIONS	RATIONALE
Pain Management (NIC)	
Independent	
Document location and intensity of pain (0 to 10, or similar coded scale) as well as quality and aggravating factors. Investigate changes in pain characteristics—numbness and tingling.	Aids in evaluating need for and effectiveness of interventions. Changes may indicate developing complications, such as necrosis or infection.
Elevate affected part by raising foot of bed slightly or using a pillow or sling for upper-limb amputation.	Lessens edema formation by enhancing venous return; reduces muscle fatigue and skin or tissue pressure. *Note:* After initial 24 hours and in absence of edema, residual limb may be extended and kept flat.
Provide or promote general comfort measures (e.g., frequent turning, back rub) and diversional activities. Encourage use of stress management techniques, such as deep-breathing exercises, visualization and guided imagery, and Therapeutic Touch.	Refocuses attention, promotes relaxation, may enhance coping abilities, and may decrease occurrence of phantom-limb pain.
Investigate reports of progressive or poorly localized pain unrelieved by analgesics.	May indicate developing compartment syndrome, especially following traumatic injury. (Refer to CP: Fractures; ND: risk for Peripheral Neurovascular Dysfunction.)
Acknowledge reality of residual limb pain and phantom pain and that various modalities will be tried for pain relief.	Residual limb pain is believed to come from injuries to bone, muscle, nerve, and skin at the amputation site (Ertl, 2012). At the ends of injured nerve fibers, neuromas send out pain impulses in a random fashion, or when trapped, as in excessive compression by other tissues such as muscle, or in the development of the infectious process. In contrast, phantom pain is thought to originate in the part of the brain that controlled the limb before it was amputated. So the client experiences pain and sensation as if the limb were still in place. Phantom pain is often described as crushing, grinding, or burning. It can occur immediately or may not start for several weeks. *Note:* Phantom pain is not well relieved by traditional pain medications.
Collaborative	
Administer medications, as indicated, such as the following:	
Opioid analgesics, for example, morphine sulfate (Astramorph, MS Contin), Fentanyl patch; combination agents: oxycodone with acetaminophen (Percocet); and anti-inflammatory agents, for example, acetaminophen (Tylenol) and ibuprofen (Motrin)	Many medications and routes of administration may be used. In acute post-amputation pain, opioid analgesics are the mainstay of pain management to reduce pain and muscle spasms.
Antidepressants, for example, amitriptyline (Elavil), nortriptyline (Pamelor), and duloxetine (Cymbalta); antiseizure drugs, for example, carbamazepine (Tegretol), gabapentin (Neurontin), and pregabalin (Lyrica); sedatives/anti-anxiety agents, for example, diazepam (Valium) and alprazolam (Xanax); and local/regional anesthetics, for example, novocaine (Marcaine) and ropivacaine (Naropin)	As surgical pain subsides, other medications will be added to manage more long-term conditions; for example, antidepressants and antiseizure medications appear to help with neuritic pain associated with phantom pain and sensations.
Instruct in, and monitor use of, patient-controlled analgesia (PCA).	PCA provides for continuous and timely drug administration, preventing fluctuations in pain level and muscle tension and spasms associated with surgical procedures.
Refer to interdisciplinary providers as appropriate—pain management specialist, physical therapist, prosthetist, orthopedic surgeon, and neurosurgeon.	A multidisciplinary approach is required, and many therapy modalities may be needed both in the acute and the long-term management of pain.
Discuss and monitor use of transcutaneous electrical nerve stimulation (TENS) of the residual limb.	For some individuals, a TENS unit may help to treat retractable phantom-limb pain, especially in combination with medications for neuropathic pain. *Note:* Stimulation of the intact (opposite) limb is often more effective. Indeed, an increase in phantom pain has occasionally been reported when TENS unit has been applied to residual limb.

NURSING DIAGNOSIS: risk for ineffective peripheral Tissue Perfusion

Risk Factors May Include

Hypovolemia; tissue edema, hematoma formation

Possibly Evidenced By

(Not applicable; presence of signs and symptoms establishes an *actual* diagnosis)

Desired Outcomes/Evaluation Criteria—Client Will

Tissue Perfusion: Peripheral (NOC)

Maintain adequate tissue perfusion as evidenced by palpable peripheral pulses; warm, dry skin; and timely wound healing.

ACTIONS/INTERVENTIONS	RATIONALE
Circulatory Precautions (NIC)	
Independent	
Monitor vital signs. Palpate peripheral pulses, noting strength and equality.	General indicators of circulatory status and adequacy of perfusion.
Perform periodic neurovascular assessments—sensation, movement, pulse, skin color, and temperature.	Amputation wound healing is a concern because most are performed for compromised circulation, for example, with peripheral vascular disease (PVD) or damaged soft tissue resulting from trauma (Ertl, 2012). Postoperative tissue edema, hematoma formation, or restrictive dressings may impair circulation to residual limb, resulting in tissue necrosis.
Note type of dressing used—soft, soft with pressure wrap, semirigid, or rigid.	Postoperative dressing varies, each with its advantages and disadvantages. For example, a soft dressing does not control edema. Adding a pressure wrap distributes pressure, but requires measures to avoid possible limb strangulation. Semirigid dressings (e.g., plaster splint, Unna paste bandage) or rigid dressings allow for decreased edema and immediate postoperative prosthesis with early ambulation but limit access to the wound, and possible excessive pressure may lead to compromised healing (Ertl, 2012).
Inspect dressings and drainage device, noting amount and characteristics of drainage, especially in client receiving antithrombotic therapy, including DVT prophylaxis.	Continued blood loss may indicate need for additional fluid replacement and evaluation for coagulation defect or surgical intervention to ligate bleeder, hematoma evacuation, or revision of stump (Nowygrod et al, 2006).
Apply direct pressure to bleeding site if hemorrhage occurs. Contact physician immediately.	Direct pressure to bleeding site may be followed by application of a bulk dressing secured with an elastic wrap once bleeding is controlled.
Investigate reports of persistent or unusual pain in operative site.	Hematoma can form in muscle pocket under the flap, compromising circulation and intensifying pain.
Evaluate nonoperated lower limb and residual limb for redness, unexplained fever, or tenderness.	Increased incidence of thrombus formation in clients with preexisting peripheral vascular disease or diabetic changes. *Note:* Research reveals that the incidence of deep vein thrombosis (DVT) is higher for above-knee amputation compared with below-knee amputation (37.5% versus 21.2%, respectively) (Matielo et al, 2008).
Encourage and assist with early ambulation.	Enhances circulation and helps prevent stasis and associated complications. Promotes sense of general well-being.
Collaborative	
Administer intravenous (IV) fluids and blood products as indicated.	Maintains circulating volume to maximize tissue perfusion.
Apply anti-embolic or sequential compression hose to nonoperated leg, as appropriate.	Enhances venous return, reducing venous pooling and risk of thrombophlebitis.
Administer low-dose anticoagulant, as indicated.	May be useful in preventing thrombus formation without increasing risk of postoperative bleeding or hematoma formation.
Monitor laboratory studies, for example:	
Hemoglobin/hematocrit (Hgb/Hct)	Indicators of hypovolemia, or dehydration, which can impair tissue perfusion.
Prothrombin time (PT)/activated partial thromboplastin time (aPTT).	Evaluates need for, and effectiveness of, anticoagulant therapy and identifies developing complication such as posttraumatic disseminated intravascular coagulation (DIC).

NURSING DIAGNOSIS: risk for Infection

Risk Factors May Include

Inadequate primary defenses—broken skin, traumatized tissue, invasive procedures

Chronic disease

Possibly Evidenced By

(Not applicable; presence of signs and symptoms establishes an *actual* diagnosis)

Desired Outcomes/Evaluation Criteria—Client Will

Wound Healing: Primary Intention (NOC)

Achieve timely wound healing, be free of purulent drainage or erythema, and be afebrile.

ACTIONS/INTERVENTIONS	RATIONALE
Wound Care (NIC)	
Independent	
Evaluate client's risk for infection.	Every client is at risk for postoperative infection; however, lower-extremity amputation is often associated with open, infected wounds and, thus, surgical wounds are classified as contaminated and associated with a high risk for surgical site infection (Kalapatapu, 2012).
Maintain strict hand hygiene measures, using soap and water or antibacterial soaps, before and after client care and after glove removal.	Hand hygiene remains the cornerstone of infection prevention and control in healthcare and community settings.
Maintain aseptic technique when changing dressings and caring for wound.	Minimizes opportunity for introduction of bacteria.
Inspect wound (noting redness and excess warmth) and dressings daily or per prescription; note characteristics of drainage, particularly in client with unexplained fever or reporting excessive stump pain.	Early detection of developing infection provides opportunity for timely intervention and prevention of more serious complications such as osteomyelitis.
Maintain patency and routinely empty drainage device.	Hemovac and Jackson-Pratt drains facilitate removal of drainage, promoting wound healing and reducing risk of infection.
Cover dressing with plastic when using the bedpan or if incontinent	Reduces risk of contamination in high-level, lower-limb amputation.
Expose residual limb to air and wash with mild soap and water after dressings are discontinued.	Maintains cleanliness, minimizes skin contaminants, and promotes healing of tender, fragile skin.
Monitor vital signs.	Temperature elevation and tachycardia may reflect developing sepsis.
Collaborative	
Obtain wound and drainage cultures and sensitivities, as appropriate.	Identifies presence of infection, specific organisms, and appropriate therapy.
Administer antibiotics, as indicated.	Wide-spectrum antibiotics may be used prophylactically, or antibiotic therapy may be geared toward specific organisms.

NURSING DIAGNOSIS: impaired physical Mobility

May Be Related To
Pain or discomfort
Decreased muscle mass/strength
Musculoskeletal impairment (e.g., loss of a limb—particularly a lower extremity)
Deconditioning; decreased endurance

Possibly Evidenced By
Limited range of motion; difficulty turning
Postural instability; gait changes

Desired Outcomes/Evaluation Criteria—Client Will

Coordinated Movement (NOC)
Increase strength and function of affected and compensatory body parts.
Move about environment safely.

Knowledge: Body Mechanics (NOC)
Verbalize understanding of individual situation and safety measures.
Demonstrate techniques and behaviors that enable resumption of activities.
Maintain position of function as evidenced by absence of contractures.

ACTIONS/INTERVENTIONS	RATIONALE
Amputation Care (NIC)	
Independent	
Provide residual limb care on a routine basis; for example, inspect the area, clean and dry it thoroughly, and rewrap the residual limb with elastic bandage or air splint. Conversely, apply a "stump shrinker" or heavy stockinette sock for "delayed" prosthesis.	Provides opportunity to evaluate healing and note complications unless covered by immediate prosthesis. Wrapping residual limb controls edema and helps form residual limb into conical shape to facilitate fitting of prosthesis. *Note:* Air splint may be preferred because it permits visual inspection of the wound.

(continues on page 622)

ACTIONS/INTERVENTIONS (continued)	RATIONALE (continued)
Measure circumference periodically.	Measurement is done to estimate shrinkage to ensure proper fit of sock and prosthesis.
Rewrap residual limb immediately with an elastic bandage; elevate if "immediate or early" cast is accidentally dislodged. Prepare for reapplication of cast.	Edema will occur rapidly, thus delaying rehabilitation.
Assist with specified range-of-motion (ROM) exercises for both the affected and unaffected limbs, beginning early in postoperative stage.	Prevents contracture deformities, which can develop rapidly and could delay prosthesis usage.
Encourage active and isometric exercises for upper torso and unaffected limbs.	Increases muscle strength to facilitate transfers and ambulation and promotes mobility and more normal lifestyle.
Provide trochanter rolls, as indicated.	Prevents external rotation of lower-limb residual limb.
Instruct client to lie in prone position, as tolerated, at least twice a day with pillow under abdomen and lower-extremity residual limb.	Strengthens extensor muscles and prevents flexion contracture of the hip, which can begin to develop within 24 hours of sustained malpositioning.
Caution against keeping pillow under lower-extremity residual limb or allowing BKA limb to hang dependently over side of bed or chair.	Use of pillows can cause permanent flexion contracture of hip; a dependent position of residual limb impairs venous return and may increase edema formation.
Demonstrate/assist with transfer techniques and use of mobility aids such as a trapeze, crutches, or a walker.	Facilitates self-care and client's independence. Proper transfer techniques prevent shearing abrasions/dermal injury related to "scooting."
Assist with ambulation based on specific prosthesis used, for example:	
Immediate postoperative fitting	Reduces potential for injury. Ambulation after lower-limb amputation depends on timing of prosthesis placement.
Early postoperative fitting	A rigid dressing is applied to the residual limb and a pylon and artificial foot are attached. Weight-bearing begins within 24 to 48 hours. Weight-bearing normally does not occur until 10 to 30 days postoperatively.
Delayed fitting	More common in areas that do not have facilities available for immediate or early application of prosthesis or when the condition of the residual limb and/or client precludes these choices. *Note:* With the advent of new medical techniques at the trauma scene, new surgical techniques, new occupational therapy techniques, and new component and prosthetic technology, such as the C-leg prosthesis that uses computer sensors and hydraulics (enabling client to move around nearly effortlessly), the initial steps for fitting begin when the stitches are removed. Client is fitted with prosthetic 2 weeks after final amputation (Schuch, 2008).
Help client continue preoperative muscle exercises as able or when allowed out of bed; for example, the client should perform abdomen-tightening exercises and knee bends; hop on foot; and stand on toes while holding on to chair for balance.	Contributes to gaining improved sense of balance and strengthens compensatory body parts.
Instruct client in residual limb-conditioning exercises, for example, pushing the residual limb against a pillow initially, then progressing to harder surface.	Hardens the residual limb by toughening the skin and altering feedback of resected nerves to facilitate use of prosthesis.
Collaborative	
Refer to rehabilitation team, for example, physical and occupational therapy and prosthetic specialists.	Provides for creation of exercise and activity program to meet individual needs and strengths and identifies mobility functional aids to promote independence. Early use of a temporary prosthesis promotes activity and enhances general well-being and a positive outlook. *Note:* Vocational counseling and/or retraining also may be indicated.
Provide foam or flotation mattress.	Reduces pressure on skin and tissues that can impair circulation, potentiating risk of tissue ischemia and breakdown.

NURSING DIAGNOSIS: Grieving

May Be Related To

Significant loss (e.g., body part, change in functional abilities, professional/family role, perception of self)

Possibly Evidenced By

Anger; suffering; psychological distress; detachment

Making meaning of loss; personal growth

Desired Outcomes/Evaluation Criteria—Client Will

Grief Resolution (NOC)

Begin to show adaptation and verbalize acceptance of self in situation (amputee).

Recognize and incorporate changes into self-concept in accurate manner without negating self-esteem.

Develop realistic plans for adapting to new role or role modifications.

ACTIONS/INTERVENTIONS	RATIONALE
Grief Work Facilitation (NIC)	
Independent	
Assess and consider client's preparation for and view of amputation.	Research shows that amputation poses serious threats to client's psychological and psychosocial adjustment. Client who views amputation as life-saving or reconstructive may be able to accept the new self more quickly. Client with sudden traumatic amputation or who considers amputation to be the result of failure in other treatments is at greater risk for disturbances in self-concept and complicated grieving.
Encourage expression of fears, negative feelings, and grief over loss of body part.	Venting emotions helps client begin to deal with the fact and reality of life without a limb.
Reinforce preoperative information, including type and location of amputation, type of prosthetic fitting if appropriate (i.e., immediate, delayed), and expected postoperative course, including pain control and rehabilitation.	Provides opportunity for client to question and assimilate information and begin to deal with changes in body image and function, which can facilitate postoperative recovery.
Assess degree of support available to client.	Sufficient support by significant other (SO) and friends can facilitate rehabilitation process and grief resolution.
Discuss client's perceptions of self, related to change, and how client sees self in usual lifestyle and role functioning.	Aids in defining concerns in relation to previous lifestyle and facilitates problem-solving. For example, client likely fears loss of independence, ability to work or express sexuality, and may experience role and/or relationship changes.
Ascertain individual strengths and identify previous positive coping behaviors.	Helpful to build on strengths that are already available for client to use in dealing with current situation.
Encourage participation in activities of daily living (ADLs). Provide opportunities to view and care for residual limb, using the moment to point out positive signs of healing.	Promotes independence and enhances feelings of self-worth. Although integration of residual limb into body image can take months or even years, looking at the residual limb and hearing positive comments made in a normal, matter-of-fact manner can help client with this acceptance.
Encourage or provide for a visit by another amputee, especially one who is successfully rehabilitating.	A peer who has been through a similar experience serves as a role model and can provide validity to comments and hope for recovery and a positive future.
Provide open environment for client to discuss concerns about sexuality.	Promotes sharing of beliefs and values about sensitive subject, and identifies misconceptions or myths that may interfere with adjustment to situation.
Note withdrawn behavior, negative self-talk, use of denial, depression, or overconcern with actual or perceived changes.	Identifies stage of grief and may indicate need for more intensive interventions. *Note:* Studies show that post-traumatic stress disorder (PTSD) develops in 20% to 22% of people who have amputations associated with combat or accidental injury (Kalapatapu, 2012).
Collaborative	
Discuss availability of various resources, for example, psychiatric or sexual counseling, a prosthetist, or a physical or occupational therapist.	May need assistance and long-term support to facilitate optimal adaptation and establish a "new" normal for future.

NURSING DIAGNOSIS: deficient Knowledge [Learning Need] regarding condition, prognosis, treatment, self-care, and discharge needs

May Be Related To

Lack of exposure or recall
Information misinterpretation
Unfamiliarity with information resources

Possibly Evidenced By

Reports the problem
Inaccurate follow-through of instructions

Desired Outcomes/Evaluation Criteria—Client Will

Knowledge: Disease Process (NOC)

Verbalize understanding of condition, disease process, and potential complications.

Knowledge: Treatment Regimen (NOC)

Verbalize understanding of therapeutic needs.
Correctly perform necessary procedures and explain reasons for the actions.
Initiate necessary lifestyle changes and participate in treatment regimen.

ACTIONS/INTERVENTIONS	RATIONALE
Amputation Care (NIC)	
Independent	
Review disease process, surgical procedure, and future expectations.	Provides knowledge base from which client can make informed choices.
Instruct in dressing and wound care, inspection of residual limb using mirror to visualize all areas, skin massage, and appropriate wrapping of the residual limb.	Promotes competent self-care, facilitates healing and fitting of prosthesis, and reduces potential for complications.
Discuss general residual limb care, for example:	
Wash daily with mild soap and water; rinse and pat dry. Do this daily, or more often if client sweats a lot or in treating a rash or infection.	Hygiene of residual limb is critical because most of the time it is enclosed in the socket or liner of the prosthesis, rendering it more prone to skin breakdown and infection.
Massage the residual limb after dressings are discontinued and suture line is healed.	Massage softens the scar and prevents adherence to the bone, decreases tenderness, and stimulates circulation.
Avoid the use of alcohol-based lotions or use of powders.	Although a small amount of lotion may be indicated if skin is dry, emollients and creams soften skin and may cause maceration when prosthesis is worn. Powder may cake, potentiating skin irritation.
Wear only properly fitted, clean, wrinkle-free limb sock.	Residual limb may continue to shrink for up to 2 years, and an improperly fitting sock or one that is mended or dirty can cause skin irritation or breakdown.
Use clean cotton T-shirt under harness for upper-limb prosthesis.	Absorbs perspiration; prevents skin irritation from harness.
Review common problems and appropriate actions.	Problems can occur even when client is taking precautions, for example, the development of a red, sore area that does not resolve when prosthesis is off, or a blister caused by pressure between socket liner and skin. These problems need early medical follow-up if home interventions are not effective.
Discuss need to report changes in pain characteristics, range of motion restrictions, warmth, and socket fitting in residual limb.	Among recent military amputees returning from combat, a high rate of heterotopic ossification (HO) has been seen in amputated residual. This complication of bone formation in soft tissue presents numerous rehabilitation challenges. For example, bone formed in soft tissues of a weight-bearing limb can result in high-pressure areas, creating a risk for skin breakdown. Skin breakdown can have devastating effects on rehabilitation because it often requires prolonged periods of non-weight-bearing and presents a risk for infection. HO can also result in complex residual limb shapes and multiple pressure-sensitive areas that can make prosthesis fitting difficult or impossible (Goff, et al, 2009).
Emphasize importance of well-balanced diet and adequate fluid intake.	Provides needed nutrients for tissue regeneration and healing, aids in maintaining circulating volume and normal organ function, and aids in maintenance of proper weight. *Note:* Weight changes affect fit of prosthesis.

ACTIONS/INTERVENTIONS (continued)	RATIONALE (continued)
Recommend cessation of smoking. Offer referral resources for cessation programs.	Smoking potentiates peripheral vasoconstriction, impairing circulation and tissue oxygenation.
Review and demonstrate care of prosthetic device. Stress importance of routine maintenance and periodic refitting.	Ensures proper fit and alignment, reduces risk of complications, and prolongs life of prosthesis.
Encourage continuation of postoperative exercise program.	Enhances circulation, healing, and function of affected part, facilitating adaptation to prosthetic device.
Identify techniques to manage phantom sensation and phantom pain. (Refer to ND: acute Pain.)	Persistent and/or recurring pain requires long-term management, with multiple strategies and modalities, including desensitization therapy, intermittent compression, medications, TENS, and nerve blocks. *Note:* Electrical stimulation offers a short-term rerouting or stimulation of different nerve pathways, thus reducing the activity of the usual pain patterns.
Encourage taking care of whole self: body, mind, and spirit. Emphasize socialization, stress management, relaxation training, or counseling.	Various techniques may be implemented, such as relaxation breathing, exercises, visualization, or biofeedback to reduce muscle tension and enhance client's control of situation and coping abilities.
Identify signs and symptoms requiring medical evaluation—edema, erythema, increased or odorous drainage from incision, changes in sensation, movement, skin color, and persistent phantom pain.	Prompt intervention may prevent serious complications and/or loss of function. *Note:* Chronic phantom-limb pain may indicate neuroma, requiring surgical resection.
Identify community and rehabilitation support, such as a certified prosthetist-orthotist, amputee groups, home-care service, and homemaker services, as needed.	Facilitates transfer to home, supports independence, and enhances coping.

POTENTIAL CONSIDERATIONS following acute hospitalization (dependent on client's age, physical condition and presence of complications, personal resources, and life responsibilities)

In addition to considerations in Surgical Intervention plan of care:

- *impaired physical Mobility*—decreased muscle mass/strength; musculoskeletal impairment; deconditioning; decreased endurance
- *risk for Trauma*—balancing difficulties, muscle weakness, reduced muscle coordination, lack of safety precautions, hazards associated with use of assistive devices
- *disturbed Body Image*—loss of body part, change in functional abilities
- *Self-Care Deficit/impaired Home Maintenance (dependent on location of amputation)*—musculoskeletal impairment, decreased strength/endurance, pain, depression

TOTAL JOINT REPLACEMENT

I. Purpose

a. Definitive treatment for advanced, irreversibly damaged joints with loss of function and unremitting pain

b. Common conditions: degenerative and rheumatoid arthritis (RA); selected fractures, such as with hip and femoral neck; joint instability; congenital hip disorders; avascular necrosis

II. Procedures

a. Performed on any joint except the spine, with hip and knee replacements the most common procedures

b. Prosthesis may be metallic, polyethylene, or ceramic, or a combination

c. Implanted with methylmethacrylate cement or may be a porous, coated implant that encourages bony ingrowth

III. Statistics

a. Morbidity: In 2006, hip and knee replacements, including revision procedures, accounted for 96% of the nearly one million inpatient arthroplasty procedures performed. Women accounted for 62% of all procedures, with a mean age (at time of procedure) of 66 to 68 years (U.S. Bone and Joint Decade, 2011).

b. Mortality: Rate is low, 0.29% in 2004, related to advanced age and comorbidities (Liu et al, 2008).

c. Cost: In 2004, annual hospital cost estimated at over $44 billion (U.S. Bone and Joint Decade, 2008). At approximately $15,000 per knee joint replacement, and with an estimated 600,000 total knee replacements performed annually in the United States, the aggregate annual cost for total knee replacement (also known as total knee arthroplasty, or TKA) is $9 billion (Cram et al, 2012). An additional estimated $15 billion is spent on hip replacement surgeries.

GLOSSARY

Arthroplasty: Reconstruction or replacement of a diseased or damaged joint.

Cemented joint replacement (cemented joint arthroplasty): Procedure in which bone cement or polymethylmethacrylate (PMMA) is used to fix the prosthesis in place in the joint.

Hemiarthroplasty: Replacement of only the femoral head.

Ingrowth, or cementless, joint replacement (ingrowth, or cementless, arthroplasty): Procedure that does not involve bone cement to fix the prosthesis in place; an anatomic or press fit with bone ingrowth into the surface of the prosthesis leads to a stable fixation.

Primary joint replacement: Initial surgical procedure.

Revision: Second or succeeding procedures to correct loose, unstable hardware or address return of pain in the joint.

THA: Total hip arthroplasty, also called total hip replacement (THR).

TJR: Total joint replacement.

TKA: Total knee arthroplasty, also called total knee replacement (TKR).

Care Setting

Client is treated in inpatient acute surgical unit and subacute or rehabilitation unit.

Related Concerns

Fractures, page 601
Psychosocial aspects of care, page 729
Rheumatoid arthritis (RA), page 709
Sepsis/septicemia, page 665
Surgical intervention, page 762
Thrombophlebitis: venous thromboembolism, page 109

Client Assessment Database

DIAGNOSTIC DIVISION MAY REPORT	MAY EXHIBIT
ACTIVITY/REST • History of occupation or participation in sports activities that wear on a particular joint • Difficulty walking • Stiffness in joints, which is worse in the morning or after a period of inactivity • Fatigue • Generalized muscle weakness • Inability to participate in occupational and/or recreational activities at desired level • Interruption of sleep, delayed falling asleep or awakened by pain • Does not feel well rested	• Decreased range of motion (ROM) of affected joints • Decreased muscle strength and tone • Gait disturbances—effort to compensate for joint pain
HYGIENE • Difficulty performing activities of daily living (ADLs) • Use of special equipment and/or mobility devices • Need for assistance with some or all activities	
NEUROSENSORY	• Soft tissue swelling, nodules • Muscle spasm, stiffness • Deformity
PAIN/DISCOMFORT • Pain—dull, aching, persistent in affected joint(s) • Pain worsened by movement	

DIAGNOSTIC DIVISION MAY REPORT (continued)	MAY EXHIBIT (continued)
SAFETY • Traumatic injury and/or fractures affecting the joint • Congenital deformities • History of inflammatory, debilitating arthritis—RA or osteoarthritis • Aseptic necrosis of the joint head	• Distorted joints • Joint or tissue swelling • Decreased ROM • Changes in gait
TEACHING/LEARNING • Current medication use—anti-inflammatories, analgesics, opioids, steroids, hormone replacement therapy (HRT), bone resorption inhibitor (e.g., donosumab [Prolia]), calcium supplements	
DISCHARGE PLAN CONSIDERATIONS • May need assistance with transportation, self-care activities, and homemaker or maintenance tasks • Possible placement in rehabilitation or extended care facility for continued therapy and assistance ➧ Refer to section at end of plan for postdischarge considerations.	

Diagnostic Studies

TEST WHY IT IS DONE	WHAT IT TELLS ME
• *Radiographs:* Visualize and evaluate skeletal changes or damage, determine treatment options, and guide orthopedic surgery.	May reveal destruction of articular cartilage, bony demineralization, fractures, soft tissue swelling, narrowing of joint space, joint subluxations, or deformity.
• *Bone scan, computed tomography (CT) scans, magnetic resonance imaging (MRI):* Assess bone loss and determine presence of comorbidities.	Determine extent of degeneration and rule out malignancy or infectious process.

Nursing Priorities

1. Alleviate pain.
2. Prevent complications.
3. Promote optimal mobility.
4. Provide information about diagnosis, prognosis, and treatment needs.

Discharge Goals

1. Mobility increased.
2. Complications prevented or minimized.
3. Pain relieved or controlled.
4. Diagnosis, prognosis, and therapeutic regimen understood.
5. Plan in place to meet needs after discharge.

NURSING DIAGNOSIS: acute Pain

May Be Related To

Physical agents (e.g., surgical procedure, muscle spasms, preexisting chronic joint diseases)
Psychological (e.g., anxiety)

Possibly Evidenced By

Verbalized/coded reports of pain distraction
Expressive behavior (e.g., restlessness, irritability)
Guarding behaviors; protective behaviors
Narrowed focus, self-focusing
Changes in vital signs

(continues on page 628)

NURSING DIAGNOSIS: acute Pain (continued)

Desired Outcomes/Evaluation Criteria—Client Will

Pain Level (NOC)
Report pain relieved or controlled.
Appear relaxed, able to rest or sleep appropriately.

Pain Control (NOC)
Demonstrate use of relaxation skills and diversional activities, as indicated by individual situation.

ACTIONS/INTERVENTIONS	RATIONALE
Pain Management (NIC)	
Independent	
Perform comprehensive assessment of pain, noting intensity (0 to 10, or similar coded scale), duration, and location. Determine if pain is at operative or different site, associated with ROM or weight-bearing, associated with vascular compromise or fever.	Provides information on which to base and monitor effectiveness of interventions.
Maintain prescribed position of operated extremity.	Reduces muscle spasm and undue tension on new prosthesis and surrounding tissues.
Provide comfort measures—frequent repositioning, back rub—and diversional activities. Encourage stress management techniques, such as progressive relaxation, guided imagery, visualization, and meditation. Provide Therapeutic Touch, as appropriate.	Reduces muscle tension, refocuses attention, promotes sense of control, and may enhance coping abilities in the management of discomfort or pain, which can persist for an extended period.
Medicate on a round-the-clock schedule initially and well before activities or therapies if getting prn dosing.	Total joint replacement (TJR) surgeries are known to be accompanied by moderate to severe pain from the reconstruction. Pain management is often complicated by client's age, comorbidities, and general deconditioned status before surgery. Effectively managing postoperative pain is essential for helping client achieve the best possible functional outcome (Rasul, 2012; D'Arcy, 2007).
Investigate reports of sudden, severe joint pain with muscle spasms and changes in joint mobility, or sudden, severe chest pain with dyspnea and restlessness.	Early recognition of developing problems, such as dislocation of prosthesis or blood or fat pulmonary emboli, provides opportunity for prompt intervention and prevention of more serious complications.
Collaborative	
Administer medications as indicated, around the clock, such as:	
Opioids—instruct in and monitor use of patient-controlled analgesia (PCA); and/or targeted analgesia, such as epidural infusion or continuous femoral blockade	Relieves surgical pain and reduces muscle tension and spasm, which contribute to overall discomfort. Opioid infusion (including epidural) may be given during the first 24 to 48 hours. The ON-Q PainBuster® ball provides continuous infusion of local anesthetic directly into surgical site for up to 5 days, decreasing need for other opioids and allowing for earlier ambulation than epidural administration (D'Arcy, 2007).
Oral analgesics (both extended release and shorter-acting formulations) such as oxycodone (OxyContin) or morphine sulfate extended release capsules (Kadian, Avinza); oxycodone and acetaminophen (Percocet), hydrocodone and acetaminophen (Vicodin, Lortab); and muscle relaxants	Oral analgesics are added to pain management program as the client progresses. *Note:* Use of ketorolac (Toradol) or other NSAID is contraindicated when client is receiving enoxaparin (Lovenox) therapy.
Apply ice packs, as indicated.	Promotes vasoconstriction to reduce bleeding and tissue edema in surgical area and lessens perception of discomfort.
Refer for/assist mobilization, such as early ambulation, transfers, gait training and other physical therapy modalities, or continuous passive motion (CPM) device (for knee joint) when used.	Improves circulation and range of motion of affected joint and muscles and can relieve muscle spasms related to disuse.

NURSING DIAGNOSIS: risk for Bleeding

Risk Factors May Include

Trauma

Treatment-related side effects (e.g., surgery, medication)

Possibly Evidenced By

(Not applicable; presence of signs and symptoms establishes an *actual* diagnosis)

Desired Outcomes/Evaluation Criteria—Client Will

Blood Loss Severity (NOC)

Be free of active bleeding or excessive blood loss as evidenced by stable vital signs, usual mentation, absence of skin pallor, and adequate urinary output

ACTIONS/INTERVENTIONS	RATIONALE
Bleeding Precautions (NIC)	
Independent	
Monitor vital signs, including pulse and blood pressure and urinary output.	Tachycardia, falling blood pressure (BP), and low urinary output may reflect hypovolemia due to blood loss.
Assess skin color and moisture. Note changes in mentation, or delay in return of usual mentation after recovery from anesthesia.	May reflect effects of anemia and hypoxemia from blood loss.
Monitor amount and characteristics of drainage on dressings and from suction device (e.g., hemovac, Jackson-Pratt drain) when used. Note swelling in operative area.	May indicate excessive bleeding or hematoma formation, which can potentiate neurovascular compromise. Note: Suction device is often discontinued the second or third day postop (Shiel, 2012).
Collaborative	
Monitor laboratory studies, such as:	
Hemaglobin (Hgb), hematocrit (Hct)	Most clients display some anemia following primary joint replacement, and many older clients are anemic prior to surgery. A Hgb drop of 4 (for hips) and 3.8 (for knees) can be expected due to intraoperative blood loss. Note: Studies show that clients who undergo a single total knee replacement consistently lose two or more units of blood. This includes the measured blood loss during surgery and that which is lost into the soft tissues from exposed bone and into the joint after wound closure (Jackson, 2010).
Administer IV fluids, and donor or autologous blood transfusions, as needed.	Restores circulating volume to maintain perfusion. *Note:* Current management of postoperative anemia in elective TJR (when preoperative anemia is diagnosed) includes infusion of client's own red blood cells (autologous donation) if donated and banked at least a month out from the procedure); or use of the hormone erythropoietin (EPO) to increase red blood count. When an anemic client has considerable perioperative blood loss, salvaged blood collected from operative site during first 6 hours following procedure may be reinfused per protocol. Research continues on this practice to determine benefit vs risk. For example, a recent prospective study showed that autotransfusion with a large volume of unwashed shed blood results in an increase of postoperative drainage due to the activation of fibrinolysis (Jackson, 2010; Matsuda et al, 2010).

NURSING DIAGNOSIS: risk for Infection

Risk Factors May Include

Inadequate primary defenses (e.g., broken skin, traumatized tissues, invasive procedures, exposure of joint, implantation of foreign body)

Inadequate secondary defenses (e.g., decreased hemoglobin, immunosuppression—long-term corticosteroid use)

Possibly Evidenced By

(Not applicable; presence of signs and symptoms establishes an *actual* diagnosis)

Desired Outcomes/Evaluation Criteria—Client Will

Infection Severity (NOC)

Achieve timely wound healing, be free of purulent drainage or erythema, and be afebrile.

ACTIONS/INTERVENTIONS	RATIONALE
Infection Protection (NIC)	
Independent	
Promote good hand washing by staff and client.	Reduces risk of cross-contamination.
Use strict aseptic or clean technique, as indicated, to reinforce or change dressings and when handling drains. Instruct client not to touch or scratch incision.	Prevents contamination and risk of wound infection, which could require removal of prosthesis.
Maintain patency of drainage devices (e.g., Hemovac, Jackson-Pratt) when present. Note characteristics of wound drainage.	Reduces risk of infection by preventing accumulation of blood and secretions in the joint space, which is a medium for bacterial growth. Purulent, nonserous, odorous drainage is indicative of infection, and continuous drainage from incision may reflect developing skin tract, which can potentiate infectious process.
Assess skin and incision color, temperature, and integrity; note presence of erythema, inflammation, and loss of wound approximation.	Provides information about status of healing process and alerts staff to early signs of infection.
Investigate reports of increased incisional pain and changes in characteristics of pain.	Deep, dull, aching pain in operative area may indicate developing infection in joint. *Note:* Infection can be devastating because once infection sets in, joint may not be salvageable and prosthetic loss may occur.
Monitor temperature. Note presence of chills.	Although temperature elevations are common in early postoperative phase, elevations occurring 5 or more days postoperatively and/or presence of chills usually require intervention to prevent more serious complications, such as sepsis, osteomyelitis, tissue necrosis, and prosthetic failure.
Encourage fluid intake coupled with a high-protein diet.	Maintains fluid and nutritional balance to support tissue perfusion and provide nutrients necessary for cellular regeneration and tissue healing.
Collaborative	
Maintain reverse or protective isolation, if appropriate.	May be done initially to reduce contact with sources of possible infection, especially in an elderly, immunosuppressed, or diabetic client.
Administer antibiotics, as indicated.	Used prophylactically in the operating room and for the first 24 hours to prevent infection. Late infections may require intravenous (IV) antibiotic treatments for several weeks, in an effort to save the prosthetic joint.

NURSING DIAGNOSIS: risk for Peripheral Neurovascular Dysfunction

Risk Factors May Include

Orthopedic surgery, immobilization, mechanical compression (e.g., dressing, brace)
Vascular obstruction

Possibly Evidenced By

(Not applicable; presence of signs and symptoms establishes an *actual* diagnosis)

Desired Outcomes/Evaluation Criteria—Client Will

Tissue Perfusion: Peripheral (NOC)

Maintain function as evidenced by sensation and movement within normal limits for individual situation.
Demonstrate adequate tissue perfusion as evidenced by palpable pulses, brisk capillary refill, warm or dry skin, and normal color.

ACTIONS/INTERVENTIONS	RATIONALE
Circulatory Care: Arterial [or] Venous Insufficiency (NIC)	
Independent	
Palpate pulses. Evaluate capillary refill and skin color and temperature. Compare with unoperated limb.	Diminished or absent pulses, delayed capillary refill time, pallor, blanching, cyanosis, and coldness of skin reflect diminished circulation or perfusion. Comparison with unoperated limb provides clues as to whether neurovascular problem is localized or generalized.
Assess motion and sensation of operated extremity.	Increasing pain, numbness or tingling, and/or inability to perform expected movements (such as flexing foot) suggest nerve injury, compromised circulation, or dislocation of prosthesis, requiring immediate intervention.

ACTIONS/INTERVENTIONS (continued)	RATIONALE (continued)
Test sensation of peroneal nerve by pinch or pinprick in the dorsal web between first and second toe, and assess ability to dorsiflex toes after hip or knee replacement.	Position and length of peroneal nerve increase risk of direct injury or compression by tissue edema or hematoma.
Ensure that stabilizing devices (such as abduction pillow or splint device) are in correct position and are not exerting undue pressure on skin and underlying tissue. Avoid use of pillow or bed knee gatch under knees.	Reduces risk of pressure on underlying nerves or compromised circulation to extremities.
Evaluate for calf tenderness, tension, and redness.	Although clinical signs are often not reliable in this population, surveillance should be carried out. Early identification of thrombus development and intervention may prevent embolus formation.
Encourage regular "foot pumps" throughout day.	Pushing the foot down, pointing toes, and pulling toes up toward the ceiling causes the calf to tighten and assists venous return to prevent blood pooling and reduce risk of deep vein thrombosis (DVT). *Note:* Blood clots (above or below the knee) following knee surgery most often occur immediately after surgery (Shiel, 2012).
Collaborative	
Monitor laboratory studies, such as:	
Coagulation studies	Evaluates presence and degree of alteration in clotting mechanisms and effects of anticoagulant or antiplatelet agents when used.
Administer medications, as indicated, for example, low-molecular-weight heparins, enoxaparin (Lovenox), or fondaparinux (Arixtra).	Anticoagulants or antiplatelet agents may be used routinely to reduce risk of thrombophlebitis and pulmonary emboli. *Note*: Without prophylaxis, the incidence of DVT after total knee replacement (TKR) is 50% to 84%, and after total hip replacement (THR), 47% to 64%. With prophylaxis, the incidence is reduced 22% to 57% after TKR and 6% to 24% after THR (Rasul, 2012).
Maintain intermittent compression stocking or foot/ankle compression boots (e.g., PlexiPulse) when used.	Promotes venous return and prevents venous stasis, reducing risk of thrombus formation.

NURSING DIAGNOSIS: impaired physical Mobility

May Be Related To
Pain/discomfort; pharmaceutical agents
Musculoskeletal impairment; joint stiffness
Decreased endurance, deconditioning
Prescribed movement restrictions

Possibly Evidenced By
Limited range of motion; difficulty turning
Slowed movement; gait changes

Desired Outcomes/Evaluation Criteria—Client Will

Mobility (NOC)
Display increased strength, ROM, and function of affected joint and limb.

Ambulation (NOC)
Ambulate with assist/assistive device as needed.

ACTIONS/INTERVENTIONS	RATIONALE
Positioning (NIC)	
Independent	
Maintain affected joint in prescribed position and body in alignment when in bed.	Provides for stabilization of prosthesis and reduces risk of injury during recovery from effects of anesthesia.
Medicate around the clock, or sufficient time before procedures and activities, so that client is able to participate.	Adequate analgesia is a priority to decrease pain, reduce muscle tension and spasm, and facilitate participation in therapy.
Turn on unoperated side using adequate number of personnel and maintaining operated extremity in prescribed alignment. Support position with pillows and wedges.	Prevents dislocation of hip prosthesis and prolonged skin and tissue pressure, reducing risk of tissue ischemia and breakdown.
Demonstrate and assist with transfer techniques and use of mobility aids, such as a trapeze, walker, crutches, or canes.	Facilitates self-care and client's independence. Proper transfer techniques prevent shearing abrasions of skin and falls.

(continues on page 632)

ACTIONS/INTERVENTIONS (continued)	RATIONALE (continued)
Determine upper body strength and need for equipment to assist with ADLs, as appropriate. Involve in exercise program.	Replacement of lower-extremity joint requires increased use of upper extremities for transfer, ADLs, and desired activities as well as use of ambulation devices.
Inspect skin; observe for reddened areas. Keep linens dry and wrinkle-free. Massage skin and bony prominences routinely. Protect operative heel, elevating whole length of leg with pillow and placing heel on water glove if burning sensation reported or area reddened.	Prevents skin irritation or breakdown.
Exercise Therapy: Joint Mobility (NIC)	
Perform or assist with ROM to unoperated joints.	Client with degenerative joint disease can quickly lose function in unoperated joints during periods of restricted activity. Contralateral joint may be nearly as painful as the surgical joint and may require careful and consistent treatment to maximize mobility.
Promote participation in rehabilitative exercise program, such as the following:	
Total hip: Quadriceps and gluteal muscle setting, isometrics, leg lifts, dorsiflexion, and plantar flexion (ankle pumps) of the foot	Strengthens muscle groups, increasing muscle tone and mass; stimulates circulation; and prevents decubitus ulcers.
Total knee: Quadriceps setting, gluteal contraction, flexion and extension exercises, and isometrics	Active use of the joint may be painful but will not injure the joint. Continuous passive motion exercise may be initiated on the knee joint postoperatively, although its use is dependent on the particular surgeon and on the individual's needs.
Observe appropriate limitations based on specific joint; for example, avoid marked flexion or rotation of hip and flexion or hyperextension of leg; adhere to weight-bearing restrictions; and wear knee immobilizer, as indicated.	Joint stress is to be avoided at all times during stabilization period to prevent dislocation of new prosthesis.
Investigate sudden increase in pain and shortening of limb as well as changes in skin color, temperature, and sensation.	May be indicative of slippage of prosthesis or other complication, requiring medical evaluation and intervention.
Encourage participation in ADLs.	Enhances self-esteem and promotes sense of control and independence.
Provide positive reinforcement for efforts.	Promotes a positive attitude and encourages involvement in therapy.
Collaborative	
Collaborate with physical and occupational therapists and rehabilitation specialist.	Client will require individualized activity and exercise program, ongoing assistance with movement, strengthening, and weight-bearing activities for an extended period of time, as well as use of adjuncts, such as walkers, crutches, canes, elevated toilet seat, pickup sticks, and so on.
Provide foam or flotation mattress.	Reduces skin and tissue pressure; limits feelings of fatigue and general discomfort.

NURSING DIAGNOSIS: risk for Constipation

Risk Factors May Include

Insufficient physical activity
Insufficient fiber or fluid intake
Decreased gastrointestinal (GI) motility, effects of medications—anesthesia, opiate analgesics
Recent environmental changes

Possibly Evidenced By

(Not applicable; presence of signs and symptoms establishes an *actual* diagnosis)

Desired Outcomes/Evaluation Criteria—Client Will

Bowel Elimination (NOC)

Maintain usual pattern of bowel functioning.
Demonstrate behaviors to prevent problem.

ACTIONS/INTERVENTIONS	RATIONALE
Bowel Management (NIC)	
Independent	
Identify individual risk factors. Determine current situation and possible impact on bowel function—surgery, new and chronic use of medications affecting intestinal functioning, age, or weakness.	Constipation is one of the most frequent complaints following surgery and during rehabilitation. If left untreated, constipation can lead to nausea and vomiting, bowel obstruction, or even sepsis, especially in the elderly.
Auscultate abdomen for presence, location, and characteristics of bowel sounds.	Reflects activity of GI tract.
Determine usual elimination pattern or frequency, characteristics of stool—color, consistency, amount—manner of constipation, and use of laxatives.	Provides baseline for comparison, promotes recognition of changes, and helps to establish a preventative plan.
Evaluate usual dietary and fluid intake; compare with current intake.	Client's usual diet and fluid intake may be marginal at best in promoting healthy bowel functioning, especially when combined with current postsurgical status.
Promote increased fluid intake, including water and high-fiber fruit juices; offer warm stimulating fluids, such as coffee, tea, and hot water.	Prevents dehydration and decreases reabsorption of water from the bowel, promoting softer stool and facilitating passage of stool.
Encourage early ambulation and exercise within client's limitation of activity. Assist with early mobility.	To stimulate and optimize GI function.
Provide privacy and routinely scheduled time for defecation based on usual pattern, as appropriate (e.g., bedside commode or toilet with elevated seat, after breakfast).	To facilitate return of normalcy in toileting routine.
Collaborative	
Consult with dietitian or nutritionist, as indicated.	Helpful in providing a diet with balanced fiber and bulk that client can continue after discharge to improve consistency of stool and facilitate its passage.
Implement bowel program: administer routine stool softeners (e.g., docusate [Colace]); stool stimulants (e.g., bisacodyl [Dulcolax]), polyethylene glycol (Miralax); sennosides (e.g., Senokot, Ex-lax); bulk-forming agents (e.g., polycarbophil [FiberCon]), psyllium (Metamucil); saline laxatives (e.g., magnesium citrate), and enemas, as indicated.	Used to prevent or treat constipation.

NURSING DIAGNOSIS: deficient Knowledge [Learning Need] regarding condition, prognosis, treatment, self-care, and discharge needs

Risk Factors May Include
Lack of exposure or recall
Information misinterpretation
Unfamiliarity with information resources

Possibly Evidenced By
Reports the problem
Inaccurate follow-through of instructions

Desired Outcomes/Evaluation Criteria—Client Will

Knowledge: Treatment Regimen (NOC)
Verbalize understanding of surgical procedure and prognosis.
Correctly perform necessary procedures and explain reasons for the actions.

ACTIONS/INTERVENTIONS	RATIONALE
Teaching: Disease Process (NIC)	
Independent	
Review disease process, surgical procedure, and future expectations.	Provides knowledge base from which client can make informed choices. The majority of total joint surgeries are elective, and preoperative education is done in some form in the surgeon's office or in the admitting facility. Postsurgical review of process and expectations may be needed or desired.
Encourage alternating rest periods with activity.	Conserves energy for healing and prevents undue fatigue, which can increase risk of injury or fall.

(continues on page 634)

ACTIONS/INTERVENTIONS (continued)	RATIONALE (continued)
Stress importance of continuing prescribed exercise and rehabilitation program within client's tolerance—crutch or cane walking, weight-bearing exercises, stationary bicycling, or hydrotherapy and swimming.	Increases muscle strength and joint mobility. Most clients will be involved in formal outpatient rehabilitation, home-care programs, or be followed in extended care facilities by physical therapists. *Note:* Client with cemented joint replacement can weight-bear as tolerated (WBAT) unless the operative procedure involved a soft tissue repair or internal fixation of bone (following fracture). Client with cementless joint replacement is put on partial weight-bearing (PWB) or toe-touch weight-bearing (TTWB) for several weeks to allow maximum bony ingrowth to take place. A knee immobilizer sometimes is worn after total knee replacement until quadriceps strength is regained. All programs will add specific range of motion and strengthening therapies as time passes after surgery (Iverson, 2012; Rasul, 2012).
Review activity limitations, depending on joint replaced: for hip or knee—sitting for long periods or in low chair or toilet seat, recliner; jogging, jumping, excessive bending, lifting, twisting, or crossing legs.	Prevents undue stress on implant. Long-term restrictions depend on individual situation and physician protocol.
Discuss need for safe environment in home, including removing scatter rugs and unnecessary furniture, and use of assistive devices, such as hand rails in tub and toilet, raised toilet seat, and cane for long walks.	Reduces risk of falls and excessive stress on joints.
Review and have client or caregiver demonstrate incisional or wound care.	Promotes independence in self-care, reducing risk of complications.
Identify signs and symptoms requiring medical evaluation: fever or chills, incisional inflammation, unusual wound drainage, pain in calf or upper thigh, or development of sore throat or dental infections.	Bacterial infections require prompt treatment to prevent progression to osteomyelitis in the operative area and prosthesis failure, which could occur at any time, even years later.
Review procedure for removal of painball catheter if not discontinued before discharge.	Medication may infuse for up to 5 days and if client removes catheter after discharge it is important to check for black marking on tip to ensure tubing is removed intact.
Review drug regimen, for example, anticoagulants or antibiotics prior to invasive procedures (e.g., tooth extraction).	Prophylactic therapy may be necessary for a prolonged period after discharge to limit risk of thromboemboli and infection. Procedures known to release bacteria into the bloodstream can lead to infection, osteomyelitis, and prosthesis failure.
Identify bleeding precautions—for example, use of soft toothbrush, electric razor, avoidance of trauma, or forceful blowing of nose—and necessity of routine laboratory follow-up.	Reduces risk of therapy-induced bleeding or hemorrhage.
Encourage intake of balanced diet, including roughage and adequate fluids.	Enhances healing and feeling of general well-being. Promotes bowel and bladder function during period of altered activity.
Discuss continuation of supplemental calcium and vitamin D, hormone replacement, bisphosphonates, and the like as indicated.	Promotes bone health in clients with decreased bone density or who are at risk for osteoporosis.

POTENTIAL CONSIDERATIONS following acute hospitalization (dependent on client's age, physical condition and presence of complications, personal resources, and life responsibilities)

In addition to considerations in Surgical Intervention plan of care:

- *risk for Falls*—postoperative conditions, impaired physical mobility, decreased lower extremity strength, impaired balance, use of assistive devices
- *risk for Constipation*—insufficient physical activity, decreased motility of gastrointestinal tract, insufficient fiber/fluid intake, side effects of medications
- *Self-Care Deficit*—musculoskeletal impairment, weakness, fatigue, pain
- *impaired Home Maintenance*—impaired functioning, inadequate support systems, unfamiliarity with neighborhood resources

Sample clinical pathway follows in Table 12.1.

TABLE 12.1 Sample CP: Total Hip Replacement, Hospital. ELOS: 3 Days Orthopedic or Surgical Unit

ND and Categories of Care	Day of Surgery ____	Day 2 ____	Day 3 ____	D/C ____
risk for Infection R/T broken skin, exposure of joint, long-term steroid use, decreased mobility	Goals: Participate in activities to reduce risk of postoperative infection	→	→	→
		Free of purulent drainage	→	→ Free of erythema
		Be afebrile	→	→
			Verbalize understanding of healthcare needs to enhance healing, promote wellness	Plan in place to meet postdischarge needs, self-care
Diagnostics	Hgb/Hct	→	Electrolytes if indicated	
	Pulse oximetry	→ D/C if stable		
Additional assessments	VS/Temp per postoperative protocol	→ q4h	→ q8h	→ bid/ D/C
	Breath sounds q8h	→	→	→ bid/ D/C
	Amount/characteristic of Hemovac drainage q8hr	→	→ D/C	
			Characteristics of wound/drainage qd and prn	→
Medications	IV antibiotics	→ D/C	→ NS lock or D/C	→ D/C lock
Allergies: ______	IV fluids/blood products	→	→	→ D/C
	Tylenol—Temp ≥101°F		Dietary needs	Wound care
Client education	Disease process/surgical procedure	S/S to report of health-care provider	Balancing rest/activity	Provide written instructions for home care
	Hand-washing technique, avoid touching of dressing/wound			
	Respiratory exercises, incentive spirometry			
Additional nursing actions	Aseptic/clean technique	→	→	→
	Reinforce dressing	→	→ Change dressing qd and prn	→ D/C if incision dry
				Clean incision bid
	Encourage PO fluids as tolerated	→	→	→
	T, C, DB, q2h	→	Per self	→
	Incentive spirometry q2h	→ q2h WA	→ q4h WA	→
	Supplemental O_2 as indicated	→ D/C if stable	High-calorie/protein diet	→
impaired physical Mobility R/T musculoskeletal impairment/discomfort, therapeutic restrictions	Maintain proper alignment and position of function	→	→	Independent in transfers
	Participate in rehabilitation/exercise program	→	→	→
				Ambulate per self w/ assistive device
				→
		Free of DVT/thromboembolic complications	→	Display increased strength/function of operated limb
				Establish regular bladder/bowel elimination

(continues on page 636)

TABLE 12.1 Sample CP: Total Hip Replacement, Hospital. ELOS: 3 Days Orthopedic or Surgical Unit (continued)

ND and Categories of Care	Day of Surgery ____	Day 2 ____	Day 3 ____	D/C ____
Referrals		PT-assistive devices if not done preop	PT-exercises/ ambulation Social Services if placement indicated	OT/rehabilitation specialist Home care
Diagnostic studies		Protime (coumadin use)	→	→ CBC w/platelets (if Lovenox used)
Additional assessments	Neurovascular status/alignment of operated leg per postoperative protocol	→ q4h	→ q8h	→ bid/ D/C
	Skin (especially heels) q8h or per protocol	→	→	→ qd
	Voiding/urinary output q8h	→	→	→ D/C
	Bowel sounds q8h	→	→ bid	→ qd
		Stool characteristics	→	→
Medications Allergies: ________	Coumadin (if Lovenox not ordered)	→ Daily order or Lovenox q12h	→	→
	Stool softener/bowel program	→	→	→
Client education	Hip precautions Use of trapeze Initial exercises—ankle pumps, quad/gluteal sets	Transfer techniques S/S to report to health-care provider	Use of mobility aids Ambulation/weight-bearing exercises Self-administer Lovenox Home exercise program Sexual concerns	Activity level/ restrictions postdischarge → Provide written instructions Coumadin dose, time, purpose, side effects, precautions, monitoring (if used)
Additional nursing actions	Bedrest/HOB elevated 30°	→ Chair/commode elevate operated leg	→ Chair × 3 ambulate with assistance	→ Ambulate with assist as needed prn
	Pillow between knees	→	→	→
	Turn per protocol q2h	→	→	→
	ROM to nonoperated side q2h	→	→ Per self	→
	Initial exercises q1h WA	CPM to tolerance	→	→ Knee exercise × 5 q1h WA/Leg strengthening
	SCDs to calves while in bed	→	→	→
	Total care	→ Assist w/care	→ Self-care	→ Shower as indicated
	Fracture pan	Elevated toilet seat	→	→
	Straight catheter if no void q8h × 2	→ Insert Foley on #3 if no void	→ D/C Foley-male	→ D/C Foley-female
	Foam/special mattress	→	→	→
acute Pain R/T therapeutic interventions, preexisting chronic joint disease	Verbalize pain within manageable level	→	→	→
			Participate in action to decrease pain	→
			Demonstrate proper use of adjunct comfort measures	Verbalize understanding of medications/ modalities for pain management

TABLE 12.1 Sample CP: Total Hip Replacement, Hospital. ELOS: 3 Days Orthopedic or Surgical Unit (continued)

ND and Categories of Care	Day of Surgery ____	Day 2 ____	Day 3 ____	D/C ____	
Additional assessments	Pain characteristics/ changes	→	→	→	→
	Response to interventions	→	→	→	
Medications Allergies: ________ ________	PCA—narcotic of choice	→ D/C, begin PO if tolerated	→	→	
	Painball	→	→	→	
	Anti-emetic prn	→ D/C	Acetaminophen prn for breakthrough pain	→	
	Muscle relaxant	→	→	→	
Client education	Orient to unit/room Proper use of PCA Reporting of pain/ effects of interventions	Relaxation techniques, guided imagery, breathing exercises	Medications: dose, time, route, purpose, side effects	Written instructions for home-care needs, equipment resources, removal of pain ball if still in place	
Additional nursing actions	Maintain position/ alignment of leg per protocol	→	→	→	
	Ice pack to operated site	→ prn	→D/C		
	Routine comfort measures prn	→	→	→	

Key: bid, twice a day; C, cough; CBC, complete blood count; CPM, continuous passive motion; DB, deep breath; D/C, discontinue; DVT, deep vein thrombosis; Hct, hematocrit; Hgb, hemoglobin; HOB, head of bed; IV, intravenous; NS, normal saline; OT, occupational therapist; PCA, patient-controlled analgesia; PO, by mouth; prn, as needed; PT, physical therapist; q1h, every 1 hour; q2h, every 2 hours; q4h, every 4 hours; q8h, every 8 hours; q12h, every 12 hours; qd, every day; ROM, range of motion; R/T, related to; SCD, sequential compression device; S/S, signs and symptoms; T, temp; VS, vital signs; WA, while awake.

CHAPTER 13

Integumentary

BURNS: THERMAL, CHEMICAL, AND ELECTRICAL—ACUTE AND CONVALESCENT PHASES

I. Pathophysiology —Local and systemic response affecting skin and/or other tissues depending on cause of burn injury and physiological response (Hettiaratchy, 2004)

a. Local responses
  i. Coagulation: Occurs at the point of maximum damage, causing irreversible tissue loss due to coagulation of the constituent proteins
  ii. Stasis: Area characterized by decreased tissue perfusion that is potentially salvageable unless additional insults, such as prolonged hypotension, infection, or edema, occur, converting this zone into an area of complete tissue loss.
  iii. Hyperemia: Outermost area has increased tissue perfusion, and tissue will recover unless severe sepsis or prolonged hypoperfusion occurs.

b. Systemic response—Cytokines and other inflammatory mediators are released at the site of burn injuries with total body surface area (TBSA) of 30% or greater.
  i. Cardiovascular: Increased capillary permeability leads to shift of intravascular proteins and fluids into the interstitial space, followed by vasoconstriction and decreased myocardial contractility; combined with fluid loss from the burn wound, systemic hypotension and organ hypoperfusion occur.
  ii. Respiratory: Bronchoconstriction occurs in response to inflammatory mediators, which, in severe inhalation injury, can cause acute respiratory distress syndrome (ARDS).
  iii. Metabolic—Rate increases up to three times the baseline rate, resulting in breakdown of muscle tissue.
  iv. Immunological—Immune suppression response occurs.

II. Classification by burn wound and depth

a. Superficial partial-thickness (first-degree) burns: affect only the epidermis; skin is often warm and dry; and wounds appear bright pink to red with minimal edema and fine blisters, if present

b. Moderate partial-thickness (second-degree) burns: include the epidermis and dermis; wounds appear red to pink with moderate edema and blisters that may be intact or draining

c. Deep partial-thickness (second-degree) burns: extend into the deep dermis; wounds are dryer than moderate partial-thickness burns and appear pale pink to pale ivory, with moderate edema and blisters

d. Full-thickness (third-degree) burns: include all layers of skin and subcutaneous fat and may involve the muscle, nerves, and blood supply; wounds have a dry, leathery texture and appearance varies from white to cherry-red to brown or black, with blistering uncommon; absence of pain in the center, but the edges of the burn wound may have heightened sensation

e. Full-thickness, subdermal (fourth-degree) burns: involve all skin layers as well as muscle, organ tissue, and bone, with charring

III. Etiology

a. Thermal burns: flame, hot fluids or gases, friction, or exposure to extremely cold objects (e.g., snow, nitrogen, dry ice); flame burns are often associated with smoke/inhalation injury. Note: It is reported that 5% to 20% of all combat injuries include burns, often of the hands and head (Hedman et al, 2008). P The majority of burn injuries in children are scald injuries resulting from hot liquids, occurring most commonly in children aged 0–4 years (Toon et al, 2011). Burns in older children and teenagers, especially boys, are often associated with risk-taking behavior, such as careless use of flammable substances and experimentation with fireworks (Reed, 2009).

b. Chemical burns: contact with a caustic substance (acid or alkaline); degree of injury dependent on type and content as well as concentration and temperature of injuring agent

c. Electrical burns: current travels through the body along the pathway of least resistance (i.e., nerves offer the least resistance and bones the greatest resistance), generating heat in proportion to resistance offered; degree of injury dependent on type/voltage of current with underlying injury more severe than visible injury. P High-voltage injuries are a serious problem in adolescent boys engaging in high-risk behavior around power lines or from lightning strikes (Tomkins, 2008).

d. Radiation burns: exposure to ionizing radiation, most commonly protracted and overexposure to ultraviolet rays—UVA and UVG (e.g., the sun, sunlamps, tanning booths), or high exposure to x-rays including radiotherapy (e.g., cancer therapy)

e. Risk factors: substance abuse, careless smoking, cultural practices, socioeconomic status (e.g., overcrowded living conditions, insufficient parental supervision of children, lack of safety precautions), and violence, including abuse and neglect, such as with those aged 4 years and under or those aged 65 years and older. P *Note*: Burn injuries account for approximately 6% to 20% of all child abuse cases (Peck, 2002), and severe burns are reported in an estimated 10% of all children suffering physical abuse (Maguire et al, 2008).

IV. Statistics (American Burn Association, 2012)

a. Morbidity: 450,000 burn injuries require medical attention in the United States annually, with approximately 40,000 requiring hospitalization, including 30,000 at hospital burn centers. (P) Burns account for the greatest length of stay of all pediatric hospital admissions for injuries (Benjamin, 2002).

b. Mortality: In 2012, the ABA reported a 96.1% survival rate in clients discharged from burn care centers but approximately 3400 deaths annually. The Federal Emergency Management Association (FEMA) report in 2011 listed approximately 4000 deaths from fires in the United States annually (Burn Injury online.com, 2011). Although mortality rate is low (<2%) (Granger, 2009) in the pediatric population, burns are the third most frequent cause of injury resulting in death, behind motor vehicle accidents and drowning (Benjamin, 2002). A direct but inverse relationship exists between age and survival for any burn size. While the mortality of a 40% TBSA burn in a 20-year-old is approximately 8%, the mortality of this same injury in someone older than 70 years is 94% (Edlich et al, 2010). (P) Respiratory failure and sepsis are the leading causes of death in severely burned children, with acute lung injury and respiratory distress syndrome (ARDS) accounting for 40% to 50% of all deaths (Williams et al, 2009).

c. Cost: In 2007, the Centers for Disease Control and Prevention (CDC) reported that $7.5 billion is spent annually for burn care in hospitals, with another $3.3 billion spent in nonhospitalized burn care (CDC, 2011).

GLOSSARY

Catabolism: Breaking down of muscle tissue.

Dermis: Inner layer of skin, which contains blood and lymph vessels, hair follicles, and glands.

Epidermis: Outermost layer of skin, made up of flat, scale-like cells called squamous cells.

Total body surface area (TBSA): The "rule of nines" estimates the extent of TBSA involved in a burn injury to guide treatment. Major anatomic areas of the body are divided into percentages: in adults, 9% for the head and neck, 9% for each upper extremity, 18% to each of the anterior and posterior portions of the trunk, 18% to each lower extremity, and 1% to the perineum and genitalia. The client's palm area represents approximately 1% of TBSA and can be helpful in calculating scattered areas of involvement.

Care Setting

The following adult clients are admitted for acute care and, during the rehabilitation phase, may be cared for in a subacute or rehabilitation unit: The American Burn Association criteria for burn center care includes any full thickness burn greater than 5%; partial thickness burn greater than 20% in people between ages 10–50; any partial thickness burn greater than 10% in children younger than 10 years and adults older than 50 years of age; any significant burns to the ears, eyes, hands, feet, or genitals (ABA, 2012; Cunha, 2007). (P) Inhalation injury is cited by some as the single most important predictor of mortality in burn victims and occurs in 50% of children less than 9 years old involved in home fires (Cunha, 2007).

Related Concerns

Disaster considerations, page 858
Fluid and electrolyte imbalances, page 885
Metabolic acidosis—primary base bicarbonate deficiency, page 450
Pediatric considerations, page 872
Psychosocial aspects of care, page 729
Respiratory acidosis (primary carbonic acid excess), page 179
Sepsis/septicemia, page 665
Surgical intervention, page 762
Total nutritional support: parenteral and enteral feeding, page 437
Upper gastrointestinal/esophageal bleeding, page 281

Client Assessment Database

Data depend on type, severity, and body surface area involved.

DIAGNOSTIC DIVISION MAY REPORT	MAY EXHIBIT
ACTIVITY/REST	• Decreased strength, endurance • Limited range of motion (ROM) of involved areas • Altered muscle mass and tone

(continues on page 640)

DIAGNOSTIC DIVISION MAY REPORT (continued)	MAY EXHIBIT (continued)
CIRCULATION (with burn injury of more than 20% TBSA)	• Hypotension (shock) • Peripheral pulses diminished distal to extremity injury; generalized peripheral vasoconstriction with loss of pulses, mottling of skin, and coolness (electrical shock) • Tachycardia (shock, anxiety, pain) • Dysrhythmias (electrical shock) • Tissue edema formation (all burns)
EGO INTEGRITY • Feeling scared, self-conscious, conspicuous, angry, embarrassed, different • Concerns about family, job, finances, disfigurement	• Anxiety, irritability • Denial, withdrawal • Crying, depression • Hostility, aggressive behavior
ELIMINATION	• Urinary output decreased or absent during emergent phase; color may be pink from damaged red blood cells (RBCs) or reddish-black if myoglobin present, indicating deep-muscle damage • Diuresis—after capillary leak sealed and fluids mobilized back into circulation • Bowel sounds decreased or absent, especially in cutaneous burns of more than 20% TBSA, because stress reduces gastric motility, peristalsis
FOOD/FLUID	• Generalized tissue edema—swelling is rapid and may be extreme in early hours after injury • Weight loss • Anorexia, nausea, vomiting
NEUROSENSORY • Mixed areas of numbness, tingling, burning pain • Changes in vision, decreased visual acuity (electrical shock)	• Changes in orientation, affect, behavior • Decreased deep tendon reflexes (DTRs), reflexes, and sensation in injured extremities • Seizure activity (electrical shock) • Corneal lacerations, retinal damage (electrical shock) • Rupture of tympanic membrane (electrical shock) • Paralysis (electrical injury to nerve pathways)
PAIN/DISCOMFORT • Pain varies—first-degree burns are extremely sensitive to touch, pressure, air movement, and temperature changes • Second-degree moderate-thickness burns are very painful, whereas pain response in second-degree deep-thickness burns is dependent on intactness of nerve endings • Third-degree burns are painless, except along the edges of the burn wound	• Guarding behavior, protective positioning • Expressive behavior, such as restlessness, moaning, crying • Self-focusing; facial mask • Changes in blood pressure (BP), pulse, respiratory rate
RESPIRATION • Confinement in a closed space, prolonged exposure (possibility of inhalation injury)	• Hoarseness, wheezy cough, carbonaceous particles on face or in sputum, drooling or inability to swallow oral secretions, and cyanosis (indicative of inhalation injury) • Thoracic excursion may be limited in presence of circumferential chest burns • Upper airway stridor, wheezes (obstruction due to laryngospasm, laryngeal edema) • Breath sounds—crackles (pulmonary edema), stridor (laryngeal edema), profuse airway secretions, wheezing (rhonchi)

DIAGNOSTIC DIVISION MAY REPORT (continued)

Safety
- Engaging in risky behavior—substance abuse, sporting activities during thunderstorm, working near high power lines
- Lack of safety practices; for example, no smoke detector, smoking in bed, wearing loose-fitting clothing around open flame, improper use or storage of caustic chemicals
- Sensory impairments limiting detection of heat or cold
- Episodes of violence or abuse
- History of previous burns or other injuries

Teaching/Learning
- Use of sedatives, alcohol, tobacco, and street drugs
- Cultural beliefs and practices

Discharge Plan Considerations
- May require assistance with treatments, wound care and supplies, self-care activities, homemaker and maintenance tasks, transportation, finances, and vocational counseling
- Changes in physical layout of home or living facility other than home during prolonged rehabilitation

➧ Refer to section at end of plan for postdischarge considerations.

MAY EXHIBIT (continued)

Skin
- *General:* Exact depth of tissue destruction may not be evident for 3 to 5 days because of the process of microvascular thrombosis in some wounds; unburned skin areas may be cool, clammy, and pale, with slow capillary refill in the presence of decreased cardiac output as a result of fluid loss or shock state
- *Flame injury:* There may be areas of mixed depth of injury because of varied intensity of heat produced by burning clothing; singed nasal hairs; dry, red mucosa of nose and mouth; blisters on posterior pharynx, circumoral and/or circumnasal edema
- *Chemical injury:* Wound appearance varies according to causative agent; skin may be yellowish-brown with soft leather-like texture; blisters, ulcers, necrosis, or thick eschar. *Note:* Injuries are generally deeper than they appear cutaneously, and tissue destruction can continue for up to 72 hours after injury.
- *Electrical injury:* The external cutaneous injury is usually much less than the underlying necrosis; appearance of wounds varies and may include entry and exit (explosive) wounds of current, arc burns from current moving in close proximity to body, and thermal burns due to ignition of clothing
- *Other:* Presence of fractures, dislocations (concurrent falls, motor vehicle accident; tetanic muscle contractions due to electrical shock)

Diagnostic Studies

WHY IT IS DONE	WHAT IT TELLS ME
Blood Tests	
• *Complete blood count (CBC):* Battery of screening tests, which typically includes hemoglobin (Hgb); hematocrit (Hct); red blood cell (RBC) count morphology, indices, and distribution width index; platelet count and size; white blood cell (WBC) count and differential.	Initial increased Hct suggests hemoconcentration due to fluid shift or loss. Later, Hct and RBCs may be decreased because of heat damage to vascular endothelium. WBCs may be elevated due to inflammatory response to injury.
• *Arterial blood gases (ABGs) and pulse oximetry:* Describe the assessment of arterial blood levels of oxygen (PaO_2) and carbon dioxide ($PaCO_2$). Typically, blood pH (acidity) is measured simultaneously with ABGs.	Baseline is especially important with suspicion of inhalation injury. Reduced PaO_2 and increased $PaCO_2$ may be seen with carbon monoxide poisoning. Acidosis may occur because of reduced renal function and loss of compensatory respiratory mechanisms.

(continues on page 642)

Diagnostic Studies (continued)

WHY IT IS DONE (continued)	WHAT IT TELLS ME (continued)
• *Carboxyhemoglobin (COHgb):* Compound that is formed when inhaled carbon monoxide combines with Hgb, binding more tightly than oxygen and rendering the Hgb incapable of transporting oxygen.	Elevated percentage reflects the extent to which normal transport of oxygen has been negatively affected. Elevation of more than 10% indicates inhalation injury in a nonsmoker. Toxic exposure with levels greater than 40% to 50 % can result in loss of consciousness, seizures, coma, and death (Serebrisky et al, 2012).
• *Serum electrolytes:* Substance that will dissociate into ions in solution and acquire the capacity to conduct electricity. Electrolytes include sodium, potassium, chloride, calcium, and phosphate.	Potassium level may be initially elevated because of injured tissues, RBC destruction, and decreased renal function; hypokalemia can occur when diuresis starts; and magnesium level may be decreased. Sodium level may initially be decreased with body water losses; hypernatremia can occur later as renal conservation occurs.
• *Serum glucose:* Simple sugar that is a major energy source for all cellular and bodily functions.	Elevation reflects stress response. P In children, hypoglycemia can occur due to decreased glycogen stores (Pham, 2008).
• *Albumin, globulin, and albumin/globulin ratio:* Albumin and globulin make up most of the protein within the body and are measured in the total protein of the blood and other body fluids. Albumin proteins are normally higher than globulin and are expressed in ratio.	Albumin/globulin ratio may be reversed because of loss of protein in edema fluid.
• *Blood urea nitrogen (BUN) and creatinine (Cr):* BUN and Cr are waste products in the blood from the breakdown of protein and are filtered by the kidneys.	Elevation reflects decreased renal perfusion or function; however, the level of Cr can become elevated because of tissue injury.
URINE TESTS	
• *Urinalysis:* Screening test to evaluate renal function and detect substances or cellular material reflecting injury.	Presence of albumin, Hgb, and myoglobin indicates deep-tissue damage and protein loss—especially seen with serious electrical burns. Reddish-black color of urine indicates presence of myoglobin.
ASSOCIATED TESTS	
• *Photographs of burns:* Documents burn wound at time of admission.	Provides baseline to evaluate healing process.
• *Laser Doppler:* Measures microvascular blood flow in dermis.	Laser Doppler flow measurements performed early after burn injury are useful in predicting the depth of burn wounds and the potential for healing. Laser Doppler flowmetry helps with selection of clients for early excision and grafting of burn wounds (Edlich et al, 2010).
• *Magnetic resonance imaging (MRI) scan:* Scan that uses magnetic fields to produce two- or three-dimensional images of organs inside the body.	Detects tissue edema—a manifestation of cell membrane damage that begins to accumulate minutes after electrical injury from increased vascular permeability and extravasation of intracellular contents.
• *Wound cultures:* Drainage or material from burn area is grown in the laboratory on nutrient-enriched media to identify presence of microorganisms such as bacteria or fungi.	May be obtained for baseline data and repeated periodically to evaluate for wound infection and/or effectiveness of antimicrobial therapies.
• *Chest x-ray:* Evaluates organs and structures within the chest for symptoms of disease.	May appear normal in early postburn period even with inhalation injury; however, a true inhalation injury presents as infiltrates, often progressing to whiteout on x-ray (ARDS) (Alexander et al, 2003).
• *Upper airway endoscopy and fiberoptic bronchoscopy—also known as direct or indirect laryngoscopy:* Direct visualization of upper airways by means of either a rigid or a flexible bronchoscope.	Useful in diagnosing extent of inhalation injury in the high-risk client; findings can include edema, hemorrhage, and/or ulceration of upper respiratory tract.
• *Pulmonary function studies—forced expiratory volume (FEV_1) and peak flow volume loop:* Evaluates respiratory status.	Provides noninvasive assessment of effects and extent of inhalation injury. Airway obstruction causes a decrease in FEV_1 and peak flow. *Note:* Full resolution of pulmonary function test result abnormalities may take several months.
• *Ventilation-perfusion lung scan:* Uses inhaled and injected radioisotopes to measure breathing and circulation in all areas of the lungs.	May be done to determine extent of inhalation injury.

WHY IT IS DONE (continued)	WHAT IT TELLS ME (continued)
• *Electrocardiogram (ECG):* Record of the electrical activity of the heart, providing important information concerning the spread of electricity to the different parts of the heart.	Signs of myocardial ischemia and dysrhythmias may occur with electrical burns.
• *Cardiac enzymes (e.g., creatinine phosphokinase [CPK] isoenzyme [MB]):* A group of enzymes normally found in heart tissue and released into the bloodstream in increased concentration when the heart muscle is damaged.	Myocardial infarction (MI) can be a complication of electrical injury or postinjury resuscitation, causing elevation of cardiac enzymes. *Note:* Acute myocardial infarction is reported but is relatively rare. Skeletal muscle cells damaged by electrical current can contain as much as 20% to 25% CK-MB fraction (McBride et al, 1986).

Nursing Priorities

1. Maintain patent airway and respiratory function.
2. Restore hemodynamic stability and circulating volume.
3. Alleviate pain.
4. Prevent complications.
5. Provide emotional support for client and significant other (SO).
6. Provide information about condition, prognosis, and treatment.

Discharge Goals

1. Homeostasis achieved.
2. Pain controlled or reduced.
3. Complications prevented or minimized.
4. Current situation dealt with realistically.
5. Condition, prognosis, and therapeutic regimen understood.
6. Plan in place to meet needs after discharge.

NURSING DIAGNOSIS: risk for ineffective Airway Clearance

Risk Factors May Include

Environmental—smoke inhalation

Obstructed airway—airway spasm, retained secretions, exudates in the alveoli

Possibly Evidenced By

(Not applicable; presence of signs and symptoms establishes an *actual* diagnosis)

Desired Outcomes/Evaluation Criteria—Client Will

Respiratory Status (NOC)

Demonstrate clear breath sounds; respiratory rate within normal range; and be free of dyspnea and cyanosis.

Display oxygen saturation within normal range.

ACTIONS/INTERVENTIONS	RATIONALE
Respiratory Monitoring (NIC)	
Independent	
Obtain history of injury. Note presence of preexisting respiratory conditions and any history of smoking.	Causative burning agent, duration of exposure, and occurrence in closed or open space predict probability of inhalation injury. Type of material burned, such as wood, plastic, or wool, suggests type of toxic gas exposure. Preexisting conditions increase the risk of respiratory complications.
Assess gag and swallow reflexes; note upper airway burns, drooling, inability to swallow, hoarseness, and wheezy cough.	Suggestive of inhalation injury, which may develop over several days.
Monitor respiratory rate, rhythm, and depth; measure pulse oximetry regularly. Note presence of pallor or cyanosis and carbonaceous or pink-tinged sputum.	Tachypnea, use of accessory muscles, decreasing oxygen level, presence of cyanosis, and changes in sputum suggest developing respiratory distress or pulmonary edema and need for medical intervention.
Auscultate lungs, noting stridor, wheezing, crackles, diminished breath sounds, and brassy cough.	Airway obstruction and respiratory distress can occur very quickly or may be delayed, for example, up to 3 days after burn.
Note presence of pallor or cherry-red color of unburned skin.	Suggests presence of hypoxemia or carbon monoxide requiring additional evaluation and prompt intervention.

(continues on page 644)

ACTIONS/INTERVENTIONS (continued)	RATIONALE (continued)
Investigate changes in behavior and mentation, such as restlessness, agitation, and confusion.	Although often related to pain, changes in consciousness may reflect developing, worsening hypoxia or effects of inhaled toxins, especially carbon monoxide.
Monitor 24-hour fluid balance, noting variations or changes.	Fluid shifts or excess fluid replacement increases risk of pulmonary edema. *Note:* Inhalation injury increases fluid demands as much as 35% or more because of edema and fluid shifts.
Airway Management (NIC)	
Elevate head of bed. Avoid use of pillow under head, as indicated.	Promotes optimal lung expansion and respiratory function. When head and neck burns are present, a pillow can inhibit respiration, cause necrosis of burned ear cartilage, and promote neck contractures.
Encourage coughing, deep-breathing exercises, and frequent position changes.	Promotes lung expansion, mobilization, and drainage of secretions.
Suction, if necessary, with extreme care, maintaining sterile technique.	Helps maintain clear airway but should be done cautiously because of mucosal edema and inflammation. Sterile technique reduces risk of infection.
Promote voice rest, but assess ability to speak and/or swallow oral secretions periodically.	Increasing hoarseness or decreased ability to swallow suggests increasing tracheal edema and may indicate need for prompt intubation.
Collaborative	
Administer humidified oxygen via appropriate mode, for example, a face mask.	Oxygen corrects hypoxemia and acidosis. Humidity decreases drying of respiratory tract and reduces viscosity of sputum.
Monitor serial ABGs.	Baseline is essential for further assessment of respiratory status and as a guide to treatment. PaO_2 less than 50, $PaCO_2$ greater than 50, and decreasing pH reflect smoke inhalation and developing pneumonia or acute respiratory distress syndrome (ARDS). *Note*: Pulse oximetry can be monitored continuously while respirations/oxygenation are compromised.
Monitor carboxyhemoglobin (COHgb) levels, if indicated.	Client with inhalation injury may be monitored for elevated carbon monoxide levels. *Note*: Hyperbaric oxygenation therapy (HOT) may be considered, in client with COHbg levels >40%, who is unconsciousness, has other neurologic findings, or has severe metabolic acidosis (pH <7.1) (Serebrisky, 2012).
Review serial chest x-rays.	Changes reflecting atelectasis or pulmonary edema may not occur for 2 to 3 days after burn.
Provide or assist with chest physiotherapy and incentive spirometry.	Chest physiotherapy drains dependent areas of the lung, and incentive spirometry may be done to improve lung expansion, thereby promoting respiratory function and reducing atelectasis. *Note:* Bronchoscopy may be done to remove endotracheal debris.
Prepare for, or assist with, intubation or tracheostomy and mechanical ventilation, as indicated.	Intubation and mechanical support is required when airway edema or circumferential burn injury interferes with respiratory function and oxygenation. If client develops signs of respiratory failure or ARDS, mechanical ventilation and intensive respiratory care is required. (Refer to CP: Ventilatory Assistance [Mechanical].)

NURSING DIAGNOSIS: risk for deficient Fluid Volume

Risk Factors May Include

Loss of fluid through abnormal routes—burn wounds
Factors influencing fluid needs—hypermetabolic state
Deviations affecting intake of fluids
Active fluid volume loss—hemorrhagic losses

Possibly Evidenced By

(Not applicable; presence of signs and symptoms establishes an *actual* diagnosis)

Desired Outcomes/Evaluation Criteria—Client Will

Fluid Balance (NOC)

Demonstrate adequate fluid balance as evidenced by appropriate urinary output with normal specific gravity, stable vital signs, and moist mucous membranes.

ACTIONS/INTERVENTIONS	RATIONALE
Shock Prevention (NIC)	
Independent	
Monitor vital signs and central venous pressure (CVP). Note capillary refill and strength of peripheral pulses.	Serves as a guide to fluid replacement needs and assesses cardiovascular response. *Note:* Systemic release of inflammatory mediators and systemic edema can result in decreased cardiac output, tissue ischemia, hypovolemia, and shock. A recent study showed that injuries greater than 60% total body surface area (TBSA) are associated with an increased hypermetabolic and inflammatory reaction as well as impaired cardiac function (Jeschke et al, 2007).
Monitor urinary output and specific gravity. Observe urine color and Hematest, as indicated.	Generally, fluid replacement should be titrated to ensure average urinary output of 30 to 50 mL/hr in the adult. Urine can appear red to black in association with massive muscle destruction because of presence of blood and release of myoglobin. If gross myoglobinuria is present, minimum urinary output should be 75 to 100 mL/hr to reduce risk of tubular damage and renal failure.
Estimate wound drainage and insensible losses.	Increased capillary permeability, protein shifts, inflammatory process, and evaporative losses greatly affect circulating volume and urinary output, especially during initial 24 to 72 hours after burn injury.
Maintain cumulative record of amount and types of fluid intake.	Massive or rapid replacement with different types of fluids and fluctuations in rate of administration require close tabulation to prevent constituent imbalances or fluid overload.
Weigh daily.	Fluid replacement formulas partly depend on admission weight and subsequent changes. A 15% to 20% weight gain can be anticipated in the first 72 hours during fluid replacement, with return to preburn weight approximately 10 days after burn.
Measure circumference of burned extremities, as indicated.	May be helpful in estimating extent of edema and fluid shifts affecting circulating volume and urinary output.
Investigate changes in mentation.	Deterioration in the level of consciousness may indicate inadequate circulating volume and reduced cerebral perfusion.
Observe for gastric distention, hematemesis, and tarry stools. Hematest nasogastric (NG) drainage and stools periodically.	Stress (Curling's) ulcer occurs in up to half of all severely burned clients and can occur as early as the first week. Clients with burns more than 20% of TBSA are at risk for mucosal bleeding in the gastrointestinal (GI) tract during the acute phase because of decreased splanchnic blood flow and reflex paralytic ileus.
Collaborative	
Insert and maintain indwelling urinary catheter.	Allows for close observation of renal function and prevents urinary retention. Retention of urine with its by-products of tissue-cell destruction can lead to renal dysfunction and infection.
Insert/maintain large-bore intravenous (IV) catheter(s).	Accommodates rapid infusion of fluids.
Administer calculated IV replacement of fluids, electrolytes, plasma, and albumin.	Fluid resuscitation replaces lost fluids and electrolytes and helps prevent complications, such as shock and acute tubular necrosis (ATN). Replacement formulas vary, such as Brooke, Evans, or Parkland, but all are based on extent of burn injury, body weight, and amount of urinary output. *Note:* Once initial fluid resuscitation has been accomplished (usually with Lactated Ringer's solution), a steady rate of fluid administration is preferred to boluses, which may increase interstitial fluid shifts and cardiopulmonary congestion. *Note:* (P) Young children require more fluid than adults and require higher maintenance fluid rates to be added to the Parkland formula (Merrill et al, 1986).
Monitor laboratory studies, such as Hgb/Hct, electrolytes, and urine sodium.	Identifies blood loss, RBC destruction, and fluid and electrolyte replacement needs. Urine sodium less than 10 mEq/L suggests inadequate fluid resuscitation. *Note:* During first 24 hours after burn, hemoconcentration is common because of fluid shifts into the interstitial space.
Administer medications, as indicated, such as the following:	
Diuretics, for example, mannitol (Osmitrol)	May be indicated to enhance urinary output and clear tubules of debris to prevent necrosis if acute renal failure (ARF) is present.

(continues on page 646)

ACTIONS/INTERVENTIONS (continued) / RATIONALE (continued)

Potassium — Although hyperkalemia often occurs during first 24 to 48 hours due to tissue destruction, subsequent replacement may be necessary because of large urinary losses.

Antacids, for example, calcium carbonate (Titralac) and magaldrate (Riopan) and histamine inhibitors, for example, cimetidine (Tagamet) and ranitidine (Zantac) — Antacids may reduce gastric acidity; histamine inhibitors decrease production of hydrochloric acid to reduce risk of gastric irritation or bleeding.

Add electrolytes to water used for wound débridement, as indicated. — Washing solution that approximates tissue fluids may minimize osmotic fluid shifts.

NURSING DIAGNOSIS: acute Pain

May Be Related To
Physical agents (e.g., destruction of skin and tissues, edema formation, wound débridement)

Possibly Evidenced By
Verbalized/coded reports of pain
Expressive behavior (e.g., irritability, restlessness, crying)
Narrowed focus; facial mask—grimacing
Guarding behaviors
Changes in vital signs

Desired Outcomes/Evaluation Criteria—Client Will

Pain Level (NOC)
Report pain reduced or controlled.
Display relaxed facial expressions and body posture.

Pain Control (NOC)
Participate in activities and sleep and rest appropriately.

ACTIONS/INTERVENTIONS / RATIONALE

Pain Management (NIC)

Independent

Assess reports of pain, noting location/character and intensity (0 to 10 or similar coded scale). — Pain is the common experience of all clients with burns—regardless of the cause, size, or depth of the burn—and the pain they experience can be among the worst known. Changes in location, character, and intensity of pain may indicate developing complications (e.g., limb ischemia) or herald improvement and return of nerve function and sensation. (P) Children with burn injuries, regardless of the depth of the burn, are often anxious and fearful, in addition to being in physical pain, and all of these emotions can exacerbate the other (Granger, 2009). Studies in 2002 indicated that children in emergency departments with burns were undermedicated for pain (Singer, 2002), but later studies showed improved practice in this area (Sullivan, 2004).

Note presence of nonverbal indicators of pain, especially in client who is unable to verbalize. — Client may not be able to verbalize pain or pain characteristics due to age, developmental level, loss of consciousness or other cognitive issues, and/or type and severity of injuries. Examples include changes in vital signs, grimacing, restlessness, trembling, or withdrawal from touch. (P) Adults and children might withdraw from contact or verbal communication; children may cry inconsolably.

Cover wounds as soon as possible unless open-air exposure burn care method required. — Temperature changes and air movement can cause great pain to exposed nerve endings.

Elevate burned extremities periodically. — Elevation may be required initially to reduce edema formation; thereafter, changes in position and elevation reduce discomfort and risk of joint contractures.

Provide bed cradle, as indicated. — Elevation of linens off wounds may help reduce pain.

Wrap digits and extremities in position of function, avoiding flexed position of affected joints, using splints and footboards as necessary. — Position of function reduces deformities and contractures and promotes comfort. Although flexed position of injured joints may feel more comfortable, it can lead to flexion contractures.

ACTIONS/INTERVENTIONS (continued)	RATIONALE (continued)
Change position frequently and assist with active and passive range-of-motion (ROM) exercises, as indicated.	Movement and exercise reduce joint stiffness and muscle fatigue, but type of exercise depends on location and extent of injury.
Maintain comfortable environmental temperature; provide heat lamps and heat-retaining body coverings.	Temperature regulation may be lost with major burns. External heat sources may be necessary to prevent chilling.
Provide adequate pain medication and adjunctive medications, such as anti-anxiety drugs, before, during, or after a procedure, such as dressing changes and débridement.	The procedure may stimulate remaining nerve fibers, resulting in greater pain than was evident during the procedure. In some cases, conscious sedation for procedural pain may be needed to reduce severe physical and emotional distress associated with painful procedures.
Encourage expression of feelings about pain.	Verbalization allows outlet for emotions and may enhance coping mechanisms.
Involve client in determining schedule for activities, treatments, and drug administration.	Enhances client's sense of control and strengthens coping mechanisms.
Explain procedures and provide frequent information as appropriate, especially during wound débridement.	Knowing what to expect provides opportunity for client to prepare self and enhances sense of control. *Note*: Burn injury often induces post-traumatic stress disorder (PTSD), which heightens the burn pain experience. PTSD can actually be triggered by wound care. For example, some topical agents used in burn wound care induce a temporary sensation of heat at the burn site, or bedside use of the portable electric cautery knife during escharotomy results in a smoky fume; such stimuli can bring the original trauma to mind (Weichman, 2004). Showing empathy and support can help alleviate pain and promote relaxation.
Provide basic comfort measures—being present, gentle touch or massage of uninjured areas, and frequent position changes.	Promotes relaxation and reduces muscle tension and general fatigue.
Instruct in and encourage use of stress management techniques, such as progressive relaxation, deep breathing, guided imagery, and visualization.	Refocuses attention, promotes relaxation, and enhances sense of control, which may enhance analgesia and/or reduce pharmacological dependency.
Provide diversional activities appropriate for age and condition.	Helps refocus attention, lessening concentration on pain experience.
Promote uninterrupted sleep periods.	Sleep deprivation can increase perception of pain and reduce coping abilities.
Collaborative	
Administer analgesics (opioid and nonopioid) as indicated, such as morphine, fentanyl (Sublimaze, Ultiva), hydrocodone (Vicodin, Hycodan), or oxycodone (OxyContin, Percocet)	The burned client may require around-the-clock medication and dose titration. IV method is often used initially to maximize drug effect. Concerns of client addiction or doubts regarding degree of pain experienced are not valid during emergent and acute phases of care, but opioids should be decreased as soon as feasible and alternative methods for pain relief initiated.
Provide and instruct in use of patient-controlled analgesia (PCA).	PCA provides for timely drug administration, preventing fluctuations in intensity of pain, often at lower total dosage than would be given by conventional methods.

NURSING DIAGNOSIS: risk for Infection

Risk Factors May Include

Inadequate primary defenses—destruction of skin barrier, traumatized tissues, invasive procedures
Environmental exposure
Inadequate secondary defenses—decreased Hgb, suppressed inflammatory response

Possibly Evidenced By

(Not applicable; presence of signs and symptoms establishes an *actual* diagnosis)

Desired Outcomes/Evaluation Criteria—Client Will

Burn Healing (NOC)
Achieve timely wound healing free of purulent exudate and be afebrile.

ACTIONS/INTERVENTIONS	RATIONALE
Infection Protection (NIC)	
Independent	
Implement appropriate isolation techniques, as indicated.	Dependent on type and extent of wounds and the choice of wound treatment (e.g., open versus closed); isolation may range from simple wound and skin to complete or reverse to reduce risk of cross-contamination and exposure to multiple bacterial flora.
Emphasize and model good hand-washing technique for all individuals coming in contact with client.	Prevents cross-contamination and reduces risk of acquired infection.
Use gowns, gloves, masks, and strict aseptic technique during direct wound care and provide sterile or freshly laundered bed linens and gowns.	Prevents exposure to infectious organisms.
Monitor and limit visitors, if necessary. Explain isolation procedure to visitors, if used. Supervise visitor adherence to protocol as indicated.	Prevents cross-contamination from visitors. Concern for risk of infection should be balanced against client's need for family support and socialization.
Wound Care (NIC)	
Shave/clip all hair from around burned areas to include a 1-inch border (excluding eyebrows). Shave facial hair (men) and shampoo head daily.	Hair is a good medium for bacterial growth; however, eyebrows act as a protective barrier for the eyes. Regular shampooing decreases bacterial fallout into burned areas.
Examine unburned areas, such as groin, neck creases, and mucous membranes, and vaginal discharge routinely.	Opportunistic infections (e.g., yeast) frequently occur because of depression of the immune system and/or proliferation of normal body flora during systemic antibiotic therapy.
Provide special care for eyes, for example, use eye covers and tear formulas as appropriate.	Eyes may be swollen shut and/or become infected by drainage from surrounding burns. If lids are burned, eye covers may be needed to prevent corneal damage.
Prevent skin-to-skin surface contact—wrap each burned finger or toe separately; do not allow burned ear to touch scalp.	Prevents adherence to the surface that it may be touching and encourages proper healing. *Note:* Ear cartilage has limited circulation and is prone to pressure necrosis.
Examine wounds daily; note and document changes in appearance, odor, or quantity of drainage.	Identifies presence of granulation tissue indicating healing and provides for early detection of burn-wound infection. Infection in a partial-thickness burn may cause conversion of burn to full-thickness injury. *Note:* A strong, sweet, musty smell at a graft site is indicative of *Pseudomonas*.
Monitor vital signs for fever and increased respiratory rate and depth in association with changes in sensorium, presence of diarrhea, decreased platelet count, and hyperglycemia with glycosuria.	Indicators of sepsis—often occurring with full-thickness burn—requiring prompt evaluation and intervention. *Note:* Changes in sensorium, bowel habits, and respiratory rate usually precede fever and alteration of laboratory studies.
Collaborative	
Remove dressings and cleanse burned areas in a hydrotherapy or whirlpool tub or in a shower stall with handheld showerhead. Maintain temperature of water at 100°F (37.8°C). Wash areas with a mild cleansing agent or surgical soap.	Water softens and aids in removal of dressings, slough layer of dead skin or tissue, and dry scabs or eschar. Sources vary as to whether bath or shower is best. Bath has advantage of water providing support for exercising extremities but may promote cross-contamination of wounds. Showering enhances wound inspection and prevents contamination from floating debris.
Excise and cover burn wounds quickly.	Early excision is known to reduce scarring and risk of infection, thereby facilitating healing.
Débride necrotic and loose tissue, including ruptured blisters, with scissors and forceps. Do not disturb intact blisters if they are smaller than 1 to 2 cm, do not interfere with joint function, and do not appear infected.	Promotes healing and prevents autocontamination. Small, intact blisters help protect skin and increase rate of re-epithelialization unless the burn injury is the result of chemicals, in which case fluid contained in blisters may continue to cause tissue destruction.
Photograph wound initially and at periodic intervals.	Provides baseline and documentation of healing process.
Infection Protection (NIC)	
Administer topical antimicrobial agents, as indicated, for example:	The following agents help control bacterial growth and prevent drying of wound, which can cause further tissue destruction.
Silver sulfadiazine (Silvadene, Flammazine)	Still the most common topical antibiotic used in burn care, Silvadene is a broad-spectrum antimicrobial that may allow the wound to heal without need for skin grafting and is relatively painless but has intermediate, somewhat delayed eschar penetration. May cause rash or depression of WBCs. *Note:* Silver sulfadiazine inhibits wound epithelialization and should be discontinued once exudates and eschar have separated from the wound, leaving a clean wound bed, which is then treated as a superficial partial-thickness burn (Hartford, 2007).

ACTIONS/INTERVENTIONS (continued)	RATIONALE (continued)
Mafenide acetate (Sulfamylon) solution or mafenide HCl cream	Antibiotic of choice with confirmed invasive burn wound infection that does not respond to Silvadene. Useful against gram-negative and gram-positive organisms and some fungal species. The solution is painless; however, the cream causes burning or pain on application and for 30 minutes thereafter. Can cause rash and is contraindicated in metabolic acidosis.
Silver-coated dressings (e.g., Acticoat, Aquacel Ag)	Nonadherent antimicrobial dressings that stay on the wound for up to 3 to 4 days, delivering a low concentration of nanocrystalline silver, with the added benefit of reduced pain with application or removal (Fong, 2005).
Aqueous silver nitrate	Effective against *Staphylococcus aureus, Escherichia coli,* and *Pseudomonas aeruginosa* but has poor eschar penetration, is painful, and may cause electrolyte imbalance. Dressings must be constantly saturated. Product stains skin and other surfaces black.
Poloxamer 188 containing bacitracin and polymixin B	This gel is effective against gram-positive organisms, does not interfere with re-epithelialization, and is generally used for tar and asphalt-based residues, other imbedded materials, and for superficial and facial burns.
Hydrogels, such as Transorb and Burnfree	Useful for partial- and full-thickness burns, in rehydrating dry wound beds, and promoting autolytic débridement. May be used when infection is present. Another gel (Plurogel) is awaiting FDA approval (Connor-Ballard, 2009).
Administer other medications, as appropriate, for example:	
Subeschar clysis/systemic antibiotics	Systemic antibiotics are given to control general infections identified by culture and sensitivity. Subeschar clysis has been found effective against pathogens in granulated tissues at the line of demarcation between viable and nonviable tissue, reducing risk of sepsis.
Tetanus toxoid or clostridial antitoxin, as appropriate.	Tissue destruction and altered defense mechanisms increase risk of developing tetanus or gas gangrene, especially in deep burns such as those caused by electricity.
Place IV and invasive lines in nonburned area.	Decreased risk of infection at insertion site with possibility of progression to septicemia.
Obtain routine cultures and sensitivities of wounds and drainage.	Allows early recognition and specific treatment of wound infection.
Assist with excisional biopsies when infection is suspected.	Bacteria can colonize the wound surface without invading the underlying tissue; therefore, biopsies may be obtained for diagnosing infection.

NURSING DIAGNOSIS: risk for Peripheral Neurovascular Dysfunction

Risk Factors May Include

Burns; immobilization

Trauma; fractures

Mechanical compression (e.g., circumferential burns/edema of extremities)

Possibly Evidenced By

(Not applicable; presence of signs and symptoms establishes an *actual* diagnosis)

Desired Outcomes/Evaluation Criteria—Client Will

Tissue Perfusion: Peripheral (NOC)

Maintain palpable peripheral pulses of equal quality and strength; good capillary refill, free of numbness or paresthesia.

ACTIONS/INTERVENTIONS	RATIONALE
Circulatory Care: Venous [or] Arterial (NIC)	
Independent	
Assess color, sensation, movement, capillary refill, and peripheral pulses via Doppler on extremities with circumferential burns.	Edema formation can readily compress blood vessels, thereby impeding circulation and increasing venous stasis and edema.
Compare with findings of unaffected limb.	Comparisons with unaffected limbs aid in differentiating localized versus systemic problems such as hypovolemia and decreased cardiac output.

(continues on page 650)

ACTIONS/INTERVENTIONS (continued)	RATIONALE (continued)
Elevate affected extremities, as appropriate. Remove jewelry or arm band. Avoid taping around a burned extremity or digit.	Promotes systemic circulation and venous return and may reduce edema or other deleterious effects of constriction of edematous tissues. *Note:* Prolonged elevation can impair arterial perfusion if BP falls or tissue pressures rise excessively.
Obtain BP in unburned extremity when possible. Remove BP cuff after each reading, as indicated.	If BP readings must be obtained on an injured extremity, leaving the cuff in place may increase edema formation, reduce perfusion, and convert partial-thickness burn to a more serious injury.
Investigate reports of deep, throbbing ache and numbness.	Indicators of decreased perfusion and/or increased pressure within enclosed space, such as may occur with a circumferential burn of an extremity (compartment syndrome).
Encourage active ROM exercises of unaffected body parts.	Promotes local and systemic circulation.
Investigate irregular pulses.	Cardiac dysrhythmias can occur as a result of electrolyte shifts, electrical injury, or release of myocardial depressant factor, compromising cardiac output and tissue perfusion.
Collaborative	
Maintain fluid replacement per protocol. (Refer to ND: risk for deficient Fluid Volume.)	Maximizes circulating volume and tissue perfusion.
Monitor electrolytes, especially sodium, potassium, and calcium. Administer replacement therapy, as indicated.	Losses or shifts of these electrolytes affect cellular membrane potential and excitability, thereby altering myocardial conductivity, potentiating risk of dysrhythmias, and reducing cardiac output and tissue perfusion.
Avoid use of intramuscular (IM) and subcutaneous (SC) injections.	Altered tissue perfusion and edema formation impair drug absorption. Injections into potential donor sites may render them unusable because of hematoma formation.
Measure intracompartmental pressures as indicated. (Refer to CP: Fractures; ND: risk for Peripheral Neurovascular Dysfunction.)	Ischemic myositis may develop because of decreased perfusion.
Assist with or prepare for escharotomy or fasciotomy, as indicated.	Enhances circulation by relieving constriction caused by rigid, nonviable tissue (eschar) or edema formation.

NURSING DIAGNOSIS imbalanced Nutrition: less than body requirements

May Be Related To

Inability to ingest food [to meet needs] (e.g., hypermetabolic state; protein catabolism) (can be as much as 50% to 60% higher than normal proportional to the severity of injury)

Possibly Evidenced By

Loss of weight; poor muscle tone

Lack of interest in food; satiety immediately after ingesting food; aversion to eating

[Development of negative nitrogen balance]

Desired Outcomes/Evaluation Criteria—Client Will

Nutritional Status (NOC)

Demonstrate nutritional intake adequate to meet metabolic needs as evidenced by stable weight and muscle-mass measurements, positive nitrogen balance, and tissue regeneration.

ACTIONS/INTERVENTIONS	RATIONALE
Nutrition Therapy (NIC)	
Independent	
Auscultate bowel sounds, noting hypoactive or absent sounds.	Ileus is often associated with postburn period but usually subsides within 36 to 48 hours, at which time oral or intragastric feedings can be initiated.
Maintain strict calorie count. Weigh daily. Reassess percentage of open body surface area and wounds weekly.	Appropriate guides to proper caloric intake include 25 kcal/kg body weight, plus 40 kcal per percentage of TBSA burn in the adult. As burn wound heals, energy needs are reevaluated to calculate prescribed dietary formulas and appropriate adjustments are made.
Monitor muscle mass and subcutaneous fat, as indicated.	Indirect calorimetry, if available, may be useful in more accurately estimating body reserves and losses and effectiveness of therapy.

ACTIONS/INTERVENTIONS (continued)	RATIONALE (continued)
Provide small, frequent meals and snacks.	Helps prevent gastric distention or discomfort and may enhance intake.
Encourage client to view diet as a treatment and to make food and beverage choices high in calories and protein.	Calories and proteins are needed to meet metabolic needs and promote wound healing.
Ascertain food likes and dislikes. Encourage SO to bring food from home, as appropriate.	Provides client/SO sense of control; enhances participation in care and may improve intake.
Encourage client to sit up for meals and visit with others.	Sitting helps prevent aspiration and aids in proper digestion of food. Socialization promotes relaxation and may enhance intake.
Provide oral hygiene before meals.	Clean mouth and clear palate enhances taste and helps promote a good appetite.
Perform fingerstick glucose and urine testing, as indicated.	Monitors for development of hyperglycemia related to hormonal changes and demands or use of hyperalimentation to meet caloric needs.
Collaborative	
Refer to dietitian or nutritional support team.	Useful in establishing individual nutritional needs based on weight and body surface area of injury and identifying appropriate routes. *Note*: Hypermetabolic state can increase caloric needs as much as 50% to 60% higher than normal proportional to the severity of injury.
Provide diet high in calories and protein with trace elements and vitamin supplements.	Calories approximating 25 kcal/kg/day, protein up to 2 g/kg/day, and vitamins are needed to meet increased metabolic needs, maintain weight, and encourage tissue regeneration. Zero fat or minimal fat is preferred during early acute phase to minimize the susceptibility to infection.
Insert and maintain small feeding tube for enteral feedings and supplements, if needed.	Provides continuous or supplemental feedings when client is unable to consume total daily calorie requirements orally. *Note:* Research supports use of early intragastric feedings as soon after admission as possible because delayed enteral feeding longer than 18 hours postinjury results in a high rate of gastroparesis and need for IV nutrition. Continuous tube feeding during the night increases calorie intake without decreasing appetite and oral intake during the day.
Administer parenteral nutritional solutions containing vitamins and minerals, as indicated.	Total parenteral nutrition (TPN) maintains nutritional intake and meets metabolic needs in presence of severe complications or sustained esophageal or gastric injuries that do not permit enteral feedings. (Refer to CP: Total Nutritional Support: Parenteral/Enteral Feeding.)
Monitor laboratory studies, such as serum albumin or prealbumin, glucose, electrolytes, magnesium, BUN/Cr, calcium, inorganic phosphorus, transaminase, and triglycerides.	Indicators of nutritional needs, and adequacy of diet and therapy.
Administer insulin, as indicated.	Elevated serum glucose levels may develop because of stress response to injury, high caloric intake, and pancreatic fatigue.

NURSING DIAGNOSIS: impaired physical Mobility

May Be Related To

Pain, discomfort; anxiety
Neuromuscular impairment; decreased muscle strength; joint stiffness; contractures
Reluctance to initiate movement; prescribed movement restrictions, limb immobilization
Decreased endurance

Possibly Evidenced By

Limited range of motion; limited ability to perform fine motor skills
Difficulty turning
Gait changes; postural instability

Desired Outcomes/Evaluation Criteria—Client Will

Immobility Consequences: Physiological (NOC)

Maintain position of function as evidenced by absence of contractures.
Maintain or increase strength and function of affected and/or compensatory body part.

Self-Care: Activities of Daily Living (ADLs) (NOC)

Demonstrate techniques and behaviors that enable resumption of activities.

ACTIONS/INTERVENTIONS	RATIONALE
Bedrest Care (NIC)	
Independent	
Maintain proper body alignment with supports or splints, especially for burns over joints.	Promotes functional positioning of extremities and prevents contractures, which are more likely over joints.
Note circulation, motion, and sensation of digits frequently.	Edema may compromise circulation to extremities, potentiating tissue necrosis and development of contractures.
Initiate the rehabilitative phase on admission.	It is easier to enlist participation when client is aware of the possibilities that exist for recovery.
Perform ROM exercises consistently, initially passive, then active.	Prevents progressively tightening scar tissue and contractures, enhances maintenance of muscle and joint functioning, and reduces loss of calcium from the bone.
Medicate for pain before activity or exercises.	Reduces muscle and tissue stiffness and tension, enabling client to be more active and facilitating participation.
Schedule treatments and care activities to provide periods of uninterrupted rest.	Increases client's strength and tolerance for activity.
Encourage family/SO support and assistance with ROM exercises.	Enables family/SO to be active in client care and provides more constant and consistent therapy.
Self-Care Assistance (NIC)	
Incorporate ADLs with physical therapy, hydrotherapy, and nursing care.	Combining activities produces improved results by enhancing effects of each.
Encourage client participation in all activities as individually able.	Promotes independence, enhances self-esteem, and facilitates recovery process.
Instruct and assist with mobility aids, such as a cane, walker, or crutches, as appropriate.	Promotes safe ambulation.
Bed Rest Care (NIC)	
Collaborative	
Provide foam or flotation mattress or kinetic therapy bed, as indicated.	Prevents prolonged pressure on tissues, reducing potential for tissue ischemia, necrosis, and decubitus ulcer formation.
Maintain pressure garment when used.	Hypertrophic scarring can develop around grafted areas or at the site of deep partial-thickness wounds. Pressure dressings minimize scar tissue by keeping it flat, soft, and pliable, enhancing movement.
Consult with rehabilitation, physical, and occupational therapists.	Normally members of the burn team, these specialists provide integrated activity and exercise programs and specific assistive devices based on individual needs. Consultation facilitates intensive long-term management of potential deficits.

NURSING DIAGNOSIS: impaired Skin Integrity [grafts]

May Be Related To

Burn injury

Possibly Evidenced By

Disruption of skin surface/layers

Desired Outcomes/Evaluation Criteria—Client Will

Burn Healing (NOC)

Demonstrate tissue granulation.

Achieve timely healing of burned areas.

ACTIONS/INTERVENTIONS	RATIONALE
Skin Care: Graft Site (NIC)	
Independent	
Preoperative	
Assess and document size, color, depth of wound, noting necrotic tissue and condition of surrounding skin.	Provides baseline information about need for skin grafting and possible clues about circulation in area to support graft.
Provide appropriate burn care and infection control measures. (Refer to ND: risk for Infection.)	Prepares tissues for grafting and reduces risk of infection and graft failure.
Collaborative	
Administer topical wound débridement ointment, as indicated, for example enzymatic products—collagenase ointment (Santyl) and papain (Accuzyme).	Early débridement of burn eschar is beneficial to wound healing, and some treatment centers suggest use of these products to promote healing. However, despite theoretical advantage, enzymatic débridement results have been highly variable.

ACTIONS/INTERVENTIONS	RATIONALE
Independent	
Postoperative	
Elevate grafted area, if possible and appropriate.	Reduces swelling and limits risk of graft separation.
Maintain desired position and immobility of area when indicated.	Movement of tissue under graft can dislodge it, interfering with optimal healing.
Maintain dressings (mesh, petroleum, nonadhesive) over newly grafted area and/or donor site, as indicated.	Areas may be covered by translucent, nonreactive surface material between graft and outer dressing to eliminate shearing of new epithelium to protect healing tissue. The donor site is usually covered for 4 to 24 hours, then bulky dressings are removed and fine mesh gauze is left in place.
Keep skin free from pressure.	Promotes circulation and prevents ischemia, necrosis, and graft failure.
Evaluate color of grafted and donor site(s); note signs of healing.	Evaluates effectiveness of circulation and identifies developing complications.
Collaborative	
Maintain wound covering (skin substitutes) as indicated, for example:	
Biosynthetic dressing (e.g., Biobrane)	Biobrane membrane contains collagenous porcine peptides that adhere to wound surface until removed or sloughed off by spontaneous skin re-epithelialization. Useful for eschar-free, partial-thickness burns awaiting autografts because it can remain in place for longer periods of time and is permeable to topical antimicrobial agents. *Note:* Studies have shown Biobrane to be as efficacious as silver sulfadiazine in wound healing without the frequency of dressing changes (Pham et al, 2007).
Human fibroblast-derived temporary skin substitute (TransCyte)	Bioengineered skin substitute used on middermal burns after débridement; in prospective trials, shows faster healing with less pain. *Note*: Studies have shown TransCyte to be superior to antibiotic creams or silver sulfadiazine in terms of healing time, infections, and scar formation, especially on facial burns (Demling, 2002).
Contact layer dressings such as Dermagraft, Apligraft.	These temporary, permanent, or adjunct dressings adhere to the tissue to support accelerated wound healing (Jones, 2002).
Prepare for/assist with surgical grafting or biological dressings, such as the following:	
Homograft (allograft)	Skin grafts obtained from living persons or cadavers are used as a temporary covering for extensive burns until individual's own skin is ready for grafting (test graft) to cover excised wounds immediately after escharotomy or to protect granulation tissue.
Heterograft (xenograft, porcine)	Skin grafts may be carried out with animal skin for the same purposes as homografts or to cover meshed autografts.
Cultured epithelial autograft (CEA) (e.g., Epicel)	Skin graft obtained from uninjured part of client's own skin and prepared in a laboratory. Can be used in client with deep dermal or full-thickness burns comprising a total body surface area of greater than or equal to 30%. It may be used in conjunction with split-thickness autografts or alone (USFDA, 2013).

NURSING DIAGNOSIS: risk for Post-Trauma Syndrome

May Be Related To

Serious accident/disaster; events outside the range of usual human experience
Serious injury to self
Survivor's role in the event

Possibly Evidenced By

(Not applicable; presence of signs and symptoms establishes an *actual* diagnosis)

Desired Outcomes/Evaluation Criteria—Client Will

Personal Resiliency (NOC)

Verbalize awareness of feelings.
Identify healthy ways to deal with feelings.
Verbalize an enhanced sense of control.
Demonstrate effective problem-solving skills.

ACTIONS/INTERVENTIONS	RATIONALE
Crisis Intervention (NIC)	
Independent	
Provide frequent explanations and information about care procedures. Repeat information as needed or desired.	Knowing what to expect usually reduces anxiety, clarifies misconceptions, and promotes cooperation. *Note:* Because of the shock of the initial trauma, many people do not recall information provided during that time.
Demonstrate willingness to listen and talk to client when free of painful procedures.	Helps client and SO know that support is available and that healthcare provider is interested in the person, not just care of the burn.
Involve client and SO in decision-making process whenever possible. Provide time for questioning and repetition of proposed treatments.	Promotes sense of control and cooperation, decreasing feelings of helplessness or hopelessness.
Assess mental status, including mood and affect, comprehension of events, and content of thoughts, such as illusions or manifestations of terror or panic.	Initially, client may use denial and repression to reduce and filter information that might be overwhelming. Some clients display calm manner and alert mental status, representing dissociation from reality, which is also a protective mechanism.
Investigate changes in mentation and presence of hypervigilance, hallucinations, sleep disturbances (e.g., nightmares), agitation or apathy, disorientation, and labile affect, all of which may vary from moment to moment.	Indicators of acute stress response or delirium state in which client is literally fighting for life. Although cause can be psychologically based, pathological life-threatening causes, such as shock, sepsis, or hypoxia, must be ruled out.
Provide constant and consistent orientation.	Helps client stay in touch with surroundings and reality.
Encourage client to talk about the burn circumstances when ready.	Client may need to tell the story of what happened over and over to make some sense out of a terrifying situation. Adjustment to the impact of the trauma and grief over losses and disfigurement can easily lead to clinical depression, psychosis, and post-traumatic stress disorder (PTSD).
Explain to client what happened. Provide opportunity for questions and give open and honest answers.	Compassionate statements reflecting the reality of the situation can help client and SO acknowledge the reality and begin to deal with what has happened.
Identify previous methods of coping with and handling stressful situations.	Past successful behavior can be used to assist in dealing with the present situation.
Create a restful environment; use guided imagery and relaxation exercises.	Clients experience severe anxiety associated with burn trauma and treatment. These interventions are soothing and helpful for positive outcomes.
Assist the family to express their feelings of grief and guilt.	The family may initially be most concerned about client's dying and/or feel guilty, believing that in some way they could have prevented the incident.
Be empathetic and nonjudgmental in dealing with client and family.	Family relationships are disrupted; financial, lifestyle, and role changes make this a difficult time for those involved with client, and they may react in many different ways.
Encourage family/SO to visit and discuss family happenings. Remind client of past and future events.	Maintains contact with a familiar reality, creating a sense of attachment and continuity of life.
Collaborative	
Involve entire burn team in care from admission to discharge, including social worker and psychiatric resources.	Provides a wide support system and promotes continuity of care and coordination of activities.
Administer mild sedation, as indicated, for example, lorazepam (Ativan), alprazolam (Xanax).	Anti-anxiety medications may be necessary for a short period of time until client is more physically stable and internal locus of control is regained.

NURSING DIAGNOSIS: disturbed Body Image

May Be Related To

Injury; trauma
Treatment regimen

Possibly Evidenced By

Reports negative feelings about body; not looking at injury
Focus on past appearance; preoccupation with change or loss
Change in social involvement; fear of reaction by others

Desired Outcomes/Evaluation Criteria—Client Will

Body Image (NOC)

Incorporate changes into self-concept without negating self-esteem.
Verbalize acceptance of self in situation.

Adjustment To Physical Disability (NOC)

Develop plan for the future to resume life—educational/employment/home responsibilities.
Modify lifestyle to accommodate situation/change.

ACTIONS/INTERVENTIONS	RATIONALE
Crisis Intervention (NIC)	
Independent	
Assess meaning of loss or change to client and SO, including future expectations and impact of cultural and religious beliefs.	Traumatic episode results in sudden, unanticipated changes, creating feelings of grief over actual or perceived losses. This necessitates support to work through to optimal resolution.
Acknowledge and accept expression of feelings of frustration, dependency, anger, grief, and hostility. Note withdrawn behavior and use of denial.	Acceptance of these feelings as a normal response to what has occurred facilitates resolution. It is not helpful or possible to push client before he or she is ready to deal with the situation. Denial may be prolonged and be an adaptive mechanism because client is not ready to cope with personal problems.
Set limits on maladaptive behavior (e.g., manipulative or aggressive). Maintain nonjudgmental attitude while giving care, and help client identify positive behaviors that will aid in recovery.	Client and SO tend to deal with this crisis in the same way in which they have dealt with problems in the past. Staff may find it difficult and frustrating to handle behavior that is disrupting and not helpful to recuperation but should realize that the behavior is usually directed toward the situation and not the care provider.
Be realistic and positive during treatments, in health teaching, and in setting goals within limitations.	Enhances trust and rapport between client and nurse.
Body Image (NOC)	
Encourage client and SO to view wounds and assist with care, as appropriate.	Promotes acceptance of reality of injury and of change in body and image of self as different.
Provide hope within parameters of individual situation; do not give false reassurance.	Promotes positive attitude and provides opportunity to set goals and plan for future based on reality.
Assist client to identify extent of actual change in appearance/body function.	Helps begin process of looking to the future and how life will be different.
Give positive reinforcement of progress and encourage endeavors toward attainment of rehabilitation goals.	Words of encouragement can support development of positive coping behaviors.
Encourage family interaction with one another and with rehabilitation team.	Maintains or opens lines of communication and provides ongoing support for client and family.
Recommend contact with survivor support person or group for client and SO, such as Survivors Offering Assistance in Recovery (SOAR). Give information about how SO can be helpful to client.	Provides a connection with a supporter who has experienced a burn injury. Talking with someone who has been directly impacted by a burn or by tissue injury can be reassuring, because he or she has had similar experiences and is familiar with what lies ahead.
Role-play social situations of concern to client.	Prepares client and SO for reactions of others and anticipates ways to deal with them.
Collaborative	
Refer to physical or occupational therapy, vocational counselor, and psychiatric counseling, for example, a psychiatric clinical nurse specialist, social services, or a psychologist, as needed.	Helpful in identifying ways and devices to regain and maintain independence. Client may need further assistance to resolve persistent emotional problems—especially post-trauma response.

NURSING DIAGNOSIS: deficient Knowledge [Learning Need] regarding condition, prognosis, treatment, self-care, and discharge needs

May Be Related To

Lack of exposure or recall
Misinterpretation of information
Unfamiliarity with resources

Possibly Evidenced By

Reports the problem
Inaccurate follow-through of instructions/performance of task

Desired Outcomes/Evaluation Criteria—Client Will

Knowledge: Disease Process (NOC)
Verbalize understanding of condition, prognosis, and potential complications.

Knowledge: Treatment Regimen (NOC)
Verbalize understanding of therapeutic needs.
Correctly perform necessary procedures and explain reasons for actions.
Initiate necessary lifestyle changes and participate in treatment regimen.

ACTIONS/INTERVENTIONS	RATIONALE
Teaching: Disease Process (NIC) *Independent*	
Review condition, prognosis, and future expectations.	Provides knowledge base from which client can make informed choices.
Discuss client's expectations of returning home, to work, and to normal activities.	Client frequently has a difficult and prolonged adjustment after discharge. Problems, such as sleep disturbances, nightmares, reliving the accident, difficulty with resumption of social interactions or intimacy and sexual activity, and emotional lability, often occur and can interfere with successful adjustment to resuming normal life.
Review and have client and SO demonstrate proper burn, skin graft, and wound care techniques. Identify appropriate sources for outpatient care and supplies.	Promotes competent self-care after discharge, enhancing independence.
Discuss skin care, such as scar massage and use of perfume-free moisturizers (e.g., Vaseline Intensive Care, Eucerin), sunscreens, and anti-itching medications (e.g., diphenhydramine [Benadryl], hydroxyzine [Atarax]).	Itching, blistering, and sensitivity of healing wounds and graft sites can be expected for an extended time, and injury can occur because of the lack of natural lubrication and fragility of the new tissue. *Note:* Sun block may be required for life because of potential for hyperpigmentation.
Explain scarring process and necessity for and proper use of silicone gel sheeting, static splint, or pressure garments when used.	Helps minimize and treat hypertrophic scarring and contracture formation. Consistent use of the pressure garment over a long period can reduce the need for reconstructive surgery to release contractures and remove scars. *Note:* (P) Remind parent that child wearing pressure garment should be evaluated periodically for proper fit due to growth.
Encourage continuation of prescribed exercise program and scheduled rest periods.	Maintains mobility, reduces complications, and prevents fatigue, facilitating recovery process.
Identify specific limitations of activity as individually appropriate.	Imposed restrictions depend on the severity and location of the injury and the stage of healing.
Emphasize importance of sustained intake of high-protein and high-calorie meals and snacks.	Optimal nutrition enhances tissue regeneration and general feeling of well-being. *Note:* Client often needs to increase caloric intake to meet calorie and protein needs for healing.
Review medications, including purpose, dosage, route, and expected or reportable side effects.	Reiteration allows opportunity for client to ask questions and be sure understanding is accurate.
Advise client and SO of potential for exhaustion, boredom, emotional lability, and adjustment problems. Provide information about possibility of discussion as well as interaction with appropriate professional counselors.	Provides perspective to some of the problems that client/SO may encounter and aids awareness that assistance is available when necessary.
Identify signs and symptoms requiring medical evaluation—inflammation, increase or changes in wound drainage, fever, chills, changes in pain characteristics, or loss of mobility or function.	Early detection of developing complications (e.g., infection, delayed healing) may prevent progression to more serious or life-threatening situations.
Emphasize necessity and importance of follow-up care and rehabilitation program.	Long-term support with continual reevaluation and changes in therapy is required to achieve optimal recovery.
Provide phone number for contact person.	Provides easy access to treatment team to reinforce teaching, clarify misconceptions, and reduce potential for complications.
Identify community resources, such as skin and wound care professionals and crisis centers; recovery groups; and mental health, Red Cross, visiting nurse, Ambli-Cab, and homemaker service.	Facilitates transition to home, provides assistance with meeting individual needs, and supports independence.

POTENTIAL CONSIDERATIONS following acute hospitalization (dependent on client's age, physical condition and presence of complications, personal resources, and life responsibilities)

- ***ineffective Coping***—situational crisis, severe/chronic pain; inadequate level of confidence in ability to cope
- ***risk for Disuse Syndrome***—severe pain, prescribed immobilization or restrictive therapies
- ***risk for situational low Self-Esteem***—functional impairment; loss; disturbed body image
- ***ineffective Self-Health Management***—complexity of therapeutic regimen; economic difficulties; added demands made on individual/family; social support deficits
- ***Post-Trauma Syndrome***—events outside the range of usual human experience; serious injury to self

WOUND CARE: COMPLICATED OR CHRONIC

I. Pathophysiology—Destruction of various layers of the integument as the result of purposeful action (surgical procedure), disease processes, impaired circulation, or incidental trauma (pressure, shearing forces)

II. Characteristics of chronic (nonhealing or impaired healing) wounds

a. Presence of necrotic or unhealthy tissue
b. Excess exudate and slough

III. Types of Wounds

a. Surgical: These are surgical wounds that failed to heal or have dehisced.
b. Traumatic: unintentional or intentional
c. Foot ulcers: Most often occurs in diabetics and are associated with polyneuropathy and injury. The lifetime risk of a person with diabetes developing a foot ulcer is estimated to be as high as 25% (Brem et al, 2006). *Note*: These wounds may be classified with Meggit-Wagner Ulcer Classification (Grades 0–5); see Glossary below.
d. Leg ulcers: Venous stasis causes about 70% of lower-extremity ulcers (Abbade, 2010); also associated with peripheral arterial disease (PAD) and sickle cell disease.
e. Pressure ulcers (also called decubitus ulcers): Occur because of prolonged ischemia-producing external pressure, usually to a soft tissue region overlying a bony prominence. Shearing forces, exposure to constant moisture, and heat buildup also are major contributing factors.
f. Irritant dermatitis: urinary or fecal incontinence, leaking tubes or drains

IV. Etiology (Baley, 2013; Salcido et al, 2012; Ayello et al, 2011; Enoch, 2004)

a. Neuropathy, such as occurs with diabetes, spinal cord injury, cerebral palsy, Hansen's disease
b. Ischemia associated with atherosclerosis, microangiopathy (such as occurs with diabetes), and any form of peripheral vascular disease
c. Peripheral edema: due to elevated venous pressure such as occurs with varicose veins or deep vein thrombosis (DVT); cardiopulmonary conditions (e.g., congestive heart failure); untreated lymphedema
d. Direct pressure, such as occurs with immobility, paralysis, poor mobility occurring due to advanced age, or dementia, terminal illness
e. Miscellaneous direct or associated causes: connective tissue disorders, vasculitis, arterio-venous malformations, pharmacological agents (e.g., corticosteroids, hydroxyurea), neoplasms/malignancy, radiation, osteomyelitis, poor nutritional status, smoking

V. Staging (EUPAP/NPUAD, 2009)

a. Stage I: intact skin, nonblanchable redness in localized area (may be difficult to detect in dark-skinned person)
b. Stage II: shiny, shallow, open ulcer without slough or bruising
c. Stage III: full-thickness tissue loss. Areas with significant subcutaneous fat can develop extremely deep ulcers. Slough may be present; may include tunneling.
d. Stage IV: full-thickness tissue loss, with exposed bone, tendon, or muscle
e. Unstageable: full-thickness tissue loss in which the base of the ulcer is covered by slough (yellow, tan, gray, green, or brown) and/or eschar (tan, brown, or black) in the wound bed
f. Deep tissue injury (DTI): purple or maroon localized area of discolored intact skin or blood-filled blister

VI. Statistics

a. Morbidity: Includes infection, sepsis, fistulas, amputation. In 2004, A National Home Care and Hospice Survey reported that of the 1.3 million clients in home health care more than 121,000 (or 9.3%) had a current diagnosis of disease of the skin and subcutaneous tissue, which includes pressure ulcers (Park-Lee, 2007).
b. Mortality: 60,000 people die each year from complications of pressure ulcers (Salcido et al, 2012).
c. Cost: Chronic wound care costs $20 billion annually (Fogg, 2009); average treatment cost for a pressure ulcer is $37,000 when client is admitted to hospital for management (Green, 2010).

GLOSSARY

Approximated: Wound edges to a surgical incision are either sutured or stapled so that edges touch, forming a thin line.

Dehisced: A break in the continuity of the surgical wound.

Deep tissue injury: Localized area of discolored (purple or maroon) skin that is either intact or a blood-filled blister.

Eschar: Hard crust or scab that is typically dark brown or black.

Meggit-Wagner Ulcer Classification: A specific classification system for diabetic foot ulcers; however, it does not capture the depth of the wound (Grade 0: preulceration lesion, healed ulcer or presence of bony deformity; Grade 1: superficial ulcer; Grade 2: ulcer penetrates through subcutaneous tissue and may have exposed bone, tendon, muscle, etc.; Grade 3: presence of osteitis, abscess, or osteomyelitis; Grade 4: gangrene of a digit; Grade 5: gangrene of the foot).

Necrosis (or necrotic tissue): Death of cells, usually within a localized area of the body, as from an interruption of the blood supply to that part.

Negative pressure wound therapy (NPWT): A sealed, air-tight vacuum wound-care system using foam dressings with the application of negative pressure in order to drain exudates and promote blood flow to the wound to enhance healing.

Peripheral arterial disease: Systemic form of atherosclerosis causing restrictive blood flow.

Periwound: Tissue immediately surrounding the wound.

Polyneuropathy: Functional disturbance or pathological changes to the nervous system that may include several systems (motor, sensory, autonomic) typically affecting the lower limbs.

Pressure ulcer: Located over a bony prominence and is a localized area of skin injury.

Slough: Necrotic tissue that is separating from the wound bed or surrounding tissue. This tissue can be yellow, tan, grey, brown, or green.

Venous stasis: Impaired venous blood flow.

Care Settings

All care settings.

Related Concerns

Surgical intervention, page 462
Total nutritional support: parenteral/enteral feeding, page 437

Client Assessment Database

Data depend on type, severity, and body surface area involved.

DIAGNOSTIC DIVISION MAY REPORT	MAY EXHIBIT
ACTIVITY/REST	
• Bedrest/wheelchair-bound, immobile, or with limited ability to reposition self	• Requires assistance for turning, repositioning, weight shifts
CIRCULATION	
• Diminished or absent dorsalis pedis or posterior tibial pulse (if foot ulcer present)	• Dependent rubor, pallor on elevation, and loss of hair on the foot or toes may be present in leg and foot ulcers • Capillary refill greater than 3 seconds • Edema of lower extremities
ELIMINATION	
	• Diarrhea, urinary incontinence (may be impacting sacral area skin)
NEUROSENSORY	
	• Paresthesias
PAIN/DISCOMFORT	
• Pain from the condition causing the wound may or may not be present or be persistent, even at rest, and chronic • Pain present during dressing changes may be acute and associated with activities of débridement	• Grimacing, withdrawal • Guarding of affected area • Emotional responses
SAFETY	
	• Elevated temperature; fever • Skin ulcerations, wounds • Decreased strength and/or range of motion (affected extremity) • Altered gait
TEACHING/LEARNING	
• History of smoking	
DISCHARGE PLAN CONSIDERATIONS	
• May require assistance with treatments, wound care and supplies, self-care activities, homemaker and maintenance tasks, transportation, finances, and vocational counseling.	

Diagnostic Studies

TEST WHY IT IS DONE	WHAT IT TELLS ME
BLOOD TESTS	
• ***Complete blood count (CBC):*** Evaluates numbers and characteristics of blood cells, including red and white blood cells, hemoglobin, hematocrit, and platelets.	Leukocytosis, anemia, and thrombocytopenia are commonly found.

TEST WHY IT IS DONE (continued)	WHAT IT TELLS ME (continued)
• ***Serum protein, albumin, pre-albumin, and transferrin levels:*** Measures types and efficiency of plasma proteins. Used to detect protein-calorie malnutrition.	May be done to evaluate the client's nutritional status in the setting of nonhealing wounds.
• *Wound cultures:* Specimens obtained from wound bed exudates are cultured to detect a wound infection and to determine which specific bacteria are present.	May be done to determine the appropriate antimicrobial therapy.
ASSOCIATED DIAGNOSTIC STUDIES	
• ***Vascular studies (e.g., plethysmography, pulse-volume recordings [PVRs]), Doppler Ankle Brachial Pressure Index (ABPI)***	May be done to evaluate hemodynamic significance of arterial occlusive disease. *Note*: Doppler ABPI may be indicated if pulse is not palpable or to assess the appropriateness of high or modified compression bandaging for venous ulcers.
• *Vascular ultrasonography:* Noninvasive procedure that uses ultrasound technology to provide information about the anatomy, physiology, and pathology of both the superficial and the deep venous systems.	May be indicated to evaluate for aneurysmal disease or deep venous occlusion.
• *Wound biopsy:* Piece of viable wound tissue obtained with scalpel or punch biopsy instrument and submitted for microscopic examination.	Recommended in the case of refractory, nonhealing ulcers or when wounds present with atypical signs *Note*: A recent study showed that approximately 10% of wounds are atypical (not originating from vascular insufficiency, neuropathy, or prolonged pressure) and are the result of infection, metabolic disorders, neoplasms, and inflammatory processes (Tang et al, 2012).

Nursing Priorities

1. Promote healing.
2. Alleviate pain.
3. Prevent complications.
4. Provide information about wound, treatment, and potential complications.

Discharge Goals

1. Wound healing progressing toward resolution.
2. Pain controlled or reduced.
3. Complications prevented or minimized.
4. Plan in place to meet discharge needs.

NURSING DIAGNOSIS: impaired Skin/Tissue Integrity

May Be Related To

Altered circulation
Nutritional factors (e.g., obesity, emaciation); skeletal prominence
Excess/deficient fluid volume; [presence of edema]
Mechanical factors (e.g., shearing forces, pressure, restraint)
Impaired physical mobility
Moisture—excretions or secretions
Extremes in age

Possibly Evidenced By

Damaged/destroyed tissue (e.g., skin layers, subcutaneous)
Invasion of body structures

Desired Outcomes/Evaluation Criteria—Client Will

Wound Healing: Secondary Intention (NOC)
Be free of signs of infection or other complications.
Display progressive improvement/healing of lesions, wounds, or pressure sores.

Self-Management: Chronic Disease (NOC)
Maintain optimal nutrition and physical well-being.
Participate in prevention measures and treatment program.

ACTIONS/INTERVENTIONS	RATIONALE
Wound Care: Nonhealing (NIC)	
Independent	
Review client factors that may delay or inhibit healing.	Client's ability to heal is affected by underlying conditions (e.g., diabetes, poor systemic circulation, or peripheral vascular disease [PVD], malnutrition/protein deficiency); persistent inflammation; use of certain medications (e.g., systemic steroids, immunosuppressive drugs, antimetabolite chemotherapy). *Note*: Chronic wounds (those with stalled healing or failure to heal) are more prevalent in older adults and are attributed to aged skin and comorbidities, such as neuropathy, arterial compromise, edema, and unrelieved pressure, in addition to factors listed above (Ayello et al, 2011; Enoch, 2004).
Determine client's age and developmental level. Note presence of compromised mobility, sensation, vision, hearing, or speech.	Factors that affect client's ability to provide for own safety needs (e.g., diabetic with impaired vision cannot satisfactorily examine own feet) or participate in care of skin/tissue wounds.
Assess nutritional status and potential for delayed healing.	Protein-calorie malnutrition and deficiencies of vitamins A, C, and zinc impair normal wound-healing mechanisms (Daley, 2013).
Review medication regimen.	Identifies medications that may impair healing (e.g., corticosteroids).
Perform routine skin inspection(s), describing observed changes. Note skin color, turgor.	Provides information about client's general nutrition and hydration status.
Ascertain if wound is acute (e.g., injury from surgery, trauma, new pressure area) or chronic (e.g., venous or arterial insufficiency, long-standing diabetic foot ulcer).	Clarifies intervention needs and priorities.
Assess, monitor, and document wound history and physical examination (using facility protocols and tools and/or using a mnemonic [MEASURE]) (Keast, 2004) if helpful:	Facilitates determination of healing and if appropriate dressing modality is being used. *Note*: Documentation of a detailed assessment is a legal requirement from both an organizational and professional standards perspective (Ayello et al, 2011).
M = measure (once/week or per protocol)	Accurate measurement of the wound provides data of wound progress. *Note*: Keast et al suggest measuring size—longest length with the widest width—at right angles.
E = exudate	Describes amount (none, scant, moderate, or heavy) and characteristics—serous, sanguineous, pustular, or combinations.
A = appearance	Describes appearance of wound bed, slough, and tissue, e.g., base: necrotic (black), fibrin (firm yellow), slough (soft yellow), or granulation tissue (pink and healthy vs red and friable = easy bleeding, unhealthy).
S = suffering	Describes pain client is experiencing from underlying condition as well as that which is occurring due to dressing changes and débridement.
U = undermining	It is suggested to measure in centimeters and use hands of clock (e.g., 2 o'clock, 6 o'clock) to document direction of undermining.
E = edge	Describes perimeter tissue (e.g., macerated, normal).
Note odors emitted from skin, wound, or dressings.	May provide information about presence of inflammation in deep tissues or wound infection.
When performing dressing changes and cleansing wound beds:	
Gently remove tape or old dressing in the direction of hair growth.	Decreases pain during removal of dressing and prevents damage to periwound skin.
Cleanse wound as needed with normal saline or prescribed solution and gently pat dry with gauze sponge.	Removal of necrotic debris facilitates removal of exudate, contaminated or infected tissue and promotes healing.
Apply wound dressing product according to manufacturer's directions.	Using the product correctly will facilitate wound healing and not result in disruption of the periwound skin.
Loosely fill wound cavity with designated product (gauze sponge, alginate), if appropriate for the wound environment.	Tightly packing the wound cavity results in slow wound healing.
Collaborative	
Review laboratory results, e.g., hemoglobin (Hgb)/hematocrit (Hct), blood glucose, albumin/proteins, etc.	These studies may reveal concerns related to underlying conditions (e.g., anemia, systemic hypoxia, diabetes, malnutrition) affecting healing.

ACTIONS/INTERVENTIONS (continued)	RATIONALE (continued)
Select wound dressing that is appropriate to the wound environment:	
Wet-to-dry	Optimal wound coverage requires wet-to-damp dressings, which support autolytic débridement, absorb exudate, and protect surrounding normal skin. *Note*: In some settings, wet-to-dry dressings are being discarded in favor of more recent forms of débridement (Dale, 2011). This change in thinking is based in part on the National Institute for Health and Clinical Excellence (NICE), United Kingdom, guideline "Surgical Site Infection: Prevention and Treatment of Surgical Site Infections," which specifically states: "do not use . . . gauze, or moist cotton gauze . . . to manage surgical wounds that are healing by secondary intention" (NICE, 2008).
Hydrogel, hydrocolloid	Useful in providing hydration to dry wound bed.
Polyvinyl film (e.g., Op-Site, Tegaderm)	Wounds that are neither dry nor highly exudative may be covered with a polyvinyl film dressing.
Absorptive dressings (e.g., alginate [Kaltostat, Curasorb], hydrocolloid [DuoDerm, Intrasite] , impregnated gauze dressings [Mesalt])	Wounds with excessive drainage require absorptive dressings.
Topical growth factor (Regranex Gel)	Wounds with eschar require débridement using collagenase (e.g., Santyl) wet-to-dry gauze dressing or products promoting autolysis (e.g., hydrocolloid, film dressing, hypertonic saline gel [Hydrogel]).
Topical growth factor (Regranex Gel)	Diabetic foot ulcers may be treated by this recently FDA-approved product (Baley, 2013; Fogg, 2009).
Negative pressure wound therapy (NPWT)	A sealed wound-care system that has been found to be useful in the treatment of large chronic wounds and acute complicated wounds. *Note*: U.S. Food and Drug Administration recommends caution when evaluating clients for NPWT use, especially regarding risk for bleeding, infection, and client/caregiver capabilities when home care considered (Mirsaidi, update 2012).

NURSING DIAGNOSIS: acute/chronic Pain

May Be Related To

Physical agent—tissue destruction
Chemical injury—excretions, secretions

Possibly Evidenced By

Verbal/coded reports of pain
Self-focus
Guarding behaviors; positioning to avoid pain
Expressive behaviors—restlessness
Changes in vital signs

Outcomes/Evaluation Criteria—Client Will

Pain Level (NOC)

Verbalize relief and/or control of pain or discomfort.
Appear relaxed; able to sleep/rest appropriately.

Pain Control (NOC)

Engage in use of nonanalgesic relief techniques such as relaxation skills and diversional activities.

ACTIONS/INTERVENTIONS	RATIONALE
Pain Management (NIC)	
Independent	
Assess pain, noting location, characteristics, and intensity (using a 0 to 10 or similar coded scale).	Helps evaluate degree of discomfort and effectiveness of analgesia or may reveal developing complications.
Determine the impact of the pain experience on quality of life.	Pain can be debilitating, causing inactivity, loss of work and/or enjoyment of life, weight loss or gain, sleep difficulties, depression, and changes in role and social functioning.

(continues on page 662)

ACTIONS/INTERVENTIONS (continued) / RATIONALE (continued)

Ensure patient receives attentive and adequate analgesic care. Anticipate pain with dressing changes or débridement and medicate accordingly.

Helps to relieve the discomfort. *Note*: Recent research has focused on pain that a client with chronic wound experiences at other times than with dressing changes. Several studies have indicated that more than 80% of people with a chronic wound reported pain at all times, with half of them rating the pain at moderate to worst pain possible (Nemeth et al, 2004).

Provide anticipatory guidance.

Client should be informed about interventions (e.g., débridement) that can increase pain and participate in decisions about type and timing of analgesia.

Teach use of relaxation techniques such as relaxation, guided imagery, and visualization. Provide diversional activities.

Helps client refocus attention and promotes coping during débridement or dressing changes, reducing pain and discomfort.

Collaborative

Administer medication, such as opioids and nonopioid analgesics, NSAIDs; antidepressants (e.g., amitriptyline [Elavil]), and anticonvulsants (e.g., carbamazepine [Tegretol]); local anesthetics, (e.g., foam dressing with local release of ibuprofen), etc. Utilize patient-controlled analgesia (PCA), as indicated.

Relieves pain, enhances comfort, and promotes rest. *Note*: Numerous agents have been found to relieve the various components of chronic pain. For example, nociceptive (deep tissue) pain may respond best to opioids and NSAIDs, while neuropathic pain (due to nerve damage) may respond better to antidepressants and anticonvulsants (Woo et al, 2008).

Apply topical analgesic, as appropriate.

May be used to decrease pain with the removal of some dressings, such as the foam used in negative wound pressure therapy.

Implement complementary therapies where indicated, such as nerve stimulation and acupuncture.

May be useful in long-term management of neuropathic pain and encourage growth of healthy tissue.

Assist client/family in developing a program of coping strategies. Encourage use of/refer to personal and community resources (e.g., assistive equipment, financial resources, home-health providers, and respite services.

Utilization of available resources to facilitate staying active even when modified activities are required, living a healthy lifestyle, encouraging client/SO to exercise own control in situation, and developing short- and long-term plans for long-term care can promote general well-being and enhance quality of life.

NURSING DIAGNOSIS: risk for Infection

Risk Factors May Include

Inadequate primary defenses—broken skin, traumatized tissue
Inadequate secondary defenses—decreased hemoglobin, leukopenia, suppressed inflammatory response
Chronic disease—diabetes mellitus, obesity; malnutrition

Possibly Evidenced By

(Not applicable; presence of signs and symptoms establishes an *actual* diagnosis)

Desired Outcomes/Evaluation Criteria—Client Will

Infection Severity (NOC)

Achieve wound healing; be free of purulent exudate or other signs of wound infection.
Verbalize understanding of individual causative or risk factors and ways to prevent complications.

ACTIONS/INTERVENTIONS / RATIONALE

Infection Protection (NIC)

Independent

Inspect condition of any surgical incision or other wound. Note risk factors for occurrence of infection.

Any wound is at risk for infection, but certain conditions can increase that risk, such as complicated surgical or contaminated traumatic wound, comorbidities (e.g., diabetes, vascular insufficiency, obesity), vulnerable age, immunosuppression, and malnutrition, placing the client at high risk for delayed healing or nonhealing of wounds.

Adhere to facility infection control policy regarding hand hygiene and prevention of cross-contamination.

Standardized practice to prevent infection.

Maintain aseptic or clean technique as is appropriate during dressing changes. Dispose of biologic waste as required.

Promotes wound healing and reduces risk of healthcare-associated infections.

Monitor for systemic and localized signs and symptoms of infection.

Early detection of infection allows for timely treatment and prevention of further complications.

Collaborative

Monitor lab studies, such as absolute granulocyte count (AGC), WBC, and differential count.

Measures the number and vitality of infection-fighting white blood cells.

NURSING DIAGNOSIS: imbalanced Nutrition: less than body requirements

May Be Related To

Biological factors (e.g., increased metabolic demands to heal wounds)

Possibly Evidenced By

Reports/observed food intake less than recommended daily allowance
Lack of interest in food; satiety immediately after ingesting food
Poor muscle tone
[Abnormal laboratory studies (e.g., decreased albumin, total proteins; electrolyte imbalances)]

Desired Outcomes/Evaluation Criteria—Client Will

Nutritional Status: Energy (NOC)

Demonstrate progress in tissue healing free of infection.
Display good muscle tone and general endurance.

Nutritional Status: Biochemical Measures (NOC)

Display normalization of laboratory values.

ACTIONS/INTERVENTIONS	RATIONALE
Nutrition Therapy (NIC)	
Independent	
Note age, body build, general strength, activity, and current health conditions (e.g., long-term immobilization, chronic diseases) and treatments.	Helps determine nutritional needs.
Weigh client and observe for emaciation, multiple bony prominences, absence of subcutaneous fat and muscle wasting, loss of hair, fissuring of nails, gum bleeding with brushing, etc.	May indicate protein-energy malnutrition especially in the setting of nonhealing wounds.
Perform calorie count; evaluate total daily food and fluid intake.	May reveal possible cause of malnutrition and changes that could be made to ensure client is receiving the required nourishment for wound healing.
Encourage foods high in protein. Offer protein-rich snacks, drinks throughout the day, especially if client eats small amounts at each meal.	The client will require protein intake of 1.25 to 1.5 g/Kg/day for adequate wound healing to occur (EPUAP/NPUAP, 2009). Adequate fluid intake is required to prevent dehydration due to increased protein intake.
Collaborative	
Assist in nutritional status assessment (e.g., Mini Nutritional Assessment [MNA], the Malnutrition Universal Screening Tool [Must] or similar tools), as indicated.	May be used to evaluate client's current status and predict nutritional needs.
Review laboratory studies (e.g., serum albumin/prealbumin, transferrin, amino acid profile, total lymphocyte count, iron stores, nitrogen balance studies, glucose, liver function tests, electrolytes).	Evaluates client's current nutritional status and response to nutritional interventions.
Collaborate in treatment of underlying conditions and factors.	Improving client's nutritional status is often multifaceted, especially if client is debilitated over long period of time. Treating infection, anemia, systemic hypotension and hypoxemia; correcting poor glucose control in diabetic or nausea associated with cancer therapies; or discontinuing medications that decrease appetite may help client regain ability to heal.
Consult registered dietitian or nutritionist, as indicated.	Aids in constructing dietary prescription with optimal amounts of protein, carbohydrates, fats, and calories within client's eating style, needs, and abilities that facilitates wound healing.
Administer vitamin and/or mineral supplements, liquid protein supplements, enteral or parenteral feedings, as needed.	Replacements needed depend on evidence of a deficiency that is impeding wound healing.

NURSING DIAGNOSIS: risk for ineffective Self-Health Management

May Be Related To

Complexity of therapeutic regimen
Deficient knowledge
Perceived barriers/benefits
Economic difficulties; excessive demands made on individual/SO

(continues on page 664)

NURSING DIAGNOSIS: risk for ineffective Self-Health Management (continued)

Possibly Evidenced By
(Not applicable; presence of signs and symptoms establishes an *actual* diagnosis)

Desired Outcomes/Evaluation Criteria—Client Will

Knowledge: Treatment Regimen (NOC)
Verbalize understanding of condition and treatment needs.
Demonstrate behaviors to maintain therapeutic regimen.
Initiate changes in lifestyle to address individual risk factors.
Identify and use available resources.

ACTIONS/INTERVENTIONS	RATIONALE
Wound Care: Nonhealing (NIC)	
Independent	
Assess complexity of client's care needs, noting whether more than one condition is present at the same time.	These factors affect view of self-care. Client may be overwhelmed, in denial, depressed, or have complications exacerbating care needs.
Ascertain client's knowledge and understanding of condition and treatment needs.	Provides baseline for planning care so that learning may begin where client is in relation to condition and current therapeutic regimen.
Identify individual perceptions and expectations of treatment plan.	May reveal misinformation, unrealistic expectations, or other factors that may interfere with client's willingness or ability to follow therapeutic regimen.
Review wound care procedures (e.g., expected tasks and how to perform them), and evaluate degree of difficulty for client:	May reveal factors that could interfere with success of self-care.
Maintaining clean technique during dressing changes	Promotes wound healing and reduces risk of infections.
Monitoring for localized signs of infection	Early detection of infection allows for prompt treatment and prevention of further complications.
Signs and symptoms to report to healthcare provider	Provides mechanism for early intervention if complications are occurring or to identify if client is being overwhelmed by complexity of treatment needs.
Refraining from smoking. (Refer for support, counseling as desired)	Smoking has been shown to decrease cutaneous blood flow by as much as 40%, which produces ischemia and impairs healing (Rayner, 2006).
Eating nutritious foods, staying well hydrated, and taking prescribed medications.	All of these measures are needed to promote wound healing and general health,
Accept client's evaluation of own strengths and limitations, working together to improve abilities. State belief in client's ability to cope and/or adapt to situation.	Client may minimize own strengths or have lack of confidence in abilities, which could be reversed with assistance and positive feedback from others.
Note availability and use of resources for assistance. Provide written information and contact numbers and encourage client/SO to seek out resources.	Client/SO may not have, be aware of, or know how to access available resources.
Mobilize support systems, including family/SO, and make appropriate referrals (e.g., social services, home-care services, medical supplies, financial assistance, and counseling).	Success of self-care may depend on support systems to reduce stress in dealing with complex and long-term needs.

POTENTIAL CONSIDERATIONS following acute hospitalization (dependent on client's age, physical condition and presence of complications, personal resources, and life responsibilities)

- ***ineffective Coping***—situational crises, vulnerability
- ***risk for Infection***—broken skin, traumatized tissue; malnutrition; chronic disease
- ***risk for disturbed Body Image***—surgery/trauma; treatment regimen

CHAPTER 14

Systemic Infections and Immunological Disorders

SEPSIS/SEPTICEMIA

I. Pathophysiology (Cunha, 2008; Latto, 2008; Wood & Lavieri, 2007; Kleinpell, 2006)

- **a.** Presence of a systemic inflammatory response to documented or presumed infection, which may progress along a continuum
  - **i.** Systemic inflammatory response syndrome (SIRS)
    1. Infection with release of endo- or exotoxins activating the inflammatory cascade—local release of cytokines into the circulation in attempt to restore homeostasis
    2. Failure of mechanism leads to destructive response with loss of circulatory integrity.
    3. Criteria (two or more)—fever higher than 100.4°F/38°C or lower than 96°F/36°C; heart rate greater than 90 beats per minute; respiration greater than 20/min or $PaCO_2$ less than 32 mm Torr; white blood cell (WBC) count greater than 12,000/μL, less than 4000/μL, or greater than 10% of bands or immature cells
  - **ii.** Severe sepsis—presence of known or suspected infection and two or more SIRS criteria; associated with organ dysfunction, hypoperfusion, hypotension with alteration of mental status, hypoxemia, lactic acidosis, and/or oliguria
  - **iii.** Septic shock—characterized by hemodynamic changes and persistent hypotension, development of perfusion abnormalities, and impaired cellular function that fails to respond to adequate fluid resuscitation
  - **iv.** Multiple organ dysfunction syndrome (MODS)—organ dysfunction leading to organ failure with inability to maintain homeostasis

II. Etiology (Cunha, 2008; Latto, 2008; Wood & Lavieri, 2007; Kleinpell, 2006)

- **a.** Multiple microorganisms associated with sepsis
  - **i.** Bacteria, fungi, viruses, or rickettsiae
  - **ii.** Common pathogens: *Streptococcus pneumoniae* or *Staphylococcus aureus, Candida, Salmonella, Escherichia coli, Legionella, Klebsiella, Pseudomonas*
- **b.** Common origin of infections
  - **i.** Abdomen: appendicitis, bowel problems (perforated diverticuli), infection of the abdominal cavity, and gallbladder or liver infections
  - **ii.** Central nervous system: infections of the brain or the spinal cord, such as encephalitis, meningitis
  - **iii.** Lungs: pneumonia
  - **iv.** Skin: wounds or cellulitis; punctures, such as from intravenous (IV) lines, intravascular devices, or catheters inserted into the body to administer or drain fluids
  - **v.** Urinary tract: kidneys or bladder (glomerulonephritis, pyelonephritis, cystitis), prostatic obstruction
- **c.** Risk factors: unsanitary and/or crowded living conditions, pollution, poor nutrition, immunosuppression, chronic health conditions, improper use of antibiotics

III. Statistics (Hall et al, 2011)

- **a.** Morbidity: Hospitalizations for septicemia or sepsis (as a first-listed or principal diagnosis) increased from 326,000 in 2000 to 727,000 in 2008, and the rate of these hospitalizations more than doubled from 11.6 per 10,000 population in 2000 to 24.0 per 10,000 population in 2008.
- **b.** Mortality: Dependent on progression of condition and degree of organ failure, presence of comorbidities, and age. In 2010, septicemia was the 11th leading cause of death in the United States with 35,539 (Centers for Disease Control [CDC], 2012); the overall rate of death in 2011 was 11.4% (Hoyert & Xu, 2012).
- **c.** Cost: Approximately $15.4 billion in 2009—$6.9 billion age 0 to 64 years, $8.5 billion age 65 and over (Strangers, 2011); averages $22,100 per case with a median of $18,000 to a high of $50,000. From 1997 to 2008, the inflation-adjusted aggregate costs for treating patients hospitalized for this condition increased on average annually by 11.9% (Hall et al, 2011).

GLOSSARY

Anaerobic infection: An infection caused by bacteria, called anaerobes, which cannot grow in the presence of oxygen.

Bacteremia: The presence of live bacteria in the bloodstream. Bacteremia is similar in some respects to viremia (the presence of a virus in the blood); parasitemia (the presence of a parasite in the blood); or fungemia (presence of a fungus in the blood).

Body substance isolation (BSI): Practice of isolating all body substances—blood, urine, feces, sputum, tears, and so on.

(continues on page 666)

GLOSSARY (continued)

Cytokines: Protein chemical messengers involved in the inflammatory process, usually from white blood cells (WBCs).

Disseminated intravascular coagulation (DIC): Hyperstimulation of coagulation pathways results in diffuse activation and consumption of coagulation factors, leading to generalized bleeding.

Endotoxins: Potentially toxic, natural compounds found inside pathogens such as bacteria.

Hyperbaric oxygen therapy: Treatment in which client is placed in a chamber and breathes oxygen at higher-than-atmospheric pressure. This high-pressure oxygen stops bacteria from growing and, at high enough pressure, destroys them.

Infection: Inflammatory response to invasion of host tissue by microorganisms.

Multiple organ dysfunction syndrome (MODS): Organ function is altered in an acutely ill individual such that homeostasis cannot be achieved without intervention and support.

Oliguria: Urine output less than 30 mL/hr.

Purpura: Hemorrhagic area in the skin, which does not blanch when touched. The area of bleeding within the skin is greater than 3 mm in diameter.

Sepsis: Systemic inflammatory response secondary to infection—symptomatic bacteremia. Sepsis is termed severe if associated with organ dysfunction, hypoperfusion, and hypotension. (Used interchangeably with septicemia).

Septicemia: Presence of rapidly multiplying microorganisms in the bloodstream, which can result in profound physiological changes. (Used interchangeably with sepsis).

Septic shock: State that produces an inability to maintain adequate tissue perfusion and oxygenation, ultimately causing cellular, and then organ system, dysfunction.

Systemic inflammatory response syndrome (SIRS): Condition in which there is inflammation throughout the body. Bacteremia may be a factor; other causes include trauma or ischemia.

Third spacing of fluid: Loss of albumin or protein from circulating blood leads to decreased oncotic pressure. Fluid can then leak from the intravascular space into the interstitial space and stay there, causing edema.

Care Setting

Although severely ill individuals will likely receive care in the intensive care unit (ICU), this plan addresses care on an inpatient acute medical-surgical unit.

Related Concerns

Acquired immunodeficiency syndrome (AIDS), page 689
Chronic obstructive pulmonary disease (COPD) and asthma, page 118
Disaster considerations, page 858
Fluid and electrolyte imbalances, page 885
Metabolic acidosis—primary base bicarbonate deficiency, page 450
Peritonitis, page 320
Pneumonia, page 129
Psychosocial aspects of care, page 729
Pulmonary tuberculosis (TB), page 170
Renal failure: acute, page 505
Surgical intervention, page 762
Total nutritional support: parenteral/enteral feeding, page 437
Ventilatory assistance (mechanical), page 157
Wound care: complicated and chronic, page 657

Client Assessment Database

Data depend on the type, location, and duration of the infective process and organ involvement.

DIAGNOSTIC DIVISION MAY REPORT	MAY EXHIBIT
ACTIVITY/REST	
• Fatigue • Malaise	• Mental status changes—withdrawn, lethargy • Respiration and heart rate increased with activity or at rest
CIRCULATION	
	• Blood pressure (BP) may be normal, slightly low to normal range—as long as cardiac output remains elevated • Profound hypotension (late-stage sign) • Peripheral pulses bounding, rapid (hyperdynamic phase), weak, thready, or easily obliterated • Heart rate elevated (greater than 90); extreme tachycardia may be present, unless blunted by beta blockers or other medications (in septic shock) • Heart sounds may include development of S_3

DIAGNOSTIC DIVISION MAY REPORT (continued)	MAY EXHIBIT (continued)
	• Dysrhythmias suggest myocardial dysfunction and effects of acidosis and electrolyte imbalance • Skin warm, dry, flushed (vasodilation) or pale, cold, clammy, mottled (vasoconstriction)
ELIMINATION • Urinary frequency, urgency • Diarrhea	• Oliguria, anuria
FOOD/FLUID • Loss of appetite, nausea, vomiting	• Weight loss • Diminished or absent bowel sounds • Extremity and generalized edema
NEUROSENSORY • Headache • Dizziness, fainting	• Restlessness, apprehension, confusion • Disorientation, delirium, or coma
PAIN/DISCOMFORT • Abdominal tenderness, localized pain or discomfort • Headache, sinus pain • Pelvic or flank pain • Localized limb pain or tenderness	
RESPIRATION	• Tachypnea (respiratory alkalosis) with decreased respiratory depth • Dyspnea, rapid labored respirations • Cough—may be productive if pneumonia is source
SAFETY • History of recent or current infection, viral illness, cancer therapies, use of corticosteroids, or other immunosuppressant medications • Presence of invasive lines or catheters	• Temperature usually elevated (greater than 100.4°F [38°C]) but may be normal in elderly or compromised client; may occasionally be lower than normal (less than 96.8°F [36°C]) • Shaking chills • Poor or delayed wound healing, purulent drainage, or localized erythema • Petechiae • Oozing or bleeding from invasive line sites, wounds, and mucous membranes (late sign)
SEXUALITY • Recent childbirth or abortion • Vaginal or urethral discharge	• Maceration of vulva or purulent vaginal drainage
TEACHING/LEARNING • Chronic, debilitating health problems—liver, renal, cardiac disease; cancer; diabetes mellitus (DM); alcoholism • History of splenectomy • Recent surgery or invasive procedures, traumatic wounds • Antibiotic use—recent or long-term	
DISCHARGE PLAN CONSIDERATIONS • May require assistance with wound care and supplies, treatments, self-care, and homemaker tasks ➧ Refer to section at end of plan for postdischarge considerations.	

Diagnostic Studies

TEST WHY IT IS DONE	WHAT IT TELLS ME
BLOOD TESTS	
• ***Complete blood count (CBC):*** Battery of screening tests, which typically includes hemoglobin (Hgb); hematocrit (Hct); red blood cell (RBC) count, morphology, indices, and distribution width index; platelet count and size; WBC count and differential, which includes neutrophils, lymphocytes, monocytes, eosinophils, and basophils.	Hct may be elevated in hypovolemic states because of hemoconcentration. Leukopenia, decreased WBCs, occurs early and may be followed by a rebound leukocytosis reflecting rapid production of immature WBCs. Neutrophils may be elevated or depressed. Platelets may be elevated initially as an acute-phase reactant but are decreased in later stages.
• ***Serum electrolytes:*** Substances that will dissociate into ions in solution and acquire the capacity to conduct electricity. Common electrolytes include sodium, potassium, chloride, calcium, and phosphate.	Various imbalances may occur because of acidosis, fluid shifts, and altered renal function.
• ***Biomarkers, such as acute-phase reactants:***	Literature review indicates that there are many biomarkers that can be used in sepsis, but none has sufficient specificity or sensitivity to be routinely employed in clinical practice. PCT and CRP have been most widely used, but even these have limited abilities to distinguish sepsis from other inflammatory conditions or to predict outcome (Clancy, 2012; Pierrakos, 2010).
• ***C-reactive protein (CRP):*** Indicator of inflammation but is not sensitive in distinguishing between causes of SIRS.	CRP is released by the liver in response to pro-inflammatory cytokines and is thought to recruit monocytes in early infection. Elevated levels may have a role in monitoring response to treatment (Burdette, 2012).
• ***Procalcitonin (PCT):*** Peptide precursor to calcitonin.	PCT rises with severity of illness and increases more rapidly than CRP in sepsis. PCT is able to differentiate between infectious and noninfectious SIRS (Burdette, 2012).
• ***Clotting studies:***	
• ***Platelets:*** Platelets play an important role in blood coagulation and hemostasis that is often altered by sepsis.	Decreased platelet levels (thrombocytopenia) can occur because of platelet aggregation.
• ***Prothrombin time (PT)/activated partial thromboplastin time (aPTT):*** Measurement of coagulation times to identify abnormalities common to sepsis and which can lead to life-threatening complications.	Both PT and aPTT may be prolonged, indicating coagulopathy associated with liver ischemia, circulating toxins, or shock state.
• ***Fibrin degradation products:*** End product of clot breakdown associated with abnormal coagulation process.	Often elevated and associated with tendency to bleed.
• ***Serum lactate:*** Product of anaerobic cellular metabolism, thus reflecting tissue hypoperfusion.	Elevated in metabolic acidosis, liver dysfunction, and shock.
• ***Serum glucose:*** Glucose is a primary energy source and necessary for cellular function.	Hyperglycemia occurs in response to insulin resistance and cellular starvation. The liver mobilizes alternative sources of glucose through gluconeogenesis and glycogenolysis. Hypoglycemia is a predictor of poor prognosis.
• ***Blood urea nitrogen (BUN)/creatinine (Cr):*** Measurement of organ involvement and indicator of early stage of endotoxin shock.	Increased levels of BUN and Cr are associated with dehydration, renal impairment or failure, and liver dysfunction or failure.
• ***Arterial blood gases (ABGs):*** Measures pH level and oxygen and carbon dioxide concentrations in arterial blood.	Early respiratory alkalosis and hypoxemia may occur. In later states, hypoxemia, respiratory acidosis, and lactic and metabolic acidosis occur because of failure of compensatory mechanisms.
OTHER DIAGNOSTIC STUDIES	
• ***Culture and sensitivity—wound, sputum, urine, blood, spinal fluid, or invasive lines:*** Determine presence of infection and microorganism(s) susceptibility or resistance to specific antimicrobials.	Identifies causative organism(s) and appropriate treatment options. However, clients can deteriorate to full-blown septic shock without an identifiable microbial agent.
• ***Urinalysis:*** Screening test for common source of infectious process.	Presence of blood cells, protein, and bacteria in the urine suggests infection.

TEST WHY IT IS DONE (continued)	WHAT IT TELLS ME (continued)
• *Imaging studies*	
• *Chest and abdominal x-rays:* Screening procedure to help determine source of infection.	Chest x-ray may reveal pneumonia, a common source of infection. Free air in the abdomen may suggest organ perforation caused by infection.
• *Abdominal ultrasound:* Imaging technique that uses high-frequency sound waves to create an image of organs.	Modality of choice when biliary tract source is suspected.
• *Computed tomography (CT) scan or CAT scan:* X-ray procedure that uses a computer to produce a detailed picture of a cross section of the body.	Modality of choice when intra-abdominal abscess or other gastrointestinal (GI) tract disorders are suspected.

Nursing Priorities

1. Eliminate infection.
2. Support tissue perfusion or circulatory volume.
3. Prevent complications.
4. Provide information about disease process, prognosis, and treatment needs.

Discharge Goals

1. Infection eliminated or controlled.
2. Homeostasis maintained.
3. Complications prevented or minimized.
4. Disease process, prognosis, and therapeutic regimen understood.
5. Plan in place to meet needs after discharge.

NURSING DIAGNOSIS: risk for Infection [progression; opportunistic/hospital-acquired]

Risk Factors May Include

Immunosuppression—pharmaceutical agents (e.g., steroids); leukopenia
Invasive procedures; increased environmental exposure

Possibly Evidenced By

(Not applicable; presence of signs and symptoms establishes an *actual* diagnosis)

Desired Outcomes/Evaluation Criteria—Client Will

Infection Severity (NOC)

Achieve timely healing; be free of purulent secretions, drainage, or erythema; and be afebrile.

ACTIONS/INTERVENTIONS	RATIONALE
Infection Control (NIC) ***Independent***	
Examine client for possible source of infection, such as sore throat, sinus pain, burning with urination, localized abdominal pain, burns, open wounds or cellulitis, presence of invasive catheters, or lines.	Respiratory tract and urinary tract infection are the most frequent causes of sepsis, followed by abdominal and soft tissue infections. The use of intravascular devices is also a well-known cause of hospital-acquired sepsis.
Ensure multidisciplinary involvement in hand hygiene. Wash hands with antibacterial soap before and after each care activity, even when gloves are used.	Hand washing and hand hygiene reduce the risk of cross-contamination. *Note:* Methicillin-resistant *Staphylococcus aureus* (MRSA) is most commonly transmitted via direct contact with healthcare workers who fail to wash hands between client contacts. Healthcare professionals must assume responsibility for reducing risk of infection spread by observing strict hand hygiene and other infection-reducing measures (Johnson et al, 2012; Bosek, 2010).
Provide isolation and monitor visitors, as indicated.	Body substance isolation (BSI) should be used for all infectious clients. Wound and linen isolation and hand washing may be all that is required for draining wounds. Clients with diseases transmitted through air may also need airborne and droplet precautions. Reverse isolation and restriction of visitors may be needed to protect the immunosuppressed client.

(continues on page 670)

ACTIONS/INTERVENTIONS (continued)	RATIONALE (continued)
Encourage or provide frequent position changes, deep-breathing and coughing exercises.	Good pulmonary toilet may reduce respiratory compromise.
Encourage client to cover mouth and nose with tissue when coughing or sneezing. Place in private room if indicated. Wear mask when providing direct care as appropriate.	Appropriate behaviors, personal protective equipment, and isolation prevent spread of infection via airborne droplets.
Limit use of invasive devices and procedures when possible. Remove lines and devices when infection is present and replace if necessary.	Reduces number of possible entry sites for opportunistic organisms.
Inspect wounds and sites of invasive devices daily, especially parenteral nutrition lines. Document signs of local inflammation and infection and changes in character of wound drainage, sputum, or urine.	Catheter-related bloodstream infections have increased where central venous catheters are used in both acute and chronic care settings. Clinical signs, such as local inflammation or phlebitis, may provide a clue to portal of entry, type of primary infecting organism(s), as well as early identification of secondary infections.
Investigate reports of pain out of proportion to visible signs.	Pressure-like pain over area of cellulitis may indicate development of necrotizing fasciitis due to group A beta hemolytic streptococci (GABS), necessitating prompt intervention.
Maintain sterile technique when changing dressings, suctioning, and providing site care, such as an invasive line or a urinary catheter.	Medical asepsis prevents or limits introduction of bacteria and reduces the risk of nosocomial infection.
Wear gloves and gowns when caring for open wounds or anticipating direct contact with secretions or excretions.	Prevents spread of infection and cross-contamination.
Dispose of soiled dressings and other materials in double bag.	Appropriate disposal of contaminated materials reduces contamination and spread of organisms.
Note temperature trends and observe for shaking chills and profuse diaphoresis.	Fever (101°F–105°F [38.5°C–40°C]) is the result of endotoxin effect on the hypothalamus and pyrogen-released endorphins. Hypothermia lower than 96°F (36°C) is a grave sign reflecting advancing shock state, decreased tissue perfusion, and/or failure of the body's ability to mount a febrile response. Chills often precede temperature spikes in presence of generalized infection.
Monitor for signs of deterioration of condition or failure to improve with therapy.	Deterioration of clinical condition or failure to improve with therapy may reflect inappropriate or inadequate antibiotic therapy or overgrowth of resistant or opportunistic organisms.
Inspect oral cavity for white plaques. Investigate reports of vaginal and perineal itching or burning.	Depression of immune system and use of antibiotics increase the risk of secondary infections, particularly yeast—thrush.
Collaborative	
Obtain specimens of urine, blood, sputum, wound, and invasive lines or tubes for culture and sensitivity, as indicated.	Identification of portal of entry and organism causing the septicemia is crucial to effective treatment based on susceptibility to specific medications.
Monitor laboratory studies, such as WBC count with neutrophils and band counts.	The normal ratio of neutrophils to total WBCs is at least 50%; however, when WBC count is markedly decreased, calculating the absolute neutrophil count is more pertinent to evaluating immune status. Likewise, an initial elevation of band cells reflects the body's attempt to mount a response to the infection, whereas a decline indicates decompensation.
Administer medications, as indicated, for example:	
Anti-infective agents: broad-spectrum antibiotics, such as imipenem and cilastatin (Primaxin), meropenem (Merrem), ticarcillin and clavulanate (Timentin), piperacillin and tazobactam (Zosyn), clindamycin (Cleocin), vancomycin (Vancocin); aminoglycosides, such as tobramycin (Nebcin), gentamicin (Garamycin); cephalosporins, such as cefepime (Maxipime); fluoroquinolones, such as levofloxacin (Levaquin), ciprofloxin (Cipro)	Specific antibiotics are determined by culture and sensitivity tests, but therapy is usually initiated before obtaining results, using broad-spectrum antibiotics and/or based on most likely infecting organisms. *Note*: Studies indicate that there is growing recognition that methicillin-resistant *S. aureus* (MRSA) is a cause of sepsis not only in hospitalized clients but also in community-dwelling individuals without recent hospitalization. For these reasons, some physicians now recommend that severely ill individuals presenting with sepsis of unclear etiology be treated with intravenous vancomycin (adjusted for renal function) until the possibility of MRSA sepsis has been excluded (Schmidt, 2013).
antifungals, such as fluconazole (Diflucan), caspofungin acetate (Cancidas)	Antifungal therapy may be considered in client who has already been treated with antibiotics, who is neutropenic, receiving total parenteral nutrition (TPN), or who has central venous access in place.
Assist with or prepare for procedures, such as removal of infected devices, incision and drainage of abscess, or débridement of infected wounds, as indicated.	Removal of infection sources promotes healing.
Prepare for hyperbaric therapy, as appropriate.	Exposing wounds to high ambient oxygen tension therapy may be done to combat anaerobic infections.

NURSING DIAGNOSIS: Hyperthermia

May Be Related To

Illness—direct effect of circulating endotoxins on the hypothalamus
Increased metabolic rate
Dehydration

Possibly Evidenced By

Increase in body temperature above normal range
Flushed skin, warm to touch
Tachypnea, tachycardia

Desired Outcomes/Evaluation Criteria—Client Will

Thermoregulation (NOC)

Demonstrate temperature within normal range and be free of chills.
Experience no associated complications.

ACTIONS/INTERVENTIONS	RATIONALE
Fever Treatment (NIC)	
Independent	
Monitor client temperature—degree and pattern. Note shaking chills or profuse diaphoresis.	Temperature of 102°F to 106°F (38.9°C–41.1°C) suggests acute infectious disease process. Fever pattern may aid in diagnosis: Sustained or continuous fever curves lasting more than 24 hours suggest pneumococcal pneumonia, scarlet or typhoid fever; remittent fever varying only a few degrees in either direction reflects pulmonary infections; and intermittent curves or fever that returns to normal once in 24-hour period suggests septic episode, septic endocarditis, or tuberculosis (TB). Chills often precede temperature spikes. *Note:* Use of antipyretics alters fever patterns and may be restricted until diagnosis is made or if fever remains higher than 102°F (38.9°C).
Monitor environmental temperature. Limit or add bed linens, as indicated.	Room temperature and linens should be altered to maintain near-normal body temperature.
Provide tepid sponge baths. Avoid use of alcohol.	Tepid sponge baths may help reduce fever. *Note:* Use of ice water or alcohol may cause chills, actually elevating temperature. Alcohol can also cause skin dehydration.
Collaborative	
Administer antipyretics, such as acetylsalicylic acid (ASA) (aspirin) or acetaminophen (Tylenol).	Antipyretics reduce fever by its central action on the hypothalamus; fever should be controlled in clients who are neutropenic or asplenic. However, fever may be beneficial in limiting growth of organisms and enhancing autodestruction of infected cells.
Provide cooling blanket, or hypothermia therapy, as indicated.	Used to reduce fever, especially when higher than 104°F to 105°F (39.5°C–40°C) and when seizures or brain damage are likely to occur.

NURSING DIAGNOSIS: risk for Shock

Risk Factors May Include

Infection; sepsis
Relative or actual hypovolemia; hypotension
Systemic inflammatory response syndrome

Possibly Evidenced By

(Not applicable; presence of signs and symptoms establishes an *actual* diagnosis)

Desired Outcomes/Evaluation Criteria—Client Will

Shock Severity: Sepsis (NOC)

Display adequate perfusion as evidenced by stable vital signs, palpable peripheral pulses, skin warm and dry, usual level of mentation, individually appropriate urinary output, and active bowel sounds.

ACTIONS/INTERVENTIONS	RATIONALE
Shock Prevention (NIC)	
Independent	
Monitor trends in blood pressure (BP), especially noting progressive hypotension and widening pulse pressure.	Hypotension develops as circulating microorganisms stimulate release and activation of chemical and hormonal substances. These endotoxins initially cause peripheral vasodilation, decreased systemic vascular resistance (SVR), and relative hypovolemia. As shock progresses, cardiac output becomes severely depressed due to major alterations in contractility, preload, and/or afterload, thus producing profound hypotension.
Monitor heart rate and rhythm. Note dysrhythmias.	Tachycardia occurs because of sympathetic nervous system stimulation secondary to stress response and to compensate for the relative hypovolemia and hypotension. Cardiac dysrhythmias can occur because of hypoxia, acid-base and electrolyte imbalance, and/or low-flow perfusion state.
Note quality and strength of peripheral pulses.	Initially, the pulse is strong and bounding because of increased cardiac output. Pulse may become weak and thready because of sustained hypotension, decreased cardiac output, and peripheral vasoconstriction if the shock state progresses.
Assess respiratory rate, depth, and quality. Note onset of severe dyspnea.	Increased respirations occur in response to direct effects of endotoxins on the respiratory center in the brain, as well as developing hypoxia, stress, and fever. Respirations become shallow as respiratory insufficiency develops, creating risk of acute respiratory failure.
Investigate changes in sensorium—mental cloudiness, agitation, restlessness, personality changes, delirium, stupor, and coma.	Changes in mentation reflect alterations in cerebral perfusion, hypoxemia, and/or acidosis.
Assess skin for changes in color, temperature, and moisture.	Vasodilation results in the warm, dry, pink skin characteristic of hyperperfusion in hyperdynamic phase of early septic shock. If shock state progresses, compensatory vasoconstriction occurs, shunting blood to vital organs, reducing peripheral blood flow, and creating cool, clammy, pale, and dusky skin.
Record hourly urinary output and specific gravity.	Decreasing urinary output with high specific gravity indicates diminished renal perfusion related to fluid shifts and selective vasoconstriction. There may be transient polyuria during hyperdynamic phase, while cardiac output is elevated, but this may progress to oliguria.
Auscultate bowel sounds.	Reduced blood flow to the mesentery (splanchnic vasoconstriction) decreases peristalsis and may lead to paralytic ileus or possibly trigger multiple organ dysfunction syndrome (MODS).
Hematest gastric secretions and stools for occult blood.	Stress of illness and use of steroids increase risk of gastric mucosal erosion and bleeding.
Evaluate lower extremities for local tissue swelling, erythema, and positive Homans' sign.	Venous stasis, changes in the coagulation processes, and infection may result in the development of thrombosis.
Maintain sequential compression devices (SCDs), as indicated.	These are preventive measures for bedfast client to reduce lower-extremity stasis complications.
Monitor for signs of bleeding: oozing from puncture sites or suture lines, petechiae, ecchymoses, hematuria, epistaxis, hemoptysis, and hematemesis.	Coagulopathies such as DIC may occur, related to accelerated clotting in the microcirculation reflecting activation of chemical mediators, vascular insufficiency, and cell destruction, creating a life-threatening hemorrhagic situation and multiple emboli.
Note drug effects, and monitor for signs of toxicity.	Massive doses of antibiotics have potentially toxic effects in clients with compromised renal and/or hepatic function.
Collaborative	
Administer parenteral fluids. (Refer to ND: risk for deficient Fluid Volume, following.)	Parenteral fluid therapy helps maintain tissue perfusion and expand circulating volume.
Administer drugs, as indicated, for example:	
Corticosteroids	Although steroid therapy remains controversial, low-dose steroids may be given for the potential advantages of decreasing capillary permeability, increasing renal perfusion, and inhibiting microemboli formation. *Note:* Adrenal insufficiency occurs in many clients with septic shock. Appropriate dosing of steroids provides support to dysfunctional adrenal glands and enhances vasomotor tone.
Inotropic agents and vasopressors, such as norepinephrine (Levophed), dopamine (Intropin), dobutamine (Dobutamine), vasopressin (Pitressin) (Mink, 2012)	Inotropic agents and vasopressors may be needed to improve organ perfusion and to maintain blood pressure during and after fluid treatment. *Note:* Client needing this level of support is critically ill and will be treated in the ICU.

ACTIONS/INTERVENTIONS (continued)	RATIONALE (continued)
Low-molecular-weight heparin, such as enoxaparin (Lovenox), dalteparin (Fragmin), and tinzaparin (Innohep); and unfractionated heparin	Low-molecular-weight heparin prevents or treats deep vein thrombosis (DVT). (Refer to CP: Thrombophlebitis: Venous Thromboembolism.)
Histamine-2 receptor blockers, such as cimetidine (Tagamet), famotidine (Pepcid AC), nizatidine (Asid), and ranitidine (Zantac)	Histamine receptor blockers prevent or treat stress ulcers.
Monitor laboratory studies, such as ABGs and lactate levels.	Circulatory collapse reduces tissue perfusion. Inadequate renal perfusion alters filtration, reabsorption, and secretion of various substances, resulting in fluid and electrolyte imbalances. ABGs and serum lactate levels indicate acid-base balance and anaerobic metabolism. Respiratory or metabolic acidosis indicates weakened compensatory mechanisms. Lactic acid accumulation is due to inadequate oxygenation and thus accumulation of anaerobic by-products or lactate.
Provide supplemental oxygen.	Supplemental oxygen improves cellular oxygenation.
Maintain stable body temperature, using adjunctive aids as necessary. (Refer to ND: Hyperthermia.)	Temperature elevations increase metabolic and oxygen demands beyond cellular resources, hastening tissue ischemia and cellular destruction.
Prepare for and transfer to critical care setting, as indicated.	Progressive deterioration requires more aggressive therapy including hemodynamic monitoring and vasoactive drug infusions.

NURSING DIAGNOSIS: risk for deficient Fluid Volume

Risk Factors May Include

Marked increase in vascular compartment, massive vasodilation

Capillary permeability with fluid leaks into the interstitial space (third spacing)

Possibly Evidenced By

(Not applicable; presence of signs and symptoms establishes an *actual* diagnosis)

Desired Outcomes/Evaluation Criteria—Client Will

Hydration (NOC)

Maintain adequate circulatory volume as evidenced by vital signs within client's normal range, palpable peripheral pulses of good quality, and individually appropriate urinary output.

ACTIONS/INTERVENTIONS	RATIONALE
Shock Prevention (NIC)	
Independent	
Measure and record urinary output and specific gravity. Note cumulative intake and output (I&O) imbalances (including insensible losses), and correlate with daily weight. Encourage oral fluids, as tolerated.	Decreasing urinary output with a high specific gravity suggests relative hypovolemia associated with vasodilation. Continued positive fluid balance with corresponding weight gain may indicate third spacing and tissue edema, suggesting need to alter fluid therapy or replacement components. *Note:* Excessive diarrhea may lead to a negative fluid balance.
Monitor BP and heart rate. Measure central venous pressure (CVP) if used.	Reduction in the circulating fluid volume reduces BP and CVP, initiating compensatory mechanisms of tachycardia to improve cardiac output and increase systemic blood pressure.
Palpate peripheral pulses.	Weak, easily obliterated pulses suggest hypovolemia.
Assess for dry mucous membranes, poor skin turgor, and thirst.	Hypovolemia and third spacing of fluid give rise to signs of dehydration.
Observe for dependent or peripheral edema in sacrum, scrotum, back, and legs.	Fluid losses from the vascular compartment into the interstitial space create tissue edema.
Collaborative	
Administer IV fluids, such as isotonic crystalloids (D_5W, normal saline [NS], lactated Ringer's [LR]), and colloids (albumin, fresh frozen plasma), as indicated.	Fluid therapy is most effective early in the course of severe sepsis because as the condition worsens, there is greater dysfunction at the cellular level. Large volumes of fluid may be required to overcome relative hypovolemia or peripheral vasodilation and replace losses from increased capillary permeability (e.g., sequestration of fluid in the peritoneal cavity) and increased insensible sources such as fever and diaphoresis (Mink, 2012).

(continues on page 674)

ACTIONS/INTERVENTIONS (continued)	RATIONALE (continued)
Monitor laboratory values, such as the following:	
Hct/RBC count	Evaluates changes in hydration/blood viscosity.
BUN/Cr	The BUN/Cr ratio could indicate dehydration or renal dysfunction and failure.
Monitor cardiac output, as indicated.	Cardiac output, and other functional parameters, such as cardiac index, preload, afterload, contractility, and cardiac work, can be measured noninvasively using thoracic electrical bioimpedance (TEB) technique. Cardiac output determination is useful in determining therapeutic needs and effectiveness.

NURSING DIAGNOSIS: risk for acute Confusion

Risk Factors May Include

Infection

Metabolic abnormalities (e.g., dehydration, electrolyte imbalance, increased blood urea nitrogen [BUN]/creatinine)

Pharmaceutical agents—multiple medications

Possibly Evidenced By

(Not applicable; presence of signs and symptoms establishes an *actual* diagnosis)

Desired Outcomes/Evaluation Criteria—Client Will

Cognition (NOC)

Maintain usual level of consciousness and cognition.

ACTIONS/INTERVENTIONS	RATIONALE
Delirium Management (NIC)	
Independent	
Note presence of factors that can contribute to confusion.	Disease process of sepsis (e.g., presence of circulating toxins, fluid and electrolyte imbalances, and fever) can contribute to confusion.
Assess mental/cognitive status, noting alertness, orientation, attention span, appropriateness of verbal responses.	Helps to identify a potential cognitive decline, possibly manifested by confusion.
Monitor temperature and note trends.	Although fever is usually present, hyperthermia can lead to confusion. It is important to determine if fever is related to the environment or to alterations in client metabolic processes.
Evaluate nutritional status.	Deficiencies of essential nutrients can affect mental status.
Note sleep/rest problems.	Sleep deprivation due to disease process or intensity of treatment interventions and environment can cause confusion.
Monitor intake and output; offer fluids accordingly.	Dehydration and electrolyte imbalances can cause or exacerbate confusion.
Encourage deep breathing or use of incentive spirometer.	Promotes respiratory function, improving oxygenation of brain tissues, which may improve cognitive function.
Collaborative	
Monitor ABGs, pulse oximetry, and end-tidal CO_2.	Identifies hypoxemia and hypercarbia, which may lead to altered cerebral functioning. Managing acid-base and metabolic imbalances can help minimize alterations in cerebral function.
Assist with treatment of underlying disease process.	As infection subsides, potential for confusion is reduced as well.
Administer fluids and electrolyte replacements as indicated.	Managing fluid, acid-base, and electrolyte imbalances can help minimize alterations in cerebral function.
Administer supplemental oxygen, as indicated.	Increases oxygen saturation and improves cerebral perfusion and function.
Administer nutritional support as indicated.	Increased metabolic rate associated with illness and fever can result in nutritional deficits especially when client is too ill for oral intake and/or gastrointestinal motility is decreased.

NURSING DIAGNOSIS: risk for impaired Gas Exchange

Risk Factors May Include

Alveolar-capillary membrane changes—increased capillary permeability leading to pulmonary congestion

[Altered O_2 supply—effects of endotoxins on the respiratory center in the medulla (resulting in hyperventilation and respiratory alkalosis); hypoventilation]

[Interference with oxygen delivery and utilization in the tissues (endotoxin-induced damage to the cells and capillaries)]

Possibly Evidenced By

(Not applicable; presence of signs and symptoms establishes an *actual* diagnosis)

Desired Outcomes/Evaluation Criteria—Client Will

Respiratory Status: Gas Exchange (NOC)

Display ABGs and respiratory rate within client's normal range, with breath sounds clear and chest x-ray clear or improving.

Experience no dyspnea or cyanosis.

ACTIONS/INTERVENTIONS	RATIONALE
Respiratory Monitoring (NIC)	
Independent	
Maintain client airway. Place client in position of comfort with head of bed elevated 30 to 45 degrees.	Elevating the head of bed enhances lung expansion and reduces respiratory effort.
Monitor respiratory rate and depth. Note use of accessory muscles or work of breathing.	Rapid, shallow respirations occur because of hypoxemia, stress, and circulating endotoxins. Hypoventilation and dyspnea reflect ineffective compensatory mechanisms and are indications that ventilatory support is needed.
Auscultate breath sounds. Note crackles, wheezes, and areas of decreased or absent ventilation.	Respiratory distress and the presence of adventitious sounds are indicators of pulmonary congestion, interstitial edema, and atelectasis. *Note:* Respiratory complications, including pneumonia and acute respiratory distress syndrome (ARDS), are prime causes of death.
Note presence of circumoral cyanosis.	Circumoral cyanosis indicates inadequate central oxygenation and hypoxemia.
Investigate alterations in sensorium: agitation, confusion, personality changes, delirium, stupor, and coma.	Cerebral function is very sensitive to decreases in oxygenation such as hypoxemia, or reduced perfusion.
Note cough and purulent sputum production.	Pneumonia is a common nosocomial infection that can occur by aspiration of oropharyngeal organisms or spread from other sites.
Reposition frequently. Encourage coughing and deep-breathing exercises. Suction, as indicated.	Good pulmonary toilet is necessary for reducing ventilation/perfusion imbalance and for mobilizing and facilitating removal of secretions to maximize gas exchange.
Oxygen Therapy (NIC)	
Collaborative	
Monitor ABGs and pulse oximetry.	Hypoxemia is related to decreased ventilation and pulmonary changes (e.g., interstitial edema, atelectasis, and pulmonary shunting) and increased oxygen demands caused by fever or infection. Respiratory acidosis (pH below 7.35 and $PaCO_2$ higher than 40 mm Hg) occurs because of hypoventilation and ventilation-perfusion imbalance. As septic condition worsens, metabolic acidosis (pH below 7.35 and HCO_3 less than 22–24 mEq/L) develops as a result of buildup of lactic acid from anaerobic metabolism.
Review serial chest x-rays.	Changes on x-ray reflect progression or resolution of pulmonary complications, such as infiltrates and edema.
Oxygen Therapy (NIC)	
Administer supplemental oxygen via appropriate route: nasal cannula, mask, or high-flow rebreathing mask.	Supplemental oxygen is necessary for correction of hypoxemia with failing respiratory effort or progressing acidosis. *Note:* Intubation and mechanical ventilation may be required if respiratory failure develops.
Administer red blood cells (RBCs), as indicated.	May be required to improve available oxygen to treat sepsis-induced hypoperfusion or when Hct is less than 30% (Kleinpell, 2006).

NURSING DIAGNOSIS: deficient Knowledge [Learning Need] regarding illness, prognosis, treatment, self-care, and discharge needs

May Be Related To

Lack of exposure or recall, information misinterpretation
Cognitive limitation

Possibly Evidenced By

Questions, request for information, statement of misconception
Inaccurate follow-through of instructions, development of preventable complications

Desired Outcomes/Evaluation Criteria—Client Will

Knowledge: Infection Management (NOC)

Verbalize understanding of disease process, prognosis, and potential complications.
Correctly perform necessary procedures and explain reasons for the actions.
Initiate necessary lifestyle changes.
Verbalize understanding of therapeutic needs.
Participate in treatment regimen.

ACTIONS/INTERVENTIONS	RATIONALE
Teaching: Disease Process (NIC)	
Independent	
Review disease process and future expectations.	Open discussion regarding the disease and clinical expectations provides knowledge base from which client can make informed choices.
Review individual risk factors, mode of transmission, and portal of entry of infections.	Awareness of means of infection transmission provides opportunity to plan for and institute protective measures.
Provide information about drug therapy, interactions, side effects, and importance of adherence to regimen.	Adequate and appropriate information promotes understanding and enhances compliance with treatment or prophylaxis and reduces risk of recurrence and complications.
Discuss need for good nutritional intake or balanced diet.	Good nutrition is necessary for optimal healing, immune system enhancement, and general well-being.
Encourage adequate rest periods with scheduled activities.	Rest prevents fatigue, conserves energy, and facilitates recovery.
Review necessity of personal hygiene and environmental cleanliness, proper cooking techniques, and food storage.	Personal hygiene and environmental cleanliness reduce exposure to pathogens.
Discuss proper use or avoidance of tampons with menstruating women, as indicated.	Superabsorbent tampons or infrequent tampon changing potentiates risk of *Staphylococcus aureus* infection and toxic shock syndrome.
Identify signs and symptoms requiring medical evaluation: persistent temperature elevation(s), tachycardia, syncope, rashes of unknown origin, unexplained fatigue, anorexia, increased thirst, and changes in bladder function.	Early recognition of developing or recurring infection allows for timely intervention and reduces risk for progression to life-threatening situation.
Emphasize importance of prophylactic immunizations and antibiotic therapy, as needed.	Prophylactic vaccines and antibiotics prevent infection, especially in high-risk groups such as those of advanced age or with chronic illness and/or a past history of infective heart disease and immunosuppression.

POTENTIAL CONSIDERATIONS following acute hospitalization (dependent on client's age, physical condition and presence of complications, personal resources, and life responsibilities)

- ***risk for recurrence/opportunistic Infection***—stasis of body fluids, decreased hemoglobin, leukopenia, suppressed inflammatory response, use of anti-infective agents, increased environmental exposure, malnutrition
- ***imbalanced Nutrition: less than body requirements***—biological factors (e.g., increased energy needs [hypermetabolic state], anorexia, continuing GI dysfunction, side effects of medication)
- ***Self-Care Deficit/impaired Home Maintenance***—fatigue, pain/discomfort, inadequate support systems, unfamiliarity with neighborhood resources

THE HIV-POSITIVE CLIENT

I. Pathophysiology

a. Infection by a subgroup of retroviruses with a high affinity for CD4 T-lymphocytes and monocytes, with viral DNA incorporating itself into host DNA (Dubin, 2008)

b. Following successful transmission of HIV, the course of subsequent infection is variable and dependent on a number of factors.

c. Main consequence of infection is damage to the immune system.

II. Stages: Continuum with progression individually variable (Health24, 2012)

a. *Infection or initial incubation period* lasts 2 to 4 weeks.
   - i. Individual asymptomatic
   - ii. HIV test negative but individual is infectious.

b. *Primary infection or acute seroconversion stage* usually occurs 4 to 8 weeks after infection.
   - i. Individual may be asymptomatic or develop flu-like symptoms—low-grade fever, sore throat, swollen lymph nodes, rash, joint and muscle pain lasting 1 to 2 weeks.
   - ii. HIV positive but immune system usually functional

c. *Latency or asymptomatic stage* can last anywhere from 2 weeks to years.
   - i. Virus remains active.
   - ii. Individual may be unaware of HIV status.

d. *Mild to moderate stage* usually occurs between 5 to 7 years after infection.
   - i. Immune system is compromised.
   - ii. Individual symptomatic—skin rashes; fatigue; night sweats; weight loss; mouth ulcers; fungal skin and nail infections, which progress to chronic oral or vaginal thrush; recurrent herpes blisters on mouth or genitals; ongoing fevers; persistent diarrhea

e. *Severe or late-stage HIV disease:* Median occurrence is 11 years' postinfection.
   - i. Viral load is very high; CD4 count is very low, thus indicating full-blown AIDS.
   - ii. Severe immune system damage and development of opportunistic infections. (Refer to CP: Acquired Immunodeficiency Syndrome (AIDS) for information.)

III. Etiology

a. Infection results from one of two similar retroviruses—HIV-1 and HIV-2—that destroy CD4 lymphocytes and impair cell-mediated immunity, thereby increasing the risk of certain infections and cancers.

b. Mode of transmission
   - i. Sexual contact—deposition of HIV on mucosal surfaces, especially the genital mucosa and intestinal epithelium (most common mode)
   - ii. Needle sharing with an infected person or use of contaminated blood products (rare in United States)
   - iii. Mother-to-baby perinatal transmission and through breast feeding (World Health Organization [WHO], 2007)

c. Worldwide, high-risk populations—sex workers, men who have sex with men, injection drug users, and prisoners (United Nations Programme on HIV/AIDS [UNAIDS] & World Health Organization [WHO], 2007)

d. Risk and severity of opportunistic infections, AIDS, and AIDS-related cancers are determined by the CD4 lymphocyte count and the client's exposure to potentially opportunistic pathogens.

e. Ability of virus to mutate has made disease management challenging, which has hindered efforts at development of a vaccine.

IV. Statistics

a. Morbidity: In 2011, there were an estimated 34 million people worldwide with HIV (Kaiser Family Foundation [KKF], 2012); in 2011, an estimated 49,273 Americans were newly diagnosed (Centers for Disease Control [CDC], 2011). New infections are still increasing in some age ranges (e.g., 13–29); among certain race/ethnicities (American Indians/Alaskan Natives); and in certain transmission categories, including male-to-male sexual contact and injection drug use (CDC, 2010). At the end of 2009, an estimated 1,148,200 persons aged 13 and older were living with HIV infection in the United States, including an estimated 207,600 persons whose infections had not yet been diagnosed (CDC, 2011).

b. Mortality: Associated with progression to AIDS; an estimated 17,774 people with AIDS died in 2009, and nearly 619,400 people with AIDS in the United States have died since the epidemic began (CDC surveillance report, 2010). Without treatment most persons with HIV develop AIDS within 10 years of infection, which results in increased morbidity and mortality (CDC, MMWR Vital Signs, 2011).

c. Cost: The average annual per patient cost of HIV treatment and care in the United States was nearly $20,000, based on 2006 figures, according to a study published in NAMAIDS (2010). Costs were highest for those with a CD4 cell count below 50 cells/mm^3 due to the high cost of inpatient care. For patients with a CD4 cell count above this level, antiretroviral therapy was the most expensive element of care. The study also makes the point that the "estimated costs do not include those associated with mental health care, treatment for drug or alcohol abuse, or social services. Moreover, the investigators caution that the ongoing costs of HIV therapy and an increase in age-related illness means that "it is likely that the aggregate costs of HIV care will continue to increase for the foreseeable future" (Gebo et al, 2010). According to the Kaiser Family Foundation (KKF), in FY 2012 the U.S. federal government spent a total of $14.8 billion on HIV care, with $5.8 billion to Medicare, $5.3 billion to Medicaid (with an additional states' share of $4.3 billion), $2.4 billion to Ryan White programs, and the rest to PEPFAR and other programs (KKF, 2013).

GLOSSARY

Acquired immunodeficiency syndrome (AIDS): Outcome of infection with a retrovirus (HIV).

Acute retroviral syndrome (ACR): Describes a group of symptoms that can resemble mononucleosis—fever, fatigue, muscle aches, loss of appetite, upset stomach, and weight loss.

CD4: Type of protein molecule in the blood that is present on the surface of immune cells. The HIV virus infects cells that have CD4 surface proteins and, as a result, depletes the number of T cells, B cells, natural killer cells, and monocytes in the blood. Most of the damage to the immune system is through destruction of CD4 lymphocytes.

Electrophoresis: Method of separating large molecules, such as DNA fragments or proteins, from a mixture of similar molecules.

Herpes simplex virus (HSV-2): Virus that has deleterious effects with co-infection of HIV.

Human immunodeficiency virus (HIV): Virus that causes a progressive disease leading to AIDS.

Seroconversion: Development of an antibody response to infection that is measurable in the serum. The HIV seropositive individual is one who is asymptomatic and who does not meet the Centers for Disease Control and Prevention definition for AIDS (CDC, 1987).

Sexually transmitted infections (STIs): Group of infections that can be transferred from one person to another through sexual contact (vaginal, anal, oral); includes chlamydia, syphilis, herpes, genital warts, and gonorrhea, among others.

T cells: Lymphocytes that originate in the thymus gland and regulate the immune system's response to infections, including HIV; CD4 lymphocytes are a subset of T lymphocytes.

Thrush: Fungal infection of the mucous membranes appearing as a patchy, raised white rash or spots.

Viral load tests: Detects viral RNA levels as low as 50 copies.

Care Setting

Client is treated in a community setting, although development of opportunistic infections may require occasional inpatient acute medical care.

Related Concerns

Acquired immunodeficiency syndrome (AIDS), page 689
Extended/long-term care, page 781
Fluid and electrolyte imbalances, page 885
Pneumonia, page 129
Psychosocial aspects of care, page 729
Sepsis/septicemia, page 665

Client Assessment Database

Although client may be asymptomatic, refer to CP: Acquired Immunodeficiency Syndrome (AIDS) for potential signs and symptoms. Refer to section at end of plan for ongoing considerations.

Diagnostic Studies

TEST WHY IT IS DONE	WHAT IT TELLS ME
BLOOD TESTS	
• ***HIV antibody test:*** Detects HIV antibodies in the blood.	Antibodies to HIV are produced by the body and can be detected in the blood about 2 to 4 weeks after exposure to the virus.
• ***Rapid HIV tests—OraQuick ADVANCE Rapid HIV-1/2 Antibody Test, MultiSpot HIV-1/HIV-2 Rapid Test, Clearview COMPLETE HIV-1/2, Clearview HIV1/2 Stat Pak, Reveal G-3Rapid HIV-1 Antibody Test, UNI-Gold Recombigen HIV (1):*** Antibody tests that are now available in the United States. In 2012 the first in-home antibody test was approved, marketed as Oraquick In Home HIV Test.	Positive results should be followed up with additional tests (Greenwald et al, 2006).
• ***Enzyme-linked immunosorbent assay (ELISA):*** Sensitive immunoassay that uses an enzyme linked to an antibody or antigen as a marker for the detection of a specific protein.	Determines exposure to a particular infectious agent, such as the HIV virus, by identifying antibodies present in a blood sample; however, it is not diagnostic because seroconversion can occur between 4 weeks and 6 months after exposure.
• ***Rapid plasma reagin test:*** Detects antibodies in the blood. Can be used as a rapid screening test, with positive results requiring confirmation by Western blot test.	During initial stage, assay test to diagnose acute HIV antibodies will be negative; however, rapid plasma reagin test may identify acute HIV infection before antibodies have developed.
• ***Western blot test:*** Technique for identifying specific antibodies or proteins in which proteins are separated by electrophoresis.	Confirms diagnosis of HIV-1 in individuals with positive ELISA screening.

TEST WHY IT IS DONE (continued)	WHAT IT TELLS ME (continued)
VIRAL LOAD TESTS	
• ***Reverse transcriptase–polymerase chain reaction (RT-PCR):*** Highly sensitive technique for detecting and quantifying viral load.	Detects viral RNA levels as low as 50 copies/mL of plasma.
• ***Branched DNA (bDNA) 3.0 assay:*** Has a wider range—50 to 500,000 copies/mL. (The RT-PCR range is 50–75,000/mL.)	Currently the leading indicator of effectiveness of therapy. Therapy can be initiated, or changes made in treatment approaches, based on rise of viral load or maintenance of a low viral load.
• ***Genotypic assays:*** Determine the nature of HIV medication resistance.	Genotype assays identify the presence of specific viral mutations that are associated with resistance to specific drugs (Durham, 2010).
• ***CD8+ (CTL) (cytopathic suppressor cells):*** Current quantitative assays allow for rapid evaluation of levels.	CD8+ (CTL) have been strongly implicated in the control of HIV-1 replications. At late stage of infection, CD8+ (CTL) numbers are reduced.
• ***CD4 lymphocyte count (previously T4 helper cells):*** CD4 cells are a target for HIV infection and destruction.	Used to diagnose HIV infection and progression and to monitor effects of drug therapy. Clients with counts below 500 benefit from antiretroviral therapy; counts equal to or below 200 define progression to AIDS. Levels are measured immediately before and again 4 to 8 weeks after initiation of antiretroviral therapy.
• ***Serum glucose:*** Monitor for development of diabetes mellitus (DM) or side effect of protease inhibitors (PIs).	Glucose levels elevated because of insulin resistance. Increased risk for developing DM in presence of HIV infection.
• ***Complete blood count (CBC):*** Battery of screening tests, which typically includes hemoglobin (Hgb); hematocrit (Hct); red blood cell (RBC) count, morphology, indices, and distribution width index; platelet count and size; white blood cell (WBC) count and differential.	Hgb and RBC counts are decreased. Abnormalities in iron metabolism can result in anemia, which occurs in some asymptomatic clients with HIV and a high percentage of clients with advanced disease.
OTHER DIAGNOSTIC STUDIES	
• ***Pap smear:*** Detects precursor lesions that can precede the diagnosis of invasive carcinoma.	Higher incidence of abnormal cells occurs in HIV-infected women.
• ***Pelvic/genital examination:*** Direct visualization of structures and mucosal membranes.	Identifies presence of lesions from STIs.
• ***Chest x-ray:*** Procedure used to evaluate organs and structures within the chest for symptoms of disease.	Abnormalities suggest presence of TB, which is common with HIV infection, or other opportunistic infections.

Nursing Priorities

1. Promote acceptance of reality of diagnosis and condition.
2. Support incorporation of behavioral and lifestyle changes to enhance well-being.
3. Provide information about disease process, prognosis, and treatment needs.
4. Assist in developing plan and strategies to meet long-term medical, behavioral, and financial needs and enhancing quality of life.

Goals of Ongoing Care

1. Dealing with current situation realistically.
2. Participating in and appropriately managing therapeutic regimen.
3. Diagnosis, prognosis, and therapeutic regimen understood.
4. Plan in place to meet medical, behavioral change, and financial needs.

NURSING DIAGNOSIS: risk-prone Health Behavior

May Be Related To

Multiple stressors
Negative attitudes toward healthcare
Inadequate social support
Smoking; excessive alcohol

(continues on page 680)

NURSING DIAGNOSIS: risk-prone Health Behavior (continued)

Possibly Evidenced By

Demonstrates nonacceptance of, or minimizes, health status change
Failure to take action that prevents health problems
Failure to achieve optimal sense of control

Desired Outcomes/Evaluation Criteria—Client Will

Acceptance: Health Status (NOC)

Verbalize reality and acceptance of condition.
Demonstrate increased trust and participation in development of plan of action.
Initiate lifestyle changes that will permit adaptation to present life situations.

ACTIONS/INTERVENTIONS	RATIONALE
Crisis Intervention (NIC)	
Independent	
Evaluate client's ability to understand events and realistically appraise situation.	Provides base to develop plan of action.
Identify real barriers to adjustment.	Promotes opportunity to deal appropriately with real problems in client's individual situation.
Encourage expression of feelings, denial, shock, and fears. Listen without judgment, accepting client's expressions. Focus on positive outcomes.	It is important to convey belief in client's fears and feelings. By focusing on positive outcomes, client is encouraged to take charge of those areas in which changes can be made, such as managing medical regimen and behavior.
Challenge morbid thoughts and reframe into positive statements: "You know why the virus is going to kill me. I deserve to die for what I've done." Response: "The virus may or may not kill you. It's not smart enough to decide when you may die. The virus is 'just there.' It does not have a mind to know what you have or have not done."	Interrupts morbid thoughts and challenges client's self-deprecating ideas. As with any potentially terminal disease, this population is likely to experience depression and is at increased risk for suicide, necessitating ongoing evaluation.
Determine available resources and programs.	Identifies client needs and what comprehensive services might be available and immediately accessible. Services may include education concerning sexual myths, HIV transmission prevention, safer sex practices, and alternate methods of expressing sexuality. Interventions and education may be needed for addictive behaviors, such as the ability of injection drug user to obtain clean "works."
Assess social system as well as presence of support, perception of losses, and stressors.	Partners, friends, and families will have individual responses depending on the individual's lifestyle, knowledge of HIV transmission, and belief systems. *Note:* Belief systems can include values or myths, which affect how the individual approaches the disease and the outcome.
Encourage client to participate in support groups.	Long-term support is critical to dealing with and effectively coping with the reality of being HIV positive and with frequent healthcare evaluations, medical treatments, and ongoing lifestyle changes.
Educate client about drug interactions, HIV, and emotions.	Fatigue and depression can be side effects of some medications and of the infection itself. Knowledge that these effects are usually of short duration can support informed choices and cooperation and promote hope.
Encourage continued or renewed use of familiar effective coping strategies.	Client is supported and given encouragement for past effective behaviors. Positive reinforcement enhances self-esteem.
Explore use and practice of new and different coping strategies.	Using new strategies is uncomfortable in the beginning, but practice fosters self-confidence.
Help client use humor to combat stigmatization of the disease.	Humor defuses the sense of secretiveness people may place on diagnosis of, and dealing with, HIV.
Reinforce structure in daily life. Include exercise as part of routine.	Routines help the client focus. Exercise improves sense of wellness and enhances immune response.
Discuss meaning of high-risk behavior, such as unprotected sexual activity, injection drug use with shared needles, and failure to take medications; and address barriers to change.	Fear of disclosure, need to change usual behaviors, and the difficulty of doing so may prevent the individual from making the changes necessary to prevent transmission of disease and to manage lifestyle.
Assist client to set limits on sexually risky behaviors and explore ways client can achieve change.	Needs for love, comfort, and companionship that are met through sexual expression must be met safely through means that carry a reduced risk of HIV transmission.

ACTIONS/INTERVENTIONS (continued)	RATIONALE (continued)
Assist client to channel anger to healthy activities.	The increased energy of anger can be used to accomplish other tasks and enhance feelings of self-esteem.
Inform client about new medical advances and treatments.	Promotes hope and helps client make informed decisions.
Discuss issues of voluntary disclosure, personal responsibility, needs of others, and federal, state, and local reporting requirements.	Understanding responsibilities and consequences of disclosure is necessary for client to make informed decisions.
Collaborative	
Refer client to nurse practitioner or clinical nurse specialist, psychologist, or social worker knowledgeable about HIV as well as specific HIV programs and resources or appropriate research programs.	Trained professionals can help client adjust to difficult situation.

NURSING DIAGNOSIS: Fatigue

May Be Related To

Disease state; poor physical condition
Negative life events; stress
Anxiety; depression

Possibly Evidenced By

Reports an unremitting, overwhelming lack of energy
Reports inability to maintain usual routines
Decreased performance; lethargic; compromised concentration

Desired Outcomes/Evaluation Criteria—Client Will

Fatigue Level (NOC)
Report improved sense of energy.
Participate in desired activities at level of ability.

Energy Conservation (NOC)
Identify individual areas of control and engage in energy conservation techniques.

ACTIONS/INTERVENTIONS	RATIONALE
Energy Management (NIC)	
Independent	
Assess sleep patterns and other factors that may be aggravating fatigue.	Multiple factors can cause and aggravate fatigue, including sleep deprivation, emotional distress, side effects of drugs, and developing central nervous system (CNS) disease.
Encourage timely evaluation of fatigue if new medications have been added to regimen.	Fatigue is present in variable degrees as part of HIV infection process but is often aggravated by nutritional deficiencies and side effects of certain medications. For example, when PIs are added or changed, fatigue may worsen.
Discuss reality of client's feelings of exhaustion and identify limitations imposed by fatigue state. Advise client to maintain a fatigue diary, and note daily energy patterns—peaks and valleys.	Helpful in planning activities within tolerance levels. Clients often expect too much of themselves, believing that they should be able to do more.
Assist client to set realistic activity goals, determining individual priorities and responsibilities.	Client may need to alter priorities and delegate some responsibilities to manage fatigue and optimize performance.
Discuss energy conservation techniques, such as sitting instead of standing for activities, as appropriate.	Enables client to become aware of ways in which energy expenditure can be maximized to complete necessary tasks.
Review importance of meeting individual nutritional needs.	Adequate nutrition is needed for optimizing energy production. (Refer to ND: imbalanced Nutrition: less than body requirements, following.)
Encourage adequate rest periods during the day, routine schedule for bedtime and arising, and scheduling activities during time of best energy.	Helps client recoup energy to manage desired activities.
Instruct in stress management techniques, such as breathing exercises, visualization, and music and light therapy.	Reduction of stress factors in client's life can minimize energy output.
Identify available resources and support systems.	May require outside assistance with homemaking and maintenance activities and child care.

NURSING DIAGNOSIS: imbalanced Nutrition: less than body requirements

Risk Factors May Include

Inability to ingest/digest food
Insufficient finances
Biological factors (e.g., co-infections—thrush)

Possibly Evidenced By

Weight loss; poor muscle tone
Reports food intake less than recommended daily allowance
Lack of interest in food; aversion to eating; reports altered taste sensation; sore buccal cavity
Lack of information; misconceptions
Abdominal cramping; diarrhea
[Abnormal laboratory studies (e.g., vitamins, minerals, protein deficiency, electrolytes)]

Desired Outcomes/Evaluation Criteria—Client Will

Nutritional Status (NOC)

Maintain stable weight.
Report improved energy level.

Nutritional Status: Biochemical Measures (NOC)

Demonstrate laboratory values within normal limits.

ACTIONS/INTERVENTIONS	RATIONALE
Nutrition Management (NIC)	
Independent	
Determine usual weight before client was diagnosed with HIV.	Early wasting is not readily determined by normal weight-to-height charts; therefore, determining current weight in relation to prediagnosis weight is more useful. Recent unexplained or involuntary weight loss may be a factor in seeking initial medical evaluation.
Weigh regularly and establish current anthropometric measurements. Measure resting energy expenditure (REE) using indirect calorimetry.	Helps assess and monitor wasting and determine nutritional needs. Indirect calorimetry is more accurate for calculating REE than the Harris-Benedict equation, which underestimates the energy needs of these clients.
Determine client's current dietary pattern and intake and knowledge of nutrition. Use an in-depth dietary assessment tool.	Identification of these factors helps plan for individual needs. Clients with HIV infection have documented vitamin (e.g., vitamin B_{12}, folate) and trace mineral (e.g., zinc, magnesium, selenium) deficits. Alcohol and drug abuse can interfere with adequate intake.
Assess presence and degree of nausea and vomiting.	The causes of nausea and vomiting are numerous and are associated with medications, functional changes in gastrointestinal (GI) system, and endocrine dysfunction. Protracted nausea and vomiting can debilitate a client, leading to loss of lean body mass, electrolyte imbalances, and further deterioration of immune function.
Ascertain current financial status and recent and/or anticipated changes in economic status. Explore related costs of a variety of foods.	Helps in planning for meeting nutritional needs, such as purchasing low-cost foods that are nutritionally rich. Client may need referral to financial aid to help with food stamps or obtaining meals.
Discuss and document nutritional side effects of medications.	Commonly used medications cause anorexia, altered taste, nausea and/or vomiting; some interfere with bone marrow production of RBCs, causing anemia. Protease inhibitors (PIs) increase the risk of developing diabetes. GI symptoms are common with over-the-counter (OTC) drugs, such as NSAIDs, which may also contribute to anorexia.
Help client plan ways to maintain/improve intake. Identify lactose-free supplements, as appropriate. Provide information about nutritionally dense high-calorie, high-protein, high-vitamin, and high-mineral foods.	Having this information helps client understand importance of a well-balanced diet. Some clients may try macrobiotic and other diets, believing the diarrhea is caused by lactose intolerance. Eliminating dairy products can have detrimental effects when these nutrient components are not replaced from other sources.
Stress importance of maintaining balanced, adequate nutritional intake and fluids rich with electrolytes, such as Gatorade or Pedialyte.	Client may be depressed and discouraged by changed health and social status and find it difficult to eat for many reasons. Knowing how important nutritionally balanced intake is to supporting the immune system and remaining healthy can motivate client to eat.

ACTIONS/INTERVENTIONS (continued)	RATIONALE (continued)
Assist client to formulate dietary plan, taking into consideration increased metabolic demands and energy needs and hyperlipidemia.	Provides guidance and feedback while promoting sense of control, enhancing self-esteem, and possibly improving intake. HIV infection is continuously stimulating the immune system, increasing metabolic rate and nutritional needs. *Note:* Use of PIs is known to elevate levels of glucose and lipids—especially triglycerides and cholesterol.
Recommend eating frequent, small meals, avoiding cooking odors if bothersome, keeping room well ventilated, and removing noxious stimuli. Suggest use of spices, marinating red meat before cooking, and/or substituting other protein sources for red meat.	Reduces possible adverse stimuli or enhances palatability of food and may improve nutritional intake, which is needed to help client restore and maintain nutritional defenses.
Recommend environment conducive to eating. Emphasize importance of sharing mealtime with others. Identify someone who can join client for meals.	A quiet, relaxed, calm, unrushed setting and socialization can enhance appetite/food intake, especially when depression, neglect of self-care, and diminished appetite are present.
Explore complementary therapies and nonpharmacological interventions, such as acupressure, progressive relaxation, and guided imagery, to manage anorexia.	The goal of these interventions is to manage distressing symptoms that interfere with optimal nutritional intake.
Discuss use of *Lactobacillus acidophilus* replacement, such as LactAid dairy products and/or tablets/capsules.	HIV infection changes the structure of the gut wall, resulting in a decreased lactose level. Intolerance causes abdominal cramping, malabsorption, a bloated feeling, and diarrhea. Also, antibiotics taken for prevention of opportunistic infections cause changes in normal bowel flora, contributing to diarrhea.
Collaborative	
Consult with dietitian and nutritional support team.	Provides assistance in planning nutritionally sound diet and identifying nutritional supplements to meet individual needs. Liquid supplements (e.g., Advera) have been specifically formulated for the GI manifestations common to the HIV-positive population.
Monitor laboratory values, such as Hgb, RBCs, albumin or prealbumin, total iron-binding capacity (TIBC), potassium, and sodium.	These laboratory tests are important in monitoring the client's nutritional immune status and in identifying nutritional therapy needs. For example, anemia may require additional interventions, such as use of epoetin (Epogen or Procrit), to stimulate RBC production.
Provide medications, as indicated, for example:	
Dronabinol (Marinol), megestrol (Megace), and cyproheptadine (Periactin)	Antiemetics or appetite stimulants can improve intake to prevent and correct dietary deficiencies. *Note:* A side effect of Megace may include impotence, necessitating change of drug as desired.
Antidiarrheal medications, such as diphenoxylate/atropine (Lomotil) and octreotide (Sandostatin)	Diarrhea may be present because of altered GI flora and side effects of anti-infective agents. Treatment can correct malabsorption and enhance oral intake.

NURSING DIAGNOSIS: deficient Knowledge [Learning Need] regarding disease, prognosis, treatment, self-care, and discharge needs

May Be Related To
Lack of exposure or recall
Information misinterpretation
Unfamiliarity with information resources
Cognitive limitation

Possibly Evidenced By
Reports the problem
Inaccurate follow-through of instructions
Inappropriate behaviors—hostile, agitated, apathetic

Desired Outcomes/Evaluation Criteria—Client Will

Knowledge: Chronic Disease Management (NOC)
Verbalize understanding of condition, disease process, and potential complications.
Identify relationship of signs and symptoms to the disease process and correlate symptoms with causative factors.
Verbalize understanding of goals of treatment.
Initiate necessary lifestyle changes.
Participate in treatment regimen.

ACTIONS/INTERVENTIONS	RATIONALE
Learning Facilitation (NIC)	
Assess emotional and intellectual ability to assimilate information and understand instructions. Respect client's need to use denial and coping techniques initially.	Initial shock and anxiety can block intake of information. Self-esteem, lifestyle, guilt, and denial of own responsibility in acquiring or transmitting disease become issues that must be dealt with. *Note:* Some initial denial may serve as a protective mechanism promoting more effective self-care.
Provide realistic, optimistic information during each contact with client.	Necessary to provide realistic hope because many clients have been exposed to some inaccurate information about AIDS or may have friends or lovers who have died of the disease.
Plan frequent short sessions for teaching. Include written information, as appropriate—a few pieces at each visit.	Client will likely feel overwhelmed and need time and repeated contacts to absorb information, the scope of, and the requirements for, treating the infection. Written materials allow for later review and reinforcement of information presented.
Include significant other (SO) and family in discussions and conferences, as appropriate.	Provides opportunity to learn information first hand, ask questions, and provide support for client.
Teaching: Disease Process (NIC)	
Determine current understanding and perception of diagnosis. Discuss difference between HIV-positive status and AIDS.	Provides opportunity to clarify misconceptions and myths and make informed choices. People often believe that if they are positive for the virus, they have AIDS; having accurate information about the difference can alleviate fears and allow for development of an individualized plan of care.
Identify and problem-solve potential or actual barriers to accessing healthcare services.	Transportation, distance, child care, work schedule, homelessness, poverty, and lack of insurance or finances are some of the issues that typically interfere with accessing needed primary care and prophylactic interventions.
Provide information about normal immune system response and how HIV affects it, transmission of the virus, behaviors, and factors believed to increase probability of progression. Encourage questions.	Client needs to be aware of own personal risk and risk to others to make immediate and long-range decisions and establish a basis for goal setting. Also, establishes rapport and provides opportunity to identify concerns and assimilate information.
Review signs and symptoms that could be a consequence of HIV infection—mild fever, anorexia, weight loss, fatigue, night sweats, diarrhea, dry cough, rashes, headaches, and sleep disturbances.	Client may experience an acute illness 2 to 6 weeks after becoming infected; however, it is common for infection to be subclinical, with the individual simply feeling unwell.
Discuss management strategies for persistent signs and symptoms.	Client involvement in care increases cooperation and satisfaction with care.
Identify signs and symptoms that require medical evaluation—persistent fever, increasing cough, swollen lymph glands, profound fatigue unrelieved by rest, weight loss of 10 pounds or more in less than 2 months, severe or persistent diarrhea, blurred vision, skin discoloration or rash that persists or spreads, open sores anywhere, and symptoms occurring with medication regimen.	Early recognition of progression of disease and development of opportunistic infections provides for timely intervention and may prevent situations that are more serious. *Note:* Most HIV-positive clients are now on medication regimens (usually at least three drugs) and must adhere to the dosages and schedules, which may be difficult and/or cause side effects that tempt client to alter or discontinue them without notifying the physician.
Stress necessity of regular follow-up care and evaluations, including routine CD4 and HIV-RNA viral load counts, and any change in medication regimen including time, frequency, and side effects.	Even though client may be asymptomatic, periodic evaluation may prevent development of complications, slow the progression of the disease, and assist with treatment decisions. *Note:* Clients who change medication dosage and/or frequency in response to side effects can create problems for medication adjustment later with increased viral load and drug resistance.
Discuss need for regular gynecological examinations.	HIV-positive women experience a high prevalence of Pap smear, vaginal, and cervical abnormalities.
Discuss family planning issues and careful selection of oral contraceptives.	Various antiretroviral drugs have differing effects on ethinyl estradiol (EE), either enhancing or decreasing protective effectiveness.
Provide preconception counseling, giving information about risk of vertical transmission and ways to reduce the possibility of perinatal transmission.	The risk of viral rebound with adverse consequences to the fetus increases in women currently receiving treatment at the time of conception. Research shows that when antiretroviral treatment is initiated early in pregnancy, the perinatal transmission rate is less than 1%.
Refer to Antiretroviral Pregnancy Registry, as appropriate.	National and international research is ongoing on the safety of Highly Active Antiretroviral Therapy (HAART) for HIV-positive pregnant woman. Research has not found strong evidence that HAART significantly increases the risk of congenital malformation (Martin, 2009). However, certain drug categories

pose a risk for mitochondrial toxicity. There is also some evidence of increased risk for preterm delivery with use of combination HAART as compared with zidovudine monotherapy. In 2012, new practice guidelines for antiretroviral therapy (ARV) during pregnancy were federally approved in the United States. All pregnant HIV-infected women should receive a combination ARV regimen regardless of plasma RNA copy numbers or CD4 count. The choice of regimen reflects current adult treatment guidelines, taking pregnancy drug recommendations into consideration. The decision when to begin the regimen would depend on HIV-RNA levels and CD4 counts as well as overall maternal condition (NIH, 2012). A woman must be counseled prior to initiating therapy. Benefits versus risks, including effects on fetus, must be weighed, especially if regimen is started in first trimester.

Teaching: Prescribed Medication (NIC)

Review drug therapies, including correct dosing and scheduling, side effects, monitoring tests and techniques, and adverse reactions as appropriate:

Teaching about drug regimen will be highly individualized, depending on the client's needs. Many clients may now be taking all-in-one combination pills (e.g., elvitegravir-cobicistat + tenofovir + emtricilabine (Stribild) once daily, especially when HIV has been diagnosed in early stages. Others may be on more complex regimens.

- Nucleoside reverse transcriptase inhibitors (NRTIs): retrovir + epivir (Combivir), lamivudine (Epivir), zidovudine vilread + emtriva (Truvada), (Retrovir, AZT), ziagen + epivir (Epzicom), stavudine (Zerit), and tenofovir (Viread) (AIDSMEDS, 2012)

In the past, zidovudine was given alone and as a first-line treatment. Presently the drug is usually given in a three-drug treatment regimen, along with another NRTI and a protease inhibitor (PI), with the combination referred to as HAART.

- Protease inhibitors (PIs), such as lopinavir and ritonavir (Kaletra), tapranavir (Aptivus), indinavir (Crixivan), ritonavir (Norvir), saquinavir (Invirase), darunavir (Prezista), atazanavir (Reyataz), and nelfinavir (Viracept) (AIDSMEDS, 2012)

When combined with NRTIs, PIs control the HIV-RNA viral load by blocking viral replication at two different target sites in the replication process. Immune function is maintained with early intervention or improved when initiated later.

- Non-nucleoside reverse transcriptase inhibitors (NNRTIs), such as rilpivirine (Edurant), etravirine (Intelence), delaviridine (Rescriptor), nevirapine (Viramune), and efavirenz (Sustiva) (AIDSMEDS, 2012)

These drugs inhibit viral replication by a different mechanism than NRTIs or PIs. They also are used in combination to reduce possibility of drug resistance.

- Entry inhibitors, including fusion inhibitors, such as enfuvirtide (Fuzeon), maraviroc (Selzentry) (AIDSMEDS, 2012)

These drugs work by preventing HIV from entering healthy CD4 cells or by blocking enzyme needed for replication.

- All-in-one combination tablets, such as elvitegravir-cobicistat + tenofovir + emtricilabine (Stribild); efacirenz + tenofovir + emtricitabine (Atripla); rilpivirine + tenofovir + embricitabine (Complera) (AIDSMEDS, 2012)

These are complete one-pill, once-daily drug regimens.

- Anti-infectives, such as trimethoprim-sulfamethoxazole/TMP/SMX (Bactrim, Septra), azithromycin (Zithromax), clarithromycin (Biaxin), foscarnet (Foscavir), rifabutin (Mycobutin), isoniazid (INH), and pyridoxine (Doxine)

These focus on prevention of commonly occurring opportunistic infections, such as Pneumocystis pneumonia (PCP), caused by *Pneumocystis jiroveci,* the distinct species that infects humans; cytomegalovirus (CMV); *Mycobacterium avium* complex (MAC); or TB; and may prolong general wellness. Primary prophylactic therapy aims to prevent or delay onset of symptoms of reactivated or newly acquired infection. The goal of secondary prophylaxis is to prevent or delay recurrent episodes of particular infection.

Provide information about clinical trials available, as individually appropriate.

Scientific research requires HIV-positive test subjects. Participation may provide individual with a sense of contributing to the body of knowledge or search for a cure in addition to no-cost monitoring and medications for those with limited financial resources.

Provide information about pharmaceutical company assistance programs.

Some medications are provided free or at reduced cost, based on income.

Risk Identification (NIC)

Assess potential for inappropriate or high-risk behavior, such as continued injection drug abuse or unsafe sexual practices. Stress need to avoid use of illicit injected drugs or, if unwilling to abstain, to avoid sharing needles and to clean works with bleach solution, rinsing carefully with water.

High levels of denial, anger, or drug addiction may cause client to continue behaviors that are high risk for spread of the virus. Even moderate changes in lifestyle may reduce exposure to other infective agents that can cause additional stress to the immune system. *Note:* Client may intensify substance abuse as a means of denial. A sense of "not me" can contribute to continuation of risky behaviors.

(continues on page 686)

ACTIONS/INTERVENTIONS (continued)	RATIONALE (continued)
Recommend exploring drug treatment resources—methadone clinics or substance abuse recovery groups or programs.	May help reduce risk of HIV transmission by reducing injection drug use when client substitutes methadone, recovers from drug use, or learns safer injection and needle use techniques. *Note:* Some women may decrease drug use or be amenable to rehabilitation in an attempt to improve relationships with children or family.
Stress necessity of, and methods for, practicing safer sex at all times.	Limits spread of virus and exposure to other STIs. A person's sexual expression and identity are threatened by the discovery of the diagnosis. Therefore, many individuals with HIV will not reveal status to potential sexual partners, contributing to ongoing transmission. Women may not follow guidelines because partner refuses to use condoms.
Discuss active changes in sexual behaviors that client can make that may satisfy sexual needs.	Learning alternative forms of expression promotes a sense of responsibility and control. May reduce sexual tensions, promote normalcy in sexual relationships, and reduce fear or guilt related to potential transmission of HIV. *Note:* Clients, particularly women, may fear partner will leave, resulting in loss of love and emotional and financial support.
Provide information about other necessary lifestyle changes and health maintenance factors:	Evidence suggests that specific dietary and lifestyle factors may slow the progression of HIV infection because they support a healthier immune system.
Avoid people with infections.	When the immune system is depressed, the person's ability to fight exposure to common communicable diseases is limited.
Exercise within ability, alternate rest periods with activity, and get adequate sleep.	Helps manage fatigue; maintains strength and sense of well-being. Exercise has also been shown to stimulate the immune system.
Eat regularly, even if appetite is reduced; try small, frequent meals and snacks high in nutritional value; and discuss ways to control nausea and vomiting and improve appetite.	Physical and psychological stressors increase metabolic needs; in addition, side effects of medication, presence of nausea or vomiting, and anorexia often limit oral intake. The result is nutritional deficits that can further impair the immune system.
Practice daily oral hygiene, use a soft toothbrush; examine mouth regularly for sores, white film, or changes in color; and have regular dental checkups every 6 months.	Poor oral hygiene and dental care can affect oral intake adversely and increase the risk of opportunistic and systemic infections.
Examine skin for rashes, bruises, and breaks in skin integrity.	May indicate developing complications and increase risk of infection.
Identify additional resources—support groups, peer counselors, mental health professionals, and case managers.	Client will experience a variety of emotional and psychological responses to the diagnosis and its consequences and may need additional assistance and periodic reinforcement to promote optimal adjustment. *Note:* In early stages of HIV infection, focus may be on social services (e.g., help with housing, employment, legal issues, and finances). Later, as disease progresses, the emphasis switches to medical and related community services.

NURSING DIAGNOSIS: risk for Social Isolation

Risk Factors May Include

Altered state of wellness, alterations in physical appearance
Unaccepted social behavior or values
Inadequate personal resources

Possibly Evidenced By

(Not applicable; presence of signs and symptoms establishes an *actual* diagnosis)

Desired Outcomes/Evaluation Criteria—Client Will

Social Support (NOC)

Identify stable support system and supportive individual(s).
Use resources for assistance, as appropriate.

Loneliness Severity (NOC)

Express sense of satisfaction with relationship(s).

ACTIONS/INTERVENTIONS	RATIONALE
Support System Enhancement (NIC)	
Independent	
Determine client's response to condition, feelings about self, concerns or fears about response of others, sense of ability to control situation, and sense of hope.	How the individual accepts and deals with the situation will help decide the plan of care and interventions.
Assess coping mechanisms and previous methods of dealing with life problems.	May reveal successful techniques that can be used in current situation.
Discuss concerns regarding employment and leisure involvement. Note potential problems involving finances, insurance, and housing.	Clients with this potentially terminal illness, which carries a stigma, face major problems with possible loss of employment, medical insurance, housing, and care sources if they become unable to independently care for themselves.
Identify availability and stability of support systems, including SO, immediate and extended family, and community.	This information is crucial to help client plan future care.
Encourage honesty in relationships, as appropriate.	As a rule, acquaintances do not need to be informed of client's health status. However, information should be shared with close relationships such as SO, family, and sexual partners. Honesty can help identify stable support persons.
Encourage contact with SO, family, and friends.	Many clients fear telling SO, family, and friends for fear of rejection, and some clients withdraw because of tumultuous feelings. Contact promotes sense of support, concern, involvement, and understanding. Supporting loved ones as they learn of the diagnosis is beneficial and can provide optimism for the long term.
Assist client to problem-solve solutions to short-term and/or imposed isolations, such as communicable disease measures or severely compromised immune system.	Anticipatory planning can defuse sense of isolation and loneliness that can accompany these situations.
Help client differentiate between isolation and loneliness or aloneness, which may be by choice.	Provides an opportunity for client to realize the control he or she has to make decisions about the choice to take care of self about these issues.
Be alert to verbal and nonverbal cues, such as withdrawal, statements of despair, and sense of aloneness. Determine presence and level of risk of suicidal thoughts.	Indicators of despair and suicidal ideation may be present. When these cues are acknowledged, client is usually willing to divulge thoughts and sense of isolation and hopelessness.
Collaborative	
Identify community resources, self-help groups, and rehabilitation or drug cessation programs, as indicated.	Provides opportunities for resolving problems that may contribute to sense of loneliness and isolation, transmission risks, and sense of guilt.
Refer to psychiatric clinical nurse specialist or psychiatrist, as needed.	May require more in-depth support to deal with feelings and manage difficult situations.

NURSING DIAGNOSIS: ineffective Self-Health Management

May Be Related To
Complexity of healthcare system; economic difficulties
Complexity of therapeutic regimen; perceived seriousness, susceptibility, or benefits
Decisional conflicts, powerlessness
Family conflict; social support deficit

Possibly Evidenced By
Reports desire to manage illness
Reports difficulty with prescribed regimens
Failure to take action to reduce risk factors
Ineffective choices in daily living for meeting health goals

Desired Outcomes/Evaluation Criteria—Client/Family Will

Self-Management: Chronic Disease (NOC)
Identify individual factors affecting management of regimen.
Accept personal responsibility for own actions and participate in problem-solving activities.
Develop contract for care with mutually agreeable goals for treatment and mechanisms for changing or terminating elements of plan.

ACTIONS/INTERVENTIONS	RATIONALE
Patient Contracting (NIC)	
Independent	
Make time to listen to client concerns.	Promotes feelings of value and may identify additional factors that affect outcome of therapy. Timing of teaching needs to consider the stage of acceptance.
Note client's stage of acceptance of the diagnosis:	
Precontemplation stage	Client has just learned of the diagnosis and may not be able to participate in any discussions.
Contemplation stage	Client can participate in, and may initiate, discussions of therapy. Encourages individual's responsibility to be involved with planning. Promotes increased sense of control and self-esteem.
Action or maintenance stage	Client is actively involved in understanding and managing own care.
Determine client's and SO's perception or understanding of regimen.	Identifies areas of confusion or conflict or lack of accurate information that may impede cooperation with regimen.
Assess perceived and actual barriers to accessing healthcare services and reasons for deviations from prescribed plan.	Provides opportunity to clarify actual problems and develop alternative plan acceptable to healthcare provider.
Instruct client carefully in all aspects of medication regimen, times, interaction with food, and side effects:	Thorough understanding may enhance cooperation with regimen and help in identifying potential for compromise.
Provide written schedule, if desired.	Helpful for keeping track of multiple drugs and changes that occur.
Suggest placing doses of medications in various locations.	When client's routine is stable, and he or she engages in activities away from home, it is helpful to keep a supply of medications in more than one location such as work or home of family and friends.
Recommend various methods to alert client to medication time, such as portable pill container or alarms.	Will assist busy or forgetful client to take medications at appropriate intervals.
Reduce dose frequency and number of pills when possible.	Increases ability to manage treatment regimen with little interference.
Emphasize importance of keeping healthcare provider informed of concerns and ability to continue prescribed medication regimen.	Drug levels quickly fall below therapeutic levels if one dose is missed. Reduces potential for drug resistance or increased viral load. Poor adherence or factors leading to discontinuation of an antiretroviral medication can impede future attempts to reduce viral load. Suboptimal drug exposure increases the potential for drug resistance.
Negotiate a therapy plan client can commit to. Include routines of awakening, meals, work schedule, and medication side effects.	The more individualized the plan is, the greater probability of adherence. *Note:* New dosing regimens are addressing the issues of pill load or number of pills in each dose, dosing frequency, dietary restrictions, and adverse events, resulting in greater individualization of the medication regimen.
Assist client to develop realistic health goals and incorporate wellness activities and practices—exercise, smoking cessation, nutrition, vitamin supplements—into daily routine.	Multiple responsibilities and demands on the client's time, especially with women, make it appear difficult to include any additional activities of self-care.
Review stress management skills.	Client must balance self-care needs and needs of other family members, which may be conflicting.
Provide anticipatory guidance and possible occurrences and choices, if any, to prevent or delay complications.	Reduces crisis events. Provides time for client to prepare for known, usual, or expected changes. Permits earlier initiation of therapies and decreases disruption of schedule.
Identify adaptive interventions valid for progressive long-term care needs.	Builds on coping strategies already effective for this individual.
Monitor adherence to prescribed medical regimen. Alter plan of care as needed.	Regimen is likely to be complicated and time-consuming. Thoughtful changes in plan may help enhance cooperation.
Evaluate short-term side effects and their interference with adherence to the medical regimen.	In the past, symptoms were considered part of having the disease and were accepted. Perception is that the side effect symptoms are the "main" effect. Improved options for better client care include the role of new HIV-1 PIs.
Support System Enhancement (NIC)	
Identify potential or actual support person(s). Include in teaching and problem-solving activities, as appropriate.	Helpful in planning for future and current needs of client and family.
Help client develop strategies that can gain supportive persons.	The more support persons there are available, the lower the risk of support burnout.
Collaborative	
Identify appropriate women's groups and services, social worker, financial resources, respite care, and other community programs.	Often female clients are single parents and caretakers for family. Groups can provide support and tangible help in dealing with issues of child care, parenting, and what to do when client is too ill to parent.
Refer to counselor, therapist, or spiritual advisor, as appropriate.	Opportunity to discuss concerns and fears may aid in problem-solving solutions and living with required changes.

POTENTIAL CONSIDERATIONS (dependent on client's age, physical condition and presence of complications, personal resources, and life responsibilities)

- ***Fatigue***—disease state; stress; depression
- ***imbalanced Nutrition: less than body requirements***—inability to ingest/digest food; insufficient finances
- ***Decisional Conflict***—unclear personal values or beliefs; perceived threat to value system; multiple or divergent sources of information; support system deficit; interference with decision making
- ***risk for Infection***— chronic disease; suppressed inflammatory response; malnutrition
- ***ineffective Self-Health Management***—complexity of healthcare system or therapeutic regimen; perceived seriousness and susceptibility, or benefits of therapy; family conflicts or crises

ACQUIRED IMMUNODEFICIENCY SYNDROME (AIDS)

I. Pathophysiology

a. End result of infection with a retrovirus—the human immunodeficiency virus (HIV)

b. Progression from HIV infection to AIDS is highly variable: In 2007, the Centers for Disease Control and Prevention (CDC) stated, "There is no one answer to this question because everyone is different. Estimates of the average length of time for progression from HIV to AIDS are being developed" (CDC, 2007). Also in 2007, the United Nations Programme on HIV/AIDS (UNAIDS) report stated, "It may take weeks to years, with median rate of 9 to 11 years after infection in the absence of antiretroviral therapy" (UNAIDS, 2007). No later data was found for this care plan.

c. Defined by the Centers for Disease Control and Prevention (CDC, 2007) as presence of HIV infection with at least one other criteria:

  i. CD4 T-cell count below 200 cells/µl

  ii. CD4 T-cell percentage of total lymphocytes at less than 14%

  iii. Presence of opportunistic infection (OI) or other AIDS-defining illness, such as HIV together with certain diseases such as tuberculosis or *Pneumocystis carinii* pneumonia (PCP). Many people are not aware of their HIV status until they seek treatment for another illness, and thus an OI becomes the initial indicator of their disease (Kaplan et al, 2009).

II. Etiology

a. Primary HIV infection: unprotected sex, anal intercourse, contaminated blood products, occupational exposure

b. OIs, while decreased in number, are still major contributors to morbidity and mortality in the HIV-infected client (Powderly, 2001)—undiagnosed HIV, CD4 T-cell count below 200 cells/µl, not taking antiretrovirals, drug resistance or failure of antiretroviral therapy.

  i. Infecting microbes: *Mycobacterium tuberculosis* (TB), *Mycobacterium avium* complex (MAC) candidiasis, coccidioidomycosis, cryptococcosis, microsporidiosis, cryptosporidiosis, cytomegalovirus (CMV), herpes simplex, syphilis, *Pneumocystis carinii* pneumonia (PCP), polyomavirus JC (causes progressive multifocal leukoencephalopathy), *salmonella* and other enterobactic microbes, *toxoplasma gondii* (causes encephalitis) (Kaplan, 2009).

  ii. Other AIDS-defining illnesses: Can be grouped into diseases affecting the central and peripheral nervous systems, malignancies, and wasting syndrome, including HIV-related encephalopathy, Kaposi's sarcoma (KS), invasive cervical cancer, Burkitt's lymphoma, among others (Kaplan, 2009; CDC, 2008).

III. Statistics (CDC, 2011)

a. Morbidity: As of 2011, an estimated 32,052 individuals were diagnosed with AIDS, with an estimated 487,692 living with AIDS in the United States at the end of 2010.

b. Mortality: In 2010, an estimated 15,529 deaths resulted from AIDS in the United States, with a cumulative estimated number of 6,367,048 deaths through 2010 since it was first diagnosed.

c. Cost: Yearly healthcare costs average $34,000 per individual with an AIDS diagnosis, with approximately $24,000 going toward antiretroviral therapy (Saag, 2002). According to the Kaiser Family Foundation (KKF), in FY 2012 the U.S. federal government spent a total of $14.8 billion on HIV care, with $5.8 billion to Medicare, $5.3 billion to Medicaid (with an additional states' share of $4.3 billion), $2.4 billion to Ryan White programs, and the rest to PEPFAR and other programs (KKF, 2013).

GLOSSARY

AIDS-defining illnesses: Group of over 20 conditions that, when coupled with a diagnosis of HIV, indicates the individual has progressed to AIDS.

AIDS dementia complex (ADC): Progressive mental disorder with different nervous system and mental symptoms—memory loss, speech problems, inability to concentrate, or poor judgment. There may be behavior changes, mood changes, and motor difficulties. ADC is considered an AIDS-defining condition in people with HIV. Also known as HIV-associated dementia.

Antigen: Substance that can stimulate the body to produce antibodies against it. Antigens include bacteria, viruses, pollen, and other foreign materials.

Antiretroviral (ARV): Medication that interferes with the ability of a retrovirus (such as HIV) to make more copies of itself.

(continues on page 690)

GLOSSARY (continued)

Co-infection: Infection with more than one virus, bacterium, or other micro-organism at a given time. For example, an HIV-infected individual may be co-infected with hepatitis C virus (HCV) or tuberculosis (TB).

Combination therapy: Two or more drugs used together to achieve optimal results in controlling HIV infection.

Highly active antiretroviral therapy (HAART): Aggressive anti-HIV treatment, using several antiretroviral drugs at one time. Also known as ART, ARV, and HART.

Immunomodulators: Drugs that strengthen the immune system and help the body to fight off infections or other diseases that attack people living with HIV/AIDS.

Immunosuppression: Inability of the immune system to function normally. May be caused by drugs, such as chemotherapy, or result from certain diseases, such as HIV infection.

Retrovirus: Type of virus that stores its genetic information in a single-stranded RNA molecule, then constructs a double-stranded DNA version of its genes using a special enzyme called reverse transcriptase. The DNA copy is then integrated into the host cell's own genetic material.

Care Setting

The interventions listed here are appropriate for community care as well as an inpatient or hospice setting. Most of the signs and symptoms and psychosocial issues happen long before inpatient care, which currently is usually of very short duration.

Related Factors

End-of-life care/hospice, page 848
Extended/long-term care, page 781
Fluid and electrolyte imbalances, page 885
The HIV-positive client, page 667
Psychosocial aspects of care, page 729
Sepsis/septicemia, page 665
Total nutritional support: parenteral/enteral feeding, page 437
Upper gastrointestinal/esophageal bleeding, page 281
Ventilatory assistance (mechanical), page 157

Client Assessment Database

Data depend on the organs and body tissues involved, the current viral load, and the specific OI or cancer.

DIAGNOSTIC DIVISION MAY REPORT	MAY EXHIBIT
ACTIVITY/REST	
• Reduced tolerance for usual activities, progressing to profound fatigue and malaise • Weakness • Altered sleep patterns	• Muscle weakness, wasting of muscle mass • Physiological response to activity— changes in blood pressure (BP), heart rate, and respirations
CIRCULATION	
• Slow healing (if anemic) • Bruising or bleeding with minor injury	• Tachycardia, postural BP changes • Decreased peripheral pulse volume • Pallor or cyanosis • Delayed capillary refill
EGO INTEGRITY	
• Stress factors related to lifestyle changes—specifically healthcare planning and regimen of multiple medications—losses, including family support, relationships, independence, financial; spiritual concerns, and change in self-concept (loss of control) • Concern about appearance—hair loss, disfiguring lesions, weight loss, altered distribution of body fat associated with protease-inhibiting drug therapy, and wrinkling of skin • Denial of diagnosis • Feelings of hopelessness, helplessness, worthlessness, guilt, depression, and powerlessness	• Denial, anxiety, depression, fear, and withdrawal • Angry behaviors, dejected body posture, crying, and poor eye contact • Failure to keep appointments or multiple appointments for similar symptoms

DIAGNOSTIC DIVISION

MAY REPORT (continued)	MAY EXHIBIT (continued)

Elimination

May Report

- Difficult and painful elimination
- Rectal pain, itching
- Intermittent, persistent, frequent diarrhea with or without abdominal cramping
- Flank pain, burning on urination

May Exhibit

- Loose-formed to watery stools with or without mucus or blood; frequent, copious diarrhea
- Abdominal tenderness
- Rectal, perianal lesions or abscesses
- Changes in urinary output, color, or character
- Urinary or bowel incontinence

Food/Fluid

May Report

- Anorexia, changes in taste of foods; food intolerance
- Nausea or vomiting
- Rapid, progressive weight loss
- Difficulty chewing and swallowing, retrosternal pain with swallowing
- Food intolerance—diarrhea after ingestions of dairy products, nausea, early satiation, or bloating

May Exhibit

- Hyperactive bowel sounds
- Abdominal distention
- Thin frame, decreased subcutaneous fat or muscle mass
- Poor skin turgor
- Lesions of the oral cavity, white patches, discoloration
- Poor dental and gum health, loss of teeth
- Edema—generalized, dependent

Hygiene

May Report

- Inability to complete activities of daily living (ADLs) independently

May Exhibit

- Deficits in many or all personal care, self-care activities

Neurosensory

May Report

- Fainting spells and dizziness
- Headache; stiff neck
- Changes in ability to solve problems, forgetfulness, poor concentration
- Impaired sensation or sense of position
- Muscle weakness, tremors
- Numbness, tingling in extremities
- Changes in vision—light flashes or floaters, photophobia; blurred visions

May Exhibit

- Mental status changes ranging from confusion to dementia, delirium with sudden onset
- Forgetfulness, poor concentration, decreased alertness, apathy, psychomotor retardation or slowed responses
- Paranoid ideation, free-floating anxiety, unrealistic expectations
- Abnormal reflexes, decreased muscle strength, ataxic gait
- Fine and/or gross motor tremors, focal motor deficits, hemiparesis
- Seizures
- Retinal hemorrhages and exudates (CMV retinitis); blindness

Pain/Discomfort

May Report

- Generalized or localized pain
- Headache
- Pleuritic chest pain

May Exhibit

- Swelling of joints, painful nodules, tenderness
- Decreased range of motion (ROM)
- Gait changes, limp
- Muscle guarding

Respiration

May Report

- Frequent, persistent upper respiratory infections (URIs)
- Progressive shortness of breath
- Cough ranging from mild to severe, nonproductive or productive of sputum; spasmodic cough on deep breathing (may be earliest sign of PCP)
- Congestion or tightness in chest
- History of exposure to or prior episode of active TB

May Exhibit

- Tachypnea, respiratory distress
- Changes in breath sounds, presence of adventitious breath sounds

Safety

May Report

- Exposure to infectious diseases, such as TB or sexually transmitted diseases (STDs)
- History of other immune deficiency diseases, such as rheumatoid arthritis, cancer
- History of frequent or multiple blood or blood product transfusions; hemophilia, major vascular surgery, traumatic incident
- History of falls, burns, episodes of fainting, slow-healing wounds
- Easy bruising, prolonged bleeding, and hemorrhage (thrombocytopenia)
- Suicidal or homicidal ideation with or without a plan
- Experiencing anger, disgust, rejection and/or violence from others

May Exhibit

- Recurrent fevers, low-grade, intermittent temperature elevations or spikes, night sweats
- Changes in skin integrity—cuts, ulcerations, rashes (eczema), exanthemas, psoriasis; discolorations; changes in size or color of moles; unexplained, easy bruising; multiple injection scars
- Rectal, perianal lesions or abscesses
- Nodules, enlarged lymph nodes in two or more areas of the body—neck, axillae, and groin, for example
- Decline in general strength, muscle tone
- Changes in gait

(continues on page 692)

DIAGNOSTIC DIVISION MAY REPORT (continued)	MAY EXHIBIT (continued)
SEXUALITY • History of high-risk behavior, such as having sex with a partner who is HIV positive, multiple sexual partners, unprotected sexual activity, and anal sex; substance use or abuse, injection drug user • Loss of libido, too sick for sex, afraid to engage in any sexual activities • Inconsistent use of condoms	• Pregnancy or risk for pregnancy (sexually active), pregnancy resulting in HIV-positive infant • Genitalia—herpes, warts, discharge
SOCIAL INTERACTION • Problems related to diagnosis and treatment—loss of family/significant other (SO), friends, support; fear of telling others, fear of rejection; loss of income • Isolation, loneliness, close friends or sexual partners who have died of, or are sick with, AIDS • Questioning of ability to remain independent, unable to plan for needs	• Changes in family or SO interaction pattern • Disorganized activities, difficulty with goal setting
TEACHING/LEARNING • Unaware of HIV infection • Failure to comply with treatment • Continued high-risk behavior (e.g., unchanged sexual behavior or injection drug use) • Injection drug use or abuse, current smoking, alcohol abuse	
DISCHARGE PLAN CONSIDERATIONS • Usually requires assistance with finances, medications and treatments, skin or wound care, equipment, supplies, transportation, food shopping and preparation, self-care, technical nursing procedures, homemaker and maintenance tasks, child care, and changes in living arrangements ➧ Refer to section at end of plan for postdischarge considerations.	

Diagnostic Studies

TEST WHY IT IS DONE	WHAT IT TELLS ME
BLOOD TESTS • ***HIV antibody test:*** Detects HIV antibodies in the blood.	Antibodies to HIV are produced by the body and can be detected in the blood about 2 to 4 weeks after exposure to the virus.
• ***Enzyme-linked immunosorbent assay (ELISA):*** Sensitive immunoassay that uses an enzyme linked to an antibody or antigen as a marker for the detection of a specific protein.	Determines exposure to a particular infectious agent, such as the HIV virus, by identifying antibodies present in a blood sample; however, it is not diagnostic.
• ***Western blot test:*** Technique for identifying specific antibodies or proteins in which proteins are separated by electrophoresis.	Confirms presence of HIV in individuals with positive ELISA screening. Based on genetic similarities, the numerous virus strains may be classified into types, groups, and subtypes. *Note:* There are two types of HIV: HIV-1 and HIV-2. Both types are transmitted through sexual contact, through blood, and from mother to child, and they appear to cause clinically indistinguishable AIDS. Worldwide, the predominant virus is HIV-1. The relatively uncommon HIV-2 type is concentrated in West Africa and is rarely found elsewhere (Avert staff, no date).

TEST WHY IT IS DONE (continued)	WHAT IT TELLS ME (continued)
VIRAL LOAD TESTS	
• ***Radioimmunoprecipitation–polymerase chain reaction (RI-PCR):*** Detects viral RNA levels as low as 50 copies/mL of plasma.	Determines progression of HIV to AIDS or onset of drug resistance.
• ***Branched DNA (bDNA):*** Currently, the leading indicator of effectiveness of therapy.	Therapy can be initiated, or changes made in treatment approaches, based on rise of viral load or maintenance of a low viral load.
• ***CD8 CTL (cytopathic suppressor cells):*** CD8 CTL has been strongly implicated in the control of HIV-1 replications.	At late stage of infection, CD8 CTL numbers are reduced.
• ***CD4 lymphocyte count (previously T4 helper cells):*** Used to diagnose HIV infection and progression and to monitor effects of drug therapy.	Client with counts below 200 defines progression to AIDS. Levels are measured immediately before and again 4 to 8 weeks after initiation of antiretroviral therapy.
• ***Complete blood count (CBC):*** Battery of screening tests, which typically includes hemoglobin (Hgb); hematocrit (Hct); red blood cell (RBC) count, morphology, indices, and distribution width index; platelet count and size; white blood cell (WBC) count and differential.	Anemia from blood loss or bone marrow infection (e.g., mycobacterium) and idiopathic thrombocytopenia (anemia occurs in up to 85% of clients with AIDS and may be profound). WBC count is low (leukopenia), and lymphocyte percentage is low (lymphopenia). Neutropenia may be drug induced.
• ***TB skin test/purified protein derivative (PPD):*** Antigen used to aid in the diagnosis of TB infection.	Determines exposure to, or active, TB disease. Outside the United States, TB is the leading cause of death among people who are HIV positive (Stop TB Partnership/WHO/UNAIDS, 2011). *Note:* PPD may be negative because of anergy.
• ***Sexually transmitted disease (STD) screening tests:*** Lifestyle behaviors may increase risk of, or exposure to, infection by STDs.	Hepatitis B (HBV) envelope and core antibodies, hepatitis C (HVC), syphilis, and other common STDs (e.g., chlamydia, gonococcus) may be positive.
OTHER DIAGNOSTIC STUDIES	
• ***Cultures:*** Specific cultures (e.g., urine, blood, stool, spinal fluid, lesions, sputum, and secretions) may be done to identify causative organism(s). Sensitivity determines microorganism susceptibility or resistance to specific antimicrobials.	Done to identify the causative organism causing the OI and to determine best therapies.
• ***Neurological studies—electroencephalogram (EEG), magnetic resonance imaging (MRI), computed tomography (CT) scans of the brain, electromyography (EMG)/nerve conduction studies:*** Indicated for persistent headache, changes in mentation, fever of undetermined origin, and/or changes in sensory or motor function.	Determines effects of HIV infection and/or OIs.
• ***Chest x-rays:*** Determines effects of disease process.	May initially be normal or may reveal progressive interstitial infiltrates secondary to advancing PCP, which is the most common opportunistic disease, or other pulmonary complications or disease processes such as TB, spontaneous pneumothorax, and hilar adenopathy.
• ***Pulmonary function tests:*** Group of tests (e.g., spirometry, lung volumes, etc.) that measure how well the lungs take in and release air and how well they move oxygen into the blood.	Useful in early detection of interstitial pneumonias.
• ***Barium swallow, endoscopy, colonoscopy:*** Tests for gastrointestinal (GI) function either by direct visualization or imaging studies.	May be done to identify OI (e.g., *Candida,* CMV) or to stage KS in the GI system.
• ***Biopsies:*** Determines presence of pathology and treatment options.	May be done for differential diagnosis of KS or other neoplastic lesions.

Nursing Priorities

1. Prevent or minimize development of new infections.
2. Maintain homeostasis.
3. Promote comfort.
4. Support psychosocial adjustment.
5. Provide information about disease process, prognosis, and treatment needs.

Discharge Goals/Goals of Care

1. Infection prevented or resolved.
2. Complications prevented or minimized.
3. Pain and discomfort alleviated or controlled.
4. Dealing with current situation realistically.
5. Diagnosis, prognosis, and therapeutic regimen understood.
6. Plan in place to meet ongoing needs.

NURSING DIAGNOSIS: risk for Infection [progression/onset of opportunistic infection]

Risk Factors May Include

Inadequate primary defenses—broken skin, traumatized tissue, stasis of body fluids
Immunosuppression; chronic disease; malnutrition
Invasive procedures

Possibly Evidenced By

(Not applicable; presence of signs and symptoms establishes an *actual* diagnosis)

Desired Outcomes/Evaluation Criteria—Client Will

Infection Severity (NOC)

Achieve timely healing of wounds or lesions.
Be afebrile and free of purulent drainage or secretions and other signs of infectious conditions.

Risk Control (NOC)

Identify and participate in behaviors to reduce risk of infection.

ACTIONS/INTERVENTIONS	RATIONALE
Infection Control (NIC)	
Independent	
Assess client knowledge and ability to maintain OI prophylactic regimen.	A multiple-medication regimen is difficult to maintain over a long period of time. Clients may adjust medication regimen based on side effects experienced, contributing to inadequate prophylaxis, active disease, and resistance. However, new medication regimens may increase adherence because they require less frequent dosing, fewer pills at each dose, and fewer side effects, thus maximizing quality of life and improving adherence to treatment.
Wash hands before and after all care contacts. Instruct client and SO to wash hands, as indicated.	Reduces risk of cross-contamination.
Provide a clean, well-ventilated environment. Screen visitors and staff for signs of infection and maintain isolation precautions as indicated.	Reduces number of pathogens presented to the immune system and reduces possibility of client contracting a nosocomial infection.
Discuss extent and rationale for isolation precautions and maintenance of personal hygiene.	Promotes cooperation with regimen and may lessen feelings of isolation.
Monitor vital signs, including temperature.	Provides information for baseline and data to track changes. Frequent temperature elevations or onset of new fever indicates that the body is responding to a new infectious process or that medications are not effectively controlling noncurable infections.
Assess respiratory rate and depth; note dry spasmodic cough on deep inspiration, changes in characteristics of sputum, and presence of wheezes or rhonchi. Initiate respiratory isolation when etiology of productive cough is unknown.	Respiratory congestion and distress may indicate developing respiratory disease, including PCP—the most common opportunistic disease in clients with CD4 count below 200. However, TB is on the rise and other fungal, viral, and bacterial infections may occur that compromise the respiratory system.
Investigate reports of headache, stiff neck, and altered vision. Note changes in mentation and behavior. Monitor for nuchal rigidity or seizure activity.	Neurological abnormalities are common and may be related to HIV or secondary infections. Symptoms may vary from subtle changes in mood or sensorium (personality changes or depression) to hallucinations, memory loss, severe dementias, seizures, and loss of vision. Central nervous system (CNS) infections (encephalitis is the most common) may be caused by protozoal and helminthic organisms or fungus.
Examine skin and oral mucous membranes for white patches or lesions. (Refer to NDs: impaired Skin Integrity; impaired Oral Mucous Membrane.)	Oral candidiasis, KS, herpes, CMV, and cryptococcosis are common opportunistic diseases affecting the cutaneous membranes.
Clean client's nails frequently. File, rather than cut, and avoid trimming cuticles.	Reduces risk of transmission of pathogens through breaks in skin. *Note:* Fungal infections along the nail plate are common.
Monitor reports of heartburn, dysphagia, retrosternal pain on swallowing, increased abdominal cramping, and profuse diarrhea.	Esophagitis may occur secondary to oral candidiasis, CMV, or herpes. Cryptosporidiosis is a parasitic infection responsible for watery diarrhea, often more than 15 L/day.
Inspect wounds and site of invasive devices, noting signs of local inflammation.	Early identification and treatment of secondary infection may prevent sepsis.

ACTIONS/INTERVENTIONS (continued)	RATIONALE (continued)
Wear gloves and gowns during direct contact with secretions or excretions or any time there is a break in skin of caregiver's hands. Wear mask and protective eyewear to protect nose, mouth, and eyes from secretions during procedures (e.g., suctioning) or when splattering of blood may occur.	Use of masks, gowns, and gloves is required by the Occupational Safety and Health Administration (OSHA, 1992) for direct contact with body fluids, such as sputum, blood or blood products, semen, or vaginal secretions.
Dispose of needles and sharps in rigid, puncture-resistant containers.	Prevents accidental inoculation of caregivers. Use of needle cutters and recapping is not to be practiced. *Note:* Accidental needlesticks should be reported immediately, with follow-up evaluations done per protocol.
Label blood bags, body fluid containers, soiled dressings or linens, and package appropriately for disposal per isolation protocol.	Prevents cross-contamination and alerts appropriate personnel to exercise specific hazardous materials procedures.
Clean up spills of body fluids or blood with bleach solution (1:10); add bleach to laundry.	Kills HIV and controls other microorganisms on surfaces.
Collaborative	
Administer medications, as indicated, for example:	The goal of pharmacotherapy is to inhibit viral replication and to reduce morbidity and development of OIs.
Nucleoside reverse transcriptase inhibitors (NRTIs): retrovir + epivir (Combivir), lamivudine (Epivir), zidovudine vilread + emtriva (Truvada), (Retrovir, AZT), ziagen + epivir (Epzicom), stavudine (Zerit), and tenofovir (Viread) (AIDSMEDS, 2012)	In the past, zidovudine was given alone and as a first-line treatment. Presently the drug is usually given in a three-drug treatment regimen, along with another NRTI and a protease inhibitor (PI) with the combination referred to as HAART.
Protease inhibitors (PIs), such as lopinavir and ritonavir (Kaletra), tapranavir (Aptivus), indinavir (Crixivan), ritonavir (Norvir), saquinavir (Invirase), darunavir (Prezista), atazanavir (Reyataz), and nelfinavir (Viracept) (AIDSMEDS, 2012)	When combined with NRTIs, PIs control the HIV-RNA viral load by blocking viral replication at two different target sites in the replication process. Immune function is maintained with early intervention or improved when initiated later.
Non-nucleoside reverse transcriptase inhibitors (NNRTIs), such as rilpivirine (Edurant), etravirine (Intelence), delaviridine (Rescriptor), nevirapine (Viramune), and efavirenz (Sustiva) (AIDSMEDS, 2012)	These drugs inhibit viral replication by a different mechanism than NRTIs or PIs. They also are used in combination to reduce possibility of drug resistance.
Entry inhibitors, including fusion inhibitors, such as enfuvirtide (Fuzeon), maraviroc (Selzentry) (AIDSMEDS, 2012).	These drugs work by preventing HIV from entering healthy CD4 cells or by blocking enzyme needed for replication.
All-in-one combination tablets, such as elvitegravir-cobicistat + tenofovir + emtricilabine (Stribild); efacirenz + tenofovir + emtricitabine (Atripla); rilpivirine + tenofovir + embricitabine (Complera) (AIDSMEDS, 2012)	These are complete one-pill, once-daily drug regimens.
Anti-infectives, such as trimethoprim-sulfamethoxazole (Bactrim), pentamidine (Pentacarinat), flucytosine (Ancobon), and clotrimazole (Femizole)	Early identification and treatment of secondary infection may prevent sepsis.
Refer to and encourage cooperation with local epidemiology agency or public health department.	This is a legal requirement. Accurate information facilitates tracking disease spread and groups affected.

NURSING DIAGNOSIS: risk for deficient Fluid Volume

Risk Factors May Include

Excessive losses through normal routes—copious diarrhea, profuse sweating, vomiting
Factors influencing fluid needs—hypermetabolic state, fever
Deviations affecting intake of fluids—nausea, anorexia, lethargy

Possibly Evidenced By

(Not applicable; presence of signs and symptoms establishes an *actual* diagnosis)

Desired Outcomes/Evaluation Criteria—Client Will

Hydration (NOC)

Maintain hydration as evidenced by moist mucous membranes, good skin turgor, stable vital signs, and individually adequate urinary output.

ACTIONS/INTERVENTIONS	RATIONALE
Fluid/Electrolyte Management (NIC)	
Independent	
Monitor vital signs, including central venous pressure (CVP) if available. Note hypotension, including postural changes.	Indicators of circulating fluid volume.
Note temperature elevation and duration of febrile episode. Administer tepid sponge baths, as indicated. Keep clothing and linens dry. Maintain comfortable environmental temperature.	Fever is one of the most frequent symptoms experienced by clients with HIV infection. Increased metabolic demands and associated excessive diaphoresis result in increased insensible fluid losses and dehydration.
Assess skin turgor, mucous membranes, and thirst.	Indirect indicators of fluid status.
Measure urinary output and specific gravity. Measure or estimate amount of diarrheal loss. Note insensible losses.	Increased specific gravity and decreasing urinary output reflects altered renal perfusion or circulating volume. *Note:* Monitoring fluid balance is difficult in the presence of excessive GI and insensible losses.
Weigh, as indicated.	Although weight loss may reflect muscle wasting, sudden fluctuations reflect state of hydration. Fluid losses associated with diarrhea can quickly create a crisis and become life-threatening.
Monitor oral intake and encourage fluids of at least 2500 mL/day.	Maintains fluid balance, reduces thirst, and keeps mucous membranes moist.
Make fluids easily accessible to client. Encourage use of fluids that are tolerable to client and that replace needed electrolytes, such as Gatorade or broth.	Enhances intake. Certain fluids such as acidic fruit juices or iced beverages may be too painful to consume because of mouth lesions.
Eliminate foods potentiating diarrhea, such as spicy or high-fat foods, nuts, cabbage, and milk products. Provide lactose-free products, such as Resource or Advera. Adjust rate or concentration of enteral feedings, if indicated.	May help reduce diarrhea. Use of lactose-free products helps control diarrhea in the lactose-intolerant client.
Encourage use of live-culture yogurt or an over-the-counter (OTC) product such as *Lactobacillus acidophilus* (Lactaid).	Antibiotic therapies disrupt normal bowel flora balance, leading to diarrhea. *Note:* Must be taken 2 hours before or after antibiotic to prevent inactivation of live culture.
Collaborative	
Administer fluids and electrolytes via feeding tube or intravenously (IV), as appropriate.	May be necessary to support or augment circulating volume, especially if oral intake is inadequate or nausea or vomiting persists.
Monitor laboratory studies, as indicated, for example:	
Serum and urine electrolytes	Alerts to possible electrolyte disturbances and determines replacement needs.
Blood urea nitrogen/creatinine (BUN/Cr)	Evaluates renal perfusion and function.
Stool specimen collection	Bowel flora changes can occur with multiple or single antibiotic therapy.
Administer medications, as indicated, for example:	
Anti-emetics, such as prochlorperazine maleate (Compazine)	Reduces incidence of vomiting to reduce further loss of fluids and electrolytes.
Antidiarrheals, such as diphenoxylate (Lomotil), loperamide (Imodium), or paregoric; or antispasmodics, such as mepenzolate bromide (Cantil)	Decreases the amount and fluidity of stool; may reduce intestinal spasm and peristalsis. *Note:* Antibiotics may also be used to treat diarrhea if caused by infection.
Antipyretics, such as acetaminophen (Tylenol)	Helps reduce fever and hypermetabolic response, decreasing insensible losses. *Note:* Studies caution that Tylenol toxicity can occur more frequently in the client with AIDS, so it needs to be used with caution
Maintain hypothermia blanket if used.	May be necessary when other measures fail to reduce excessive fever and insensible fluid losses.

NURSING DIAGNOSIS: ineffective Breathing Pattern

May Be Related To

Respiratory muscle fatigue—wasting of respiratory musculature

Fatigue

Possibly Evidenced By

Alterations in depth of breathing—shallow respirations

Dyspnea; use of accessory muscles for breathing

Desired Outcomes/Evaluation Criteria—Client Will

Respiratory Status (NOC)

Maintain effective respiratory pattern.

Experience no dyspnea or cyanosis, with breath sounds and chest x-ray clear or improving and arterial blood gases (ABGs) within client's normal range.

ACTIONS/INTERVENTIONS	RATIONALE
Respiratory Monitoring (NIC)	
Independent	
Auscultate breath sounds, noting areas of decreased or absent ventilation and presence of adventitious sounds—crackles, wheezes, and rhonchi.	Suggests developing pulmonary complications or infections, such as atelectasis or pneumonia. *Note:* PCP is often advanced before changes in breath sounds occur.
Note rate and depth of respiration, use of accessory muscles, increased work of breathing, and presence of dyspnea, anxiety, and cyanosis.	Tachypnea, cyanosis, restlessness, and increased work of breathing reflect respiratory distress and need for increased surveillance or medical intervention.
Assess changes in level of consciousness.	Hypoxemia can result in changes ranging from anxiety and confusion to unresponsiveness.
Investigate reports of chest pain.	Pleuritic chest pain may reflect nonspecific pneumonitis or pleural effusions associated with malignancies.
Ventilation Assistance (NIC)	
Elevate head of bed. Have client turn, cough, and deep breathe as indicated.	Promotes optimal pulmonary function and reduces incidence of aspiration or infection due to atelectasis.
Suction airways as indicated, using sterile technique and observing safety precautions—mask, protective eyewear.	Assists in clearing the ventilatory passages, thereby facilitating gas exchange and preventing respiratory complications.
Allow adequate rest periods between care activities. Maintain a quiet environment.	Reduces oxygen consumption.
Collaborative	
Monitor and graph serial ABGs or pulse oximetry.	Indicators of respiratory status and treatment needs and effectiveness.
Review serial chest x-rays.	Presence of diffuse infiltrates may suggest pneumonia, whereas areas of congestion or consolidation may reflect other pulmonary complications, such as atelectasis or KS lesions.
Assist with and instruct in use of incentive spirometer. Provide chest physiotherapy—percussion, vibration, and postural drainage.	Encourages proper breathing technique and improves lung expansion. Loosens secretions and dislodges mucous plugs to promote airway clearance. *Note:* In the event of multiple skin lesions, chest physiotherapy may be discontinued.
Provide humidified supplemental oxygen via appropriate means—cannula, mask, or intubation with mechanical ventilation.	Maintains effective ventilation and oxygenation to prevent or correct respiratory crisis.
Administer medications, as indicated, for example:	Choice of therapy depends on individual situation and infecting organism(s).
Bronchodilators, expectorants, and cough suppressants	May be needed to improve or maintain airway patency or help clear secretions.
Antimicrobials, such as clarithromycin (Bixian), azithromycin (Zithromax), or ethambutol (Myambutol)	Clarithromycin (Biaxin) or azithromycin (Zithromax) may be used prophylactically for prevention of *Mycobacterium avium* complex (MAC), or one drug may be used in combination with ethambutol (Myambutol) as treatment of choice for MAC.
Prepare for and assist with procedures as indicated, such as bronchoscopy, lavage, and biopsy.	May be required to clear mucous plugs or obtain specimens for diagnosis.

NURSING DIAGNOSIS: risk for Bleeding

Risk Factors May Include

Impaired liver function

[Abnormal blood profile—decreased vitamin K absorption, presence of autoimmune antiplatelet antibodies, malignancies (KS), and/or circulating endotoxins (sepsis)]

Possibly Evidenced By

(Not applicable; presence of signs and symptoms establishes an *actual* diagnosis)

Desired Outcomes/Evaluation Criteria—Client Will

Blood Loss Severity (NOC)

Display homeostasis as evidenced by absence of bleeding.

ACTIONS/INTERVENTIONS	RATIONALE
Bleeding Precautions (NIC)	
Independent	
Avoid injections and rectal temperatures and rectal tubes; administer rectal suppositories with caution.	Protects client from procedure-related causes of bleeding; for example, insertion of thermometers or rectal tubes can damage or tear rectal mucosa. *Note:* Some medications may need to be given via suppository in spite of risk.
Maintain a safe environment—keep all necessary objects and call bell within client's reach and keep bed in low position.	Reduces accidental injury, which could result in bleeding.
Maintain bedrest or chair rest when platelets are low, or as individually appropriate. Assess medication regimen.	Reduces possibility of injury, although activity needs to be maintained. May need to discontinue or reduce dosage of a drug. *Note:* Client can have a surprisingly low platelet count without bleeding.
Hematest body fluids—urine, stool, and vomitus—for occult blood.	Prompt detection of bleeding and initiation of therapy may prevent critical loss of blood.
Observe for and report epistaxis, hemoptysis, hematuria, nonmenstrual vaginal bleeding, or oozing from lesions, body orifices, or IV insertion sites.	Spontaneous bleeding may indicate development of disseminated intravascular coagulation (DIC) or immune thrombocytopenia, necessitating further evaluation and prompt intervention.
Monitor for changes in vital signs and skin color, such as BP, pulse, respirations, and skin pallor or discoloration.	Presence of bleeding or hemorrhage may lead to circulatory failure and shock.
Evaluate change in level of consciousness.	May reflect cerebral bleeding.
Collaborative	
Review laboratory studies, such as prothrombin time (PT), International Normalized Ratio (INR), activated partial thromboplastin time (aPTT), clotting time, platelets, and Hgb and Hct.	Detects alterations in clotting capability; identifies therapy needs. *Note:* Many individuals display platelet counts below 50,000 and may be asymptomatic, necessitating regular monitoring.
Administer blood products, as indicated.	Transfusions may be required in the event of persistent or massive spontaneous bleeding.
Avoid use of aspirin products and NSAIDs, especially in presence of gastric lesions.	These medications reduce platelet aggregation, prolonging the coagulation process, and may cause further gastric irritation, increasing risk of bleeding. *Note:* Aspirin is contraindicated even in the short term because of its nonreversible effect on platelets.

NURSING DIAGNOSIS: imbalanced Nutrition: less than body requirements

May Be Related To

Inability to ingest/digest food—nausea, vomiting, hyperactive gag reflex, fatigue
Inability to absorb nutrients—intestinal disturbances, GI tract infections

Possibly Evidenced By

Weight loss; poor muscle tone
Lack of interest in food; aversion to eating; sore buccal cavity
Reports altered taste sensation
Abdominal cramping, diarrhea
[Abnormal laboratory results—vitamin, mineral, and protein deficiencies, electrolyte imbalances]

Desired Outcomes/Evaluation Criteria—Client Will

Nutritional Status (NOC)

Maintain weight or display weight gain toward desired goal.

Nutritional Status: Biochemical Measures (NOC)

Demonstrate positive nitrogen balance, be free of signs of malnutrition, and display improved energy level.

ACTIONS/INTERVENTIONS	RATIONALE
Nutritional Monitoring (NIC)	
Independent	
Assess ability to chew, taste, and swallow.	Lesions of the mouth, throat, and esophagus are often caused by candidiasis, herpes simplex, hairy leukoplakia, or KS and other cancers; and metallic or other taste changes caused by medications may cause dysphagia, limiting client's ability to ingest food and reducing desire to eat.

ACTIONS/INTERVENTIONS (continued)	RATIONALE (continued)
Auscultate bowel sounds.	Hypermotility of intestinal tract is common and is associated with vomiting and diarrhea, which may affect choice of diet or route. *Note:* Lactose intolerance and malabsorption, such as associated with CMV, MAC, or cryptosporidiosis, contribute to diarrhea and may necessitate change in diet or supplemental formula, such as Advera or Resource.
Weigh, as indicated. Evaluate weight in terms of premorbid weight. Compare serial weights and anthropometric measurements.	Indicator of nutritional needs and adequacy of intake. *Note:* Because of immune suppression, some blood tests normally used for testing nutritional status are not useful.
Note drug side effects.	Prophylactic and therapeutic medications can have side effects affecting nutrition, such as altered taste, nausea, and vomiting associated with ZDV; anorexia, glucose intolerance, or glossitis associated with Bactrim; altered taste and smell, nausea, vomiting, and glucose intolerance associated with Pentam; or elevated lipids and blood sugar secondary to insulin resistance associated with PIs.
Nutritional Therapy (NIC)	
Plan diet with client and SO, incorporating foods client likes or food from home. Encourage small, frequent meals and snacks of nutritionally dense foods and nonacidic foods and beverages, with choice of foods palatable to client. Encourage high-calorie, nutritious foods, some of which may be considered appetite stimulants. Note time of day when appetite is best, and try to serve a larger meal at that time.	Including client in planning gives a sense of control of environment and may enhance intake. Fulfilling cravings for desired food may also improve intake. *Note:* In this population, foods with a higher fat content may be recommended as tolerated to enhance taste and oral intake.
Limit food(s) that induce nausea or vomiting or are poorly tolerated by client with mouth sores or dysphagia. Avoid serving very hot liquids and foods. Serve foods that are easy to swallow, such as eggs, ice cream, or cooked vegetables.	Pain in the mouth or fear of irritating oral lesions may cause client to be reluctant to eat. These measures may be helpful in increasing food intake.
Schedule medications between meals if tolerated and limit fluid intake with meals, unless fluid has nutritional value.	Gastric fullness diminishes appetite and food intake.
Encourage as much physical activity as possible.	May improve appetite and general feelings of well-being.
Provide frequent mouth care, observing secretion precautions. Avoid alcohol-containing mouthwashes.	Reduces discomfort associated with nausea or vomiting, oral lesions, mucosal dryness, and halitosis. A clean mouth may enhance appetite.
Provide rest period before meals. Avoid stressful procedures close to mealtime.	Minimizes fatigue; increases energy available for work of eating.
Remove existing noxious environmental stimuli or conditions that aggravate gag reflex.	Reduces stimulus of the vomiting center in the medulla.
Encourage client to sit up for meals.	Facilitates swallowing and reduces risk of aspiration.
Record ongoing caloric intake.	Identifies need for supplements or alternative feeding methods.
Collaborative	
Review laboratory studies, such as BUN, glucose, liver function studies, electrolytes, protein, and albumin or prealbumin.	Indicates nutritional status and organ function and identifies replacement needs. *Note:* Nutritional tests can be altered because of disease processes and response to some medications or therapies. *Note:* Multiple medications are metabolized by the liver and have potential for synergistic damage.
Maintain nothing by mouth (NPO) status when appropriate.	May be needed to reduce nausea or vomiting.
Insert and maintain nasogastric (NG) tube, as indicated.	May be required to reduce vomiting or to administer tube feedings. *Note:* Esophageal irritation from existing infection, such as *Candida,* herpes, or KS, may provide site for secondary infections or trauma; therefore, NG tube should be used with caution.
Consult with dietitian or nutritional support team.	Provides for diet based on nutritional needs and appropriate route.
Administer enteral or parenteral feedings, as indicated.	Enteral feedings are preferred because they cost less and carry less risk of exacerbating endocrine dysfunction than total parenteral nutrition (TPN). However, TPN may be required when oral or enteral feedings are not tolerated. TPN is reserved for those whose gut cannot absorb even an elemental formula, such as Vivonex, or those with severe refractory diarrhea.
Administer medications, as indicated, for example:	
Anti-emetics, such as prochlorperazine (Compazine)	Reduces incidence of nausea and vomiting, possibly enhancing oral intake.

(continues on page 700)

ACTIONS/INTERVENTIONS (continued) / RATIONALE (continued)

Gastric protective agents such as sucralfate (Carafate) suspension; oral suspension sometimes known as Magic (Mouthwash), which is a mixture of Maalox, diphenhydramine (Benadryl), and lidocaine (Xylocaine)
— Given with meals—swish and hold in mouth—to relieve mouth pain and enhance intake. Mixture may be swallowed in presence of pharyngeal or esophageal lesions.

Vitamin supplements
— Corrects vitamin deficiencies resulting from decreased food intake and/or disorders of digestion and absorption in the GI system. *Note:* Avoid megadoses; suggested supplemental level is two times the recommended daily allowance (RDA).

Appetite stimulants, such as dronabinol (Marinol), megestrol (Megace), or oxandrolone (Oxandrin)
— Marinol, an anti-emetic, and Megace, an antineoplastic, act as appetite stimulants in the presence of AIDS. Oxandrin is currently being studied in clinical trials to boost appetite and improve muscle mass and strength.

Antidiarrheals, such as diphenoxylate (Lomotil), loperamide (Imodium), or octreotide (Sandostatin)
— These drugs inhibit GI motility, subsequently decreasing diarrhea. Imodium or Sandostatin is an effective treatment for secretory diarrhea with secretion of water and electrolytes by intestinal epithelium.

Antifungals, such as ketoconazole (Nizoral) or fluconazole (Diflucan)
— These may be given to treat or prevent infections involving the GI tract.

NURSING DIAGNOSIS: acute/chronic Pain

May Be Related To

Physical agents—tissue inflammation or destruction (e.g., infections, internal or external cutaneous lesions, rectal excoriation, malignancies, necrosis); peripheral neuropathies

Possibly Evidenced By

Verbal/coded reports of pain; restlessness
Self-focusing, narrowed focus; reduced interaction with people
Guarding behavior
Changes in appetite, sleep pattern
Changes in vital signs (acute)

Desired Outcomes/Evaluation Criteria—Client Will

Pain Level (NOC)
Report pain relieved or controlled.
Demonstrate relaxed posture and facial expression.
Be able to sleep or rest appropriately.

ACTIONS/INTERVENTIONS / RATIONALE

Pain Management (NIC)
Independent

Assess pain reports, noting location, intensity (0–10 or similar coded scale), frequency, and time of onset. Note nonverbal cues, such as restlessness, tachycardia, or grimacing.
— Indicates need for, and effectiveness of, interventions and may signal development or resolution of complications. *Note:* Chronic pain does not produce autonomic changes; however, acute and chronic pain can coexist.

Encourage client to report pain as it develops rather than waiting until level is severe.
— Efficacy of comfort measures and medications is improved with timely intervention.

Encourage verbalization of feelings.
— Can reduce anxiety and fear and thereby reduce perception of intensity of pain.

Provide diversional activities, such as reading, visiting, music, and television.
— Refocuses attention; may enhance coping abilities.

Perform palliative measures—repositioning, massage, or ROM exercises of affected joints.
— Promotes relaxation and decreases muscle tension.

Instruct client in, and encourage use of, visualization, guided imagery, progressive relaxation, deep-breathing techniques, meditation, and mindfulness.
— Promotes relaxation and feeling of well-being. May decrease the need for opioid analgesics (CNS depressants) when a neurological or motor degenerative process is already involved. May not be successful in presence of dementia, even when dementia is minor. *Note:* Mindfulness is the skill of staying in the here and now.

Provide oral care. (Refer to ND: impaired Oral Mucous Membrane.)
— Oral ulcerations or lesions may cause severe discomfort.

Apply warm, moist packs to pentamidine injection or IV sites for 20 minutes after administration.
— These injections are known to cause pain and sterile abscesses.

ACTIONS/INTERVENTIONS (continued)	RATIONALE (continued)
Collaborative	
Administer analgesics, antipyretics, or opioid analgesics. Use patient-controlled analgesia (PCA) or provide around-the-clock analgesia with rescue doses, as needed.	Provides relief of pain and discomfort; reduces fever. PCA or around-the-clock medication keeps the blood level of analgesia stable, preventing cyclic undermedication or overmedication.

NURSING DIAGNOSIS: impaired Skin Integrity

May Be Related To

Immunological deficit
Imbalanced nutritional state (e.g., malnutrition)
Changes in turgor; skeletal prominence
Impaired sensation
Excretions; moisture

Possibly Evidenced By

Destruction of skin surface/layers

Desired Outcomes/Evaluation Criteria—Client Will

Wound Healing: Secondary Intention (NOC)

Be free of or display improvement in wound or lesion healing.

Risk Control (NOC)

Demonstrate behaviors or techniques to prevent skin breakdown and promote healing.

ACTIONS/INTERVENTIONS	RATIONALE
Skin Surveillance (NIC)	
Independent	
Assess skin daily. Note color, turgor, circulation, and sensation. Describe and measure lesions and observe changes.	Establishes comparative baseline providing opportunity for timely intervention.
Provide and instruct in good skin hygiene—wash thoroughly, pat dry carefully, and gently massage with lotion or appropriate cream.	Maintaining clean, dry skin provides a barrier to infection. Patting skin dry instead of rubbing reduces risk of dermal trauma to dry, fragile skin. Massaging increases circulation to the skin and promotes comfort. *Note:* Isolation precautions are required when extensive or open cutaneous lesions are present.
Reposition frequently. Use turn sheet as needed. Encourage periodic weight shifts. Protect bony prominences with pillows, heel and elbow pads, or sheepskin.	Reduces stress on pressure points, improves blood flow to tissues, and promotes healing.
Maintain clean, dry, wrinkle-free linen, preferably soft cotton fabric.	Skin friction caused by movement over wet, wrinkled, or rough sheets leads to irritation of fragile skin and increases risk of infection.
Encourage ambulation as tolerated.	Decreases pressure on skin from prolonged bedrest.
Cleanse perianal area by removing stool with water and mineral oil or commercial product. Avoid use of toilet paper if vesicles are present. Apply protective creams—zinc oxide or A & D ointment.	Prevents maceration caused by diarrhea and keeps perianal lesions dry. *Note:* Use of toilet paper may abrade lesions.
File nails regularly.	Long or rough nails increase risk of dermal damage.
Wound Care (NIC)	
Cover open pressure ulcers with sterile dressings or protective barrier, such as Tegaderm or DuoDerm, as indicated.	May reduce bacterial contamination and promote healing.
Collaborative	
Provide foam, flotation, or alternate pressure mattress or bed.	Reduces pressure on skin, tissue, and lesions, decreasing tissue ischemia.
Obtain cultures of open skin lesions.	Identifies pathogens and appropriate treatment choices.
Apply topical or administer systemic drugs, as indicated.	Used in treatment of skin lesions. Use of agents, such as Prederm spray, can stimulate circulation, enhancing healing process. *Note:* When multidose ointments are used, care must be taken to avoid cross-contamination.

(continues on page 702)

ACTIONS/INTERVENTIONS (continued)	RATIONALE (continued)
Provide wound care, as indicated:	
Cover ulcerated KS lesions with wet-to-wet dressings or antibiotic ointment and nonstick dressing such as Telfa.	Protects ulcerated areas from contamination and promotes healing.
Apply Tegasorb Thin or other absorbing product, as indicated.	If the wound or ulcer is moist with exudate, these products keep the wound slightly moist with no maceration of periwound tissue. (Refer to CP: Wounds: Complicated and Chronic, as indicated.)
Refer to physical therapy for regular exercise program.	Promotes improved muscle tone and skin health.

NURSING DIAGNOSIS: impaired Oral Mucous Membrane

May Be Related To

Immunocompromised; stress
Dehydration; malnutrition
Ineffective oral hygiene
Treatment-related side effects—pharmaceutical agents, chemotherapy

Possibly Evidenced By

Open lesions/ulcers; vesicles
Oral pain or discomfort
Stomatitis; white patches; gingivitis
Difficulty eating/swallowing

Desired Outcomes/Evaluation Criteria—Client Will

Oral Hygiene (NOC)

Display intact mucous membranes, which are pink, moist, and free of inflammation or ulcerations.

Risk Control (NOC)

Demonstrate techniques to restore or maintain integrity of oral mucosa.

ACTIONS/INTERVENTIONS	RATIONALE
Oral Health Restoration (NIC)	
Independent	
Assess mucous membranes and document all oral lesions. Note reports of pain, swelling, and difficulty with chewing or swallowing.	Edema, open lesions, and crusting on oral mucous membranes and throat may cause pain and difficulty with chewing or swallowing.
Provide oral care daily and after food intake, using soft toothbrush, nonabrasive toothpaste, nonalcoholic mouthwash, floss, and lip moisturizer.	Alleviates discomfort, prevents acid formation associated with retained food particles, and promotes feeling of well-being.
Rinse oral mucosal lesions with saline or dilute hydrogen peroxide or baking soda solutions.	Reduces spread of lesions and encrustations from candidiasis and promotes comfort.
Suggest use of sugarless gum or candy or commercial salivary substitute.	Stimulates flow of saliva to neutralize acids and protect mucous membranes. Sorbitol in some artificially sweetened products can increase risk for loose stools.
Plan diet to avoid salty, spicy, abrasive, and acidic foods or beverages. Check for temperature tolerance of foods. Offer cool or cold smooth foods.	Abrasive foods may open healing lesions. Open lesions are painful and aggravated by salt, spices, and acidic foods and beverages. Extreme cold or heat can cause pain to sensitive mucous membranes.
Encourage oral intake of at least 2500 mL/day.	Maintains hydration; prevents drying of oral mucous membranes.
Encourage client to refrain from smoking.	Smoke is drying and irritating to mucous membranes.
Collaborative	
Obtain culture specimens of lesions.	Reveals causative agents and identifies appropriate therapies.
Administer medications, as indicated, such as nystatin (Mycostatin) or ketoconazole (Nizoral).	Specific drug choice depends on particular infecting organism(s), such as *Candida*.
Apply Magic Mouthwash (mixture of Maalox, diphenhydramine [Benadryl], and lidocaine [Xylocaine]), or similar product to oral lesions, as prescribed.	Reduces local pain of *Candida* and other oral lesions.
Refer for dental consultation, if appropriate.	May require additional therapy to prevent dental losses.

NURSING DIAGNOSIS: Fatigue

May Be Related To

Disease state; malnutrition
Stress; depression
Sleep deprivation

Possibly Evidenced By

Reports unremitting, overwhelming lack of energy; inability to maintain usual routines
Decreased performance; compromised concentration
Disinterest in surroundings; lethargic; listless

Desired Outcomes/Evaluation Criteria—Client Will

Fatigue Level (NOC)

Report improved sense of energy.
Perform ADLs, with assistance as necessary.
Participate in desired activities at level of ability.

In addition to interventions in CP: HIV-Positive Client; ND: Fatigue.

ACTIONS/INTERVENTIONS	RATIONALE
Energy Management (NIC)	
Independent	
Recommend scheduling activities for periods when client has most energy. Plan care to allow for rest periods. Involve client and SO in schedule planning.	Planning allows client to be active during times when energy level is higher, which may restore a feeling of well-being and a sense of control. Frequent rest periods are needed to restore or conserve energy.
Encourage client to do whatever possible, such as perform self-care, sit in chair, or take short walks. Provide assistance, as needed. Increase activity level, as indicated.	Prevents severe deconditioning and may conserve strength, increase stamina, and enable client to become more active. *Note:* Weakness may make ADLs almost impossible for client to complete.
Monitor physiological response to activity, such as changes in BP, respiratory rate, or heart rate.	Tolerance varies greatly, depending on the stage of the disease process, nutrition state, fluid balance, and number and type of opportunistic diseases.
Collaborative	
Refer to physical and/or occupational therapy.	Programmed daily exercises and activities help client maintain or increase strength and muscle tone and enhance sense of well-being.
Refer to community resources, such as grocery delivery, Meals on Wheels, house cleaning or home maintenance services, or home-care agency.	Provides assistance in areas of individual need as ability to care for self becomes more difficult.
Provide supplemental oxygen, as indicated.	Presence of anemia and hypoxemia reduces oxygen available for cellular uptake and contributes to fatigue.

NURSING DIAGNOSIS: risk for acute/chronic Confusion

Risk Factors May Include

Infection (CNS)
Metabolic abnormalities—dehydration, malnutrition, electrolyte imbalance, increased blood urea nitrogen (BUN)/creatinine
Pharmaceutical agents—multiple medications

Possibly Evidenced By

(Not applicable; presence of signs and symptoms establishes an *actual* diagnosis)

Desired Outcomes/Evaluation Criteria—Client Will

Cognition (NOC)

Maintain usual reality orientation and optimal cognitive functioning.

ACTIONS/INTERVENTIONS	RATIONALE
Cognitive Stimulation (NIC)	
Independent	
Assess mental and neurological status using appropriate tools.	Establishes functional level at time of admission and provides baseline for future comparison.
Consider effects of emotional distress, such as anxiety, grief, and anger.	May contribute to reduced alertness, confusion, withdrawal, and hypoactivity, requiring further evaluation and intervention.
Monitor medication regimen and usage.	Actions and interactions of various medications, prolonged drug half-life, and altered excretion rates result in cumulative effects, potentiating risk of toxic reactions. Some drugs may have adverse side effects, such as haloperidol (Haldol), which can seriously impair motor function in clients with AIDS dementia complex.
Investigate changes in personality, response to stimuli, orientation, and level of consciousness; or development of headache, nuchal rigidity, vomiting, fever, or seizure activity.	Changes may occur for numerous reasons, including development or exacerbation of opportunistic diseases or CNS infection. *Note:* Early detection and treatment of CNS infection may limit permanent impairment of cognition.
Maintain a pleasant environment with appropriate auditory, visual, and cognitive stimuli.	Providing normal environmental stimuli can help in maintaining some sense of reality orientation.
Provide cues for reorientation such as radio, television, calendars, clocks, or a room with an outside view. Use client's name; identify yourself. Maintain consistent personnel and structured schedules, as appropriate.	Frequent reorientation to place and time may be necessary, especially during fever or acute CNS involvement. Sense of continuity may reduce associated anxiety.
Discuss use of datebooks, lists, and other devices to keep track of activities.	These techniques help client manage problems of forgetfulness.
Encourage family/SO to socialize and provide reorientation with current news and family events.	Familiar contacts are often helpful in maintaining reality orientation, especially if client is hallucinating.
Encourage client to do as much as possible, such as dressing and grooming and visiting with friends.	Can help maintain mental abilities for longer period.
Provide support for SO. Encourage discussion of concerns and fears.	Bizarre behavior or deterioration of abilities may be very frightening for SO and makes management of care and dealing with situation difficult. SO may feel a loss of control as stress, anxiety, burnout, and anticipatory grieving impair coping abilities.
Provide information about care on an ongoing basis. Answer questions simply and honestly. Repeat explanations as needed.	Can reduce anxiety and fear of unknown; can enhance client's understanding, involvement, and cooperation in treatment when possible.
Cognitive Restructuring (NIC)	
Reduce provocative or noxious stimuli. Maintain bedrest in quiet, darkened room, if indicated.	If client is prone to agitation, violent behavior, or seizures, reducing external stimuli may be helpful.
Decrease noise, especially at night.	Promotes sleep, reducing cognitive symptoms and effects of sleep deprivation.
Set limits on maladaptive or abusive behavior; avoid open-ended choices.	Provides sense of security and stability in an otherwise confusing situation.
Maintain safe environment, such as excess furniture out of the way, call bell within client's reach, bed in low position, rails up; restriction of smoking unless monitored by caregiver and SO; seizure precautions; and soft restraints, if indicated.	Decreases the possibility of client injury.
Discuss future expectations and treatment if dementia is diagnosed. Use concrete terms.	Obtaining information that some medications have been shown to improve cognition can provide hope.
Collaborative	
Assist with diagnostic studies, such as MRI, CT scan, and spinal tap, and monitor laboratory studies (BUN/Cr, electrolytes, ABGs), as indicated.	Choice of tests or studies depends on clinical manifestations and index of suspicion, because changes in mental status may reflect a wide variety of causative factors, such as CMV meningitis or encephalitis, drug toxicity, electrolyte imbalances, and altered organ function.
Administer medications, as indicated, for example:	
Amphotericin B (Fungizone)	Antifungal useful in treatment of cryptococcosis meningitis.
ZDV (Retrovir) and other antiretrovirals alone or in combination	Shown to improve neurological and mental functioning for undetermined period of time.
Antipsychotics, such as haloperidol (Haldol), and/or antianxiety agents, such as lorazepam (Ativan)	Cautious use may help with problems of sleeplessness, emotional lability, hallucinations, suspiciousness, and agitation.
Provide controlled environment and behavioral management.	Team approach may be required to protect client when mental impairment, especially delusions, threatens client safety.
Refer to counseling, as indicated.	May help client gain control in presence of thought disturbances or psychotic symptoms.

NURSING DIAGNOSIS: Death Anxiety

May Be Related To

Confronting the reality of terminal disease
Anticipating pain, suffering
Uncertainty about life after death, encounter with a higher power
Anticipating impact of death on others

Possibly Evidenced By

Reports negative thoughts related to death and dying, deep sadness
Reports feeling powerless over dying
Reports fear of pain or suffering related to dying, or prolonged dying

Desired Outcomes/Evaluation Criteria—Client Will

Dignified Life Closure (NOC)

Verbalize acceptance of reality of situation.
Express hopefulness and sense of control.
Appear calm and peaceful.
Participate in decisions about care and death.

ACTIONS/INTERVENTIONS	RATIONALE
Dying Care (NIC)	
Independent	
Assure client of confidentiality within limits of situation.	Provides reassurance and opportunity for client to problem-solve solutions to anticipated situations.
Maintain frequent contact with client. Talk with and touch client. Limit use of isolation clothing and masks.	Provides assurance that client is not alone or rejected; conveys respect for and acceptance of the person, fostering trust.
Provide accurate, consistent information regarding prognosis. Avoid arguing about client's perceptions of the situation.	Can reduce anxiety and enable client to make decisions or choices based on realities.
Be alert to signs of denial or depression, including withdrawal or angry, inappropriate remarks. Determine presence of suicidal ideation and assess potential on a scale of 1 to 10.	Client may use defense mechanism of denial and continue to hope that diagnosis is inaccurate. Feelings of guilt and spiritual distress may cause client to become withdrawn and believe that suicide is a viable alternative. Although client may be too "sick" to have enough energy to implement thoughts, ideation must be taken seriously and appropriate intervention initiated.
Provide open environment in which client feels safe to discuss feelings or to refrain from talking.	Helps client feel accepted in present condition without feeling judged and promotes sense of dignity and control.
Permit expressions of anger, fear, and despair without confrontation. Give information that feelings are normal and are to be appropriately expressed.	Acceptance of feelings allows client to begin to deal with situation.
Recognize and support the stage client and family are at in the grieving process. (Refer to CP: Cancer, ND: Grieving.)	Choice of interventions is dictated by stage of grief and coping behaviors, such as anger, withdrawal, and denial.
Explain procedures, providing opportunity for questions and honest answers. Arrange for someone to stay with client during anxiety-producing procedures and consultations.	Accurate information allows client to deal more effectively with the reality of the situation, thereby reducing anxiety and fear of the unknown.
Identify and encourage client interaction with support systems. Encourage verbalization and interaction with family and SO.	Reduces feelings of isolation. If family support systems are not available, outside sources such as local AIDS task force may be needed.
Provide reliable and consistent information and support for SO.	Allows for better interpersonal interaction and reduction of anxiety and fear.
Include SO as indicated when major decisions are to be made.	Ensures a support system for client and allows SO the chance to participate in client's life. *Note:* If client, family, and SO are in conflict, separate care consultations and visiting times may be needed.
Discuss advance directives and end-of-life desires and needs. Review specific wishes and explain various options clearly.	May assist client and SO to plan realistically for terminal stages and death. *Note:* Many individuals do not understand medical terminology or options such as percutaneous endoscopic gastrostomy (PEG) tube for short- or long-term feeding and pain management techniques.
Collaborative	
Refer to counseling—psychiatric clinical nurse specialist, psychiatrist, or social worker.	May require further assistance in dealing with diagnosis/prognosis, especially when suicidal thoughts are present.

(continues on page 706)

ACTIONS/INTERVENTIONS (continued)	RATIONALE (continued)
Provide contact with other resources, as indicated:	
Spiritual advisor	Provides opportunity for addressing spiritual concerns.
Hospice staff	May help relieve anxiety regarding end-of-life care and provide physical and emotional support for client and SO.

NURSING DIAGNOSIS: Social Isolation

May Be Related To

Altered state of wellness
Alterations in physical appearance, mental status
Unacceptable social behavior or values
Inadequate personal resources or support systems

Possibly Evidenced By

Reports feelings of aloneness imposed by others, feelings of rejection
Absence of supportive SO(s)—partners, family, acquaintances, or friends

Desired Outcomes/Evaluation Criteria—Client Will

Loneliness Severity (NOC)
Express sense of satisfaction with relationship(s).
Reports sense of acceptance or belonging.

Social Support (NOC)
Identify supportive individual(s).
Develop stable support system.
Use resources for assistance, as appropriate.

ACTIONS/INTERVENTIONS	RATIONALE
Support System Enhancement (NIC)	
Independent	
Ascertain client's perception of situation.	Isolation may be partly self-imposed because client fears rejection or reaction of others.
Spend time talking with client during and between care activities. Be supportive, allowing for verbalization. Treat with dignity and regard for client's feelings.	Client may experience physical isolation as a result of current medical status and some degree of social isolation secondary to diagnosis of AIDS.
Limit or avoid use of mask, gown, and gloves when possible, such as when talking to client.	Reduces client's sense of physical isolation and provides positive social contact, which may enhance self-esteem and decrease negative behaviors.
Identify support systems available to client, including presence of, relationship with, immediate and extended family.	When client has assistance from SO, feelings of loneliness and rejection are diminished. However, for some homosexual clients this may be the first time that the family has been made aware that client lives an alternative lifestyle. *Note:* Client may not receive needed support for coping with life-threatening illness and associated grief because of discrimination, fear, and lack of understanding—AIDS hysteria.
Explain isolation precautions and procedures to client and SO.	Gloves, gowns, and mask are not routinely required with a diagnosis of AIDS, except when contact with secretions or excretions is expected. Misuse of these barriers enhances feelings of emotional and physical isolation. When precautions are necessary, explanations help client understand reasons for procedure and provide feeling of inclusion in what is happening.
Encourage open visitation, as appropriate, telephone contacts, and social activities within level of tolerance.	Participation with others can foster a feeling of belonging.
Encourage active role of contact with SO.	Helps reestablish a feeling of participation in a social relationship. May lessen likelihood of suicide attempts.
Develop a plan of action with client that looks at available resources and supports healthy behaviors. Help client problem-solve solution to short-term or imposed isolation.	Having a plan promotes a sense of control over own life and gives client something to look forward to and actions to accomplish.
Be alert to verbal and nonverbal cues, including withdrawal, statements of despair, and sense of aloneness. Ask client if thoughts of suicide are being entertained.	Indicators of despair and suicidal ideation are often present. When these cues are acknowledged by the caregiver, client is usually willing to talk about thoughts of suicide and sense of isolation and hopelessness.

ACTIONS/INTERVENTIONS (continued)	RATIONALE (continued)
Collaborative	
Refer to resources, such as social services counselors and local and national AIDS organizations.	Establishes support systems; may reduce feelings of isolation.
Provide for placement in sheltered community when necessary.	May need more specific care when unable to be maintained at home or when SO cannot manage care.

NURSING DIAGNOSIS: Powerlessness

May Be Related To

Illness-related regimen
Unsatisfying interpersonal interactions

Possibly Evidenced By

Depression over physical deterioration
Reports lack of control
Reports frustration over inability to perform previous activities
Dependence on others

Desired Outcomes/Evaluation Criteria—Client Will

Acceptance: Health Status (NOC)

Express positive self-regard.
Make choices related to healthcare.
Engage in self-care activities.

Health Beliefs: Perceived Control (NOC)

Acknowledge feelings and healthy ways to deal with them.
Verbalize some sense of control over present situation.

ACTIONS/INTERVENTIONS	RATIONALE
Self-Responsibility Facilitation (NIC)	
Independent	
Identify factors that contribute to client's feelings of powerlessness—diagnosis of a terminal illness, lack of support systems, and lack of knowledge about present situation.	Powerlessness is most prevalent in a client newly diagnosed with HIV and when dying with AIDS. Fear of AIDS (by the general population and the client's family/SO) is the most profound cause of client's isolation. Multiple medications and inconvenient dosing regimens can also reduce a person's sense of control, independence, and general quality of life.
Assess degree of feelings of helplessness, noting verbal and nonverbal expressions indicating lack of control ("It won't make any difference"), flat affect, or lack of communication.	Determines the status of the individual client and allows for appropriate intervention when client is immobilized by depressed feelings.
Encourage active role in planning activities, establishing realistic and attainable goals. Encourage client control and responsibility as much as possible. Assist client to identify things that client can and cannot control.	May enhance feelings of control and self-worth and sense of personal responsibility.
Encourage advance directives or living will and durable medical power of attorney documents, with specific and precise instructions regarding acceptable and unacceptable procedures to prolong life.	Many factors associated with the treatments used in this debilitating and often fatal disease process place client at the mercy of medical personnel and other unknown people who may be making decisions for and about client without regard for client's wishes, increasing loss of independence.
Discuss desires and assist with planning for funeral, as appropriate.	The individual can gain a sense of completion and value to his or her life when he or she decides to be involved in planning this final ceremony. This provides an opportunity to include things that are of importance to the client.

NURSING DIAGNOSIS: ineffective Self-Health Management

May Be Related To

Complexity of therapeutic regimen
Economic difficulties; perceived barriers/benefits
Powerlessness
Family conflict; social support deficit

Possibly Evidenced By

Reports difficulty with prescribed regimen
Failure to include treatment regimen in daily living
Ineffective choices in daily living for meeting health goals

Desired Outcomes/Evaluation Criteria—Client Will

Self-Management: Chronic Disease (NOC)

Verbalize understanding of condition, disease process, and potential complications.
Identify relationship of signs and symptoms to the disease process and correlate symptoms with causative factors.
Engage in behaviors/precautions to limit progression of disease.
Identify strategies to cope with effects of disease.

ACTIONS/INTERVENTIONS	RATIONALE
Teaching: Disease Process (NIC)	
Independent	
Review disease process and future expectations.	Provides knowledge base from which client can make informed choices. *Note:* Clients with AIDS are usually aware of the current literature and prognosis unless newly diagnosed.
Determine level of dependence and physical condition. Note extent of care and support available from family and SO and need for supplemental caregivers.	Helps plan amount of care and symptom management required and need for additional resources.
Review modes of transmission of disease, especially if newly diagnosed.	Corrects myths and misconceptions; promotes safety for client and others. Accurate epidemiological data are important in targeting prevention interventions.
Instruct client and caregivers concerning infection control: Using good hand-washing techniques for everyone, including client, family, and caregivers; Using gloves when handling bedpans, dressings, and soiled linens; Wearing mask if client has productive cough; Placing soiled or wet linens in plastic bag and separating them from family laundry; washing with detergent and hot water; Cleaning surfaces with bleach and water solution of 1:10 ratio, disinfecting toilet bowl or bedpan with full-strength bleach; Preparing client's food in clean area; washing dishes and utensils in hot, soapy water—can be washed with the family dishes	Reduces risk of transmission of diseases; promotes wellness in presence of reduced ability of immune system to control level of flora.
Stress necessity of daily skin care, including inspecting skinfolds, pressure points, and perineum, and of providing adequate cleansing and protective measures such as ointments and padding.	Healthy skin provides barrier to infection. Measures to prevent skin disruption and associated complications are critical.
Ascertain that client/SO can perform necessary oral and dental care. Review procedures, as indicated. Encourage regular dental care.	The oral mucosa can quickly exhibit severe, progressive complications; therefore, preventative and early intervention measures are critical. *Note:* Recent studies indicate that 30% of HIV/AIDS clients experience some oral symptoms at least once during their illness. The decrease in occurrence is attributed to increased dental screening and success of antiretroviral therapy (Fox et al, 2012).
Review high-protein and high-calorie dietary needs and ways to improve intake when anorexia, diarrhea, weakness, or depression interfere with intake.	Promotes adequate nutrition necessary for healing and support of immune system and enhances feeling of well-being.
Discuss medication regimen, interactions, and side effects.	Enhances cooperation and increases probability of success with therapeutic regimen.
Provide information about and assist in developing a plan for symptom management that complements medical regimen; for example, client experiencing intermittent diarrhea should take diphenoxylate (Lomotil) before going to a social event.	Quality of life is an important issue in the management of symptoms of severe HIV infection, such as anemia, pain, fatigue, weakness, sleep disorders, or GI symptoms, and/or the side effects of medications. Having a plan provides client with increased sense of control, reduces risk of embarrassment, and promotes comfort.

ACTIONS/INTERVENTIONS (continued)	RATIONALE (continued)
Emphasize importance of adequate rest.	Helps manage fatigue; enhances coping abilities and energy level.
Encourage activity and exercise at level that client can tolerate.	Stimulates release of endorphins in the brain, enhancing sense of well-being.
Stress necessity of continued healthcare and follow-up.	Provides opportunity for altering regimen to meet individual changing needs.
Recommend cessation of smoking.	Smoking increases risk of respiratory infections and can further impair immune system.
Identify signs and symptoms requiring medical evaluation: persistent fever or night sweats, swollen glands, continued weight loss, diarrhea, skin blotches or lesions, headache, and chest pain or dyspnea.	Early recognition of developing complications and timely interventions may prevent progression to life-threatening situation.
Identify community resources such as hospice or residential care centers, visiting nurse, home-care services, Meals on Wheels, and peer group support.	Facilitates transfer from acute care setting for recovery and independence or end-of-life care.

POTENTIAL CONSIDERATIONS in addition to the nursing diagnoses listed in the plan of care.
- ***Grieving***—loss of significant object (e.g., job, status, significant others/family, processes of body)
- ***ineffective Protection***—abnormal blood profile (e.g., anemia, thrombocytopenia, coagulation), inadequate nutrition, pharmaceutical agents (e.g., antineoplastic, immune), cancer
- ***Caregiver Role Strain***—illness severity of care receiver, increasing care needs, amount/complexity of activities, history of family dysfunction, lack of respite for caregiver, caregiver's competing role commitments

RHEUMATOID ARTHRITIS (RA)

I. Pathophysiology (Bingham, 2012)

a. Systemic inflammatory process originating in the synovium or synovial fluid involving connective tissue and characterized by destruction and proliferation of the synovial membrane
b. Phagocytosis produces enzymes within the joint, causing inflammation.
c. Collagen is destroyed over time and pannus formations occur, narrowing the joint space.
d. May result in joint destruction, ankylosis, and deformity, with loss of articulation and joint motion
e. Inflammatory process can also affect the spine, blood vessels, the pleural membrane of the lungs, or the pericardial sac.
f. Condition may be short-lived and limited or progressive and severe.
g. Spontaneous remissions and unpredictable exacerbations can occur.

II. Classification: (Centers for Disease Control and Prevention [CDC] 2011)

a. Monocyclic: One episode which ends within 2 to 5 years of initial diagnosis and does not recur. This may result from early diagnosis and/or aggressive treatment.
b. Polycyclic: Levels of disease activity fluctuate over the course of the condition.
c. Progressive: Disease activity continues to increase in severity and is unremitting.

III. Etiology (Temprano, 2013)

a. Systemic inflammatory disease
b. Specific cause unknown
c. Associated factors: infectious triggers, genetic predisposition, autoimmune response
d. Other possible factors: more common in females, with ratio to males approximately 3:1; hormone interaction; psychological stress; heavy, long-term smoking; history of blood transfusions

IV. Statistics

a. Morbidity: In 2005, an estimated 1.3 to 1.5 million U.S. adults aged ≥18 (0.6%) had RA (Helmick et al, 2008; Arthritis Foundation, 2008); peak incidence occurs at ages 35–50 years (Temprano, 2013).
b. Mortality: Dependent on overall deterioration in health and secondary organ dysfunction, primarily cardiovascular conditions. One source states that "over the past 50 years, many studies have found mortality to be increased in persons with established RA in comparison with the general population" (Symmons, 2011). One source stated that between 1979 to 1998 RA accounted for 22% of all deaths from arthritis and other rheumatic conditions (Sacks, 2004).
c. Cost: Arthritis and related conditions, such as RA, cost the U.S. economy nearly $128 billion per year in medical care and indirect expenses, including lost wages and productivity (Arthritis Foundation, 2008).

GLOSSARY

Arthrodesis (fusion): Surgical procedure that involves removing the joint and fusing the bones into one immobile unit. Although the procedure limits movement, it can be useful for increasing stability and relieving pain in affected joints. The most commonly fused joints are the ankles and wrists and joints of the fingers and toes.

Disease-modifying antirheumatic drugs (DMARDs): A class of medications used in the treatment of RA; they often slow or stop the course of the disease to help prevent joint destruction.

Pannus: Inflamed synovial granulation tissue reflecting chronic RA.

Phagocytosis: Cellular process involved in the acquisition of nutrients for certain cells; major mechanism used to remove pathogens and cell debris.

Raynaud's phenomenon: Condition in which cold temperatures or strong emotions cause blood vessel spasms that block blood flow to the fingers, toes, ears, and nose. This causes intermittent pallor, cyanosis, and then redness before color returns to normal.

Sjögren's syndrome: Chronic disorder that causes insufficient moisture production in certain glands of the body. This leads to impaired secretion of saliva and tears and results in the sicca complex: dry mouth (xerostomia) and dry eyes (keratoconjunctivitis sicca). Secondary Sjögren's syndrome is often associated with other autoimmune disorders, including RA.

Synovial fluid: A thick, straw-colored substance found in small amounts in joints, bursae, and tendon sheaths.

Synovial membrane: Tissue that lines a joint.

Synovitis: Inflammation of the lining of a joint.

Tendon reconstruction: RA can damage and even rupture tendons, the tissues that attach muscle to bone. This surgery, which is used most frequently on the hands to restore function, reconstructs the damaged tendon by attaching an intact tendon to it.

Care Settings

Client is treated at community level unless surgical procedure is required.

Related Concerns

Psychosocial aspects of care, page 729
Total joint replacement, page 625

Client Assessment Database

Data depend on severity and involvement of other organs (e.g., eyes, heart, lungs, kidneys), stage (i.e., acute exacerbation or remission), and coexistence of other forms of arthritis and autoimmune diseases.

DIAGNOSTIC DIVISION MAY REPORT	MAY EXHIBIT
ACTIVITY/REST	
• Joint pain and tenderness, usually symmetrical, worsened by movement • Morning stiffness often lasting 1 hour or more, and that does not improve with movement • Generalized weakness (possible effect of anemia) • Fatigue; sleep disturbances • Functional limitations affecting desired lifestyle, leisure time, and occupation	• Malaise • Impaired ROM of joints, particularly hands—fingers and wrist, hips, knees, ankles, elbows, and shoulders • Altered gait and posture • Muscle weakness, contractures, and atrophy • Joint deformities
CARDIOVASCULAR	
• Changes in color of fingers, toes	• Raynaud's phenomenon
EGO INTEGRITY	
• Acute and/or chronic stress factors, including financial, employment, disability, and relationship • Hopelessness and powerlessness over incapacitating situation • Threat to self-concept, body image, and personal identity	• Dependence on others
FOOD/FLUID	
• Inability to consume adequate food and fluids (temporomandibular joint [TMJ] involvement) • Anorexia, nausea	• Weight loss • Dryness of oral mucous membranes, decreased oral secretions, and dental caries
HYGIENE	
• Varying difficulty performing self-care activities • Dependence on others	

DIAGNOSTIC DIVISION MAY REPORT (continued)	MAY EXHIBIT (continued)
NEUROSENSORY • Numbness, tingling of hands and feet • Loss of sensation or burning in fingers	• Symmetrical joint swelling
PAIN/DISCOMFORT • Acute episodes of pain that may or may not be accompanied by soft tissue swelling in joints • Symmetrical pattern of pain involving joints on both sides of the body • Chronic aching pain and stiffness with mornings most difficult	• Red, swollen, hot joints (during acute exacerbations) • Pain limiting ability to perform tasks, such as lifting, using hands, or walking
SAFETY • Persistent low-grade fever • Dryness of eyes and mucous membranes • Difficulty managing homemaker or maintenance tasks	• Pale, shiny, taut skin • May have skin problems, especially under nails; or skin rash, ulcers, blisters (reflects a more serious case of RA in general) • Subcutaneous rounded, nontender nodules on pressure points of elbows, feet, knees • Decreased muscle strength, altered gait, reduced ROM • Palpation of joint reveals spongy tissue • Lymph node enlargement
SEXUALITY • Difficulty engaging in sexual activity as desired; abstinence • Risk for pregnancy complications	
SOCIAL INTERACTION • Impaired interactions with family and others • Change in roles, responsibilities • Isolation	
TEACHING/LEARNING • Familial history of RA (in juvenile onset) • Higher risk of heart and lung disorders, including pericarditis, valvular lesions, pulmonary fibrosis, pleuritis • Use of health foods, vitamins, untested arthritis "cures"	
DISCHARGE PLAN CONSIDERATIONS • May require assistance with transportation, self-care activities, homemaker/maintenance tasks, and changes in physical layout of home ➧ Refer to section at end of plan for postdischarge considerations.	

Diagnostic Studies

TEST WHY IT IS DONE	WHAT IT TELLS ME
BLOOD TESTS	
• ***Rheumatoid factor (RF):*** Macroglobulin type of antibody found in blood of individuals with RA. RF antibodies are usually immunoglobulin (Ig) M, but may also be IGG or IGA (Van Leeuwen et al, 2006).	Rheumatoid factors are not specific for the diagnosis of RA (seen in many other inflammatory and autoimmune conditions); however, the tests is positive in 70% to 80% of cases and may turn positive later in disease process than the AACP (Ruffing, 2012).
• ***Inflammatory markers: Cyclic citrullinated peptide antibody test (also called anti-CCP [ACCP]):*** Useful in early detection of RA.	More specific marker for RA. If both anti-CCP and rheumatoid factor (RF) are positive, it is likely the client has a more severe form of the disease.

(continues on page 712)

Diagnostic Studies (continued)

TEST WHY IT IS DONE (continued)	WHAT IT TELLS ME (continued)
• *Erythrocyte sedimentation rate (ESR):* Measures the speed at which red blood cells (RBCs) fall to the bottom of a test tube.	A high ESR indicates inflammation, and the higher it is, the more severe the RA. *Note:* Only about 60% of people with RA have an elevated ESR (Arthritis Foundation, 2007).
• *Antinuclear antibody (ANA) titer:* Presence of ANA indicates presence of collagen vascular and immune complex disorders such as RA.	Elevated in 30% to 40% of clients with RA (Arthritis Foundation, 2007). Follow-up tests are needed to pinpoint/diagnose the specific rheumatic disorder.
• *C-reactive protein (CRP):* Glycoprotein produced by the body in response to inflammation.	May be elevated with RA but is not specific to RA.
• *Complement C_3 and C_4:* Act as enzymes that aid in the immunologic and inflammatory response and are used to detect autoimmune disease.	C_3 and C_4 are increased in acute onset RA. Normal C_4 and decreased C_3 may be present in chronic RA (Van Leeuwen et al, 2006). Immune disorder or exhaustion results in depressed total complement levels.
• *Complete blood count (CBC):* Battery of screening tests, which typically includes hemoglobin (Hgb); hematocrit (Hct); RBC count and morphology, indices, and distribution width index; platelet count and size; white blood cell (WBC) count and differential.	Hgb may be decreased, revealing anemia, which is a common problem in clients with RA (Ruffing, 2012). Platelet count may be elevated when inflammation is present or low because of certain medications. WBCs are elevated when infectious processes are present.
OTHER DIAGNOSTIC STUDIES	
• *X-rays/radiographs:* Identify early indicators of RA and changes over time.	Reveals soft tissue swelling, erosion of bone, destruction of cartilage, osteoporosis of adjacent bone, as well as progression to bone cyst formation, narrowing of joint space, and subluxation. Concurrent osteoarthritic changes may also be noted. *Note:* Radiographic erosion is typically fastest in the first year of disease (Graudal, 1998).
• *Joint ultrasound; power Doppler ultrasonography (PDUS); quantitative ultrasound (QUS):* Uses high-energy sound waves bounced off internal tissues to detect arthritis by identifying the presence of fluid in the joints.	Can reveal joint inflammation before x-rays show damage and document early evidence of RA. PDUS may be reliable for monitoring inflammatory activity in the joint. QUS, which is used for osteoporosis, can detect bone loss in fingers, which may prove to be a good indicator of early RA.
• *Computed tomography (CT) scan:* X-ray procedure that produces cross-sectional images of the body layer by layer.	Provides preoperative assessment as to the main indications for surgical intervention, namely, neurological deficit and severe pain.
• *Magnetic resonance imaging (MRI):* Diagnostic technique that provides cross-sectional images of structures within the body without x-ray or other forms of radiation.	MRI can detect early inflammation in the hands before it is even visible on x-ray and is particularly accurate at pinpointing synovitis.
• *Direct arthroscopy:* Surgical technique where a tubelike instrument is inserted into a joint to inspect, diagnose, and repair tissues.	Visualization of area reveals bone irregularities and degeneration of joint.
• *Synovial fluid aspirate:* Needle aspiration of joint fluid to note volume, clarity, and presence of cells (red and white cells), crystals, and bacteria to aid in diagnosing joint-related problems and determining treatment options.	May reveal volume greater than normal; may be opaque, cloudy, or yellow due to inflammatory response, bleeding, or degenerative waste products. WBCs and leukocytes are increased, whereas viscosity and complement (C_3 and C_4) are decreased.

Nursing Priorities

1. Alleviate pain.
2. Increase mobility.
3. Promote positive self-concept.
4. Support independence.
5. Provide information about disease process, prognosis, and treatment needs.

Discharge Goals

1. Pain relieved or controlled.
2. Dealing realistically with current situation.
3. Managing activities of daily living (ADLs) by self or with assistance, as appropriate.
4. Disease process, prognosis, and therapeutic regimen understood.
5. Plan in place to meet needs after discharge.

NURSING DIAGNOSIS: acute/chronic Pain

May Be Related To

Physical agents—accumulation of fluid/inflammatory process, destruction of joint

Possibly Evidenced By

Verbal/coded reports of pain; fatigue
Narrowed focus
Expressive behaviors (e.g., restlessness, irritability)
Guarding behavior; protective gestures
Changes in vital signs (acute)

Desired Outcomes/Evaluation Criteria—Client Will

Pain Control (NOC)

Report pain is relieved or controlled.
Follow prescribed pharmacological regimen.
Incorporate relaxation skills and diversional activities into pain control program.

Pain: Disruptive Behaviors (NOC)

Appear relaxed and able to sleep or rest appropriately.
Participate in activities of daily living at level of ability.

ACTIONS/INTERVENTIONS	RATIONALE
Pain Management (NIC)	
Independent	
Investigate reports of pain, noting location, and intensity using a 0 to 10 or similar coded scale. Note precipitating factors and nonverbal pain cues.	Self-report should be the primary source of pain assessment in determining pain management needs and effectiveness of program.
Suggest client assume position of comfort while in bed or sitting in chair. Promote bedrest when indicated, but resume movement as soon as possible.	In severe disease or acute exacerbation, total bedrest may be necessary until objective and subjective improvements are noted to limit pain and injury to joint. *Note:* Immobility is known to worsen arthritis pain and stiffness.
Place and monitor use of pillows, sandbags, trochanter rolls, splints, and orthotics.	Stabilizes joint, decreasing joint movement and associated pain. *Note:* Orthotic devices play an important role in rehabilitation management to decrease pain and inflammation, improve function, reduce deformity, and correct biomechanical malalignment (Temprano, 2013).
Encourage frequent changes of position.	Prevents general fatigue and joint stiffness.
Recommend that client take warm bath or shower on arising and/or at bedtime. Apply warm, moist compresses to affected joints several times a day. Monitor water temperature.	Heat promotes muscle relaxation and mobility, decreases pain, and relieves morning stiffness. Sensitivity to heat may be diminished and dermal injury may occur.
Provide gentle massage.	Promotes relaxation and reduces muscle tension.
Encourage use of stress management techniques, such as progressive relaxation, biofeedback, visualization, guided imagery, self-hypnosis, and controlled breathing. Provide Therapeutic Touch, if desired.	Promotes relaxation, provides sense of control, and may enhance coping abilities.
Involve client in diversional activities appropriate for individual situation.	Refocuses attention, provides stimulation, and enhances self-esteem and feelings of general well-being.
Medicate before planned activities and exercises, as indicated.	Promotes relaxation, reduces muscle tension and spasms, facilitating participation in therapy.
Monitor for development of skin rash in clients using cyclooxgenase-2 (COX-2) inhibitors, especially those allergic to sulfa.	Severe, life-threatening skin reactions, such as toxic epidermal necrolysis, Stevens-Johnson syndrome, and erythema multiforme, may develop within the first 2 weeks of treatment or later on, indicating need for prompt discontinuation of medication.
Collaborative	
Administer medications, as indicated, for example:	Because irreversible joint damage occurs within the first 2 years, early diagnosis and intervention are necessary. Medications are the mainstay of treatment with a goal of (1) managing pain, (2) slowing joint destruction, and (3) preserving joint function.
Analgesics: NSAIDS, such as aspirin and acetaminophen (Tylenol Arthritis, Panadol); ibuprofen (Advil, Motrin); naproxen (Alleve); meloxicam (Mobic), etodolac (Lodine), and nabumetone (Relafen); indomethacin (Indocin) and Ketoprofen (Orudis)	These drugs control mild to moderate pain and inflammation by inhibition of prostaglandin synthesis and allow for improvement in mobility and function.

(continues on page 714)

ACTIONS/INTERVENTIONS (continued)	RATIONALE (continued)
COX-2 inhibitors, such as celecoxib (Celebrex)	The NSAID class of COX-2 inhibitors is also effective in controlling inflammation. However, Celebrex is the only one currently available in the United States due to Food and Drug Administration (FDA) findings of potential for adverse cardiovascular side effects with other COX-2 drugs (Buffing, 2012), including Viox and Bextra (Flynn & Johnson, 2008).
Disease-modifying antirheumatic drugs (DMARDS), such as:	Although both NSAIDs and DMARDs improve symptoms of active RA, only DMARDs have been shown to alter the disease course and improve radiographic outcomes.
Methotrexate (Rheumatrex, Trexall), sulfasalazine (Azulfidine), leflunomide (Arava), hydroxychloroquine (Plaquenil), and minocycline (Singh et al, 2012)	Methotrexate is considered the first-line DMARD agent for most individuals with RA. *Note:* Current DMARD therapy typically includes combinations of two or three drugs, most of which are methotrexate based (e.g., methotrexate + hydroxychloroquine, or methotrexate + hydroxychloroquine + sulfasalazine (Singh et al, 2012).
Tumor necrosis factor inhibitors, such as non-tumor necrosis factor (non-TNF) biologics (includes abatacept [Orencia], rituximab [Rituxan] (see below) and interleukin-6 [IL-6] drug toxilizumab [Actemra]); and anti-tumor necrosis factor (anti-TNF) biologics (e.g., adalimumab [Humira], etanercept [Enbrel], infliximab [Remicade], certolizumab pegol [Cimzia], golimumab [Simponi])	Tumor necrosis factor (TNF) is a pro-inflammatory cytokine produced by the immune system. Excess levels of TNF are associated with inflammatory diseases such as rheumatoid arthritis. Anti-TNFs reduce TNF to control inflammation and have been used for more than 10 years to treat inflammatory conditions. Given by injection or infusion, these drugs are able to stop disease progression. Non- TNFs use other mechanisms to interrupt the inflammatory autoimmune response. *Note:* Because of the effect of these drugs on the immune system, the client is at greater risk for infections. Therefore, screening for tuberculosis is recommended for all clients who are beginning or currently receiving biologic agents. And vaccinations are recommended for all clients taking DMARDs or biologic agents: pneumococcal, influenza, hepatitis B, human papillomavirus (HPV), and herpes zoster (Singh et al, 2012).
T-cell costimulatory blocker, such as Abatacept (Orencia)	This first-in-class agent works by interfering with the interactions between antigen-presenting cells and T lymphocytes and is specifically indicated for use in the client that has not responded well to TNF inhibitors and methotrexate.
B-cell reducer, such as Rituximab (Rituxan)	The depletion of specific B cells has been shown to limit the immune system's attack, effectively reducing pain and symptoms of RA and slowing radiographic progression.
Immunomodulatory and cytotoxic agents, such as Azathioprine (Imuran) and cyclosporine (Neoral)	Immune suppressants may be used for treatment of severe cases of RA when other medications have failed.
Corticosteroids, such as prednisone (Deltasone) and methylprednisolone (Medrol)	These drugs have both anti-inflammatory and immunoregulatory activity and are useful in early disease as temporary adjunctive therapy. Corticosteroids may also be used as chronic adjunctive therapy in clients with severe disease not well controlled by NSAIDs and DMARDs. These drugs selectively block parts of the immune system.
Topical skin products, e.g., diclofenac (Voltaren)	Topical gel approved for osteoarthritis at a dosage of 32 g/day applied over all affected joints has also been used to provide analgesic effects in patients with RA (Temprano, 2013).
Assist with physical therapies, such as paraffin gloves or whirlpool baths.	Provides sustained heat to reduce pain and improve ROM of affected joints.
Apply ice or cold packs when indicated.	Cold may relieve pain and swelling during acute episodes.
Instruct in use and monitor effect of transcutaneous electrical nerve stimulator (TENS) unit, if used.	Constant low-level electrical stimulus blocks transmission of pain sensations.
Assist with other modalities, as indicated, such as blood filtration.	Prosorba Column is a device similar to a kidney dialysis machine that removes substances from blood plasma that contribute to joint swelling and pain. The plasma is then returned to the client's bloodstream. The offending antibodies are gone, decreasing the immune response.
Prepare for surgical interventions, such as tendon realignment and repair, tunnel release procedures, total joint replacement, joint fusion.	Corrective surgical procedures may be indicated to reduce pain and/or improve joint function and mobility.

NURSING DIAGNOSIS: impaired physical Mobility

May Be Related To
Musculoskeletal impairment; joint stiffness
Pain
Decreased endurance
Reluctance to initiate movement

Possibly Evidenced By
Limited range of motion; slowed movement
Gait changes; difficulty turning

Desired Outcomes/Evaluation Criteria—Client Will

Joint Movement (NOC)
Maintain or increase strength and function of affected joint(s).
Maintain position of function with absence or limitation of contractures.

Ambulation (NOC)
Engage in techniques or behaviors that enhance ability to ambulate.

ACTIONS/INTERVENTIONS	RATIONALE
Exercise Therapy: Joint Mobility (NIC)	
Independent	
Evaluate and then continuously monitor degree of joint inflammation and pain.	Level of activity and exercise depends on progression or resolution of inflammatory process.
Maintain bedrest or chair rest when indicated. Schedule activities providing frequent rest periods and uninterrupted nighttime sleep.	Person with RA needs a good balance between rest and exercise, with more rest when disease is active and more exercise when it is not. Systemic rest is mandatory during acute exacerbations and important throughout all phases of disease to reduce fatigue and improve strength.
Assist with active, or perform passive, ROM and resistive exercises and isometrics when able.	Maintains and may improve joint function, muscle strength, and general stamina. *Note:* Inadequate exercise leads to joint stiffening, whereas excessive activity can damage joints.
Encourage client to maintain upright and erect posture when sitting, standing, and walking.	Maximizes joint function and maintains mobility.
Discuss and provide safety needs, such as raised chairs and toilet seat, use of handrails in tub or shower and toilet, proper use of mobility aids or wheelchair safety.	Helps prevent accidental injuries and falls.
Positioning (NIC)	
Reposition frequently using adequate personnel. Demonstrate and assist with transfer techniques and use of mobility aids, such as walker, cane, or trapeze.	Relieves pressure on tissues and promotes circulation. Facilitates self-care and client's independence. Proper transfer techniques prevent shearing abrasions of skin.
Position with pillows, sandbags, or trochanter roll. Provide joint support with splints.	Promotes joint stability, reducing risk of injury, and maintains proper joint position and body alignment, minimizing contractures.
Suggest using small or thin pillow under neck.	Prevents flexion of neck.
Collaborative	
Provide foam or alternating pressure mattress.	Decreases pressure on fragile tissues to reduce risks of immobility and development of decubitus ulcers.
Exercise Therapy: Joint Mobility (NIC)	
Consult with physical and occupational therapists and vocational specialist.	Helps with formulating exercise and activity program based on individual needs in identifying and reducing impairments in ROM, flexibility, strength, and endurance, and to instruct in joint protection strategies and mobility devices and adjuncts.
Self-Care Assistance: Instrumental Activities of Daily Living (IADLs) (NIC)	
Determine appropriateness of, and ability to use, scooter or special enhancements to automobile such as hand controls and wide mirrors.	Facilitates movement within the environment, decreases fatigue, and promotes independence.

NURSING DIAGNOSIS: ineffective Role Performance

May Be Related To

Pain
Fatigue; depression
Job schedule demands
Lack of resources; inadequate support system

Possibly Evidenced By

Change in capacity to resume role
Inadequate external support for role enactment
Powerlessness

Desired Outcomes/Evaluation Criteria—Client Will

Role Performance (NOC)

Talk with family/employer about changes or limitations imposed by condition.
Verbalize acceptance of self in changed role.
Formulate realistic plans for adapting to role change.

ACTIONS/INTERVENTIONS	RATIONALE
Role Enhancement (NIC)	
Independent	
Encourage verbalization about concerns of disease process and future expectations.	Provides opportunity to identify fears or misconceptions and deal with them directly.
Discuss meaning of loss or change to client and SO as appropriate. Ascertain how client views self in usual lifestyle functioning, including home, employment, and sexual aspects.	Identifying how illness affects perception of self and interactions with others will determine need for further intervention or counseling.
Discuss client's perception of how SO perceives limitations.	Verbal and nonverbal cues from SO may have a major impact on how client views self.
Acknowledge and accept feelings of grief, hostility, and dependency.	Constant pain is wearing, and feelings of anger and hostility are common. Acceptance provides feedback that feelings are normal.
Note withdrawn behavior, use of denial, or overconcern with changes.	May suggest emotional exhaustion or maladaptive coping methods, requiring more in-depth intervention and psychological support.
Set limits on maladaptive behavior. Assist client to identify positive behaviors that will aid in coping.	Helps client maintain self-control, enhancing self-esteem.
Involve client in planning care and scheduling activities.	Enhances feelings of competency and self-worth and encourages independence and participation in therapy.
Give positive reinforcement for accomplishments.	Allows client to feel good about self. Reinforces positive behavior. Enhances confidence.
Collaborative	
Identify community resources, local and national support groups, disability advocate as appropriate.	Provides role models and assistance with problem-solving and adapting to changes as they occur. Disability advocates provide additional support when dealing with problems within the community.
Recommend vocational/employment counselors as indicated.	Employment counselors provide client with information regarding available assistive devices and appropriate worksite accommodations or modifications.
Refer to psychiatric counseling, such as psychiatric clinical nurse specialist, psychiatrist/psychologist, or social worker.	Client/SO may require ongoing support to deal with long-term debilitating process.
Administer medications as indicated, such as anti-anxiety and mood-elevating drugs.	May be needed in presence of severe depression until client develops more effective coping skills.

NURSING DIAGNOSIS: Self-Care Deficit (specify)

May Be Related To

Pain, discomfort
Fatigue
Musculoskeletal impairment; weakness
Environmental barriers

Possibly Evidenced By

Inability to manage ADLs—feeding, bathing, dressing, and/or toileting

NURSING DIAGNOSIS: Self-Care Deficit (specify) (continued)

Desired Outcomes/Evaluation Criteria—Client Will

Self-Care: Status (NOC)

Perform self-care activities at a level consistent with individual capabilities.
Demonstrate techniques and lifestyle changes to meet self-care needs.
Identify personal and community resources that can provide needed assistance.

ACTIONS/INTERVENTIONS	RATIONALE
Self-Care Assistance (NIC)	
Independent	
Determine usual level of functioning using Functional Level Classification 0–4 for status before onset or exacerbation of illness and potential changes now anticipated.	May be able to continue usual activities with necessary adaptations to current limitations.
Maintain mobility, pain control, and exercise program.	Supports physical and emotional independence.
Allow client sufficient time to complete tasks to fullest extent of ability. Capitalize on individual strengths.	May need more time to complete tasks by self but provides an opportunity for greater sense of self-confidence and self-worth.
Assess barriers to participation in self-care. Identify and plan for environmental modifications.	Prepares for increased independence, which enhances self-esteem.
Identify sources for necessary equipment such as lifts, elevated toilet seat, wheelchair, or scooter.	Provides opportunity to acquire equipment before discharge.
Collaborative	
Consult with rehabilitation specialists, such as occupational therapist.	Helpful in determining assistive devices to meet individual needs, such as buttonhooks, long-handled shoehorn, reacher, and handheld showerhead.
Arrange for consult with other agencies, such as Meals on Wheels, home-care service, or nutritionist.	May need additional kinds of assistance to continue in home setting.

NURSING DIAGNOSIS: risk for impaired Home Maintenance

Risk Factors May Include

Disease; impaired functioning
Inadequate family organization or planning
Insufficient finances
Unfamiliarity with neighborhood resources

Possibly Evidenced By

(Not applicable; presence of signs and symptoms establishes an *actual* diagnosis)

Desired Outcomes/Evaluation Criteria—Client Will

Safe Home Environment (NOC)

Maintain safe, health-promoting environment.
Demonstrate appropriate, effective use of resources.

ACTIONS/INTERVENTIONS	RATIONALE
Home Maintenance Assistance (NIC)	
Independent	
Determine level of physical functioning using Functional Level Classification 0 to 4.	Identifies degree of assistance and support required. For example, the level 0 client is completely able to perform usual ADLs, including self-care, vocational, and avocational, whereas the level 4 client is limited in all these areas and does not participate in activity.
Discuss client's/SO's perception of current environmental needs and ability to maintain safe surroundings.	Determines feasibility of remaining in and changing home layout to meet individual needs.
Determine financial resources to meet needs of individual situation. Identify support systems available to client, such as extended family, friends, and neighbors.	Availability of personal resources and community supports will affect ability to problem-solve and choice of solutions.

(continues on page 718)

ACTIONS/INTERVENTIONS (continued)	RATIONALE (continued)
Develop plan for restoring/maintaining a clean, healthy environment, such as sharing of household repairs and other tasks among family members or by contract services.	Some problems may be immediate (e.g., lack of heat, failed roof, stairs preventing entry to or access to parts of home) or ongoing needs such as lawn care, snow removal, pest control, and general repairs. Planning helps ensure that needs will be met on an ongoing basis.
Collaborative	
Coordinate home evaluation by occupational therapist and rehabilitation team as indicated.	Helpful in identifying potential or existing health and safety hazards and to determine adaptations that may be required (e.g., chair or stair lifts, wheelchair-accessible doors and hallways, clean water available, timely trash removal).
Identify sources for necessary home repairs or modifications.	Provides opportunity to schedule or perform necessary home repairs or upgrades in a timely manor.
Identify and meet with community resources, such as visiting nurse, homemaker service, social services, and senior citizens' groups.	Can facilitate transfer to, and support continuation in, home setting.

NURSING DIAGNOSIS: risk for ineffective Self-Health Management

May Be Related To

Complexity of therapeutic regimen; perceived barriers/benefits
Economic difficulties
Excessive demands made (e.g., family, employment)
Social support deficits

Possibly Evidenced By

(Not applicable; presence of signs and symptoms establishes an *actual* diagnosis)

Desired Outcomes/Evaluation Criteria—Client Will

Self-Management: Chronic Disease (NOC)

Verbalize understanding of condition, prognosis, and potential complications.
Verbalize understanding of therapeutic needs.
Develop a plan for self-care, including lifestyle modifications consistent with mobility and/or activity restrictions.

ACTIONS/INTERVENTIONS	RATIONALE
Teaching: Disease Process (NIC)	
Independent	
Review disease process, prognosis, and future expectations.	Provides knowledge base from which client can make informed choices.
Discuss client's role in management of disease process through nutrition, medication, and balanced program of exercise and rest.	Goal of disease control is to suppress inflammation in joints and other tissues to maintain joint function and prevent deformities.
Assist in planning a realistic and integrated schedule of activity, rest, personal care, drug administration, physical therapy, and stress management.	Provides structure and defuses anxiety when managing a complex chronic disease process.
Identify individually appropriate exercise program components, such as swimming, stationary bike, or nonimpact aerobics.	Can increase client's energy level and mental alertness and minimize functional limitations. Program needs to be customized based on joints involved and client's general condition to maximize effect and reduce risk of injury.
Stress importance of continued pharmacotherapeutic management.	Benefits of drug therapy depend on correct regimen, dosage, timing, and continuation without gaps
Recommend use of enteric-coated or buffered aspirin or nonacetylated salicylates, such as choline salicylate (Arthropan) or choline magnesium trisalicylate (Trilisate).	These preparations, ingested with food, minimize gastric irritation, reducing risk of gastric bleeding. *Note:* Nonacetylated products have a longer half-life, requiring less frequent administration in addition to producing less gastric irritation.
Suggest taking medications, such as NSAIDs, with meals, milk products, or antacids and at bedtime.	Limits gastric irritation. Reduction of pain at bedtime enhances sleep and increased blood level decreases early-morning stiffness.
Identify adverse drug effects, such as tinnitus, gastric intolerance, gastrointestinal (GI) bleeding, or purpuric rash.	Prolonged, maximal doses of aspirin may result in overdose. Tinnitus usually indicates high therapeutic blood levels. If tinnitus occurs, the dosage is usually decreased by one tablet every 2 to 3 days until it stops.

ACTIONS/INTERVENTIONS (continued)	RATIONALE (continued)
Emphasize importance of reading product labels and refraining from over-the-counter (OTC) drug usage without prior medical approval.	Many products, such as cold remedies or antidiarrheals, contain hidden salicylates that increase risk of drug overdose and harmful side effects.
Review importance of balanced diet with foods high in vitamins, protein, and iron.	Promotes general well-being and tissue repair or regeneration.
Encourage obese client to lose weight and supply with weight reduction information, as appropriate.	Weight loss reduces stress on joints, especially hips, knees, ankles, and feet.
Provide information about and resources for assistive devices, such as wheeled dolly or wagon for moving items, pickup sticks, lightweight dishes and pans, raised toilet seat, and safety handlebars.	Reduces force exerted on joints and enables individual to participate more comfortably in needed or desired activities.
Discuss energy-saving techniques, such as sitting instead of standing to prepare meals, shower, shave, or apply make-up.	Prevents fatigue; facilitates self-care and independence.
Encourage maintenance of correct body position and posture both at rest and during activity—keeping joints extended, not flexed, wearing splints for prescribed periods, avoiding remaining in a single position for extended periods, positioning hands near center of body during use, and sliding rather than lifting objects when possible.	Good body mechanics must become a part of client's lifestyle to lessen joint stress and pain.
Review safety issues related to mobility devices, especially electric scooters. Suggest use of a pennant when traveling on open streets.	Ability to travel over uneven surfaces, gravel, or soft ground is dependent upon specific scooter model. In addition, speed and safe maneuvering are equally important for the driver and other individuals in the vicinity. A pennant can be seen by other motorists.
Review necessity of frequent inspection of skin and meticulous skin care under splints, casts, and supporting devices. Demonstrate proper padding.	Reduces risk of skin irritation and breakdown.
Discuss necessity of medical follow-up and laboratory studies.	Drug therapy requires frequent assessment and refinement to ensure optimal effect and to prevent overdose or dangerous side effects.
Provide for sexual and childbirth counseling, as necessary.	Information about different positions and techniques and/or other options for sexual fulfillment may enhance personal relationships and feelings of self-worth and self-esteem. *Note:* A large number of clients with RA are in childbearing years and need counseling, support, and medical interventions.
Identify community resources, such as chapters of the National Institute of Arthritis and Muscular and Skin Diseases (NIAMS) and the Arthritis Foundation.	Assistance and support from others promote maximal recovery.

POTENTIAL CONSIDERATIONS following acute hospitalization (dependent on client's age, physical condition and presence of complications, personal resources, and life responsibilities)

- ***Fatigue***—disease state, poor physical condition, stress, depression
- ***chronic Pain***—chronic physical disability
- ***impaired physical Mobility***—pain, joint stiffness, disuse, decreased endurance, reluctance to initiate movement
- ***Self-Care Deficit***—pain, musculoskeletal impairment, weakness, fatigue, environmental barriers

TRANSPLANTATION CONSIDERATIONS—POSTOPERATIVE AND LIFELONG

I. Procedure

a. Transfer of whole or partial organs—including heart, lung, kidney, liver, pancreas, and intestines—and tissues or cells from one location to another

b. Long considered experimental, heart and other transplant procedures are successfully moving to domain of conventional therapy; however, others, such as hand and limb transplants, are still at the experimental stage.

c. Bone, bone marrow, heart valve, cartilage, vein, pancreatic islet, cornea, and stem cell transplantations are also performed on a daily basis (Sharma, 2006).

  i. Stem cell use is being investigated for treating a wide range of diseases, tissue damage, or both.

  ii. Two types of stem cells: human embryonic stem cells (hES) and adult somatic stem cells (ASSC), which is the source currently being used in research (Sullivan, 2007)

(continues on page 720)

d. Major concerns (Workman, 2006)
   i. Immunological response of the client to donor tissues and the ability of the immune system to distinguish self from nonself leading to rejection of the transplant
   ii. Special considerations necessitate meticulous measures to prevent infection and identify early signs of rejection.

II. **Types**—characterized according to the genetic relationship between the donor and recipient or the anatomical site of the implantation
   a. Genetic relationship characterized into four classes (Sharma, 2006)
      i. Autograft
      ii. Isograft or syngeneic graft
      iii. Allograft or homograft
      iv. Xenograft or heterograft
   b. Site of implantation (Sharma, 2006)
      i. Orthotropic: tissue implanted in the anatomically correct position
      ii. Heterotopic: relocation of the implant at a site different from the normal anatomy

III. **Statistics** (U.S. Organ Procurement and Transplant Network [OPTN], 2013)
   a. Morbidity: In 2012, 28,063 transplants were performed in all categories—heart, lung, kidney, pancreas, liver, intestine, and multi-organ—in the United States; kidney transplant is the most common (more than 16,000), followed by liver (more than 6000) and heart (more than 2300).
   b. Mortality: Dependent on type of transplant, level of match and human leukocyte antigen (HLA) status, recipient's age at transplant, preoperative condition, presence of comorbidities (Parimon et al, 2005). For example, Lucey et al reported, "Today, death attributable to acute or chronic allograft rejection is uncommon throughout the first 10 years after [liver] transplantation" (Lucey et al, 2013). Another study showed that 7-year survival rates for heart transplant recipients transplanted between 2000 and 2007 were 59%, 62%, and 65%, respectively (UnitedHealth Group, 2012).
   c. Cost: Varies according to procedure; the 2011 estimated average medical charges for 30 days pretransplant through 180 days post-transplant (including outpatient immunosuppressants and other medications) per transplant episode for kidney, $262,900; heart, $997,700; single lung, $561,200; double lung, $797,300; heart-lung, $1,148,400; pancreas, $289,400; liver, $577,100; intestine, $1,206,800 (Bentley, 2011).

GLOSSARY

Acute rejection: Usually occurs within 3 to 6 months and is diagnosed through laboratory testing and biopsy of the donated organ. Drug management of the host immune responses may limit damage to the organ so that it can be retained.

Allograft or homograft: Organ or tissue donor and recipient are genetically unrelated but belong to the same species.

Antibody: Protein molecule produced by the immune system in response to a foreign body, such as a transplanted organ.

Antirejection drugs: Drugs that are used to prevent and/or treat rejection of a transplanted organ; also called immunosuppressive therapies.

Autograft: Donor and recipient are the same individual.

Chronic rejection: May occur months or years after transplant and is similar to chronic inflammation and scarring where functional tissue of the donated organ is replaced by fibrotic tissue, thus hindering organ function. The process is gradual and can be delayed with drug management of host immune responses. However, if fibrosis causes the donated organ to fail, the only cure is reimplantation.

Donor: Someone from whom at least one organ or tissue is recovered for the purpose of transplantation. A deceased donor is a person who has been declared dead using either brain death or cardiac death criteria, from whom at least one vascularized solid organ is recovered for the purpose of organ transplantation. A living donor is one who donates an organ or segment of an organ for the intent of transplantation.

Graft: Transplanted organ or tissue.

Heterotopic transplantation: Relocation of the implant in the recipient at a site different from the normal anatomy, such as positioning the donor heart so that the chambers and blood vessels of both hearts are joined.

Human leukocyte antigens (HLAs): Genetic markers found on all cells of the body that determine white blood cell (WBC) types. HLA tissue types are used to match donated organs or bone marrow with transplant recipients.

Hyperactive or hyperacute rejection: Process where an antibody-remediated reaction occurs within minutes to hours and causes widespread clotting in the new organ. It occurs most frequently in transplanted kidneys and requires removal of the rejected organ.

Immune response: Body's natural defense against foreign objects or organisms, such as bacteria, viruses, or transplanted organs or tissue.

Isograft or syngeneic graft: Donor and recipient are genetically identical.

Match: Compatibility between the donor and the recipient. The more appropriate the match is, the greater the chance of a successful transplant.

Orthotopic transplantation: Donor tissue is implanted in the anatomically correct position in the recipient.

Retransplantation: Due to rejection or failure of a transplanted organ, some patients receive another transplant.

Stem cell: An unspecialized cell that is capable of replicating or self-renewing itself and developing into specialized cells of a variety of cell types.

Xenograft or heterograft: Organ or tissue procured from a different species for transplantation into a human—use of pig heart valve in humans.

Care Setting

Post-intensive care unit (ICU) plan of care addresses early recovery and long-term postdischarge community or clinic follow-up phases.

Related Concerns

Refer to (1) specific surgical plans of care for general considerations (e.g., cardiac surgery) and (2) organ-specific plans (e.g., heart failure, renal failure, cirrhosis, hepatitis) relative to issues of target organ problems following transplantation.

Peritonitis, page 320
Psychosocial aspects of care, page 729
Sepsis/septicemia, page 665
Surgical intervention, page 762
Thrombophlebitis: venous thromboembolism, page 109

Client Assessment Database

Refer to specific plans of care for data reflecting specific organ failure necessitating transplantation.

DIAGNOSTIC DIVISION MAY REPORT	MAY EXHIBIT
EGO INTEGRITY	
• Feelings of anxiety, fearfulness	• Anxiety, delirium, depression
• Multiple stressors—impact of condition on personal relationships, ability to perform expected or needed roles, loss of control, required lifestyle changes, financial concerns, cost of procedure and future treatment needs, uncertainty of outcomes, personal mortality, spiritual conflicts, waiting period for suitable donation	• Cognitive and emotional behavioral changes
• Concerns about changes in appearance—bloating, jaundice, major scars, esthetic side effects of immunosuppressant medications	
• Spiritual questioning, such as "Why me?" or "Why should I benefit from someone else's death?"	
SEXUALITY	
• Loss of libido	
• Concerns regarding sexual activity	
SOCIAL INTERACTIONS	
• Reactions of family members	
• Conflicts regarding family member(s) ability and willingness to participate—financial, organ or bone marrow donation, postprocedure support	
• Concern about benefiting from other person's death	
• Concern for family member who must take on new responsibilities as roles shift	
TEACHING/LEARNING	
• Previous illnesses, hospitalizations, surgeries	
• Lack of improvement or deterioration in condition	
• Beliefs about transplantation; previous noncompliance with medical treatment	
• History of abuse or current dependency on alcohol or other drug(s) resulting in organ failure	
DISCHARGE PLAN CONSIDERATIONS	
• May need assistance with activities of daily living (ADLs); shopping, transportation, ambulation; managing medication regimen	
➧ Refer to section at end of plan for postdischarge considerations.	

Diagnostic Studies (dependent on specific organ involvement)

General preoperative screening studies include the following.

TEST WHY IT IS DONE	WHAT IT TELLS ME
BLOOD TESTS	
• Blood tests to determine blood type, clotting ability, and biochemical status of blood and to gauge renal and liver function.	Help to predict success of procedure and to identify treatment needs.
• *Serology screening tests:* Tests for potentially transmissible infections.	Detect presence and type of hepatitis, HIV, or viruses (e.g., cytomegalovirus [CMV], herpes).
• *Complete blood count (CBC):* Battery of screening tests, which typically includes hemoglobin (Hgb); hematocrit (Hct); red blood cell (RBC) count, morphology, indices, and distribution width index; platelet count and size; and WBC count and differential.	Determines adequacy of RBCs, including oxygen-binding capacity that may affect recovery. WBCs, specifically leukocytes (made up of granulocytes, lymphocytes, and monocytes), are crucial to immune defense.
OTHER DIAGNOSTIC STUDIES	
• *Donor-recipient matching:* Studies include three distinct areas: (1) blood type, (2) tissue type matching, and (3) crossmatching.	
• *Blood typing:* Initial screening for compatibility, which is repeated just prior to surgery to verify that recipient has not developed new antibodies that would cause rejection of transplant.	There are four major blood types—A, B, AB, and O. Example of a match is type O for both parties; or recipient with type AB is a positive match for donor with AB, A, B, or O blood type. Another factor, the Rh factor, adds a plus or a minus following the above blood type letter, such as A+ or B–, and so on.
• *Tissue matching:* Complex testing relates to genetic matching between donors and recipients. Prior to a graft or transplant, tissue types of the donor and recipient are examined for compatibility by testing antigens, such as HLAs.	A six-antigen match is not always necessary because rejection can be overcome through the use of immunosuppressive drugs. However, if the recipient has already been exposed to one or more of the donor's HLAs, as might occur due to a previous blood transfusion, there may be antibodies already present that would increase the chances of rejection (Twynman, 2003).
• *Crossmatching:* Involves a mixing of cells and serum.	Positive result indicates donor and recipient are incompatible, resulting in immediate loss of transplant.
• *Computed tomography (CT)/magnetic resonance imaging (MRI) scans:* Uses x-ray or magnetic energy to generate images of organs.	Reveals status of body systems and organs, including size, shape, and general function of major blood vessels; organ size for best match with donor organ; and potential sources of postoperative complications. Rules out presence of cancer, which would contraindicate transplantation.
• *Total-body bone scan:* Evaluates status of skeletal system.	Determines presence or absence of bone cancer.
• *Electrocardiogram (ECG):* Measures the electrical activity of the heart.	Screens for cardiac dysrhythmias, infarcts, and hypertrophy.
• *Pulmonary function studies (PFTs):* Battery of studies or maneuvers, including spirometry, lung volume measurement, diffusing capacity for carbon monoxide, and arterial blood gases (ABGs).	Determines lung function and ability to exchange oxygen and carbon dioxide.
• *Renal function studies (e.g., intravenous [IV] pyelogram, creatinine clearance):* Determines functional status of kidneys.	Presence of preexisting renal problems may alter options or medication choices as research suggests an increased risk for developing chronic renal failure following nonkidney transplants and progressing to end-stage renal disease even in individuals with normal renal function preoperatively (Ojo et al, 2003).
• *Dental evaluation:* Rules out oral infection or abscessed teeth.	Dental work may be required prior to transplantation procedures.

Nursing Priorities

1. Prevent infection.
2. Maximize organ function.
3. Promote independent functioning.
4. Support family involvement and coping.

Discharge Goals

1. Free of signs of infection.
2. Signs of rejection absent or controlled.
3. New organ function adequate.
4. Usual activities resumed.
5. Client and family education plan established.
6. Plan in place to meet individual needs following discharge.

NURSING DIAGNOSIS: risk for Infection

Risk Factors May Include

Immunosuppression, suppressed inflammatory response
Invasive procedures; broken skin, traumatized tissue
Chronic disease

Possibly Evidenced By

(Not applicable; presence of signs and symptoms establishes an *actual* diagnosis)

Desired Outcomes/Evaluation Criteria—Client Will

Infection Severity (NOC)

Be free of signs of infection.
Achieve timely wound healing.

Client/Caregiver Will

Risk Control (NOC)

Demonstrate techniques and lifestyle changes to promote safe environment.

ACTIONS/INTERVENTIONS	RATIONALE
Infection Protection (NIC)	
Independent	
Screen visitors and staff for signs of infection; make sure nurse caring for client with new transplant is not caring for another client with infection. Maintain protective isolation, as indicated.	Isolation precautions reduce possibility of client's contracting a nosocomial infection. *Note:* Total isolation is usually restricted to clients with lung transplants or individuals with neutropenia.
Demonstrate and emphasize importance of proper hand-washing techniques by client and caregivers.	Hand washing is the first-line of defense against infection and cross-contamination.
Inspect all incisions and puncture sites. Evaluate healing progress.	Frequent assessment of incisions and puncture sites promotes early identification of onset of infection and prompt intervention.
Provide meticulous care of invasive lines, incisions, and wounds. Remove invasive devices as soon as possible.	Minimizes potential for bacteria to reduce exposure and risk of infection.
Encourage deep breathing and coughing.	Mobilizes respiratory secretions and reduces risk of respiratory problems.
Provide or assist with frequent oral hygiene.	Meticulous oral hygiene reduces the risk for opportunistic infections in clients who are on antibiotic therapy or who are immunocompromised.
Obtain culture specimens of wound drainage, as appropriate.	Identifying organism allows for appropriate treatment.
Collaborative	
Monitor laboratory tests, such as WBC count and blood glucose.	Elevated WBC count signals inflammation or infection. However, reduced WBC levels may result from severe immunosuppression and viral infection. *Note:* Use of some medications such as corticosteroids increases risk of insulin resistance. Tight glucose control is required to reduce risk of deep wound infections during the postoperative period.
Administer antimicrobials, as indicated, such as levofloxacin (Levaquin), cefazolin (Ancef), cefepime (Maxipime), vancomycin (Lyphocin), or ciprofloxacin (Cipro).	Antibiotics may be used to treat infections; however, they must be closely monitored for side effects and drug interaction with cyclosporine and other immunosuppressants.

NURSING DIAGNOSIS: Anxiety [specify level]

May Be Related To

Threat of death
Unconscious conflict about essential values or goals of life
Situational crises; stress; interpersonal transmission or contagion
Change in economic status, role function

Possibly Evidenced By

Reports concerns due to change in life events
Increased tension; apprehensive, uncertainty, worried

(continues on page 724)

NURSING DIAGNOSIS: Anxiety [specify level] (continued)

Focus on self
Sleep disturbance; fatigue
Change in vital signs

Desired Outcomes/Evaluation Criteria—Client Will

Anxiety Self-Control (NOC)
Appear relaxed and report anxiety is reduced to a manageable level.
Verbalize awareness of feelings.
Identify healthy ways to deal with anxiety.
Use resources and support systems effectively.

ACTIONS/INTERVENTIONS	RATIONALE
Anxiety Reduction (NIC)	
Independent	
Discuss client's post-transplant expectations and fears, including physical appearance, lifestyle changes, and concern about recurrence of disease or condition that precipitated the need for the transplant.	Depending on past experience and exposure to others with transplants, client may have unrealistic ideas and real concerns about what may happen, for example, rejection of received organ, effects of required medications, or limitations associated with immunosuppression. Even with effective preoperative teaching, client will continue to have new concerns or suppressed thoughts and beliefs, which can surface during recovery. For example, client may fear recurrence of disease, such as hepatitis C, in the transplanted organ or chronic rejection.
Encourage client to discuss feelings and concerns about situation and to express fears.	Open discussion helps identify issues and can lead to problem-solving. Client may experience anxiety about many things, such as physical limitations, cognitive changes, or role changes in the family. These anxieties change frequently; some are persistent, and new ones arise. Serious anxiety, delirium, and depression are the most commonly reported postoperative psychiatric problems.
Discuss beliefs and concerns that are commonly held regarding source of organ.	Cultural or spiritual beliefs may lead client to question whether organ from someone of another race or particular group may change own sense of self-identity or sexuality. *Note:* Some clients may use denial to deal with concerns about the organ donor.
Answer client's questions about donor honestly but refrain from providing unrequested information.	Excess information may add to survivor guilt that could distract the client from focusing on business of recovery.
Identify and encourage use of previously successful coping behaviors.	Prolonged nature of stressors can erode coping abilities. Discussion regarding previous successes may promote repetition of more effective behaviors.
Help client focus on one problem at a time.	Dealing with one issue at a time seems to make it more manageable. Provides sense of success and opportunity to build on each success.
Discuss possibility and normalcy of mood swings.	Feelings of euphoria and depression are not uncommon, especially in the early postoperative period, and can be managed to a large extent by presence, quiet environment, and rest. Medication may be required to promote client safety and comfort.
Encourage open communication between significant other (SO)/family and client within safe environment.	Free expression of feelings and beliefs can lead to clarification and problem-solving of different views. When concerns or beliefs are hidden from one another, additional stress and adverse effects may result.
Provide opportunity for client and SO/family to meet with other(s) that have experienced a similar and successful transplant.	Sharing experiences and hearing about successes and universal problems can lessen client's and SO's anxieties, promote hope, and provide a role model.
Identify possible actions to limit physical effects or manifestations of long-term steroid or cyclosporine use.	Learning about clothing styles, makeup techniques, and the use of bleach or mild depilatory to reduce facial hair can enhance client's appearance and reduce anxiety about social rejection.
Collaborative	
Refer to spiritual advisor, as indicated.	Facing one's mortality may provoke feelings of anxiety and questions about one's spiritual beliefs and practices.
Refer to social worker and other professionals, as indicated.	Provides assistance with readjustment to life following major life event.

NURSING DIAGNOSIS: risk for compromised family Coping

Risk Factors May Include

Prolonged disease that exhausts supportive capacity of significant people
Little support provided by client, in turn, for primary person
Temporary family role changes, disorganization

Possibly Evidenced By

(Not applicable; presence of signs and symptoms establishes an *actual* diagnosis)

Desired Outcomes/Evaluation Criteria—Family Will

Family Coping (NOC)

Assess current situation accurately.
Verbalize awareness of own coping abilities.
Meet psychological needs as evidenced by appropriate expression of feelings, identifying options and resources.

Family Support During Treatment (NOC)

Identify ways to assist client.
Provide support and encouragement to client.
Participate in planning care and preparation for discharge.

ACTIONS/INTERVENTIONS	RATIONALE
Family Integrity Promotion (NIC) *Independent*	
Encourage and support client and family in evaluating lifestyle. Discuss implications for the future.	Transplant clients sometimes cannot evaluate the seriousness of their condition or do not comprehend the risks or benefits involved in transplantation. Acceptance into a transplant program is often a major stressful event as it signals a "last treatment option." Additionally, there may be denial about the impact of long-term post-transplantation treatment requirements—use of immunosuppressant drugs, biopsies, blood tests, and clinic visits. *Note:* A meta-analysis of 147 studies found high nonadherence rates for aspects of the post-transplant regimen, including taking immunosuppressant medications (22.6% overall), following dietary (25.0%) and exercise (19.1%) recommendations, and monitoring vital signs (20.0%) (Dew et al, 2007). The consequences of nonadherence, particularly to the medication regimen, can be devastating for transplant clients, resulting in acute rejection, graft loss, decreased quality of life, and even death. Nonadherence is costly as well, leading to hospital readmissions, biopsies, additional immunosuppression, and retransplantation (O'Grady et al, 2010).
Assess client's and family's current functional status, and note how transplant is affecting ability to cope.	Provides a starting point to identify needs and plan care. The client's SO/family have been dealing with client's chronic disease, experiencing the uncertainty of organ waiting period, and protracted postoperative recovery course. They are the family members who also face a complicated medical regimen after the client's discharge, factors that place demands on their life routines, time, energy, finances, and relationships.
Determine additional outside stressors—family, social, work environment, or healthcare management.	Illness and treatment demands may affect all areas of life, and problems need to be addressed to enable client and SO to manage current situation optimally.
Provide ongoing information about expected progression of recuperation and potential course of recovery. Encourage family participation in care and planning for discharge needs as appropriate.	Knowing what to expect helps individuals cope more effectively and encourages planning for future needs and lifestyle changes. *Note:* These clients normally require a longer postoperative recovery period because of effects of medication regimen, opportunistic infections, or episodes of acute organ rejection.
Discuss normalcy of, and monitor progression through, states of acceptance of transplanted organ:	Movement through stages is variable and regression is common, especially during early post-transplant period.
Foreign body stage—organ feels strange, separate from own body. Partial internalization stage—protective of organ, restricts movement or activity, excessive concern regarding organ function or fragility.	Sense that organ is "outside" body can be very frightening, while fixation on organ can be irritating to others. Understanding normalcy of feelings is reassuring. *Note*: Movement through stages is variable and regression is common, especially, during early post-transplant period.

(continues on page 726)

ACTIONS/INTERVENTIONS (continued)	RATIONALE (continued)
Complete internalization—acceptance of organ into self-concept, discusses organ only in response to direct questioning.	
Have client and SO list previous methods of dealing with life problems and outcomes of actions.	Identifying previously successful life strategies promotes problem-solving in current situation and allows client to build on past successes.
Active-listen and identify individual's perceptions of what is happening and how transplant has affected view of self and family member.	Helps those involved to recognize own feelings and concerns regarding use of an organ from someone who died.
Encourage discussion between client and family regarding future expectations.	Period of dependence during illness and concerns over possible acute or chronic organ rejection and other life-threatening complications may lead to conflicts regarding client's return to an independent role.
Collaborative	
Involve in individual and family support groups.	Support groups serve as resources for practical advice and emotional sharing.
Refer to spiritual resource and/or psychiatric clinical nurse specialist, psychiatrist, or social worker, as indicated.	Spiritual and psychological guidance may be helpful in resolving lingering or difficult concerns. *Note:* During waiting period for transplant, relationships may be strained due to various stressors.

NURSING DIAGNOSIS: deficient Knowledge [Learning Need] regarding prognosis, therapeutic regimen, self-care, and discharge needs

May Be Related To
Lack of exposure or recall
Information misinterpretation
Unfamiliarity with information resources
Cognitive limitation

Possibly Evidenced By
Report of problem
Inappropriate behaviors—agitated, apathetic

Desired Outcomes/Evaluation Criteria—Client Will

Knowledge: Chronic Disease Management (NOC)
Describe measures to reduce individual risk factors to recovery and general well-being.
Initiate necessary lifestyle changes and participate in treatment regimen.
Identify community resources.
Develop plan to meet follow-up care needs.
Assume responsibility for own learning and begin to look for information and ask questions.

For routine postoperative instructions, refer to CP: Surgical Intervention.

ACTIONS/INTERVENTIONS	RATIONALE
Teaching: Disease Process (NIC)	
Independent	
Assess client's and SO's learning needs, readiness to learn, learning styles, and potential barriers to learning.	Teaching plan should concentrate on individualized behavioral outcomes and address client's needs. *Note:* Common learning barriers in the transplant population are the clients' emotional and mental status, their pretransplant physical health, and the critical care environment (Frank-Bader, 2011).
Include transplant team, client, SO, and family in teaching.	Successful recovery and long-term wellness require a coordinated effort by client and those regularly involved with client.
Provide information via multiple media, including written format, depending on level of comprehension. Include presentations by various members of the transplant team, as appropriate.	Multiple forms of information enhance learning experience and provide references for postdischarge review and recall. Use of team members, such as dietitian and physical and occupational therapists, provides for personalization of teaching plan to meet individual needs.

ACTIONS/INTERVENTIONS (continued)	RATIONALE (continued)
Review general signs and symptoms of rejection and infection, such as general malaise, fatigue, dyspnea, sudden weight gain, fever, chills, sore throat, delayed healing of wound, nausea, vomiting, and syncope. Review indicators specific to transplanted organ (e.g., liver rejection: pain in liver or back, lighter-colored stools, jaundice, dark-colored urine).	Prompt recognition and timely intervention may limit severity of complication. Acute rejection usually develops within days of transplant or may be delayed for a number of months. If detected early, rejection process can be minimized or reversed with changes in drug regimen. *Note:* Chronic rejection developing after months or years is generally irreversible.
Emphasize necessity for, and verify client's ability to adhere to, medical regimen and appropriate follow-up, including periodic laboratory tests such as drug levels, lipid panels, and organ function studies. Routine examinations, including dental and gynecologic, or specialty examinations, such as ophthalmologic or gastroenterologic, may also be required. Anticipate problems and participate in problem-solving with client and SO.	Because the incidence of medication noncompliance is a major cause of post-transplant complications and mortality, the client and SO need to understand that adherence to regimen is imperative—dosing, timing, length of time after transplant, and addition of this medication regimen to others that client requires; and physical and cognitive demands of routine. Routine follow-up care by healthcare providers is necessary to maximize general well-being and to monitor effects of long-term medication regimen on other organ systems, such as nephrotoxic effects. Specialty examinations aid in monitoring new organ function and effect on other systems. Additionally, steroid use may cause changes in visual acuity or development of cataracts or glaucoma.
Recommend that results of laboratory tests and diagnostic studies done locally be faxed to transplant center.	Long-term care is very complex and requires coordination and cooperation among all healthcare providers.
Discuss need to seek prompt medical attention.	Generally a "wait-and-see" attitude can be detrimental because a delay in treatment could result in organ damage or rejection.
Discuss managing immunosuppressant therapy, including "do's and don'ts" of specific medications, anticipated and adverse effects, interaction with other drugs, appropriate use of over-the-counter (OTC) products; adjustment of prescribed medication dosage during periods of stress, or with gradual decrease in immunosuppression over months or years, as appropriate.	Multiple medications such as a triple therapy regimen of cyclosporine (Sandimmune), tacrolimus (Prograf), and sirolimus (Rapamune) are typically required after liver transplant on an ongoing, lifelong basis to prevent or manage organ rejection (Guillen et al, 2005). Additional drugs or other drug regimens may be needed (depending on particular organ/tissue transplanted). Drugs are also often needed to manage side and adverse effects of immunosuppressant therapy, such as infection, weight gain, nausea, diarrhea, osteoporosis, peptic ulcers, and hypertension.
Encourage client and SO to maintain a working relationship with transplant team. Include family members and caregivers in education sessions and discharge planning, as appropriate.	Good working relationships among the client, SO, family, and transplant team promote understanding, cooperation, goal setting, and achievement of outcomes.
Recommend wearing an ID medical alert bracelet or necklace.	In emergencies, provides immediate information to care providers relative to surgical and transplant history and medication regimen.
Identify community resources, including transplant club or other support groups.	Community resources provide opportunity for client and SO to share experiences with others who are going through the same process. Providing anticipatory guidance may enhance problem-solving.
Discuss self-monitoring routine and record keeping, such as chart temperature per protocol (twice a day before meals and when not feeling well), weigh daily before breakfast in like clothing using same scale; record blood pressure and pulse, changes in medication dosage, and changes in health status and functional ability.	Self-monitoring helps identify individual needs and onset of preventable complications.
Recommend frequent oral and dental care and periodic visual inspection of oral mucosa and gums.	Immunosuppression increases susceptibility to common opportunistic infections affecting the mouth (e.g., *Candida,* herpes simplex). Ongoing drug regimen can cause hypertrophy of gums (cyclosporine) or ulcerations of the oral mucosa (Rapamune).
Review dietary needs. Determine optimal weight and discuss expected changes associated with medication regimen.	Requirements of normal healing, as well as effects of current stress, medications, and preoperative debilitation, can exacerbate nutritional deficiencies and cause excessive weight loss; however, undesired weight gain can also occur because food tastes better, dietary restrictions are eliminated, and prednisone stimulates appetite.
Identify risk factors and safety concerns relative to infections, such as avoid changing cat litter box or use of live virus vaccines, use gloves when gardening, and take proper care of wounds and tissue trauma.	Awareness of possible risks including unusual sources enables client and family/SO to plan for avoidance. Cat litter can transmit infectious agents such as *Listeria.* Steroid-induced skin fragility increases risk of injury from minor trauma as a result of thinning of the skin and immunosuppression.

(continues on page 728)

ACTIONS/INTERVENTIONS (continued)	RATIONALE (continued)
Discuss necessity of handling skin carefully, avoiding strong sunlight and using sunblock with sun protection factor (SPF) of 15 or higher.	Steroid therapy results in skin fragility, sun sensitivity, and risk of developing skin cancers.
Review common postoperative care needs, such as routine wound care and need for adequate rest; avoidance of heavy lifting, physical labor or exercise including contact sports, and activities that stretch or put pressure on incision; when and how to resume driving and sexual activity; and dietary and fluid needs or restrictions.	Reduces likelihood of complications, aids client and SO in determining appropriateness of activities, and enhances client's sense of control and personal responsibility for altering activity level.
Provide information about potential sexual dysfunction and encourage open communication for future discussion and support, as needed.	Decreased libido, erectile dysfunction, and impaired orgasmic ability often occur because of medication regimen, low hormone levels, impaired blood flow, fear of harm to transplanted organ, or emotional disturbances. Initially, client may be too focused on survival to address sexual issues or concerns.
Encourage continuation of pre-illness daily routines and activities, as appropriate.	Continuation of pre-illness activities enhances general well-being, promotes focus on returning to "normal life," and reduces the sense of "everything is different now."
Discuss participation in planned endurance and strength training exercise programs and inform about Transplant Olympics, as appropriate and desired.	Endurance and strength training restores strength, promotes sense of well-being and self-esteem, reduces risk of osteoporosis and inappropriate weight gain, and decreases hypertension.
Identify employment concerns and risks specific to particular transplanted organ, job responsibilities, and workplace environment.	Provides opportunity to problem-solve, plan for modifications, or seek alternative options.
Discuss travel needs, including notifying team contact person in advance regarding plans, hand-carrying medications when traveling by airplane, and locating transplant center nearest to travel destination before leaving home.	Transplant clients must carefully integrate their health needs when traveling.
Stress importance of notifying future care providers of medication regimen.	Status of immune system functioning may require prophylactic therapy for procedures (such as antibiotics with dental care).

POTENTIAL CONSIDERATIONS following acute hospitalization (depending on client's age, physical condition and presence of complications, personal resources, and life responsibilities)

- ***ineffective Self-Health Management***—complexity of therapeutic regimen, perceived barriers, economic difficulties, excessive demands made
- ***risk for Infection***—immunosuppression, invasive procedures, chronic disease
- ***ineffective Protection***—pharmaceutical agents (corticosteroid, immune)
- ***readiness for enhanced Family Coping***—chooses experiences that optimize wellness; individual expresses interest in making contact with others who have experienced a similar situation

CHAPTER 15

General

PSYCHOSOCIAL ASPECTS OF CARE

I. Mind-Body-Spirit Connection

a. When a physiological response occurs, there is a corresponding psychological response (Anandarajah, 2001).
   i. Emotional instability associated with steroid therapy or Cushing's syndrome
   ii. Irritability of hypoglycemia
   iii. Anxiety associated with impaired oxygenation
a. Emotional response during illness is of extreme importance.
   i. The stress of illness is well recognized; however, the effect on the individual is unpredictable.
   ii. The client's perception of, and response to, the event may result in unmet psychological needs that drain energy resources needed for healing.
   iii. Values brought to the interactions between clients, families, and healthcare providers affect the care that a client expects and receives.

II. Psychoneuroimmunology (PNI) provides new information about how interactions between the mind and the neuroendocrine and immune systems influence health and healing.

a. Negative emotions or stressful experiences can intensify health threats, contribute to prolonged infection, and result in delayed healing (Kiecolt-Glaser et al, 1999).
   i. Chronic stress: decreased T and B cells, decreased natural killer (NK) cells, increased blood levels of Epstein-Barr virus
   ii. Depression: decreased T cells, decreased number and function of lymphocytes, decreased NK cells
   iii. Grieving: decreased lymphocyte proliferation
a. Positive emotions can enhance immune response, facilitate healing, and slow disease progression.
   i. Personal sharing of traumatic experience: increased lymphocyte response
   ii. Support group intervention: increased NK cells and activity, increased lymphocyte count
   iii. Humor and laughter: increased immunoglobulin A, increased lymphocyte count and activity

GLOSSARY

Active-listening: Reflecting the underlying feelings in the message that is heard.

Eye movement desensitization and reprocessing (EMDR): Information-processing psychotherapy technique that integrates elements of psychodynamic, cognitive-behavioral, interpersonal, experiential, and body-centered therapies to assist individuals to deal with anxious feelings and stress associated with traumatic memories.

Guided imagery: Method of helping an individual relax by means of guiding them in a vision of tranquil places.

I-messages: Expression of feelings stated as "I feel . . ." in a nonblameful way.

Implosive therapy (flooding): The individual is "flooded" with a continuous presentation of the phobic stimulus until it no longer elicits anxiety.

Labile affect: Excessive emotional reactivity associated with frequent changes or swings in emotions and mood.

Locus of control: Site of control in an individual, which may be internal or external.

Mindfulness: Method of staying in the moment.

Natural killer (NK) cells: Cytotoxic lymphocytes play a major role in suppressing cancer cells and killing cells infected by viruses.

Psychoneuroimmunology (PNI): Field of study that focuses on relationship between psychosocial processes and nervous, endocrine, and immune system functioning.

Psychosocial: Theory of development proposed by Eric Erickson (1963).

Religiosity: Excessive demonstration of or obsession with religious ideas and behavior.

Tapping: A healing method using ancient Chinese acupressure and modern psychology (Ortner, 2013).

Therapeutic Touch: Method of healing by use of the hands moving through the energy field.

Care Setting

Any setting in which nursing contact occurs and care is provided.

Related Concerns

This is an aspect of all care and plans of care.

Assessment Factors to Be Considered

SUBJECTIVE	OBJECTIVE
INDIVIDUAL • Level of knowledge and education, how the individual accesses and incorporates information—auditory, visual, kinesthetic • Religious affiliation—church attendance, importance of religion in client's life, belief in life after death • Perception of body and its functions in health, illness, current situation • Past experience with illness, hospitalization, and healthcare systems • Emotional reactions in feeling (sensory) terms, for example, client states, "I feel scared"	• Age and gender • Client's dominant language, literacy, knowledge and use of other languages, style of speech • Patterns of communication with significant others (SOs), with healthcare givers • How is client experiencing illness versus what illness actually is • Emotional response to current treatment or hospitalization • Behavior when anxious, afraid, impatient, withdrawn, or angry
SIGNIFICANT OTHERS (SOs) • Marital status, SOs, nuclear and extended family, recurring or patterned relationships • Client's role in family tasks and functions • How are SOs affected by the illness and prognosis? • Lifestyle preferences to be considered: dietary, spiritual, sexual preference, other community—religious order, commune, retirement center	• Family development cycle—just married; young, adolescent children, leaving or returning home; retired • Interaction processes within the family may not be supportive.
SOCIOECONOMIC • Employment; finances • Environmental factors—residence, work, and recreation; out of usual environment such as on vacation, visiting	• Social class, value system • Social acceptability of disease or condition—sexually transmitted infections (STIs), HIV, obesity, substance abuse
CULTURAL • Ethnic background, heritage, and residence or locale • Beliefs regarding caring and curing • Values related to health and treatment • Cultural factors related to illness in general and to pain response	• Health-seeking behaviors, illness referral system
DISEASE (ILLNESS) • Kind and cause of illness; how has it been treated and how should it be treated? • Anticipated response to treatment; client's and SO's expectations • If terminal illness, what do the client and SO know and anticipate?	• Is this an acute or chronic condition, is it inherited, what is the threat to self or others? • Is the condition "appropriate" to the afflicted individual, for example, multiple sclerosis, diabetes mellitus (DM), cancer? (*Note:* Some theories suggest certain personalities are more prone to certain illnesses.) (Jongward & James, 1996) • Illness related to personality factors, such as type A (may be myth or valid relative to management of stressors); high-risk behaviors
NURSE RELATED • Basic knowledge of human responses and how the current situation is related to response of the individual • Basic knowledge of biological, psychological, social, cultural, and religious issues • Knowledge of own value and belief systems, including prejudices and biases	• Knowledge and use of therapeutic communication skills • Willingness to look at own behavior in relation to interaction with others and make changes as necessary • Respect of client's privacy, confidentiality, human needs

Nursing Priorities

1. Encourage effective coping skills of client and SO.
2. Reduce emotional distress.
3. Facilitate integration of self-concept and body-image changes.
4. Support grieving process.
5. Promote safe environment and client well-being.

Discharge Goals

1. Client and family dealing realistically with current situation.
2. Anxiety or fear manageable.
3. Progressing through stages of grieving.
4. Safe environment maintained.
5. Plan in place to meet needs after discharge.

NURSING DIAGNOSIS: ineffective Coping

May Be Related To

Situational crises; high degree of threat
Disturbance in pattern of appraisal of threat
Disturbance in pattern of tension release
Inadequate resources available
Gender differences in coping strategies

Possibly Evidenced By

Poor concentration; difficulty organizing information
Use of forms of coping that impede adaptive behavior
Change in usual communication patterns
Fatigue

Desired Outcomes/Evaluation Criteria—Client Will

Coping (NOC)
Identify ineffective coping behaviors and consequences.
Verbalize awareness of own coping and problem-solving abilities.
Meet psychological needs as evidenced by appropriate expression of feelings, identification of options, and use of resources.

Decision Making (NOC)
Make decisions and express satisfaction with choices.

ACTIONS/INTERVENTIONS	RATIONALE
Coping Enhancement (NIC) *Independent*	
Review pathophysiology affecting the client and extent of feelings of hopelessness, helplessness, and loss of control over life; level of anxiety, and perception of situation.	Indicators of degree of disequilibrium and need for intervention to prevent or resolve the crisis. Studies suggest that 20% to 40% of physically ill individuals are depressed (Robinson, 2002). Impairment of normal functioning for more than 2 weeks, especially in presence of chronic condition, may reflect depression, requiring further evaluation. *Note:* In contrast, depression is believed to contribute to the development and progression of some physical illnesses, such as heart or vascular disease or certain viral infections (Thomas, 2010).
Establish therapeutic nurse-client relationship.	Client may feel less inhibited in the context of this relationship to verbalize feelings of helplessness and powerlessness and feel more freedom to discuss changes that may be necessary in the client's life to improve situation.
Assess presence of positive coping skills and inner strengths, such as use of relaxation techniques, willingness to express feelings, and use of support systems.	When the individual has coping skills that have been successful in the past, they may be used in the current situation to relieve tension and preserve the individual's sense of control. However, limitations of condition may impact choices available to client; for example, playing a musical instrument to relieve stress may not be possible for individual with tremors or hemiparesis, but listening to tapes or CDs may provide some degree of comfort.
Encourage client to talk about what is happening at this time and what has occurred to precipitate feelings of helplessness and anxiety.	Provides clues to assist client to develop coping and regain equilibrium.
Provide quiet, nonstimulating environment. Determine what client needs, and provide, if possible. Give simple, factual information about what client can expect and repeat as necessary.	Decreases anxiety and provides control for the client during crisis situation.

(continues on page 732)

ACTIONS/INTERVENTIONS (continued)	RATIONALE (continued)
Allow client to be dependent in the beginning, with gradual resumption of independence in ADLs, self-care, and other activities. Make opportunities for client to make simple decisions about care and other activities when possible, accepting choice not to do so.	Promotes feelings of security—client knows nurse will provide safety. As control is regained, client has the opportunity to develop adaptive coping and problem-solving skills.
Accept verbal expressions of anger, setting limits on maladaptive behavior.	Verbalizing angry feelings is an important process for resolution of grief and loss. However, preventing destructive actions, such as striking out at others, preserves client's self-esteem.
Discuss feelings of self-blame or projection of blame on others.	Although these mechanisms may be protective at the moment of crisis, they eventually are counterproductive and intensify feelings of helplessness and hopelessness.
Note expressions of inability to find meaning in life or reason for living and feelings of futility or alienation from God.	Crisis situation may evoke questioning of spiritual beliefs, affecting ability to cope with current situation and plan for the future.
Promote safe and hopeful environment, as needed. Identify positive aspects of this experience and assist client to view it as a learning opportunity.	May be helpful while client regains inner control. The ability to learn from the current situation can provide skills for moving forward.
Provide for gradual implementation and continuation of necessary behaviors or lifestyle changes. Reinforce positive adaptation and new coping behaviors.	Reduces anxiety of sudden change and allows for developing new and creative solutions.
Collaborative	
Refer to other resources as necessary, such as clergy, psychiatric clinical nurse specialist, psychiatrist, family or marital therapist, and addiction support groups.	Additional assistance may be needed to help client resolve problems or make decisions. *Note:* If untreated, depression may complicate recovery from physical illness (Robinson, 2002).

NURSING DIAGNOSIS: Decisional Conflict (specify)

May Be Related To
Divergent sources of information
Lack of experience with decision making
Lack of relevant information
Moral obligations require performing or not performing action

Possibly Evidenced By
Delayed decision making; vacillation among alternative choices
Physical signs of tension; self-focusing
Questioning moral principles while attempting a decision
Verbalizes undesired consequences of alternative actions being considered

Desired Outcomes/Evaluation Criteria: Client Will

Decision Making (NOC)
Verbalize awareness of problem-solving abilities.
Use relevant information, and cultural/social considerations as appropriate, to make decisions.
Identify alternatives and potential consequences.
Verbalize satisfaction with decisions made.

ACTIONS/INTERVENTIONS	RATIONALE
Decision-Making Support (NIC)	
Independent	
Establish therapeutic nurse-client relationship.	Client may feel less inhibited in the context of this relationship to verbalize feelings of helplessness and powerlessness and feel more freedom to discuss changes that may be necessary in the client's life to improve situation.
Note expressions of indecision, dependence on others, and inability to manage own activities of daily living (ADLs).	May indicate need to lean on others for a time. Early recognition and intervention can help client regain equilibrium.
Evaluate ability to understand events. Correct misperceptions and provide factual information.	Assists in identification and correction of perception of reality and enables problem-solving to begin.
Active-listen; identify reason for indecisiveness.	Helps client to clarify problem and begin looking for resolution, alternative choices.
Identify cultural values and beliefs or moral obligations that may be creating conflict for client.	These issues must be addressed before client can be at peace with the decision that is made.

ACTIONS/INTERVENTIONS (continued)	RATIONALE (continued)
Provide support for client to problem-solve solutions for current situation. Provide information and reinforce reality as client begins to ask questions and look at what is happening.	Helping client and SO to brainstorm possible solutions and giving consideration to the pros and cons of each promotes feelings of self-control and strengthens self-esteem.
Collaborative	
Refer to other resources as necessary, such as clergy, psychiatric clinical nurse specialist, psychiatrist, family or marital therapist, and addiction support groups.	Additional assistance may be needed to help client resolve problems or make decisions. *Note:* If untreated, depression may complicate recovery from physical illness (Robinson, 2002).

NURSING DIAGNOSIS: risk for compromised family Coping

May Be Related To

Temporary family disorganization or role change
Exhaustion of supportive capacity of significant people
Lack of reciprocal support
Incorrect understanding of information by a primary person

Possibly Evidenced By

(Not applicable; presence of signs and symptoms establishes an *actual* diagnosis)

Desired Outcomes/Evaluation Criteria—Family Will

Family Coping (NOC)

Identify resources within themselves to deal with situation.
Visit regularly and participate positively in care of client, within limits of abilities.
Express more realistic understanding and expectations of the client.
Provide opportunity for client to deal with situation in own way.

ACTIONS/INTERVENTIONS	RATIONALE
Family Involvement Promotion (NIC)	
Independent	
Establish rapport and acknowledge difficulty of the situation for the family.	May assist family to accept what is happening and be willing to share problems with caregivers.
Determine current knowledge and perception of the situation.	Lack of information or unrealistic perceptions can interfere with family members' and client's response to illness situation.
Assess level of anxiety present in family and SO.	Anxiety level needs to be dealt with before problem-solving can begin. Individuals may be so preoccupied with own reactions to situation that they are unable to respond to another's needs.
Evaluate pre-illness and current behaviors that are interfering with care or recovery of the client.	Information about family problems, such as divorce or separation, financial limitations, and substance use, will be helpful in determining options and developing an appropriate plan of care.
Discuss underlying reasons for client behaviors with family.	When family members know why client is behaving in different ways, it helps them understand and accept or deal with situation.
Assist family/client to understand "who owns the problem" and who is responsible for resolution. Avoid placing blame or guilt (Gordon, 2000).	When these boundaries are defined, each individual can begin to take care of own self and stop taking care of others in inappropriate ways.
Reframe negative expressions into positives whenever possible.	Promotes more hopeful attitude and helps family and client look toward the future.
Involve SO in information giving, problem-solving, and care of client as feasible. Identify other ways of demonstrating support while maintaining client's independence.	Information can reduce feelings of helplessness. Involvement in care enhances feelings of control and self-worth.
Collaborative	
Refer to appropriate resources for assistance, as indicated, such as counseling, psychotherapy, and financial and spiritual support.	May need additional assistance in resolving family issues.

NURSING DIAGNOSIS: readiness for enhanced family Coping

Possibly Evidenced By

Individual expresses interest in making contact with others who have experienced a similar situation
Chooses experiences that optimize wellness
Significant person attempts to describe growth impact of crisis
Significant person moves in direction of health promotion, enriching lifestyle

Desired Outcomes/Evaluation Criteria—Family Will

Family Resiliency (NOC)

Express willingness to look at own role in family's growth.
Use community resources for support or assistance as needed.
Undertake tasks leading to change.
Verbalize feelings of self-confidence and satisfaction with progress being made.

ACTIONS/INTERVENTIONS	RATIONALE
Family Support (NIC)	
Independent	
Provide opportunities for family to talk with client and/or caregiver(s).	Reduces anxiety and allows expression of what has been learned and how they are managing as well as opportunity to make plans for the future and share support.
Listen to family's expressions of hope, planning, effect on relationships and life, and change of values.	Provides clues to avenues to explore for assistance with growth.
Provide opportunities for, and instruction in, how SOs can care for client. Discuss ways in which they can support client in meeting own needs.	Enhances feelings of control and involvement in situation in which SOs cannot do many things. Also provides opportunity to learn how to be most helpful when client is discharged from care.
Provide a role model with which family may identify.	Having a positive example can help with adoption of new behaviors to promote growth.
Discuss importance of open communication. Role play effective communication skills of active-listening, "I-messages," and problem-solving.	Helps individuals to express needs and wants in ways that will develop family cohesiveness. Promotes solutions in which everyone wins.
Encourage family to learn new and effective ways of dealing with feelings.	Effective recognition and expression of feelings clarify situation for involved individuals.
Encourage seeking support appropriately. Give information about available persons and agencies.	Permission to seek help as needed allows them to choose to take advantage of available assistance and resources.
Collaborative	
Refer to specific support group(s) as indicated.	Provides opportunities for sharing experiences, provides mutual support and practical problem-solving, and can aid in decreasing alienation and helplessness.

NURSING DIAGNOSIS: Anxiety [specify level]

May Be Related To

Change in health status, economic status, or role function
Situational crisis; stress
Unconscious conflict about essential values or goals of life

Possibly Evidenced By

Reports concerns due to change in life events
Apprehensive; distressed; increased tension
Focus on self
Changes in vital signs
Diminished ability to problem-solve

Desired Outcomes/Evaluation Criteria—Client Will

Anxiety Self-Control (NOC)

Acknowledge and discuss fears and concerns.
Verbalize awareness of feelings of anxiety and healthy ways to deal with them.
Demonstrate problem-solving and use resources effectively.

Anxiety Level (NOC)

Appear relaxed and report anxiety is reduced to a manageable level.

ACTIONS/INTERVENTIONS	RATIONALE
Anxiety Reduction (NIC)	
Independent	
Note palpitations and elevated pulse or respiratory rate.	Changes in vital signs may suggest the degree of anxiety the client is experiencing or reflect the impact of physiological factors such as pain or endocrine imbalances.
Acknowledge presence of anxiety. Validate observations with client, for example, "You seem to be afraid."	Feelings are real, and it is helpful to bring them out in the open so they can be discussed and dealt with.
Assess degree and reality of threat to client and level of anxiety—mild, moderate, severe—by observing behavior, such as clenched hands, wide eyes, startle response, furrowed brow, clinging to family and staff, or physical and verbal lashing out.	Individual responses can vary according to cultural beliefs and traditions and culturally learned patterns. Distorted perceptions of the situation may magnify feelings.
Note narrowed focus of attention and client concentrating on one thing at a time.	Narrowed focus usually reflects extreme fear or panic.
Observe speech content, vocabulary, and communication patterns, such as rapid or slow, pressured speech; words commonly used, repetition, use of humor or laughter, and swearing.	Provides clues about such factors as the level of anxiety, ability to comprehend what is currently happening, cognition difficulties, and possible language differences.
Assess severity of pain when present. Delay gathering of information if pain is severe.	Severe pain and anxiety leave little energy for critical thinking and other activities.
Determine client's and SO's perception(s) of the situation.	Regardless of the reality of the situation, perception affects how each individual deals with the illness and stress.
Acknowledge reality of the situation as the client sees it, without challenging the belief.	Client may need to deny reality until ready to deal with it. It is not helpful to force the client to face facts.
Evaluate coping and defense mechanisms being used to deal with the perceived or real threat.	May be dealing well with the situation at the moment; for example, denial and regression may be helpful coping mechanisms for a time. However, use of such mechanisms diverts energy the client needs for healing, and problems need to be dealt with at some point in time.
Review coping mechanisms used in the past, such as problem-solving skills and recognizing and asking for help.	Provides opportunity to build on resources the client and SO may have used successfully.
Assist client to use the energy of anxiety for coping with the situation when possible.	Moderate anxiety heightens awareness and can help motivate the client to focus on dealing with problems.
Maintain frequent contact with the client and SO. Be available for listening and talking, as needed.	Establishes rapport, promotes expression of feelings, and helps client and SO look at realities of the illness and treatment without confronting issues they are not ready to deal with.
Acknowledge feelings, as expressed, using active-listening or reflection. If actions are unacceptable, take necessary steps to control or deal with behavior. (Refer to ND: risk for Violence.)	Often acknowledging feelings enables client to deal more appropriately with situation. May need chemical or physical control for brief periods.
Identify ways in which client can get help when needed, including telephone numbers of contact persons.	Provides assurance that staff and resources are available for assistance/support.
Stay with or arrange to have someone stay with client, as indicated.	Continuous support may help client regain internal locus of control and reduce anxiety and fear to a manageable level.
Provide accurate information as appropriate and when requested by the client and SO. Answer questions freely and honestly and in language that is understandable by all. Repeat information as necessary; correct misconceptions.	Complex and/or anxiety-provoking information can be given in manageable amounts over an extended period. As opportunities arise and facts are given, individuals will accept what they are ready for. *Note:* Words and phrases may have different meanings for each individual; therefore, clarification is necessary to ensure understanding.
Avoid empty reassurances, with statements of "everything will be all right." Instead, provide specific information, such as "Your heart rate is regular, your pain is being easily controlled, and that is what we want," or "Your CD4 count has been stable for the last three visits."	It is not possible for the nurse to know how the specific situation will be resolved, and false reassurances may be interpreted as lack of understanding or honesty, further isolating the client. Sharing observations used in assessing condition and prognosis provides opportunity for client and SO to feel reassured.
Note expressions of concern or anger about treatment or staff.	Anxiety about self and outcome may be masked by comments or angry outbursts directed at therapy or caregivers.
Ask client and SO to identify what he or she can or cannot do about what is happening.	Assists in identifying areas in which control can be exercised and those in which control is not possible.
Provide as much order and predictability as possible in scheduling care, activities, and visitors.	Helps client anticipate and prepare for difficult treatments or movements, as well as look forward to pleasant occurrences.
Instruct in ways to use positive self-talk: "I can manage this pain for now," or "My cancer is shrinking."	Internal dialogue is often negative. When this is shared out loud, the client becomes aware and can be directed in the use of positive self-talk, which can help reduce anxiety.
Encourage client to develop regular exercise and activity program.	Has been shown to raise endorphin levels to enhance sense of well-being and help reduce level of anxiety.

(continues on page 736)

ACTIONS/INTERVENTIONS (continued)	RATIONALE (continued)
Encourage and instruct in guided imagery or other relaxation methods, such as imagining a pleasant place, use of music, deep breathing, meditation, and mindfulness (Healthwise Staff, 2011).	Promotes release of endorphins and aids in developing internal locus of control, reducing anxiety. May enhance coping skills, allowing body to go about its work of healing.
Collaborative	
Provide touch, Therapeutic Touch, massage, and other adjunctive therapies as indicated (Kreiger, 1998).	Aids in meeting basic human need, decreasing sense of isolation and assisting client to feel less anxious. *Note:* Therapeutic Touch requires the nurse to have specific knowledge and experience to use the hands to correct energy field disturbances by redirecting human energies to help or heal.
Collaborative	
Administer medications, as needed, for example: Anti-anxiety agents, such as diazepam (Valium), clorazepate (Tranxene), or chlordiazepoxide (Librium) Benzodiazepines, such as palprazolam (Xanax), oxazepam (Serax), lorazepam (Ativan), or temazepam (Restoril) Selective serotonin reuptake inhibitors (SSRIs), such as fluoxetine (Prozac), sertraline (Zoloft), fluvoxamine (Luvox), citalopram HAABr (Celexa), or paroxetine HCL (Paxil) Other drugs, such as buspirone (BuSpar) or doxepin (Adapin, Sinequan)	Anti-anxiety agents and/or antidepressants may be useful for brief periods to assist the client and SO to reduce anxiety to manageable levels, providing opportunity for initiation of client's own coping skills. *Note:* Use of SSRIs, such as Prozac or Zoloft, has been associated with sexual function complaints. Alternatives may need to be considered. Also, ethnic variations affecting psychotropic drugs require close monitoring to determine therapeutic dosage. For example, East Asians and blacks may be more sensitive or react faster, have higher plasma drug levels, and have increased risk of side effects, necessitating lower dosage than whites in general (Munoz, 2005).

NURSING DIAGNOSIS: risk for situational low Self-Esteem

May Be Related To

Decreased control over environment
Physical illness; functional impairment
Disturbed body image

Possibly Evidenced By

(Not applicable; presence of signs and symptoms establishes an *actual* diagnosis)

Desired Outcomes/Evaluation Criteria—Client Will

Self-Esteem (NOC)

Verbalize realistic view and acceptance of self in situation.
Identify existing strengths and view self as capable person.
Recognize and incorporate change into self-concept in accurate manner without negating self-worth.
Demonstrate adaptation to changes or events that have occurred as evidenced by setting of realistic goals and active participation in work, play, and personal relationships.

ACTIONS/INTERVENTIONS	RATIONALE
Self-Esteem Enhancement (NIC)	
Independent	
Ask how the client would like to be addressed.	Shows courtesy and respect and acknowledges person.
Identify SO from whom the client derives comfort and who should be notified in case of emergency.	Allows provisions to be made for specific person(s) to visit or remain close and provides needed support for client. *Note:* May or may not be legal next of kin.
Identify basic sense of self-esteem and image client has of existential, physical, psychological self. Identify locus of control.	May provide insight into whether this is a single episode or recurrent or chronic situation and can help determine needs and treatment plan. Determining whether the individual's locus of control is internal or external facilitates choosing most effective interventions.
Determine client's perception of threat to self.	Client's perception is more important than what is really happening and needs to be dealt with before reality can be addressed.
Active-listen client concerns and fears.	Conveys sense of caring and can be helpful in identifying the client's needs, problems, and coping strategies and how effective they are. Provides opportunity to develop and begin a problem-solving process.

ACTIONS/INTERVENTIONS (continued)	RATIONALE (continued)
Encourage verbalization of feelings, accepting what is said.	Helps client and SO begin to adapt to change and reduces anxiety about altered function or lifestyle.
Discuss stages of grief and the importance of grief work. (Refer to ND: Grieving [specify].)	Grieving is a necessary step for integration of change or loss into self-concept.
Provide nonthreatening environment; listen and accept client as presented.	Promotes feelings of safety, encouraging verbalization.
Observe nonverbal communication including body posture and movements, eye contact, gestures, and use of touch.	Nonverbal language is a large portion of communication and therefore is extremely important. How the person uses touch provides information about how it is accepted and how comfortable the individual is with being touched.
Reflect back to the client what has been said, for example, "You were upset when he told you that."	Clarification and verification of what has been heard promotes understanding and allows client to validate information; otherwise, assumptions may be inaccurate.
Observe and describe behavior in objective terms.	All behavior has meaning, some of which is obvious and some of which needs to be identified. This is a process of educated guesswork and requires validation by the client.
Identify age and developmental level.	Age is an indicator of the stage of life client is experiencing, whether it be adolescence or middle age. However, developmental level may be more important than chronological age in anticipating and identifying some of the client's needs. Some degree of regression occurs during illness, depending on many factors, such as the normal coping skills of the individual, the severity of the illness, and family and cultural expectations.
Discuss client's view of body image and how illness or condition might affect it.	The client's perception of a change in body image may occur suddenly or over time, such as actual loss of a body part through injury or surgery, or a perceived loss, such as a heart attack; or be a continuous subtle process, such as chronic illness, eating disorders, or aging. Awareness can alert the nurse to the need for appropriate interventions tailored to the individual need.
Encourage discussion of physical changes in a simple, direct, and factual manner. Give realistic feedback and discuss future options such as rehabilitation services.	Provides opportunity to begin incorporating actual changes in an accepting and hopeful atmosphere.
Acknowledge efforts at problem-solving, resolution of current situation, and future planning.	Provides encouragement and reinforces continuation of desired behaviors.
Recognize client's pace for adaptation to demands of current situation.	Failure to acknowledge client's need to take time and/or pressuring client to "get on with it" conveys a lack of acceptance of the person as an individual and may result in feelings of lowered self-esteem.
Introduce tasks at client's level of functioning, progressing to more complex activities as tolerated.	Provides opportunity for client to experience successes, reaffirming capabilities and enhancing self-worth.
Ascertain how the client sees own role within the family system: breadwinner, homemaker, or husband or wife.	Illness may create a temporary or permanent problem in role expectations. Sexual role and how the client views self in relation to the current illness also play important parts in recovery.
Assist client and SO with clarifying expected roles and those that may need to be relinquished or altered.	Provides opportunity to identify misconceptions and begin to look at options; promotes reality orientation.
Determine client awareness of own responsibility for dealing with situation and personal growth.	Conveys confidence in client's ability to cope. When client acknowledges own part in planning and carrying out treatment plan, he or she has more investment in following through on decisions that have been made.
Assess impact of condition, surgery, or medication regimen on sexuality.	Sexuality encompasses the whole person in the total environment. Many times problems of illness are superimposed on already existing problems of sexuality and can affect client's sense of self-worth. Some problems are more obvious than others, such as illness involving the reproductive parts of the body. Others are less obvious, such as sexual values and role in family: mother, wage earner, or single parent.
Be alert to comments and innuendos, which may mean the client has a concern in the area of sexuality.	People are often reluctant and/or embarrassed to ask direct questions about sexual or sexuality concerns.
Be aware of caregiver's feelings about dealing with the subject of sexuality.	Nurses and caregivers are often as reluctant and embarrassed in dealing with sexuality issues as most clients. (Refer to CP: Extended Care; ND: Sexual Dysfunction.)

(continues on page 738)

ACTIONS/INTERVENTIONS	RATIONALE
Collaborative	
Provide information and referral to community resources.	Enables client and SO to be in contact with interested groups with access to assistive and supportive devices, services, and counseling.
Support participation in group or community activities, such as assertiveness classes, volunteer work, and support groups.	Promotes skills of coping and sense of self-worth. Provides role models and facilitates problem-solving.
Refer to psychiatric support or therapy group and social services, as indicated.	May be needed to assist client and SO to achieve optimal recovery.
Refer to appropriate resources for sexuality counseling as need indicates.	May be someone with comfort level and knowledge who is available, or it may be necessary to refer to professional resources for additional guidance and support.

NURSING DIAGNOSIS: Grieving [specify]

May Be Related To

Anticipation or actual loss of significant object (e.g., parts or processes of body, status, job, home)
Lack of social support

Possibly Evidenced By

Alteration in activity level
Disturbed sleep pattern
Anger; blame; psychological distress

Desired Outcomes/Evaluation Criteria—Client Will

Grief Resolution (NOC)

Identify and express feelings freely and effectively.
Verbalize a sense of progress toward acceptance of loss.
Function at an acceptable level and participate in work and ADLs, as appropriate.

ACTIONS/INTERVENTIONS	RATIONALE
Grief Work Facilitation (NIC)	
Independent	
Provide open environment in which client feels free to realistically discuss feelings and concerns.	Therapeutic communication skills, such as active-listening, silence, being available, and acceptance, provide opportunity and encourage the client to talk freely and deal with the perceived or actual loss (Evesham, 2011).
Determine client perception and meaning of loss—current and past. Note cultural or religious factors and expectations.	Affects client's responses and needs to be acknowledged in planning care.
Identify stage of grieving and effect on functioning:	Awareness allows for appropriate choice of interventions because individuals handle grief in many different ways.
Denial: Be aware of avoidance behaviors, such as anger and/or withdrawal; allow client to talk about what he or she chooses, and do not try to force client to "face the facts."	Denying the reality of diagnosis and/or prognosis is an important phase in which the client protects self from the pain and reality of the threat of loss. Each person does this in an individual manner based on previous experiences with loss and cultural or religious factors.
Anger: Note behaviors of withdrawal, lack of cooperation, and direct expression of anger; be alert to body language and check meaning with client, noting congruency with verbalizations; encourage, and provide opportunity for, verbalization of anger; and acknowledge feelings and set limits regarding destructive behavior.	Denial gives way to feelings of anger, rage, guilt, and resentment. Client may find it difficult to express anger directly and may feel guilty about normal feelings of anger. Although staff may have difficulty dealing with angry behaviors, acceptance allows client to work through the anger and move on to more effective coping behaviors.
Bargaining: Be aware of statements such as ". . . if God will just . . . I will do . . ."; allow verbalization without confrontation about realities.	Bargaining with care providers or God often occurs and may be helpful in beginning resolution and acceptance. Client may be working through feelings of guilt about things done or undone.
Depression: Give client permission to be where he or she is; provide hope within parameters of individual situation without giving false reassurance; and provide comfort and availability as well as caring for physical needs.	When client can no longer deny the reality of the loss, feelings of helplessness and hopelessness replace feelings of anger. The client needs information that this is a normal progression of feelings.
Acceptance: Respect client's needs and wishes for quiet, privacy, and/or talking.	Having worked through the denial, anger, and depression stages, client often prefers to be alone and may not want to talk much at this point. Client may still cling to hope, which can be sustaining through whatever is currently happening.

ACTIONS/INTERVENTIONS (continued)	RATIONALE (continued)
Active-listen client's concerns and be available for support, as necessary (Evesham, 2011).	The process of grieving does not proceed in an orderly fashion, but fluctuates with various aspects of all stages present at one time or another. If process is dysfunctional or prolonged, more aggressive interventions may be required to facilitate the process.
Determine quality of interactions with others, including family members.	Although periods of withdrawal and loneliness usually accompany grieving, persistent isolation may indicate deepening depression, necessitating further evaluation and intervention. *Note:* Family/SO may not be dysfunctional but may be intolerant of client's behaviors.
Identify and problem-solve solutions to existing physical responses, such as eating, sleeping, activity levels, and sexual desire.	May need additional assistance to deal with the physical aspects of grieving.
Assess needs of SO and assist, as indicated.	Identification of problems indicating dysfunctional grieving allows for individual interventions.
Include family/SO, as appropriate, when determining future needs.	Depending on client's desires and legal requirements, choices regarding future plans (e.g., living situation, continuation of care, end-of-life decisions, funeral arrangements) can provide guidance and peace of mind.
Discuss healthy ways of dealing with difficult situation.	Provides opportunity to look toward the future and plan for family's/SO's needs (e.g., for life after loss).
Collaborative	
Refer to other resources, such as support groups, counseling, spiritual or pastoral care, and psychotherapy, as indicated.	May need additional help to resolve grief, make plans, and look toward the future.

NURSING DIAGNOSIS: risk for impaired Religiosity

Risk Factors May Include

Illness; hospitalization
Life transitions
Barriers to practicing religion; lack of transportation
Ineffective support; social isolation

Possibly Evidenced By

(Not applicable; presence of signs and symptoms establishes an *actual* diagnosis)

Desired Outcomes/Evaluation Criteria—Client Will

Spiritual Health (NOC)
Participate in beliefs and rituals of desired religion.
Discuss beliefs and values about spiritual or religious issues.
Attend religious or worship services of choice as desired.

ACTIONS/INTERVENTIONS	RATIONALE
Spiritual Support (NIC)	
Independent	
Listen to client's and SO's reports and expressions of anger and concern or alienation from God. Note sense of guilt or retribution.	May be suffering from severe or terminal illness or accident straining resources and affecting client's ability to cope. Perception of guilt may cause spiritual crisis or suffering resulting in rejection of religious activities and symbols.
Discuss differences between grief and guilt and help client to identify and deal with each. Point out consequences of actions based on guilt.	As client recognizes consequences of actions, they can be discussed, and desire to change may enhance new coping skills, avoid acting out of false guilt, and enable client to resume desired religious activities.
Use therapeutic communication skills of reflection and active-listening.	Communicates acceptance and enables client to find own solutions to concerns.
Determine sense of futility, feelings of hopelessness, and lack of motivation to help self.	Indicators that client may see no, or only limited, options or personal choices available and lack energy to deal with situation.
Assess extent of depression client may be experiencing.	Some studies suggest that a focus on religion may protect against depression.

(continues on page 740)

ACTIONS/INTERVENTIONS (continued)	RATIONALE (continued)
Note recent changes in behavior, such as withdrawal from others and religious activities and dependence on alcohol or medications.	Helpful in determining severity and duration of situation and possible need for additional referrals, such as substance withdrawal. Lack of connectedness with self or others impairs ability to trust others or feel worthy of trust from others or God.
Suggest use of journaling and/or reminiscence.	Promotes life review. Can assist in clarifying values and ideas, recognizing and resolving feelings and situation, and identifying reasons for resuming desired religious activities.
Encourage client to identify SO(s) and others such as spiritual advisor or parish nurse who can provide needed support.	Ongoing support is required to enhance sense of connectedness and strengthen religious ties as desired.
Religious Ritual Enhancement (NIC)	
Identify client's religious affiliation, associated rituals, and beliefs.	Helps determine individual's needs and possible resources, if desired.
Make time for nonjudgmental discussion of philosophical issues related to religious belief patterns and customs.	Open communication can assist client to check reality of perceptions and identify personal options and willingness to resume desired activities.
Discuss desire to continue or reconnect with previous belief patterns and customs.	Enables client to identify barriers to participating in desired activities and take appropriate actions to resume them.
Involve client in refining healthcare goals and therapeutic regimen, as appropriate.	Identifies role illness is playing in current concerns about ability to or appropriateness of participating in desired religious activities.
Provide privacy for meditation, prayer, or performance of rituals, as appropriate.	Allows client to engage in spiritual activities in own way without fear of interruption or judgment of others.
Explore alternatives to, or modifications for, ritual based on setting and individual needs or limitations.	Assists client to develop new ways of expressing religious beliefs and satisfying these needs.
Collaborative	
Refer to spiritual resources, such as spiritual advisor—who has qualifications and experience in dealing with specific problems individual is concerned about—or to facility's chaplain or visiting clergy and parish nurse.	Provides answers to spiritual questions, assists in the journey of self-discovery, helps client learn to accept, forgive self, and engage in desired rituals.

NURSING DIAGNOSIS: ineffective Self-Health Management

May Be Related To

Complexity of therapeutic regimen
Economic difficulties
Perceived barriers/benefits
Decisional conflicts
Family conflict, patterns of healthcare
Social support deficit

Possibly Evidenced By

Reports difficulty with prescribed regimens
Failure to include treatment regimens in daily living
Ineffective choices in daily living for meeting health goals

Desired Outcomes/Evaluation Criteria—Client Will

Knowledge: Acute Illness [or] Chronic Disease Management (NOC)

Participate in the development of goals and treatment plan.
Verbalize accurate knowledge of disease, prognosis, and potential complications.
Demonstrate behaviors or changes in lifestyle necessary to incorporate or maintain therapeutic regimen in daily life.
Identify and use available resources.

ACTIONS/INTERVENTIONS	RATIONALE
Values Clarification (NIC)	
Independent	
Review client's and SO's knowledge and understanding of the need for treatment or medication as well as consequences of actions and choices. Note ability to comprehend information, including literacy, level of education, and primary language.	Provides opportunities to clarify viewpoints or misconceptions. Verifies that client and SO have accurate and factual information with which to make informed choices.
Be aware of developmental and chronological age.	Impacts ability to understand own needs and incorporate into treatment regimen.

ACTIONS/INTERVENTIONS (continued)	RATIONALE (continued)
Determine cultural, spiritual, and health beliefs and ethical concerns.	Provides insight into thoughts and factors related to individual situation. Beliefs will affect client's perception of situation and participation in treatment regimen. Treatment may be incongruent with client's social and cultural lifestyle and perceived role/responsibilities.
Self-Modification Assistance (NIC)	
Review treatment plan with client and SO.	Provides opportunities to exchange accurate information and to clarify viewpoints or misconceptions.
Contract with client for participation in care.	Client who agrees to own responsibility is more apt to adhere to treatment plan.
Establish graduated goals or modified regimen as necessary; work out alternate solutions.	Promotes client involvement and independence; provides opportunity for compromise and may enhance cooperation with regimen. When client participates in setting goals, there is a sense of investment that encourages cooperation and willingness to follow through with the program.
Assess availability and use of support systems. Identify additional resources, as appropriate.	Access to and proper use of helpful resources can assist client in meeting treatment goals and provide purpose for living. Presence of caring, empathic family/SO(s) can help client in process of recovery.
Determine problems that may, or do, interfere with treatment, including lack of financial or personal resources or lack of availability of providers. Assess level of anxiety, locus of control, and sense of powerlessness.	Many factors may be involved in behavior that is disruptive to the treatment regimen, such as fear of hospitalization or treatment; denial of situation consequences; suspicion about healthcare system; and physical factors such as pain, hypoxemia, and chemical imbalance.
Note length of illness and prognosis.	Clients tend to become passive and dependent in long-term, debilitating illness.
Active-listen client's reports and comments (Evesham, 2011).	Conveys message of concern and belief in individual's capabilities to resolve situation in positive manner.
Develop a system for self-monitoring. Share data pertinent to client's condition such as laboratory results or blood pressure (BP) readings.	Provides a sense of control; enables client to follow own progress and make informed choices.
Have same personnel care for client as much as possible.	Enables relationship to develop in which the client can begin to trust and participate in care.
Accept client's choice or point of view even if it appears to be self-destructive, such as a decision to continue smoking.	Client has the right to make own decisions, and acceptance may give a sense of control, which can help client look more clearly at consequences. Confrontation is not beneficial and may actually be detrimental to future cooperation and goal achievement.
Be aware of own and caregiver's response to client's treatment choices such as refusal of blood or chemotherapy and living will or advance directive choices.	Negative feelings regarding these choices may create power struggles and be expressed in judgmental behaviors that block or interfere with client's wishes, comfort, and/or care. *Note:* If resolution cannot be found, providers have the right to terminate their services with appropriate notice.

NURSING DIAGNOSIS: risk for self- or other-directed Violence

Risk Factors May Include

Physical health problems; neurological impairment; cognitive impairment
Emotional problems (e.g., hopelessness, despair, increased anxiety, hostility)
Employment problems; lack of social resources
Impulsivity; history of violence; suicidal behavior
Psychotic symptomatology (e.g., hallucinations, delusions, illogical thought processes)

Possibly Evidenced By

(Not applicable; presence of signs and symptoms establishes an *actual* diagnosis)

Desired Outcomes/Evaluation Criteria—Client Will

Impulse Self-Control (NOC)

Acknowledge realities of the situation.
Verbalize understanding of reason(s) for behavior/precipitating factors.
Express increased self-concept.

Agitation Level (NOC)

Demonstrate self-control, as evidenced by relaxed posture and nonviolent behavior.

ACTIONS/INTERVENTIONS	RATIONALE
Mood Management (NIC)	
Independent	
Observe for early signs of distress and investigate possible causes.	Irritability, pacing, shouting or cursing, lack of cooperation, and demanding behavior may all be signs of increasing anxiety or indicate change in health status of confused client that requires further evaluation.
Identify conditions that may interfere with ability to control own behavior.	Acute or chronic brain syndrome or drug-induced or postsurgical confusion may precipitate violent behavior that is difficult to control.
Assume that the client has control and is responsible for own behavior.	Often enables the individual to exercise control. *Note:* When violent behavior is the result of drug use, client may not be able to respond appropriately.
Remain calm and state limits on behavior in a firm manner. Be truthful and nonjudgmental.	Understanding that helplessness and fear underlie this behavior aids in choosing appropriate response.
Accept client's anger without reacting on an emotional basis.	Responding with anger is not helpful in resolving the situation and may result in escalating client's behavior. Anger is usually not directed at the nurse, but at the situation and feelings of powerlessness.
Maintain straightforward communication and assist client to learn assertive rather than manipulative, nonassertive, or aggressive behavior.	Avoids reinforcing manipulative behavior and enhances positive interactions with others, accomplishing the goal of getting needs met in acceptable ways.
Help client identify more adequate solutions and behaviors such as motor activities or exercise. Redirect and provide directions for actions client can take.	Promotes release of energies in acceptable ways. Redirecting confused client can minimize escalation of agitation. (Refer to CP: Dementia of the Alzheimer's Type/Vascular Dementia.)
Give as much autonomy as is possible in the situation.	Enhances feelings of power and control in a situation in which many things are not within individual's control.
Monitor for suicidal or homicidal ideation, for example, morbid or anxious feelings while with the client; thoughts expressed by, or warning from, the client, "It doesn't matter, I'd be better off dead"; and mood swings, putting affairs in order, and previous suicide attempt.	Indicators of need for further assessment and intervention or psychiatric care.
Assess suicidal intent (scale of 1 to 10) by asking directly if client is thinking of killing self, has plan, means, and so on.	Provides guidelines for necessity and urgency of interventions. Direct questioning is most helpful when done in a caring, concerned manner.
Acknowledge reality of suicide or homicide as an option. Discuss consequences of actions if client were to follow through on intent. Ask how it will help client resolve problems.	Client may focus on suicide, or possibly homicide, as the "only" option and this response provides an opening to look at and discuss other options. *Note:* Be aware of own responsibility under Tarasoff's rule to warn possible victim(s) when client is expressing homicidal ideation. (Under Tarasoff's rule, the counselor/care provider has a legal responsibility to notify a third party of a credible threat made by the client.) (Tarasoff v. Regents of the University of California—17 Cal.3d 425 [1976]).
Environmental Management: Violence Prevention (NIC)	
Provide protection within the environment such as constant observation and removal of objects that might be used to harm self and others.	May need more structure to maintain control until own internal locus of control is regained.
Tell client to stop.	May be sufficient to help client control own actions if exhibiting hostile actions. *Note:* Client is often afraid of own actions and wants staff to set limits.
Use an organized team approach when necessary to subdue client with force. Tell client clearly and concisely what is happening.	Knowing and practicing these actions before they are needed helps prevent untoward problems. Keeping client informed can help client to regain internal control.
Hold client; place in restraints or seclusion if necessary. Do so in a calm, positive, nonstimulating, and nonpunitive manner.	As a last resort, physical restraint may be necessary while the client regains control. *Note:* These measures are meant to protect client, not punish the behavior.
Apply and adjust restraint devices properly.	It is important to maintain body alignment and client safety and comfort.
Document precise reason for restraints, actions taken, and doctor's order. Check restraints frequently per facility protocol, each time documenting the condition and how long the restraints are used.	Restraints are to be used for very specific reasons, which need to be clearly documented to avoid overuse or misuse, and to ensure client safety.
Collaborative	
Administer medications, such as anti-anxiety or antipsychotic agents, sedatives, and narcotics, as appropriate.	May be indicated to quiet or control behavior. *Note:* May need to be withheld if they are suspected to be the cause of, or contribute to, the behavior.

ACTIONS/INTERVENTIONS	RATIONALE
Refer to psychiatric resource(s): psychiatric clinical nurse specialist, psychiatrist, psychologist, social worker.	More in-depth assistance may be needed to deal with client and defuse situation. Learning new ways to deal with feelings can provide opportunity for individual to manage life in a more optimal way.
Encourage participation in classes such as anger management. Discuss what client is learning about dealing with anger.	Attending class helps individual to learn positive ways to handle anger instead of usual acting-out.

DEMENTIA OF THE ALZHEIMER'S TYPE/ VASCULAR DEMENTIA/LEWY BODY DISEASE

I. Pathophysiology (Alzheimer's Association, 2012; Nelson-Marsh, 2005)

- **a.** Cognitive disorder characterized by impaired memory, language, thinking, and perception
- **b.** Alzheimer's, vascular, and Lewy body dementias are irreversible and share common symptomology and therapeutic intervention.
- **c.** Criteria for dementia diagnosis
  - **i.** Decline in memory and at least one of the following cognitive abilities:
    - **1.** Coherent speech, understand spoken or written language
    - **2.** Recognize or identify objects, assuming intact sensory function
    - **3.** Execute motor activities, assuming intact motor abilities, sensory function, and comprehension of the required task
    - **4.** Abstract thinking, make sound judgments, plan, and carry out complex tasks
  - **ii.** Decline in cognitive abilities must be severe enough to interfere with daily life.

II. Classification

- **a.** Dementia of the Alzheimer's type (DAT) (Alzheimer's Association, 2012; Trahan et al, 2011; Hausman, 2006; Nelson-Marsh, 2005)
  - **i.** Accounts for 60% to 80 % of dementia diagnoses
  - **ii.** The three stages of Alzheimer's disease identified in the 2011 criteria and guidelines are (1) preclinical Alzheimer's disease, (2) mild cognitive impairment (MCI) due to Alzheimer's disease, and (3) dementia due to Alzheimer's disease.
    - **1.** Characterized by structural and chemical changes in the brain, causing a steady and global decline in function
    - **2.** Degenerative process occurring primarily in the cells located at the base of the forebrain that sends information to the cerebral cortex and hippocampus
    - **3.** Decrease in acetylcholine production reduces the amount of neurotransmitter released to cells in the cortex, hippocampus, and nucleus basalis, resulting in a disruption of memory processes.
    - **4.** Enzyme required to produce acetylcholine is dramatically reduced, especially in the area of the brain where neuritic plaques and neurofibrillary tangles occur in the greatest numbers.
    - **5.** Formation of plaques composed of beta-amyloid and tangles appears to be related to the cholesterol-transporting protein apolipoprotein-E (ApoE).
- **b. Vascular dementia**
  - **i.** Vascular dementia accounts for 17% of cases.
  - **ii.** Referred to as multi-infarct, post-stroke dementia, or vascular cognitive impairment, resulting in decreased blood flow to parts of the brain
  - **iii.** Multiple infarcts to various areas of the brain result in a pattern of intermittent deterioration determined by the area of the brain that is affected.
- **c. Lewy body disease** (Mayo Clinic Staff, 2013; National Institute of Neurological Disorders and Stroke [NINDS], 2013; Otto, 2013; Lewy Body Dementia Association, [LBDA] 2012)
  - **i.** Umbrella term for two related diagnoses, Parkinson's disease dementia (PDD) and dementia with Lewy bodies (DLB).
  - **ii.** Lewy body diseases (LBDs) are the second most common type of progressive dementia after Alzheimer's.
  - **iii.** Protein bodies (alpha synuclein) develop in nerve cells in the areas of the brain involved with thinking, memory, and movement.
  - **iv.** Differentiated from Alzheimer's disease or other non-synucleinopathies by the diagnosis of REM sleep behavior disorder (RBD)
  - **v.** The central feature of DLB is progressive cognitive decline, combined with three additional defining features: (1) pronounced fluctuations in alertness and attention, (2) recurrent visual hallucinations, and (3) parkinsonian type motor symptoms, such as rigidity and the loss of spontaneous movement.

III. Etiology

- **a.** DAT: Exact cause unknown; most likely due to multiple factors rather than a single cause (Alzheimer's Association, 2012)
  - **i.** Lifelong process—Incidence increases with longevity, and changes in the brain may develop decades before the onset of dementia.
  - **ii.** Genetics—Familial pattern four times greater than general population (Nelson-Marsh, 2005)
    - **1.** Familial or early-onset Alzheimer's is linked to defects on genes on chromosome 1, 14, or 21 with some families exhibiting a pattern of inheritance suggesting possible autosomal dominant gene transmission (Anderson, 2013).
    - **2.** Down syndrome: presents with an extra chromosome 21; may have a relationship to Alzheimer's disease
      - **A.** At autopsy, both disorders have many of the same pathophysiological changes.

(continues on page 744)

B. High percentage of individuals with Down syndrome who survive to adulthood develop Alzheimer's lesions by late 40s or early 50s (Alvarez, 2012).

3. Studies suggest that autoantibodies are produced in the brain, reflecting a possible alteration in the body's immune system.

iii. Known risk factors: Age and genetics. Familial Alzheimer's is a rare form of early onset disease and is known to be caused by mutations on one of three chromosomes: 1, 14, and 21 (Benetti, 2012).

iv. Proposed risk factors: Studies to date have not confirmed causal relationship; however, various factors that have been suggested include cardiovascular disease, type 2 diabetes, oxidative damage. Inflammation occurs as protein plaques appear, but it is not known whether inflammation is a cause or result. Other factors that may contribute are prior severe head trauma, low educational level, female gender. Aluminum has been disproven as a cause.

b. Vascular dementia

i. Predisposing factors: Various diseases and conditions that interfere with blood circulation, including cerebral and systemic vascular disease, hypertension, cerebral hypoxia, hypoglycemia, cerebral embolism, and severe head injury. Sometimes called "mixed dementia" (Mayo Clinic Staff, 2011).

IV. Statistics (Alzheimer's Association, 2013; Centers for Disease Control and Prevention [CDC], 2012)

a. Morbidity: In 2013, an estimated 5.2 million people in the United States are living with Alzheimer's disease. By 2025, the number of people age 65 and older with Alzheimer's disease is estimated to reach 7.1 million.

b. Mortality: DAT is the sixth-leading cause of death, and the fifth leading cause of death for people age 65 and older. In 2010, 83,494 Americans died, the most recent year for which final data are available (CDC, 2012).

c. Cost: In 2013, the direct costs of caring for Alzheimer's patients will total an estimated $203 billion in direct medical costs, including $142 billion in costs to Medicare and Medicaid for Alzheimer's and other dementias. Total payments for healthcare, long-term care, and hospice for people with Alzheimer's and other dementias are projected to increase from $203 billion in 2013 to $1.2 trillion in 2050 (in current dollars). This dramatic rise includes a 500% increase in combined Medicare and Medicaid spending and $36.5 billion in indirect costs to businesses. It is estimated that, in 2012, 15.4 million family, friends, and neighbors provided 17.5 billion hours of unpaid care, a contribution valued at $216.4 billion. Due to the physical and emotional toll of caregiving, Alzheimer's and dementia caregivers had $9.1 billion in additional healthcare costs of their own in 2012 (Alzheimer's Association, 2013).

GLOSSARY

apolipoprotein-E (ApoE): Lipoprotein with three isoforms with the $ApoE_4$ variant associated with an earlier-than-average age of onset for the common form of Alzheimer's disease.

Amyloid plaque: Buildup of amyloid protein and a primary hallmark of Alzheimer's disease.

Atrophy: Wasting or a decrease in the size of an organ or tissue.

Beta-amyloid: Insoluble protein that is an abnormal breakdown product of the cell membrane constituent amyloid precursor protein (APP) and is a component of the neurofibrillary tangles and plaques characteristic of Alzheimer's disease.

Catastrophic reactions: Extreme outbursts of emotion, most often anger or agitation. Also called "challenging behaviors," "disruptive behaviors," "behavioral symptoms related to dementia," "Alzheimer's behaviors," "behavioral issues," "behavioral and psychological symptoms of dementia" (BPSD) (Marsh, 2010).

Emotional lability: Excessive emotional reactivity associated with frequent changes or swings in emotions or mood.

Hippocampus: Part of the limbic system of the brain and one of several structures involved with emotion, memory, and learning.

Hypermetamorphosis: Compulsive exploration of environment, including touching.

Hyperorality: Consists of unexplained movements of the mouth and tongue and the act of placing nonfood items in the mouth.

Lewy bodies: Abnormal protein deposits that disrupt the brain's normal functioning, found in an area of the brainstem where they deplete the neurotransmitter dopamine. In Lewy body disease, these abnormal proteins are diffuse throughout other areas of the brain, including the cerebral cortex. The brain chemical acetylcholine is depleted, causing disruption of perception, thinking, and behavior (Lewy Body Dementia Association [LBDA], 2012).

Neuritic plaques: Extracellular abnormalities composed of beta-amyloid in the gray matter of the brain.

Neurofibrillary tangles: Masses of fine fibrous elements found in cytoplasm signaling an abnormality of the hippocampus and neurons of the cerebral cortex that occurs especially in Alzheimer's disease. Classic finding at autopsy in the brain of client with DAT.

Proprioception: Awareness of posture; movement; changes in equilibrium; and the knowledge of position, weight, and resistance of objects in relation to the body.

Sundowner's syndrome (also called sundowning syndrome): Increased restlessness, wandering, aggression, or exacerbation of behavioral symptoms of Alzheimer's disease in the afternoon and evening.

Synucleinopathies: Alpha [α] synuclein is the primary structural component of Lewy body fibrils. It is an unstructured soluble protein that mutates in pathological conditions characterized by Lewy bodies, such as Parkinson's disease, dementia with Lewy bodies, and multiple system atrophy. These disorders are known as synucleinopathies (Arima et al, 1999).

Tau: Protein that channels chemical messages inside nerve cells.

Care Setting

Client is cared for primarily in the home or assisted living/extended care; however, inpatient care may be required for treatment of other health problems.

Related Concerns

End-of-life care/hospice, page 848
Extended/long-term care, page 781
Pneumonia, page 129
Psychosocial aspects of care, page 729
Sepsis/septicemia, page 665
Total nutritional support: parenteral/enteral feeding, page 437

Client Assessment Database

DIAGNOSTIC DIVISION MAY REPORT	MAY EXHIBIT
ACTIVITY/REST	
• Feeling tired • Decreased interest in usual activities, hobbies; inability to recall what is read or follow plot of television program • Forced to retire from work	• Day-night reversal • Wakefulness disturbance of sleep rhythms • Lethargy • Impaired motor skills • Inability to carry out familiar, purposeful movements • Content sitting and watching others • Repetitive motions, such as folding, unfolding, refolding linen • Wandering
CIRCULATION	
• History of systemic vascular disease, cerebral vascular disease, hypertension, embolic episodes (may be predisposing factors)	
EGO INTEGRITY	
• Anxiety, depression—usually during early stages related to the knowledge that cognitive abilities are deteriorating • Multiple losses, such as changes in body image and self-esteem	• Inconsistent behavior • Verbal and nonverbal communication and behavior may be incongruent • Suspicious or fearful of imaginary people and situations • May cling to significant others SO(s) • Misperception of environment, misidentification of objects and people • Hoarding objects • Belief that misplaced objects are stolen • Emotional lability—may cry easily or laugh inappropriately • Variable mood changes, such as apathy, lethargy, restlessness, short attention span, or irritability • Catastrophic reactions • May deny significance of early changes and symptoms, especially cognitive changes • May conceal limitations, such as make excuses for not being able to perform tasks, redirect conversation, or avoid direct answers to questions • Feelings of helplessness; strong, depressive overlay; delusions; or paranoia
ELIMINATION	
	• Incontinence • Diarrhea—related to impaction
FOOD/FLUID	
• Changes in taste, appetite • Denial of hunger, refusal to eat—may be trying to conceal lost skills	• Hypoglycemic episodes—predisposing factor • Lack of interest in or forgetting mealtimes • Dependence on others for food cooking and preparation at table, feeding, or using utensils

(continues on page 746)

DIAGNOSTIC DIVISION MAY REPORT (continued)	MAY EXHIBIT (continued)
	• Loss of ability to chew—silent aspiration concerns • Weight loss • Decreased muscle mass; emaciation in advanced stage
HYGIENE • Dependence on others to meet basic hygiene needs	• Disheveled, unkempt appearance • Body odor • Poor personal habits • Inappropriate clothing for situation or weather conditions • Misinterpretation of, or ignoring, internal cues • Forgetting steps involved in toileting self, or inability to find the bathroom
NEUROSENSORY • Family members may report a gradual decrease in cognitive abilities, impaired judgment, or inappropriate decisions; impaired recent memory but good remote memory; behavioral changes and altered or exaggerated individual personality traits	• Concealing inabilities, may make excuses not to perform task or may thumb through a book without actually reading • Loss of proprioception • Primitive reflexes such as positive snout, suck, and palmar reflexes may be present • Facial signs or symptoms dependent on degree of vascular insults • Seizure activity secondary to associated brain damage • Disorientation to time initially then place; usually oriented to person until late in disease process • Impaired recent memory, progressive loss of remote memory • May change answers during the interview • Difficulty in comprehension, abstract thinking • Unable to do simple calculations or repeat the names of three objects; short attention span • Hallucinations, delusions, severe depression, or mania may occur in advanced stage • May have impaired communication—difficulty finding correct words, especially nouns; conversation repetitive or scattered with substituted meaningless words; speech may become inaudible; gradually loses ability to write or read
SAFETY • Predisposing or factors that may accelerate the condition, such as a history of recent viral illness or serious head trauma, drug toxicity, stress, or nutritional deficits • Incidental trauma such as falls or burns	• Forgets how to negotiate places when away from home • Ignores safety issues • Presence of bruises, lacerations, or other evidence of falling • Disturbance of gait • Striking out or violence directed toward others
SOCIAL INTERACTIONS • Difficulty in relating to others	• Fragmented speech, aphasia, and dysphasia • Demonstrates inappropriate behavior and ignores rules of social conduct • Behavioral pattern alterations related to prior psychosocial factors and individuality and personality • Family roles possibly altered/reversed as individual becomes more dependent
TEACHING/LEARNING • Family history of DAT • May present a total healthy picture, with exception of memory or behavioral changes	

DIAGNOSTIC DIVISION MAY REPORT (continued)	MAY EXHIBIT (continued)
• Use or misuse of medications, over-the-counter (OTC) drugs, including alcohol • Difficulty managing medications **Discharge Plan Considerations** • May require support and legal services, financial assistance, caregiver support groups, respite and home health care ➧ Following inpatient acute care, refer to underlying condition requiring admission for postdischarge considerations.	

Diagnostic Studies

Although no diagnostic studies are specific for Alzheimer's disease, these studies are used to rule out reversible problems that may be confused with these types of dementia.

TEST WHY IT IS DONE	WHAT IT TELLS ME
Blood Tests	
• *Antibodies:* Tests for marker for amyloid-â peptide and receptor for advanced glycation end products (Medical College of Georgia, 2004).	Abnormally high levels may be found, leading to a theory of an immunological defect. Investigation of the neuritic plaques gives rise to the possibility that the body has turned against itself.
• *ApoE$_4$:* Tests for a variant form of ApoE$_4$, a low penetrance mutation believed to be associated with an increased likelihood of Alzheimer's disease.	Screens for the presence of a genetic defect associated with the common form of DAT. In rare families, an autosomal dominant inheritance of early onset Alzheimer's disease occurs due to high penetrance mutations. Genetic testing may be helpful in such families.
Other Diagnostic Studies	
• *Neurological mental status examination:* The client is asked to perform maneuvers or answer questions that are designed to elicit information about the condition of specific parts of the brain or peripheral nerves. Testing assesses mental status and alertness, muscle strength, reflexes, sensory-perception, language skills, and coordination.	Many tests may be administered to evaluate client's brain functioning, each measuring a different aspect. One such test, the 7-minute screen (7MS), appears to be highly sensitive to Alzheimer's disease by differentiating between cognitive changes related to the normal aging process and those related to Alzheimer's disease (Solomon et al, 1998).
• *Electroencephalogram (EEG):* Measures electrical activity of the brain.	May reveal slow-wave delta activity indicative of later stages of Alzheimer's disease. May also reveal focal vascular lesions associated with vascular dementia.
• *Skull x-rays:* Determine presence of structural injury.	Usually normal but may reveal signs of head trauma.
• *Positron-emission tomography (PET) scan:* Three-dimensional, computer-enhanced, full-color image of the brain.	Traces a positron-emitting chemical that binds effectively to abnormal protein plaques and tangles, thus detecting these Alzheimer markers.
• *Computed tomography (CT) or CAT scan:* X-ray procedure that uses a computer to produce a detailed picture of a cross section of the brain.	May show widening of ventricles or cerebral atrophy. These studies are also used to rule out other central nervous system (CNS) disease.
• *Cerebrospinal fluid (CSF):* Fluid produced within the brain, which surrounds the brain and spinal cord. Samples are obtained by means of lumbar puncture and evaluated for abnormal proteins.	Evidence supports that some cases of mild cognitive impairment may be an early form of Alzheimer's disease. Individuals likely to progress can be identified by measuring Aβ42, T-tau, and P-tau in the CSF (Mattson et al, 2009).

Nursing Priorities

1. Provide safe environment and prevent injury.
2. Promote socially acceptable responses and limit inappropriate behavior.
3. Maintain reality orientation and prevent sensory deprivation or overload.
4. Encourage participation in self-care within individual abilities.
5. Promote coping mechanisms of client/SO(s).
6. Support client and family in grieving process.
7. Provide information about disease process, prognosis, and resources available for assistance.

Discharge Goals

Not indicated in home or community setting. Following inpatient care, based on underlying condition requiring admission.

NURSING DIAGNOSIS: impaired Environmental Interpretation Syndrome

May Be Related To
Dementia

Possibly Evidenced By
Consistent disorientation
Inability to reason or concentrate
Inability to follow commands

Desired Outcomes/Evaluation Criteria—Family/Caregiver(s) Will

Safe Home Environment (NOC)
Identify and correct environmental factors that increase risk of injury to client.

Client Will

Physical Injury Severity (NOC)
Be free of injury.

Safe Wandering (NOC)
Ambulate freely in environment without harm to self or others.
Accept redirection from unsafe activities.

ACTIONS/INTERVENTIONS	RATIONALE
Environmental Management: Safety (NIC)	
Independent	
Assess degree of impairment in ability and competence and presence of impulsive behavior.	Identifies potential risks in the environment and heightens awareness of risks so caregivers are more alert to dangers. Clients demonstrating impulsive behavior are at increased risk of injury because they are less able to control their own behavior/actions.
Assist caregiver to identify any risks or potential hazards and visual-perceptual deficits that may be present.	Visual-perceptual deficits increase the risk of falls.
Eliminate or minimize identified hazards in the environment.	A person with cognitive impairment and perceptual disturbances is prone to accidental injury because of the inability to take responsibility for basic safety needs or to evaluate the unforeseen consequences, such as lighting a stove or cigarette and forgetting about it, mistaking plastic fruit for the real thing and eating it, or misjudging distance involving chairs and stairs. Preventive measures can contain client without constant supervision. Activities promote involvement and keep client occupied.
Lock outside doors as appropriate, especially in evening and night. Do not allow access to stairwell or exit. Provide supervision and activities for client who is regularly awake during the night. Recommend use of "child-proof locks"; secure such items as medications, cleaning products, poisonous substances, tools, and sharp objects. Remove stove knobs and burners.	As the disease worsens, the client may compulsively handle or fidget with objects, including locks, or put small items in mouth, which potentiates possibility of accidental injury and death.

ACTIONS/INTERVENTIONS (continued)	RATIONALE (continued)
Dementia Management (NIC)	
Monitor behavior routinely; note timing of behavioral changes, increasing confusion, and hyperactivity. Initiate least restrictive interventions before behavior escalates.	Early identification of negative behaviors with appropriate action can prevent need for more stringent measures. *Note:* Sundowner's syndrome develops in late afternoon or early evening, requiring programmed interventions and closer monitoring at this time to redirect and protect client.
Distract or redirect client's attention when behavior is agitated or dangerous, for example, climbing out of bed. Place bed in low position and mattress on floor, as indicated.	Maintains safety while avoiding a confrontation that could escalate behavior or increase risk of injury.
Obtain and have client wear identification jewelry, such as bracelet or necklace showing name, phone number, and diagnosis.	Facilitates safe return of client if lost. Because of poor verbal ability and confusion, these persons may be unable to state name, address, and phone number. Client may wander, exhibit poor judgment, and be detained by police, appearing confused, irritable, or having violent outbursts.
Dress according to physical environment and individual need.	The general slowing of metabolic processes results in lowered body heat. The hypothalamic gland may be affected by the disease process or by aging, causing client to feel cold. Client may have seasonal disorientation and may wander out in the cold. *Note:* Leading causes of death in these clients include pneumonia and accidents (Neergard, 2013).
Be attentive to nonverbal physiological symptoms.	Because of sensory loss and language dysfunction, client may express needs nonverbally such as thirst by panting and pain by sweating or doubling over. *Note:* Wandering may be a coping mechanism as client seeks a change in environment if too hot or cold, bored, or overstimulated; or searches for food or relief from discomfort.
Be alert to underlying meaning of verbal statements.	May direct a question to another, such as, "Are you cold or tired?" meaning client is cold or tired.
Monitor for medication side effects and signs of overmedication—extrapyramidal signs, orthostatic hypotension, visual disturbances, and gastrointestinal (GI) upsets.	Client may not be able to report signs or symptoms, and drugs can easily build up to toxic levels in the elderly. Dosages or drug choice may need to be altered.
Provide quiet room and reduced activity.	Overstimulation increases irritability and agitation, which can escalate to violent outbursts.
Avoid use of restraints. Have SO or others stay with client during periods of acute agitation.	Endangers the individual who succeeds in partial removal of restraints. May increase agitation and potentiate fall risk and fractures in the elderly.
Collaborative	
Administer medications as appropriate, such as:	
risperidone (Risperdal), olanzapine (Zyprexa), quetiapine (Seroquel), or ziprasidone (Geodon), memantine (Namenda), galantamine (Razadyne), rivastigmine (Exelon), donepezil (Aricept).	Some antipsychotics are favored to control agitation, aggression, hallucinations, thought disturbances, and wandering because of their lower propensity to cause anticholinergic and extrapyramidal side effects. *Note:* May help moderate "sundowning," a condition related to deterioration of the hypothalamus, which controls the sleep–wake cycle. Other drugs, such as rivastigmine (Exelon), donepezil (Aricept), prevent the breakdown of acetylcholine in the brain.

NURSING DIAGNOSIS: chronic Confusion

May Be Related To

Alzheimer's disease; multi-infarct dementia

Possibly Evidenced By

Altered interpretation or response to stimuli
Altered personality; impaired socialization
Progressive, long-standing cognitive impairment
Clinical evidence of organic impairment

Desired Outcomes/Evaluation Criteria— Client Will

Dementia Level (NOC)

Experience a decrease in level of frustration, especially when participating in daily activities.

(continues on page 750)

NURSING DIAGNOSIS: chronic Confusion (continued)

Family/Caregiver Will

Caregiver Performance: Direct Care (NOC)

Verbalize understanding of disease process and client's needs.
Identify and participate in interventions to deal effectively with situation.
Provide for maximal independence while meeting safety needs of client.
Initiate behaviors or lifestyle changes to maximize client's cognitive functioning.

ACTIONS/INTERVENTIONS	RATIONALE
Dementia Management (NIC)	
Independent	
Assess degree of cognitive impairment, including changes in orientation to person, place, and time and attention span and thinking ability. Talk with SO and caregiver about changes from usual behavior and length of time problem has existed.	Provides baseline for future evaluation and comparison and influences choice of interventions. *Note:* Repeated evaluation of orientation may actually heighten negative responses and client's level of frustration.
Maintain a pleasant, quiet environment.	Reduces distorted input, whereas crowds, clutter, and noise generate sensory overload that stresses the impaired neurons.
Approach in a slow, calm manner.	This nonverbal gesture lessens the chance of misinterpretation and potential agitation. Hurried approaches can startle and threaten the confused client who misinterprets or feels threatened by imaginary people and/or situations.
Face the individual when conversing.	Maintains reality, expresses interest, and arouses attention, particularly in persons with perceptual disturbances.
Address client by name.	Names form our self-identity and establish reality and individual recognition. Client may respond to own name long after failing to recognize family or caregiver.
Use lower voice register and speak slowly to client.	Increases the chance for comprehension. High-pitched, loud tones convey stress and anger, which may trigger memory of previous confrontations and provoke an angry response.
Give simple directions, one at a time, or step-by-step instructions, using short words and simple sentences.	As the disease progresses, the communication centers in the brain become impaired, hindering the individual's ability to process and comprehend complex messages. Simplicity is the key to communicating, both verbally and nonverbally, with the cognitively impaired person.
Pause between phrases or questions.	Invites a verbal response and may increase comprehension.
Give hints and use open-ended phrases when possible.	Hints stimulate communication and give the person a chance for a positive experience.
Listen with regard despite content of client's speech.	Conveys interest and worth to the individual.
Interpret statements, meanings, and words. If possible, supply the correct word.	Assisting the client with word processing aids in decreasing frustration.
Reduce provocative stimuli, such as negative criticism, arguments, and confrontations.	Any provocation decreases self-esteem and may be interpreted as a threat, which may trigger agitation or increase inappropriate behavior.
Use distraction. Talk about real people and real events when client begins ruminating about false ideas, unless talking realistically increases anxiety or agitation.	Rumination promotes disorientation. Reality orientation increases client's sense of reality, self-worth, and personal dignity.
Change the subject if current topic increases anxiety or agitation.	Enables the client to focus on another topic and decreases anxiety.
Refrain from forcing activities and communications.	Force decreases cooperation and may increase suspiciousness and delusions.
Change activity if client loses interest in present activity.	Changing activity maintains interest and reduces restlessness and possibility of confrontation.
Use humor with interactions.	Laughter can assist in communication.
Focus on appropriate behavior. Give verbal feedback and positive reinforcement such as a pat on the back or applause. Use touch judiciously and respect individual's personal space and response.	Reinforces correctness and appropriate behavior. A focus on inappropriate behavior can encourage repetition. Although touch frequently transcends verbal interchange and conveys warmth and acceptance, the individual may misinterpret the meaning of touch. Intrusion into personal space may be interpreted as threatening because of the client's distorted perceptions.
Respect individuality and evaluate individual needs.	Persons experiencing a cognitive decline deserve respect, dignity, and recognition of worth as an individual. Client's past and background are important in maintaining self-concept, planning activities, and communication.

ACTIONS/INTERVENTIONS (continued)	RATIONALE (continued)
Allow personal belongings.	Familiarity enhances security, sense of self, and decreases feelings of loss and deprivation.
Permit hoarding of safe objects.	This activity may preserve security and counterbalances irrevocable losses.
Create simple, noncompetitive activities paced to the individual's abilities. Provide entertaining, memory-stimulating music, videos, and TV programs. Engage in old hobbies and preferred activities, such as arts and crafts, music, supervised cooking, gardening, and spiritual programs.	Motivates client in ways that will reinforce usefulness and self-worth and stimulate reality.
Make useful activities or jobs out of hoarding and repetitive motions, such as collecting junk mail, creating scrapbook, folding and unfolding linen, bouncing balls, dusting, or sweeping floors.	May decrease restlessness and provide option for pleasurable activity. Having a "job" helps client feel useful.
Provide several drawers or baskets that are acceptable to rummage through. Fill with safe items that would be of interest to client, such as yarn balls, quilt blocks, fabrics with different textures and colors, baby clothes, pictures, costume jewelry (without pins), small tools, or sports magazines.	Availability of this kind of assortment provides stimulation that enhances the sense and promotes memories of past life experiences.
Help client find misplaced items; label drawers and belongings. Do not challenge client.	May decrease defensiveness when client believes he or she is being accused of stealing a misplaced, hoarded, or hidden item. To refute the accusation will not change the belief and may invite anger.
Monitor phone use closely. Post significant phone numbers in prominent place and secure long-distance numbers.	Can be used as reality orientation. However, client may forget time of day when making calls or may try to call dead relative. Impaired judgment does not allow for distinguishing long-distance numbers and makes client easy prey for phone sales pitches.
Evaluate sleep and rest pattern and adequacy. Note lethargy, increasing irritability or confusion, frequent yawning, and dark circles under eyes.	Lack of sleep can impair cognitive function and coping abilities. Fatigue may increase severity of symptoms, especially as evening approaches. (Refer to ND: disturbed Sleep Pattern.)
Monitor for medication side effects and signs of overmedication.	Drugs can easily build up to toxic levels in the elderly, aggravating confusion. Dosages or drug choice may need to be altered.
Collaborative	
Administer medications, as individually indicated, for example:	
Acetylcholinesterase (AChE) inhibitors, such as donepezil (Aricept), rivastigmine (Exelon), or galantamine (Razadyne)	Cholinesterase inhibitors prevent the breakdown of acetylcholine, a chemical messenger important for learning and memory. These medications are being used for the treatment of mild to moderate cognitive impairment by delaying progression of symptoms in Alzheimer's disease (Anderson, 2013).
N-methyl-D-aspartate (NMDA) inhibitors, such as memantine (Namenda, Axura)	This class of drugs works by regulating the activity of glutamate, a different messenger chemical involved in learning and memory. This medication was approved by the Food and Drug Administration (FDA) in 2003 for treatment of moderate to severe Alzheimer's disease. It slows the progression of the disease and has been shown to improve cognitive and physical abilities in the later stages of the disease (Anderson, 2013).
Antipsychotic agents, such as aripiprazole (Abilify), clozapine (Clozaril), haloperidol (Haldol), quetiapine (Seroquel), or ziprasidone (Geodon)	Psychotic symptoms, such as hallucinations, delusions, aggression, agitation, and hostility may respond to neuroleptic management in most clients with dementia.
Anxiolytic agents, such as buspirone (BuSpar), lorazepam (Ativan), or oxazepam (Serax)	These drugs may be useful for management of anxiety, restlessness, verbally disruptive behavior, and resistance.
Investigational drugs approved for other uses, for example, NSAIDs, such as ibuprofen (Motrin), estrogen, Ginkgo biloba, vitamin E, selegiline (Eldepryl), and prednisone	These drugs are being studied for possible benefit of treatment or for delaying the onset and progression of DAT (NIA, 2008).

NURSING DIAGNOSIS: [disturbed Sensory Perception (specify)]

May Be Related To

Altered sensory reception or integration

Possibly Evidenced By

Change in usual response to stimuli; change in behavior
Restlessness; irritability
Change in sensory acuity; hallucinations

Desired Outcomes/Evaluation Criteria—Client Will

Sensory Function Status (NOC)

Demonstrate improved or appropriate response to stimuli.

Caregivers Will

Risk Control (NOC)

Identify and control external factors that contribute to alterations in sensory and/or perceptual abilities.

ACTIONS/INTERVENTIONS	RATIONALE
Reality Orientation (NIC)	
Independent	
Assess degree of impairment and how it affects the individual, including hearing or visual deficits.	Although brain involvement is usually global, a small percentage of clients may exhibit asymmetrical involvement, which may cause unilateral neglect. Client may not be able to access internal cues, recognize hunger or thirst, perceive external pain, or locate body within the environment (Tales, 2012).
Encourage use of corrective lenses and hearing aids, as appropriate.	May enhance sensory input and limit or reduce misinterpretation of stimuli.
Maintain a reality-oriented relationship and environment.	Reduces confusion and promotes coping with the frustrating struggles of misperception and being disoriented or confused.
Provide clues for 24-hour reality orientation with calendars, clocks, notes, cards, signs, music, seasonal hues, and scenic pictures; color-code rooms.	Dysfunction in visual-spatial perception interferes with the ability to recognize directions and patterns, and the client may become lost even in familiar surroundings. Clues are tangible reminders that aid recognition and may permeate memory gaps, increasing independence.
Provide quiet, nondistracting environment when indicated, including soft music or room with plain but colorful wallpaper or paint.	Helps to avoid visual or auditory overload by emphasizing qualities of calmness and consistency. *Note:* Patterned wallpaper may be disturbing to the client.
Provide touch in a caring way.	May enhance perception to self and body boundaries.
Engage client in individually meaningful activities, supporting remaining abilities and minimizing failures. Examples include meal preparation, setup and cleaning activities, making bed, and gardening or watering plants.	Supports client's dignity, familiarizes individual with home and community events, and enables him or her to experience satisfaction and pleasure (Cascians, 2008).
Use sensory games to stimulate reality, such as smelling mentholated ointment may prompt client to tell of the time mother used it on client; use of spring or fall nature boxes may stimulate reality.	Communicates reality through multiple channels (Cascians, 2008).
Indulge in periodic reminiscence, such as listening to old music; recalling historical events; and looking at photos, mementoes, or videos.	Stimulates recollections, awakens memories, aids in the preservation of self and individuality via past accomplishments, and increases feelings of security. Helpful in easing adaptation to a changed environment (Cascians, 2008).
Provide intellectual stimulation activities, such as word games, review of current events, storytime, or travel discussions.	Stimulates remaining cognitive abilities and provides a sense of normalcy.
Include in Bible study group, church activities, and TV services for shut-ins; or arrange for visitation by clergy or spiritual advisor, as appropriate.	Provides opportunity to meet spiritual needs and to maintain connection with religious beliefs; may help reduce sense of isolation from humanity.
Encourage simple outings and short walks. Monitor activity.	Outings refresh reality and provide pleasurable sensory stimuli, which may reduce suspiciousness or hallucinations caused by feelings of imprisonment. Motor functioning may be decreased because nerve degeneration results in weakness, decreasing stamina.
Promote balanced physiological functions tossing colorful foam or beach balls or beanbags, marching, dancing, or arm dancing with music.	Preserves mobility by reducing the potential for bone loss and muscle atrophy; provides diversional activity and opportunity for interaction with others.

ACTIONS/INTERVENTIONS (continued)	RATIONALE (continued)
Involve in activities with others as dictated by individual situation—one-to-one visitors; animal visitation; socialization groups at an Alzheimer center; or occupational therapy including crafts, painting or finger paints, and modeling clay.	Provides opportunity for the stimulation of participation with others and may maintain some level of social interaction.

NURSING DIAGNOSIS: Anxiety

May Be Related To

Change in health status
Threat to self-concept
Unmet needs

Possibly Evidenced By

Extraneous movement, restlessness, vigilance
Apprehensive, irritability, increased wariness
Increased tension; sleep disturbance

Desired Outcomes/Evaluation Criteria—Client Will

Anxiety Level (NOC)

Display decreased muscle tension and restlessness.
Demonstrate more appropriate range of feelings and lessened anxiety.

ACTIONS/INTERVENTIONS	RATIONALE
Anxiety Reduction (NIC) *Independent*	
Note change of behavior, suspiciousness, irritability, and defensiveness.	Change in moods may be one of the first signs of cognitive decline, and the client, fearing helplessness, tries to hide the increasing inability to remember and engage in normal activities.
Identify strengths the individual had previously.	Facilitates assistance with communication and management of current deficits.
Deal with aggressive behavior by imposing calm, firm limits.	Acceptance can reduce fear and lessen progression of aggressive behavior.
Provide safe containment when necessary.	Safety of client and staff is important for avoidance of injury.
Provide clear, honest information about actions and events.	Assists in maintaining trust and orientation as long as possible. When the client knows the truth about what is happening, coping is often enhanced, and guilt over what is imagined is decreased.
Discuss feelings of SO and caregivers. Acknowledge normalcy of feelings and concerns and provide information as needed.	Client senses but may not understand reaction of others. This may heighten client's sense of anxiety and fear.

NURSING DIAGNOSIS: Grieving

May Be Related To

Anticipatory loss (e.g., decline in memory, loss of job, status, and independence)
Family perception of potential loss of loved one

Possibly Evidenced By

Psychological distress; anger
Despair; suffering
Alteration in activity level, disturbed sleep pattern

Desired Outcomes/Evaluation Criteria—Client/Family Will

Grief Resolution (NOC)

Express feelings, concerns openly, as able.
Acknowledge difficulty of dealing with impaired cognition.
Discuss sense of loss with significant others.

ACTIONS/INTERVENTIONS	RATIONALE
Grief Work Facilitation (NIC)	
Independent	
Assess degree of deterioration or level of coping.	Information is helpful to understand how much the client is capable of doing to maintain highest level of independence and to provide encouragement to help individuals deal with losses.
Provide open environment for discussion. Use therapeutic communication skills of active-listening and acknowledgment.	Encourages client and caregivers to discuss feelings and concerns realistically.
Note statements of despair, hopelessness, "nothing to live for," and expressions of anger.	May be indicative of suicidal ideation. Angry behavior may be client's way of dealing with feelings of despair.
Respect desire not to talk.	May not be ready to deal with or share grief.
Be honest; do not give false reassurances or dire predictions about the future.	Honesty promotes a trusting relationship. Expressions of gloom, such as "You'll spend the rest of your life in a nursing home," are not helpful because no one knows what the future holds.
Discuss with client and SOs ways they can plan together for the future.	Having a part in problem-solving and planning can provide a sense of control over anticipated events.
Assist client and SO to identify positive aspects of the situation.	Ongoing research, possibility of slow progression may offer some hope for the future.
Identify strengths client and SO see in self and situation and support systems available.	Recognizing these resources provides opportunity to work through feelings of grief.
Collaborative	
Refer to other resources, such as support groups, counseling, and spiritual advisor.	May need additional support or assistance to resolve feelings.

NURSING DIAGNOSIS: Sleep Deprivation

May Be Related To
Dementia, sundowner's syndrome
Aging-related sleep stage shifts
Inadequate daytime activity

Possibly Evidenced By
Irritability; agitation
Fatigue; daytime drowsiness; lethargy

Desired Outcomes/Evaluation Criteria—Client Will

Sleep (NOC)
Establish adequate sleep pattern, with wandering reduced.
Report or appear rested.

ACTIONS/INTERVENTIONS	RATIONALE
Sleep Enhancement (NIC)	
Independent	
Provide for adequate rest. Restrict daytime sleep as appropriate; increase interaction time between client and family and staff during the day, then reduce mental activity late in the day.	Although prolonged physical and mental activity results in fatigue, which can increase confusion, programmed activity without overstimulation promotes sleep.
Avoid use of continuous restraints.	Restraints may potentiate sensory deprivation, agitation, and restrict rest. *Note:* The Health Care Financing Administration's (HCFA) guidelines of 1999 require that clients be free from chemical or mechanical restraint unless warranted by a medical diagnosis; that when used, restraints must be used for a specified period of time; and that the least restrictive means of control be used.
Evaluate level of stress and orientation as day progresses.	Increasing confusion, disorientation, and uncooperative behaviors may interfere with attaining restful sleep pattern.
Adhere to regular bedtime schedule and rituals. Tell client that it is time to sleep.	Reinforces that it is bedtime and maintains stability of environment. *Note:* Later-than-normal bedtime may be indicated to allow client to dissipate excess energy and facilitate falling asleep.
Provide evening snack, warm milk, bath, or back rub or general massage with lotion.	Promotes relaxation and drowsiness and helps to address skin-care needs.

ACTIONS/INTERVENTIONS (continued)	RATIONALE (continued)
Reduce fluid intake in the evening. Toilet before retiring.	Decreases need to get up to go to the bathroom/incontinence during the night.
Provide soft music or "white noise."	Reduces sensory stimulation by blocking out other environmental sounds that could interfere with restful sleep.
Allow to sleep in shoes or clothing, if client demands.	Provided no harm is done, altering the "normal" lessens the rebellion and allows rest.
Collaborative	
Administer medications, as indicated for sleep, for example:	
Antidepressants, such as trazadone (Desyrel) or quetiapine (Seroquel)	May be effective in treating pseudodementia or depression, thus improving ability to sleep.
Sedative-hypnotics, such as zolpidem (Ambien) or zaleplon (Sonata)	Used sparingly, low-dose, short-acting, rapid-onset hypnotics may be effective in treating insomnia or sundowner's syndrome.
Avoid use of diphenhydramine (Benadryl).	Once used for sleep, this drug is now contraindicated because it interferes with the production of acetylcholine, which is already inhibited in the brains of clients with DAT.

NURSING DIAGNOSIS: Self-Care Deficit (specify type/level)

May Be Related To

Cognitive impairment

Fatigue; decreased motivation

Possibly Evidenced By

Impaired ability to perform activities of daily living (ADLs)—misuse or misidentification of objects; inability to bring food from receptacle to mouth; inability to wash body part(s), regulate water temperature; impaired ability to put on/take off clothing; difficulty completing toileting tasks

Desired Outcomes/Evaluation Criteria—Client Will

Self-Care Status (NOC)

Perform self-care activities within level of own ability.

Caregiver Will

Caregiver Performance: Direct Care (NIC)

Identify and use personal and community resources to provide necessary assistance; support client's independence.

ACTIONS/INTERVENTIONS	RATIONALE
Self-Care Assistance: [specify] (NIC)	
Independent	
Identify reason for difficulty in self-care related to physical limitations in motion, depression, cognitive decline, or environment.	Underlying cause affects choice of interventions and strategies. Clients reported to be unable to perform specific ADLs are often able to do so given the right circumstances, such as adequate and knowledgeable caregiver support.
Determine hygienic needs and provide assistance as needed with activities, including care of hair, nails, and skin; brushing teeth; and cleaning glasses.	As the disease progresses, basic hygienic needs may be forgotten. Infection, gum disease, disheveled appearance, or harm may occur when client or caregivers become frustrated, irritated, or intimidated by degree of care required.
Inspect skin regularly.	Presence of such lesions as ecchymoses, lacerations, or rashes may require treatment as well as signal the need for closer monitoring and protective interventions.
Incorporate usual routine into activity schedule as possible. Wait or change the time to initiate dressing and hygiene if a problem arises.	Maintaining routine may prevent worsening of confusion and enhance cooperation. Because anger is quickly forgotten, another time or approach may be successful.
Be attentive to nonverbal physiological symptoms.	Sensory loss and language dysfunction may cause client to express self-care needs in nonverbal manner, such as thirst by panting, need to void by holding self or fidgeting, and pain by facial grimacing.
Be alert to underlying meaning of verbal statements.	May direct a question to another, such as "Are you cold?" meaning "I am cold and need additional clothing."
Supervise but allow as much autonomy as possible.	Eases the frustration over lost independence.

(continues on page 756)

ACTIONS/INTERVENTIONS (continued)	RATIONALE (continued)
Allot plenty of time to perform tasks.	Tasks that were once easy, such as dressing or bathing, are now complicated by decreased motor skills or cognitive and physical changes. Time and patience can reduce chaos resulting from trying to hasten this process.
Assist with neat dressing and provide colorful clothes.	Enhances esteem; may diminish sense of sensory loss and convey aliveness.
Offer one item of clothing at a time in sequential order. Talk client through each step of the task. Allow the wearing of extra clothing if client demands.	Simplicity reduces frustration and the potential for rage and despair. Guidance reduces confusion and allows autonomy. Altering the "normal" may lessen rebellion.
Provide reminders for elimination needs. Involve in bowel and bladder program, as appropriate.	Loss of control and independence in this self-care activity can have a great impact on self-esteem and may limit socialization. (Refer to ND: Constipation.)
Assist with and provide reminders for pericare after toileting or incontinence.	Good hygiene promotes cleanliness and reduces risks of skin irritation and infection.

NURSING DIAGNOSIS: risk for imbalanced Nutrition: less/more than body requirements

Risk Factors May Include

Inability to ingest food (e.g., regressed habits, inability to feed self)
Psychological factors (e.g., agitation, forgetfulness, impaired judgment)

Possibly Evidenced By

(Not applicable; presence of signs and symptoms establishes an *actual* diagnosis)

Desired Outcomes/Evaluation Criteria—Client Will

Nutritional Status (NOC)

Ingest nutritionally balanced diet.
Maintain or regain appropriate weight.

ACTIONS/INTERVENTIONS	RATIONALE
Nutrition Management (NIC) *Independent*	
Assess caregiver's and client's knowledge of nutritional needs.	Identifies needs to assist in formulating individual teaching plan. Role-reversals may occur: a child now cooks for a parent, or a husband taking over "duties" of his wife, increasing the need for information.
Perform Edinburgh Feeding Evaluation in Dementia (EdFED) scale, as appropriate, if client demonstrates weight loss or decline in mealtime function. Schedule regular repeat reviews at same time of day and in same environment, as needed.	Helps establish baseline and monitors behaviors in moderate-to-severe dementia and determines level of assistance required (Stockdell, 2008).
Determine amount of exercise or pacing client does.	Nutritional intake may need to be adjusted to meet needs related to individual energy expenditure.
Offer or provide assistance in menu selection.	Poor judgment may lead to poor choices; client may be indecisive or overwhelmed by choices and/or unaware of the need to maintain elemental nutrition. *Note:* In general, metabolic rate decreases with age, requiring caloric adjustment that must be balanced with activity.
Provide privacy when eating habits become an insoluble problem. Accept eating with hands, spills, and whimsical mixtures such as salad dressing in milk or salt and pepper on ice cream. Avoid solo dining or separating client from other people too early in the disease process.	Socially unacceptable and embarrassing eating habits develop as the disease progresses. Acceptance preserves esteem and decreases irritability or refusal to eat as a result of anger or frustration. Early separation can result in client feeling upset and rejected and can actually result in decreased food intake.
Offer small meals and/or snacks of one or two foods around the clock, as indicated.	Large feedings may overwhelm the client, resulting either in complete abstinence or gorging. Small feedings may enhance appropriate intake. Limiting number of foods offered at a single time reduces confusion regarding which food to choose.
Simplify steps of eating and serve food in courses.	Promotes autonomy and independence; decreases potential frustration or anger over lost abilities.
Anticipate needs, cut foods, and provide soft or finger foods.	Coordination decreases as the disease progresses, which impairs the client's ability to chew and handle utensils.

ACTIONS/INTERVENTIONS (continued)	RATIONALE (continued)
Provide ample time for eating.	A leisurely approach aids digestion and decreases the chance of anger precipitated by rushing.
Place food items in pita bread or paper sack for the client who paces.	Carrying food may encourage client to eat.
Avoid baby food and excessively hot foods.	Baby foods lack adequate nutritional content, fiber, and taste for adults and can add to client's humiliation. Hot foods may result in mouth burns and/or refusal to eat.
Observe swallowing ability; monitor oral cavity.	Diminished abilities may result in client or caregiver repeatedly placing food in client's mouth, which is not swallowed, increasing risk of aspiration.
Stimulate oral-suck reflex by gentle stroking of the cheeks or stimulating the mouth with a spoon.	As the disease progresses, the client may clench teeth and refuse to eat. Stimulating the reflex may increase cooperation and intake.
Collaborative	
Refer to dietitian or nutritionist, as indicated.	Assistance may be needed to develop nutritionally balanced diet individualized to meet client needs or food preferences.

NURSING DIAGNOSIS: Bowel Incontinence/impaired Urinary Elimination

May Be Related To

Multiple causality (e.g., impaired cognition, inability to locate bathroom or recognize need; general decline in muscle tone)

Possibly Evidenced By

Inability to recognize or inattention to urge to defecate/void

Urgency; incontinence

Desired Outcomes/Evaluation Criteria—Client Will

Bowel [or] Urinary Elimination (NOC)

Establish adequate or appropriate pattern of elimination.

ACTIONS/INTERVENTIONS	RATIONALE
Urinary Elimination [or] Bowel Management (NIC)	
Independent	
Assess prior pattern and compare with current situation.	Provides information about changes that may require further assessment and intervention.
Establish bowel and bladder training program. Promote client participation to level of ability.	Stimulates awareness, enhances regulation of body function, and helps to avoid accidents.
Monitor appearance and color of urine. Note amount and consistency of stool.	Detection of changes provides opportunity to alter interventions to prevent complications or acquire treatment, as indicated. *Note:* Although it is difficult, the caregiver must try to monitor frequency of bowel movements during the stage of the illness when the client is still toileting self. It is not enough to ask client, "Did you have a bowel movement today?" Client cannot remember. Monitoring is essential to prevent constipation and potential for impaction.
Encourage adequate fluid intake during the day, with diet high in fiber and fruit juices. Limit intake during the late evening and at bedtime.	Essential for bodily functions and prevents potential dehydration and constipation. Restricting intake in evening may reduce frequency and incontinence during the night.
Self-Care Assistance: Toileting (NIC)	
Locate bed near a bathroom when possible; make signs or color code door. Place a picture of a commode on the door. Provide adequate lighting, particularly at night.	Promotes orientation and increases success in finding bathroom. Incontinence may be attributed to inability to find a toilet.
Take client to the toilet at regular intervals. Dictate each step one at a time and use positive reinforcement.	Adherence to a daily and regular schedule may prevent accidents. Frequently, the problem is forgetting how to toilet, such as pushing pants down or positioning.
Avoid a sense of hurrying or being rushed.	Hurrying may be perceived as intrusion, which leads to anger and lack of cooperation with activity.
Be alert to nonverbal cues, such as restlessness, holding self, or picking at clothes.	May signal urgency or inattention to cues and/or inability to locate bathroom.
Be discreet and respect client's privacy.	Although the client is confused, a sense of modesty is often retained.

(continues on page 758)

ACTIONS/INTERVENTIONS	RATIONALE
Convey acceptance when incontinence occurs. Change promptly; provide good skin care.	Acceptance is important to decrease the embarrassment and feelings of helplessness that may occur during the changing process. Prompt changing reduces risk of skin irritation and breakdown.
Collaborative	
Administer stool softeners, bulk expanders (e.g., Metamucil), or glycerin suppository, as indicated.	May be necessary to facilitate or stimulate regular bowel movement.

NURSING DIAGNOSIS: risk for Sexual Dysfunction

Risk Factors May Include

Biopsychosocial alteration of sexuality (e.g., progression of disease—decrease in habit or control of behavior, confusion, forgetfulness, and disorientation to place or person)

Lack of privacy; lack of significant other

Possibly Evidenced By

(Not applicable; presence of signs and symptoms establishes an *actual* diagnosis)

Desired Outcomes/Evaluation Criteria—Client Will

Sexual Functioning (NOC)

Meet sexuality needs in an acceptable manner.

Experience fewer or no episodes of inappropriate behavior.

ACTIONS/INTERVENTIONS	RATIONALE
Sexual Counseling (NIC)	
Independent	
Assess individual needs, desires, and abilities of client and partner.	Alternative methods need to be designed for the individual situation to fulfill the need for intimacy and closeness.
Encourage partner to show affection and acceptance.	The cognitively impaired person retains the basic needs for affection, love, acceptance, and sexual expression.
Ensure privacy or encourage home visitation for residential client, as appropriate.	Sexual expression or behaviors may differ. The individual may masturbate or expose self. Privacy allows sexual expression without embarrassment and the objections of others.
Use distraction, as indicated. Remind client that, when in a public area, sexual behavior is unacceptable.	This tool is useful when there is inappropriate or objectionable behavior, such as self-exposure.
Provide time to listen to and discuss concerns of partner.	Partner may need information and/or counseling about alternatives for sexual activity and ways to deal with problems, such as impotence or sexual aggression.

NURSING DIAGNOSIS: compromised family Coping

May Be Related To

Prolonged disease that exhausts supportive capacity of significant person

Little support provided by client, in turn, for primary person

Coexisting situations affecting the significant other

Possibly Evidenced By

Significant person attempts assistive/supportive behaviors with unsatisfactory results

Significant person enters into limited personal communication or withdraws from client

Desired Outcomes/Evaluation Criteria—Family Will

Family Coping (NOC)

Identify strategies/resources within themselves to deal with the situation.

Demonstrate positive coping behaviors in dealing with problems.

Use outside support systems/resources effectively.

ACTIONS/INTERVENTIONS	RATIONALE
Family Support (NIC)	
Independent	
Include family in teaching and planning for home care.	Can ease the burden of home management and increase adaptation. A comfortable and familiar lifestyle at home helps preserve the client's need for belonging.
Review past life experiences, role changes, and coping skills.	Identifies skills that may help individuals cope with grief of current situation more effectively.
Focus on specific problems as they occur, the "here and now."	Disease progression follows no set pattern. A premature focus on the possibility of long-term care or possible incontinence, for example, impairs the ability to cope with present issues.
Establish priorities.	Helps to create a sense of order and facilitates problem-solving.
Be realistic and honest in all matters.	Decreases stress that surrounds false hopes, such as that client may regain past level of functioning from advertised or unproven medication.
Reassess family's ability to care for client at home on an ongoing basis.	Behaviors like hoarding, clinging, unjust accusations, and angry outbursts can precipitate family burnout and interfere with ability to provide effective care.
Provide time to listen with regard to concerns and anxieties.	SO and caregiver require constant support with the multifaceted problems that arise during the course of this illness to ease the process of adaptation and grieving.
Help caregiver/family understand the importance of maintaining psychosocial functioning.	Embarrassing behavior and the demands of care may cause withdrawal from social contact.
Discuss possibility of isolation. Reinforce need for support systems.	The belief that a single individual can meet all the needs of the client increases the potential for physical or mental illness due to caregiver role strain. *Note:* Mortality rate for primary caregivers is actually higher than for the client with DAT.
Provide positive feedback for efforts.	Reassures individuals that they are doing their best and provides reinforcement to continue efforts.
Acknowledge concerns generated by consideration or decision to place client in long-term care facility. Answer questions honestly and explore options, as appropriate.	Constant care requirements may be more than can be managed by the caregiver and support systems. Support is needed for this difficult, guilt-producing decision, which may create a financial burden as well as family disruption and dissension.
Encourage visitation by extended family and friends as tolerated by client.	Familiarity forms a base of reality and can provide a reassuring freedom from loneliness. Recurrent contact helps family members realize and accept situation. *Note:* Family members may require ongoing support in dealing with visitation and issues of client's deterioration and their own personal needs.
Collaborative	
Involve SO and family members in planning care and problem-solving. Verify presence of advance directives and durable medical power of attorney.	Consensus may be more readily achieved when family participates in decision making. It is important, however, to keep client's wishes in mind when making choices and to be aware of who actually has the power to make decisions for the cognitively impaired client.
Refer to local resources such as adult day care, respite care, homemaker services, or a local chapter of Alzheimer's Disease Education and Referral (ADEAR) and the National Family Caregivers Association (NFCA).	Coping with these clients is a full-time, frustrating task. Respite and day care may lighten the burden, reduce potential social isolation, and prevent family burnout and caregiver role strain. ADEAR provides group support and family teaching and promotes research. Local groups provide a social outlet for sharing grief and promote problem-solving with such matters as financial or legal advice and home care. NFCA also provides programs for educating caregivers and healthcare providers and a quarterly publication.
Refer for family counseling or to appropriate ethical committee, as indicated.	Differing opinions regarding client care and placement can result in conflict requiring professional mediation.

NURSING DIAGNOSIS: ineffective Health Maintenance

May Be Related To

Cognitive impairment
Diminished gross and/or fine motor skills
Inability to make appropriate judgments
Ineffective individual or family coping
Insufficient resources

Possibly Evidenced By

Inability to take responsibility for meeting basic health practices
Impairment of personal support system

Desired Outcomes/Evaluation Criteria—Family/Caregiver(s) Will

Health-Promoting Behavior (NOC)

Identify factors related to difficulty in maintaining a safe, healthy environment.
Assume responsibility for and initiate behaviors and screenings supporting client healthcare goals.
Demonstrate effective use of resources such as respite or home health care services, homemakers, and other resources.

ACTIONS/INTERVENTIONS	RATIONALE
Health System Guidance (NIC)	
Independent	
Evaluate level of cognitive, emotional, and physical functioning, including level of independence.	Identifies strengths, areas of need, and how much responsibility the client may be expected to assume. (Refer to ND: Self-Care Deficit.)
Assess environment, noting unhealthy factors and ability of client to care for self.	Determines what changes need to be made to accommodate disabilities. (Refer to ND: impaired Environmental Interpretation Syndrome.)
Assist client to develop plan for keeping track of and dealing with health needs.	Schedule can be helpful to maintain system for managing routine healthcare services.
Identify support systems available to client and SO, including other family members and friends.	Planning and constant care is necessary to maintain this client at home. If family system is unavailable or unaware, client health needs, such as nutrition, dental care, or eye exams, can be neglected. Primary caregiver can benefit from sharing responsibilities and constant care with others. (Refer to ND: risk for Caregiver Role Strain, following.)
Evaluate coping abilities, effectiveness, and commitment of caregiver(s) and support persons.	Progressive debilitation taxes caregiver(s) and may alter ability to meet client's and own needs. (Refer to ND: disabled family Coping.)
Collaborative	
Identify senior services such as Meals on Wheels and community resources for homemaking and cleaning or handyman tasks.	As client's condition worsens, caregiver will require additional support to maintain healthy environment for client and self, especially if family support is limited or not available.
Refer to supportive services, as needed.	Medical and social services consultant may be needed to develop ongoing plan or identify resources as needs change.
Identify in-home healthcare options including medical, dental, and diagnostic services.	Delivery of healthcare needs "on site" may prevent exacerbation of confusion, increase cooperation, and provide more accurate picture of client's status.

NURSING DIAGNOSIS: risk for Caregiver Role Strain

Risk Factors May Include

Illness severity of the care receiver, duration of caregiving required, complexity or amount of caregiving tasks
Caregiver is female, spouse
Care receiver exhibits deviant, bizarre behavior
Family/caregiver isolation; lack of respite or recreation for caregiver

Possibly Evidenced By

(Not applicable; presence of signs and symptoms establishes an *actual* diagnosis)

Desired Outcomes/Evaluation Criteria—Caregiver Will

Caregiver Role Endurance (NOC)

Demonstrate effective use of family and community resources to assist in meeting client's needs.
Engage in behaviors or lifestyle changes to promote own well-being.

ACTIONS/INTERVENTIONS	RATIONALE
Caregiver Support (NIC)	
Independent	
Determine family/caregiver's understanding of condition and expectations for the future.	Identifies teaching needs. Provides opportunity to update information and clarify misconceptions. During the prolonged caregiving experience, 7 of 10 clients with Alzheimer's continue to live at home, where family and friends provide almost 75% of their care. As the individual descends into the disease, he or she cannot translate a thought into a motor action, thus full-time supervision and care is required. For some family members and care partners, this supervision becomes overwhelming and exhausting (Rentz, 2008).
Provide bibliotherapy.	Materials that can be reviewed as time permits or questions arise can be very helpful in expanding knowledge and providing ongoing support.
Identify strengths of caregiver and care receiver.	Helps to use positive aspects of each individual to the best of abilities in daily activities.
Facilitate family conference to share responsibilities as indicated and to stress importance of self-nurturing for caregiver, including such factors as pursuing self-development interests, personal needs, hobbies, and social activities.	Helps family to focus on needs of caregiver as well as care receiver. When others are involved in care, the risk of one person becoming overwhelmed is lessened.
Determine available supports and resources currently used.	Organizations including Alzheimer's Foundation of America, Alzheimer's Association, NFCA, or local support groups can provide information regarding adequacy of supports, identify needs, and suggest possible options.
Identify alternate-care sources such as sitter or day-care facility; senior care services such as Meals on Wheels and respite care; and Alzheimer's programs or a home-care agency.	As client's condition worsens, caregiver may need additional help from several sources to maintain client at home, even on a part-time basis.

Refer to CP: Multiple Sclerosis, ND: risk for Caregiver Role Strain for additional interventions.

NURSING DIAGNOSIS: risk for Relocation Stress Syndrome

Risk Factors May Include

Decreased health status
Moderate-to-high degree of environmental change
Lack of predeparture counseling

Possibly Evidenced By

(Not applicable; presence of signs and symptoms establishes an *actual* diagnosis)

Desired Outcomes/Evaluation Criteria—Client Will

Stress Level (NOC)

Experience minimal disruption of usual activities.
Display limited increase in agitation or emotional lability.

Family/Caregiver Will

Family Participation in Professional Care (NOC)

Engage in proactive planning to match client care needs with available resources.
Include client in prior planning and decision-making process to level of ability.
Recognize need to provide stability for client during adaptation period.

ACTIONS/INTERVENTIONS	RATIONALE
Relocation Stress Reduction (NIC)	
Independent	
Discuss ramifications of move to new surroundings.	Discussing pros and cons of this decision helps those involved to reach an informed decision and feel better about and plan for the future.
Encourage visitation to facility prior to planned move.	Familiarizes family and client with new options to enable them to make informed decision.
Provide clear, honest information about actions and events.	Decreases "surprises." Assists in maintaining trust and orientation. When the client knows the truth about what is happening, coping may be enhanced.

Refer to CP: Extended Care, ND: risk for Relocation Stress Syndrome for additional interventions.

POTENTIAL CONSIDERATIONS following acute hospitalization (dependent on underlying cause for admission and comorbidities). Refer to appropriate care plan.

SURGICAL INTERVENTION

I. Procedure—Therapeutic manipulation or use of instruments to diagnose or remedy physical disorders or defects

- **a.** Indications
  - **i.** Diagnose or cure a specific disease process
  - **ii.** Correct a structural deformity
  - **iii.** Restore a functional process
  - **iv.** Reduce the level of dysfunction or pain
- **b.** Classification
  - **i.** Generally elective or preplanned
    1. Inpatient procedure
    2. Ambulatory or outpatient
  - **ii.** Potentially life-threatening conditions can arise requiring emergent intervention.

II. Pathophysiology—Dependent upon the type of injury or disease process that the client has experienced

GLOSSARY

Ambulatory surgery: Refers to surgical procedures performed on an outpatient basis in a hospital or freestanding ambulatory surgery center's general or main operating rooms, satellite operating rooms, cystoscopy rooms, endoscopy rooms, cardiac catheterization labs, or laser procedure rooms.

Atelectasis: Collapsed or airless condition of the lung or lung segment.

Bronchospasm: Abnormal narrowing with partial obstruction of the lumen of the bronchi due to spasm of the peribronchial smooth muscle.

Cephalad diffusion: Movement toward the head, in context of spinal anesthesia, indicates advancement of drug effect generally beyond desired level.

Cubital: Refers to the ulna or the forearm.

Dehiscence: Bursting open or separation of surgical incision or wound.

Electrocautery: Cauterization using a variety of electrical modalities to create thermal energy, including a directly heated metallic applicator or bipolar or monopolar electrodes.

Fasciculation: Involuntary contraction or twitching of muscle fibers, which are visible under the skin.

Hemostasis: Arrest or cessation of bleeding from an injured vessel.

Hypercoagulation: Increased ability of blood, for example, to coagulate.

Hypoxia: An oxygen deficiency in body tissues.

Intraoperatively: Occurring during surgery.

Laryngospasm: Spasm of the laryngeal muscles that may be life-threatening.

Perioperative: Period of time that constitutes the surgical experience; includes the preoperative, intraoperative, and postoperative phases of nursing care.

Postoperative: Period of time that begins with admission to the postanesthesia care unit (PACU) and ends after a follow-up evaluation in the clinical setting or home.

Preoperative: Period of time from when the decision for surgical intervention is made to when the individual is transferred to the operating room table.

Prophylactically: Any agent or regimen that contributes to the prevention of infection or disease.

Surgical Care Improvement Project: Multiyear, national quality partnership of organizations called the Surgical Care Improvement Project, or SCIP, with the goal of decreasing surgical complications. The focuses being reported for SCIP areas (as of 2011) are: infection prevention (administration of antibiotics, monitoring blood glucose levels, appropriate hair removal, removal of urinary catheters, and perioperative temperature management), cardiac care, and venous thromboembolism (VTE) prevention (QualityNet Specifications Manual, 2011).

Time-out protocol: Procedure for ensuring final verification of the correct client, procedure, site, and, if applicable, implants. Includes active communication among all members of the surgical team; procedure is not started until this has occurred.

Care Setting

Client may be inpatient on a surgical unit or outpatient or have a short stay in an ambulatory surgical setting.

Related Concerns

Also refer to plan of care for specific surgical procedure performed.

Client Assessment Database

Data depend on the duration and severity of underlying problem and involvement of other body systems. Refer to specific plans of care for data and diagnostic studies relevant to the procedure and additional nursing diagnoses.

DIAGNOSTIC DIVISION MAY REPORT	MAY EXHIBIT
CIRCULATION	
• History of cardiac problems, heart failure (HF), pulmonary edema, peripheral vascular disease, or vascular stasis, which increase risk of thrombus formation	• Changes in heart rate due to sympathetic stimulation
EGO INTEGRITY	
• Feelings of anxiety, fear, anger, apathy • Multiple stress factors related to financial, relationship, lifestyle issues	• Restlessness, increased tension or irritability • Sympathetic stimulation—changes in heart or respiratory rate
ELIMINATION	
• History of kidney or bladder conditions • Use of diuretics and/or laxatives • Change in bowel habits	• Abdominal tenderness, distention • Absence of bowel elimination • Decreased or absent urinary elimination
FOOD/FLUID	
• History of pancreatic insufficiency or diabetes mellitus (DM), which may predispose client to hypoglycemia or ketoacidosis • Use of diuretics	• Malnutrition, including obesity • Dry mucous membranes due to limited intake or nothing-by-mouth (NPO) status preoperatively
PAIN/DISCOMFORT	
• History of painful body area—often the reason for surgical procedure—due to disease, inflammation, infection, or trauma	• Guarding behavior, facial mask, sleep disturbance, restlessness, moaning
RESPIRATION	
• History or presence of respiratory infections • Chronic lung conditions • Past and/or current smoking	• Changes in respiratory rate (respiratory pathology, pain, or sympathetic stimulation)
SAFETY	
• Differences in personal identifiers, procedure type, and/or site when compared to verification tools, such as the consent form, history and physical examination, surgery schedule • Allergies or sensitivities to medications, iodine, food, tape, latex, and solution(s)	• Presence of existing infectious process • Fever • Advanced age

(continues on page 764)

DIAGNOSTIC DIVISION MAY REPORT (continued)	MAY EXHIBIT (continued)
• Immune deficiencies—increased risk of systemic infections and delayed healing • Presence of cancer or recent cancer therapy • Family history of malignant hyperthermia or reaction to anesthesia, autoimmune diseases • History of hepatic disease, which might affect drug detoxification and may alter coagulation • History of blood transfusion(s) or transfusion reaction **TEACHING/LEARNING** • Use of medications, such as anticoagulants, steroids, NSAIDs, antibiotics, antihypertensives, cardiotonic glycosides, antidysrhythmics, bronchodilators, diuretics, decongestants, analgesics, anti-inflammatory drugs, anticonvulsants, or antipsychotics and anti-anxiety agents as well as over-the-counter (OTC) medications, herbal supplements (e.g., garlic, ginseng, ginkgo biloba, ginger, and feverfew present risk of excessive postoperative bleeding), or alcohol or other drugs of abuse, with risk of liver damage affecting coagulation and choice of anesthesia as well as potential for postoperative withdrawal **DISCHARGE PLAN CONSIDERATIONS** • May require temporary assistance with transportation, dressing(s), supplies, self-care, and homemaker or maintenance tasks • Possible placement in rehabilitation or extended care facility ➧ Refer to section at end of plan for postdischarge considerations.	

Diagnostic Studies

Studies depend on type of operative procedure, underlying medical conditions, current medications, age, and weight. Deviations from normal should be corrected, if possible, for safe administration of anesthetic agents.

TEST WHY IT IS DONE	WHAT IT TELLS ME
BLOOD TESTS	
• ***Complete blood count (CBC):*** Battery of screening tests, which typically includes hemoglobin (Hgb); hematocrit (Hct); red blood cell (RBC) count, morphology, indices, and distribution width index; platelet count and size; and white blood cell (WBC) count and differential.	An elevated WBC count is indicative of inflammatory process. It may be diagnostic, as in appendicitis. A decreased WBC count suggests viral processes, requiring further evaluation because immune system may be dysfunctional. Low Hgb suggests anemia or blood loss, which impairs tissue oxygenation and decreases the amount of Hgb available to bind with inhalation anesthetics. It may suggest need for crossmatch for possible blood transfusion. An elevated Hct may indicate dehydration, whereas decreased Hct suggests fluid overload.
• ***Electrolytes:*** Substances that dissociate into ions in solution and acquire the capacity to conduct electricity. Common electrolytes include sodium, potassium, chloride, calcium, and phosphate.	Imbalances impair organ function; for example, decreased potassium affects cardiac muscle contractility, leading to decreased cardiac output.
• ***Arterial blood gases (ABGs):*** Measurement of the pH level and the oxygen and carbon dioxide concentrations in arterial blood.	Evaluates current respiratory status, which may be especially important in smokers or clients with chronic lung diseases.
• ***Bleeding or coagulation studies—prothrombin time (PT) and activated partial thromboplastin time (aPTT):*** Screening for coagulation problems indicated with history of abnormal bleeding, liver or kidney disease, use of anticoagluants, or when	May be prolonged, interfering with intraoperative and/or postoperative hemostasis. Hypercoagulation increases risk of thrombosis formation, especially in conjunction with dehydration and decreased mobility associated with surgery.

TEST WHY IT IS DONE (continued)	WHAT IT TELLS ME (continued)
medical history is not available as well as for high-risk procedures, such as peripheral vascular surgery, cardiopulmonary bypass, or prostatectomy.	
OTHER DIAGNOSTIC STUDIES	
• *Chest x-ray:* Procedure used to evaluate organs and structures within the chest for symptoms of disease.	Should be free of infiltrates or pneumonia. Used for identification of masses and chronic obstructive pulmonary disease (COPD).
• *Electrocardiogram (ECG):* Record of the electrical activity of the heart.	Abnormal findings require attention before administering anesthetics.
• *Urinalysis:* Examination of urine for various cells and chemicals such as RBCs, WBCs, infection, or excessive protein.	Presence of WBCs or bacteria indicates infection. Elevated specific gravity may reflect dehydration.
• *Pregnancy test:* Recommended in presence of recently absent or irregular menses, unreliable use of contraception, or for gynecological procedures to limit fetal exposure to teratogenic agents.	Positive results affect timing of procedure and choice of pharmacological agents.

Nursing Priorities

1. Assure correct client, procedure, and site.
2. Reduce anxiety and emotional trauma.
3. Provide for physical safety.
4. Prevent complications.
5. Alleviate pain.
6. Facilitate recovery process.
7. Provide information about disease process, surgical procedure, prognosis, and treatment needs.

Discharge Goals

1. Client dealing realistically with current situation.
2. Injury prevented.
3. Complications prevented or minimized.
4. Pain relieved or controlled.
5. Wound healing and organ function progressing toward normal.
6. Disease process, surgical procedure, prognosis, and therapeutic regimen understood.
7. Plan in place to meet needs after discharge.

Perioperative

NURSING DIAGNOSIS: deficient Knowledge [Learning Need] regarding condition, prognosis, treatment, self-care, and discharge needs

May Be Related To

Lack of exposure or recall, information misinterpretation
Unfamiliarity with information resources

Possibly Evidenced By

Reports the problem
Inappropriate, exaggerated behaviors—agitated, apathetic, hostile
Inaccurate follow-through of instructions

Desired Outcomes/Evaluation Criteria—Client Will

Knowledge: Treatment Procedure(s) (NOC)

Verbalize understanding of disease process, perioperative process, and postoperative expectations.
Correctly perform necessary procedures and explain reasons for the actions.
Initiate necessary lifestyle changes and participate in treatment regimen.

ACTIONS/INTERVENTIONS	RATIONALE
Teaching: Preoperative (NIC)	
Independent	
Assess client's level of understanding.	Facilitates planning of preoperative teaching program and identifies content needs.
Review specific pathology and anticipated surgical procedure. Verify correct client, procedure, and marked site and that appropriate consent has been signed.	Provides knowledge base from which client can make informed therapy choices and consent appropriate for correct procedure and site. Presents opportunity to clarify misconceptions.
Use institution's protocol for Preventing Wrong Site, Wrong Procedure, and Wrong Person Surgery and resource teaching materials and audiovisuals, as available.	Completion of specific checklists will minimize risk of error. Specifically designed materials can facilitate the client's learning.
Implement individualized preoperative teaching program:	Enhances client's understanding and control and can relieve stress related to the unknown or unexpected.
Preoperative and postoperative procedures and expectations, urinary and bowel changes, dietary considerations, activity levels, transfers, respiratory and cardiovascular exercises; anticipated intravenous (IV) lines and tubes such as nasogastric (NG) tubes, drains, and catheters	Absence or limitation of preoperative preparation and teaching increases the need for postoperative support in addition to managing underlying medical conditions.
Preoperative instructions including bowel prep, NPO time, antibacterial soap shower and other skin preparation, which routine medications to take or hold—prophylactic antibiotics or anticoagulants; anesthesia premedication	Helps reduce the possibility of postoperative complications and promotes a rapid return to normal body function. *Note:* In some instances, liquids and medications are allowed up to 2 hours before scheduled procedure.
Intraoperative client safety—positional needs due to arthritis, previous injury, or current mobility; not crossing legs during procedures performed under local or light anesthesia	Reduced risk of complications or untoward outcomes, such as muscular, nerve (e.g., injury to the peroneal and tibial nerves with postoperative pain in the calves and feet), or joint soreness.
Expected or transient reactions such as low backache, localized numbness, and reddening or skin indentations	Minor effects of immobilization or positioning should resolve in 24 hours. If they persist, medical evaluation is required.
Inform client and SO about timely arrival on surgical day, itinerary, and physician-SO communications.	Logistical information about preoperative preparation time, operating room (OR) schedule and locations (e.g., recovery room, postoperative room assignment), as well as where and when the surgeon will communicate with SO relieves stress and miscommunications, preventing confusion and doubt over client's well-being.
Discuss and develop individual postoperative pain-management plan. Identify misconceptions client may have and provide appropriate information. Review use of 0 to 10 or similar pain assessment scale.	Increases likelihood of successful pain management. Some clients may expect to be pain-free or fear becoming addicted to opioid agents.
Provide opportunity to practice coughing, deep-breathing exercises, possible use of incentive spirometry, and muscular exercises.	Enhances learning and continuation of activity postoperatively.

NURSING DIAGNOSIS: Fear/Anxiety [specify level]

May Be Related To

Situational crisis (e.g., wrong client, procedure or site error; unfamiliarity with environment)
Change in health status, threat of death
Separation from usual support systems

Possibly Evidenced By

Increased tension, apprehension, decreased self-assurance, fear
Reports concerns due to change in life events, being scared
Facial tension, restlessness, focus on self
Sympathetic stimulation

Desired Outcomes/Evaluation Criteria—Client Will

Anxiety [or] Fear Self-Control (NOC)

Acknowledge feelings and identify healthy ways to deal with them.
Appear relaxed and be able to rest or sleep appropriately.
Report decreased fear and anxiety reduced to a manageable level.
Demonstrate ability to carry out procedure requirements.

ACTIONS/INTERVENTIONS	RATIONALE
Preoperative Coordination (NIC)	
Independent	
Provide preoperative education, including intentional repetitive verification of client identifiers, procedure, marked site steps, and surgical "time out" process. Visit with OR personnel before surgery when possible. Discuss or demonstrate routine procedures and processes that may frighten or concern client, such as masks, lights, IVs, blood pressure (BP) cuff, electrodes, bovie pad, feel of oxygen cannula or mask on nose or face, autoclave and suction noises, or child crying.	Can provide reassurance that client safety precautions are constantly ongoing, alleviate client's anxiety, as well as provide information for formulating intraoperative care. Acknowledges that foreign environment may be frightening and alleviates associated fears. Decreased anxiety level reduces elevation of glucocorticosteroid levels, which can interfere with healing.
Inform client and SO of nurse's intraoperative advocate role.	Develops trust and rapport, decreasing fear of loss of control in a foreign environment. Provides client and SO with contact person.
Assure client anticipating conscious sedation or spinal anesthesia that drowsiness or sleep occurs, that more sedation may be requested and will be given if needed, and that surgical drapes will block view of the operative field.	Reduces concerns that client may "see" the procedure.
Surgical Preparation (NIC)	
Identify fear levels that may necessitate postponement of surgical procedure.	Overwhelming or persistent fears result in excessive stress reaction and increasing glucocorticosteroid levels, potentiating risk of adverse reaction to procedure and anesthetic agents and impairing healing.
Validate source of fear. Provide accurate factual information. Active-listen concerns.	Identification of specific fear helps client deal realistically with fears, such as misidentification or wrong operation, dismemberment, disfigurement, loss of dignity and control, or being awake or aware with local anesthesia. Client may have misinterpreted preoperative information or have misinformation regarding surgery or disease process. Fears regarding previous experiences of self, family, or acquaintances may be unresolved.
Note expressions of distress or feelings of helplessness, preoccupation with anticipated change or loss, and choked feelings.	Client may already be grieving for the loss represented by the anticipated surgical procedure, diagnosis, or prognosis of illness.
Introduce client to staff at time of transfer to operating suite.	Establishes rapport and psychological comfort with operative team.
Verbalize and document client identifiers to surgery schedule, client identification band, chart, marked site, and signed operative consent for surgical procedure according to facility's protocol and checklist.	Provides for positive identification, reducing fear that wrong procedure may be done as well as minimizing risk for wrong procedure and site.
Prevent unnecessary body exposure during transfer to and in OR suite.	Preserves client's modesty, reduces fear of loss of dignity and inability to exercise control, and reinforces nurse advocacy role.
Give simple, concise directions and explanations to sedated client. Review environmental concerns, as needed.	Impairment of thought processes makes it difficult for client to understand lengthy instructions.
Control external stimuli.	Extraneous noises and commotion may accelerate anxiety.
Collaborative	
Refer to surgeon, anesthesiologist, clinical manager, pastoral spiritual care, psychiatric clinical nurse specialist, or psychiatric counseling, if indicated.	Further evaluation, information, or counseling may be desired or required for client to deal with fear, especially concerning life-threatening conditions and serious and/or high-risk procedures.
Discuss postponement or cancellation of surgery with physician, anesthesiologist, client, and family, as appropriate.	May be necessary if overwhelming fears are not reduced or resolved.
Refer wrong client, procedure, site, or implant discrepancies to surgeon, anesthesiologist, and appropriate persons.	Discrepancies must be corrected and verified by surgeon, client, and SO prior to OR entry.
Administer medications, as indicated, for example:	
Sedatives and hypnotics	Used to promote sleep the evening before surgery; may enhance coping abilities.
IV anti-anxiety agents	May be provided in the outpatient admitting or preoperative holding area to reduce nervousness and provide comfort. *Note:* Respiratory depression or bradycardia may occur, necessitating prompt intervention.
Antacids and H_2 blocker, preoperatively as indicated	Neutralizes gastric acidity and may reduce risk of aspiration or severity of pneumonia should aspiration occur, especially in obese or pregnant clients in whom there is an 85% risk of mortality with aspiration. *Note:* Ranitidine (Zantac) has been found to reduce postoperative infections in acute colorectal surgery.

NURSING DIAGNOSIS: risk for Perioperative Positioning Injury

Risk Factors May Include

Disorientation, sensory/perceptual disturbances due to anesthesia
Immobilization, muscle weakness
Obesity, emaciation, edema

Possibly Evidenced By

(Not applicable; presence of signs and symptoms establishes an *actual* diagnosis)

Desired Outcomes/Evaluation Criteria—Client Will

Physical Injury Severity (NOC)

Be free of injury related to perioperative disorientation.
Be free of untoward skin or tissue injury or changes lasting beyond 24 to 48 hours following procedure.
Report resolution of localized numbness, tingling, or changes in sensation related to positioning within 24 to 48 hours, as appropriate.

ACTIONS/INTERVENTIONS	RATIONALE
Positioning Intraoperative (NIC)	
Independent	
Note anticipated length of procedure and customary position. Provide for potential complications.	Supine position may cause low back pain and skin pressure at heels, elbows, and sacrum; lateral chest position can cause shoulder and neck pain as well as eye and ear injury on the client's downside.
Review client's history, noting age, weight, height, nutritional status, and physical limitation or preexisting conditions that may affect choice of position and skin and tissue integrity during surgery.	Many conditions, such as lack of subcutaneous padding in elderly person, arthritis, thoracic outlet or cubital tunnel syndrome, diabetes, obesity, presence of abdominal stoma, peripheral vascular disease, level of hydration, and temperature of extremities, can make individual prone to injury.
Stabilize both client cart and OR table when transferring client to and from OR table, using an adequate number of personnel for transfer and support of extremities.	Unstabilized cart or table can separate, causing client to fall. Both side rails must be in the down position for caregiver(s) to assist client transfer and prevent loss of balance.
Anticipate movement of extraneous lines and tubes during the transfer and secure or guide them into position.	Prevents undue tension and dislocation of IV lines, NG tubes, catheters, and chest tubes; maintains gravity drainage when appropriate.
Secure client on OR table with safety belt and arm protection as appropriate, explaining necessity for safety precautions.	OR tables and arm boards are narrow, placing client at risk for injury, especially during fasciculation. Client may become resistive or combative when sedated or emerging from anesthesia, furthering potential for injury.
Protect body from contact with metal parts of the operating table.	Reduces risk of electrical injury.
Prepare equipment and padding for required position, according to operative procedure and client's specific needs. Pay special attention to pressure points of bony prominences on arms and ankles and neurovascular pressure points and soft tissues such as breasts and knees.	Depending on individual client's size, weight, and preexisting conditions, extra padding materials may be required to protect bony prominences, prevent circulatory compromise or nerve pressure, or to allow for optimal chest expansion for ventilation.
Position extremities so they may be periodically checked for safety, circulation, nerve pressure, and alignment. Monitor peripheral pulses and skin color and temperature.	Prevents accidental trauma to hands, fingers, and toes, which could inadvertently be scraped, pinched, or amputated by moving table attachments. Reduces risk of positional pressure on brachial plexus, peroneal, and ulnar nerves, which can cause serious neurovascular impairment in extremities; or prolonged plantar flexion, which may result in footdrop.
Place legs in stirrups simultaneously when lithotomy position used, adjusting stirrup height to client's legs, maintaining symmetrical position. Pad popliteal space and heels and feet, as indicated.	Prevents muscle strain and reduces risk of hip dislocation in elderly clients. Padding helps prevent peroneal and tibial nerve damage. *Note:* Prolonged positioning in stirrups may lead to compartment syndrome in calf muscles.
Provide foot board, elevate drapes off toes, and decrease blanket weight on extremities. Avoid or monitor equipment and instrumentation placement on trunk or extremities during procedure.	Pressure may cause neural, circulatory, and skin integrity disruption.
Reposition slowly at transfer from table and to bed.	Myocardial depressant effect of various agents increases risk of hypotension and/or bradycardia. Controlling movement enhances volume accommodation.

ACTIONS/INTERVENTIONS (continued)	RATIONALE (continued)
Determine specific postoperative positioning guidelines, such as elevation of head of bed following spinal anesthesia or nose and throat surgery, or turning to unoperated side following pneumonectomy.	Reduces risk of postoperative complications, such as headache associated with migration of spinal anesthesia, or loss of maximal respiratory effort.
Collaborative	
Recommend position changes to anesthesiologist and/or surgeon, as appropriate.	Close attention to proper positioning can prevent muscle strain, nerve damage, circulatory compromise, and undue pressure on skin and bony prominences. Although the anesthesiologist is responsible for positioning, the nurse may be able to see or have more time to note client needs and provide assistance.

NURSING DIAGNOSIS: risk for Injury

Risk Factors May Include

Wrong client, procedure, site, implants, equipment, or materials
Interactive conditions between individual and environment
External environment—physical design, structure of environment, exposure to equipment, instrumentation, positioning, use of pharmaceutical agents
Internal environment—tissue hypoxia, abnormal blood profile or altered clotting factors, broken skin

Possibly Evidenced By

(Not applicable; presence of signs and symptoms establishes an *actual* diagnosis)

Desired Outcomes/Evaluation Criteria—Care Provider Will

Safe Health Care Environment (NOC)
Implement surgical Universal "Time Out" Protocol.
Identify individual risk factors.
Modify environment, as indicated, to enhance safety and use resources appropriately.

Desired Outcomes/Evaluation Criteria—Client Will

Physical Injury Severity (NOC)
Be free of injury.

ACTIONS/INTERVENTIONS	RATIONALE
Surgical Precautions (NIC)	
Independent	
Verify client identity and scheduled operative procedure by comparing client chart, arm band, and surgical schedule. Verbally ascertain correct name, procedure, operative site, and physician.	Ensures correct client, procedure, and appropriate extremity or side.
Remove dentures, partial plates, or bridges preoperatively per protocol. Inform anesthesiologist of problems with natural teeth such as loose teeth.	Foreign bodies may be aspirated during endotracheal intubation and extubation.
Remove prosthetics or other devices preoperatively or after induction, depending on sensory or perceptual alterations and mobility impairment.	Contact lenses may cause corneal abrasions while under anesthesia; eyeglasses and hearing aids are obstructive and may break; however, clients may feel more in control of environment if hearing and visual aids are left on as long as possible. Artificial limbs may be damaged and skin integrity impaired if left on.
Remove jewelry preoperatively. Tape over, or isolate from skin, according to institution protocol. Remove piercing hardware.	Metals conduct electrical current and provide an electrocautery hazard. Piercings may be "snagged," resulting in soft tissue injury. In addition, loss or damage to client's personal property can easily occur in the foreign environment. *Note:* In some cases (e.g., arthritic knuckles), it may not be possible to remove rings without cutting them off. In this situation, applying tape over the ring may prevent client from "catching" ring and prevent loss of stone or damage to finger and decrease psychological loss because of damage to personal property.

(continues on page 770)

ACTIONS/INTERVENTIONS (continued)	RATIONALE (continued)
Document allergies, including risk for adverse reaction to latex, tape, and prep solutions.	Reduces risk for allergic responses that may impair skin integrity or lead to life-threatening systemic reactions.
Give simple and concise directions to the sedated client.	Impairment of thought process makes it difficult for client to understand lengthy directions.
Prevent pooling of skin prep solutions under and around client.	Antiseptic solutions may chemically burn skin as well as conduct electricity.
Assist with induction as needed, for example, standing by to apply cricoid pressure during intubation or stabilizing position during lumbar puncture for spinal block.	Facilitates safe administration of anesthesia.
Verify electrical safety of equipment used in surgical procedure, which includes intact cords, grounds, and medical engineering verification labels.	Malfunction of equipment can occur during the operative procedure, causing not only delays and unnecessary anesthesia but also injury or death. Short circuits, faulty grounds, laser malfunctions, or laser misalignment could occur. Periodic electrical safety checks are imperative for all OR equipment.
Place dispersive electrode or electrocautery pad over largest available muscle mass closest to surgical site, ensuring its contact.	Provides for shortest distance and maximum conductivity to ground to prevent electrical burns.
Confirm and document correct sponge, instrument, needle, and blade counts.	Foreign bodies remaining in body cavities at closure may result in inflammation, infection, perforation, abscess formation, and disastrous complications that can lead to death.
Laser Precautions (NIC)	
Verify credentials of laser operators for specific wavelength laser required for particular procedure.	Because of the potential hazards of lasers, physician and equipment operators must be certified in the use and safety requirements of specific wavelength laser and procedure including open, endoscopic, abdominal, laryngeal, and intrauterine procedures.
Confirm presence of fire extinguishers and wet fire smothering materials when lasers are used intraoperatively.	Laser beam may inadvertently contact and ignite combustibles outside of surgical site such as drapes and sponges.
Apply client and personnel eye protection before laser activation.	Eye protection for specific laser wavelength must be used to prevent injury.
Protect surrounding skin and anatomy appropriately utilizing wet towels, sponges, dams, and cottonoids.	Prevents inadvertent skin integrity disruption, hair ignition, and adjacent anatomy injury in area of laser beam use.
Specimen Management (NIC)	
Handle, label, and document specimens appropriately, ensuring proper medium and transport for tests required.	The OR nurse advocate must properly identify specimens to client, site, and test to ensure validity and maximum client outcome. Loss or mislabeling of specimens renders the surgical procedure fruitless and grossly compromises further treatment and client outcome. Frozen sections, preserved or fresh examination, and cultures all have different medium and transfer requirements.
Fluid Management (NIC)	
Observe intake and output (I&O) during procedure. Anticipate need for volume replacement or rapid infusion via infusion pumps and set up appropriately. Ascertain that pumps are functioning accurately.	Potential for fluid volume deficit or excess exists, affecting safety of anesthesia, tissue perfusion, organ function, and client well-being.
Collaborative	
Administer IV fluids, blood or blood components, as indicated.	Maintains homeostasis and adequate level of sedation and muscle relaxation to produce optimal surgical outcome.
Collect autologous blood intraoperatively, as appropriate.	Blood lost intraoperatively may be collected, filtered, and reinfused either intraoperatively or postoperatively. A continuous, closed circuit must be maintained for the procedure to be acceptable for use by Jehovah's Witnesses. *Note:* Alternatively, red blood cell (RBC) production may be increased by the administration of epoetin (Epogen, Procrit) for up to 3 weeks preoperatively, reducing the need for blood transfusion whether autologous or donated.
Surgical Precautions (NIC)	
Validate surgical field medications and dosages with surgeon and anesthesiologist, including local anesthetics with or without epinephrine in regional blocks.	Prevents administration of contraindicated medications or inappropriate dosages. *Note:* Excessive doses of local anesthetic agents may potentiate cardiovascular compromise.

NURSING DIAGNOSIS: risk for Infection

Risk Factors May Include

Broken skin, traumatized tissues, stasis of body fluids
Presence of pathogens or contaminants, environmental exposure, invasive procedures

Possibly Evidenced By

(Not applicable; presence of signs and symptoms establishes an *actual* diagnosis)

Desired Outcomes/Evaluation Criteria—Care Provider Will

Knowledge: Infection Control (NOC)

Identify individual risk factors and interventions to reduce potential for infection.
Maintain safe aseptic environment.

Desired Outcomes/Evaluation Criteria—Client Will

Infection Severity (NOC)

Be free of signs of healthcare-acquired infection.

ACTIONS/INTERVENTIONS	RATIONALE
Infection Control: Intraoperative (NIC) ***Independent***	
Adhere to surgical care policies and procedures.	These policies have been established nationwide for inpatient and outpatient surgeries to prevent or reduce infections. *Note:* The Surgical Care Improvement Project (SCIP) is currently focused on reduction of surgically related infections. Infection prevention includes (1) administration of antibiotics (includes timeliness of preoperative dose prior to cutting, correct dosing following surgery, and early and appropriate discontinuation time); (2) monitoring of blood glucose levels; (3) appropriate hair removal (nicks from shaving may increase infection potential); (4) early removal of urinary catheters; (5) perioperative temperature management); (6) cardiac care; and (7) venous thromboembolism (VTE) prevention (QualityNet Specifications Manual, 2011).
Verify sterility of all items used in procedure as event related.	Prepackaged items may appear to be sterile; however, each item must be scrutinized for manufacturer's sterility statement or central sterile processing indicators, package integrity, environmental effect on package, and delivery techniques. *Note:* Package sterilization and expiration dates and lot and serial numbers must be documented on implant items for further follow-up if necessary.
Review laboratory studies for systemic infections and scrutinize operative area for possibility of localized infections.	Increased WBC count may indicate ongoing infection, which the operative procedure will alleviate, such as appendicitis, abscess, and inflammation from trauma. Presence of local or systemic infection such as an upper respiratory infection (URI), urinary tract infection (UTI), skin lesions, or unknown infections may contraindicate or adversely affect the surgical procedure and/or anesthesia.
Verify that preoperative skin, vaginal, and bowel cleansing procedures have been done, as needed, depending on specific surgical procedure.	Cleansing reduces bacterial counts on the skin, vaginal mucosa, and alimentary tract.
Prepare operative site according to specific procedures (e.g., scrubbing with liquid antibacterial soap, swabbing with betadine prep).	Minimizes bacterial counts at operative site.
Maintain normal client temperature range as much as possible.	One study found that patients who experienced mild hypothermia during surgery were three times more likely to have positive cultures from the surgical site (The Association of periOperative Registered Nurses [AORN], 2011).
Examine skin for breaks or irritation and signs of infection.	Disruptions of skin integrity at or near the operative site are sources of contamination to the incision. Careful shaving or clipping as close as possible to incision time will prevent skin cuts or abrasions, which provide potential entry for bacteria. *Note*: AORN recommendations state that hair at the surgical site should be left in place whenever possible. If

(continues on page 772)

Maintain dependent gravity drainage of indwelling catheters, tubes, and/or positive pressure of parenteral or irrigation lines.
: hair must be removed, remove only the hair at the surgical site (AORN, 2011). Prevents stasis and reflux of body fluids.

Identify breaks in aseptic technique and resolve immediately upon occurrence.
: Contamination by environmental or personnel contact renders the sterile field unsterile, thereby increasing the risk of infection.

Utilize Universal Precautions, contain contaminated fluids or materials to specific site in operating room suite, and dispose of them according to facility protocol.
: Containment of blood and body fluids, tissue, and materials in contact with an infected wound or client will prevent spread of infection to environment and other clients or personnel.

Apply sterile dressing.
: Prevents environmental contamination of fresh wound.

Monitor blood glucose levels of diabetic clients, and maintain tight glycemic control, as indicated.
: Depending on length of procedure and type of IV fluids infused, intervention may be required to maintain preferred glucose levels. *Note*: Studies have supported that control of blood glucose contributes to better outcomes in critically ill and surgical patients (Frangou, 2008).

Collaborative

Provide and document copious wound irrigation with saline, water, antibiotic, or antiseptic solution.
: May be used intraoperatively to reduce bacterial counts at surgical site and cleanse the wound of bone, ischemic tissue, bowel contaminants, toxins, or other debris.

Obtain specimens for cultures and Gram stain.
: Immediate identification of infective organism type by Gram stain allows prompt treatment, whereas more specific identification by cultures can be obtained in hours or days.

Administer appropriate antibiotics in timely manner, as indicated.
: Antibiotics may be given prophylactically for selected elective surgical procedures or planned in client at high-risk for infection or when procedures need to be performed in the setting of known or suspected wound contamination. SCIP guidelines require the antibiotic to be administered within 1 hour of cut time (any time skin integrity is disrupted, such as in laparoscopic procedures) with the belief that it provides opportunity for the medication to travel through the body and be available at the surgical site at the time of incision (van Kasterin et al, 2007).

NURSING DIAGNOSIS: risk for imbalanced Body Temperature

Risk Factors May Include

[Exposure to cool environment]
Pharmaceutical agents causing vasodilation/vasoconstriction; sedation
Extremes of age, weight; dehydration

Possibly Evidenced By

(Not applicable; presence of signs and symptoms establishes an *actual* diagnosis)

Desired Outcomes/Evaluation Criteria—Client Will

Thermoregulation (NOC)

Maintain body temperature within normal range.

ACTIONS/INTERVENTIONS — RATIONALE

Temperature Regulation: Perioperative (NIC)

Independent

Note preoperative temperature related to age and disease process.
: Used as baseline for monitoring intraoperative temperature. Preoperative temperature elevations may be indicative of disease process, such as appendicitis, abscess, or systemic disease requiring perioperative treatment. *Note:* Effects of aging on hypothalamus may decrease fever response to infection in the older adult client.

Assess environmental temperature and modify, as needed, by providing warming blankets or increasing room temperature.
: Manipulating ambient air around client will prevent heat loss.

Cover exposed areas outside of operative field.
: Heat losses will occur as skin on head, arms, and legs are exposed to cool environmental temperatures.

ACTIONS/INTERVENTIONS (continued)	RATIONALE (continued)
Provide cooling measures for client with preoperative or intraoperative temperature elevations.	Cool irrigations, exposure of skin surfaces to air, or cooling blanket may be required to decrease temperature.
Increase ambient room temperature (e.g., to 78°F or 80°F [25.6°C to 26.7°C]) at conclusion of procedure.	Minimizes client heat loss when drapes are removed and client is prepared for transfer.
Apply warming blankets at emergence from anesthesia.	Inhalation anesthetics depress the hypothalamus, resulting in poor body temperature regulation.
Collaborative	
Monitor temperature throughout intraoperative phase.	Continuous warm or cool humidified inhalation anesthetics are used to maintain humidity and temperature balance within the tracheobronchial tree. Temperature fluctuations may indicate adverse response to anesthesia. *Note:* Use of atropine or scopolamine may further increase temperature.
Malignant Hyperthermia Precautions (NIC)	
Respond promptly to symptoms of malignant hyperthermia (MH)—rapid temperature elevation and persistent high fever:	Prompt recognition and immediate action to control temperature is necessary to prevent serious complications or death.
Provide iced saline to all body surfaces and orifices.	Iced solution lavage of body surfaces and cavities will reduce body temperature.
Obtain dantrolene (Dantrium) for IV administration per protocol.	Immediate action to control temperature is necessary to prevent intense catabolic process associated with MH.

Postoperative

NURSING DIAGNOSIS: ineffective Breathing Pattern

May Be Related To

Neuromuscular dysfunction (e.g., sedation)
Pain
[Tracheobronchial obstruction]

Possibly Evidenced By

Alterations in depth of breathing; reduced vital capacity
Bradypnea

Desired Outcomes/Evaluation Criteria—Client Will

Respiratory Status: Ventilation (NOC)

Establish an effective respiratory pattern free of cyanosis or other signs of hypoxia.

ACTIONS/INTERVENTIONS	RATIONALE
Postanesthesia Care (NIC)	
Independent	
Maintain client airway by head tilt, jaw hyperextension, or oral pharyngeal airway.	Prevents airway obstruction.
Auscultate breath sounds. Listen for gurgling, wheezing, crowing, and/or silence after extubation.	Lack of breath sounds is indicative of obstruction by mucus or tongue and may be corrected by positioning and/or suctioning. Diminished breath sounds suggest atelectasis. Wheezing indicates bronchospasm, whereas crowing or silence reflects partial to total laryngospasm.
Observe respiratory rate and depth, chest expansion, use of accessory muscles, retraction or flaring of nostrils, and skin color; note airflow.	Ascertains effectiveness of respirations immediately so that corrective measures can be initiated.
Monitor vital signs continuously.	Increased respirations, tachycardia, and/or bradycardia suggest hypoxia.
Position client appropriately, depending on respiratory effort and type of surgery.	Head elevation and left lateral Sims' position prevents aspiration of secretions or vomitus, enhances ventilation to lower lobes, and relieves pressure on diaphragm.
Observe for return of muscle function, especially respiratory.	After administration of intraoperative muscle relaxants, return of muscle function occurs first to the diaphragm, intercostals, and larynx; followed by large muscle groups, neck, shoulders, and abdominal muscles; then by midsize muscles, tongue, pharynx, extensors, and flexors; and finally, by eyes, mouth, face, and fingers.

(continues on page 774)

ACTIONS/INTERVENTIONS (continued)	RATIONALE (continued)
Initiate "stir-up" regimen—turn, cough, deep breathe—as soon as client is reactive and continue in the postoperative period.	Active deep ventilation inflates alveoli, breaks up secretions, increases O_2 transfer, and removes anesthetic gases; coughing enhances removal of secretions from the pulmonary system. *Note:* Respiratory muscles weaken and atrophy with age, possibly hampering elderly client's ability to cough or deep-breathe effectively.
Observe for excessive somnolence.	Opioid-induced respiratory depression or action of muscle relaxants in the body may be cyclical in recurrence, creating sine-wave pattern of depression and reemergence from anesthesia. In addition, thiopental sodium (Pentothal) is absorbed in the fatty tissues, and, as circulation improves, it may be redistributed throughout the bloodstream.
Elevate head of bed as appropriate to surgical procedure. Get out of bed as soon as possible.	Promotes maximal expansion of lungs, decreasing risk of pulmonary complications.
Suction, as necessary.	Airway obstruction can occur as a result of blood or mucus in throat or trachea.
Collaborative	
Administer supplemental O_2, as indicated.	Maximizes oxygen for uptake to bind with Hgb in place of anesthetic gases to enhance removal of inhalation agents.
Administer IV medications, such as naloxone (Narcan), doxapram (Dopram), or neostigmine (Prostigmin).	Narcan reverses opioid-induced central nervous system (CNS) depression; Dopram stimulates respiratory muscles. The effects of both drugs are cyclic in nature and respiratory depression may return. Prostigmin reverses nonpolarizing muscle blockers.
Provide and maintain ventilator assistance, as indicated.	Depending on cause of respiratory depression or type of surgery (e.g., pulmonary, extensive abdominal, cardiac), endotracheal tube (ET) may be left in place and mechanical ventilation continued for a time.
Assist with use of respiratory aids such as incentive spirometer.	Maximal respiratory efforts reduce potential for atelectasis and pulmonary infection. Client may need to be reminded and coached to reach specific goal.

NURSING DIAGNOSIS: [disturbed Sensory Perception (specify)]

May Be Related To
Chemical alteration—use of pharmaceutical agents, hypoxia
Therapeutically restricted environments; excessive sensory stimuli
Physiological stress

Possibly Evidenced By
Disorientation (e.g., person, place, time); hallucinations
Change in usual response to stimuli
Change in problem-solving ability
Motor incoordination

Desired Outcomes/Evaluation Criteria—Client Will

Cognition (NOC)
Regain usual level of consciousness and mentation.
Recognize limitations and seek assistance as necessary.

ACTIONS/INTERVENTIONS	RATIONALE
Postanesthesia Care (NIC)	
Independent	
Reorient client continuously when emerging from anesthesia; confirm that surgery is completed.	As client regains consciousness, support and assurance of current physical status will help alleviate anxiety.
Speak in normal, clear voice without shouting, being aware of what you are saying. Minimize discussion of negatives about the client or personal or work-related problems within client's hearing. Explain procedures and environmental events even if client does not seem aware.	The nurse cannot tell when client is aware, but it is thought that the sense of hearing returns before client appears fully awake, so it is important not to say things that may be misinterpreted. Providing factual information helps client preserve dignity and prepare for next recuperative activity.
Evaluate sensation and movement of extremities and trunk, as appropriate.	Return of function following local or spinal nerve blocks depends on type and amount of agent used and duration of procedure.

ACTIONS/INTERVENTIONS (continued)	RATIONALE (continued)
Use bed rail padding, other medical protective devices as necessary.	Provides for client safety and protection from environment during emergence state. Prevents injury if client becomes combative while disoriented.
Secure parenteral lines, ET tube, and catheters, if present, and check for patency.	Disoriented client may pull on lines and drainage systems, disconnecting or kinking them.
Maintain quiet, calm environment.	External stimuli, such as noise, lights, and touch, may cause psychic aberrations when dissociative anesthetics (e.g., ketamine, tiletamine [Telazol]) have been administered.
Investigate changes in sensorium.	Continued confusion, specific to pediatric and geriatric age groups, may reflect drug interactions, hypoxia, anxiety, pain, electrolyte imbalances, or fear.
Observe for hallucinations, delusions, depression, or an excited state.	May develop following trauma and indicate delirium or may reflect sundowner's syndrome in elderly client. In client who has used alcohol or other drugs to excess, may suggest impending delirium tremens.
Reassess sensory, motor, and cognitive function thoroughly before discharge.	Phase II recovery or ambulatory surgical client must be able to care for self with the help of SO, if available, to prevent personal injury after discharge.
Collaborative	
Evaluate need for extended stay in postoperative recovery area or need for additional nursing care before discharge, as appropriate.	Disorientation may persist, and SO may not be able to protect the client at home.
Contact or refer to case manager for alternate care options.	May not be ready or able to care for self, especially if no SO and family member is available to provide necessary assistance.

NURSING DIAGNOSIS: risk for deficient Fluid Volume

Risk Factors May Include

Deviations affecting intake of fluids (e.g., sedation, nausea)
Loss of fluid through abnormal routes—indwelling tubes, drains; through normal routes—vomiting
Active fluid loss (bleeding)
Extremes of age and weight

Possibly Evidenced By

(Not applicable; presence of signs and symptoms establishes an *actual* diagnosis)

Desired Outcomes/Evaluation Criteria—Client Will

Hydration (NOC)

Demonstrate adequate fluid balance, as evidenced by stable vital signs, palpable pulses of good quality, normal skin turgor, moist mucous membranes, and individually appropriate urinary output.

ACTIONS/INTERVENTIONS	RATIONALE
Fluid Management (NIC)	
Independent	
Measure and record I&O including tubes and drains. Calculate urine specific gravity, as appropriate. Review intraoperative record for potential causes of imbalance.	Accurate documentation helps identify fluid losses and replacement needs and influences choice of interventions. *Note:* Ability to concentrate urine declines with age, increasing renal losses despite general fluid deficit.
Assess urinary output specifically for type of operative procedure done.	May be decreased or absent after procedures on the genitourinary system and/or adjacent structures, such as ureteroplasty, ureterolithotomy, and abdominal or vaginal hysterectomy, indicating malfunction or obstruction of the urinary system.
Provide voiding assistance measures as needed such as privacy, sitting position, running water in sink, and pouring warm water over perineum, as needed.	Promotes relaxation of perineal muscles and may facilitate voiding efforts.
Monitor vital signs, noting changes in BP, heart rate and rhythm, and respirations. Calculate pulse pressure.	Hypotension, tachycardia, and increased respirations may indicate fluid deficit—dehydration or hypovolemia. Although a drop in BP is generally a late sign of fluid deficit or hemorrhagic loss, widening of the pulse pressure may occur early, followed by narrowing as bleeding continues and systolic BP begins to fall.

(continues on page 776)

ACTIONS/INTERVENTIONS (continued)	RATIONALE (continued)
Note presence of nausea or vomiting.	Women, obese individuals, and those prone to motion sickness have a higher risk of postoperative nausea and vomiting. In addition, the longer the duration of anesthesia, the greater the risk for nausea. *Note:* Nausea occurring during first 12 to 24 hours postoperatively is frequently related to anesthesia (including regional anesthesia). Nausea persisting more than 3 days postoperatively may be related to the choice of opioid for pain control or other drug therapy.
Inspect dressings and drainage devices at regular intervals. Assess wound for swelling.	Excessive bleeding can lead to hypovolemia and circulatory collapse. Local swelling may indicate hematoma formation or hemorrhage. *Note:* Bleeding into a cavity (e.g., retroperitoneal) may be hidden and diagnosed only via vital sign depression or client reports of pressure sensation in affected area.
Monitor skin temperature; palpate peripheral pulses.	Cool or clammy skin and/or weak pulses indicate decreased peripheral circulation and need for additional fluid replacement.
Collaborative	
Administer parenteral fluids, blood products including autologous collection, and/or plasma expanders, as indicated. Increase IV rate, if needed.	Replaces documented fluid loss. Timely replacement of circulating volume decreases potential for complications of deficit including electrolyte imbalance, dehydration, and cardiovascular collapse. *Note:* Increased volume may be required initially to support circulating volume and prevent hypotension because of decreased vasomotor tone following halothane (Fluothane) administration.
Insert and maintain urinary catheter with or without urimeter, as necessary.	Provides mechanism for accurate monitoring of urinary output.
Resume oral intake gradually, or begin enteral feeding, as indicated.	Following surgical procedures not involving the gastrointestional (GI) tract, the small bowel may be capable of absorbing nutrients regardless of absence of bowel sounds reflecting GI motility. If there is no evidence of abdominal distention, mechanical obstruction, or GI bleeding, early enteral feeding can hasten resolution of postoperative ileus and reduce risk of infection. As ileus resolves, oral fluids can be started.
Administer medications, as appropriate, for example: Anti-emetics	Relieves nausea and vomiting, which may impair intake and add to fluid deficit. *Note:* Naloxone (Narcan) may relieve nausea related to use of anesthetic agents such as morphine (Duramorph) or fentanyl citrate (Sublimaze).
Epoetin alfa, vitamins B_{12} and C, and folic acid.	Medications used to stimulate production of RBCs are begun preoperatively, when needed, and may be administered postoperatively as well.
Monitor laboratory studies, such as Hgb and Hct or electrolytes. Compare preoperative and postoperative blood studies.	Indicators of hydration and circulating volume. Preoperative anemia and/or low Hct combined with unreplaced fluid losses intraoperatively will further potentiate deficit.

NURSING DIAGNOSIS: acute Pain

May Be Related To

Physical agents (e.g., disruption of skin, tissue, and muscle integrity; musculoskeletal or bone trauma; presence of tubes and drains)

Possibly Evidenced By

Verbal/coded report of pain
Expressive behavior (e.g., restlessness, irritability)
Guarding behavior; protective gestures
Self-focus; narrowed focus
Changes in vital signs

Desired Outcomes/Evaluation Criteria—Client Will

Pain Level (NOC)
Report pain relieved or controlled.
Appear relaxed, able to rest or sleep and participate in activities appropriately.

ACTIONS/INTERVENTIONS	RATIONALE
Pain Management (NIC)	
Independent	
Note client's age, weight, coexisting medical or psychological conditions, idiosyncratic sensitivity to analgesics, and intraoperative course, including size and location of incision, drain placement, and anesthetic agents used.	Approach to postoperative pain management is based on multiple variable factors.
Review intraoperative and recovery room record for type of anesthesia and medications administered.	Presence of opioids and droperidol in system potentiates opioid analgesia, whereas inhalation anesthetics have no analgesic effects. In addition, intraoperative local and regional blocks have varying duration based on drug choice and dose.
Evaluate pain frequently in immediate postoperative phase and regularly (e.g., hourly per protocol) following transfer, noting characteristics, location, and intensity (0 to 10 [or similar] scale).	Provides information about need for, and effectiveness of, interventions. *Note:* It may not always be possible to eliminate pain; however, analgesics should reduce pain to a tolerable level. A frontal and/or occipital headache may develop 24 to 72 hours following spinal anesthesia, necessitating recumbent position, increased fluid intake, and notification of the anesthesiologist for alternative pain relief plan.
Note presence of anxiety or fear, and relate with nature of and preparation for procedure.	Concern about the unknown, such as outcome of a biopsy and/or inadequate preparation due to emergent procedure, can heighten client's perception of pain.
Assess causes of possible discomfort other than operative procedure.	Discomfort can be caused or aggravated by other factors (e.g., presence of indwelling catheter causing bladder pain, NG tube resulting in gastric fluid and gas accumulation, or parenteral lines that have infiltrated IV fluids or medications).
Provide information about transitory nature of discomfort, as appropriate.	Understanding the cause of the transitory discomfort, such as sore muscles from administration of succinylcholine, which may persist up to 48 hours postoperatively; sinus headache, which may be associated with nitrous oxide; or sore throat, which may be due to intubation, provides emotional reassurance. *Note:* Paresthesia of body parts suggests nerve injury. Symptoms may last hours or months and require additional evaluation.
Reposition as indicated, such as semi-Fowler's or lateral Sims'.	May relieve pain and enhance circulation. Semi-Fowler's position relieves abdominal muscle tension and arthritic back muscle tension, whereas lateral Sims' will relieve dorsal pressures.
Provide additional comfort measures such as backrub and heat or cold applications.	Improves circulation, reduces muscle tension and anxiety associated with pain. Enhances sense of well-being.
Encourage use of relaxation techniques such as deep-breathing exercises, guided imagery, visualization, or music.	Relieves muscle and emotional tension; enhances sense of control and may improve coping abilities.
Provide regular oral care, occasional ice chips or sips of fluids as tolerated.	Reduces discomfort associated with dry mucous membranes due to anesthetic agents and oral restrictions.
Document effectiveness and side or adverse effects of analgesia.	Respirations may decrease on administration of opioid, or synergistic effects with anesthetic agents may occur. *Note:* Migration of epidural analgesia toward head may cause respiratory depression or excessive sedation.
Collaborative	
Administer medications, as indicated, for example:	
IV analgesics after reviewing anesthesia record for contraindications and/or presence of agents that may potentiate analgesia	Analgesics given IV reach the pain centers immediately, providing more effective relief with smaller doses of medication. *Note:* Initial opioid dosage should be reduced by one-fourth to one-third after use of fentanyl (Innovar) or droperidol (Inapsine) to prevent respiratory depressant effects (Deglin & Valler, 2005).
Around-the-clock analgesia via patient-controlled analgesia (PCA) or epidural analgesia (PCEA) with intermittent rescue doses, as needed	Research supports need to administer analgesics around the clock initially to prevent rather than merely treat pain. Use of PCA necessitates detailed client instruction. PCA is considered very effective in managing acute postoperative pain with smaller amounts of opioid and increased client satisfaction. *Note:* Continuous epidural infusions may be used for 1 to 5 days following procedures that are known to cause severe pain such as certain types of thoracic or abdominal procedures.
Regional anesthetics, such as epidural block	Analgesics may be injected into the operative site, or nerves to the site may be kept blocked in the immediate postoperative phase to prevent severe pain. *Note:* Continuous

(continues on page 778)

ACTIONS/INTERVENTIONS (continued)	RATIONALE (continued)
	epidural infusions may be used for 1 to 5 days following procedures that are known to cause severe pain such as certain types of thoracic or abdominal surgeries.
NSAIDs, such as ketorolate (Toradol), diflunisal (Dolobid), or naproxen (Anaprox)	Useful for mild to moderate pain or as adjuncts to opioid therapy in moderate to severe pain. Allows for a lower dosage of opioids, reducing potential for side effects. Use alternating schedule with NSAIDs administered between opioid doses so peak effect occurs at a different time.
Monitor use and effectiveness of transcutaneous electrical nerve stimulation (TENS) unit when used.	TENS may be useful in reducing pain and amount of medication required postoperatively.

NURSING DIAGNOSIS: impaired Tissue Integrity

May Be Related To

Mechanical factors (e.g., pressure, shear, friction; [surgical trauma to tissues])

Impaired physical mobility

Altered circulation

Possibly Evidenced By

Damaged tissues (e.g., integumentary, subcutaneous, muscle)

Desired Outcomes/Evaluation Criteria—Client Will

Wound Healing: Primary Intention (NOC)

Achieve timely wound healing.

Knowledge: Treatment Regimen (NOC)

Demonstrate behaviors or techniques to promote healing and prevent complications.

ACTIONS/INTERVENTIONS	RATIONALE
Incision Site Care (NIC)	
Independent	
Ascertain if client is at risk for delayed healing.	Presence of comorbidities (e.g., diabetes, COPD, anemia, obesity, malnutrition, alcohol withdrawal; use of steroid therapy) and extremes of age can impact healing.
Inspect incision regularly, noting characteristics and integrity.	Early recognition of delayed healing or developing complications may prevent a more serious situation. Incisions may heal more slowly in clients with comorbidity or the elderly, in whom reduced cardiac output decreases capillary blood flow.
Observe initial surgical dressings, noting accumulation of blood/other drainage. Reinforce initial dressing or change, as indicated, using clean or sterile technique per protocol or surgeon preference.	Close observation of surgical dressings promotes early identification of problems, such as hematoma formation, outright bleeding.
Gently remove tape in direction of hair growth and dressings when changing.	Reduces risk of skin trauma and disruption of wound.
Apply skin sealants or barriers before tape, if needed. Use hypoallergenic tape, Montgomery straps, or elastic netting for dressings requiring frequent changing.	Reduces potential for skin trauma or abrasions and provides additional protection for delicate skin and tissues.
Check tension of dressings. Apply tape at center of incision to outer margin of dressing. Avoid wrapping tape around extremity.	Prevents tape skin abrasions. Wrapping tape can impair or occlude circulation to wound and to distal portion of extremity.
Assess amounts and characteristics of drainage.	Decreasing drainage suggests evolution of healing process, whereas continued drainage or presence of bloody or odoriferous exudate suggests complications, which may include hemorrhage, infection, and fistula formation.
Maintain patency of drainage tubes; apply collection bag over drains or incisions in presence of copious or caustic drainage.	Facilitates approximation of wound edges; reduces risk of infection and chemical injury to skin and tissues.
Elevate operative area, as appropriate.	Promotes venous return and limits edema formation. *Note:* Elevation in presence of venous insufficiency may be detrimental.
Splint abdominal and chest incisions or area with pillow or pad during coughing and movement.	Equalizes pressure on the wound, minimizing risk of dehiscence—especially important during stage I healing during the first 3 to 4 days—and for incisions closed with adhesives.

ACTIONS/INTERVENTIONS (continued)	RATIONALE (continued)
Caution client not to touch incision.	Prevents contamination of area.
Cleanse skin surface, if needed, with running water and mild soap after incision is sealed.	Reduces skin contaminants; aids in removal of drainage or exudate.
Monitor blood glucose levels of diabetic clients, as indicated.	These clients are at higher risk for healthcare-associated infections and delayed healing, and the risk increases if glucose level exceeds 220 mg/dL on the first postoperative day.
Collaborative	
Apply ice, if appropriate.	Reduces edema formation that may cause undue pressure on incision during initial postoperative period.
Use abdominal binder, if indicated.	Provides additional support for high-risk incisions, especially in obese clients.
Wound Care (NIC)	
Irrigate open wounds; assist with débridement as needed.	Removes infectious exudate and necrotic tissue to promote healing.
Monitor and maintain dressings, whether hydrogel, vacuum dressing, or other types.	May be used to hasten healing in large, draining wound or fistula, to increase client comfort, and to reduce frequency of dressing changes. Also allows drainage to be measured more accurately and analyzed for pH and electrolyte content, as appropriate. (Refer to CP: Wound Care—Complicated or Chronic)

NURSING DIAGNOSIS: risk for ineffective Tissue Perfusion (specify)

Risk Factors May Include

Hypovolemia
[Interruption of flow—arterial, venous]

Possibly Evidenced By

(Not applicable; presence of signs and symptoms establishes an *actual* diagnosis)

Desired Outcomes/Evaluation Criteria—Client Will

Circulation Status (NOC)

Demonstrate adequate perfusion evidenced by stable vital signs, peripheral pulses present and strong, warm and dry skin, usual mentation, and individually appropriate urinary output.

ACTIONS/INTERVENTIONS	RATIONALE
Hypovolemia Management (NIC)	
Independent	
Change position slowly initially.	Vasoconstrictor mechanisms are depressed and quick movement may lead to orthostatic hypotension, especially in the early postoperative period.
Monitor vital signs; palpate peripheral pulses; and note skin temperature, color, and capillary refill. Evaluate urinary output and time of voiding. Document dysrhythmias.	Indicators of adequacy of circulating volume and tissue perfusion or organ function. Effects of medications and electrolyte imbalances may create dysrhythmias, impairing cardiac output and tissue perfusion.
Investigate changes in mentation or failure to achieve usual mental state.	May reflect a number of problems, such as inadequate clearance of anesthetic agent, oversedation with pain medication, hypoventilation, hypovolemia, or intraoperative complications such as emboli.
Embolus Precautions (NIC)	
Determine client's risk and assess for development of venous thromboembolism (VTE) symptoms (e.g., warm, red, painful lower leg; sudden-onset dyspnea with chest pain and cough).	Preventing complications of thromboembolic phenomena is part of improved surgical care according to the Surgical Care Improvement Project (Drake, 2011). Risk factors for VTE (which includes both deep vein thrombosis and pulmonary embolism) include the specific type of surgery (e.g., higher risk with hip or knee surgery), trauma to lower extremities, increasing age (older than age 40), hormonal therapy, chemotherapy, central line catheter placement, immobility, obesity, varicose veins, and pregnancy. (Refer to CP: Thrombophlebitis.)

(continues on page 780)

ACTIONS/INTERVENTIONS (continued)	RATIONALE (continued)
Assist with range-of-motion (ROM) exercises, including active ankle and leg exercises.	Stimulates peripheral circulation; aids in preventing venous stasis to reduce risk of thrombus formation.
Encourage and assist with early ambulation.	Enhances circulation and return of normal organ function.
Avoid use of knee gatch or pillow under knees. Caution client against crossing legs or sitting with legs dependent for prolonged period.	Prevents stasis of venous circulation and reduces risk of thrombophlebitis.
Assess lower extremities for erythema, edema, and calf tenderness.	Circulation may be restricted by some positions used during surgery, whereas anesthetics and decreased activity alter vasomotor tone, potentiating vascular pooling and increasing risks of thrombus formation.
Collaborative	
Apply antiembolic hose or sequential compression device (SCDs), as indicated.	Promotes venous return and prevents venous stasis of legs to reduce risk of thrombosis.
Administer low-dose-unfractionated or low-molecular-weight heparin, as indicated.	Client identified as moderate or high risk will receive pharmacologic intervention to prevent or treat VTE (Drake, 2011).
Hypovolemia Management (NIC)	
Administer IV fluids and/or blood products, as needed.	Maintains circulating volume and supports perfusion.

NURSING DIAGNOSIS: deficient Knowledge [Learning Need] regarding condition/situation, prognosis, treatment, self-care, and discharge needs

May Be Related To

Lack of exposure or recall, information misinterpretation
Unfamiliarity with information resources
Cognitive limitation

Possibly Evidenced By

Reports the problem
Inaccurate follow-through of instructions

Desired Outcomes/Evaluation Criteria—Client Will

Knowledge: Disease Process (NOC)

Verbalize understanding of condition, effects of procedure, and potential complications.

Knowledge: Treatment Regimen (NOC)

Verbalize understanding of therapeutic needs.
Correctly perform necessary procedures and explain reasons for actions.
Initiate necessary lifestyle changes and participate in treatment regimen.

ACTIONS/INTERVENTIONS	RATIONALE
Treatment: Disease Process (NIC)	
Independent	
Ascertain client's readiness and ability to receive information about self-care management following surgery. Note barriers to learning, such as short hospitalization for surgical procedure; client's pain and fatigue; complexity and number of tasks client must perform at home (e.g., simple dressing change vs. open wound care); client's developmental and cognitive abilities and health literacy; access and use of support and resources.	Throughout the postoperative recovery period, the nurse has a professional obligation to plan for discharge. This includes providing information to clients and their families to help them come to terms with their current condition and to prepare them for the future, in order to prevent complications. The length of the hospital stay is usually short; this impacts the time available for client/SO teaching and also means that much of the postoperative care and monitoring is done at home by clients and their families. Potential problems that may occur after discharge have little chance of getting addressed if not identified during the discharge planning process (Bowles, 2011; Bednarski et al, 2006).
Determine amount and type of information desired, and utilize desired teaching style, considering client's personal preferences and values, family situation and lifestyles, and cultural traditions.	These factors are involved in client-centered care. Studies have shown that certain aspects of postoperative care are important to clients (e.g., understanding their health progress [67%], appropriate activity level [66%], knowledge of insurance coverage [61%], information regarding medications and side effects [52%], understanding pain management [51%], and knowing when to consult the physician [49%]) (Boyle, 1992).

ACTIONS/INTERVENTIONS (continued)	RATIONALE (continued)
Review specific surgery or procedure performed and future expectations.	Provides knowledge base from which client can make informed choices.
Review and have client and SO demonstrate dressing change and incision and tube care, when indicated. Identify source for supplies.	Promotes competent self-care and enhances independence. *Note:* For incisions closed with a surgical zipper, client should be instructed as to when it is appropriate to peel off the device.
Emphasize avoidance of environmental risk factors including exposure to crowds or persons with infections.	Reduces potential for acquired infections.
Discuss drug therapy, including use of prescribed and OTC analgesics and resumption of herbal supplements.	Enhances cooperation with regimen, reduces risk of adverse reactions or untoward effects. *Note:* Herbal preparations such as garlic, ginseng, ginkgo biloba, ginger, and feverfew increase the risk of postoperative bleeding and are contraindicated for several days following surgery.
Identify specific activity limitations.	Prevents undue strain on operative site.
Recommend planned, progressive exercise program.	Promotes return of normal function and enhances feelings of general well-being.
Schedule adequate rest periods.	Prevents fatigue and conserves energy for healing.
Review importance of nutritious diet and adequate fluid intake.	Provides elements necessary for tissue regeneration and healing and support of tissue perfusion and organ function.
Encourage cessation of smoking.	Smoking increases risk of pulmonary infections, causes vasoconstriction, and reduces oxygen-binding capacity of blood, affecting cellular perfusion and potentially impairing healing.
Identify signs and symptoms requiring medical evaluation, such as nausea or vomiting; difficulty voiding; fever; continued or odoriferous wound drainage; incisional swelling, erythema, or separation of edges; and unresolved pain or changes in characteristics of pain.	Early recognition and treatment of developing complications, which may include ileus, urinary retention, infection, and delayed healing, and may prevent progression to more serious or life-threatening situation.
Emphasize necessity of follow-up visits with providers, including therapists and laboratory.	Monitors progress of healing and evaluates effectiveness of regimen.
Include SO in teaching program and discharge planning. Provide written instructions and teaching materials in client's dominant language. Instruct in use of and arrange for special equipment.	Provides additional resources for reference after discharge. Promotes effective self-care.
Identify available resources, including home-care services, visiting nurse, Meals on Wheels, outpatient therapy, and contact phone number for questions.	Enhances support for client during recovery period and provides additional evaluation of ongoing needs or new concerns.

POTENTIAL CONSIDERATIONS following surgical procedure (dependent on client's age, physical condition and presence of complications, personal resources, and life responsibilities)

- ***Fatigue***—disease states, anemia, stress
- ***risk for Infection***—broken skin, traumatized tissues, stasis of body fluids, increased environmental exposure to pathogens, invasive procedures
- ***Self-Care Deficit***—pain or discomfort, weakness, decreased motivation

Refer also to appropriate plans of care regarding underlying condition/specific surgical procedure for additional considerations.

EXTENDED/LONG-TERM CARE

I. Indications

a. Level of care and needs of the client are frequently the deciding factors in the choice of placement.

b. Short-term rehabilitation—individuals requiring services postdischarge from acute care setting

c. Long-term nursing care—individuals requiring assistance with activities of daily living (ADLs)

  i. Elderly individuals are the primary population requiring assistance with (on average) 4 to 6 ADLs.

  ii. Increasing numbers of younger individuals are requiring care for debilitating conditions when they cannot be managed in the home setting (Family Caregiver Alliance, 2005).

II. Statistics (Centers for Disease Control [CDC], 2006)

a. Population: In 2004, 1.5 million people resided in nursing homes nationally, of which almost 75% were women. One recent study released by the National Center for Health Statistics' Long-Term Care Surveys states, "About 45% of nursing home residents in 2004 … were 85 years and older, white, and women…. More than two-thirds of the oldest nursing home residents, home health care patients, and discharged hospice care patients needed assistance in performing three or more activities of daily living (ADLs) and were bladder incontinent" (Park-Lee et al, 2013).

(continues on page 782)

b. Cost: In 2004, spending on long-term care services exceeded $115.2 billion and accounted for 7.4% of national healthcare expenditures (Stewart, Grabowski, Lakdawalla, 2009). In 2010, the average daily rate for a private room in a skilled nursing facility was $229, or $83,580 annually; for a semiprivate room, $205, or $74,820 annually, according to data from the U.S. Department of Health and Human Services (HHS, 2010). Studies published by insurance companies in 2012 showed that national average rates for a private room increased 4.4% over the 2010 figures to $239 daily or $87,235 annually; rates for a semiprivate room rose to $214 daily, or $78,110 annually.

GLOSSARY

Activities of daily living (ADLs): Basic everyday self-care activities, including bathing, grooming, dressing, feeding, toileting, hygiene, and personal safety.

Instrumental activities of daily living (IADLs): Activities needed to function independently in the home or community, including shopping, meal preparation, housekeeping/home maintenance, laundry, managing medications and health maintenance, use of transportation, and money management.

Long-term or extended care facility: Provision of custodial or personal care services, with ongoing supervision and coordination of care by licensed nurses (RN or LPN/LVN).

Polypharmacy: Occurs when "more medications are used or prescribed than are clinically indicated" (Lee, 1998).

Short-term rehabilitation or skilled nursing facility: Provision of registered nursing and rehabilitation services, such as physical, occupational, and/or speech therapies; intravenous (IV) antibiotics or chemotherapy; complicated wound care; and respiratory and nutritional support.

Related Concerns

Acquired immunodeficiency syndrome (AIDS), page 689
Cancer, page 827
Cerebrovascular accident (CVA)/stroke, page 214
Craniocerebral trauma—acute rehabilitative phase, page 197
Dementia of the Alzheimer's type/vascular dementia/Lewy body disease, page 743
End-of-life care/hospice, page 848
Multiple sclerosis, page 266
Psychosocial aspects of care, page 729
Spinal cord injury, page 248
Surgical intervention, page 762
Ventilatory assistance (mechanical), page 157

Client Assessment Database

Data depend on underlying physical and psychosocial conditions necessitating continuation of structured care.

DIAGNOSTIC DIVISION MAY REPORT	MAY EXHIBIT
TEACHING/LEARNING • ***Discharge plan considerations:*** May require assistance with treatments, self-care activities, health maintenance, and nutritional support ➧ Refer to section at end of plan for postdischarge considerations.	

Diagnostic Studies

Dependent on age, general health, and medical condition. Individuals are often transferred to facility or admitted following an acute care episode where diagnostic studies were previously performed.

TEST WHY IT IS DONE	WHAT IT TELLS ME
TESTS	
• ***Complete blood count (CBC):*** Battery of screening tests, which typically includes hemoglobin (Hgb); hematocrit (Hct); red blood cell (RBC) count, morphology, indices, and distribution width index; platelet count and size; and white blood cell (WBC) count and differential.	Hgb suggests anemia. Elevated Hct may indicate dehydration, whereas decreased Hct suggests fluid overload. An elevated WBC count is indicative of inflammatory process. Decreased WBC count suggests viral processes, requiring further evaluation because immune system may be dysfunctional.

TEST WHY IT IS DONE (continued)	WHAT IT TELLS ME (continued)
• *Chemistry profile:* Evaluates general organ function and imbalances.	Age-related changes include decreased serum albumin, up to 20% increase in alkaline phosphatase, and decreased urine creatinine clearance.
OTHER DIAGNOSTIC TESTS	
• *Urinalysis:* Provides information about kidney function.	Determines presence of urinary tract infection (UTI) or diabetes mellitus (DM). *Note:* Bacteria are common in some populations, especially the elderly and bedridden, reflecting urinary stasis.
• *Pulse oximetry:* Determines oxygenation and respiratory function.	Decreased levels indicate need for supplemental oxygen therapy. Testing identifies treatment needs and provides for safety of staff and other residents.
• *Communicable disease screens:* Rule out tuberculosis (TB), HIV, venereal disease, and hepatitis.	Testing identifies treatment needs and provides for safety of staff and other residents.
• *Drug screen:* As indicated by usage to identify therapeutic or toxic levels.	Therapeutic drug monitoring aids in establishing individually appropriate drug dosage and frequency to maintain steady state for maximal drug effect and with minimal side effects.
• *Visual acuity testing:* Assesses sight and health of the eyes.	Identifies cataracts or other vision problems.
• *Tonometer test:* Measures intraocular pressure.	Elevation indicates glaucoma.
• *Chest x-rays:* Procedure used to evaluate organs and structures within the chest for symptoms of disease.	Reveals size of heart and lung abnormalities or disease conditions, or changes of the large blood vessels and bony structure of the chest.
• *Electrocardiogram (ECG):* Provides baseline data; detects abnormalities.	ST-segment and T-wave changes, atrial and ventricular dysrhythmias, and various heart blocks are common in the elderly population.

Nursing Priorities

1. Promote physiological and psychological well-being.
2. Provide for security and safety.
3. Prevent complications of disease and/or aging process.
4. Promote effective coping skills and independence.
5. Encourage continuation of healthy habits and participation in plan of care to meet individual needs and wishes.

Discharge Goals

1. Client dealing realistically with current situation.
2. Homeostasis maintained.
3. Injury prevented.
4. Complications prevented or minimized.
5. Client performing ADLs by self or with assistance, as necessary.
6. Plan in place to meet needs after discharge, as appropriate.

NURSING DIAGNOSIS: risk for Relocation Stress Syndrome

Risk Factors May Include

Decreased health status
Moderate-to-high degree of environmental change
Losses
Feelings of powerlessness
Lack of predeparture counseling
Unpredictability of experience

Possibly Evidenced By

(Not applicable; presence of signs and symptoms establishes an *actual* diagnosis)

Desired Outcomes/Evaluation Criteria—Client Will

Anxiety Level (NOC)
Demonstrate appropriate range of feelings and appear relaxed.

Psychosocial Adjustment: Life Change (NOC)
Verbalize understanding of reasons for change as able.
Participate in routine and special or social events as capable.
Verbalize acceptance of situation.

ACTIONS/INTERVENTIONS	RATIONALE
Relocation Stress Reduction (NIC)	
Independent	
Ascertain if client has completed an advance directive. Provide information, as appropriate.	Assures client/family wishes will be known to provide direction to caregivers.
Determine client's and SO's attitude toward admission to facility and expectations for the future.	If this is expected to be a temporary placement, client's and SO's concerns will be different than if placement is permanent. When client is giving up own home and way of life, feelings of helplessness, loss, and grief are to be expected.
Help family and SO to be honest with client regarding admission. Be clear about actions and events.	Family may have difficulty dealing with decision and reality of permanent placement and may avoid discussing situation with client. Honesty decreases "surprises," assists in maintaining trust, and may enhance coping.
Identify support person(s) important to client and include in care activities, mealtime, and so on, as appropriate.	During adjustment period and times of stress, client may benefit from presence of trusted individual who can provide reassurance and reduce sense of isolation.
Assess level of anxiety and discuss reasons when possible.	Identifying specific problems enables individual to deal more realistically with them and care provider to intervene as necessary; for example, a client who is being neglected or abused or has unrelieved pain may be very anxious and afraid or unable to verbalize.
Develop nurse-client relationship.	Trusting relationships among client, SO, and staff promotes optimal care and support.
Make time to listen to client about concerns, and encourage free expression of feelings, including anger, hostility, fear, and loneliness.	Being available in this way allows client to feel accepted and begin to acknowledge and deal with feelings related to circumstances of admission.
Acknowledge reality of situation and feelings of client. Accept expressions of anger while limiting aggressive, acting-out behavior.	Permission to express feelings allows for beginning of resolution. Acceptance promotes sense of self-worth. *Note:* Psychosocial and/or physiological disturbances can occur as a result of transfer from one environment to another, especially if the move is unexpected or involuntary.
Assist client to identify strengths and successful coping behaviors and incorporate into problem-solving.	Building on past successes increases likelihood of positive outcome in present situation. Enhances sense of control and management of current deficits.
Orient to physical aspects of facility, schedules, and activities. Introduce to roommate(s) and staff. Give explanation of roles.	Getting acquainted is an important part of admission. Knowledge of where things are and from whom client can expect assistance can be helpful in reducing anxiety.
Determine client's usual schedule and incorporate into facility routine as much as possible.	Consistency provides reassurance and may lessen confusion and enhance cooperation.
Provide above information in written or audiovisual form as well.	Overload of information is difficult to handle. Client can refer to written or audiovisual materials as needed to refresh memory or learn new information.
Give careful thought to room placement. Provide help and encouragement in placing client's own belongings around room. Do not transfer from one room to another without client approval and documentable need.	Location, roommate compatibility, and place for personal belongings are important considerations for helping the client feel "at home." Changes are often met with resistance and can result in emotional upset and decline in physical condition. *Note:* Persons with severe behavioral problems or cognitive dysfunctions may require a private room.
Note behavior, presence of suspiciousness or paranoia, irritability, and defensiveness. Compare to SO's description of client's customary responses.	Increased stress, physical discomfort, and fatigue may temporarily exacerbate mental deterioration and cognitive decline and further impair communication and social inaccessibility. This represents a catastrophic episode that can escalate into a panic state and violence.
Be aware of escalating anxiety and presence of delirium. Look for possible causes.	Common causes of delirium include drug toxicity, electrolyte imbalances, withdrawal from alcohol and other drugs, pain, and trauma—especially hip fractures and advanced disease resulting in organ failure.
Collaborative	
Refer to social service or other appropriate agency for assistance. Have case manager or social worker discuss ramifications of Medicare and/or Medicaid if client is eligible for these resources.	Client may not be aware of the resources available, and sources of support can assist with adjustment in new situation.

NURSING DIAGNOSIS: Grieving

May Be Related To

Loss of significant object (e.g., processes of body, job, status, home, possessions)

Possibly Evidenced By

Psychological distress; suffering; despair

Alterations in activity level; disturbed sleep pattern

Desired Outcomes/Evaluation Criteria—Client Will

Grief Resolution (NOC)

Identify and express feelings appropriately.

Progress through the grieving process.

Enjoy the present and plan for the future one day at a time.

ACTIONS/INTERVENTIONS	RATIONALE
Grief Work Facilitation (NIC)	
Independent	
Assess emotional state. Note cultural beliefs and expectations.	Anxiety and depression are common reactions to changes and losses associated with long-term illness or debilitating condition. In addition, changes in neurotransmitter levels, such as increased monoamine oxidase (MAO) and serotonin levels with decreased norepinephrine, may potentiate depression in elderly clients. Personal expectations may affect response to change.
Make time to listen to the client. Encourage free expression of hopeless feelings and desire to die.	Allowing these feelings to be expressed, rather than denying or ignoring them, provides a sounding board for the client to hear and reflect on own thoughts, start to deal with the feelings, and consider alternatives.
Assess suicidal potential.	May be related to physical disease, social isolation, and grief. *Note:* Statistics show that suicide is the eighth leading cause of death among older adults; and elderly males (age 75 and older) are disproportionately more likely than women to die by suicide (CDC Web-based Injury Statistics Query and Reporting System [WISQARS], 2012).
Involve SO in discussions and activities to the level of their willingness.	When SOs are involved, there is more potential for successful problem-solving. *Note:* SO may not be available or may choose not to be involved.
Provide liberal touching and hugs as individually accepted.	Conveys sense of concern and closeness to reduce feelings of isolation and enhance sense of self-worth. *Note:* Touch may be viewed as a threat by some clients and escalate feelings of anger or fear.
Identify spiritual concerns. Discuss available resources and encourage participation in religious activities, as appropriate.	Search for meaning is common to those facing changes in life. Participation in religious or spiritual activities can provide sense of direction and peace of mind.
Assist with planning for specifics as necessary, including advance directives to determine code status, living will wishes, making of will, and funeral arrangements, if appropriate.	Having these issues resolved can help client and SO deal with the grieving process and may provide peace of mind.
Collaborative	
Refer to other resources as indicated, such as a spiritual advisor, parish nurse, case manager, or social worker.	May need further assistance to resolve some problems.

NURSING DIAGNOSIS: impaired Memory

May Be Related To

Neurological disturbances

Possibly Evidenced By

Inability to recall events or factual information

Forgets to perform a behavior at a scheduled time or recall if a behavior was performed

Inability to learn new information

(continues on page 786)

NURSING DIAGNOSIS: impaired Memory (continued)

Desired Outcomes/Evaluation Criteria—Client Will

Cognition (NOC)

Maintain usual cognitive orientation.
Demonstrate appropriate information processing.
Engage in effective decision making.

ACTIONS/INTERVENTIONS	RATIONALE
Cognitive Stimulation (NIC)	
Independent	
Allow adequate time for client to respond to questions or comments and to make decisions.	Reaction time may be slowed with aging due to changes in metabolism and cerebral blood flow or with brain injuries and some neuromuscular conditions.
Discuss happenings of the past. Place familiar objects in room. Encourage the display of photographs and photo albums and frequent visits from SO and friends.	Events of the past may be more readily recalled by the elderly client because long-term memory usually remains intact. Reminiscence or life review and companionship are beneficial to clients.
Note presence of short-term memory loss, and provide with such aids as calendars, clocks, room signs, and pictures.	Short-term memory loss presents a challenge for nursing care, especially if the client cannot remember such things as how to use the call bell or how to get to the bathroom. This problem is not in client's control but may be less frustrating if simple reminders are used to assist in providing continual reorientation. It may be helpful for older person and their family to know that short-term memory loss is common and is not necessarily a sign of "senility."
Evaluate individual stress level and deal with it appropriately.	Stress level may be greatly increased because of recent losses, such as poor health, death of spouse or companion, or loss of home. In addition, some conflicts that occur with age come from previously unresolved problems that may need to be dealt with now.
Assess physical status and psychiatric symptoms, especially in presence of recent change in mentation or development of confusion. Institute interventions appropriate to findings.	Not all mental changes are the result of aging, and it is important to rule out physical causes before accepting these as unchangeable. Possibilities include pain that is often unreported and underestimated, metabolic imbalances, adverse toxic medication levels, drug-induced side effects (e.g., anti-Parkinsonian agents, tricyclic antidepressants), or the result of infectious, cardiac, or respiratory disorders (Amella, 2004).
Reorient to person, place, and time, as appropriate.	Helps client maintain focus.
Have client repeat verbal or written instructions, when indicated.	Verifies hearing and ability to read and comprehend.
Note cyclic changes in mentation or behavior, such as evening confusion, picking at bedclothes, pacing, shouting or angry outbursts, or wandering aimlessly.	"Sundowner syndrome" may occur in response to visual and/or hearing deficits enhanced by declining light or an accumulation of all the sensory stimulation during the day, fatigue, inflexible institution schedules, peak-and-trough drug levels, dehydration, and electrolyte imbalances.
Involve in regular exercise, activity, and diversional programs.	Promotes release of endorphins, enhancing sense of well-being, and can improve thinking abilities.
Schedule at least one rest period per day.	Prevents fatigue; enhances general well-being.
Provide brighter lighting in room and common areas by midafternoon (e.g., 3 p.m.) or earlier on cloudy or winter days.	Maximizes visual perception; may limit evening confusion.
Turn off lights at bedtime. Provide night lights where appropriate.	Reinforces "sleep time" while meeting safety needs.
Support client's involvement in own care. Provide opportunity for choices on a daily basis.	Choice is a necessary component in everyday life. Cognitively impaired clients may respond with aggressive behavior as they lose control in their lives.
Collaborative	
Review results of laboratory and diagnostic tests, such as electrolytes, thyroid studies, or full drug screen and computerized tomography (CT) scan.	Aids in establishing cause of changes in mentation and determining treatment options.
Administer medications as indicated, such as donepazil (Aricept), rivastigmine (Exelon), galantamine (Razadyne), and memantine (Namenda).	Aricept, Exelon, and Razadyne are cholinesterase inhibitors used to treat mild to moderate dementia, whereas Namenda, which regulates glutamine activation, is prescribed for the treatment of moderate to severe dementia (National Institute on Aging [NIA], 2010). (Refer to CP: Dementia of the Alzheimer's Type/Vascular Dementia/Lewy Body Disease.)

NURSING DIAGNOSIS: compromised family Coping

May Be Related To
Prolonged disease that exhausts supportive capacity of significant people
Little support provided by client, in turn, for primary person
Coexisting situations affecting the significant person

Possibly Evidenced By
Significant person reports preoccupation with personal reactions (e.g., fear, anticipatory grief, guilt, anxiety) to client's need
Significant person attempts assistive or supportive behaviors with unsatisfactory results
Significant person withdraws from client
Significant person displays protective behavior disproportionate—too little or too much—to client's abilities or need for autonomy

Desired Outcomes/Evaluation Criteria—Family Will

Family Coping (NOC)
Identify resources within themselves to deal with the situation.
Interact appropriately with the client and staff, providing support and assistance, as indicated.
Verbalize knowledge and understanding of situation.
Participate in planning for discharge, as appropriate.

ACTIONS/INTERVENTIONS	RATIONALE
Family Support (NIC)	
Independent	
Introduce staff and provide SO with information about facility and care. Be available for questions. Provide tour of facility.	Helpful to establish beginning relationships. Offers opportunities for enhancing feelings of involvement.
Determine involvement and availability of family and SO.	Clarifies expectations and abilities and identifies needs.
Encourage SO participation in care at level of desire and capability and within limits of safety. Include in social events and celebrations.	Helps family to feel at ease and allows them to feel supportive and a part of the client's life.
Accept choices of SO/family regarding level of involvement in care.	Families may choose to ignore client or may project feelings of guilt regarding placing client in facility by criticizing staff. *Note:* Feelings of dissatisfaction with the staff may be transferred back to the client.
Evaluate SO's and caregiver's level of stress and coping abilities, especially before planning for discharge.	Caring for and about client with chronic or debilitating conditions places a heavy strain on SO. Recognizing own strengths and areas for improvement provides opportunity for personal growth, enhancing potential for success if client returns home.
Support the caregiver with attention, compassion, time, respect, honesty, advocacy, and understanding.	Nursing interventions need to prepare the caregivers for the challenges they face and meet their needs for compassion and caring.
Identify availability and use of community support systems.	Helps determine areas of need and provides information regarding additional resources to enhance coping.
Be aware of staff's own feelings of anger and frustration about client's and SO's choices and goals that differ from those of staff, and deal with them appropriately.	Group care conferences or individual counseling may be helpful in problem-solving.
Collaborative	
Inform SO of services available to them such as meal tickets, family cooking time or celebrations, group care conference, visiting nurse, caseworker, and other social services.	Promotes feeling of involvement; eases transition in adjustment to client's admission to home care or facility care.
Advise caregivers of resources available, such as Eldercare Locator, Seniornet, Today's Caregiver, and Caregiver Network, Inc.	Helps nurses, clients, and caregivers feel supported and able to provide more skillful care.
Refer SO and caregivers to stress management classes, as indicated.	Although support groups may be very helpful, learning stress management techniques may be more effective in strengthening individual coping as the focus is on the SO rather than the SO-client relationship.

NURSING DIAGNOSIS: risk for Poisoning [drug toxicity]

Risk Factors May Include

[Reduced metabolism; impaired circulation; chronic diseases, organ involvement]
[Use of multiple prescribed and/or over-the-counter (OTC) drugs]

Possibly Evidenced By

(Not applicable; presence of signs and symptoms establishes an *actual* diagnosis)

Desired Outcomes/Evaluation Criteria—Client Will

Risk Control: Drug Use (NOC)
Maintain prescribed drug regimen free of untoward side effects.

ACTIONS/INTERVENTIONS	RATIONALE
Medication Management (NIC)	
Independent	
Review client's drug regimen on routine basis. Refer to physician for assessment of medications that could be reduced in dose or discontinued.	Reduces risk of client taking too many medications at once (polypharmacy), with attendant problems. *Note:* Studies support that older adults are more prone to adverse drug reactions (ADRs) and drug-drug interactions due to physiological changes and multiple comorbidities. These reactions are compounded by polypharmacy (Ziere et al, 2006).
Determine allergies, medication, and other drug use history.	Helps avoid repetition or creation of problems.
Review resources such as drug manuals or pharmacist for information about toxic symptoms and side effects. List drug actions and interactions and idiosyncrasies, such as medications that are given with or without foods, as well as those that should not be crushed.	Provides information about drugs being taken and identifies possible interactions. Toxicity can be increased in the debilitated and older client with symptoms not as apparent.
Discuss self-administration of, or access to, OTC products.	Limits interference with prescribed regimen, desired drug action, and organ function. May prevent inadvertent overdosing or toxic reactions. *Note:* Appropriate use of OTC products kept at bedside or via free access at nurses' station fosters independence and enhances sense of control and self-esteem.
Identify swallowing problems or reluctance to take tablets or capsules.	May not be able to or want to take medication.
Give pills in a spoonful of soft foods, such as applesauce or ice cream; or use liquid form of medication if available.	Ensures proper dosage if client is unable, or does not like, to swallow pills.
Open capsules or crush tablets only when appropriate.	Should not be done unless absolutely necessary because this may alter absorption of medications; for example, enteric-coated tablets may be absorbed in the stomach when crushed, instead of in the intestines.
Make sure client swallows medication.	Ensures effective therapeutic use of medication and prevents pill hoarding.
Observe for changes in condition or behavior.	Behavior may be only indication of drug toxicity, and early identification of problems provides for appropriate intervention. *Note:* Elderly individuals have increased sensitivity to anticholinergic effects of medications; therefore, use of anticholinergics, antiparkinson agents, benzodiazepines, central nervous system (CNS) depressants, and tricyclic antidepressants may cause delirium or confusion.
Use discretion in the administration of sedatives.	A quiet place where the client can pace or be secluded may be more helpful. If client is destructive or excessively disruptive, pharmacological or mechanical control measures may be required. Convenience of the staff is never a reason for sedating client; however, client safety and rights of other clients need to be taken into consideration.
Collaborative	
Review drug regimen routinely with physician and pharmacist.	Provides opportunity to alter therapy by reducing dosage or discontinue medications as client's needs and organ functions change, affecting drug absorption, distribution, and renal clearance (Amella, 2004).
Obtain serum drug levels, as indicated.	Determines therapeutic or toxic levels.

NURSING DIAGNOSIS: impaired verbal Communication

May Be Related To

Alteration of central nervous system (e.g., Parkinson disease, Alzheimer's disease)
Physical barrier (e.g., laryngectomy or tracheostomy)
Decreased circulation to brain (e.g., stroke, traumatic brain injury)

Possibly Evidenced By

Difficulty expressing thoughts (e.g., aphasia, dysphasia)
Difficulty forming words or sentences
Partial/total visual or hearing deficit

Desired Outcomes/Evaluation Criteria—Client Will

Communication (NOC)

Establish method of communication by which needs can be expressed.
Demonstrate congruent verbal and nonverbal communication.

ACTIONS/INTERVENTIONS	RATIONALE
Communication Enhancement: Speech Deficit (NIC)	
Independent	
Assess reason for lack of communication, including CNS and neuromuscular functioning, gag and swallow reflexes, hearing, and teeth and mouth problems.	Identification of the problem is essential to appropriate intervention. Sometimes clients do not want to talk, may think they talk when they do not, may expect others to know what they want, or may not be able to comprehend or be understood.
Determine whether client is bilingual and what language is primary.	With declining cerebral function or diminished thought processes and increased level of stress, client may mix languages or revert to original language.
Investigate how SO communicates with the client.	Provides opportunity to develop or continue effective communication patterns that have already been established.
Assess client knowledge base and level of comprehension. Treat the client as an adult, avoiding pity and impatience.	Knowing how much to expect of the client can help to avoid frustration and unreasonable demands for performance. However, having an expectation that the client will understand may help raise level of performance.
Establish therapeutic nurse-client relationship through active-listening, being available for problem-solving.	Aids in dealing with communication problems.
Make client aware of presence when entering the room by speaking, turning a light off and on, or touching client, as appropriate.	Getting clients' attention is the first step in communication.
Make eye contact, place self at or below client's level, and speak face to face.	Conveys interest and promotes contact.
Speak slowly and distinctly, using simple sentences and yes-or-no questions. Avoid speaking loudly or shouting. Supplement with written communication when possible or needed. Allow sufficient time for reply; remain relaxed with client.	Assists in comprehension and overall communication. Client may respond poorly to high-pitched sounds; shouting also obscures consonants and amplifies vowels.
Use other creative measures to assist in communication, such as picture chart or alphabet board, sign language, or lip reading, when appropriate.	Many options are available, depending on individual situation. *Note:* Sign language also may be used effectively with other than hearing-impaired individuals.
Communication Enhancement: Hearing Deficit (NIC)	
Check ears for excess cerumen.	Hardened earwax may decrease hearing acuity and cause tinnitus.
Ascertain if client has or uses hearing aid.	Client may have, but not use, a hearing aid because it may not fit well or it may need batteries.
Be aware that behavioral problems may be associated with hearing loss.	Anger, explosive temper outbursts, frustration, embarrassment, depression, withdrawal, and paranoia may be attempts to deal with communication problems.
Collaborative	
Refer to speech therapists, ear-nose-throat physician, or for audiometry, as needed.	Determines extent of hearing loss and whether a hearing aid is appropriate. May be helpful to a client and staff in improving communication. *Note:* Some sources believe 90% of the clients in extended care facilities have some degree of hearing loss because this is a common age change. Hearing aids are most effective with conductive losses and may help with sensorineural losses.

NURSING DIAGNOSIS: disturbed Sleep Pattern

May Be Related To

Lack of sleep privacy; sleep partner/roommate
Ambient temperature; noise; interruptions (facility routines)

Possibly Evidenced By

Change in normal sleep pattern
Reports not feeling well rested; dissatisfaction with sleep
Decreased ability to function

Desired Outcomes/Evaluation Criteria—Client Will

Sleep (NOC)

Report improvement in sleep or rest pattern.
Verbalize increased sense of well-being and feeling rested.

ACTIONS/INTERVENTIONS	RATIONALE
Sleep Enhancement (NIC)	
Independent	
Ascertain usual sleep habits and changes that are occurring.	Determines need for action and helps identify appropriate interventions.
Provide comfortable bedding and some of own possessions, such as a pillow or an afghan.	Increases comfort for sleep; provides physiological and psychological support.
Establish new sleep routine incorporating old pattern and new environment.	When new routine contains as many aspects of old habits as possible, stress and related anxiety may be reduced, enhancing sleep.
Match with roommate who has similar sleep patterns and nocturnal needs.	Decreases likelihood that "night owl" roommate may delay client's falling asleep or create interruptions that cause awakening.
Encourage some light physical activity during the day. Make sure client stops activity several hours before bedtime, as individually appropriate.	Daytime activity can help client expend energy and be ready for nighttime sleep; however, continuation of activity close to bedtime may act as a stimulant, delaying sleep.
Promote bedtime comfort regimens such as warm bath, massage, a glass of warm milk, or small amount wine or brandy at bedtime.	Promotes a relaxing, soothing effect. *Note:* Milk has soporific qualities, enhancing synthesis of serotonin, a neurotransmitter that helps client fall asleep faster and sleep longer.
Instruct in relaxation measures.	Helps induce sleep.
Reduce noise and light.	Provides atmosphere conducive to sleep.
Encourage position of comfort and assist in turning, if needed.	Repositioning reduces pressure on tissues, enhances muscle relaxation, and promotes rest.
Lower bed and position one side against wall when possible. Avoid use of side rails.	May have fear of falling because of change in size and height of bed. *Note:* Side rails place client at risk for falling when climbing over rails or for possible entrapment.
Avoid or limit interruptions such as awakening for medications or therapies.	Uninterrupted sleep is more restful, and client may be unable to return to sleep when wakened.
Collaborative	
Administer sedatives and hypnotics with caution, as indicated.	May be given to help client sleep or rest during transition period from home to new setting. *Note:* Avoid habitual use because these drugs decrease REM (rapid eye movement) sleep time.

NURSING DIAGNOSIS: imbalanced Nutrition: less [or] more than body requirements

May Be Related To

Inability to ingest food (e.g., impaired dentition, inability to feed self effectively)
Biological factors (dulling of senses of smell and taste)
Excessive intake in relation to physical activity/metabolic need

Possibly Evidenced By

Dysfunctional eating pattern
Weight under or over ideal for height and frame
Poor muscle tone, pale mucous membranes
Sedentary lifestyle
[Signs and symptoms of vitamin and protein deficits, electrolyte imbalances]

NURSING DIAGNOSIS: imbalanced Nutrition: less [or] more than body requirements (continued)

Desired Outcomes/Evaluation Criteria—Client Will

Nutritional Status (NOC)

Maintain normal weight or progress toward weight goal with normalization of laboratory values and be free of signs of malnutrition and obesity.

Demonstrate eating patterns or behaviors to maintain appropriate weight.

ACTIONS/INTERVENTIONS	RATIONALE
Nutrition Management (NIC)	
Independent	
Perform initial nutritional assessment—admission height, weight, and body mass index (BMI); ability to feed self, chew, and swallow; and eating preferences.	Provides baseline evaluation to help determine dietary needs and formulate dietary plan (Henkel, 2004).
Evaluate activity pattern.	Extremes of exercise, such as sedentary life and continuous pacing, affect caloric needs.
Incorporate favorite foods and maintain as near-normal food consistency as possible, such as soft or finely ground food with gravy or liquid added. Avoid pureed or baby food whenever possible.	Aids in maintaining intake, especially when mouth and dental problems exist. Baby food is often unpalatable and can decrease appetite and lower self-esteem.
Encourage the use of spices, other than sodium, to client's personal taste.	Reduction in number and acuity of taste buds results in food tasting bland and decreases enjoyment of food and desire to eat.
Provide small, frequent feedings, as indicated.	Decreased gastric motility causes client to feel full and reduces intake.
Serve hot foods hot and cold foods cold.	Foods served at the proper temperature are more palatable, and enjoyment may increase appetite.
Promote a pleasant environment for eating in dining room or with company, if possible.	Eating is, in part, a social event and appetite can improve with increased socialization.
Have healthy snack foods, such as cheese, crackers, soup, and fruit available on a 24-hour basis.	Helps meet individual needs and enhances intake with caloric recommendations.
Plan for social events and provide for snacks even when working to reduce total calories.	Eating is part of socialization, and being able to respond to body's needs enhances sense of control and willingness to participate in dietary program.
Weigh on a regular basis—preferably, same time of day and in similar clothing.	Monitors nutritional state and effectiveness of interventions.
Assess causes of weight loss or gain, such as dysphagia due to decreased saliva production, neurogenic or psychogenic disturbances, tumors, muscular dysfunction, altered senses of smell and taste, or dysfunctional eating patterns related to depression or dementia.	Aids in adjusting plan of care and choice of interventions. *Note:* In elderly clients, saliva secretion may be decreased by as much as 66%, taste buds atrophy with reduced sensitivity to sweet and salt.
Review medication regimen for potential effects on food intake.	Drug side effects can impact client's intake; for example, corticosteroids may increase intake; angiotensin-converting enzyme (ACE) inhibitors and antihistamines cause change in taste; antidepressants, NSAIDs, and ferrous sulfate can decrease appetite or cause dysphagia; NSAIDs, antibiotics, digoxin, opiates, and chemotherapeutic agents can cause gastrointestinal (GI) distress, nausea, constipation, or mucositis (Henkel, 2004).
Check state of client's dental health periodically, including fit and condition of dentures, if present.	Oral infections and dental problems, shrinking gums, reaction of client's oral mucous membranes and saliva (associated with some medications or treatments), loss of teeth or ill-fitting dentures can all decrease client's ability to chew.
Monitor total caloric intake, as indicated.	If dietary plan is ineffective in meeting individual goals, calorie count or food diary may help identify problem areas.
Observe condition of skin; note muscle wasting; brittle nails; dry, lifeless hair; and signs of poor healing.	Reflects lack of adequate nutrition.
Encourage exercise and activity program within individual ability.	Promotes sense of well-being and may improve appetite.
Collaborative	
Consult with dietitian.	Aids in establishing specific nutritional program to meet individual client needs.

(continues on page 792)

ACTIONS/INTERVENTIONS (continued) / RATIONALE (continued)

ACTIONS/INTERVENTIONS	RATIONALE
Provide balanced diet with individually appropriate protein, complex carbohydrates, and calories. Include supplements between meals, as indicated.	Adjustments may be needed to deal with the body's decreased ability to process protein, as well as decreased metabolic rate and levels of activity. *Note:* Reduced production of salivary ptyalin inhibits digestion of complex carbohydrates in elderly individuals, affecting dietary plan. In addition, delayed insulin release by the pancreas and reduced peripheral sensitivity to insulin decrease glucose tolerance.
Administer vitamin and mineral supplements, as appropriate.	With age, renal and other regulatory systems cannot compensate as well for errors in intake. Mineral requirements change as hormone levels, metabolism, and GI function change. In addition, absorption can be impaired by medication use and chronic illness.
Refer to speech therapist for swallowing evaluation, as indicated.	Information useful in determining diet type or consistency, need for special exercises to strengthen muscles for swallowing, and/or inclusion in a restorative dining program (Henkel, 2004).
Refer for dental care routinely and as needed.	Maintenance of oral and dental health and good dentition can enhance intake.

NURSING DIAGNOSIS: Self-Care Deficit: [specify]

May Be Related To
Cognitive or perceptual impairment; decreased motivation
Neuromuscular or musculoskeletal impairment; weakness
Pain, discomfort
Fatigue

Possibly Evidenced By
Inability to perform ADLs

Desired Outcomes/Evaluation Criteria—Client Will

Self-Care: Status (NOC)
Perform self-care activities within level of own ability.
Demonstrate techniques or lifestyle changes to meet own needs.
Use resources effectively.

ACTIONS/INTERVENTIONS / RATIONALE

Self-Care Assistance (NIC)

Independent

ACTIONS/INTERVENTIONS	RATIONALE
Determine current capabilities (using 0 to 4 scale) and barriers to participation in self-care.	Comprehensive functional assessment includes independent performance of basic ADLs, social activities, sensory abilities, cognition, and ability to ambulate.
Involve client in formulation of plan of care at level of ability.	Enhances sense of control and aids in cooperation and maintenance of independence.
Encourage self-care. Work within present abilities; do not pressure client, but encourage client to reach beyond current capabilities. Provide adequate time for client to complete tasks. Have expectation of improvement and assist as needed.	Doing for oneself enhances feeling of self-worth. Failure can produce discouragement and depression.
Provide and promote privacy, including during bathing or showering.	Modesty may lead to reluctance to participate in care or perform activities in the presence of others.
Use specialized equipment as needed, such as tub transfer seat, grab bars, or raised toilet seat.	Enhances ability to move and perform activities safely.
Give tub bath, using walk-in tub, or two-person or mechanical lift if necessary. Use shower chair and spray attachment, as appropriate. Avoid chilling.	Provides safety for those who cannot get into the tub alone. Shower may be more feasible for some clients, though it may be less beneficial or desirable to the client. Elderly or debilitated clients are more prone to chilling.
Shampoo and style hair, as needed. Provide or assist with manicure.	Aids in maintaining appearance. Shampooing may be required more or less frequently than bathing schedule.
Encourage use of barber or beauty salon if client is able.	Enhances self-image and self-esteem, preserving dignity of the client.
Acquire clothing with modified fasteners, as indicated.	Use of Velcro instead of buttons or shoelaces can facilitate process of dressing, undressing, and toileting.

ACTIONS/INTERVENTIONS	RATIONALE
Encourage and assist with routine mouth and teeth care daily. Promote, or provide, denture care on a regular basis—cleaning, disinfecting, storage, repair, and use of dental adhesive. Use alternate oral hygiene measures as indicated, such as suction toothbrush, backward-bent toothbrush, chlorhexidine and fluoride mouth rinses, and regular suctioning.	Reduces risk of gum disease and tooth loss, enhances oral health, and promotes proper fitting and use of dentures.
Collaborative	
Consult with physical and/or occupational therapists and rehabilitation specialist.	Useful in establishing exercise and activity program, identifying assistive devices to meet individual needs and safety concerns, and facilitating independence.

NURSING DIAGNOSIS: risk for impaired Skin Integrity

Risk Factors May Include

Mechanical factors (e.g., shearing forces, pressure, restraint)
Impaired circulation, sensation
Moisture (bladder or bowel incontinence)
Imbalanced nutritional state (e.g., obesity, emaciation); skeletal prominence
Extremes of age

Possibly Evidenced By

(Not applicable; presence of signs and symptoms establishes an *actual* diagnosis)

Desired Outcomes/Evaluation Criteria—Client Will

Risk Control (NOC)

Maintain intact skin.
Identify individual risk factors.
Demonstrate behaviors or techniques to prevent skin breakdown or facilitate healing.

ACTIONS/INTERVENTIONS	RATIONALE
Skin Surveillance (NIC)	
Independent	
Assess for presence of conditions that may impact skin health.	Client's age and general health can impact skin health; however, other conditions may have more impact (e.g., older client who is smoking, or presence of diabetes, impaired kidney function, vascular insufficiency, incontinence, high risk for falls).
Inspect skin, tissues, and mucous membranes routinely. Observe for dry skin, rashes, evidence of pruritus (e.g., redness, scratches), any type of lesion, skin tears.	Provides opportunity for early intervention in high-risk population, which has less elastic and more fragile skin and tissues.
Anticipate and use preventive measures in clients who are at risk for skin breakdown, such as anyone who is thin, obese, aging, or debilitated.	Decubitus ulcers are difficult to heal, and prevention is the best treatment.
Assess nutritional status and initiate corrective measures, as indicated. Provide balanced diet with adequate protein, vitamins, and minerals.	A positive nitrogen balance and improved nutritional state can help prevent skin breakdown and promote ulcer healing. *Note:* May need additional calories and protein if draining ulcer is present.
Encourage adequate fluid intake especially in presence of cognitive impairment or dementia.	Prevention of dehydration is necessary to maintain circulating volume and tissue perfusion, moist mucous membranes, and good skin turgor to reduce risk of ulcer formation.
Maintain skin hygiene, using mild, nondetergent soap (e.g., Dove), drying gently and thoroughly, and lubricating.	A daily bath is usually not necessary in elderly clients because there is atrophy of sebaceous and sweat glands, and bathing may create dry skin problems. However, as epidermis thins with age, cleansing and use of moisturizing agents (containing occlusive ingredients [e.g., Vaseline, lanolin], humectants [e.g., glycerin, sorbitol], and emollients) is needed to keep skin soft, smooth, and pliable and to protect susceptible skin from breakdown (Haroun, 2003).
Change position frequently in bed and chair. Recommend 10 minutes of exercise each hour and/or perform passive ROM.	Improves circulation, muscle tone, and joint motion and promotes client participation.

(continues on page 794)

ACTIONS/INTERVENTIONS (continued)	RATIONALE (continued)
Use a rotation schedule in turning client. Use draw or turn sheet. Pay close attention to client's comfort level.	Allows for longer periods free of pressure; prevents shearing or tearing motions that can damage fragile tissues. *Note:* Use of prone position depends on client tolerance and should be maintained for only a short time.
Keep sheets and bedclothes clean, dry, and free from wrinkles, crumbs, and other irritating material.	Avoids friction or abrasion injury of skin.
Use elbow and heel protectors and foam, water, or gel pads for positioning in bed and when up in chair. Avoid use of plastic sheet protectors or incontinent pads.	Reduces risk of tissue abrasions and decreases pressure that can impair cellular blood flow. Promotes circulation of air along skin surface to dissipate heat and moisture. Plastic can actually trap heat and moisture against fragile tissues, increasing risk of tissue irritation and breakdown.
Provide for safety during ambulation, using appropriate adaptive devices, such as a walker or cane.	Loss of muscle strength and flexibility and physical disease process or debilitation may result in impaired coordination.
Limit exposure to temperature extremes and use of heating pad or ice pack.	Decreased sensitivity to pain, heat, or cold increases risk of tissue trauma.
Examine feet and nails routinely and provide foot and nail care as indicated:	Foot problems are common among clients who are elderly, diabetic, bedfast, and/or debilitated.
Keep nails cut short and smooth.	Jagged, rough nails can cause tissue damage and infection.
Use lotion or softening cream on feet.	Prevents drying or cracking of skin; promotes maintenance of healthy skin.
Check for fissures between toes, swab with hydrogen peroxide or dust with antiseptic powder, and place a wisp of cotton between the toes.	Prevents spread of infection and/or tissue injury.
Rub feet with witch hazel or a mentholated preparation and have client wear lightweight cotton socks.	Even though rash may not be present, burning and itching may be a problem. *Note:* Witch hazel may be contraindicated if skin is dry.
Inspect bony prominences, skin surface and folds routinely, especially when incontinence pad or pants are used. Increase preventive measures when reddened areas are noticed.	Skin breakdown can occur quickly with potential for infection and necrosis, possibly involving muscle and bone. There is increased risk of redness and irritation around legs due to elastic bands in adult incontinence pads or pants.
Continue regimen for redness and irritation when break in skin occurs.	Aggressive measures are important because decubitus ulcers can develop in a matter of a few hours.
Observe for decubitus ulcer development, and treat immediately according to protocol.	Timely intervention may prevent extensive damage.
Collaborative	
Provide waterbed, alternating-pressure, egg-crate, or gel mattress and pad for chair.	Provides protection and improved circulation by decreasing amount of pressure on tissues.
Monitor Hgb and Hct and blood glucose levels.	Anemia, dehydration, and elevated glucose levels are factors in skin breakdown and can impair healing.
Refer to podiatrist, as indicated.	May need professional care for such problems as ingrown toenails, corns, bony changes, and skin or tissue ulceration.
Assist with topical applications, such as hydrogel dressings, skin barrier dressings (Duoderm, Op-Site), collagenase therapy, absorbable gelatin sponges (Gelfoam), and aerosol sprays.	Although there are differing opinions about the efficacy of these agents, individual or combination use may enhance healing.
Administer nutritional supplements and vitamins, as indicated.	Aids in healing and cellular regeneration.
Prepare for skin grafting. (Refer to CP: Wound Care: Complicated or Chronic; Burns, ND: impaired Skin/Tissue Integrity.)	May be required to close large ulcers.

NURSING DIAGNOSIS: risk for impaired Urinary Elimination

Risk Factors May Include

Multiple causality (e.g., changes in fluid or nutritional pattern; perceptual or cognitive impairment)
Urinary tract infection

Possibly Evidenced By

(Not applicable; presence of signs and symptoms establishes an *actual* diagnosis)

Outcomes/Evaluation Criteria—Client Will

Urinary Elimination (NOC)

Maintain or regain effective pattern of elimination.
Initiate necessary lifestyle changes.
Participate in treatment regimen to correct or control situation, such as bladder training program or use of indwelling catheter.

ACTIONS/INTERVENTIONS	RATIONALE
Elimination Management (NIC)	
Independent	
Monitor voiding pattern. Identify possible reasons for changes, such as disorientation, neuromuscular impairment, and psychotropic medications.	This information is essential to plan for care and influences choice of individual interventions. Nocturia, frequency, and urgency are common because bladder capacity and/or tone are affected. Bladder pelvic muscles and sphincter tone may also be affected. *Note:* Urinary incontinence occurs more frequently in older adults but is not considered a normal part of aging (Dowling-Castronovo, update 2012).
Palpate bladder. Observe for "overflow" voiding and determine frequency and timing of dribbling or voiding.	Bladder distention indicates urinary retention, which may cause incontinence and infection.
Promote fluid intake of 2000 to 3000 mL/day within cardiac tolerance; include fruit juices, especially cranberry juice. Schedule fluid intake times appropriately.	Maintains adequate hydration and promotes kidney function (Dowling-Castronovo, 2012). Acid-ash juices act as an internal pH acidifier, retarding bacterial growth. *Note:* Client may decrease fluid intake in an attempt to control incontinence and become dehydrated. Instead, fluids may be scheduled to decrease frequency of incontinence, such as limiting fluids after 6 p.m. to reduce need to void during the night.
Institute bladder program, including scheduled voiding times and Kegel's exercises, involving client and staff in a positive manner.	Regular toileting times may help control incontinence. Program is more apt to be successful when positive attitudes and cooperation are present.
Assist client to sit upright on bedside commode, or bedpan, if not able to use toilet.	Provides functional position for voiding.
Provide, or encourage, perineal care daily and as needed.	Reduces risk of contamination and ascending infection.
Use adult incontinence pads or pants during day if needed based on individual type and amount of incontinence. Keep client clean and dry. Provide frequent skin care.	When training is unsuccessful, this is the preferred method of management (Dowling-Castronovo, 2012). *Note:* Avoiding use of incontinence pads during night exposes skin to air, reducing risk of irritation.
Avoid verbal or nonverbal signs of rejection, disgust, or disapproval over failures.	Expressions of disapproval lower self-esteem and are not helpful to a successful program.
Provide regular catheter care with soap and water, keep collecting bag below level of bladder, and maintain patency of system when indwelling catheter is present.	Reduces risk of ascending infection and/or minimizes reflux (Umscheid et al, 2009; Cravens, 2000).
Collaborative	
Administer medications as indicated, such as the following:	
Oxybutynin chloride (Ditropan) and tolterodine tartrate (Detrol)	Promotes bladder sphincter control.
Vitamin C and methenamine mandelate (Mandelamine)	Bladder pH acidifiers retard bacterial growth (Cravens & Zweig, 2000).
Maintain condom or indwelling catheter, or provide intermittent catheterization, if needed, using aseptic technique.	Catheterization for maintenance of continence should be avoided if at all possible, unless needed during healing of sacral or perineal wounds or for client with prolonged immobilization (e.g., spinal cord injury) or to improve comfort at end-of-life (Umscheid, 2012). *Note:* A single catheter insertion may lead to bacteriuria in up to 20% of elderly clients, and "chronic indwelling catheterization is not a substitute for good nursing care in the management of incontinence" (Cravens, 2000).

NURSING DIAGNOSIS: risk for Constipation/Diarrhea

Risk Factors May Include

Inadequate toileting
Insufficient fluid/fiber intake; poor eating habits
Decreased motility of gastrointestinal tract
Adverse effects of pharmaceutical agents
Mental confusion
Tube feedings

Possibly Evidenced By

(Not applicable; presence of signs and symptoms establishes an *actual* diagnosis)

Desired Outcomes/Evaluation Criteria—Client Will

Bowel Elimination (NOC)

Establish or maintain normal pattern of bowel functioning.
Demonstrate changes in lifestyle as necessitated by risk or contributing factors.
Participate in bowel program as able.

ACTIONS/INTERVENTIONS	RATIONALE
Bowel Management (NIC)	
Independent	
Review medical, surgical, and social history to identify conditions commonly associated with elimination difficulties.	Elimination problems may be multifactorial, and include: (1) physical conditions of the gut (e.g., diverticulitis, obstructions, anal fissures; (2) limited physical activity; (3) chronic pain and use of opoid analgesics; (4) neurological disorders (e.g., stroke); (5) poor eating habits, poor diet, food intolerances, malnutrition; (6) use of multiple medications, reaction to medication (e.g., diarrhea caused by antibiotic); (7) age and developmental issues; (8) cognitive decline or dementia with failure to attend to elimination needs; and (9) emotional/psychological issues, such as depression, distress over loss of privacy; inability to adjust to new surroundings and routines.
Ascertain usual bowel pattern and aids used, including previous long-term laxative use. Compare with current routine.	Determines extent of problem and indicates type of interventions required. Many clients may already be laxative-dependent, and it is important to reestablish as near-normal functioning as possible.
Assess reasons for elimination problems; rule out medical causes such as hemorrhoids, drug effect, impaction, bowel obstruction, and cancer.	Identification and treatment of underlying medical condition is necessary to achieve optimal bowel function.
Determine presence of food and/or drug sensitivities.	May contribute to diarrhea.
Institute individualized program of exercise, rest, diet, and elimination.	Depends on the needs of the client. Loss of muscular tone reduces peristalsis or may impair control of rectal sphincter.
Provide diet high in bulk in the form of whole-grain cereals, breads, and fresh fruits—especially prunes and plums.	Improves stool consistency and promotes evacuation.
Encourage increased fluid intake.	Promotes normal stool consistency.
Use adult incontinence pads or pants, if needed. Keep client clean and dry. Provide frequent perineal care. Apply skin protective ointment to anal area.	Prevents skin breakdown.
Keep air freshener in room, at bedside, or in bathroom, as needed.	Limits noxious odors and may help reduce client embarrassment and concern.
Give emotional support to client. Avoid "blaming" talk or actions if incontinence occurs.	Decreases feelings of frustration and embarrassment that can diminish self-esteem.
Collaborative	
Administer medications, as indicated, for example:	If nonpharmacologic treatments are inadequate in managing constipation, laxatives may be added to the treatment regimen (Gallagher, 2008; Ginsberg et al, 2007).
Bulk-forming laxatives, (e.g., psyllium seed [Metamucil], methylcellulose [Citrucel])	These agents absorb water, adding to the size of the fecal mass.
Osmotic laxatives (e.g., low-dose polyethylene glycol [Miralax] and saline laxatives [Ceo-Two, Fleet Enema, Milk of Magnesia])	These agents aren't absorbed in the intestine; instead, they pull water into the fecal mass to create more watery stool.
Stimulant laxatives (e.g., senna [Ex-Lax, Fletchers Castoria, Senokot]; bisacodyl [Correctol, Dulcolax])	These agents irritate the bowel to increase peristalsis.
Stool softeners or surfactants (e.g., docusate [Colase, Surfak]),	These agents cause more water and fat to be absorbed into the stool.
Miscellaneous agents (e.g., mineral oil)	These agents act by lubricating the stool and colon mucosa.
Administer antidiarrheal medications as indicated, for example: Loperidol (Immodium), atropine/diphenoxylate (Lomotil)	May be needed on a short-term basis for persistent diarrhea.

NURSING DIAGNOSIS: impaired physical Mobility

May Be Related To

Decreased endurance, deconditioning
Decreased muscle mass/control; joint stiffness; musculoskeletal impairment
Pain or discomfort
Cognitive impairment

Possibly Evidenced By

Limited range of motion
Gait changes; postural instability
Slowed movement

NURSING DIAGNOSIS: impaired physical Mobility (continued)

Desired Outcomes/Evaluation Criteria—Client Will

Mobility (NOC)

Maintain or increase strength and function of affected body parts.
Verbalize willingness to, and participate in, desired activities.
Demonstrate techniques or behaviors that enable continuation or resumption of activities.

ACTIONS/INTERVENTIONS	RATIONALE
Environmental Management (NIC)	
Independent	
Determine functional ability using a scale of 0 to 4 and reasons for impairment.	Identifies need for and degree of intervention required.
Note emotional and behavioral responses to altered ability.	Physical changes and loss of independence often create feelings of anxiety, anger, frustration, and depression that may be manifested as reluctance to engage in activity.
Plan activities and visits with adequate rest periods as necessary.	Can limit or prevent fatigue; conserve energy for continued participation.
Encourage participation in self-care, occupational or recreational activities.	Promotes independence and self-esteem; may enhance willingness to participate.
Provide chairs with firm, high seats and lifting chairs, when indicated.	Facilitates rising from seated position.
Fall Prevention (NIC)	
Perform initial and ongoing fall-risk assessment, including fall history, gait and balance assessment, cognition, use of mobility adjuncts, and environmental conditions.	Information can help determine client's potential for falling and identify which risk factors can be modified, such as medications, uncorrected sensory impairments, or poorly fitting shoes.
Assist with transfers and ambulation if indicated; show client and SO ways to move safely.	Prevents accidental falls and injury, especially in the client with altered gait, generalized weakness, orthostatic hypotension, fatigue, and vision disturbances.
Obtain supportive shoes and well-fitting, nonskid slippers.	Assists client to walk with a firm step, maintains sense of balance, and prevents slipping.
Remove clutter, wires or cords, scatter rugs, and extraneous furniture from pathways. Keep floors dry.	Reduces risk of falling and injuring self.
Encourage use of hand rails in hallway, stairwells, and bathrooms. Keep bed height in low position.	Promotes independence in mobility; reduces risk of falls.
Review safe use of mobility aids and adjunctive devices such as walker, braces, and prosthetics.	Facilitates activity and reduces risk of injury.
Provide for environmental changes to meet visual deficiencies:	Prevents accidents and reduces sense of sensory deprivation. If client is visually impaired, may need assistance and ongoing orientation to surroundings.
Keep areas well lighted. Accompany and keep close to client when in unfamiliar areas.	Provides for safety and psychological comfort.
Avoid use of physical restraints.	Studies show that older adults who are restrained, particularly when visually or cognitively impaired, are more likely to experience a fall than those who are not restrained.
Speak to client when entering the room, and let client know when leaving.	Special actions help client who cannot see to know when someone is there.
Encourage client with glasses or contacts to wear them. Be sure glasses are kept clean. Determine reason if glasses are not being worn.	Optimal visual acuity facilitates participation in activities and reduces risk of falls and injury. Client may not be wearing glasses because they need adjustment or change in correction.
Collaborative	
Arrange for regular eye examinations.	Identifies development or progression of vision problem such as myopia, hyperopia, presbyopia, astigmatism, cataract, glaucoma, tunnel vision, loss of peripheral fields, and blindness and specific options for care.
Consult with physical and occupational therapists and rehabilitation specialist.	Useful in creating individual exercise and activity program and identifying adjunctive aids. *Note:* Even in the elderly population, inclusion of moderate weight-lifting in the exercise program can improve and maintain the cardiovascular system; decrease obesity and blood pressure; and improve bone density, balance, and muscle tone and strength.

NURSING DIAGNOSIS: deficient Diversional Activity

May Be Related To

Environmental lack of diversional activity
[Depression, cognitive impairment]

Possibly Evidenced By

Reports feeling bored
Usual hobbies cannot be undertaken in the current setting

Desired Outcomes/Evaluation Criteria—Client Will

Leisure Participation (NOC)

Recognize own response and initiate appropriate coping actions.
Engage in satisfying activities within personal limitations.

ACTIONS/INTERVENTIONS	RATIONALE
Activity Therapy (NIC)	
Independent	
Determine avocation and hobbies client previously pursued. Incorporate activities, if appropriate, into present program.	Encourages involvement and helps to stimulate client mentally and physically to improve overall condition and sense of well-being.
Encourage participation in mix of activities and stimuli, such as music, news program, educational presentations, crafts, and social interactions, as appropriate.	Offering different activities helps client to try out new ideas and develop new interests. Activities need to be personally meaningful for the client to derive the most enjoyment from them, such as talking or Braille books for the blind and closed-caption TV broadcasts for the deaf or hearing impaired.
Provide change of scenery when possible, alter personal environment, encourage trips to shop or participate in local and family events.	Stimulates energy and provides new outlook for client.
Collaborative	
Refer to occupational therapist or activity director.	Can introduce and design new programs to provide positive stimuli for the client.

NURSING DIAGNOSIS: risk for Sexual Dysfunction

Risk Factors May Include

Altered body function (e.g., disease process, drugs, surgery)
Biopsychosocial alteration of sexuality
Lack of privacy and/or significant other

Possibly Evidenced By

(Not applicable; presence of signs and symptoms establishes an *actual* diagnosis)

Desired Outcomes/Evaluation Criteria—Client Will

Sexual Functioning (NOC)

Verbalize knowledge and understanding of sexual limitations, difficulties, or changes that have occurred.
Demonstrate improved communication and relationship skills.
Identify appropriate options to meet needs.

ACTIONS/INTERVENTIONS	RATIONALE
Sexual Counseling (NIC)	
Independent	
Note client's and SO's cues regarding sexuality.	May be concerned that condition or environmental restrictions may interfere with sexual function or ability but is afraid to ask directly.
Determine cultural and religious values and conflicts or other factors that may be present.	Affects client's perception of existing problems and response of others—family, staff, and other residents. Provides starting point for discussion and problem-solving.
Assess developmental and lifestyle issues.	Factors such as menopause and aging, adolescence, and young adulthood need to be taken into consideration with regard to sexual concerns about illness and long-term care.

ACTIONS/INTERVENTIONS (continued) — RATIONALE (continued)

Provide atmosphere in which discussion of sexuality is permitted and encouraged.
— When concerns are identified and discussed, problem-solving can begin.

Provide privacy for client and SO.
— Demonstrates acceptance of need for intimacy and provides opportunity to continue previous patterns of interaction as much as possible.

Collaborative

Refer to sex counselor or therapist and family therapy when indicated.
— May require additional assistance for resolution of problems.

NURSING DIAGNOSIS: ineffective Self-Health Maintenance

May Be Related To

Deficient knowledge
Decisional conflicts
Inadequate number of cues to action
Perceived seriousness/benefits

Possibly Evidenced By

Failure to take action to reduce risk factors
Ineffective choices in daily living for meeting health goals
Demonstrated lack of behaviors adaptive to internal or external environmental changes

Desired Outcomes/Evaluation Criteria—Client/Caregiver Will

Participation in Health Care Decisions (NOC)

Verbalize understanding of factors contributing to current situation.
Adopt lifestyle changes supporting individual healthcare goals.
Assume responsibility for own healthcare needs when possible.

ACTIONS/INTERVENTIONS — RATIONALE

Health Education (NIC)

Independent

Assess level of adaptive behavior, knowledge, and skills about health maintenance, environment, and safety.
— Identifies areas of concern or need and aids in choice of interventions.

Provide information about individual healthcare needs.
— Provides knowledge base and encourages participation in decision making.

Develop plan with client and SO for self-care incorporating existing disabilities and adapting and organizing care.
— Assists client and caregiver to maintain and manage desired level of independence when possible.

Maintain adequate hydration and balanced diet with sufficient protein intake.
— Promotes general well-being and aids in disease prevention.

Schedule adequate rest with progressive activity program.
— Prevents fatigue and enhances general well-being.

Promote good hand washing and personal hygiene. Use aseptic techniques as necessary.
— Prevents contamination or cross-contamination, reducing risk of illness or infection.

Protect from exposure to infections and avoid extremes of temperature. Recommend the wearing of masks, monitor staff and visitors, and provide other interventions, as indicated.
— With age, immune protective responses slow down and physiological reactions to temperature extremes may be impaired. As organ function decreases, especially the thymus gland, and natural antibodies decline, clients are at increased risk for infection. Staff and/or visitors with colds or other infections may expose client to these illnesses. *Note:* Nursing home acquired pneumonia (NHAP) is a common cause of infection in chronic care facilities and is a significant cause of mortality (Cunha, 2013).

Encourage cessation of smoking.
— Smokers are prone to bronchitis and ineffective clearing of secretions.

Encourage reporting of signs and symptoms as they occur.
— Provides opportunity for early recognition of developing complications and timely intervention to prevent serious illness.

Health System Guidance (NIC)

Note client's previous use of professional services, and continue as appropriate. Include in choice of new healthcare providers as able.
— Preserves continuity and promotes independence in meeting own healthcare needs.

Observe for and monitor changes in vital signs such as temperature elevation.
— Early identification of onset of illness allows for timely intervention and may prevent serious complications. *Note:* Elderly

(continues on page 800)

ACTIONS/INTERVENTIONS (continued)	RATIONALE (continued)
	persons often display subnormal temperatures, so presence of a low-grade fever may be of serious concern.
Collaborative	
Identify resources for, or administer medications, as indicated, for example:	Reduces risk of acquiring contagious, potentially life-threatening diseases.
Immunizations, such as *Haemophilus influenzae* (flu) and pneumonia	
Antibiotics	May be used prophylactically, depending on individual disease process or risk factors, and to treat infections.
Schedule preventive and routine healthcare appointments based on individual needs with cardiologist, podiatrist, ophthalmologist, or dentist.	Promotes optimal recovery and maintenance of health.
Refer to support services as indicated, such as home health care agency, durable medical equipment company, Senior Resources, social services, national hospice organization, Alzheimer's Disease and Related Disorders Association, American Association of Retired Persons (AARP), Center for Health Care Ethics, Choice in Dying, American Bar Association, Commission on Legal Problems of the Elderly, Internet resources, and Adult Protective Services.	Many community resources are available, and often untapped, to make life and care of the individual easier.

POTENTIAL CONSIDERATIONS following discharge from care facility.
Refer to plan of care for diagnosis that required admission.

ALCOHOL: ACUTE WITHDRAWAL

I. Pathophysiology (McKeown, 2012)

a. Alcohol intoxication and withdrawal—complex mechanism
b. Most clinical effects explained by the interaction of ethanol with various neurotransmitters and neuroreceptors in the brain
c. Resulting changes in the inhibitory and excitatory neurotransmitters disrupt the neurochemical balance in the brain, causing symptoms of withdrawal if alcohol is suddenly stopped or decreased after extended usage (Donnelly, 2012; Burton, 2010).

II. Stages of Alcohol Withdrawal (McKeown, 2012)

a. Stage I: autonomic hyperactivity
b. Stage II: hallucinations
c. Stage III: neuronal excitation
d. Stage IV: delirium tremens (DTs)

III. Etiology

a. Individual's desire to repeatedly reach a state of feeling high; numb, negative feelings
b. Associated with serious mental health disorders—anxiety, mood disorders, or major depression
c. Personality traits—dependency more common in isolation, loneliness, shyness, depression, dependency, hostile and self-destructive impulsivity, and sexual immaturity (Ali et al, 2013)
d. Environment—frequently come from a broken home and have a disturbed relationship with their parents
e. Genetics—incidence of alcoholism is higher in biological children of alcoholics, and some people who become alcoholics are less easily intoxicated, having a higher threshold for central nervous system (CNS) effects.

IV. Statistics

a. Morbidity: In 2007, Approximately 463,000 hospital discharge episodes in the United States for persons ages 15 and older had a principal (first-listed) alcohol-related diagnosis (National Institute on Alcohol Abuse and Alcoholism [NIAAA], 2010); approximately 5% of individuals who have alcohol withdrawal progress to DTs (McKeown, 2012).
b. Mortality: There are approximately 80,000 deaths related to health consequences of alcohol abuse annually (Centers for Disease Control [CDC], 2012). This figure includes every type of alcohol-attributable condition or event, including acute causes (e.g., alcohol poisoning, vehicle crashes, fall injuries, homicide) and chronic causes (e.g., alcoholic liver disease, alcoholism, various cancers, pancreatitis, fetal alcohol syndrome). In 2010, 16,634 deaths were attributed to alcoholic liver disease alone (Hoyert & Xu, 2010). Despite appropriate treatment, DTs are reported to have a 5% to 15% mortality rate (McKeown, 2012).
c. Cost: According to a 2011 study published by the CDC, in 2006 the cost of excessive alcohol consumption reached $223.5 billion. Researchers found that about $94.2 billion of the total economic costs was borne by federal, state, and local governments, while $92.9 billion (41.5%) was borne by excessive drinkers and their family members. Further analysis showed that the costs largely resulted from losses in workplace productivity (72% of the total cost), healthcare expenses for problems caused by excessive drinking (11% of the total cost), law enforcement and other criminal justice expenses related to excessive alcohol consumption (9% of the total cost), and motor vehicle crash costs from impaired driving (6% of the total cost).

GLOSSARY

Addiction: Dependence on a substance (such as alcohol or other drugs) or an activity to the point that stopping is very difficult and causes severe physical and mental reactions.

Alcohol withdrawal syndrome (AWS): The neurological, psychiatric, and cardiovascular manifestations that result when a person accustomed to consuming large quantities of alcohol suddenly becomes abstinent or reduces alcohol intake (Burton, 2010).

Arcus senilis: White or gray ring-like opacity of the cornea.

Ataxia: Gross incoordination of voluntary muscle movement, reflecting loss of proprioception in chronic alcohol abuse.

Autonomic hyperactivity stage: Usually occurs within 24 hours of the last drink. Symptoms may be mild, characterized by tremulousness, insomnia, anxiety, diaphoresis, mild tachycardia, and gastrointestinal (GI) upset.

Binge: Uninterrupted consumption of a drug for several hours or days.

Blackout: Amnesia for events occurring during the period of alcoholic intoxication, even though consciousness is still maintained during that time.

Delirium tremens (DTs): Potentially fatal form of alcohol withdrawal characterized by disorientation, confusion, impaired attention, pronounced autonomic hyperactivity, and visual and auditory hallucinations. Usually begins at 48 to 72 hours but can be delayed up to 4 to 5 days. Death is usually due to cardiovascular or respiratory collapse.

Detoxification: Process of removing alcohol or other drugs from the body. This is the initial period addicts must go through to become drug-free. Withdrawal symptoms appear early during this process. Depending on the drug, detoxification lasts for a few days to a week or more.

Gluconeogenesis: Conversion of glycogen to glucose in the liver.

Hallucination stage: Development of false visual (most common), olfactory, or auditory perceptions that have no relation to reality, usually occurring 24 to 36 hours after the cessation of alcohol intake.

Hepatic encephalopathy: Condition used to describe the deleterious effects of liver failure on the central nervous system (CNS). Features include confusion ranging to coma, with alcoholic cirrhosis being the most common cause.

Myelosuppression: Decrease in the production by the bone marrow of red blood cells (RBCs), platelets, and some white blood cells (WBCs).

Neuronal excitation stage: Development of autonomic hyperactivity or seizures occurring within 48 hours after cessation of alcohol consumption.

Nystagmus: Unintentional jittery movement of the eyes. Nystagmus usually involves both eyes and is often exaggerated by looking in a particular direction.

Thrombocytopenia: Low platelet count, which can lead to impaired blood clotting and spontaneous bleeding.

Wernicke's syndrome or Wernicke encephalopathy: Neurological disease characterized by the clinical triad of confusion, inability to coordinate voluntary movement, and eye abnormalities.

Care Setting

Client may be inpatient on a behavioral unit, at a substance abuse rehabilitation facility, or outpatient in community programs. Although clients are not generally admitted to the acute care setting with this diagnosis, withdrawal from alcohol may occur secondarily during hospitalization for other illnesses or conditions (Riddle et al, 2010). An alcohol screening should be done for all hospitalized clients (Burton, 2010; Daly, 2009). A short hospital stay may be required during the acute phase because of severity of general condition or comorbidities, or a delayed discharge from acute care can be the result of alcohol withdrawal beginning within 6 to 48 hours of admission.

Related Concerns

Cirrhosis of the liver, page 412
Heart failure: chronic, page 43
Psychosocial aspects of care, page 729
Substance use disorders (SUDs), page 815
Upper gastrointestinal/esophageal bleeding, page 281

Client Assessment Database

Data depend on the duration and extent of use of alcohol, concurrent use of other drugs, degree of organ involvement, and presence of other pathology.

DIAGNOSTIC DIVISION MAY REPORT	MAY EXHIBIT
ACTIVITY/REST • Insomnia, difficulty sleeping, not feeling well rested • Fatigue or weakness	• Abnormal heart rate or blood pressure (BP) in response to activity

(continues on page 802)

DIAGNOSTIC DIVISION MAY REPORT (continued)	MAY EXHIBIT (continued)
CIRCULATION	• Tachycardia common during acute withdrawal • Numerous dysrhythmias may be identified, especially atrial fibrillation • Hypertension common in early withdrawal stage; may become labile or progress to hypotension • Peripheral pulses weak, irregular, or rapid
EGO INTEGRITY • Feelings of guilt, shame; defensiveness about drinking • Denial, rationalization • Multiple stressors or losses— relationships, employment, finances • Use of alcohol to deal with life stressors, boredom	• Anxiety, fear • Irritability • Antisocial behavior
ELIMINATION • Diarrhea	• Bowel sounds varied (may reflect gastric complications such as hemorrhage)
FOOD/FLUID • Nausea, vomiting; food intolerance • Anorexia	• Gastric distention, ascites, liver and spleen enlargement (seen in cirrhosis) • Muscle wasting; dry, dull hair; swollen salivary glands; inflamed buccal cavity; capillary fragility (malnutrition) • Bowel sounds varied (reflecting malnutrition, electrolyte imbalances, general bowel dysfunction)

NEUROSENSORY
• "Internal shakes"
• Headache, dizziness, blurred vision
• Blackouts
	• Psychopathology—paranoia, schizophrenia, major depression, neurosis (may indicate dual diagnosis)
	• Level of consciousness (LOC) and orientation varied—confusion, stupor, hyperactivity, distorted thought processes, slurred, incoherent speech
	• Memory loss, confabulation
	• Affect/mood/behavior—fearful, anxious, easily startled, inappropriate, silly, euphoric, irritable, physically or verbally abusive, depressed, and/or paranoid
	• Hallucinations may be visual, tactile, olfactory, or auditory; for example, client may be picking items out of the air or responding verbally to unseen person or voices
	• ***Eye examination:***
	  • Nystagmus—associated with cranial nerve palsy
	  • Pupil constriction (may indicate CNS depression)
	  • Arcus senilis (normal in aging populations, suggests alcohol-related changes in younger individuals)
	• Fine-motor tremors of face, tongue, and hands
	• Seizure—grand mal or partial that is usually brief, generalized, tonic-clonic in nature, and without an aura, occurs in a cluster of 1 to 3 seizures with a short postictal period; in 20% to 50% of individuals, the seizures progress to DTs (McKeown, 2012; Riddle et al, 2010).
	• Gait unsteady (ataxia), which may be due to thiamine deficiency or cerebellar degeneration associated with Wernicke's encephalopathy (Riddle et al, 2010).

DIAGNOSTIC DIVISION MAY REPORT (continued)	MAY EXHIBIT (continued)
PAIN/DISCOMFORT • Constant upper abdominal pain and tenderness radiating to the back (pancreatic inflammation) • Headache (may be "pulsating")	• Guarding affected area • Narrowed focus
RESPIRATION • History of smoking • Chronic respiratory problems	• Tachypnea, hyperventilation • Breath sounds diminished, adventitious sounds (suggests pulmonary complications such as respiratory depression or pneumonia)
SAFETY • History of recurrent trauma—falls, fractures, lacerations, burns, or motor vehicle crashes • Violence toward self or others	• Skin—flushed face and palms of hands; scars, ecchymotic areas; fissures at corners of mouth (vitamin deficiency) • Fractures healed or new—signs of recent or recurrent trauma • Temperature elevation, flushing, diaphoresis • Suicidal ideation; alcohol is a major risk factor in suicide (Ali et al, 2013; Davies, 2012).
SEXUALITY • Loss of sexual desire • Not achieving sexual satisfaction, or needing alcohol for satisfying sex • Actual or perceived limitation imposed by disease	• Alteration in relationship with partner
SOCIAL INTERACTION • Frequent sick days off from work or school, fighting with others, arrests for disorderly conduct, or motor vehicle violations such as driving under the influence (DUI) • Denial that alcohol intake has any significant effect on present condition • Dysfunctional family system of origin (generational involvement), problems in current relationships, often alienated from family when problem is chronic • Mood changes affecting interactions with others	• Speech unintelligible or slurred • Family interactions and communications strained and difficult. Alcohol is often the cause of social decline, which includes failed marriages, loss of employment, and severed family ties (Ali et al, 2013).
TEACHING/LEARNING • Family history of alcoholism • History of alcohol and/or other drug use or abuse, tobacco use • Ignorance and/or denial of addiction to alcohol, or inability to cut down or stop drinking despite repeated efforts, previous periods of abstinence or withdrawal • History of daily alcohol use for at least 3 months • Large amount of alcohol consumed in last 24 to 48 hours ("bingeing") • Previous hospitalizations for alcoholism or alcohol-related diseases such as cirrhosis and esophageal varices	• Acting annoyed when people ask client about drinking (McPeake, 2013)
DISCHARGE PLAN CONSIDERATIONS • May require assistance to maintain abstinence and begin to participate in rehabilitation program ➧ Refer to section at end of plan for postdischarge considerations.	

Diagnostic Studies

TEST WHY IT IS DONE	WHAT IT TELLS ME
BLOOD TESTS	
• ***Blood alcohol level (BAL):*** Measures level of alcohol in the blood.	BAL may or may not be severely elevated, depending on amount consumed, time between consumption and testing, and the degree of tolerance, which varies widely. In the absence of elevated alcohol tolerance, blood levels of 100 mg/dL are associated with loss of control of fine motor movements and confusion when faced with tasks requiring thinking; at 200 mg/dL, very slurred speech, ataxia, and lethargy; at 400 mg/dL, coma and respiratory depression; at 500 mg/dL, death is possible due to respiratory arrest, severe hypotension, and aspiration (Balentine, 2013).
• ***Complete blood count (CBC):*** Battery of screening tests, which typically includes hemoglobin (Hgb); hematocrit (Hct); RBC count, morphology, indices, and distribution width index; platelet count and size; WBC count and differential.	Blood loss from the GI tract and nutritional deficiencies producing anemia are common in alcohol withdrawal. In addition, alcohol ingestion leads to myelosuppression with a slight reduction in all cell lines. Thrombocytopenia is common. Increased mean corpuscular volume (MCV) suggests anemia based on deficiencies in vitamin B_{12} and folate. WBC count may be increased with infection or decreased if client is immunosuppressed.
• ***Glucose and ketones:*** Determines ability of liver to manage simple sugars and end products of sugar metabolism.	Clients with liver disease due to alcoholism have reduced glycogen stores, and alcohol impairs gluconeogenesis. As a consequence, these clients are susceptible to hypoglycemia (McKeown, 2012). Ketoacidosis may be present with or without metabolic acidosis. Alcoholic ketoacidosis (AKA) can occur in chronic alcohol abuse with history of recent binge drinking, decreased food intake, and persistent vomiting (López et al, 2012).
• ***Electrolytes:*** Substances that dissociate into ions in solution and acquire the capacity to conduct electricity. Common electrolytes include sodium, potassium, chloride, calcium, and phosphate.	Alcoholics with liver disease frequently have abnormal sodium serum concentrations, with hyponatremia (low plasma sodium concentration) as the most common alteration. Decreased serum potassium concentration may be associated with respiratory alkalosis, elevated insulin levels, and elevated epinephrine levels resulting from alcohol withdrawal. Client with chronic alcoholism usually has dietary magnesium deficiency and possibly concurrent alcoholic hepatitis. Alcoholic pancreatitis may cause hypocalcemia.
• ***Liver function tests—lactate dehydrogenase (LDH), alanine aminotransferase (ALT), lipase, and amylase:*** Determine level of liver and pancreatic dysfunction.	May be elevated, reflecting liver or pancreatic damage.
• ***Blood ammonia:*** Helps evaluate the cause of the change in consciousness.	Level is elevated if hepatic encephalopathy is present.
• ***Nutritional tests—albumin or prealbumin, total protein, carbohydrate-deficient transferrin (CDT), iron, vitamins D and B_{12}, and folate:*** Evaluates nutritional status, identifies deficiencies and treatment needs.	Albumin and total protein may be decreased. CDT, a protein molecule involved in iron transport, is a relatively new test that is sometimes used to help identify chronic, heavy drinking. Vitamin deficiencies are usually present, reflecting malnutrition or malabsorption.
OTHER DIAGNOSTIC STUDIES	
• ***Urinalysis:*** Detects and measures various compounds that pass through the urine.	Increased WBCs and/or protein may indicate infection; ketones may be present related to breakdown of fatty acids in malnutrition (pseudodiabetic condition).
• ***Chest x-ray:*** Procedure used to evaluate organs and structures within the chest for symptoms of disease.	May reveal right lower lobe pneumonia, a common manifestation which may be related to malnutrition, depressed immune system, and aspiration. X-ray may also reveal evidence of chronic lung disorders associated with heavy tobacco use, also common in alcoholics.

TEST WHY IT IS DONE (continued)	WHAT IT TELLS ME (continued)
• *Electrocardiogram (ECG):* Record of the electrical activity of the heart.	Dysrhythmias, cardiomyopathies, and/or ischemia may be present because of direct effect of alcohol on the cardiac muscle and/or conduction system, as well as effects of electrolyte imbalance. The adrenergic storm produced by alcohol withdrawal increases cardiac demand, which may precipitate infarction in susceptible individuals. Atrial fibrillation is the most common cardiac symptom seen in the alcoholic (Burton, 2010).
• *Computed tomography (CT) scan of the head:* X-ray procedure that uses a computer to produce a detailed picture of a cross section of the body.	May be obtained in clients with depressed LOC, in those with multiple seizures or signs of head trauma, and in those with failure to respond to treatment. *Note:* Client with AWS is at risk for intracranial bleeding because of frequent falls, cortical atrophy, and coagulopathy.
• *Clinical Institute Withdrawal Assessment (CIWA):* Clinical rating tool that provides a numerical rating for 10 factors, including nausea and vomiting, tactile disturbances, tremor, auditory and visual disturbances, sweating, anxiety, headache agitation, and orientation (Donnelly, Kent-Wilkinson, & Rush, 2012).	Provides a clinical quantification of the severity of the alcohol withdrawal syndrome and can be rapidly administered at the bedside. Scores of 9 to 15 points correspond with moderate withdrawal, and scores greater than 15 correspond to severe withdrawal symptoms and increased risk of DTs and seizures.
• *Addiction severity index (ASI):* A 161-item multidimensional clinical and research tool that produces a "problem severity profile" of the client, including chemical, medical, psychological, legal, family and social, and employment and support aspects, indicating areas of treatment needs.	Provides basic diagnostic information on a client prior to, during, and after treatment for substance use-related problems as well as for the assessment of change in client status and treatment outcome.

Nursing Priorities

1. Maintain physiological stability during acute withdrawal phase.
2. Promote client safety.
3. Provide appropriate referral and follow-up.
4. Encourage and support significant other (SO) involvement in "intervention" or confrontation process.
5. Provide information about condition, prognosis, and treatment needs.

Discharge Goals

1. Homeostasis achieved.
2. Complications prevented or resolved.
3. Sobriety maintained on a day-to-day basis.
4. Ongoing participation in rehabilitation program or group therapy, such as Alcoholics Anonymous (AA).
5. Condition, prognosis, and therapeutic regimen understood.
6. Plan in place to meet needs after discharge.

This plan of care is to be used in conjunction with CP: Substance Use Disorders.

NURSING DIAGNOSIS: risk for ineffective Breathing Pattern

Risk Factors May Include

Neuromuscular dysfunction (e.g., direct effect of alcohol toxicity on respiratory center and/or sedative drugs given to decrease alcohol withdrawal symptoms)
Fatigue
[Tracheobronchial obstruction]

Possibly Evidenced By

(Not applicable; presence of signs and symptoms establishes an *actual* diagnosis)

Desired Outcomes/Evaluation Criteria—Client Will

Respiratory Status: Ventilation (NOC)
Maintain effective breathing pattern with respiratory rate within normal range, lungs clear, and free of cyanosis or other signs and symptoms of hypoxia.

ACTIONS/INTERVENTIONS	RATIONALE
Respiratory Monitoring (NIC)	
Independent	
Monitor respiratory rate, depth, and pattern as indicated. Note periods of apnea and Cheyne-Stokes respirations.	Frequent assessment is important because toxicity levels may change rapidly. Hyperventilation is common during acute withdrawal phase. Kussmaul's respirations are sometimes present because of acidotic state associated with vomiting and malnutrition. However, marked respiratory depression can occur because of CNS depressant effects of alcohol if acute intoxication is present. This may be compounded by drugs used to control AWS.
Auscultate breath sounds. Note presence of adventitious sounds such as rhonchi, wheezes.	Client is at risk for atelectasis related to hypoventilation and pneumonia.
Airway Management (NIC)	
Elevate head of bed.	Decreases potential for aspiration; lowers diaphragm, enhancing lung inflation.
Encourage coughing, deep-breathing exercises, and frequent position changes.	Facilitates lung expansion and mobilization of secretions to reduce complications from atelectasis or pneumonia.
Have suction equipment and airway adjuncts available.	Sedative effects of alcohol potentiate risk of aspiration, relaxation of oropharyngeal muscles, and respiratory depression, requiring intervention to prevent respiratory arrest.
Collaborative	
Administer supplemental oxygen, if necessary.	Hypoxia may occur with respiratory depression and chronic anemia.
Review serial chest x-rays, arterial blood gases (ABGs), or pulse oximetry, as indicated.	Monitors presence of secondary complications, evaluates effectiveness of respiratory effort, and identifies therapy needs. *Note:* Right lower lobe pneumonia is common in alcohol-debilitated clients and is often due to chronic aspiration. Chronic lung diseases, such as emphysema or bronchitis, are also common.

NURSING DIAGNOSIS: risk for decreased Cardiac Output

Risk Factors May Include
Altered contractility (e.g., direct effect of alcohol on the heart muscle)
Altered afterload—systemic vascular resistance
Altered rhythm

Possibly Evidenced By
(Not applicable; presence of signs and symptoms establishes an *actual* diagnosis)

Desired Outcomes/Evaluation Criteria—Client Will

Circulation Status (NOC)
Display vital signs within client's normal range; absence, or reduced frequency, of dysrhythmias.
Demonstrate an increase in activity tolerance.

ACTIONS/INTERVENTIONS	RATIONALE
Hemodynamic Regulation (NIC)	
Independent	
Monitor vital signs frequently during acute withdrawal.	Hypertension frequently occurs in acute withdrawal phase. Extreme hyperexcitability, accompanied by catecholamine release and increased peripheral vascular resistance, raises BP and heart rate; however, BP may become labile and progress to hypotension. *Note:* Client may have underlying cardiovascular disease, which is compounded by alcohol withdrawal.
Monitor cardiac rate and rhythm. Document irregularities and dysrhythmias.	Long-term alcohol abuse may result in cardiomyopathy and heart failure (HF). Tachycardia is common because of sympathetic response to increased circulating catecholamines. Dysrhythmias may develop with electrolyte imbalance. All of these may have an adverse effect on cardiac output.
Monitor body temperature.	Elevation may occur because of sympathetic stimulation, dehydration, and/or infections, causing vasodilation and compromising venous return and cardiac output.

ACTIONS/INTERVENTIONS (continued)	RATIONALE (continued)
Monitor intake and output (I&O). Note 24-hour fluid balance.	Preexisting dehydration, vomiting, fever, and diaphoresis may result in decreased circulating volume that can compromise cardiovascular function. *Note:* Hydration is difficult to assess in the alcoholic client because the usual indicators are not reliable, and overhydration is a risk in the presence of compromised cardiac function.
Be prepared for and assist in cardiopulmonary resuscitation.	Causes of death during acute withdrawal stages include cardiac dysrhythmias, respiratory depression and arrest, oversedation, excessive psychomotor activity, severe dehydration or overhydration, and massive infections. Mortality for DTs may be as high as 20% to 25% (McKoewn, 2012; Riddle et al, 2010).
Collaborative	
Monitor laboratory studies, such as serum electrolyte levels, RBCs, Hgb and Hct, and platelets.	Potassium and magnesium imbalances potentiate risk of cardiac dysrhythmias. Anemia may be present and platelets can be decreased in late-stage alcoholism due to liver dysfunction.
Administer fluids and electrolytes, as indicated.	Severe alcohol withdrawal causes the client to be susceptible to excessive fluid losses associated with fever, diaphoresis, and vomiting; electrolyte imbalances, especially potassium and magnesium.
Administer medications, as indicated, for example:	
Clonidine (Catapres) or atenolol (Tenormin)	Although the use of benzodiazepines is often sufficient to control hypertension during initial withdrawal from alcohol, some clients may require more specific therapy. *Note:* Atenolol and other beta-adrenergic blockers may speed up the withdrawal process and eliminate tremors as well as lower the heart rate, BP, and body temperature.
Potassium	Corrects deficits that can result in life-threatening dysrhythmias.

NURSING DIAGNOSIS: risk for Injury [specify]

Risk Factors May Include

Biochemical dysfunction (e.g., cessation of alcohol use with varied autonomic nervous responses; thiamine deficiency)
Physical (e.g., equilibrium/balancing difficulties, seizures activity, reduced muscle and hand–eye coordination)

Possibly Evidenced By

(Not applicable; presence of signs and symptoms establishes an *actual* diagnosis)

Desired Outcomes/Evaluation Criteria—Client Will

Physical Injury Severity (NOC)

Demonstrate absence of untoward effects of withdrawal.
Experience no physical injury.

ACTIONS/INTERVENTIONS	RATIONALE
Substance Use Treatment: Alcohol Withdrawal (NIC)	
Independent	
Identify stage of AWS using CIWA. Stage I is associated with signs and symptoms of hyperactivity, such as tremors, sleeplessness, nausea, vomiting, diaphoresis, tachycardia, and hypertension; stage II is manifested by increased hyperactivity plus hallucinations and/or seizure activity; stage III symptoms include DTs and extreme autonomic hyperactivity with profound confusion, anxiety, insomnia, and fever.	AWS usually begins 3 to 36 hours after the last drink. Prompt recognition and intervention may halt progression of symptoms and enhance recovery, improving prognosis. In addition, progression of symptoms indicates need for changes in drug therapy and more intense treatment to prevent death. DTs may not present until 2 to 3 days after last alcohol intake, usually lasting 1 to 5 days.
Monitor and document seizure activity. Maintain patent airway. Provide environmental safety such as padded side rails and bed in low position.	Grand mal seizures are most common and may be related to decreased magnesium levels, hypoglycemia, elevated blood alcohol, or history of head trauma or preexisting seizure disorder. *Note:* In absence of history of seizures or other pathology causing them, they usually stop spontaneously or with magnesium replacement, which reduces CNS excitability (Burns, 2013).

(continues on page 808)

ACTIONS/INTERVENTIONS (continued) / RATIONALE (continued)

Check deep-tendon reflexes (DTRs). Assess gait, if possible. Palpate upper arm to discern actual withdrawal versus medication-seeking behavior.

Reflexes may be depressed, absent, or hyperactive. Peripheral neuropathies are common, especially in malnourished client. Ataxia is associated with Wernicke's syndrome (thiamine deficiency) and cerebellar degeneration. Three ways to assess whether the client is having actual withdrawal tremors are (1) have the client stick out his or her tongue—it will be tremulous; (2) feel the client's upper arm—withdrawal tremors can be felt bone deep; and (3) have the client visually track a pencil—there will be observable nystagmus.

Assist with ambulation and self-care activities, as needed.

Prevents falls with resultant injury.

Provide for environmental safety when indicated. (Refer to ND: [disturbed Sensory Perception], following.)

May be required when equilibrium and hand–eye coordination problems exist.

Collaborative

Administer medications, as indicated, for example:

Benzodiazepines (BZDs), such as chlordiazepoxide (Librium), diazepam (Valium), lorazepam (Ativan), oxazepam (Serax), or clonidine (Catapess)

BZDs are commonly used to control neuronal hyperactivity because of their minimal respiratory and cardiac depression and anticonvulsant properties. Studies have also shown that these drugs can prevent progression to more severe states of withdrawal. Intravenous (IV) or oral (PO) administration is preferred route because intramuscular (IM) absorption is unpredictable. Muscle-relaxant qualities are particularly helpful to client in controlling "the shakes," trembling, and ataxic quality of movements.

Haloperidol (Haldol)

May be used in conjunction with BZDs for clients experiencing agitation and hallucinations, although should be used with caution as it can lower seizure threshold.

Thiamine

Thiamine deficiency may lead to neuritis, Wernecke's syndrome (abnormal gait and paralysis of eye muscles as well as cognitive deficits), and/or Korsakoff's psychosis (Riddle, 2010).

Magnesium sulfate

Reduces tremors and seizure activity by decreasing neuromuscular excitability.

NURSING DIAGNOSIS: [disturbed Sensory Perception (specify)]

May Be Related To

Biochemical imbalances (e.g., sudden cessation of alcohol consumption, electrolyte imbalance, elevated ammonia and blood urea nitrogen [BUN])

Psychological stress—anxiety, fear

[Sleep deprivation]

Possibly Evidenced By

Disorientation; sensory distortions; visual/auditory hallucinations

Changes in usual response to stimuli; change in behavior pattern

Restlessness; irritability

Desired Outcomes/Evaluation Criteria—Client Will

Cognition (NOC)

Regain or maintain usual LOC.

Distorted Thought Self-Control (NOC)

Report absence of, or reduced, hallucinations.

Identify external factors that affect sensory-perceptual abilities.

ACTIONS/INTERVENTIONS / RATIONALE

Substance Use Treatment: Alcohol Withdrawal (NIC)

Independent

Assess LOC, ability to speak, and response to stimuli and commands.

Speech may be garbled, confused, or slurred. Response to commands may reveal inability to concentrate, impaired judgment, or muscle coordination deficits.

Observe for behavioral responses such as hyperactivity, disorientation, confusion, sleeplessness, and irritability.

Hyperactivity related to CNS disturbances may escalate rapidly. Sleeplessness is common due to loss of sedative effect gained from alcohol usually consumed before bedtime. Sleep deprivation may aggravate disorientation or

ACTIONS/INTERVENTIONS (continued)	RATIONALE (continued)
	confusion. Progression of symptoms may indicate impending hallucinations (stage II) or DTs (stage IV).
Note onset of hallucinations and document as auditory, visual, and/or tactile.	Auditory hallucinations are reported to be more frightening and threatening to client. Visual hallucinations occur more at night and often include insects, animals, or faces of friends or enemies. Clients are frequently observed "picking the air." Yelling may occur if client is calling for help from perceived threat, which is usually seen in stage III of AWS.
Provide quiet environment. Speak in calm, quiet voice. Regulate lighting, as indicated. Turn off radio or TV during sleep.	Reduces external stimuli during hyperactive stage. Client may become more delirious when surroundings cannot be seen, but some respond better to quiet, darkened room.
Encourage SO to stay with client whenever possible.	Promotes recognition of caregivers and a sense of consistency, which may reduce fear.
Reorient frequently to person, place, time, and surrounding environment, as indicated.	May have a calming effect, and may provide a reorienting influence. May reduce confusion; prevent or limit misinterpretation of external stimuli.
Avoid bedside discussion about client or topics unrelated to the client that do not include the client.	Client may hear and misinterpret conversation, which can aggravate hallucinations.
Provide environmental safety as indicated; for example, place bed in low position, leave doors in full open or closed position, observe frequently, place call light/bell within reach, and remove articles that can harm client.	Client may have distorted sense of reality or be fearful or suicidal, requiring protection from self.
Collaborative	
Provide seclusion and restraints as necessary, adhering to facility policy regarding restraints.	Clients with excessive psychomotor activity, severe hallucinations, violent behavior, and/or suicidal gestures may respond better to seclusion. Restraints are usually ineffective and add to client's agitation but occasionally may be required to prevent self-harm.
Monitor laboratory studies such as electrolytes, magnesium levels, liver function studies, ammonia, BUN, glucose, and ABGs.	Changes in organ function may precipitate or potentiate sensory-perceptual deficits. Electrolyte imbalance is common. Liver function is often impaired in the chronic alcoholic, and ammonia intoxication can occur if the liver is unable to convert ammonia to urea. Ketoacidosis is sometimes present without glycosuria; however, hyperglycemia or hypoglycemia may occur, suggesting pancreatitis or impaired gluconeogenesis in the liver. Hypoxemia and hypercarbia are common manifestations in chronic alcoholics who are also heavy smokers.
Replace fluids and continue to monitor electrolytes (Riddle et al, 2010).	Alcohol induces diuresis leading to dehydration and electrolyte imbalances.
Administer medications, as indicated, for example:	
Anti-anxiety agents as indicated. (Refer to ND: Anxiety [severe/panic], following.)	Reduces hyperactivity, promoting relaxation and sleep. Drugs that have little effect on dreaming may be desired to allow dream recovery or rapid eye movement (REM) rebound to occur, which has previously been suppressed by alcohol use.
Thiamine, vitamins C and B complex, multivitamins, and Stresstabs	Vitamins may be depleted because of insufficient intake and malabsorption. Vitamin deficiency, especially thiamine, is associated with ataxia, loss of eye movement and pupillary response, palpitations, postural hypotension, and exertional dyspnea.

NURSING DIAGNOSIS: Anxiety [severe/panic]

May Be Related To
Exposure to toxins—alcohol intake
Situational crisis—hospitalization
Change in health status; threat to self-concept

Possibly Evidenced By
Restlessness; fidgeting; irritability
Increased tension; apprehension
Feelings of inadequacy; increased helplessness; tendency to blame others
Fear of unspecified consequences

(continues on page 810)

NURSING DIAGNOSIS: Anxiety [severe/panic] (continued)

Desired Outcomes/Evaluation Criteria—Client Will

Anxiety Self-Control (NOC)

Verbalize reduction of fear and anxiety to an acceptable and manageable level.

Express sense of regaining some control of situation and life.

Demonstrate problem-solving skills and use resources effectively.

ACTIONS/INTERVENTIONS	RATIONALE
Anxiety Reduction (NIC)	
Independent	
Identify cause of anxiety, involving client in the process. Explain that alcohol withdrawal increases anxiety and uneasiness. Reassess level of anxiety on an ongoing basis.	Persons in acute phase of withdrawal may be unable to identify and/or accept what is happening. Anxiety may be physiologically or environmentally caused. *Note:* Individuals with alcohol use disorders often also have post-traumatic stress disorder (PTSD) (U.S. Department of Veterans Affairs, 2011).
Develop a trusting relationship through frequent contact and being honest and nonjudgmental. Project an accepting attitude about alcoholism.	Provides client with a sense of humanness, helping to decrease paranoia and distrust. Client will be able to detect biased or condescending attitude of caregivers.
Inform client about what you plan to do and why. Include client in planning process and provide choices when possible.	Enhances sense of trust, and explanation may increase cooperation and reduce anxiety. Provides sense of control over self in circumstance where loss of control is a significant factor. *Note:* Feelings of self-worth are intensified when one is treated as a worthwhile person.
Reorient frequently. (Refer to ND: [disturbed Sensory Perception].)	Client may experience periods of confusion, resulting in increased anxiety.
Collaborative	
Administer medications, as indicated, for example:	
Benzodiazepines, such as chlordiazepoxide (Librium) and diazepam (Valium)	Anti-anxiety agents are given during acute withdrawal to help client relax, be less hyperactive, and feel more in control.
Barbiturates, such as phenobarbital, or possibly secobarbital (Seconal) or pentobarbital (Nembutal)	These drugs are sometimes used to treat or prevent alcohol withdrawal seizures but need to be used with caution because they are respiratory depressants and REM sleep cycle inhibitors.
Arrange "intervention" or confrontation in controlled setting, when client has recovered sufficiently from withdrawal to address addiction issues.	Process wherein SO and family members, supported by staff, provide information about how client's drinking and behavior have affected each one of them; helps client acknowledge that drinking is a problem and has resulted in current situational crisis.
Provide consultation or referral to detoxification or crisis center for ongoing treatment program as soon as medically stable (e.g., oriented to reality).	Client is more likely to contract for treatment while still hurting and experiencing fear and anxiety from last drinking episode. Motivation decreases as well-being increases and person again feels able to control the problem. Direct contact with available treatment resources provides realistic picture of help. Decreases time for client to "think about it," change mind, or restructure and strengthen denial systems.

POTENTIAL CONSIDERATIONS following acute care (dependent on client's age, physical condition and presence of complications, personal resources, and life responsibilities)

Refer to: Substance Use Disorders (SUDs) plan of care, and plans of care for any specific underlying medical condition(s).

Sample clinical pathway follows in Table 15.1.

TABLE 15.1 Sample CP: Alcohol Withdrawal Program. ELOS: 4 Days Behavioral Unit

ND and Categories of Care	Time Dimension	Goals/Actions	Time Dimension	Goals/Actions	Time Dimension	Goals/Actions
Risk for injury R/T biochemical dysfunction, balancing difficulties, seizure activity	Day 1	Verbalize understanding of safety concerns relative to individual needs	Day 3	Vital signs stable I&O balanced	Day D/C	Be free of injury resulting from ETOH withdrawal
		Cooperate with therapeutic regimen	Day 4	Display marked decrease in objective symptoms		Display no objective symptoms of withdrawal
Referrals	Day 1	RN-NP or MD If indicated: Internist Cardiologist Neurologist				
Diagnostic studies	Day 1	BA level Drug screen If indicated: CXR Pulse oximetry ECG	Day 2 Serum Mg, amylase	CMP 20 RPR UA	Day 4	Repeat of selected studies as indicated
Additional assessments	Day 1	VS, temp, respiratory status/breath sounds q4h	Day 2–3	VS q8h if stable	Day 4–D/C	VS gd
	Day 1–4	I&O q8h Motor activity, body language, verbalizations, need for/type of restraint				
	Ongoing	Withdrawal symptoms:				
	Stage I	Tremors, N/V, hypertension, tachycardia, diaphoresis, sleeplessness				
	Stage II	Increased hyperactivity, hallucinations, seizure activity				
	Stage III	Extreme autonomic hyperactivity, profound confusion, anxiety, fever				

(continues on page 812)

TABLE 15.1 Sample CP: Alcohol Withdrawal Program. ELOS: 4 Days Behavioral Unit (continued)

ND and Categories of Care	Time Dimension	Goals/Actions	Time Dimension	Goals/Actions	Time Dimension	Goals/Actions
Medications	Day 1	Librium 200 mg PO	Day 3	Librium 120 mg PO	Day D/C	Librium 40 mg PO
Allergies:	Day 1-D/C	Thiamine 100 mg IM				
________	Day 1–4	Thiamine 100 mg IM	Day 4	Librium 80 mg PO		
________	Day 2	Librium 160 mg PO				
Client education	Day 1	Orient to room/unit, schedule, procedures	Day 3–4	Need for ongoing therapy Goals/availability of AA program	Day D/C	Schedule of follow-up visits if indicated
Additional nursing actions	Day 1	Bedrest 12 hours if in withdrawal Position change, HOB elevated; C, DB exercises if on bedrest	Day 3–D/C	Activity as tolerated		
	Day 1–2	Assist with ambulation, self-care as needed Encourage fluids if free of N/V				
	Ongoing	Provide environmental safety measures, seizure precautions as indicated Reorient as needed				
Ineffective coping R/T situational crisis, inadequate level of confidence in ability to cope, inadequate social support	Day 1–D/C	Participate in development and evaluation of treatment plan	Day 3	Verbalize understanding of relationship of ETOH abuse to current situation	Day D/C	Plan in place to meet needs postdischarge
	Day 2–D/C	Interact in group sessions	Day 4	Identify/make contact with potential resources, support groups		
Referrals	Day 1 Day 2–D/C	Psychiatrist group sessions	Day 4	Community classes: Assertiveness training Stress management		
Additional assessments	Day 1	Understanding of current situation; drinking pattern, previous withdrawal; other drug use, attitudes toward substance use	Day 2–3	Previous coping strategies/consequences Perception of drug use on life, employment, legal issues		
		History of violence	Day 3–D/C	Congruency of actions based on insight		

	Day 1–2	Relationships with others: personal, work/school Readiness for group activities				
Medications					Day D/C	Naltrexone 50 mg/day if indicated
Client education	Day 1	Physical effects of ETOH abuse	Day 3–D/C	Human behavior and interactions with others	Day D/C	Medication dose, frequency, side effects
	Day 1–2	Types/use of relaxation techniques	Day 4–D/C	Community resources for self/family		Written instructions for therapeutic program
	Day 2	Consequences of ETOH abuse		Identify goals for change		
Additional nursing actions	Day 1–D/C	Support client's taking responsibility for own recovery Provide consistent approach/expectations for behavior Set limits/confront inappropriate behaviors	Day 2–D/C	Discuss alternative solutions Provide positive feedback for efforts Support during confrontation by peer group Encourage verbalization of feelings, personal reflection		
Imbalanced nutrition: less than body requirements R/T poor intake, effects of ETOH on digestive system, and hypermetabolic response to withdrawal; insufficient finances	Day 2–D/C	Select foods appropriately to meet individual dietary needs	Day 4	Verbalize understandings of effects of ETOH abuse and reduced dietary intake on nutritional status	Day D/C	Display stable weight or initial weight gain as appropriate, and laboratory results WNL
Referrals	Day 1 and prn	Dietitian				
Diagnostic studies	Day 1	CBC, liver function studies, random blood glucose Serum albumin, transferrin	Day 2–D/C	Fingerstick glucose prn		
Additional assessments	Day 1	Weight, skin turgor, condition of mucous membranes, muscle tone			Day D/C	Weight

(continues on page 814)

TABLE 15.1 Sample CP: Alcohol Withdrawal Program. ELOS: 4 Days Behavioral Unit (continued)

ND and Categories of Care	Time Dimension	Goals/Actions	Time Dimension	Goals/Actions	Time Dimension	Goals/Actions
	Day 1–2	Bowel sounds, characteristics of stools				
	Day 1–D/C	Appetite, dietary intake				
Medications	Day 1–D/C	Antacid ac and hs Imodium 2 mg prn	Day 2–D/C	Multivitamin 1 tab/qd		
Client education	Day 1–2	Individual nutritional needs	Day 4	Principles of nutrition, foods for maintenance of wellness		
Additional nursing actions	Day 1	Liquid/bland diet as tolerated				
	Day 1–D/C	Encourage small, frequent, nutritious meals/snacks Encourage good oral hygiene pc and hs	Day 2–D/C	Advance diet as tolerated		

Key: AA, Alcoholics Anonymous; ac, after meals; BA, blood alcohol; C, cough; CBC, complete blood count; CMP, comprehensive metabolic panel; CXR, chext x-ray; D/C, discharge; DM, diabetes mellitus; ECG, electrocardiogram; ELOS, estimated length of stay; ETOH, ethyl alcohol; HOB, head of bed; hs, hour of sleep; IM, intramuscular; I&O, intake and output; N/V, nausea and vomiting; pc, after meals; PO, by mouth; prn, as needed; q4h, every 4 hours; q8h, every 8 hours; qd, every day; RPR, rapid plasma reagin; R/T, related to; tab, tablet; UA, urinalysis; VS, vital signs; WNL, within normal limits.

SUBSTANCE USE DISORDERS (SUDs)

I. Pathophysiology

a. Considered a continuum of phases incorporating a cluster of cognitive, behavioral, and physiological symptoms, including loss of control over use of the substance and a continued use of the substance to reach a state of feeling high despite adverse consequences—effects on all body systems, relationship problems, financial difficulties, self- or other-directed violence, exposure to criminal element and activities, legal consequences

b. All commonly abused drugs stimulate the brain's limbic system, elevating dopamine levels and affecting level of alertness, perceptions, emotions, judgment, attention, movement, and sleep (Ali et al, 2013; Crews, 2011).

c. Prescription drug abuse is the fastest-growing type of drug abuse in the United States and deaths from prescription drugs is reaching epidemic proportions (Garcia, 2013; Phillips, 2013).

d. The following is a recently compiled list of commonly misused substances in descending order according to the number of people affected (National Institute on Drug Abuse [NIDA], 2013):

   i. Alcohol: An estimated 20 million adults in the United States abuse alcohol. P More than half of these alcoholics started drinking heavily when they were teenagers (American Academy of Child and Adolescent Psychiatry, 2012)

   ii. Bath Salts (synthetic cathinones): New family of drugs containing one or more man-made chemicals related to cathinone, an amphetamine-like stimulant found naturally in the khat plant. P Teens and young adults are gravitating to these easy-to-access drugs, as they incorrectly believe them to be legal and harmless (Lohmann, 2012).

   iii. Club Drugs: Includes methamphetamines (e.g., "speed, crystal, meth, crank"), methamphetamine-derivative methylenedioxymethamphetamine (MDMA, Ecstasy), and other stimulant drugs such as methylphenidate (Ritalin), phencyclidine (PCP), and ketamine (Special K). P Club drugs are not only popular in raves (all-night dance parties with loud, pounding music and flashing lights stimulating vigorous dancing) but are often used in other social settings frequented by adolescents and young adults (Dryden-Edwards, 2012).

   iv. Cocaine: The National Survey on Drug Use and Health (NSDUH) estimated in 2008 that there were 1.9 million current (past-month) cocaine users, of which approximately 359,000 were current crack users. Young adults aged 18 to 25 years have a higher rate of current cocaine use than any other age group (NIDA, 2010).

   v. Heroin: In 2011, 4.2 million Americans aged 12 or older had used heroin at least once in their lives. P Although heroin abuse has trended downward during the past several years, its prevalence is still higher than in the early 1990s, especially among school-age youth (NIDA, 2013).

   vi. Inhalants: Includes volatile solvents (e.g., paint thinner, nail-polish remover); aerosols (e.g., spray paint, hair or deodorant spray); gases (e.g., butane lighters, nitrous oxide [laughing gas]); and hydrocarbons (e.g., fluorinated hydrocarbons, found in whipped cream dispensers called "whippits"). P Data from national and state surveys suggest that inhalant abuse is most common among 7th through 9th graders (National Institute for Drug Abuse [NIDA] for Teens, 2012).

   vii. K2/Spice (also called synthetic marijuana, fake weed, Yucatan Fire, Skunk, Moon Rocks): Wide variety of herbal mixtures that produce experiences similar to marijuana. P Of the illicit drugs most used by high school seniors, K2 is secondary only to marijuana (NIDA, 2012).

   viii. LSD (acid) and other hallucinogens such as psilocybin (mushrooms, "shrooms"), phencyclidine (PCP): P In 2007, the National Survey on Drug Use and Health (NSDUH) states that approximately 1.1 million persons aged 12 or older reported using hallucinogens for the first time within the past 12 months (NIDA, 2009).

   ix. Marijuana (e.g., pot, grass, weed, reefer, mary jane):. P In 2012, 6.5% of 12th graders reported using marijuana daily, compared to 5.1% in 2007 (NIDA, 2012).

   x. Tobacco (street names for tobacco delivery methods include "smokes, cigs, chew, dip, snuff"): P In 2012, smoking was at historically low levels among young people, according to NIDA's Monitoring the Future study (reported as 4.9% for 8th graders and 17.1% for 12th graders) (NIDA, 2012).

   xi. Prescription drugs: In 2010, the National Institute on Drug Abuse reported that an estimated 52 million people (20% of those aged 12 and older) have used prescription drugs for nonmedical reasons at least once in their lifetimes. P Young people are strongly represented in using this group of drugs (NIDA, 2013 and 2010), which include:

      1. Opioids, such as fentanyl (Duragesic), hydrocodone (Vicodin), oxycodone (OxyContin, Percocet), oxymorphone (Opana), propoxyphene (Darvon), hydromophone (Dilaudid), meperidine (Demerol), morphine (Kadian, Avenza), diphenoxylate (Lomotil).
      2. Central nervous system (CNS) depressants, such as pentobarbital sodium (Nembutal), diazepam (Valium), alprazolam (Xanax).
      3. Stimulants such as dextroamphetamine (Dexedrine), methylphenidate (Ritalin and Concerta), amphetamines (Adderall).

II. Etiology

a. No single theory developed to date explains condition.

b. Multiple predisposing factors implicated in abuse of substances (Claros, 2012)

   i. Biological—genetic predisposition, chronic pain, illness, trauma

   ii. Biochemical—properties of psychoactive drugs, individual's higher threshold for central nervous system (CNS) effects

   iii. Psychological—depression; psychosis (Charles, 2010); personality traits including isolation, low self-esteem, passivity, impulsivity, sexual immaturity, lack of emotional intelligence (Claros, 2012); comorbidity with schizophrenia in 50% of cases (Bridgman, 2013)

   iv. Sociocultural—unstable home environment, disturbed relationship with parental figures, peer or group pressure, conditioning, availability of substance, childhood sexual abuse (Sartor et al, 2013)

(continues on page 816)

v. Cultural and ethnic influences—attitudes toward alcohol or drug use, expectation that substance can safely relieve distress

III. Statistics

a. Morbidity: Excessive alcohol use, either in the form of heavy drinking or binge drinking, occurs in approximately 15% of the U.S. population in 2010 (Centers for Disease Control and Prevention [CDC], 2010). That same year, illicit drugs with the highest levels of past-year dependence or abuse were marijuana (an estimated 4.5 million people), pain relievers (1.9 million), and cocaine (1 million) (Center for Behavioral Health Statistics and Quality [CBHSQ], 2011). In 2011, there were 5.1 million drug-related emergency department (ED) visits; about one-half (49%) were attributed to drug misuse or abuse. Among visits involving drug misuse or abuse, 1.4 million visits involved pharmaceuticals and 1.3 million involved illicit drugs (Substance Abuse and Mental Health Services Administration [SAMHSA], 2011). Only 11.2% of people who were found to need substance use treatment received such treatment in a specialty facility (CBHSQ, 2011).

b. Mortality: In 2011, 40,239 persons died of drug-induced causes in the United States, which includes deaths from use of either legal or illegal drugs and poisoning from medically prescribed and other drugs (Hoyert, 2012).

c. Cost: According to a survey published in 2011 by the U.S. Department of Justice, use of illicit drugs in 2007 (the most recent year for which data were available) cost $11 billion for healthcare and more than $193 billion overall, with the majority share attributable to lost productivity (Department of Justice [DOJ], 2011).

GLOSSARY

Addiction: Chronic relapsing brain disorder characterized by compulsive drug seeking and use and by long-lasting chemical changes in the brain.

ATOD: Stands for alcohol, tobacco and other drug—acronym used for addressing substance use in interviews.

CAGE Screening tool: A questionnaire focusing on individual's attempts to Cut down on drinking (or drug use), Annoyance with criticism from others regarding use, Guilt about substance use, and using alcohol (or drug) as an Eye opener or to counter negative effects of withdrawal.

Compulsive: Type of behavior a person exhibits that is overpowering, repeated, and, often, irrational.

Craving: Powerful desire for a substance that cannot be ignored.

Detoxification: Medically supervised treatment for alcohol or drug addiction designed to purge the body of intoxicating or addictive substances.

Dual diagnosis: Co-occurring mental illness and substance abuse.

Enabling: Doing for the client what he or she needs to do for self—rescuing. Due to shame and fear, significant others (SOs) and family member(s) often allow the drug or alcohol user to continue disruptive, irrational behavior patterns.

Harm reduction: Program that accepts the reality of drug use while attempting to reduce its harmful consequences to individuals and society. An example could be a "clean-needle program" for intravenous (IV) drug users.

Peer support: Structured relationship in which people meet to provide or exchange emotional support with others facing similar challenges. Peer-to-peer groups, such as Alcoholics Anonymous (AA), Narcotics Anonymous (NA), Smart Recovery, and online forums.

Substance use disorder (SUD): Condition that is used to describe a person dependent on or abusing alcohol and/or drugs, including the nonmedical use of prescription drugs.

Care Setting

Client is treated inpatient on behavioral unit or outpatient in a day program or community agency.

Related Concerns

Alcohol: acute withdrawal, page 800
Psychosocial aspects of care, page 729

Client Assessment Database

Data depend on substances involved, duration of use, and organs affected.

MAY REPORT	MAY EXHIBIT
ADDITIONAL DATA REQUIREMENTS • Family issues—discipline, conflict, attitudes • Peer and individual—the individual's delinquency, perception of risk, friends' attitudes and use of substances • (P) Adolescent children are at high risk for drug abuse due to incomplete brain development, which may lead to poor decision making and risk-taking (Winters, 2011).	• Family issues—communication • Community—availability of substances, attitudes regarding use • Work or school—attendance, performance or grades • Risk-taking behaviors
TEACHING/LEARNING • ***Discharge plan considerations:*** May need assistance with long-range plan for recovery ➧ Refer to section at end of plan for postdischarge considerations.	

Diagnostic Studies

TEST WHY IT IS DONE	WHAT IT TELLS ME
DRUG SCREENS	
• ***Drug screens:*** Serum, urine, saliva, sweat, and/or hair may be tested.	Identifies drug(s) being used, including usual drugs of abuse—alcohol, heroin, marijuana, cocaine, and inhalants.
• ***Screening for use or relapse:*** Variety of tools may be used, such as Alcohol Use Disorders Identification Test (AUDIT), CAGE survey, Drug Abuse Screening Test (DAST), and brief Michigan Alcoholism Screening Test (BMAST).	Useful in determining patterns reflecting social, vocational, or family problems associated with alcohol intake or abuse of other drugs. MAST has a geriatric version and (P) DAST has an adolescent version.
• ***Addiction Severity Index (ASI) assessment tool:*** Produces a "problem severity profile" of the client, including chemical, medical, psychological, legal, family and social, and employment and support aspects.	Reveals treatment needs and areas to be addressed.
• ***Other screening studies (e.g., hepatitis, HIV, tuberculosis [TB]):*** Depends on general condition, individual risk factors, and care setting.	Reveals organ involvement and presence of comorbidities.

Nursing Priorities

1. Provide support for decision to stop substance use and harm reduction.
2. Strengthen individual coping skills.
3. Facilitate learning of new ways to reduce anxiety.
4. Promote family involvement in rehabilitation program.
5. Facilitate family growth and development.
6. Provide information about condition, prognosis, and treatment needs.

Discharge Goals

1. Responsibility for own life and behavior assumed.
2. Plan to maintain substance-free life formulated.
3. Family relationships and enabling issues being addressed.
4. Treatment program successfully begun.
5. Condition, prognosis, and therapeutic regimen understood.
6. Plan in place to meet needs after discharge.

NURSING DIAGNOSIS: ineffective Denial

May Be Related To

Anxiety; threat of unpleasant reality
Lack of competency in using effective coping mechanisms
Lack of control of life situation

Possibly Evidenced By

Delays in seeking or refuses healthcare attention; minimizes symptoms
Unable to admit impact of condition on life pattern
Makes dismissive comments or gestures when speaking of distressing events

Desired Outcomes/Evaluation Criteria—Client Will

Acceptance: Health Status (NOC)
Verbalize awareness of relationship of substance use to current situation.
Engage in therapeutic program.
Verbalize acceptance of responsibility for own behavior.

ACTIONS/INTERVENTIONS	RATIONALE
Behavior Modification (NIC) ***Independent***	
(P) Ask client (including pediatric client) about alcohol, tobacco, and other drug (ATOD) use at each contact.	Although client may deny or minimize actions, healthcare provider can open the door to obtaining help and treatment for client by asking broad questions in initial interview. (P) *Note:* In one study of underage drinking, 1 in 4 seventh graders reported drinking (MA Youth Alcohol Prevention Task Force, 2002). In 2012, 6.5% of 8th graders, 17.0% of

(continues on page 818)

ACTIONS/INTERVENTIONS (continued)	RATIONALE (continued)
	10th graders, and 22.9% of 12th graders used marijuana in the past month. This source also reported that in 2012, 14.8% of high school seniors used a prescription drug nonmedically in the past year (National Institute on Drug Abuse, 2012).
Convey attitude of acceptance, separating individual from unacceptable behavior.	Promotes feelings of dignity and self-worth.
Ascertain reason for beginning abstinence and involvement in therapy.	Provides insight into client's willingness to commit to long-term behavioral change and whether client even believes that he or she can change. *Note:* Denial is one of the strongest and most resistant manifestations of SUD. The decision to quit is an important step to success in therapy.
Review definition of drug dependence and use with categories of symptoms, including risk factors, patterns of use, impairment caused by use, tolerance to substance.	This information helps client make decisions regarding acceptance of problem and treatment choices. P *Note*: The risk of becoming a drug abuser involves the relationship among the number and type of risk factors (e.g., deviant attitudes and behaviors) and protective factors (e.g., parental support). Early intervention with risk factors (e.g., aggressive behavior and poor self-control) often has a greater impact than later intervention by changing a child's life path (trajectory) away from problems and toward positive behaviors (Hawkins et al, 2008).
Answer questions honestly and provide factual information. Keep your word when agreements are made.	Creates trust, which is the basis of the therapeutic relationship.
Provide information about addictive use versus experimental, occasional use; biochemical and genetic disorder theory—genetic predisposition, use activated by environment; and compulsive desire.	Progression of use continuum ranges from experimental or recreational to addictive use. Comprehending this process is important in combating denial. Education may relieve client's guilt and blame and may help awareness of recurring addictive characteristics.
Discuss current life situation and impact of substance use.	First step in decreasing use of denial is for client to see the relationship between substance use and personal problems.
Confront and examine denial and rationalization in peer group. Use confrontation with caring attitude.	Because denial is the major defense mechanism in addictive disease, confrontation by peers can help the client accept the reality of adverse consequences of behaviors and that drug use is a major problem. Caring attitude preserves self-concept and helps decrease defensive response.
Provide information regarding effects of addiction on mood and personality.	Individuals often mistake effects of addiction and use this to justify or excuse drug use.
Remain nonjudgmental. Be alert to changes in behavior such as restlessness and increased tension.	Confrontation can lead to increased agitation, which may compromise safety of client and staff.
Provide positive feedback for expressing awareness of denial in self and others.	Necessary to enhance self-esteem and to reinforce insight into behavior.
Maintain firm expectation that client attends recovery support and therapy groups regularly.	Attendance is related to admitting need for help; to working with denial; and for maintaining long-term, substance-free existence.
Encourage and support client's taking responsibility for own recovery, such as development of alternative behaviors to drug urge and use. Assist client to learn own responsibility for recovering.	Denial can be replaced with positive action when client accepts the reality of own responsibility.
Be aware of own enabling behaviors. Understand professional boundaries needed to be therapeutic with client experiencing a SUD (Tsai et al, 2010).	Caregiving lends itself to "taking care" of clients that can backfire in substance abuse treatment.

NURSING DIAGNOSIS: ineffective Coping

May Be Related To

Situational crisis; uncertainty
Inadequate level of confidence in ability to cope
Inadequate social support created by characteristics of relationships

Possibly evidenced by

Inadequate problem-solving; lack of resolution of problem
Use of forms of coping that impede adaptive behavior
Destructive behavior toward self; substance abuse
Reports inability to cope or ask for help

NURSING DIAGNOSIS: ineffective Coping (continued)

Desired Outcomes/Evaluation Criteria—Client Will

Substance Addiction Consequences (NOC)
Identify consequences of using substance as a method of coping.

Coping (NOC)
Identify other ineffective coping behaviors.
Engage in effective coping skills and problem-solving.
Initiate necessary lifestyle changes.

ACTIONS/INTERVENTIONS	RATIONALE
Substance Use Treatment (NIC)	
Independent	
Review program rules and philosophy expectations.	Having information provides opportunity for client to cooperate and function as a member of the group or milieu, enhancing sense of control and sense of success.
Determine understanding of current situation and previous or other methods of coping with life's problems.	Provides information about degree of denial, acceptance of personal responsibility and commitment to change; identifies coping skills that may be used in present situation.
Set limits and confront efforts to get caregiver to grant special privileges, making excuses for not following through on agreed-upon behaviors, and attempting to continue drug use. Avoid use of labels, such as lying.	Client has learned manipulative behavior throughout life and needs to learn a new way of getting needs met. Following through on consequences of failure to maintain limits can help the client to change ineffective behaviors. Use of labels promotes negative attitudes that can impede therapeutic relationships.
Be aware of staff attitudes, feelings, and enabling behaviors.	Lack of understanding and judgmental or enabling behaviors can result in inaccurate data collection and nontherapeutic approaches.
Encourage verbalization of feelings, fears, and anxiety.	May help client begin to come to terms with long-unresolved issues.
Explore alternative coping strategies.	Client may have little or no knowledge of adaptive responses to stress and needs to learn other options for managing time, feelings, and relationships without drugs.
Assist client to learn and encourage use of relaxation skills, guided imagery, and visualizations.	Helps client relax and develop new ways to deal with stress and to problem-solve.
Structure diversional activity that relates to recovery such as social activity within support group, wherein issues of being chemically free are examined.	Discovery of alternative methods of coping with drug hunger can remind client that addiction is a lifelong process and opportunity for changing patterns is available.
Use peer support to examine ways of coping with drug hunger.	Self-help groups, such as Alcoholics Anonymous (AA), Narcotics Anonymous (NA), and Crystal Methamphetamine Anonymous (CMA), are valuable for learning and promoting abstinence in each member by using understanding and support as well as peer pressure.
Identify possible and actual triggers for relapse. Encourage client to use the acronym HALT—"Am I hungry, angry, lonely, or tired?"	Employment and financial stressors, isolation, unhealthy relationships, being around substance-using friends, hearing certain songs, premenstrual syndrome—the list of possibilities depends on the individual. Being aware of the triggers provides an opportunity to plan for ways to avoid and deal with them.
Encourage involvement in therapeutic writing. Have client begin journaling or writing autobiography.	Therapeutic writing or journaling can enhance participation in treatment; serves as a release for grief, anger, and stress; provides a useful tool for monitoring client's safety; and can be used to evaluate client's progress. Autobiographical activity provides an opportunity for client to remember and identify sequence of events in his or her life that relate to current situation.
Discuss client's plans for living without drugs.	Provides opportunity to develop and refine plans. Devising a comprehensive strategy for avoiding relapses helps client into maintenance phase of behavioral change.
Collaborative	
Administer medications, as indicated, for example:	
Disulfiram (Antabuse)	This drug can be helpful in maintaining abstinence from alcohol while other therapy is undertaken. By inhibiting alcohol oxidation, the drug leads to an accumulation of acetaldehyde with a highly unpleasant reaction if alcohol is consumed.

(continues on page 820)

ACTIONS/INTERVENTIONS (continued)	RATIONALE (continued)
Metronidazole (Flagyl)	Increasingly used to maintain abstinence from alcohol instead of Antabuse. It has the same gastrointestinal (GI) distress effects but fewer cardiac concerns and lower cost.
Acamprosate (Campral EC)	Helps prevent relapses in alcoholism by lowering receptors for the excitatory neurotransmitter glutamate. This agent may become drug of choice because it does not make the user sick if alcohol is consumed; it has no sedative, anti-anxiety, muscle-relaxant, or antidepressant properties and produces no withdrawal symptoms.
Buprenorphine (Buprex, Subutex, Suboxone)	Used in the treatment of opioid addiction. At low doses it produces sufficient agonist effect to enable opioid-addicted individuals to discontinue the misuse of opioids without experiencing withdrawal symptoms. This drug carries a lower risk of abuse, dependence, and side effects compared to full opioid agonists (Liberto, 2013).
Methadone (Dolophine) and levo-acetymethadol (LAAM)	Methadone is thought to blunt the craving for or diminish the effects of opioids and is used to assist in withdrawal and long-term maintenance programs. It can allow the individual to maintain daily activities and ultimately withdraw from drug use. LAAM, a long-acting synthetic μ agonist, is an effective alternative to methadone maintenance and only has to be taken three times a week. Harm reduction needs to be considered versus the possibility of exchanging one addiction for another (Tetrault, 2012).
Naltrexone (Trexan) and nalmefine (Revex).	Used to suppress craving for opioids and may help prevent relapse in the client abusing alcohol. Current research suggests that naltrexone suppresses urge to continue drinking by interfering with alcohol-induced release of endorphins (Tetrault, 2012).
Encourage involvement with self-help associations such as AA, NA, or CMA.	Puts client in direct contact with support system necessary for managing sobriety and drug-free life.
Refer to community or social resources such as housing assistance, employment agencies, childcare, food stamps, or alternative schooling.	Dealing with life problems in a proactive way enhances coping abilities, reduces sense of isolation and hopelessness, and decreases risk of relapse.

NURSING DIAGNOSIS: Powerlessness

May Be Related To

Unsatisfactory interpersonal interactions
Illness-related regimen

Possibly Evidenced By

Reports lack of control
[Constantly thinking about drug and/or obtaining drug]

Desired Outcomes/Evaluation Criteria—Client Will

Health Beliefs: Perceived Threat (NOC)

Admit inability to control drug habit and surrender to powerlessness over addiction.
Verbalize acceptance of need for treatment and awareness that willpower alone cannot control abstinence.

Acceptance: Health Status (NOC)

Demonstrate active participation in program.
Regain and maintain healthy state with a drug-free lifestyle.

ACTIONS/INTERVENTIONS	RATIONALE
Self-Responsibility Facilitation (NIC)	
Independent	
Use crisis intervention techniques to initiate behavior changes:	May need to use emergency commitments or other legal holds for the client's safety. Client may be more amenable to acceptance of need for treatment at this time.
Assist client to recognize problem exists. Discuss in a caring, nonjudgmental manner how drug has interfered with life.	In the precontemplation phase, the client has not yet identified that drug use is problematic. While client is hurting, it is easier to admit substance use has created negative consequences.

ACTIONS/INTERVENTIONS (continued)	RATIONALE (continued)
Involve client in development of treatment plan, using problem-solving process in which client identifies goals for change and agrees to desired outcomes.	During the contemplation phase, the client realizes a problem exists and is thinking about a change of behavior. The client is committed to the outcomes when the decision-making process involves solutions that are promulgated by the individual.
Discuss alternative solutions.	Brainstorming helps creatively identify possibilities and provides sense of control. During the preparation phase, minor action may be taken as individual organizes resources for definitive change.
Assist in selecting most appropriate alternative.	As possibilities are discussed, the most useful solution becomes clear.
Support decision and implementation of selected alternative(s).	Helps the client persevere in process of change. During the action phase, the client engages in a sustained effort to maintain sobriety and mechanisms are put in place to support abstinence.
Explore support in peer group. Encourage sharing about drug hunger, situations that increase the desire to indulge, and ways that substance has influenced life.	Client may need assistance in expressing self, speaking about powerlessness, and admitting need for help in order to face up to problem and begin resolution.
Assist client to learn ways to enhance health and structure healthy diversion from drug use, including maintaining a balanced diet; getting adequate rest; exercise such as walking; slow or long distance running; and acupuncture, biofeedback, or deep meditative techniques.	Learning to empower self in constructive areas can strengthen ability to continue recovery. These activities help restore natural biochemical balance; aid detoxification; and manage stress, anxiety, and use of free time. These diversions can increase self-confidence, thereby improving self-esteem. *Note:* Exercise promotes release of endorphins, creating a feeling of well-being.
Provide information regarding understanding of human behavior and interactions with others, such as transactional analysis.	Understanding these concepts can help the client to begin to deal with past problems and losses and prevent repeating ineffective coping behaviors and self-fulfilling prophecies.
Assist client in self-examination of spirituality and faith.	Although not mandatory for recovery, surrendering to and faith in a power greater than oneself has been found to be effective for many individuals in substance recovery; may decrease sense of powerlessness.
Instruct in and role-play assertive communication skills.	Effective in helping refrain from use, to stop contact with users and dealers, to build healthy relationships, and to regain control of own life.
Provide treatment information on an ongoing basis.	Helps client know what to expect, and creates opportunity for client to be a part of what is happening and make informed choices about participation and outcomes.
Collaborative	
Refer to, or assist with making contact with, programs for ongoing treatment needs—partial hospitalization drug treatment programs, NA, AA, CMA, or peer support groups.	Continuing treatment is essential to positive outcome. Follow-through may be easier once initial contact has been made.

NURSING DIAGNOSIS: imbalanced Nutrition: less than body requirements

May Be Related To
Insufficient dietary intake—psychological, physiological, or insufficient finances

Possibly Evidenced By
Weight loss; body weight below norm for height and body build
Reports altered taste sensation; food intake less than recommended daily allowance; lack of interest in food
Poor muscle tone; sore buccal cavity
[Laboratory evidence of protein and vitamin deficiencies]

Desired Outcomes/Evaluation Criteria—Client Will

Nutritional Status (NOC)
Demonstrate progressive weight gain toward goal with normalization of laboratory values and absence of signs of malnutrition.

Knowledge: Treatment Regimen (NOC)
Verbalize understanding of effects of substance abuse and reduced dietary intake on nutritional status.
Demonstrate behaviors or lifestyle changes to regain and maintain appropriate weight.

ACTIONS/INTERVENTIONS	RATIONALE
Nutrition Therapy (NIC)	
Independent	
Assess height, weight, age, body build, strength, and activity and rest levels. Note condition of oral cavity.	Provides information on which to base individual caloric needs and dietary plan. Type of foods may be affected by condition of mucous membranes and teeth.
Take anthropometric measurements, such as midarm muscle circumference, triceps skinfold, and percentage of body fat, when available.	Calculates subcutaneous fat and muscle mass to aid in determining dietary needs.
Note total daily calorie intake. Recommend client maintain a diary of intake, as well as times and patterns of eating.	Information will help identify nutritional deficiencies.
Evaluate energy expenditure (e.g., pacing or sedentary), and establish an individualized exercise program.	Activity level affects nutritional needs. Exercise enhances muscle tone and may stimulate appetite.
Provide opportunity to choose foods and snacks to meet dietary plan.	Enhances sense of control, may promote resolution of nutritional deficiencies, and helps evaluate client's understanding of dietary teaching.
Recommend monitoring weight weekly.	Provides information regarding effectiveness of dietary plan.
Collaborative	
Consult with dietitian.	Useful in establishing individual dietary needs and plan, and provides additional resource for learning.
Review laboratory studies as indicated, such as glucose, serum albumin or prealbumin, and electrolytes.	Identifies anemias, electrolyte imbalances, and other abnormalities that may be present, requiring specific therapy.
Refer for dental consultation as necessary.	Teeth are essential to good nutritional intake, and oral hygiene and dental care are often a neglected area in this population.

NURSING DIAGNOSIS: chronic low Self-Esteem

May Be Related To

Repeated failures, negative reinforcement
Perceived lack of respect from others, lack of belonging
Perceived discrepancy between self and cultural norms

Possibly Evidenced By

Evaluation of self as unable to deal with events
Frequent lack of success in life events
Rejects positive feedback about self
Reports feelings of guilt, shame

Desired Outcomes/Evaluation Criteria—Client Will

Self-Esteem (NOC)

Identify feelings and underlying dynamics for negative perception of self.
Verbalize acceptance of self as is and an increased sense of self-worth.
Set goals and participate in realistic planning for lifestyle changes necessary to live without drugs.

ACTIONS/INTERVENTIONS	RATIONALE
Self-Esteem Enhancement (NIC)	
Independent	
Provide opportunity for and encourage verbalization and discussion of individual situation.	Client often has difficulty expressing self, even more difficulty accepting the degree of importance substance has assumed in life and its relationship to present situation.
Assess mental status. Note presence of other psychiatric disorders.	Many clients use substances in an attempt to obtain relief from depression or anxiety, which may predate use and/or be the result of substance use. Approximately 60% of substance-dependent clients have underlying psychological problems or a dual diagnosis, and treatment for both is imperative to achieve and maintain abstinence.
Spend time with client. Discuss client's behavior and use of substance in a nonjudgmental way.	The nurse's presence conveys acceptance of the individual as a worthwhile person.
Provide grief counseling, as indicated.	Discussion provides opportunity for insight into the problems substance abuse has created for the client. Life losses secondary to alcohol or other drug use problems need to be addressed to enable client to move forward with rehabilitation.

ACTIONS/INTERVENTIONS (continued)	RATIONALE (continued)
Provide reinforcement for positive actions and encourage client to accept this input.	Failure and lack of self-esteem have been problems for this client, who needs to learn to accept self as an individual with positive attributes.
Observe family interactions and SO dynamics and level of support.	Substance abuse is a family disease, and how the members act and react to the client's behavior affects the course of the disease and how client sees self. Many unconsciously become "enablers," helping the individual to cover up the consequences of the abuse. (Refer to ND: dysfunctional Family Processes, following.)
Encourage expression of feelings of guilt, shame, and anger.	The client often has lost respect for self and believes that the situation is hopeless. Expression of these feelings helps client begin to accept responsibility for self and take steps to make changes.
Help client acknowledge that substance use is the problem and that problems can be dealt with without the use of drugs. Confront the use of defenses—denial, projection, and rationalization.	When drugs can no longer be blamed for the problems that exist, client can begin to deal with the problems and live without substance use. Confrontation helps client accept the reality of the problems as they exist.
Ask client to list and review past accomplishments and positive happenings.	There are things in everyone's life that have been successful. Often when self-esteem is low, it is difficult to remember these successes or to view them as successes.
Use techniques of role rehearsal.	Assists client to practice developing skills to cope with new role as a person who no longer uses or needs drugs to handle life's problems.
Collaborative	
Involve client in group therapy.	Group sharing helps encourage verbalization because other members of the group are in various stages of abstinence from drugs and can address the client's concerns or denial. The client can gain new skills, hope, and a sense of family or community from group participation.
Formulate plan to treat other mental illness problems.	Clients who seek relief for other mental health problems through drugs will continue to do so once discharged. Both the substance use and the mental health problems need to be treated together to maximize abstinence potential. Treatment may be difficult because of difficulty of taking initiative, thinking realistically, and problem-solving. Behavioral methods seem to be most helpful.
Administer antipsychotic medications, such as quetiapine (Seroquel) or olanzapine (Zyprexa or Zydis), as necessary.	Prolonged or profound psychosis following lysergic acid diethylamide (LSD) or phencyclidine (PCP) use can be treated with these drugs because it is probably the result of an underlying functional psychosis that has now emerged. Methamphetamine psychosis often does not reverse. *Note:* Avoid the use of phenothiazines because they may decrease seizure threshold and cause hypotension in the presence of LSD or PCP use.
Monitor for diabetes, weight gain, and dyslipidemia.	Atypical antipsychotics (e.g., Zyprexa) are associated with these effects and should be monitored closely for changes in glucose control. Measurement of fasting blood glucose at the beginning of therapy and periodical monitoring during therapy are recommended.

NURSING DIAGNOSIS: dysfunctional Family Processes

May Be Related To

Substance abuse; addictive personality
Family history of substance abuse, resistance to treatment
Addictive personality
Inadequate coping skills; lack of problem-solving skills

Possibly Evidenced By

Feelings: anxiety, anger, suppressed rage, shame, embarrassment, emotional isolation, loneliness, vulnerability, repressed emotions
Roles and responsibilities: disturbed family dynamics, closed communication systems, ineffective spouse communication, marital problems, altered role function, disrupted family roles
Behavioral: manipulation, dependency, criticizing, rationalization, denial of problems, enabling maintenance of substance abuse pattern, refusal to get help, inability to accept help or receive help appropriately

(continues on page 824)

NURSING DIAGNOSIS: dysfunctional Family Processes (continued)

Desired Outcomes/Evaluation Criteria—Family Will

Family Coping (NOC)

Verbalize understanding of dynamics of enabling behaviors.
Participate in individual family programs.
Identify ineffective coping behaviors and consequences.
Initiate and plan for necessary lifestyle changes.
Take action to change self-destructive behaviors and alter behaviors that contribute to partner's/SO's addiction.

ACTIONS/INTERVENTIONS	RATIONALE
Substance Use Treatment (NIC) *Independent*	
Review family history and explore roles of family members, circumstances involving drug use, strengths, and areas for growth.	Determines areas for focus and potential for change.
Explore how the SO has coped with the client's habit—use of denial, repression, rationalization, projection, feelings of hurt, and loneliness.	The person who enables also suffers from the same feelings as the client and uses ineffective methods for dealing with the situation, necessitating help in learning new, more effective coping skills.
Determine understanding of current situation and previous methods of coping with life's problems.	Provides information on which to base present plan of care.
Assess current level of functioning of family members.	Affects individual's ability to cope with situation.
Determine extent of enabling behaviors being evidenced by family members and explore with each individual and client.	People want to be helpful and do not want to feel powerless to help their loved one stop substance use and change the behavior that is so destructive. However, the substance user often relies on others to rescue them by covering up own inability to cope with daily responsibilities.
Provide information about enabling behavior, addictive disease characteristics for both user and nonuser.	Awareness and knowledge of behaviors such as avoiding and shielding, taking over responsibilities, rationalizing, and subserving provide opportunity for individuals to begin the process of change.
Identify and discuss sabotage behaviors of family members.	Even though family member(s) may verbalize a desire for the individual to become substance-free, the reality of interactive dynamics is that they may unconsciously not want the individual to recover because this would affect their own role in the relationship. Additionally, they may receive sympathy and attention from others—secondary gain.
Encourage participation in therapeutic writing, such as journaling (narrative) or guided or focused writing.	Serves as a release for feelings such as anger, grief, and stress and helps move individuals forward in treatment process.
Provide factual information to client and family about the effects of addictive behaviors on the family and what to expect after discharge.	Many clients and SOs are not aware of the nature of addiction. If client is using legally obtained drugs, he or she may believe this does not constitute abuse.
Encourage family members to be aware of their own feelings and look at the situation with perspective and objectivity. They can ask themselves, "Am I being conned? Am I acting out of fear, shame, guilt, or anger? Do I have a need to control?"	When the enabling family members become aware of their own actions that perpetuate the addict's problems, they need to decide to change themselves. If they change, the client can then face the consequences of his or her own actions and may choose to get well.
Provide support for enabling partner(s). Encourage group work.	Families and SOs need support to produce change as much as the person who is addicted.
Assist the client's partner to become aware that client's abstinence and drug use are not the partner's responsibility.	Partners need to learn that user's habit may or may not change despite partner's involvement in treatment.
Help the recovering partner who is enabling to distinguish between destructive aspects of behavior and genuine motivation to aid the user.	Enabling behavior can be partner's attempts at personal survival.
Note how partner relates to the treatment team.	Determines enabling style. A parallel exists between how partner relates to user and to staff, based on partner's feelings about self and situation.
Explore conflicting feelings the enabling partner may have about treatment, such as feelings similar to those of abuser—blend of anger, guilt, fear, exhaustion, embarrassment, loneliness, distrust, grief, and possibly relief.	Useful in establishing the need for therapy for the partner. This individual's own identity may have been lost; she or he may fear self-disclosure to staff and may have difficulty giving up the dependent relationship.
Involve family in discharge referral plans.	Drug abuse is a family illness. Because the family has been so involved in dealing with the substance use behavior, family members need help adjusting to the new behavior of sobriety

ACTIONS/INTERVENTIONS (continued)	RATIONALE (continued)
	and abstinence. Incidence of recovery is almost doubled when the family is treated along with the client.
Be aware of staff's enabling behaviors and feelings about client and enabling partners.	Lack of understanding of enabling can result in nontherapeutic approaches to clients and their families.
Collaborative	
Involve in substance abuse prevention or treatment plan, as indicated.	Can be voluntary, court ordered, or via the Department of Human Services (DHS) involvement. (P) Prevention programs should address all forms of drug use, alone or in combination, including the underage use of legal drugs (e.g., tobacco or alcohol); the use of illegal drugs (e.g., marijuana [real and counterfeit (such as 9K2, Spice)], meth, cocaine, other designer drugs, including Ecstasy); and the inappropriate use of legally obtained substances (e.g., inhalants), prescription medications, or over-the-counter drugs (Johnston, 2002).
Encourage involvement with self-help associations, AA or NA, Al-Anon, Alateen, and professional family therapy.	Puts client and family in direct contact with support systems necessary for continued sobriety and to assist with problem resolution.

NURSING DIAGNOSIS: Sexual Dysfunction

May Be Related To

Altered body function (e.g., neurological damage, debilitating effects of drug use—particularly alcohol and opiates)

Possibly Evidenced By

Verbalization of problem
Inability to achieve desired satisfaction

Desired Outcomes/Evaluation Criteria—Client Will

Substance Addiction Consequences (NOC)
Verbally acknowledge effects of drug use on sexual functioning and reproduction.

Sexual Functioning (NOC)
Identify interventions to correct and overcome individual situation.

ACTIONS/INTERVENTIONS	RATIONALE
Sexual Counseling (NIC)	
Independent	
Ascertain client's beliefs and expectations. Have client describe problem in own words.	Determines level of knowledge, identifies misperceptions, level of concern regarding sexually transmitted infections (STIs), level of risk reduction, and specific learning needs.
Encourage and accept individual expressions of concern.	Most people find it difficult to talk about this sensitive subject and may not ask directly for information.
Provide educational opportunities such as pamphlets or consultation with appropriate persons regarding effects of drug on sexual functioning.	Much of denial and hesitancy to seek treatment may be reduced as a result of sufficient and appropriate information.
Provide information about individual's condition.	Sexual functioning may have been affected by the drug itself and/or by psychological factors, such as stress or depression. Information can assist client to understand own situation and identify actions to be taken.
Assess drinking and drug history of pregnant client. Provide information about effects of substance abuse on the reproductive system and fetus, including increased risk of premature birth, brain damage, and fetal malformation.	Awareness of the negative effects of alcohol and other drugs on reproduction may motivate client to stop using substance. When client is pregnant, identification of potential problems aids in identifying concerns and planning for future fetal needs.
Discuss prognosis for sexual dysfunction, such as impotence or low sexual desire.	Impotence may be reversed with abstinence from drug(s) for many individuals; however, for some erectile dysfunction will be permanent.
Collaborative	
Refer for sexual counseling, if indicated.	Couple may need additional assistance to resolve more severe problems or situations. Client may have difficulty adjusting if drug has improved sexual experience, such as heroin,

(continues on page 826)

ACTIONS/INTERVENTIONS (continued)	RATIONALE (continued)
	which decreases dyspareunia in women and premature ejaculation in men. Furthermore, the client may have engaged enjoyably in bizarre, erotic sexual behavior under influence of the stimulant drug; client may have found no substitute for the drug, may have driven a partner away, and may have no motivation to adjust to sexual experience without drugs.
Review results of sonogram if pregnant.	Assesses fetal growth and development to identify possibility of fetal alcohol syndrome or other harmful drug effects and future needs. There are concerns about placental abruption with the use of methamphetamine and cocaine.

NURSING DIAGNOSIS: deficient Knowledge [Learning Need] regarding condition, prognosis, treatment, self-care, and discharge needs

May Be Related To

Lack of information, information misinterpretation, lack of recall
Cognitive limitation

Possibly Evidenced By

Reports the problem
Inaccurate follow-through of instructions
Inappropriate behavior (e.g., hostile, apathetic)

Desired Outcomes/Evaluation Criteria—Client Will

Knowledge: Substance Abuse Control (NOC)

Verbalize understanding of own condition or disease process, prognosis, and potential complications.
Verbalize understanding of therapeutic needs.
Identify and initiate necessary lifestyle changes to remain drug-free.
Participate in treatment program including plan for follow-up and long-term care.

ACTIONS/INTERVENTIONS	RATIONALE
Learning Facilitation (NIC)	
Independent	
Be aware of and deal with anxiety of client and family members.	Anxiety can interfere with ability to hear and assimilate information.
Provide an active role for the client and SO in the learning process using discussions, group participation, and role-playing.	Learning is enhanced when persons are actively involved.
Provide written and verbal information as indicated. Include list of articles, books, Internet resources, and special TV programs related to client and family needs and encourage reading and discussing what they learn.	Helps client and SO make informed choices about future and can be a useful addition to other therapeutic approaches.
Assess client's knowledge of own situation, including disease process, prognosis, complications, and needed changes in lifestyle.	Assists in planning for long-range changes necessary for maintaining sobriety and drug-free status. Client may have street knowledge of the drug but be ignorant of medical facts.
Pace learning activities to individual needs.	Facilitates learning because information is more readily assimilated when timing is considered.
Teaching: Disease Process (NIC)	
Review condition, prognosis, and future expectations.	Provides knowledge base from which client can make informed choices.
Discuss relationship of drug use to current situation.	Often client has misperception or denial of real reason for admission to the medical or psychiatric care setting.
Educate about effects of specific drug(s) used; for example, PCP is deposited in body fat and may reactivate, causing flashbacks even after long interval of abstinence; alcohol use may result in mental deterioration and liver involvement or damage; cocaine can damage postcapillary vessels and increase platelet aggregation, promoting thromboses and infarction of skin or internal organs, causing localized atrophie blanche or sclerodermatous lesions.	Information will help client understand possible long-term effects of drug use.

ACTIONS/INTERVENTIONS (continued)	RATIONALE (continued)
Discuss potential for reemergence of withdrawal symptoms in stimulant abuse as early as 3 months or as late as 9 to 12 months after discontinuing use.	Even though intoxication may have passed, client may manifest denial, drug hunger, and periods of "flare-up," wherein there is a delayed recurrence of withdrawal symptoms such as anxiety, depression, irritability, sleep disturbance, or compulsiveness with food, especially sugars.
Inform client of effects of disulfiram (Antabuse) in combination with alcohol intake and importance of avoiding use of alcohol-containing products such as cough syrups, foods, candy, mouthwash, aftershave, and cologne.	Interaction of alcohol and Antabuse results in nausea and hypotension, which may produce fatal shock. Individuals on Antabuse are sensitive to alcohol on a continuum, with some being able to drink while taking the drug and others having a reaction with only slight exposure. Reactions also appear to be dose related.
Review specific aftercare needs; for example, PCP user should drink cranberry juice and continue use of ascorbic acid; alcohol abuser with liver damage should refrain from drugs, anesthetics, or use of household cleaning products that are detoxified in the liver.	Promotes individualized care related to specific situation. Cranberry juice and ascorbic acid enhance clearance of PCP from the system. Substances that have the potential for liver damage are more dangerous in the presence of an already damaged liver.
Discuss variety of helpful organizations and programs that are available for assistance or referral such as AA, Dual Recovery Anonymous (DRA), or NA.	Long-term support is necessary to maintain optimal recovery. Psychosocial needs and other issues may need to be addressed.

POTENTIAL CONSIDERATIONS following acute care (dependent on client's age, physical condition and presence of complications, personal resources, and life responsibilities)

- ***ineffective Self-Health Management/ineffective family Therapeutic Regimen Management***—decisional conflicts, excessive demands made on individual or family, family conflict, perceived seriousness/benefits
- ***ineffective Coping***—situational crises, inadequate level of confidence in ability to cope, inadequate level of perception of control
- ***readiness for enhanced family Coping***—significant person moves in direction of health promotion, chooses experiences that optimize wellness

Physical needs depend on substance effect on organ systems—refer to appropriate medical plans of care for additional considerations.

CANCER—GENERAL CONSIDERATIONS

I. Pathophysiology

a. General term describing a disturbance of cellular growth and referring to a group of 150 different known diseases or types
b. Genetic and genomic factors underlie the etiology of all cancer. The alteration of genes manifests in abnormal cellular proliferation. Genes and genomic alterations often occur due to multifactorial genetic, infectious, radiation, environmental, hormonal, or lifestyle factors (Santos et al, 2013).
c. The metastatic behavior or "natural history" of cancer varies according to the primary site of diagnosis—metastatic pattern for primary breast cancer may be from the breast to the bone, lung, liver, and/or brain.

II. Classification

a. Four main classifications of cancer according to tissue type:
   i. Lymphomas: cancers originating in infection-fighting organs
   ii. Leukemias: cancers originating in blood-forming organs
   iii. Sarcomas: cancers originating in bones, muscle, or connective tissue
   iv. Carcinomas: cancers originating in epithelial cells
b. Within these broad categories, a cancer is classified by histology, stage, and grade (tumor profiling).

III. Etiology

a. Cellular disease that can arise from any body tissue with manifestations that result from failure to control the proliferation and maturation of cells
b. Multiple risk factors or cancer-causing agents:
   i. Chemicals
   ii. Radiation
   iii. Viruses
   iv. Human behaviors and lifestyles that affect cancer risk
   v. Tobacco use
   vi. Poor nutrition
   vii. Inactivity, obesity
   viii. Sun exposure
   ix. Workplace or occupational exposure
   x. Pollution—air, water, soil
c. Biological factors that may increase or reduce risk:
   i. Inflammation
   ii. DNA repair mechanisms
   iii. Immunologic responses
   iv. Heredity
      1. 75% of cancers are sporadic or manifest in one body organ at an expected age.
      2. 10% to 15% are familial, or two or more siblings are diagnosed with the same cancer at a specific age.
      3. 5% to 10% of cancers are hereditary or the result of a single gene expression (Santos et al., 2013).

IV. Statistics

a. Morbidity: In 2011, the American Cancer Society (ACS) projected 1,660,290 new cancer cases in the United States. In 2010, cancer was the first-listed diagnosis in 1.2 million

(continues on page 828)

hospital discharges (Centers for Disease Control and Prevention [CDC], 2010).

b. Mortality: In 2011, there were an estimated 575,313 deaths from all types of cancers in the United States (Hoyert, 2012).

c. Cost: In a study released January 2011, researchers at the National Cancer Institute put the total direct medical costs for all cancers in 2010 at $124.5 billion, projecting direct costs to reach at least $158 billion by 2020.

GLOSSARY

Adenocarcinoma: Cancer arising in gland-forming tissue. An example is breast cancer.

Adjuvant therapy: Treatment given in addition to the primary treatment.

Alopecia: Hair loss.

Biotherapy: Treatment to boost or restore the ability of the immune system to fight cancer. Also used to decrease the side effects caused by some cancer treatments. Agents used in biotherapy include monoclonal antibodies, growth factors, and vaccines.

Cachexia: Loss of body weight and muscle mass as a result of anorexia, nausea and vomiting, or hypermetabolism.

Cancer-related fatigue (CRF): Persistent and subjective sense of tiredness that can occur with cancer or cancer treatment, which interferes with usual functioning and can drastically affect the client's quality of life.

Carcinogen: Any substance that causes cancer.

Carcinoma: Cancer that begins in the lining or covering of an organ.

Desquamation: Shedding of the skin as a reaction to radiotherapy. In its mildest form, it is "dry" when the skin flakes in a powdery form. In a more severe form ("wet"), the deeper layers of the skin are exposed.

Genome: The expanded study of genetics that no longer focuses on specific genes but on a person's entire genetic content and interacting factors that regulate or modify gene expression (Santos et al, 2013).

Holistic Needs Assessment (HNA): Specific terminology to describe assessing all aspects of the life of a client diagnosed with cancer (Taylor, 2012). In the United States, this term is synonymous with palliative needs assessment.

Metastasis: Spread of cancer to another organ, usually through the bloodstream.

Mucositis: A complication of some cancer therapies in which the lining of the digestive system becomes inflamed; often seen as sores in the mouth.

Nadir: Period of time following chemotherapy treatment when blood counts generally are at their lowest levels and client is at greatest risk of developing infection and other blood-related side effects.

Palliative care: "An approach that improves the quality of life of patients and their families facing the problems associated with life-limiting illness, through the prevention and relief of suffering by means of early identification and impeccable assessment and treatment of pain and other problems, physical, psychosocial and spiritual"(World Health Organization [WHO], 2002).

Peripheral progenitor cell (stem cell) transplant: Method of replacing blood-forming cells destroyed by cancer treatment. Immature blood cells (stem cells) in the circulating blood that are similar to those in the bone marrow are given to the client after treatment.

Radiation dermatitis: Skin condition that is a common side effect of radiation therapy. The affected skin becomes painful, red, itchy, and blistered.

Staging: Classification of the primary tumor (T), lymph node involvement (N), combined with tests to see if the cancer has metastasized (M).

Stomatitis: Inflammation of the mucous membranes of the mouth.

Superior vena cava syndrome (SVCS): Condition in which a tumor presses against the superior vena cava—the large vein that carries blood from the head, neck, arms, and chest to the heart. This pressure blocks blood flow to the heart and may cause coughing; difficulty in breathing; and swelling of the face, neck, and upper arms.

Tumor: An abnormal mass of tissue, either benign (noncancerous) or malignant (cancerous).

Tumor marker: Substance detectable in the blood or urine that suggests the presence of cancer.

Vein flare: Painless local allergic reaction identified by redness along the vein used to infuse chemotherapeutic agent; urticaria or hives may also be present. Usually subsides within 30 to 60 minutes without treatment.

Weight-related distress (WDR) and/or eating-related distress (ERD): Syndrome, common in advanced cancer, and characterized by resistance to eating, poor and capricious appetite, a disconnection of oral intake and ability to gain weight, or continuous efforts to eat. The client's SOs may have feelings of deep concern, frustration, and insufficiency in their efforts to prepare appealing food and be more concerned about client's weight loss than is the client (also sometimes known as "anorexia-cachexia syndrome") (Hopkinson, 2013; Strasser et al, 2007).

Care Setting

Cancer centers may focus on staging and major treatment modalities for complex cancers. Treatment for managing adverse effects, such as malnutrition and infection, may take place in short-stay, ambulatory, or community setting. More cancer clients are receiving care at home because of personal choice and healthcare costs. P Cancer treatment needs to be age and life-stage appropriate. Over 70% of children diagnosed with cancer mature into adulthood and present with special nursing needs (McInally, 2013).

Related Concerns

Adult leukemias, page 484
End-of-life care/hospice, page 848
Hysterectomy, page 581
Lung cancer: postoperative care, page 141
Lymphomas, page 494
Mastectomy, page 589
Pediatric considerations, page 872
Prostatectomy, page 566
Psychosocial aspects of care, page 729
Sepsis/septicemia, page 665
Total nutritional support: parenteral/enteral feeding, page 437
Urinary diversions/urostomy (postoperative care), page 548

Client Assessment Database

Data depend on organs or tissues involved and stage of disease. A holistic needs assessment (HNA) should be completed for every client/family diagnosed with cancer to prioritize care (Taylor, 2012). Refer to appropriate plans of care for additional assessment information.

DIAGNOSTIC DIVISION MAY REPORT	MAY EXHIBIT
ACTIVITY/REST	
• Weakness and fatigue (most prevelant problems reported by clients with advanced cancer) (Girgis et al, 2006) • Changes in rest pattern and usual hours of sleep per night • Presence of factors affecting sleep, such as pain, anxiety, night sweats, more frequent elimination needs • Limitations of participation in hobbies, exercise, usual activities	• Inability to maintain usual routines or desired level of activity or work • Lack of energy • Disinterest in surroundings • Compromised concentration
CIRCULATION	
• Palpitations • Chest pain on exertion	• Changes in blood pressure (BP) • Fluctuations in heart rate
EGO INTEGRITY	
• Stress factors—financial, job, role changes • Ways of handling stress—smoking, drinking, delay in seeking treatment, religious or spiritual crisis • Concern about changes in body image (e.g., alopecia, disfiguring lesions, surgery, profound weight loss, edema, weight gain, or rash) • Denial of diagnosis • Feelings of powerlessness, hopelessness, helplessness, worthlessness, guilt, loss of control • Eating-related distress (ERD) or weight-related distress (WRD): Client and caregivers may express feelings of frustration, hopelessness, pressure, failure to meet exceptions (Hopkinson, 2013; Strasser et al, 2007).	• Denial, withdrawal, anger • Depression
ELIMINATION	
• Changes in bowel pattern—blood in stools, pain with defecation, constipation, or diarrhea • Changes in urinary elimination—pain or burning on urination, hematuria, frequent urination or nocturia	• Changes in bowel sounds • Abdominal distention • Diarrhea • Dysuria, frequency, incontinence

(continues on page 830)

DIAGNOSTIC DIVISION MAY REPORT (continued)	MAY EXHIBIT (continued)
FOOD/FLUID • Poor dietary habits, • Anorexia, resistance to eating, poor or capricious appetite (ERD, WRD) • Altered sense of taste • Nausea and vomiting • Difficulty swallowing, mouth sores • Food intolerances	• Changes in weight, severe weight loss, cachexia • Wasting of muscle mass • Changes in skin moisture or turgor • Edema • Ulcerations of oral mucosa
NEUROSENSORY • Dizziness, syncope • Lack of coordination, unstable balance • Numbness or tingling of extremities • Sensation of coldness • Difficulty performing fine motor skills such as buttoning shirt	

PAIN/DISCOMFORT
• Varying degrees of pain from mild discomfort to severe pain. Younger age (<65) may be associated with a higher prevalence of pain and may also be associated with severity of pain (Girgis et al, 2006).
• Pain localized in a specific area
• Quality or description
  • Stabbing, throbbing, dull, aching (somatic pain often present with surgery or metastases in bone)
  • Pressure-like, cramping, gnawing, squeezing—visceral pain that may be referred from one site to another
  • Sharp, burning, shooting pain; may be accompanied by numbness and tingling in extremities—neuropathic pain caused from damage to nervous system
	• Guarding behaviors, positioning to avoid pain
	• Facial mask
	• Sleep disturbance
	• Restlessness, moaning, crying, irritability, lethargy
	• Self-focusing; narrowed focus
	• Reduced interaction with others
	• Depression

RESPIRATION • Dyspnea with exertion • History of chronic respiratory disease • Smoking—tobacco, marijuana • Living with someone who smokes • Asbestos or dust exposure—coal, sandstone, silica, and the like	
SAFETY • Occupational, professional, or environmental exposure to toxic chemicals, carcinogens • Excessive or prolonged sun exposure	• Skin rashes, ulcerations • Dry, leather-like skin
SEXUALITY • Sexual concerns such as impact on relationship, change in level of satisfaction, impotence, menopausal symptoms • Nulligravida greater than 30 years of age, multigravida • Multiple sex partners, early sexual activity, genital herpes • Exposure to human papillomavirus (HPV)	
SOCIAL INTERACTION • Inadequate or weak support system • Marital history regarding in-home satisfaction, support, or help • Concerns about role function and responsibility	

DIAGNOSTIC DIVISION MAY REPORT (continued)	MAY EXHIBIT (continued)
TEACHING/LEARNING • Family history of cancer, for example, multiple family members—mother, grandmother, aunt, or sister—with breast cancer (Santos et al, 2013) • Primary site, date discovered or diagnosed • Metastatic disease—additional sites involved (if none, natural history of primary will provide important information for looking for metastasis) • Treatment history—previous treatment for cancer—place and treatments given	
DISCHARGE PLAN CONSIDERATIONS • May require assistance with finances, medications, treatments, wound care and supplies, transportation, food shopping and preparation, self-care, homemaker or maintenance tasks, provision for child care, changes in living facilities, or hospice ➧ Refer to section at end of plan for postdischarge considerations.	

Diagnostic Studies

Test selection depends on history, clinical manifestations, and index of suspicion for a particular cancer.

TEST WHY IT IS DONE	WHAT IT TELLS ME
BLOOD TESTS	
• ***Tumor markers:*** Substances produced and secreted by tumor cells and found in serum; for example, carcinoembryonic antigen (CEA), prostate-specific antigen (PSA), (-fetoprotein (AFP), human chorionic gonadotropin (hCG), CA15-3, CA19-9, and CA125.	Helpful in diagnosing cancer but more useful as prognostic indicator and/or therapeutic monitor. For example, CA125 levels are monitored in ovarian cancer, with levels often high prior to surgery but should be lower after surgery or with a response to chemotherapy. If the cancer begins to grow, the CA125 level will usually begin to increase before any other signs or symptoms are evident.
• ***Hormone receptors:*** Estrogen and progesterone receptor assay done on breast tissue.	Provides information about whether or not hormonal manipulation can be therapeutic in breast cancer treatment.
• ***Her-2/neu amplification:*** Cellular proto-oncogene that stimulates cell growth.	Amplification (a large number of these receptors found on the cell surface) results in more aggressive breast cancers and, usually, a worse prognosis with earlier appearance of metastatic disease.
• ***Gene mutations:*** BRCA-1 and BRCA-2 function as tumor suppressor genes.	If these genes are mutated, there may be an increased lifetime risk of acquiring breast, ovarian, prostatic, and possibly other cancers.
• ***Immunohistochemistry (IHC) tumor profiling:*** Staining of cells/biopsied tissues with specific antibodies.	IHC is helpful in determining the stage and grade of a tumor, as well as cell type and origin of metastasis to identify primary site (American Cancer Society, 2013).
• ***Complete blood count (CBC):*** Battery of screening tests, which typically includes hemoglobin (Hgb); hematocrit (Hct); red blood cell (RBC) count, morphology, indices, and distribution width index; platelet count and size; and white blood cell (WBC) count and differential.	May reveal anemia, changes in RBCs and WBCs, and reduced or increased platelets.
OTHER DIAGNOSTIC STUDIES	
• ***Scans—magnetic resonance imaging (MRI), computed tomography (CT), positron emission tomography (PET), or ultrasound:*** May be done for diagnostic purposes, identification of metastasis, and evaluation of response to treatment.	Knowledge of the etiology and natural history or pattern of metastasis of a cancer type is important in planning the client's care and in evaluating the client's progress, prognosis, and physical complaints.
• ***Biopsy—fine-needle aspiration (FNA), needle core, incisional or excisional:*** May be taken from various sites, such as bone marrow (e.g., leukemia), skin, or organ.	Differentiates diagnosis and delineates treatment options.

Nursing Priorities

1. Support adaptation and independence.
2. Promote comfort.
3. Maintain optimal physiological functioning.
4. Prevent complications.
5. Provide information about disease process, condition, prognosis, and treatment needs.

Discharge Goals

1. Dealing with current situation realistically.
2. Pain alleviated or controlled.
3. Homeostasis achieved.
4. Complications prevented or minimized.
5. Disease process, condition, prognosis, and therapeutic choices and regimen understood.
6. Plan in place to meet needs after discharge.

NURSING DIAGNOSIS: Fear/Anxiety [specify level]

May Be Related To

Situational crisis
Threat to, or change in, health status, economic status, role function, interaction patterns
Threat of death
Separation from support systems in potentially stressful situation (e.g., hospitalization, procedures)
Interpersonal transmission or contagion of feelings

Possibly Evidenced By

Increased tension, shakiness; apprehension, distressed, fear
Reports concerns due to changes in life events; restlessness, insomnia
Feelings of inadequacy
Changes in BP, pulse, respirations

Desired Outcomes/Evaluation Criteria—Client Will

Fear [or] Anxiety Self-Control (NOC)

Display appropriate range of feelings and lessened fear.
Appear relaxed and report anxiety is reduced to a manageable level.
Demonstrate use of effective coping mechanisms and active participation in treatment regimen.

ACTIONS/INTERVENTIONS	RATIONALE
Anxiety Reduction (NIC)	
Independent	
Review client's and significant other's (SO's) previous experience with cancer. Determine what the doctor has told client and what conclusion client has reached.	Clarifies client's perceptions; assists in identification of fear(s) and misconceptions based on diagnosis and experience with cancer.
Encourage client to share thoughts and feelings.	Provides opportunity to examine realistic fears and misconceptions about diagnosis.
Provide open environment in which client feels safe to discuss feelings or to refrain from talking.	Helps client feel accepted in present condition without feeling judged and promotes sense of dignity and control.
Maintain frequent contact with client. Talk with and touch client, as appropriate.	Provides assurance that the client is not alone or rejected; conveys respect for and acceptance of the person, fostering trust.
Be aware of effects of isolation on client when required by immunosuppression or radiation implant. Limit use of isolation clothing, as possible.	Sensory deprivation may result when sufficient stimulation is not available and may intensify feelings of anxiety, fear, and alienation.
Assist client and SO in recognizing and clarifying fears to begin developing coping strategies for dealing with these fears.	Coping skills are often stressed after diagnosis and during different phases of treatment. Support and counseling are often necessary to enable individual to recognize and deal with fear and to realize that control and coping strategies are available.
Provide accurate, consistent information regarding diagnosis and prognosis. Avoid arguing about client's perceptions of situation.	Can reduce anxiety and enable client to make decisions and choices based on realities.
Permit expressions of anger, fear, and despair without confrontation. Give information that feelings are normal and are to be appropriately expressed.	Acceptance of feelings allows client to begin to deal with situation.
Explain the recommended treatment, its purpose, and potential side effects. Help client prepare for treatments.	The goal of cancer treatment is to destroy malignant cells while minimizing damage to normal ones. Treatment may include curative, preventive, or palliative surgery as well as chemotherapy, internal or external radiation, or newer, organ-specific treatments such as whole-body

ACTIONS/INTERVENTIONS (continued)	RATIONALE (continued)
	hyperthermia or biotherapy. Bone marrow or peripheral progenitor cell transplant may be recommended for some types of cancer.
Explain procedures, providing opportunity for questions and honest answers. Stay with client during anxiety-producing procedures and consultations.	Accurate information allows client to deal more effectively with reality of situation, thereby reducing anxiety and fear of the unknown.
Provide primary and consistent caregivers whenever possible.	May help reduce anxiety by fostering therapeutic relationship and facilitating continuity of care.
Provide calm, quiet environment.	Facilitates rest, conserves energy, and may enhance coping abilities.
Identify stage and degree of grief client and SO are currently experiencing. (Refer to ND: Grieving, following.)	Choice of interventions is dictated by stage of grief and negative coping behaviors, such as anger, withdrawal, and denial.
Note ineffective coping such as poor social interactions, helplessness, giving up everyday functions and usual sources of gratification.	Identifies individual problems and provides support for client and SO in using effective coping skills. *Note:* Studies have found that clients with unmet needs in physical symptom control, occupational functioning, nutrition, sleep, and personal care demonstrate higher symptom distress and psychological distress (Girgis et al, 2006).
Be alert to signs of denial or depression, such as withdrawal and anger or making inappropriate remarks. Determine presence of suicidal ideation and assess potential on a scale of 1 to 10.	Client may use defense mechanism of denial and express hope that diagnosis is inaccurate. Feelings of guilt, spiritual distress, physical symptoms, or lack of cure may cause the client to become withdrawn and believe that suicide is a viable alternative.
Encourage and foster client interaction with support systems, including counselors, spiritual leader, and local cancer resources.	Reduces feelings of isolation. If family support systems are not available, outside sources may be needed immediately.
Provide reliable and consistent information and support for SO.	Allows for better interpersonal interaction and reduction of anxiety and fear.
Include SO as indicated and client desires when major decisions are to be made.	Provides a support system for the client and allows the SO to be involved appropriately.
Collaborative	
Administer anti-anxiety medications, such as lorazepam (Ativan) or alprazolam (Xanax), as indicated.	May be useful for brief periods of time to help client handle feelings of anxiety related to diagnosis or situation during periods of high stress, to assist client with diagnostic procedures, such as lying still during scan, and/or to minimize nausea.
Refer to additional resources for counseling and support as needed.	May be useful from time to time to assist client and SO in dealing with anxiety.

NURSING DIAGNOSIS: Grieving

May Be Related To
Anticipated loss of significant object—body part and processes of body
Potential of death

Possibly Evidenced By
Psychological distress; suffering
Alteration in activity level; disturbed sleep pattern
Despair; anger; blame

Desired Outcomes/Evaluation Criteria—Client Will

Grief Resolution (NOC)
Identify and express feelings appropriately.
Continue normal life activities, looking toward and planning for the future, one day at a time.
Verbalize reality and acceptance of situation.

ACTIONS/INTERVENTIONS	RATIONALE
Grief Work Facilitation (NIC)	
Independent	
Expect initial shock and disbelief following diagnosis of cancer and/or traumatizing procedures such as disfiguring surgery, colostomy, and amputation.	Few clients are fully prepared for the reality of the changes that can occur.
Assess client and SO for stage of grief currently being experienced. Explain process, as appropriate.	Knowledge about the grieving process reinforces the normalcy of feelings and reactions being experienced, helping client deal more effectively with them.
Provide open, nonjudgmental environment. Use therapeutic communication skills of active-listening, acknowledgment, and so on.	Promotes and encourages realistic dialogue about feelings and concerns.
Encourage verbalization of thoughts and concerns, accepting expressions of sadness, anger, and rejection. Acknowledge normalcy of these feelings.	Client may feel supported in expression of feelings by the understanding that deep and often conflicting emotions are normal and experienced by others in this difficult situation.
Be aware of mood swings, evidence of conflict, expressions of anger or hostility, and other acting-out behavior. Set limits on inappropriate behavior and redirect negative thinking.	May be client's way of expressing or dealing with feelings of despair and spiritual distress, reflecting ineffective coping and need for additional interventions. Preventing destructive actions enables client to maintain control and sense of self-esteem.
Note signs of debilitating depression. Ask client direct questions about state of mind. Listen for statements of despair, guilt, and hopelessness, such as "There's nothing to live for."	Studies show that clients with physical illnesses are at higher risk for suicide (Taur et al, 2013; Aiello-Laws, 2010). They are especially vulnerable when recently diagnosed and/or discharged from hospital.
Reinforce teaching regarding disease process and treatments. Be honest; do not give false hope while providing emotional support.	Client and SO benefit from factual information. Honest answers promote trust and provide reassurance that correct information will be given.
Review past life experiences, role changes, and coping skills.	Opportunity to identify skills that may help individuals cope with grief of current situation more effectively.
Hope Instillation (NIC)	
Identify positive aspects of the situation.	Possibility of remission and slow progression of disease and/or new therapies can offer hope for the future.
Discuss ways client and SO can plan together for the future. Encourage setting of realistic goals.	Having a part in problem-solving and planning can provide a sense of control over anticipated events.
Assist client and SO to identify strengths in self, situation, and support systems.	Recognizing these resources provides opportunity to work through feelings of grief.
Encourage participation in care and treatment decisions.	Allows client to retain some control over life.
Refer to appropriate counselor as needed, such as psychiatric clinical nurse specialist, social worker, hospice counselor, psychologist, and clergy.	Can help alleviate distress or palliate feelings of grief to facilitate coping and foster growth.
Collaborative	
Refer to visiting nurse, home health agency as needed, or hospice program, if appropriate.	Provides support in meeting physical and emotional needs of client and SO and can supplement the care family and friends are able to give.

Refer to CP: End-of-life care/hospice; ND: Grieving/Death Anxiety for additional interventions.

NURSING DIAGNOSIS: risk for situational low Self-Esteem

May Be Related To

Physical illness
Disturbed body image; functional impairment
Decreased control over environment

Possibly Evidenced By

(Not applicable; presence of signs and symptoms establishes an *actual* diagnosis)

Desired Outcomes/Evaluation Criteria—Client Will

Self-Esteem (NOC)

Verbalize understanding of body changes, acceptance of self in situation.
Begin to develop coping mechanisms to deal effectively with problems.
Demonstrate adaptation to changes and events that have occurred as evidenced by setting of realistic goals and active participation in work, play, and personal relationships, as appropriate.

ACTIONS/INTERVENTIONS	RATIONALE
Chemotherapy [or] Radiation Therapy Management (NIC)	
Independent	
Discuss with client and SO how the diagnosis and treatment are affecting the client's personal life and home and work activities.	Aids in defining concerns to begin problem-solving process.
Review anticipated side effects associated with a particular treatment, such as alopecia or disfiguring surgery, including possible effects on sexual activity and sense of attractiveness or desirability. Tell client that not all side effects occur and that others may be minimized.	Anticipatory guidance can help client and SO begin the process of adaptation to new state and to prepare for some side effects, such as buying a wig before radiation and scheduling time off from work, as indicated. (Refer to ND: risk for Sexual Dysfunction.)
Prechemotherapy group sessions led by nurses are improving client and family cancer treatment experiences and outcomes.	Group information sessions ensure consistent information is provided and establishes an early support system for clients and families (Sullivan et al, 2013).
Encourage discussion of and problem-solve concerns about effects of cancer or cancer treatments on role as homemaker, wage earner, or parent.	May help reduce problems that interfere with acceptance of treatment or aggravate progression of disease.
Acknowledge difficulties client may be experiencing. Give information that counseling is often necessary and important in the adaptation process.	Validates reality of client's feelings and gives permission to take whatever measures are necessary to cope with what is happening.
Evaluate support structures available to and used by client and SO.	Helps with planning for care while hospitalized and after discharge.
Provide emotional support for client and SO during diagnostic tests and treatment phase.	Although some clients adjust to cancer effects or side effects of therapy, many need additional support during this period.
Use touch during interactions, if acceptable to client, and maintain eye contact.	Affirmation of individuality and acceptance is important in reducing client's feelings of insecurity and self-doubt.
Collaborative	
Refer client and SO to supportive group programs, such as I Can Cope, Reach to Recovery, Man to Man Prostate Cancer Group, or Leukemia/Lymphoma Society.	Group support is usually very beneficial for both client and SO, providing contact with other clients with cancer at various levels of treatment and/or recovery, validating feelings, and assisting with problem-solving.
Refer for professional counseling as indicated.	May be necessary to regain and maintain a positive psychosocial structure if client and SO support systems are deteriorating.

NURSING DIAGNOSIS: acute/chronic Pain

May Be Related To

Physical agents (e.g., compression or destruction of nerve tissue, infiltration of nerves or their vascular supply, obstruction of a nerve pathway, inflammation, metastasis to bones)

Chemical agent (e.g., chemotherapy, radiation therapy)

Possibly Evidenced By

Verbal/coded report of pain

Expressive behaviors—restlessness, irritability; positioning to avoid pain

Self-focus; narrowed focus

Changes in vital signs (acute pain)

Desired Outcomes/Evaluation Criteria—Client Will

Pain Level (NOC)

Report maximal pain relief or control with minimal interference with activities of daily living (ADLs).

Pain Control (NOC)

Follow prescribed pharmacological regimen.

Demonstrate use of relaxation skills and diversional activities as indicated for individual situation.

ACTIONS/INTERVENTIONS	RATIONALE
Pain Management (NIC)	
Independent	
Determine pain history, for example, location of pain, frequency, duration, and intensity using a rating scale (scale of 0 to 10) or verbal rating scale—"no pain" to "excruciating pain"—and relief measures used. Believe client's report.	Information provides baseline data to evaluate need for, and effectiveness of, interventions. Pain of more than 6 months' duration constitutes chronic pain, which may affect therapeutic choices. Recurrent episodes of acute pain can occur within chronic pain, requiring increased level of intervention. *Note:* The pain experience is an individualized one composed of both physical and emotional responses.
Determine timing and precipitants of "breakthrough" pain when using around-the-clock agents, whether oral, intravenous (IV), topical, transmucosal, epidural, or patch medications.	Pain may occur near the end of the dose interval, indicating need for higher dose or shorter dose interval. Pain may be precipitated by identifiable triggers or occur spontaneously, requiring use of short half-life agents for rescue or supplemental doses.
Evaluate painful effects of particular therapies, such as surgery, radiation, chemotherapy, or biotherapy. Provide information to client and SO about what to expect.	A wide range of discomforts are common, such as incisional pain, burning skin, low back pain, mouth sores, or headaches, depending on the procedure or agent being used. Pain is also associated with invasive procedures to diagnose or treat cancer.
Provide nonpharmacological comfort measures, such as massage, repositioning, and back rub, as well as diversional activities, such as music, reading, and TV.	Promotes relaxation and helps refocus attention.
Encourage use of stress management skills and complementary therapies, such as relaxation techniques, visualization, guided imagery, biofeedback, laughter, music, aromatherapy, and Therapeutic Touch.	Enables client to participate actively in nondrug treatment of pain and enhances sense of control. Pain produces stress and, in conjunction with muscle tension and internal stressors, increases client's focus on self, which in turn increases the level of pain.
Provide cutaneous stimulation, such as heat and cold packs, or massage.	May decrease inflammation, muscle spasms, reducing associated pain.
Be aware of barriers to cancer pain management related to client as well as to the healthcare system.	Clients may be reluctant to report pain for reasons such as fear that disease is worse; worry about unmanageable side effects of pain medications; belief that pain has meaning, such as "God wills it," and they should overcome it; or that pain is merited or deserved for some reason. Healthcare system problems include factors such as inadequate assessment of pain, concern about controlled substances or client addiction, inadequate reimbursement, and cost of treatment modalities.
Evaluate pain relief at regular intervals. Adjust medication regimen as necessary.	Goal is maximum pain control with minimum interference with ADLs.
Inform client and SO of the expected therapeutic effects and discuss management of side effects.	This information helps establish realistic expectations and confidence in own ability to handle what happens.
Collaborative	
Discuss use of alternative or complementary therapies, such as acupuncture, if client desires.	May provide reduction or relief of pain without drug-related side effects.
Develop individualized pain-management plan with the client and physician. Provide written copy of plan to client, family and SO, and care providers.	An organized plan beginning with the simplest dosage schedules and least invasive modalities improves chance for pain control. Particularly with chronic pain, client and SO must be active participants in pain management, and all care providers need to be consistent.
Administer analgesics, as indicated, for example:	A wide range of analgesics and associated agents may be employed around the clock to manage pain. *Note:* Addiction to or dependency on drug is not a concern.
Opioids such as codeine, morphine (MSContin, Kadian), oxycodone (oxycontin), hydrocodone (Vicodin), hydromorphone (Dilaudid), methadone (Dolophine), fentanyl (Duragesic, Actiq, Fentora), or oxymorphone (Numorphan, Opana)	Effective for localized and generalized moderate to severe pain, with long-acting or controlled-release forms available. Routes of administration include oral; transmucosal; transdermal; nasal; rectal; and subcutaneous, IV, epidural, and intrathecal infusions, which may be delivered via patient-controlled analgesia (PCA). Fentanyl citrate (Oralet) is available as a transmucosal agent that is absorbed through the mucosa of the inner cheek. *Note:* Intramuscular (IM) route is not recommended for pain medications because absorption is not reliable, in addition to being painful and inconvenient.
Acetaminophen (Tylenol) and NSAIDs, including aspirin, ibuprofen (Motrin, Advil), peroxicam (Feldene), or indomethacin (Indocin)	Adjuvant drugs are useful for mild to moderate pain and can be combined with opioid and other modalities.

ACTIONS/INTERVENTIONS (continued)	RATIONALE (continued)
Neuraxial techniques (intrathecal or epidural) or nerve blocks (neurolytic techniques)	These techniques are used to target the pathophysiologic origin of pain that is not relieved by conventional pain relief methods (McHugh et al, 2012).
Corticosteroids, such as dexamethasone (Decadron) or prednisone	May be effective in controlling pain associated with inflammatory process including metastatic bone pain, acute spinal cord compression, and neuropathic pain.
Anticonvulsants, such as phenytoin (Dilantin), valproic acid (Depakote), clonazepam (Klonopin), gabapentin (Neurontin), or pregabalin (Lyrica)	Useful for peripheral pain syndromes associated with neuropathic pain, especially shooting pain, postherpetic neuralgia.
Antidepressants, such as amitriptyline (Elavil), imipramine (Tofranil), doxepin (Sinequan), trazodone (Desyrel), or duloxetine (Cymbalta)	Effective for neuropathic pain (e.g., tingling, burning pain) and pain resulting from surgery, chemotherapy, or nerve infiltration.
Antihistamines, such as hydroxyzine (Atarax, Vistaril)	Mild anxiolytic agent with sedative and analgesic properties. May produce additive analgesia with therapeutic doses of opioids and may be beneficial in limiting opioid-induced nausea or vomiting.
Radioisotopes, such as strontium-89 (Metastron) or Samarium SM 153 lexidronam (Quadramet)	Effective in treating pain resulting from osteoblastic metastatic bone lesions. Drug onset is about 1 week with duration of 2 to 4 months. May help reduce dosage of opioid analgesics. *Note:* Bone marrow, WBC, and platelet counts may be suppressed for up to 8 weeks after administration of the drug.
Bisphosphonates, such as Pamidronate (Aredia) or zoledronic acid (Zometa)	Specific inhibitors of osteoclastic activity that treat hypercalcemia and reduce bone pain and fractures especially in multiple myeloma, breast, and prostate cancers.
Provide and instruct in use of PCA, as appropriate.	Provides for timely drug administration, preventing fluctuations in intensity of pain, often at lower total dosage than would be given by conventional methods.
Instruct in use of electrical stimulation (e.g., transcutaneous electrical nerve stimulation [TENS]) unit.	TENS blocks nerve transmission of pain stimulus, providing reduction and relief of pain without drug-related side effects. Can be used in combination with other modalities.
Prepare for and assist with procedures such as nerve blocks, cordotomy, commissural myelotomy, or radiation therapy.	May be used in severe, intractable pain unresponsive to other measures. *Note:* Radiation is especially useful for bone metastasis and may provide fast onset of pain relief even with only one treatment.
Refer to structured support group, psychiatric clinical nurse specialist, psychologist, or spiritual advisor for counseling, as indicated.	May be necessary to reduce anxiety and enhance client's coping skills, decreasing level of pain. *Note:* Hypnosis can heighten awareness and help to focus concentration to decrease perception of pain.

NURSING DIAGNOSIS: imbalanced Nutrition: less than body requirements

May Be Related To
Biological factors (e.g., hypermetabolic state, fatigue)
Inability to ingest food (e.g., anorexia, gastric irritation, taste distortions, nausea)
Psychological factors (e.g., emotional distress, poorly controlled pain)

Possibly Evidenced By
Reports food intake less than recommended daily allowance
Reports altered taste sensation; lack of interest in food; aversion to eating
Body weight 20% or more under ideal for height and frame
Abdominal cramping; sore buccal cavity

Desired Outcomes/Evaluation Criteria—Client Will

Nutritional Status (NOC)
Demonstrate stable weight or progressive weight gain toward goal with normalization of laboratory values and be free of signs of malnutrition.

Adherence Behavior: Healthy Diet (NOC)
Verbalize understanding of individual interferences to adequate intake.
Participate in specific interventions to stimulate appetite and increase dietary intake.

ACTIONS/INTERVENTIONS	RATIONALE
Nutrition Therapy (NIC)	
Independent	
Monitor daily food intake and have client keep food diary, as indicated.	Identifies nutritional strengths and deficiencies.
Measure height, weight, and skinfold thickness or other anthropometric measurements, as appropriate. Ascertain amount of recent weight loss. Weigh daily or as indicated.	If these measurements fall below minimum standards, client's chief source of stored energy, fat tissue, is depleted.
Assess skin and mucous membranes for pallor, delayed wound healing, and enlarged parotid glands.	Helps in identification of protein-calorie malnutrition, especially when weight and anthropometric measurements are less than normal.
Encourage client to eat high-calorie, nutrient-rich diet, with adequate fluid intake. Encourage use of supplements and frequent, smaller meals spaced throughout the day.	Hypermetabolic state and treatment requires increased nutrients and fluids to promote healing and elimination of toxins. Supplements can play an important role in maintaining adequate caloric and protein intake. *Note:* Early studies regarding eating-related distress indicates there is currently no evidence that people with advanced cancer can improve their survival or quality of life by changing what they eat. Therefore, the goal of psychosocial intervention may need to change from optimizing nutritional intake to mitigating weight- and eating-related distress when the focus of treatment and care shifts from achieving cure to optimizing quality of life (Hopkinson et al, 2006; Brown, 2002).
Create pleasant dining atmosphere; encourage client to share meals with family and friends.	Makes mealtime more enjoyable, which may enhance intake.
Encourage open communication regarding anorexia and cachexia.	Often a source of emotional distress, especially for SO who wants to feed client frequently. When client refuses to eat, SO may feel rejected or frustrated.
Chemotherapy Management (NIC)	
Adjust diet before and immediately after treatments (e.g., clear, cool liquids; light or bland foods; candied ginger; dry crackers; toast; and carbonated drinks). Offer liquids 1 hour before or 1 hour after meals.	The effectiveness of diet adjustment is individualized in relief of post-therapy nausea. Client must experiment to find best solution and combinations. Avoiding fluids during meals minimizes becoming "full" too quickly.
Control environmental factors, such as strong or noxious odors and noise. Avoid overly sweet, fatty, or spicy foods.	Can trigger nausea and vomiting response.
Encourage use of relaxation techniques, visualization, guided imagery, and moderate exercise before meals.	May prevent onset or reduce severity of nausea, decrease anorexia, and enable client to increase oral intake.
Identify the client who experiences anticipatory nausea or vomiting, and take appropriate measures.	Psychogenic nausea and vomiting occurring before chemotherapy generally does not respond to anti-emetic drugs. Change of treatment environment or client routine on treatment day may be effective.
Evaluate effectiveness of anti-emetic agents.	Individuals respond differently to all medications. First-line anti-emetics may not work, requiring alteration in or use of combination drug therapy.
Hematest stools and gastric secretions.	Certain therapies, such as antimetabolites, inhibit renewal of epithelial cells lining the gastrointestinal (GI) tract, which may cause changes ranging from mild erythema to severe ulceration with bleeding.
Collaborative	
Review laboratory studies, as indicated, such as total lymphocyte count, serum transferrin, and albumin or prealbumin.	Helps identify the degree of biochemical imbalance or malnutrition and influences choice of dietary interventions. *Note:* Anticancer treatments can also alter nutrition studies, so all results must be correlated with the client's clinical status.
Administer medications, as indicated, for example:	
5-HT3 receptor antagonists, such as ondansetron (Zofran), granisetron (Kytril), dolasetron (Anzemet), and palonosetron (Aloxi); NK-1 receptor antagonist aprepitant (Emend); phenothiazines, such as prochlorperazine (Compazine) and thiethylperazine (Torecan); antidopaminergics, such as metoclopramide (Reglan); antihistamines, such as diphenhydramine (Benadryl); and cannabinoids, such as dronabinol (Marinol)	Most anti-emetics act to interfere with stimulation of true vomiting center, and chemoreceptor trigger zone agents also act peripherally to inhibit reverse peristalsis. These medications are often prescribed routinely before, during, and after chemotherapy to prevent nausea and vomiting.
Corticosteroids, such as dexamethasone (Decadron); benzodiazepines, such as lorazepam (Ativan); and butyrophenones, such as haloperidol (Haldol) or droperidol (Inapsine)	Combination therapy such as Compazine with Decadron and/or Ativan is often more effective than single agents.
Vitamins, especially A, D, and B_6	Prevents deficit related to decreased absorption of fat-soluble vitamins. Deficiency of B_6 can contribute to or exacerbate

ACTIONS/INTERVENTIONS (continued)	RATIONALE (continued)
	depression, irritability, and neuropathy. *Note:* Some medical providers recommend avoiding such antioxidants as E and C because they may interfere with chemotherapy and radiation.
Antacids and/or proton pump inhibitors, such as esomeprazole (Nexium), lansoprazole (Prevacid), or pantoprazole (Protonix)	Minimizes gastric irritation, decreases nausea, and reduces risk of mucosal ulceration.
Administer anti-emetic on a regular schedule before or during and after administration of antineoplastic agent and radiation, as appropriate.	Nausea and vomiting are frequently the most disabling and psychologically stressful side effects of chemotherapy.
Provide support and psychosocial interventions to deal with WRD and ERD experienced by clients and families.	Psychosocial interventions are beginning to be used to directly deal with eating- and weight-related distress manifestations experienced by 80% of clients with advanced cancer disease (Hopkinson, 2013). For many clients, mitigation of distress is likely to be achieved by supporting them in optimizing their nutritional intake within the confines of their small appetite and other obstacles to eating (considered to be a psychosocial intervention) (Hopkinson, 2002).
Nutrition Therapy (NIC)	
Refer to dietitian or nutritional support team.	Provides for specific dietary plan to meet individual needs and reduce problems associated with protein or calorie malnutrition and micronutrient deficiencies.
Insert and maintain nasogastric (NG) or feeding tube for enteric feedings or central line for total parenteral nutrition (TPN), if indicated.	In the presence of severe malnutrition (and when the client is not currently terminal) (e.g., loss of 25% to 30% body weight) or if client has been nothing-by-mouth status (NPO) for 5 days and is unlikely to be able to eat for another week, tube feeding or TPN may be necessary to meet nutritional needs.

NURSING DIAGNOSIS: risk for deficient Fluid Volume

Risk Factors May Include

Excessive losses through normal routes—vomiting, diarrhea; and/or abnormal routes—indwelling tubes, wounds, fistulas
Factors influencing fluid needs (e.g., hypermetabolic state)
Deviations affecting intake of fluids (e.g., nausea)

Possibly Evidenced By

(Not applicable; presence of signs and symptoms establishes an *actual* diagnosis)

Desired Outcomes/Evaluation Criteria—Client Will

Hydration (NOC)

Display adequate fluid balance as evidenced by stable vital signs, moist mucous membranes, good skin turgor, prompt capillary refill, and individually adequate urinary output.

ACTIONS/INTERVENTIONS	RATIONALE
Fluid/Electrolyte Management (NIC)	
Independent	
Monitor intake and output (I&O) and specific gravity. Include all output sources, such as emesis, diarrhea, or draining wounds. Calculate 24-hour balance.	Continued negative fluid balance, decreasing renal output, and concentration of urine suggest developing dehydration and need for increased fluid replacement.
Weigh, as indicated.	Sensitive measurement of fluctuations in fluid balance.
Monitor vital signs. Evaluate peripheral pulses and capillary refill.	Reflects adequacy of circulating volume.
Assess skin turgor and moisture of mucous membranes. Note reports of thirst.	Indirect indicators of hydration status and degree of deficit.
Encourage increased fluid intake as individually appropriate and tolerated.	Assists in maintenance of fluid requirements and reduces risk of harmful side effects such as hemorrhagic cystitis in client receiving cyclophosphamide (Cytoxan).
Observe for bleeding tendencies, such as oozing from mucous membranes or puncture sites and presence of ecchymosis or petechiae.	Early identification of problems that may occur as a result of cancer and/or therapies allows for prompt intervention.

(continues on page 840)

ACTIONS/INTERVENTIONS (continued)	RATIONALE (continued)
Minimize venipunctures such as combining IV starts with blood draws. Encourage client to consider central or peripheral venous catheter placement.	Reduces potential for hemorrhage and infection associated with repeated venous puncture.
Avoid trauma and apply pressure to puncture sites.	Reduces potential for bleeding and hematoma formation.
Collaborative	
Provide IV fluids as indicated.	Given for general hydration and to dilute antineoplastic drugs and reduce adverse side effects—nausea, vomiting, or nephrotoxicity.
Administer anti-emetic therapy. (Refer to ND: imbalanced Nutrition: less than body requirements.)	Alleviation of nausea and vomiting decreases gastric losses and allows for increased oral intake.
Monitor laboratory studies, such as CBC, electrolytes, and serum albumin.	Provides information about level of hydration and corresponding deficits. *Note:* Malnutrition and effects of decreased albumin levels potentiates fluid shifts or edema formation.
Administer transfusions, as indicated:	
RBCs	May be needed to restore blood count and prevent manifestations of anemia often present in cancer clients, such as tachycardia, tachypnea, dizziness, and weakness.
Platelets	Thrombocytopenia may occur as a side effect of chemotherapy, radiation, or cancer process, increasing the risk of bleeding from mucous membranes and other body sites. Spontaneous bleeding may occur with platelet count of 5000.
Avoid use of aspirin, gastric irritants, platelet inhibitors, or herbs such as ginseng, green tea, garlic, ginger, ginkgo, or willow bark.	These substances can negatively affect clotting mechanism and/or potentiate risk of bleeding.

NURSING DIAGNOSIS: Fatigue

May Be Related To

Disease states; anemia; malnutrition

Anxiety; depression

[Altered body chemistry—side effects of pain and other medications, chemotherapy, radiation therapy, biotherapy]

Possibly Evidenced By

Reports an unremitting, overwhelming lack of energy; inability to maintain usual routines

Decreased performance, compromised concentration

Lethargy; listlessness; disinterest in surroundings

Desired Outcomes/Evaluation Criteria—Client Will

Endurance (NOC)

Report improved sense of energy.

Perform ADLs and participate in desired activities at level of ability.

ACTIONS/INTERVENTIONS	RATIONALE
Energy Management (NIC)	
Independent	
Have client rate fatigue, using a numeric scale, such as the Multidimensional Fatigue Inventory (MFI), if possible, and the time of day when it is most severe.	Helps in developing a plan for managing CRF to improve client's quality of life (Horneber et al, 2012).
Plan care to allow for rest and uninterrupted sleep periods. Schedule activities for periods when client has most energy. Involve client and SO in schedule planning.	Frequent rest periods and/or naps are needed to conserve and restore energy. Planning will allow client to be active during times when energy level is higher, which may restore a feeling of well-being and a sense of control.
Establish realistic activity goals with client.	Provides for a sense of control and feelings of accomplishment.
Assist with self-care needs when indicated; keep bed in low position and pathways clear of furniture and assist with ambulation.	Weakness may make ADLs difficult to complete or place the client at risk for injury during activities.
Encourage client to do whatever possible, such as self-bathing, sitting up in chair, and walking. Increase activity level as individual is able.	Enhances strength and stamina and enables client to become more active without undue fatigue.
Encourage aerobic exercise, as client is able, with goal of 30 minutes per day.	Aerobic exercise minimizes fatigue, increases strength and stamina, and stimulates release of natural endorphins, which promotes sense of well-being.

ACTIONS/INTERVENTIONS (continued)	RATIONALE (continued)
Monitor physiological response to activity, such as changes in BP or heart and respiratory rate.	Tolerance varies greatly depending on the stage of the disease process, nutrition state, fluid balance, and reaction to therapeutic regimen.
Perform pain assessment and provide pain management.	Poorly managed cancer pain can contribute to fatigue.
Encourage nutritional intake. (Refer to ND: imbalanced Nutrition: less than body requirements.)	Adequate intake and use of nutrients is necessary to meet energy needs and build energy reserves for activity.
Encourage adequate fluid intake. (Refer to ND: risk for deficient Fluid Volume.)	Prevents dehydration, which increases fatigue.
Collaborative	
Provide supplemental oxygen, as indicated.	Presence of anemia or hypoxemia reduces O_2 available for cellular uptake and contributes to fatigue.
Refer to physical and occupational therapy.	Programmed daily exercises and activities help client maintain or increase strength and muscle tone and enhance sense of well-being. Use of adaptive devices may help conserve energy.

NURSING DIAGNOSIS: risk for Infection

Risk Factors May Include

Inadequate secondary defenses—immunosuppression, pharmaceutical agents
Malnutrition; chronic disease
Invasive procedures

Possibly Evidenced By

(Not applicable; presence of signs and symptoms establishes an *actual* diagnosis)

Desired Outcomes/Evaluation Criteria—Client Will

Infection Severity (NOC)
Remain afebrile.
Achieve timely healing, as appropriate.

Knowledge: Infection Control (NOC)
Identify and participate in interventions to prevent and reduce risk of infection.

ACTIONS/INTERVENTIONS	RATIONALE
Infection Protection (NIC)	
Independent	
Promote good hand-washing procedures by staff and visitors. Screen and limit visitors who may have infections.	Protects client from sources of infection, such as visitors and staff who may have an upper respiratory infection (URI).
Emphasize personal hygiene.	Limits potential sources of infection.
Monitor temperature.	Temperature elevation may occur, if not masked by corticosteroids or anti-inflammatory drugs, because of various factors, including chemotherapy side effects, disease process, or infection. Early identification of infectious process enables appropriate therapy to be started promptly.
Encourage fluids. (Refer to ND: risk for deficient Fluid Volume.)	Adequate fluid intake enhances immune system and aids natural defense mechanisms.
Assess all systems (e.g., skin, respiratory, genitourinary) for signs and symptoms of infection on a continual basis.	Early recognition and intervention may prevent progression to more serious situation such as sepsis.
Reposition frequently; keep linens dry and wrinkle-free.	Reduces pressure and irritation to tissues and may prevent skin breakdown.
Promote adequate rest and exercise periods.	Limits fatigue, yet encourages sufficient movement to prevent stasis complications—pneumonia, decubitus ulcers, or thrombus formation.
Stress importance of good oral hygiene.	Development of stomatitis increases risk of infection and secondary overgrowth.
Avoid or limit invasive procedures, as possible. Adhere to aseptic techniques.	Reduces risk of contamination and limits portal of entry for infectious agents.
Collaborative	
Monitor CBC with differential WBC and granulocyte count and platelets, as indicated.	Bone marrow activity may be inhibited by effects of chemotherapy, the disease state, or radiation therapy. Monitoring status of myelosuppression is important for preventing further

(continues on page 842)

ACTIONS/INTERVENTIONS (continued)	RATIONALE (continued)
	complications, such as infection, anemia, or hemorrhage, and scheduling drug delivery. *Note:* The nadir is usually seen 7 to 10 days after administration of chemotherapy.
Obtain cultures, as indicated.	Identifies causative organism(s) and appropriate therapy.
Administer antibiotics, as indicated. Provide antibiotics within 1 hour, as ordered for neutropenic sepsis (Davis, 2013).	May be used to treat identified infection or given prophylactically in immunocompromised client.

NURSING DIAGNOSIS: risk for impaired Oral Mucous Membrane

Risk Factors May Include

Treatment-related side effects (e.g., chemotherapy; radiation therapy)
Nil by mouth (NPO) for more than 24 hours; dehydration; malnutrition

Possibly Evidenced By

(Not applicable; presence of signs and symptoms establishes an *actual* diagnosis)

Desired Outcomes/Evaluation Criteria—Client Will

Oral Health (NOC)

Display intact mucous membranes, which are pink, moist, and free of inflammation or ulcerations.

Self-Care Oral Hygiene (NOC)

Verbalize understanding of causative factors.
Demonstrate techniques to maintain or restore integrity of oral mucosa.

ACTIONS/INTERVENTIONS	RATIONALE
Oral Health Maintenance (NIC)	
Independent	
Assess dental health and oral hygiene periodically.	Identifies prophylactic treatment needs before initiation of chemotherapy or radiation and provides baseline data of current oral hygiene for future comparison.
Encourage client to assess oral cavity daily, noting changes in mucous membrane integrity. Note reports of burning in the mouth, changes in voice quality, ability to swallow, sense of taste, development of thick saliva, or blood-tinged emesis.	Stomatitis generally occurs 7 to 14 days after treatment begins, but signs may be seen as early as day 3 or 4, especially if there are any preexisting oral problems. The range of response extends from mild erythema to severe ulceration and may extend the length of the GI tract, which can be very painful, can inhibit oral intake, and is potentially life-threatening. Early identification enables prompt treatment.
Discuss with client areas needing improvement and demonstrate methods for good oral care.	Good care is critical during treatment to control stomatitis complications.
Initiate and recommend oral hygiene program to include the following:	
Avoidance of commercial mouthwashes and lemon or glycerin swabs	Products containing alcohol or phenol may exacerbate mucous membrane dryness or irritation.
Use of mouthwash made from warm water with salt and baking soda; dilute solution of hydrogen peroxide may be used for bleeding or infected tissue	May be soothing to the membranes. Rinsing before meals may improve the client's sense of taste. Rinsing after meals and at bedtime dilutes oral acids and relieves xerostomia.
Brushing with soft toothbrush or foam swab	Prevents trauma to delicate, fragile tissues. *Note:* Toothbrush should be changed every month.
Flossing gently or use WaterPik cautiously	Removes food particles that can promote bacterial growth. *Note:* Water under pressure has the potential to injure gums and force bacteria under gum line.
Keeping lips moist with lip gloss or balm, K-Y Jelly, Chapstick	Promotes comfort and prevents drying and cracking of tissues.
Use of mints, other hard candy or artificial saliva (Ora-Lube, Salivart), as indicated	Stimulates secretions and provides moisture to maintain integrity of mucous membranes, especially in presence of dehydration and reduced saliva production.
Instruct regarding dietary changes, such as avoiding hot or spicy foods and acidic juices; suggest use of straw; ingest soft or blenderized foods, popsicles, and ice cream, as tolerated.	Severe stomatitis may interfere with nutritional and fluid intake leading to negative nitrogen balance or dehydration. Dietary modifications may make foods easier to swallow and may feel soothing.
Encourage fluid intake as individually tolerated.	Adequate hydration helps keep mucous membranes moist, preventing drying and cracking.

ACTIONS/INTERVENTIONS (continued) | RATIONALE (continued)

Discuss effects of smoking and alcohol intake, if indicated, and address concerns.
May cause further irritation and dryness of mucous membranes.

Monitor for, and explain to client, signs of oral super infection such as thrush.
Early recognition provides opportunity for prompt treatment.

Collaborative

Refer to dentist before initiating chemotherapy or head and neck radiation.
Prophylactic examination and repair work before therapy reduce risk of infection.

Culture suspicious oral lesions.
Identifies organism(s) responsible for oral infections and suggests appropriate drug therapy.

Administer medications, as indicated, for example:

- Analgesic rinses, such as GelClair, mixture of Koatin, pectin, diphenhydramine [Benadryl], and topical lidocaine [Xylocaine]
  Aggressive analgesia program may be required to relieve intense pain. *Note:* Rinse should be used as a swish-and-spit rather than a gargle, which could anesthetize client's gag reflex.
- Antifungal mouthwash preparation, such as nystatin (Mycostatin) and antibacterial Biotane
  May be needed to treat or prevent secondary oral infections, such as *Candida, Pseudomonas,* and herpes simplex.
- Antinausea agents, such as dolasetron (Anzemet), granisetron (Kytril)
  When given before beginning mouth care regimen, may prevent nausea associated with oral stimulation, especially when client is receiving a chemotherapy regimen.
- Opioid analgesics, such as hydromophone (Dilaudid) or morphine
  May be required for acute episodes of moderate to severe oral pain.

NURSING DIAGNOSIS: risk for impaired Skin/Tissue Integrity

Risk Factors May Include

Medications (e.g., chemotherapy); radiation
Immunological factors
Nutritional factors (e.g., malnutrition; anemia)

Possibly Evidenced By

(Not applicable; presence of signs and symptoms establishes an *actual* diagnosis)

Desired Outcomes/Evaluation Criteria—Client Will

Risk Control (NOC)

Identify interventions appropriate for specific condition.
Participate in techniques to prevent complications and promote healing, as appropriate.

ACTIONS/INTERVENTIONS | RATIONALE

Chemotherapy [or] Radiation Therapy Management (NIC)

Independent

Assess skin frequently for side effects of cancer therapy; note breakdown and delayed wound healing. Emphasize importance of reporting open areas to caregiver.
A reddening and/or tanning effect called radiation dermatitis may develop within the field of radiation. Dry desquamation with dryness and pruritus, moist desquamation with blistering, ulceration, hair loss, and loss of dermis and sweat glands may also be noted. In addition, skin reactions—allergic rashes, hyperpigmentation, pruritus, increased risk of sunburn, acne-like skin eruptions, and alopecia—may occur with some chemotherapy agents.

Bathe with lukewarm water and mild soap.
Maintains cleanliness without irritating the skin.

Encourage client to avoid vigorous rubbing and scratching and to pat skin dry instead of rubbing.
Helps prevent skin friction or trauma to sensitive tissues.

Turn or reposition frequently.
Promotes circulation and prevents undue pressure on skin and tissues.

Review skin care protocol for client receiving radiation therapy:
Designed to minimize trauma to area of radiation therapy.

- Avoid rubbing or use of soap, lotions, creams, ointments, powders, or deodorants on area; avoid applying heat or attempting to wash off marks or tattoos placed on skin to pinpoint location for radiation therapy.
  These factors can potentiate or otherwise interfere with radiation delivery and may actually increase reaction.
- Recommend wearing soft, loose cotton clothing; have female client avoid wearing bra if it creates pressure.
  Skin is very sensitive during and after treatment, and all irritation should be avoided to prevent dermal injury.
- Apply cornstarch, Aquaphor, Lubriderm, Eucerin, or other water-soluble moisturizing gel to area twice daily or more frequently, as needed.
  Helps control dampness or pruritus. Maintenance care is required until skin and tissues have regenerated and are back to normal.

(continues on page 844)

ACTIONS/INTERVENTIONS (continued)	RATIONALE (continued)
Encourage liberal use of sunblock and breathable, protective clothing.	Protects skin from ultraviolet rays and reduces risk of recall reactions.
Review skin care protocol for client receiving chemotherapy:	
Use appropriate peripheral or central venous catheter, dilute anticancer drug per protocol, and ascertain that IV is infusing well.	Reduces risk of tissue irritation or extravasation of agent into tissues.
Instruct client to notify caregiver promptly of discomfort at IV insertion site.	Development of irritation indicates need for alteration of rate or dilution of chemotherapy and/or change of IV site to prevent more serious reaction.
Assess skin, IV site, and vein for erythema, edema, tenderness, weltlike patches, itching, burning, swelling, soreness, and blisters progressing to ulceration or tissue necrosis.	Presence of phlebitis or extravasation requires immediate discontinuation of antineoplastic agent and medical intervention. *Note:* Vein flare, a localized reaction, may resolve without intervention based on individual reaction.
Wash skin immediately with soap and water if antineoplastic agents are spilled on unprotected skin of client or caregiver.	Dilutes drug to reduce risk of skin irritation and chemical burn.
Advise clients receiving 5-fluorouracil (5-FU) and methotrexate to avoid sun exposure. Withhold methotrexate if sunburn is present.	Sun can cause exacerbation of burn spotting, a side effect of 5-FU, or can cause a red "flash" area with methotrexate, which can exacerbate drug's effect.
Review expected dermatological side effects seen with chemotherapy, such as rash, hyperpigmentation, acne-like eruptions, and peeling of skin on palms.	Anticipatory guidance helps decrease concern if side effects do occur.
Inform client that if alopecia occurs, hair could grow back after completion of chemotherapy but may or may not grow back after radiation therapy.	Anticipatory guidance may help adjustment to, or preparation for, baldness. Men are often as sensitive to hair loss as women. Radiation's effect on hair follicles may be permanent, depending on radiation dosage.
Collaborative	
Administer appropriate antidote if extravasation of IV should occur, for example:	
Dimethyl sulfoxide (DMSO)	Some studies suggest benefit with topical DMSO for mitomycin and doxorubicin (Adriamycin). *Note:* Injection of diphenhydramine (Benadryl) may relieve urticaria of vein flare.
Hyaluronidase (Wydase)	Injected subcutaneously for vincristine (Oncovin), vinblastine (Velban), etoposide (VP16), vindesine (Eldisine), vinorelbine (Navelbine), teniposide (Vm26), or paclitaxel (Taxol) infiltration.
Thiosulfate	Injected subcutaneously for nitrogen mustard and large amounts, greater than 20 mL, of concentrated cisplatin.
Apply ice pack or warm compresses per protocol.	Controversial intervention depends on type of agent used. Ice restricts blood flow, keeping drug localized, whereas heat enhances dispersion of neoplastic drug or antidote, minimizing tissue damage.

NURSING DIAGNOSIS: risk for Constipation/Diarrhea

Risk Factors May Include

Change in eating patterns; change in usual foods; insufficient fiber/fluids
Adverse effects of pharmaceutical agents; radiation
Malabsorption of fat

Possibly Evidenced By

(Not applicable; presence of signs and symptoms establishes an *actual* diagnosis)

Desired Outcomes/Evaluation Criteria—Client Will

Bowel Elimination (NOC)

Maintain usual bowel consistency and pattern.
Verbalize understanding of factors and appropriate interventions or solutions related to individual situation.

ACTIONS/INTERVENTIONS	RATIONALE
Bowel Management (NIC)	
Independent	
Ascertain usual elimination habits.	Data required as baseline for future evaluation of therapeutic needs and effectiveness.
Assess bowel sounds and monitor and record bowel movements (BMs) including frequency and consistency—particularly during first 3 to 5 days of vinca alkaloid therapy and when on pain and/or nausea medications.	Defines problem—diarrhea or constipation. *Note:* Constipation is one of the earliest manifestations of neurotoxicity.
Monitor I&O and weight.	Dehydration, weight loss, and electrolyte imbalance are complications of diarrhea. Inadequate fluid intake may potentiate constipation.
Encourage adequate fluid intake, increased fiber in diet, and regular exercise.	May reduce potential for constipation by improving stool consistency and stimulating peristalsis; can prevent dehydration associated with diarrhea.
Provide small, frequent meals of foods low in residue if not contraindicated, maintaining needed protein and carbohydrates, such as eggs, cooked cereal (oatmeal), or bland cooked vegetables.	Reduces gastric irritation. Use of low-fiber foods can decrease irritability and provide bowel rest when diarrhea present.
Adjust diet as appropriate—avoid foods high in fat, such as butter, fried foods, and nuts; foods with high-fiber content and those known to cause diarrhea or gas, including cabbage, baked beans, and chili; food or fluids high in caffeine; or extremely hot or cold food and fluids.	GI stimulants that may increase gastric motility and frequency of stools.
Check for impaction if client has not had BM in 3 days or if abdominal distention, cramping, and headache are present.	Further interventions and alternative bowel care may be needed.
Collaborative	
Monitor laboratory studies, such as electrolytes, as indicated.	Electrolyte imbalances may be the result of, or contribute to, altered GI function.
Administer the following, as indicated:	
IV fluids.	Prevents dehydration and dilutes chemotherapy agents to diminish side effects.
Antidiarrheal agents	May be indicated to control severe diarrhea.
Stool softeners and laxatives	Prophylactic use may prevent further complications in some clients, such as those who will receive vinca alkaloid, have poor bowel pattern before treatment, or have decreased motility. *Note:* Enemas and suppositories are to be avoided when possible as they increase the potential for infection and are uncomfortable and unpleasant for the client.

NURSING DIAGNOSIS: risk for Sexual Dysfunction

Risk Factors May Include

Altered body function or structure (e.g., disease process, drugs, surgery, radiation)

Lack of privacy or significant other

Possibly Evidenced By

(Not applicable; presence of signs and symptoms establishes an *actual* diagnosis)

Desired Outcomes/Evaluation Criteria—Client Will

Sexual Functioning (NOC)

Verbalize understanding of effects of cancer and therapeutic regimen on sexuality and measures to correct or deal with problems.

Maintain sexual activity at a desired level, as possible.

ACTIONS/INTERVENTIONS	RATIONALE
Sexual Counseling (NIC)	
Independent	
Discuss with client and SO the nature of sexuality and reactions when it is altered or threatened. Provide information about normality of these problems and that many people find it helpful to seek assistance with adaptation process.	Acknowledges legitimacy of the problem. Sexuality encompasses the way men and women view themselves as individuals and how they relate between and among themselves in every area of life.
Advise client of side effects of prescribed cancer treatment that are known to affect sexuality.	Anticipatory guidance can help client and SO begin the process of adaptation to new state.

(continues on page 846)

ACTIONS/INTERVENTIONS (continued)	RATIONALE (continued)
Provide private time for hospitalized client. Knock on door and receive permission from client and SO before entering.	Sexual needs do not end because the client is hospitalized. Intimacy needs continue, and an open and accepting attitude for the expression of those needs is essential.
Collaborative	
Refer to sex therapist, as indicated.	May require additional assistance in dealing with situation.

NURSING DIAGNOSIS: risk for interrupted Family Processes

Risk Factors May Include

Situational crises; shift in health status of a family member

Shift in family roles; modification in family finances

Possibly Evidenced By

(Not applicable; presence of signs and symptoms establishes an *actual* diagnosis)

Desired Outcomes/Evaluation Criteria—Family Will

Family Resiliency (NOC)

Express feelings freely.

Demonstrate individual involvement in problem-solving process directed at appropriate solutions for the situation.

Encourage and allow member who is ill to handle situation in own way.

ACTIONS/INTERVENTIONS	RATIONALE
Family Process Maintenance (NIC)	
Independent	
Note components of family, presence of extended family, and others, including friends and neighbors.	Helps client and caregiver know who is available to assist with care and provide respite and support.
Identify patterns of communication in family and patterns of interaction between family members.	Provides information about effectiveness of communication and identifies problems that may interfere with family's ability to assist client and adjust positively to diagnosis and treatment of cancer.
Assess role expectations of family members and encourage discussion about them.	Each person may see the situation in own individual manner, and clear identification and sharing of these expectations promote understanding.
Assess energy direction: Are efforts at resolution or problem-solving purposeful or scattered?	Provides clues about interventions that may be appropriate to assist client and family in directing energies in a more effective manner.
Note cultural and religious beliefs.	Affects client and SO reaction and adjustment to diagnosis, treatment, and outcome of cancer.
Listen for expressions of helplessness.	Helpless feelings may contribute to difficulty adjusting to diagnosis of cancer and cooperating with treatment regimen.
Deal with family members in a warm, caring, respectful way. Provide verbal and written information and reinforce, as necessary.	Provides feelings of empathy and promotes individual's sense of worth and competence in ability to handle current situation.
Encourage appropriate expressions of anger without reacting negatively to them.	Feelings of anger are to be expected when individuals are dealing with the difficult, potentially fatal illness of cancer. Appropriate expression enables progress toward resolution of the stages of the grieving process.
Acknowledge difficulties of the situation, such as the diagnosis and treatment of cancer, or possibility of death.	Communicates acceptance of the reality the client and family are facing.
Identify and encourage use of previously successful coping behaviors.	Most people have developed effective coping skills that can be useful in dealing with current situation.
Emphasize importance of continuous open dialogue between family members.	Promotes understanding and assists family members to maintain clear communication and resolve problems effectively.
Collaborative	
Refer to support groups, clergy, and family therapy, as indicated.	May need additional assistance to resolve problems of disorganization that may accompany diagnosis of potentially terminal illness.

NURSING DIAGNOSIS: deficient Knowledge [Learning Need] regarding illness, prognosis, treatment, self-care, and discharge needs

May Be Related To
Lack of exposure or recall; information misinterpretation
Unfamiliarity with information resources
Cognitive limitation

Possibly Evidenced By
Reports the problem
Inaccurate follow-through of instructions

Desired Outcomes/Evaluation Criteria—Client Will

Knowledge: Cancer Management (NOC)

Verbalize accurate information about diagnosis, prognosis, and potential complications at own level of readiness.
Verbalize understanding of therapeutic needs.
Correctly perform necessary procedures and explain reasons for the actions.
Initiate necessary lifestyle changes and participate in treatment regimen.
Identify and use available resources appropriately.

ACTIONS/INTERVENTIONS	RATIONALE
Teaching: Disease Process (NIC)	
Independent	
Review with client and SO understanding of specific diagnosis, treatment alternatives, and future expectations.	Validates current level of understanding, identifies learning needs, and provides knowledge base from which client can make informed decisions.
Determine client's perception of cancer and cancer treatment(s). Ask about client's own or previous experience or experience with other people who have, or had, cancer.	Aids in identification of ideas, attitudes, fears, misconceptions, and gaps in knowledge about cancer.
Provide clear, accurate information in a factual but sensitive manner. Answer questions specifically, but do not bombard with nonessential details.	Helps with adjustment to the diagnosis of cancer by providing needed information along with time to absorb it. *Note:* Rate and method of giving information may need to be altered to decrease client's anxiety and enhance ability to assimilate information.
Provide anticipatory guidance with client and SO regarding treatment protocol, length of therapy, expected results, and possible side effects. Be honest with client.	Client has the "right to know" and participate in decisions. Accurate and concise information helps to dispel fears and anxiety, helps clarify the expected routine, and enables client to maintain some degree of control.
Provide written materials about cancer, treatment, and available support systems.	Anxiety and preoccupation with thoughts about life and death often interfere with client's ability to assimilate adequate information. Written materials provide reinforcement and clarification about information as client needs it.
Ask client for verbal feedback, and correct misconceptions about individual's type of cancer and treatment choices.	Misconceptions about cancer may be more disturbing than facts and can interfere with treatments or delay healing.
Review specific medication regimen and use of over-the-counter (OTC) drugs.	Enhances ability to manage self-care and avoid potential complications and drug reactions or interactions.
Outline normally expected limitations, if any, on ADLs, including difficulty cooking meals when nauseated or fatigued and loss of work time because of effects of treatments.	Enables client and SO to begin to put limitations into perspective and plan for, or adapt, as indicated.
Address specific home-care needs such as ability to live alone, perform necessary treatments or procedures, and acquire supplies.	Provides information regarding changes that may be needed in current plan of care to meet therapeutic needs.
Do predischarge home evaluation, as indicated.	Aids in transition to home setting by providing information about needed changes in physical layout and the acquisition of needed supplies.
Refer to community resources, as indicated, such as social services, home health agencies, Meals on Wheels, local chapter of American Cancer Society, respite care, hospice center, or other services.	Promotes competent self-care and optimal independence. Maintains client in home or desired setting.
Review with client and SO the importance of maintaining optimal nutritional status.	Promotes well-being, facilitates recovery, and is critical in enabling the client to tolerate treatments.
Encourage diet variations and experimentation in meal planning and food preparation, such as cooking with sweet juices or wine and serving foods cold or at room temperature, as appropriate.	Creativity may enhance flavor and intake, especially when protein foods taste bitter.

(continues on page 848)

ACTIONS/INTERVENTIONS (continued)	RATIONALE (continued)
Recommend cookbooks that are designed for cancer clients.	Helps provide specific menu and recipe ideas.
Recommend increased fluid intake and fiber in diet, as well as routine exercise.	Improves consistency of stool and stimulates peristalsis.
Instruct client to assess oral mucous membranes routinely, noting erythema or ulceration.	Early recognition of problems promotes early intervention, minimizing complications that may impair oral intake and provide avenue for systemic infection.
Initiate medical and support referrals for smoking or alcohol cessation program if client desires.	Decreases irritation to mucous membranes, enhances healing, and promotes general well-being.
Advise client concerning skin and hair care: avoid harsh shampoos, hair dyes, permanents, salt water, and chlorinated water; avoid exposure to strong wind and extreme heat or cold; avoid sun exposure to target area for 1 year after end of radiation treatments; and regularly apply sunblock (SPF 15 or greater).	Prevents additional hair damage and skin irritation and may prevent recall reactions.
Review signs and symptoms requiring medical evaluation, such as infection, delayed healing, drug reactions, and increased pain; or swelling of face or hands and arms that may worsen when lying down, dyspnea, cough, headache, and visual disturbances suggestive of SVCS.	Early identification and treatment may limit severity of complications. *Note:* The use of central venous access devices for various therapies—chemotherapy, TPN, or antibiotic administration—may cause local vein trauma leading to SVCS days, months, or even years after catheter insertion.
Stress importance of continuing medical follow-up.	Provides ongoing monitoring of progression or resolution of disease process and opportunity for timely diagnosis and treatment of complications and early detection of second malignancies. *Note:* Some complications can develop long after therapy is completed, such as pathological fractures, radiation cystitis, or pneumonitis. Periodic thyroid function tests are indicated for clients with radiation to the neck and upper chest because hypothyroidism may develop.
Encourage periodic review of advance directives. Promote inclusion of family and SO in decision-making process.	Client, family, and SO need to reevaluate choices as condition changes and treatment options become available or are exhausted.
Refer to community palliative care if needed.	Palliative care will address pain control, long-term support, and end-of-life care if indicated (Leadbeater, 2013).

POTENTIAL CONSIDERATIONS following acute hospitalization (dependent on client's age, physical condition and presence of complications, personal resources, and life responsibilities)

In addition to Potential Considerations in specific plans of care such as leukemia, mastectomy:

- ***ineffective Coping***—situational crises; uncertainty; high degree of threat
- ***Self-Care Deficit/impaired Home Maintenance***—disease; pain, discomfort; weakness, impaired functioning; fatigue; insufficient finances; unfamiliarity with neighborhood resources; inadequate support systems
- ***risk for Caregiver Role Strain***—illness severity of care receiver; presence of situational stressors that normally affect families (e.g., crisis, economic vulnerability); unpredictable illness course; amount/complexity of caregiving tasks
- ***acute/chronic Pain***—physical agents (e.g., disease process, compression or destruction of nerve tissue, infiltration of nerves or their vascular supply, obstruction of a nerve pathway, inflammation)
- ***ineffective Self-Health Management***—complexity of therapeutic regimen; economic difficulties; decisional conflicts; perceived barriers; powerlessness; social support deficit

END-OF-LIFE CARE/HOSPICE

I. Purpose—provides care and support to the client and family in the client's final stage of a terminal illness when a return to physical health is not possible. Hospice care focuses on comfort and quality of life, rather than curative treatments. *Note*: Pain relief and other measures intended to improve quality of life and mood may result in extending life (Temel, 2010), and on occasion some clients may improve enough to "graduate" from hospice care for a period of time.

II. Indications

a. Criteria (Allen, 2008):

i. Physician certification of terminal illness

ii. Life expectancy of 6 months or less

iii. Presence of a family member or other caregiver continuously in the home when the client is no longer able to safely care for self

b. Care of the dying person encompasses several dimensions (Malloy et al, 2008).

i. Management of pain and other physical symptoms—nausea, vomiting, fatigue, anorexia, functional decline

ii. Psychological and spiritual support

1. Provide client and family the opportunity to consider the meaning of their lives.

2. Encourage participation in making plans and shaping the course of their living while preparing for death.

iii. Bereavement support after death for family

III. Trajectories of Death Appropriate for Hospice Care (Glaser & Strauss, 1968; Lunney, 2007)
- **a.** Steady decline, short terminal phase, as may occur with certain cancers
- **b.** Slow decline with periodic crises and then death, as may occur with chronic obstructive pulmonary disease (COPD), heart or kidney failure
- **c.** Lingering, expected death as expected in frail elderly, dementias, stroke, Parkinson disease

IV. Barriers to Using Hospice Services (Malloy et al, 2008)
- **a.** Influence of managed care on end-of-life care
  - **i.** Lack of understanding of hospice goals and services provided
  - **ii.** Delay in referral to services
- **b.** Client's or family member's denial or avoidance of death; negative perception of hospice
- **c.** Access to care
  - **i.** Limitations of insurance coverage
  - **ii.** Medicare payment source requires care be provided by a Medicare-certified hospice program.
- **d.** Lack of continuity of care across care settings
- **e.** Caregiver fatigue (psychological and physical) that can compromise the care provided in the home

V. Statistics (National Hospice and Palliative Care Organization [NHPCO]
- **a.** Availability: In 2011, there were more than 3600 certified hospice agencies and an estimated 1.65 million patients received services from hospice (NHPCO, 2012).
- **b.** Mortality: There were 2.5 million deaths in the United States in 2011 (National Vital Statistics, 2012); 42% of those were served by hospice (NHPCO, 2011).
- **c.** Cost: In 2010, Medicare expenditures for hospice services were $13 billion (MedPac, 2012).

GLOSSARY

Advance directives: Used to give other people, including health-care providers, information about client's wishes for medical care at a time when client is not physically or mentally able to speak for self. The most common types of advance directives are the living will and the durable power of attorney for healthcare.

End-of-life care: General term that refers to the comprehensive care given in the advanced or terminal stages of illness.

Hospice care: Type of care designed to help clients and their families during the final stages of a terminal illness. Hospice treatment is concentrated primarily on maintaining comfort.

Locus of control: The site of control in an individual—internal or external.

Mindfulness: Method of staying in the moment.

Palliative care: Philosophy of care with the goal of improving the quality of life of clients and their families facing life-threatening illness, through the prevention and relief from suffering. This type of care can encompass treatment of disease processes; provides more than comfort care.

Care Setting

Although much of the care of the dying is still provided by nurses in hospitals (primarily in oncology and critical care areas), hospice care is more common in the home, assisted living, extended care facilities, or hospice inpatient units.

Related Concerns

Cancer, page 827
Extended/long-term care, page 781
Psychosocial aspects of care, page 729

Client Assessment Database

Data depend on underlying terminal condition, involvement of other body systems, and stage of dying process. Refer to care plan(s) reflecting underlying pathology of terminal condition for specific assessments related to that condition.

DIAGNOSTIC DIVISION MAY REPORT	MAY EXHIBIT
ACTIVITY/REST • Fatigue • General weakness • Sleep disturbances	
ELIMINATION • Abdominal discomfort	• *End stage:* • Constipation (effect of opioids, decreased fluids) • Dark urine, oliguria

(continues on page 850)

Client Assessment Database (continued)

DIAGNOSTIC DIVISION MAY REPORT (continued)	MAY EXHIBIT (continued)
EGO INTEGRITY	
• Inability to care for self and decision to accept hospice services • Feelings of helplessness, hopelessness, sorrow, anger; choked feelings • Fear of the dying process, loss of physical and/or mental abilities • Concern about impact of death on significant other (SO) and family; difficulty coping—client and/or family • Inner conflict about beliefs, meaning of life and death; moral distress • Financial concerns, lack of preparation (e.g., will, power of attorney, funeral)	• Deep sadness, crying, anxiety • Apathy, social isolation, withdrawal • Grieving • Spiritual distress
FOOD/FLUID	
• Decreasing appetite • Nausea • Anorexia	• Weight loss • Decreased muscle mass, subcutaneous fat • Poor skin turgor, dry mucous membranes • Difficulty swallowing
NEUROLOGICAL	

	• *End stage:*
	  • Decreasing level of consciousness (LOC)
	  • Agitation, restlessness
	  • Terminal delirium

PAIN/DISCOMFORT	
• Acute or chronic pain	• Muscle tension, restlessness • Facial grimacing
RESPIRATION	

	• *End stage:*
	  • Adventitious breath sounds—rhonchi, wheezes
	  • Abnormal breathing patterns

SAFETY	
	• Erythema over body prominences • Skin breakdown, pressure ulcers • Perineal infection—candidiasis
SOCIAL INTERACTION	
• Apprehension about caregiver's ability to provide care • Changes in family roles and usual patterns of responsibility • Loneliness • Deep sadness • Apathy, withdrawal	• Altered communication pattern • Difficulty adapting to changes imposed by condition and dying process • Family coping concerns

Nursing Priorities

1. Control pain.
2. Prevent or manage complications.
3. Maintain quality of life as possible.
4. Plans in place to meet client's and family's last wishes such as care setting, advance directives, will, and funeral.

NURSING DIAGNOSIS: acute/chronic Pain

May Be Related To
Physical agents (e.g., disease process; chronic physical disability)
Psychological agent (e.g., stress, anxiety)

Possibly Evidenced By
Verbal/coded report of pain; restlessness, irritability
Changes in appetite; anorexia; sleep pattern disturbance; fatigue
Altered ability to continue previous activities
Changes in vital signs (acute pain)

Desired Outcomes/Evaluation Criteria—Client Will

Pain Control (NOC)
Report pain is relieved or controlled, using self-report pain tool.
Demonstrate reduction in pain-related behaviors if unable to provide self-report.
Identify and use nonpharmacological methods that provide relief.
Follow prescribed pharmacological regimen.

Family/SO(s) Will
Cooperate in pain-management program.

ACTIONS/INTERVENTIONS	RATIONALE
Pain Management (NIC)	
Independent	
Perform a comprehensive pain evaluation, including location, characteristics, onset, duration, frequency, quality, severity using a 0 to 10 (or similar) scale, and precipitating or aggravating factors. Note cultural issues impacting reporting and expression of pain. Determine client's acceptable comfort-function level.	Provides baseline information from which a realistic plan can be developed, keeping in mind that verbal and behavioral cues may have little direct relationship to the degree of pain perceived. If self-report is not possible, behavior or physical responses may be helpful (Bjoro, 2008). *Note:* Often client does not feel the need to be completely pain-free but is able to be more functional when pain is at lower level on the pain scale.
Determine possible pathophysiological and psychological causes of pain, such as may be caused by inflammation, fractures, cancer process, surgery, grief, fear, anxiety, or delirium.	Pain is associated with many factors that may be interactive and increase the degree of pain experienced.
Assess client's perception of pain, being aware of client's cognitive status along with behavioral and psychological responses. Determine client's attitude toward, and use of, pain medications and locus of control—internal or external.	Helps identify client's needs, ability to adequately express self, and pain control methods found to be helpful or not helpful in the past. *Note:* Individuals with external locus of control may take little or no responsibility for pain management.
Encourage client and family to express feelings and concerns about opioid use.	Inaccurate information regarding drug use, fear of addiction, or oversedation could impair pain-management efforts.
Verify current and past analgesic and drug use, including alcohol.	May provide insight into what has or has not worked in the past or may impact therapy plan.
Assess degree of personal adjustment to diagnosis, such as anger, irritability, withdrawal, and acceptance.	These factors are variable and often affect the perception of pain, ability to cope, and pain management.
Discuss with SO(s) ways in which they can assist client and reduce precipitating factors.	Promotes involvement in care and belief that there are things they can do to help.
Identify specific signs and symptoms and changes in pain requiring notification of healthcare provider and medical intervention.	Unrelieved pain may be associated with progression of terminal disease process or with complications that require medical management.
Involve caregivers in identifying effective comfort measures for client, such as use of nonacidic fluids, oral swabs, lip salve, and suctioning; skin and perineal care; and use of laxatives. Instruct in use of any needed equipment, such as suction and oxygen.	Managing troubling symptoms, such as nausea, dry mouth, dyspnea, and constipation, can reduce client's suffering and family anxiety, thus improving quality of life and allowing client and family to focus on other issues.
Demonstrate and encourage use of relaxation techniques, such as guided imagery, music, and meditation.	Can supplement analgesic therapy, especially during periods when client desires to minimize sedative effects of medication.
Monitor for, and discuss possibility of, changes in mental status, such as agitation, confusion, and restlessness.	Although causes of deterioration are numerous in terminal stages, early recognition and management of the psychological component are integral parts of pain management.

(continues on page 852)

ACTIONS/INTERVENTIONS (continued)	RATIONALE (continued)
Collaborative	
Establish pain-management plan with client, family, and healthcare providers, including options for management of breakthrough pain.	Inadequate pain management remains one of the most significant deficiencies in the care of the dying client. A stepwise plan or analgesic ladder developed in advance increases client's level of trust that comfort will be maintained, reducing anxiety.
Schedule and administer analgesics, as indicated, to maximal dosage. Use various modalties such as patch, lollipop, sublingal, or combinations of medications, as indicated.	Helps maintain "acceptable" level of pain. Various drugs, dosages, and combinations allow for smaller doses and fewer side effects.
Plan for aggressive pain management, as indicated. Notify physician if regimen is inadequate to meet pain control goal.	Primary goal is for client to be comfortable. Sometimes frequent alterations are required in achieving this, but medications and comfort measures must be sufficient to ensure that client is not suffering.
Instruct client, family, and caregiver in use of sustained-release formulations, around-the-clock dosing, and breakthrough pain management and technology, such as pump or patient-controlled analgesia (PCA) for pain control.	By understanding and managing these factors, pain relief can be enhanced and quality of life improved.
Review medicinal options to treat constipation.	Various "cocktails" are available to manage constipation associated with use of opioid pain medications, reduced peristalsis, and lack of food intake. This is a frequent problem that must be managed to reduce client discomfort.

Refer to CP: Cancer; ND: acute/chronic Pain for additional interventions.

NURSING DIAGNOSIS: Fatigue

May Be Related To
Disease states; anemia; malnutrition
Stress; anxiety; depression; negative life events

Possibly Evidenced By
Report feeling tired, unable to restore energy even after sleep
Lack of energy; lethargic; drowsy; increase in rest requirements
Decreased performance; reports inability to maintain usual routines
Disinterest in surroundings; introspection

Desired Outcomes/Evaluation Criteria—Client Will

Energy Conservation (NOC)
Identify negative factors affecting performance and eliminate or reduce their effects when possible.
Adapt lifestyle to energy level.
Verbalize understanding of potential loss of ability in relation to existing condition.

Fatigue Level (NOC)
Maintain or achieve slight increase in activity tolerance evidenced by manageable level of fatigue or weakness.

ACTIONS/INTERVENTIONS	RATIONALE
Energy Management (NIC)	
Independent	
Assess severity of fatigue on 0 to 10 or similar coded scale.	The fatigue experienced by the terminally ill can arise from both physical and psychological causes. This fatigue has multiple components, including symptoms of tiredness, a general lack of energy not relieved by rest, diminished mental capacity and subjective weakness associated with difficulty in performing activities of daily living (Girgis et al, 2007; Portenoy, 1999).
Assess sleep patterns and note changes in thought processes and behaviors.	Multiple factors can aggravate fatigue, including sleep deprivation, emotional distress, cognitive impairment (may be related to effects or side effects of medications/therapies, or progression of disease process).
Recommend scheduling activities for periods when client has most energy. Adjust activities as necessary, reducing intensity level or discontinuing activities, as indicated.	Prevents overexertion and allows for some activity within client's ability.

ACTIONS/INTERVENTIONS (continued)	RATIONALE (continued)
Encourage client to do whatever possible, for example, self-care, sit in chair, or visit with family and friends. Plan for shorter activities.	Provides for sense of control and feeling of accomplishment.
Instruct client, family, and caregiver in energy conservation techniques. Emphasize necessity of allowing for frequent rest periods following activities.	Enhances performance while conserving limited energy and preventing increase in level of fatigue.
Plan family and friend visits around client's increased sleep time and shorter periods of alertness.	Client may become tired easily and will sleep more. In addition, client may have periods of unresponsiveness or confusion or seem to be in a dream state. This may be distressing to families/visitors.
Demonstrate proper performance of/assist with activities of daily living (ADLs), ambulation, and position changes. Emphasize safety measures such as use of assistive devices, temperature of bath water, and keeping pathways clear of furniture.	Protects client and caregiver from injury during activities.
Encourage nutritional intake and use of supplements, as appropriate.	Client may or may not want to eat, but food can be offered, if client is able to eat. Easy-to-digest foods that client enjoys may help meet energy needs for activity.
Discuss future plans regarding food and fluid, as indicated. Help client's family understand that forced eating and drinking may harm instead of help.	As the body starts the natural process of dying, the need for food and fluids decreases due to the shutdown of body systems. At this point, dehydration associated with the dying process actually causes analgesic effects (Allen, 2008). Intravenous (IV) fluids and enteral feedings do not prolong life of the dying person. In fact, they may increase discomfort and hasten death. For example, IV fluids can cause edema, increased pain from inflammation, and fluid overload, whereas enteral feedings can cause pulmonary congestion and pneumonia (Suter et al, 2008).
Document cardiopulmonary response to activity—weakness, fatigue, dyspnea, arrhythmias, and diaphoresis.	Can provide guidelines for participation in activities and changes in the plan of care and level of assistance required.
Monitor breath sounds. Note feelings of panic or air hunger.	Hypoxemia increases sense of fatigue and impairs ability to function.
Collaborative	
Collaborate in identifying causes of fatigue that can be treated (e.g., medication effects, electrolyte levels, anemia, pain, depression).	If an etiology for fatigue can be determined, the condition should be treated appropriately.
Provide supplemental oxygen as indicated and monitor response.	Increases oxygenation, reducing anxious feelings. Evaluates effectiveness of therapy.

NURSING DIAGNOSIS: Grieving/Death Anxiety

May Be Related To
Anticipating pain, suffering; loss of body processes
Anticipating impact of death on others
Confronting the reality of terminal disease; perceived proximity of death
Uncertainty about the existence of/encounter with a higher power

Possibly Evidenced By
Reports fear of pain/suffering related to dying
Reports negative thoughts related to death and dying
Reports worry about the impact of one's own death on significant others
Anger; despair; blame; psychological distress

Desired Outcomes/Evaluation Criteria—Client Will

Grief Resolution (NOC)
Verbalize understanding of the dying process.
Discuss spiritual concerns or unresolved conflicts.

Dignified Life Closure (NOC)
Identify and express feelings appropriately.
Participate in decisions regarding basic care and dying process.
Verbalize sense of control over remaining time.

Family Will

Grief Resolution (NOC)
Ventilate conflicts and feelings related to illness and death.
Verbalize understanding of, and progress through, the stages of grief and loss.

ACTIONS/INTERVENTIONS	RATIONALE
Grief Work Facilitation (NIC)	
Independent	
Facilitate development of a trusting relationship with client and family.	Trust is necessary before client and family can feel free to open personal lines of communication with the hospice team and address sensitive issues.
Assess client and SO for stage of grief currently being experienced. Explain process, as appropriate.	Knowledge about the grieving process reinforces the normalcy of feelings and reactions being experienced and can help client deal more effectively with them.
Provide open, nonjudgmental environment. Use therapeutic communication skills of active-listening and acknowledgment.	Promotes and encourages realistic dialogue about feelings and concerns.
Encourage verbalization of thoughts and concerns. Accept expressions of sadness, anger, and rejection. Acknowledge normalcy of these feelings.	Client may feel supported in expression of feelings by the understanding that deep and often conflicting emotions are normal and experienced by others in this difficult situation (Otis-Green, 2008b).
Be aware of mood swings, hostility, and other acting-out behavior. Set limits on inappropriate behavior and redirect negative thinking.	Indicators of ineffective coping and need for additional interventions. Preventing destructive actions enables client to maintain control and sense of self-esteem.
Monitor for signs of debilitating depression such as statements of hopelessness, desire to "end it now." Ask client direct questions about state of mind.	Client may be especially vulnerable when recently diagnosed with end-stage disease process and/or when discharged from hospital. Fear of loss of control or concerns about managing pain effectively may cause client to consider suicide.
Reinforce teaching regarding disease process and provide information as requested and appropriate about dying. Be honest; do not give false hope while providing emotional support.	Client and SO benefit from factual information. Individuals may ask direct questions about death, and honest answers promote trust and provide reassurance that correct information will be given.
Review past life experiences, role changes, sexuality concerns, and coping skills. Promote an environment conducive to talking about things that interest client.	This is an opportunity to identify skills that may help individuals cope with grief of current situation more effectively. *Note:* Issues of sexuality remain important at this stage, such as feelings of masculinity or femininity, giving up caretaker or provider role within family, and ability to maintain sexual activity or closeness, if desired.
Investigate evidence of conflict; expressions of anger; and statements of despair, guilt, hopelessness, and inability to grieve.	Interpersonal conflicts and angry behavior may be client's and SO's way of expressing or dealing with feelings of despair or spiritual distress, necessitating further evaluation and support.
Determine way that client and SO understand and respond to death—cultural expectations; learned behaviors; experience with death of close family members or friends; and beliefs about life after death, spirituality, or faith in a higher power.	These factors affect how each individual faces death and influences how he or she may respond and interact.
Assist client and SO to identify strengths in self or situation and support systems.	Recognizing these resources provides opportunity to work through feelings of grief.
Be aware of own feelings about death. Accept whatever methods client and SO have chosen to help each other through the process.	Caregiver's anxiety and unwillingness to accept reality of possibility of own death may block ability to be helpful to client and SO, necessitating enlisting the aid of others to provide needed support.
Dying Care (NIC)	
Provide open environment for discussion with client and SO, when appropriate, about desires and plans pertaining to death, including making a will, burial arrangements, tissue donation, death benefits, insurance, time for family gatherings, and how to spend remaining time.	If client and SO are mutually aware of impending death, they may more easily deal with unfinished business or desired activities. Having a part in problem-solving and planning can provide a sense of control over anticipated events.
Encourage participation in care decisions.	Allows client to retain some control over life.
Visit frequently and provide physical contact as appropriate and desired, or provide frequent phone support as appropriate for setting. Arrange for care provider or support person to stay with client, as needed.	Helps reduce feelings of isolation and abandonment. Provides respite and time for SO and family to meet own needs and complete required activities.
Allow SO to be physically close, giving permission, instruction, and opportunities to touch the client.	Family and SO may need encouragement to touch the client, which is therapeutic to both the patient and the SO.
Provide time for acceptance, final farewell, and arrangements for memorial or funeral service according to individual spiritual, cultural, and ethnic needs.	Accommodation of personal and family wishes helps reduce anxiety and may promote sense of peace.
Collaborative	
Determine spiritual needs and/or conflicts and refer to appropriate team members, including clergy or spiritual advisor and parish nurse.	Providing for spiritual needs, forgiveness, prayer, devotional materials, or sacraments as requested can relieve spiritual pain and provide a sense of peace. (Refer to ND: risk for Spiritual Distress.)

ACTIONS/INTERVENTIONS (continued)	RATIONALE (continued)
Refer to appropriate counselor, as needed, such as psychiatric clinical nurse specialist, social worker, psychologist, and pastoral support.	Compassion and support can help alleviate distress or palliate feelings of grief to facilitate coping and foster growth.
Refer to visiting nurse or home-health agency if hospice services not available.	Provides support in meeting physical and emotional needs of client and SO and can supplement the care family and friends are able to give.
Identify need for and appropriate timing of antidepressants or anti-anxiety medications.	May alleviate distress and enhance coping, especially for clients not requiring analgesics.

NURSING DIAGNOSIS: compromised family Coping

May Be Related To

Prolonged disease that exhausts the supportive capacity of significant people
Inadequate/incorrect understanding of information by a primary person
Temporary family disorganization, role changes

Possibly Evidenced By

Significant person attempts assistive or supportive behaviors with less than satisfactory results
Client reports a concern about significant person's response to health problem
Significant person enters into limited personal communication with client/withdraws from client

Desired Outcomes/Evaluation Criteria—Family Will

Family Coping (NOC)

Express feelings freely among family members.
Use available support system/community resources.
Engage in decision making for resolution of identified problems.
Share responsibility for family duties and care tasks as appropriate.

ACTIONS/INTERVENTIONS	RATIONALE
Family Involvement Promotion (NIC)	
Independent	
Assess level of anxiety present in family and SO.	Anxiety level needs to be dealt with before problem-solving can begin. Individuals may be so preoccupied with own reactions to situation that they are unable to respond to another's needs.
Establish rapport and acknowledge difficulty of the situation for the family.	May assist SO to accept what is happening and be willing to share problems with healthcare providers.
Determine level of coping impairment. Evaluate current behaviors that may be interfering with the care of client.	Information about family problems such as divorce or separation, alcoholism, other drug use, or abusive situation will be helpful in determining options and developing an appropriate plan of care.
Note client's emotional and behavioral responses resulting from increasing weakness and dependency, such as depression, withdrawal, hostility, hallucinations, and delusions.	Approaching death is most stressful when client and family coping responses are strained, resulting in increased frustration, guilt, and anguish.
Discuss underlying reasons for client behaviors with family.	When family members know why client is behaving differently, it may help them understand, accept, and deal with unusual behaviors.
Assist family and client to understand "who owns the problem" and who is responsible for resolution. Avoid placing blame or guilt.	When these boundaries are defined, each individual can begin to take care of own self and stop taking care of others in inappropriate ways.
Determine current knowledge and perceptions of the situation.	Provides information on which to begin planning care and making informed decisions. Lack of information or unrealistic perceptions can interfere with individual's responses to illness situation.
Assess current actions of SO and how they are received by client.	SO may be trying to be helpful, but actions are not perceived as such by client. SO may be withdrawn or too protective.
Facilitate family conference; include all family members, as appropriate. Provide and reinforce information about terminal illness, death, and future family needs.	Knowledge can help the family prepare for eventualities and deal with the actual death process. Increases understanding of necessary activities and steps to be taken to deal with funeral preparations, legal and financial concerns, and survivor issues.
Collaborative	
Refer to appropriate resources for assistance, as indicated, including family counseling, psychotherapy, community support groups, and respite care.	May need additional assistance in resolving family issues, making peace, and maintaining personal well-being.

NURSING DIAGNOSIS: risk for Spiritual Distress

Risk Factors May Include

Anxiety; stress; depression
Separated from support systems
Blocks to experiencing love; low self-esteem; inability to forgive

Possibly Evidenced By

(Not applicable; presence of signs and symptoms establishes an *actual* diagnosis)

Desired Outcomes/Evaluation Criteria—Client Will

Spiritual Health (NOC)

Identify meaning and purpose in own life.
Report sense of connectedness with self/others.
Verbalize feelings of peacefulness or spiritual contentment.

ACTIONS/INTERVENTIONS	RATIONALE
Spiritual Support (NIC)	
Independent	
Listen to client's and SO's reports and expressions of anger or concern.	May reveal many conflicting thoughts and beliefs, for example, that illness or situation is a punishment for wrongdoing or that death is desirable or feared. Dying client faces momentous losses of physical control and function, of independence, of relationships, of possibilities, and ultimately of life itself. To family members and friends, the loss of a loved one causes great stress and temporarily impairs concentration, decision making, and work performance.
Determine client's religious or spiritual orientation, current involvement, and presence of conflicts in current circumstances.	Provides insight as to where client currently is and what hopes for the future may be. *Note:* Individuals reporting high spirituality were less hopeless, had less desire to hasten their deaths, and had less suicidal ideation.
Assess sense of self-concept, worth, and ability to enter into or maintain loving relationships.	Necessary to provide firm foundation for growth and guiding client and family through life closure and completion tasks.
Explore interpretation and relationship of spirituality, concept of life, and death and illness to client's spiritual centeredness.	Identifying the meaning of these issues may be helpful in forming or stating a belief system that enables client to move forward. Comfort can be gained when family and friends share client's beliefs and support search for spiritual knowledge.
Explore ways that spirituality or religious practices, such as music, prayer, meditation, and rituals, have affected client's life.	Allows client to explore spiritual needs and decide what fits own view, and provides support for dealing with current situation.
Determine support systems available to and used by client and SO.	May help identify strengths and weaknesses in relationship dynamics that the client and SOs may want to address, such as expressing love, forgiveness, and support.
Encourage client to be introspective in search for peace and harmony.	Finding peace within will carry over to relationships with others and one's outlook on life and death.
Establish environment that promotes free expression of feelings and concerns.	May help identify the real need of the day. For example, the dying person may not hope for cure or postponement of death, but rather that on the next day he or she will feel better with fewer physical and emotional discomforts.
Have client and SO identify and prioritize current and immediate needs regarding faith, influence, and community.	Helps client and SO focus on what needs to be done and identify manageable steps to take.
Make time for nonjudgmental discussion of cultural and philosophical issues and questions about spiritual impact of illness and/or impending death.	Spiritual or religious practices, customs, and rituals often play important roles, especially at a time of such significant transition in life.
Discuss difference between grief and guilt and help client to identify and deal with each, assuming responsibility for own actions.	Identifies persons at risk for complicated grief and bereavement and its associated depression and complications. May provide opportunities for resolution.
Use therapeutic communication skills of gentle stillness, reflection, conveying respect through tone of voice and body language, and active-listening.	Encourages client and SO to identify and express end-of-life concerns, hopes, fears, and expectations openly and honestly in a caring milieu.
Review coping skills used and their effectiveness in current situation.	Helps client and SO remember and call upon strengths that have been helpful in other situations. May free the client to be "more" creative, loving, and into the experience of well-being.

ACTIONS/INTERVENTIONS (continued)	RATIONALE (continued)
Suggest use of storytelling, journaling, or taping thoughts.	Helps client explore and find own solutions to concerns. Identifies strengths to incorporate into plan and techniques needing revision.
Determine how involved in physical care the family members want to be. Establish with client and SO wishes for the moment of death.	Clarification of specific wishes can be helpful in reducing stress and allow for needed differences in response.
Collaborative	
Encourage participation in desired religious activities, prayer, meditation, or contact with minister, spiritual advisor, or grief counselor.	May prove beneficial to both client and family members in reflecting on life and death issues. Can assist in clarifying values and ideas, recognizing and resolving feelings, and promoting comfort. Validating one's beliefs in an external way can support and strengthen the inner self.

Refer to CP: Psychosocial Aspects of Care; ND: risk for impaired Religiosity for additional interventions.

NURSING DIAGNOSIS: risk for Caregiver Role Strain

Risk Factors May Include

Amount/complexity of caregiving tasks; duration of caregiving required
Presence of situational stressors that normally affect families (e.g., major life event, crisis, significant loss)
Caregiver is spouse; lack of respite for caregiver

Possibly Evidenced By

(Not applicable; presence of signs and symptoms establishes an *actual* diagnosis)

Desired Outcomes/Evaluation Criteria—Caregiver Will

Caregiver Role Endurance (NOC)

Demonstrate mastery of direct/indirect care tasks.
Share responsibility for caregiving tasks with family members/support system.
Engage in appropriate leisure activities/respite.

ACTIONS/INTERVENTIONS	RATIONALE
Caregiver Support (NIC)	
Independent	
Determine caregiver's health, level of commitment, responsibility, and involvement in care. Use assessment tool, such as Burden Interview, to further clarify caregiver's abilities, when appropriate.	Terminal care taxes caregiver and may alter ability to meet client's and own needs (Otis-Green, 2008a).
Ascertain caregiver's understanding and acceptance of client's wishes and advance directives.	If caregiver is not in total agreement with client's wishes, role strain may be intensified as specific decisions are made regarding care and termination of therapies.
Involve SO in information giving, problem-solving, and care of client, as appropriate. Instruct in medication administration techniques, needed treatments, and appropriate complementary and alternative therapies, such as massage, herbs, aromatherapy, and relaxation techniques. Ascertain adeptness with required equipment.	Information can reduce feelings of helplessness and uselessness. Helping a client and family find comfort is often more important than adhering to strict routines. However, family caregivers need to feel confident with specific care activities and equipment. *Note:* Use of complementary and alternative medicine is increasing for pain and symptom relief with lessened side effects.
Provide positive feedback for efforts.	Helps caregiver recognize and feel valued for contribution to care.
Emphasize importance of self-nurturing, personal needs, and social contacts.	Taking time for self can help lessen risk of being overwhelmed by situation.
Identify and schedule alternative care resources, such as family, friends, sitter, and respite services, as needed.	As client's condition worsens, primary caregiver will require additional help from other sources to maintain client at home as desired while still meeting own needs for rest and personal time.
Collaborative	
Refer to community resources to address specific needs, as indicated, such as insurance/financial services and hospice/respite care.	May need additional assistance to facilitate client's wishes for end-of-life care and to support caregiver's well-being.
Arrange for appropriate prescriptions for SO (e.g., sedative, hypnotic).	Mild medication may be beneficial in reducing anxiety and promoting sleep, which, in turn, can enhance coping ability.

DISASTER CONSIDERATIONS

I. Problem

a. The bigger the disaster or catastrophe, the greater the number of people involved and the wider the effect.

b. Physical effects of a catastrophic event can vary depending on the type of disaster.
   - i. Explosive devices, transportation accidents, hurricanes, or floods—burns, traumatic brain and crush injuries, amputations
   - ii. Release of chemical agents—burns, pulmonary or other organ damage, neurological impairment
   - iii. Biological weapons or infections/disease outbreaks (e.g., avian flu or pandemic influenza)
   - iv. Radioactive contamination or exposure—burns, radiation sickness, cancer (long-term concern)

c. Disaster classifications and examples:
   - i. Time-limited—tornado
   - ii. Evolving—wildfires, floods, hurricanes
   - iii. Prolonged—drought
   - iv. Recurrent—wildfire followed by spring flood

II. Consequences

a. Following any disaster, those involved—victims, rescuers, and the surrounding community—suffer from a variety of responses.

a. Disaster or extreme events can have indirect health-related effects.
   - i. Exacerbation of chronic condition, such as heart or respiratory problems
   - ii. Precipitation of emergent conditions such as premature births, seizures, or mental health conditions

c. Psychological ramifications
   - i. Immediate stressors may cause anxiety or panic disorders.
   - ii. The playing and replaying of the events in one's mind may lead to suicidal thoughts and post-traumatic stress disorder (PTSD).
   - iii. Repeated media coverage can magnify the effects; people far removed from the scene may also suffer.

GLOSSARY

Acute stress disorder (ASD): Symptoms of ASR last more than 2 days but less than 1 month after exposure to traumatic event.

Acute stress reaction (ASR): Refers to a range of transient conditions that develop in response to a traumatic event. Onset of some signs and symptoms may occur within minutes of the event and in most cases will disappear within days or even hours.

Biological agents: Viruses (smallpox), bacteria (anthrax, *Salmonella*), other agents including toxins (botulism), that can cause illness or death.

Chemical agents: Poisonous gases, liquids, or solids, including nerve agents (sarin), biotoxins (ricine), choking or pulmonary agents (chlorine, ammonia), blood agents (cyanide), caustics (hydrofluoric acid), visicants or blister agents (lewisite, mustard gas), or long-acting anticoagulants (super warfarin) that can cause serious injury or death.

Disaster: Generally refers to a catastrophic natural or man-made event affecting a large population resulting in injury, death, and destruction of property that overwhelms local resources.

Eye movement desensitization and reprocessing (EMDR): Information-processing psychotherapy technique integrating elements of psychodynamic, cognitive-behavioral, interpersonal, experiential, and body-centered therapies to assist individuals to deal with anxious feelings and stress associated with traumatic memories (EMDR Institute, 2004).

Post-traumatic stress disorder (PTSD): Intense physical and psychological distress that ensues following a traumatic event, manifested by horrifying memories, reexperiencing the event or flashbacks, recurring fears, and feelings of helplessness. May be acute—beginning within 6 months and not lasting longer than 6 months; chronic—lasting longer than 6 months; or delayed—period of latency of 6 months or more.

Psychological first aid: An evidenced-based set of skills to help children, adolescents, adults, and families immediately following a disaster event to reduce the associated distress and to foster short- and long-term adaptive coping by providing information, support, comfort, and safety. It is the behavioral health correlation to physical first aid with the goal being to "stop the bleeding" (Brymer, 2006).

Care Setting

Wherever disaster occurs and includes triage areas, aid stations, clinics, hospital and emergency centers, and community shelters.

Related Concerns

Burns: thermal, chemical, and electrical—acute and convalescent phases, 638
Craniocerebral trauma—acute rehabilitative phase, page 197
Fractures, page 601
Pediatric considerations, page 872
Pneumonia, page 129
Psychosocial aspects of care, page 729
Sepsis/septicemia, page 665

Client Assessment Database

Data depend on specific injuries incurred and presence of chronic conditions (refer to specific plans of care for appropriate data, such as burns, multiple trauma, cardiac and respiratory conditions, and so forth) and timing of presentation for care.

DIAGNOSTIC DIVISION MAY REPORT	MAY EXHIBIT
ACTIVITY/REST	
• Sleep disturbances—recurrent intrusive dreams of the event, nightmares, difficulty in falling or staying asleep; hypersomnia with intrusive thoughts, flashbacks • Fatigue	• Listlessness
CIRCULATION	
• Palpitations • Hot flashes or chills	• Tachycardia • Sweating • Cold, clammy hands • Elevated blood pressure (BP) (anxiety) • Decreased BP (dehydration, hypovolemia)
EGO INTEGRITY	
• Excessive worry about event • Avoidance of circumstances or locations associated with incident • Sense of inner turmoil • Dry mouth, upset stomach, lump in throat • Perceived threat to physical integrity or self-concept • Questioning of God's purpose, abandonment	• Facial expression in keeping with level of anxiety—furrowed brow, strained face, eyelid twitch • Labile emotions • Inappropriate humor
ELIMINATION	
• Frequent urination • Diarrhea	
FOOD/FLUID	
• Lack of interest in food, dysfunctional eating pattern—decreased or increased intake • Nausea, vomiting, gastric distress	
NEUROSENSORY	
• Lightheadedness, dizziness • Anticipation of misfortune to self or others • Feeling stuck • Absence of other mental disorder	• Confusion, memory loss • Motor tension, shakiness, jitteriness, trembling, easily startled • Apprehensive expectation, rumination • Excessive vigilance, hyperattentiveness • Distractibility, difficulty concentrating or making decisions, shortened attention span • Irritability, impatience • Psychic numbing
PAIN/DISCOMFORT	
• Muscle aches, tension headaches, chest pain • Pain related to physical injuries or comorbid conditions	• Guarding or distraction behaviors
RESPIRATORY	
• Shortness of breath • Smothering sensation	• Increased respiratory rate
SAFETY	
• Increased smoking, substance use or abuse • Fear of harm to self or others	
SEXUALITY	
• Decreased libido	

(continues on page 860)

Client Assessment Database (continued)

DIAGNOSTIC DIVISION MAY REPORT (continued)	MAY EXHIBIT (continued)
SOCIAL INTERACTIONS • Concern for well-being of others • Questioning own actions, survival • Difficulty participating in social settings • Reluctance to engage in usual activities, work	• Withdrawal
TEACHING/LEARNING • *Discharge plan considerations:* Dependent on individual situation, level of support, and available resources	

Diagnostic Studies

Dependent on injuring agent and exposure and availability of resources for testing and procedures.

Nursing Priorities

1. Prevent or treat life-threatening conditions.
2. Prevent further injury and spread of infection.
3. Support efforts to cope with situation.
4. Facilitate integration of event.
5. Assist community in recovery process and preparing for future occurrences.

Discharge Goals

1. Free of preventable complications.
2. Anxiety reduced to a manageable level.
3. Beginning to cope effectively with situation.
4. Plan in place to meet needs after discharge.
5. Community preparedness enhanced.

NURSING DIAGNOSIS: risk for Injury—Trauma, Suffocation, or Poisoning

Risk Factors May Include

Biological—immunization level of community, presence of microorganism
Chemical—contact with chemical pollutants, poisonous agents
Exposure to open flame or flammable material
Acceleration and deceleration forces
Contamination of food or water

Possibly Evidenced By

(Not applicable; presence of signs and symptoms establishes an *actual* diagnosis)

Desired Outcomes/Evaluation Criteria—Client/Caregivers Will

Physical Injury Severity (NOC)
Minimize degree of and prevent further injury.

Personal Safety Behavior (NOC)
Verbalize understanding of condition and specific needs.
Identify interventions appropriate to situation.
Demonstrate behaviors necessary to protect self from further injury.
Accept responsibility for own care and follow up as individually able.

ACTIONS/INTERVENTIONS	RATIONALE
Triage: Disaster (NIC)	
Independent	
Acquire information about nature of emergency, accident, or disaster.	Identifies basic resource needs and helps to prepare staff for appropriate level of response based on customary injuries and healthcare needs usually associated with specific event.
Prepare area and equipment; check and restock supplies.	Assists in providing safe medical and nursing care in anticipation of emergency need.

ACTIONS/INTERVENTIONS (continued)	RATIONALE (continued)
Assist in prioritizing (triaging) clients for treatment, including decontamination. Monitor for and treat life-threatening injuries.	Promotes efficient care of those who can be medically treated and maximizes use of resources. *Note:* In routine emergency situations, the goal is to do the best for each individual. However, in a disaster, the focus of treatment shifts to do the greatest good for the greatest number.
Determine primary needs and specific complaints of client. Check for medical alert tag.	Information necessary for triaging to appropriate services. (P) *Note:* Pediatric clients are better able to compensate during early hypovolemic shock than adults, creating a false impression of normalcy (American Academy of Pediatrics [AAP], 2006).
Obtain additional medical information, including preexisting conditions, allergies, and current medication. Perform more in-depth assessment as time allows and condition warrants.	Provides for assessment and treatment of conditions that might not be evident initially.
Determine client's developmental level, decision-making ability, level of cognition, and competence.	Affects treatment plan regarding issues of informed consent, self-care, client teaching, and discharge.
Evaluate individual's response to event, mood, coping abilities, and personal vulnerability.	People react to traumatic situations in many ways and may exhibit a wide range of responses—from no visible response to wild emotions. This may result in carelessness or increased risk-taking without considerations of consequences or inability to act on own behalf, including protecting self.
Ascertain knowledge of needs and injury prevention and motivation to prevent further injury.	Indicator of need for information and assistance with making positive changes, promoting safety and sense of security.
Discuss importance of self-monitoring of conditions and emotions that can contribute to occurrence of injury—shock state, ignoring basic needs, fatigue, anger, and irritability.	Recognizing these factors and dealing with them appropriately, including seeking support and assistance, can reduce individual risks.
Note socioeconomic status and availability and use of resources.	May determine ability to access help for identified problems.
Collaborative	
Work with other agencies, such as law enforcement, fire department, Red Cross, and ambulance and EMTs, as indicated. Follow prearranged roles when participating in a community disaster plan.	During a disaster, many people are involved with care of victims. Most communities have disaster plans in which nurses will participate.
Triage: Emergency Care (NIC)	
Identify and manage life-threatening situations—airway problems, bleeding, and diminished consciousness.	Stabilization of medical condition is necessary before proceeding with additional therapies. (P) *Note:* Children are at greater risk than adults when exposed to chemical agents/poisonous gases because of (1) higher minute volume, (2) increased skin permeability, (3) greater body surface to weight ratio, (4) less intravascular volume increasing risk of hypovolemic shock, (5) shorter stature increasing exposure to greatest gas vapor density at ground level (Foltin, 2006).
Obtain and assist with diagnostic studies, as indicated.	Choice of studies is dependent on individual situation and availability of resources.
Provide therapeutic interventions as individually appropriate. (Refer to specific CPs; e.g., Burns, Fractures, Craniocerebral Trauma, Myocardial Infarction, Chronic Obstructive Pulmonary Disease [COPD], Ventilatory Assistance [Mechanical].)	Specific needs of client and the level of care available at a particular site determine response.
Provide written instructions and list of resources for later review.	Client and significant other(s) (SO[s]) are generally not able to assimilate information at time of crisis and may need reinforcement or want additional information.
Identify community resources, including shelter, neighbors, friends, and government agencies available for assistance.	May need assistance or ongoing monitoring postdischarge to deal with self-care needs as well as safe housing and other life requirements. *Note:* Release of client without active support increases personal risk because of possibility of unrecognized or subacute injury or delayed psychological response.
Refer to other resources, as indicated, such as counseling and psychotherapy.	Immediate "debriefing" or counseling is beneficial for dealing with crisis to enhance ability to meet own needs.

NURSING DIAGNOSIS: risk for Infection

Risk Factors May Include

Increased environmental exposure, inadequate acquired immunity, inadequate vaccination
Inadequate primary defenses—broken skin, tissue destruction, invasive procedures
Chronic disease, malnutrition

Possibly Evidenced By

(Not applicable; presence of signs and symptoms establishes an *actual* diagnosis)

Desired Outcomes/Evaluation Criteria—Client Will

Risk Control (NOC)

Verbalize understanding of individual exposure and risk factor(s).
Identify interventions to prevent and reduce risk of infection.

Infection Severity (NOC)

Be free of or demonstrate resolution of infection.

ACTIONS/INTERVENTIONS	RATIONALE
Infection Control (NIC)	
Independent	
Note risk factors for occurrence of infection—environmental exposure (including other individuals sharing close quarters such as shelter residents), compromised host, traumatic injury, loss of skin integrity. Determine client's proximity to incident. Be aware of incubation period for various diseases.	Understanding nature and properties of infectious agents and individual's exposure determines choice of therapeutic intervention. *Note:* Those upwind of an aerosol release of a biological agent may have little or no exposure to the agent. (Refer to Table 15.2, at the end of plan of care, for pertinent information.)
Observe for signs and symptoms of infective agent and systemic infection—fever, chills, diaphoresis, altered level of consciousness (LOC), and positive blood cultures. Investigate presence of rash.	Initial symptoms of some agents include fever, fatigue, joint aches, and headache similar to influenza. The infection may even be misdiagnosed as an influenza-like infection (ILI), unless healthcare providers maintain an index of suspicion and obtain additional diagnostic studies. *Note:* (P) The immature immunological system of children places them at higher risk for developing infections (AAP, 2006).
Practice and demonstrate proper hand hygiene.	First-line defense to limit spread of infections.
Provide for infection precautions or isolation, as indicated—standard precautions of gown, gloves, face shield or goggles, respiratory mask or filter, and reverse or negative pressure room, when available.	Reduces risk of cross-contamination to staff, visitors, and other clients.
Group or cohort individuals in facility/shelter with same diagnosis or exposure as resources require.	Limited resources may dictate open ward-like environment, but need to control spread of infection still exists.
Monitor visitors/shelter residents, caregivers, and volunteers for infectious diseases.	Prevents exposure of client to further infection and may reveal additional cases.
Review individual nutritional needs, appropriate exercise program, and need for rest.	Essential for well-being and recovery.
Instruct client/SO(s) in techniques to prevent spread of infection, protect the integrity of skin, and care for wounds or lesions.	Self-care activities that may provide protection for client and others.
Emphasize necessity of taking antibiotics as directed, especially dosage and length of therapy.	Premature discontinuation of treatment when client begins to feel well may result in return of infection. However, unnecessary use of antibiotics may result in development of secondary infections or resistant organisms.
Monitor cleanliness of shelter, food storage and preparation.	Proper food-handling techniques and disposal of waste/diapers and incontinent pads/briefs as well as medical waste such as dressings reduces risk of spread of infection.
Involve community/shelter residents in education programs geared to increasing awareness of spread and prevention of communicable diseases.	Helps to reduce incidence of disease in the community as well as manage the dissemination of information.
Collaborative	
Obtain appropriate specimens for observation and culture and sensitivities testing—nose and throat swabs, sputum, blood, urine, or feces.	Provides information to diagnose infection and determine appropriate therapeutic interventions.
Assist with medical procedures, such as incision and drainage of abscess, bronchoscopy, or wound care, as indicated.	Helps determine causative factors for appropriate treatment and facilitates recovery.
Administer and monitor medication regimen (e.g., antimicrobials, topical antibiotics) and note client's response.	Determines effectiveness of therapy and presence of side effects.

ACTIONS/INTERVENTIONS (continued) — RATIONALE (continued)

Provide passive protection such as immune globulin, active protection (e.g., vaccination), or chemoprophylaxis, as appropriate.

May prevent development of infection following exposure or reduce the likelihood of acquiring disease in the future. (Refer to Table 15.3 at the end of plan of care.)

Alert proper authorities to presence of specific infectious agent and number of cases.

Diseases that could be caused by biological releases or that spread rapidly through populations have reporting requirements to local, state, and national agencies, such as the state health department or the Centers for Disease Control and Prevention (CDC). These agencies, in turn, have responsibilities for the public safety and welfare.

NURSING DIAGNOSIS: [severe/panic] Anxiety

May Be Related To

Situational crisis; exposure to toxins
Threat to health status; threat of death
Interpersonal transmission (e.g., of concerns or fears)
Unconscious conflict about essential values, beliefs
Unmet needs

Possibly Evidenced By

Reports concerns due to change in life events
Distressed, apprehensive, irritability, worried, focus on self, fear
Scanning, vigilance, restlessness
Cardiovascular excitation; changes in vital signs
Impaired attention; difficulty concentrating; rumination

Desired Outcomes/Evaluation Criteria—Client Will

Anxiety Self-Control (NOC)

Acknowledge and discuss feelings.
Verbalize accurate knowledge of current situation and potential outcomes.
Identify healthy ways to successfully deal with stress.
Report anxiety is reduced to a manageable level.
Demonstrate problem-solving skills appropriate for individual situation.
Use resources and support systems effectively.

ACTIONS/INTERVENTIONS — RATIONALE

Crisis Intervention (NIC)

Independent

Perform screening/needs assessment for all individuals following event.

Initial reactions following event are varied, complex, and can be unstable. Acute stress reaction (ASR) is a transient condition developing within minutes or hours and although usually resolving within 2–3 days; early intervention (such as psychological first aid) may reduce progression to a more serious stress disorder (VA/DoD, 2010).

Determine degree of anxiety or fear present; associated behaviors, such as laughter, crying, calm or agitation, excited or hysterical behavior; expressions of disbelief and/or self-blame; and reality of perceived threat.

Clearly understanding client's perception is pivotal to providing appropriate assistance in dealing with anxiety. Individual may be agitated or totally overwhelmed. Severe anxiety increases risk for client's own safety as well as the safety of others in the environment. *Note:* (P) Children are affected by their own reaction to the event as well as the transmission of anxiety or fear being experienced by parents and care providers, thus magnifying the psychological impact on the child (AAP, 2006).

Note cultural factors that may influence anxiety and response to event.

Individual responses are influenced by cultural values and beliefs and culturally learned patterns of one's family of origin impacting how the individual expresses emotions and attitudes toward assistance from others/government agencies or counseling services (Brymer, 2006). *Note*: Cultural or religious affiliations may impact responses of others client comes in contact with.

(continues on page 864)

ACTIONS/INTERVENTIONS (continued)	RATIONALE (continued)
Note degree of disorganization.	Client may be unable to handle activities of daily living (ADLs) or work requirements and may need more intensive evaluation and intervention. P Children may regress—girls may express anxiety and sadness, whereas boys are more likely to display behavioral problems (AAP, 2006).
Maintain and respect client's personal space boundaries—approximately 4-foot circle around client.	Entering client's personal space without permission or invitation could result in an overwhelming anxiety response and, possibly, an overt act of violence. Respecting personal space helps client to feel safe, which is an important factor in client regaining or maintaining pre-event status (VA/DoD, 2010).
Create quiet area as able. Maintain a calm, confident manner. Speak in even tone using short, simple sentences.	Decreases sense of confusion, overstimulation, and enhances sense of safety. Helps client focus on what is said and reduces transmission of anxiety.
Develop trusting relationship with client.	Trust is the basis of a therapeutic nurse-client relationship and enables them to work together effectively.
Identify whether incident has reactivated preexisting or coexisting situations—physical or psychological.	Concerns or psychological issues will be recycled every time trauma is re-experienced and affect how the client views the current situation.
Determine presence of physical symptoms, such as numbness, headache, chest tightness, nausea, and pounding heart.	Physical problems need to be differentiated from anxiety symptoms so that appropriate treatment can be given.
Identify psychological responses—anger, shock, acute anxiety, panic, confusion, and denial. Record emotional changes.	Although these are normal responses at the time of the trauma, they will recycle again and again until they are dealt with adequately.
Discuss with client perception of what is causing anxiety or panic.	Increases ability to connect symptoms to subjective feeling of anxiety, providing opportunity to gain insight and control, and make desired changes.
Assist client to correct any distortions being experienced.	Provides opportunity to clarify misperceptions, including possibility of survivor's guilt. Perceptions based on reality will help to decrease fearfulness.
P Use developmentally appropriate language to discuss event and its meaning to child.	P Younger children usually have less understanding of abstract concepts and benefit from direct and simple language. Approaching adolescents "adult-to-adult" reinforces that you respect their feelings and concerns (Brymer, 2006).
Explore with client and SO the manner in which the client has coped with anxiety-producing events before the trauma.	May help client regain sense of control and recognize significance of trauma.
Engage client in learning new coping behaviors, such as progressive muscle relaxation and thought stopping.	Replacing maladaptive behaviors can enhance ability to manage and deal with stress. Interrupting obsessive thinking allows client to use energy to address underlying anxiety, while continued rumination about the incident can actually retard recovery.
Demonstrate and encourage use of techniques to reduce or manage stress and vent emotions such as anger and hostility.	Reduces likelihood of eruptions that can result in abusive behavior.
Give positive feedback when client demonstrates better ways to manage anxiety and is able to calmly and/or realistically appraise own situation.	Provides acknowledgment and reinforcement, encouraging use of new coping strategies. Enhances ability to deal with fearful feelings and gain control over situation, promoting future successes.
Engage client in simple tasks and advance responsibilities as appropriate.	Encourages individual to focus attention other than on self, enhancing sense of control and self-worth.
Collaborative	
Administer medications, as indicated, for example:	
Anti-anxiety agents, such as Diazepam (Valium), buspirone (BuSpar), alprazolam (Xanax), and oxazepam (Serax)	Provides temporary relief of anxiety symptoms, enhancing client's ability to cope with situation. Also useful for alleviating feelings of panic and intrusive nightmares.
Antidepressants, such as Fluoxetine (Prozac), paroxetine (Paxil), and bupropion (Wellbutrin)	Used to decrease anxiety, lift mood, aid in management of behavior, and ensure rest until client regains control of own self. Helpful in suppressing intrusive thoughts and explosive anger.
Refer for additional therapies, such as hypnosis, EMDR, or Thought Reprocessing Therapy, as appropriate.	When used by trained therapist, these short-term therapies are particularly effective with individuals who have been traumatized or who have problems with anxiety and depression. Systematic desensitization, reframing, and reinterpretation of memories may be achieved through hypnosis.
Coordinate release or discharge to family, friend, or emergency services, as indicated.	Triaging and maximum use of resources may limit time allotted for care, and client may not be ready to meet own needs or assume full responsibility for self.

ACTIONS/INTERVENTIONS (continued)	RATIONALE (continued)
Educate victims and public about risks and steps being taken to deal with problem. Include other members of healthcare teams, stressing risks to themselves. Refer to such resources as the CDC or specific Web sites.	Nurses have a role in community education because they are close to the individuals affected. Providing accurate information and credible resources helps limit level of concern and transmission of anxiety. Current, timely information regarding biological concerns and healthcare needs can be accessed through such Web sites as www.cdc.gov, www.hhs.gov, and www.fbi.gov.

NURSING DIAGNOSIS: Spiritual Distress

May Be Related To

Natural disasters; environmental/life changes
Anxiety; stress; depression
Separated support system; loss

Possibly Evidenced By

(Not applicable; presence of signs and symptoms establishes an *actual* diagnosis)

Desired Outcomes/Evaluation Criteria—Client Will

Spiritual Health (NOC)

Verbalize increased sense of self-concept and hope for future.
Discuss beliefs and values about spiritual issues.
Verbalize acceptance of self as being worthy.

ACTIONS/INTERVENTIONS	RATIONALE
Spiritual Support (NIC)	
Independent	
Determine client's religious or spiritual orientation, current involvement, and presence of conflicts.	Provides baseline for planning care and accessing appropriate resources.
Establish environment that promotes free expression of feelings and concerns. Provide calm, peaceful setting when possible.	Promotes awareness and identification of feelings so they can be dealt with.
Listen to client's and SO's reports or expressions of anger, concern, alienation from God, and/or belief that situation is a punishment for wrongdoing.	Helpful to understand client's and SO's point of view and how they are questioning their faith in the face of tragedy.
Note sense of futility, feelings of hopelessness and helplessness, and lack of motivation to help self.	These thoughts and feelings can result in the client feeling paralyzed and unable to move forward to resolve the situation.
Listen to expressions of inability to find meaning in life or reason for living. Evaluate for suicidal ideation.	May indicate need for further intervention to prevent suicide attempt.
Determine support systems available to client and SO(s).	Presence or lack of support systems can affect client's recovery.
Ask how you can be most helpful. Convey acceptance of client's spiritual beliefs and concerns.	Promotes trust and comfort, encouraging client to be open about sensitive matters.
Make time for nonjudgmental discussion of philosophical issues or questions about spiritual impact of events and current situation.	Helps client to begin to look at basis for spiritual confusion. *Note:* There is a potential for care provider's belief system to interfere with client finding own way. Therefore, it is most beneficial to remain neutral and not espouse own beliefs.
Discuss difference between grief and guilt and help client to identify and deal with each, assuming responsibility for own actions and expressing awareness of the consequences of acting out of false guilt.	Blaming self for what has happened impedes dealing with the grief process and needs to be discussed and dealt with.
Use therapeutic communication skills of reflection and active-listening.	Helps client find own solutions to concerns.
Discuss use of, and provide opportunities for, client and SO to experience meditation, prayer, and forgiveness. Provide information that anger with God is a normal part of the grieving process.	Can help to heal past and present pain.
Assist client to develop goals for dealing with life situation.	Enhances commitment to goal, optimizing outcomes and promoting sense of hope.
Collaborative	
Identify and refer to resources that can be helpful, such as pastoral or parish nurse, religious counselor, crisis counselor, psychotherapy, and Alcoholics or Narcotics Anonymous.	Specific assistance to resolve life stressors such as relationship problems, substance use, or suicidal ideation are important to advance recovery process.
Encourage participation in support groups.	Discussing concerns and questions with others can help client resolve feelings.

NURSING DIAGNOSIS: risk for Post-Trauma Syndrome

Risk Factors May Include

Events outside the range of usual human experience
Serious threat or injury to self or loved ones, witnessing violent death or tragic events
Disasters; destruction of one's home or community; epidemics
Exaggerated sense of responsibility and survivor's role in the event

Possibly Evidenced By

(Not applicable; presence of signs and symptoms establishes an *actual* diagnosis)

Desired Outcomes/Evaluation Criteria—Client/Caregivers Will

Personal Resiliency (NOC)

Express own feelings and reactions openly, avoiding projection.
Demonstrate ability to deal with emotional reactions in an individually appropriate manner.

Anxiety Level (NOC)

Report absence of physical manifestations such as pain, nightmares, flashbacks, or fatigue associated with the event.

ACTIONS/INTERVENTIONS	RATIONALE
Crisis Intervention (NIC)	
Independent	
Determine involvement in event— survivor, SO, and family, rescue or aid worker, healthcare provider, or family member of responder.	All those concerned with a traumatic event are at risk for emotional trauma and have needs related to their situation and involvement in the event. *Note:* Close involvement with victims or survivors affects individual responses and may prolong emotional suffering.
Evaluate life factors and stressors currently or recently occurring, such as displacement from home due to catastrophic event—illness, injury, natural disaster, or terrorist attack. Identify how client's past experiences may affect current situation.	Affects client's reaction to current event and is basis for planning care and identifying appropriate supports and resources.
Listen for comments of taking on responsibility such as "I should have been more careful . . . or gone back to get her."	Indicators of "survivor's guilt" and blaming self for actions that can delay recovery and impair general well-being.
Identify client's current coping mechanisms.	Noting positive or negative skills provides direction for care.
Determine availability and usefulness of client's support systems—family, social, and community.	Family and others close to the client may also be at risk and require assistance to cope with the trauma.
Provide information about signs and symptoms of post-trauma response, especially if individual is involved in a high-risk occupation.	Awareness of these factors helps individual identify need for assistance when they occur.
Identify and discuss client's strengths as well as vulnerabilities.	Provides information to build on for coping with traumatic experience.
Evaluate individual's perceptions of events and personal significance, for example, a rescue worker trained to provide lifesaving assistance but recovering only dead bodies.	Events that trigger feelings of despair and hopelessness may be more difficult to deal with and require long-term interventions.
Provide emotional and physical presence by sitting with client and SO and offering solace.	Strengthens coping abilities.
Encourage expression of feelings. Note whether feelings expressed appear congruent with events experienced.	It is important to talk about the incident repeatedly. Incongruencies may indicate deeper conflict and can impede resolution.
Note presence of nightmares, reliving the incident, loss of appetite, irritability, numbness and crying, and family or relationship disruption.	These responses are normal in the early postincident time frame. If prolonged and persistent, they may indicate need for more intensive therapy.
Provide a calm, safe environment.	Helps client deal with the disruption in personal life.
Encourage and assist client in learning stress management techniques.	Promotes relaxation and helps individual exercise control over self and what has happened.
Collaborative	
Recommend participation in debriefing sessions that may be provided following major disaster events.	Dealing with the stresses promptly may facilitate recovery from event and prevent exacerbation.
Identify employment and community resource groups.	Provides opportunity for ongoing support to deal with recurrent feelings related to the trauma.
Administer medications, as indicated, such as the following:	
Antipsychotics, for example, phenothiazines such as chlorpromazine (Thorazine) and haloperidol (Haldol)	Low doses may be used for reduction of psychotic symptoms when loss of contact with reality occurs, usually for clients with especially disturbing flashbacks.
Carbamazepine (Tegretol)	Used to alleviate intrusive recollections and flashbacks, impulsivity, and violent behavior.

NURSING DIAGNOSIS: ineffective community Coping

May Be Related To

Natural or human-made disasters—earthquakes, floods, reemerging infectious agents, terrorist activity
Deficits in social support services and resources
Ineffective or nonexistent community systems such as lack of, or inadequate, emergency medical system, transportation system, or disaster planning systems

Possibly Evidenced By

Deficits of community participation; community does not meet its own expectations
Expressed vulnerability; community powerlessness; excessive community conflicts
Stressors perceived as excessive
High illness rates

Desired Outcomes/Evaluation Criteria—Community Will

Community Competence (NOC)

Recognize negative and positive factors affecting community's ability to meet its own demands or needs.
Identify alternatives to inappropriate activities for adaptation and problem-solving.
Report a measurable increase in necessary or desired activities to improve community functioning.

ACTIONS/INTERVENTIONS	RATIONALE
Community Disaster Preparedness (NIC)	
Independent	
Evaluate community activities as related to meeting collective needs within the community itself and between the community and the larger society. Note immediate needs, including healthcare, food, shelter, and funds.	Provides a baseline to determine community needs in relation to current concerns or threats.
Note community reports of functioning, including areas of weakness or conflict.	Provides a view of how the community itself sees these areas.
Identify effects of related factors on community activities.	In the face of a current threat, local or national, community resources need to be evaluated, updated, and given priority to meet the identified need.
Determine availability and use of resources. Identify unmet demands or needs of the community.	Information necessary to identify what else is needed to meet the current situation.
Determine community strengths.	Promotes understanding of the ways in which the community is already meeting the identified needs.
Encourage community members and groups to engage in problem-solving activities.	Promotes a sense of working together to meet the needs.
Develop a plan jointly with the members of the community to address immediate needs.	Deals with deficits in support of identified goals.
Create plans managing interactions within the community itself and between the community and the larger society.	Meets collective needs when the concerns or threats are shared beyond a local community.
Make information accessible to the public. Provide channels for dissemination of information to the community as a whole, including print media, radio and television, reports and community bulletin boards, Internet resources, speaker's bureau, reports to committees, councils, or advisory boards.	Readily available accurate information can help citizens make informed decisions to deal with the situation.
Make information available in different modalities and geared to differing educational levels and cultures within the community.	Using languages other than English and making written materials accessible to all members of the community will promote understanding.
Seek out and evaluate needs of underserved populations.	The homeless and those residing in lower-income areas may have special needs requiring additional resources.

NURSING DIAGNOSIS: readiness for enhanced community Coping

May Be Related To

Social support available; resources available for problem-solving
Community has a sense of power to manage stressors

Possibly Evidenced By

Active planning by community for predicted stressors
Active problem-solving by community when faced with issues
Positive communication among community members and between community and aggregates and larger community
Resources sufficient for managing stressors

(continues on page 868)

NURSING DIAGNOSIS: readiness for enhanced community Coping (continued)

Desired Outcomes/Evaluation Criteria—Community Will

Community Competence (NOC)

Identify positive and negative factors affecting management of current and future problems or stressors.
Have an established plan in place to deal with various contingencies.
Report a measurable increase in ability to deal with potential events.

ACTIONS/INTERVENTIONS	RATIONALE
Program Development (NIC) *Independent*	
Review community plans to monitor for and deal with untoward events.	Provides a baseline for comparison of preparedness with other communities and developing plan to address concerns.
Assess effects of related factors on management of problems or stressors.	Identifies areas that need to be addressed to enhance community coping.
Determine community strengths and weaknesses. Identify limitations in current pattern of community activities that can be improved through adaptation and problem-solving.	Plan can be built on strengths, and areas of weakness can be addressed.
Evaluate community activities as related to management of problems or stressors within the community itself and between the community and the larger society.	Disasters occurring in the community or the country affect the local community and need to be recognized and addressed.
Define and discuss current needs and anticipated or projected concerns.	Agreement on scope and parameters of needs is essential for effective planning.
Identify and prioritize community goals.	Helps to bring the community together to meet a common concern or threat. Helps maintain focus and facilitates accomplishment.
Promote community awareness about the problems of design of buildings, equipment, transportation systems, and workplace practices that may compound disaster or impact disaster response.	Provides opportunity for making changes that promote safety.
Identify available resources—persons, groups, financial, governmental, as well as other communities.	Important to work together to meet goals. Major catastrophes affect more than local community, and communities need to work together to deal with and accomplish growth.
Seek out and involve underserved and at-risk groups within the community.	Supports communication and commitment of community as a whole.
Assist the community to form partnerships within the community and between the community and the larger society.	Promotes long-term developmental growth of the community.
Establish mechanism for self-monitoring of community needs and evaluation of efforts.	Facilitates proactive rather than reactive responses by the community.
Participate in exercises and activities to test preparedness.	Provides opportunities to verify appropriateness of plans and problem-solve deficiencies.
Use multiple formats—TV, radio, print media, billboards, computer bulletin boards, speaker's bureau, and reports to community leaders and groups on file that are accessible to the public.	Keeps the community informed and involved regarding plans, needs, and outcomes of tests of the plans.

TABLE 15.2 Clinical Characteristics of Critical Biological Agents—7/1/00

Disease	Signs and Symptoms	Physical Exam	Clinical Test	Key Differential Diagnosis	Incubation Period	Duration of Illness	Case Fatality	U.S. Epidemiology
Inhalational anthrax	Fever, malaise, cough, mild chest discomfort, possible short recovery phase then onset of dyspnea, diaphoresis, stridor, cyanosis, shock. Death 24–36 hours after onset of severe symptoms. Hemor-rhagic meningitis in up to 50%.	Nonspecific physical findings.	Serology, gram stain, culture, polymerase chain reaction (PCR); chest x-ray (CXR)—widened mediastinum. Rarely pneumonia.	Hantavirus pulmonary syndrome (HPS), dissecting aortic aneurysm (no fever)	1–6 days (up to 45 days)	3–5 days	Usually fatal if untreated	None
Pneumonic plague	High fever, chills, headache, hemoptysis and toxemia, rapid progression to dyspnea, stridor, and cyanosis. Death from respiratory failure, shock, and bleeding.	Rales, hemoptysis, purpura	Gram stain, culture, serum immunoassay for capsular antigen, PCR, immunohistochemical stains (IHC)	HPS, tuberculosis (TB), community acquired pneumonia (CAP), meningococcemia, rickettsioses	1–7 days Usually 2–5 days	1–6 days	High unless treated in 12–24 hours	2–3 cases/yr, mainly in SW U.S.
Tularemia	Typhoidal–aerosol, gastrointestinal, and intradermal challenge. Fever, headache, malaise, chest discomfort, anorexia, nonproductive cough. Pneumonia in 30%–80%. Oculoglandular from inoculation of conjunctiva with periorbital edema.	No adenopathy with typhoidal illness	Serology, culture, PCR, IHC; CXR—pneumonia, mediastinal lymphadenopathy, or pleural effusion	Atypical CAP, Q fever, brucellosis	1–21 days (average 3–5 days)	≥2 wks	Moderate if untreated	150 case/yr, transmitted by ticks/deer flies or contact with infected animals

(continues on page 870)

TABLE 15.2 Clinical Characteristics of Critical Biological Agents—7/1/00 (continued)

Disease	Signs and Symptoms	Physical Exam	Clinical Test	Key Differential Diagnosis	Incubation Period	Duration of Illness	Case Fatality	U.S. Epidemiology
Smallpox	Fever, back pain, vomiting, malaise, headache, rigors. Papules 2–3 days later, progressing to pustular vesicles. Abundant on face and extremities initially.	Papules, pustules, or scabs of similar stage, many on face/ extremities, palms/soles	Guamierl bodies on Glemsa or modified silver stain, virions on electron microscopy, PCR, viral isolation, IHC	Varicella, vaccinia, monkeypox, cowpox, disseminated herpes zoster	7–17days (average 12 days)	4 wks	High to moderate	None
Botulism	Ptosis, blurred vision, diplopia, generalized weakness, dizziness, dysarthria, dysphonia, dysphagia, followed by symmetrical descending flaccid paralysis and respiratory failure	No fever, client alert, postural hypotension, pupils unreactive, normal sensation, variable muscle weaknesss	Serology, toxin assays/anaerobic cultures of blood/stool; electromyography studies	Guillain Barré, myasthenia gravis, tick paralysis, Mg^{++} intoxication, organophosphate poisoning, polio	12 hours–5 days	Death 24–72 hours, lasts months if not lethal	High mortality without respiratory support	30 cases/yr; food intoxication, wound infections, or honey ingestion (infants)
Viral Hemorrhagic Fever								
Filoviruses (Marburg, Ebola)	Fever, severe headache, malaise, myalgia, maculopapular rash day 5; progression to pharyngitis, hematemasis, melena, uncontrolled bleeding; shock/ death 6–9 days	Petechia, ecchymoses, conjunctivitis, uncontrolled bleeding	Serology, PCR, IHC, electron microscopy (EM); elevated liver enzymes, thrombocytopenia	Meningococcemia, malaria, typhus, leptospirosis, borreliosis, thrombotic thrombocytopenic purpura (TTP), rickettsiosis, hemolytic uremic syndrome	2–19 days (average 4–10 days)	Days to weeks	Marburg 23%–70% Ebola 50%–90%	None
Arenaviruses (Lassa, Junin, Sabia, Machupo, Guanarito)	Fever, malaise, headache, N/V, pharyngitis, cough, retro-intestinal pain, bleeding, tremors of tongue and hands (Junin), shock, aspetic meningitis, coma, hearing loss in some	Conjunctivitis, petechia, ecchymoses, flushing over head and upper torso	Serology, viral isolation, PCR, IHC; leukopenia, thrombocytopenia, proteinuria	Leptospirosis, meningococcemia, malaria, typhus, borreliosis, rickettsiosis, TTP, HUS, filoviruses	5–21 days Lassa; 7–16 days Sabia, Junin, Machapo, Guanarito	7–15 days	Lassa 1%–2% Junin 30% Machupo 25%–35%	None

Source: Adapted from Medical Management of Biological Casualties Handbook, 7th ed. U.S. Army Medical Research Institute of Infectious Diseases, September 2010.

TABLE 15.3 BW Agents: Vaccine, Therapeutics, and Prophylaxis

Disease	Vaccine	Chemotherapy	Chemoprophylaxis (PX)	Comments
Anthrax	Bioport vaccine (licensed) 0.5 mL IM at 0, 2, 4 wk; 6, 12, 18 mo then annually	Ciprofloxacin 400 mg IV q 12 h	Ciprofloxacin 500 mg PO bid × 60 days if unvaccinated, begin initial doses of vaccine	Plus one or two additional Rx: clindamycin rifampicin, gentamicin, macrolides, vancomycin, imipenem, and chloramphenicol
		Doxycycline 200 mg IV, then 100 mg IV q 12 h Penicillin G 4 million units IV q2h	Doxycycline 100 mg PO bid × 60 days plus vaccination	PCN for sensitive organisms only
Plague	Greer inactivated vaccine (FDA licensed) is no longer available	Streptomycin 1 g IM q 12 h × 10 d (or gentamicin) Doxycycline 200 mg IV then 100 mg IV bid × 10–14 d Chloramphenicol 25 mg/kg IV qid × 14 d	Doxycycline 100 mg PO bid × 7 or duration of exposure Ciprofloxacin 500 mg PO bid × 7 d Doxycycline 100 mg PO bid × 7 d Tetracycline 500 mg PO qid × 7 d	Plague vaccine not protective against aerosol challenge in animal studies. Alternate Rx: trimethoprim-sulfamethoxazole Chloramphenicol for plague meningitis
Tularemia	IND—live attenuated vaccine: one dose by scarification	Streptomycin 1 g IM bid × 10–14 d Gentamicin 5 mg/kg/d IM or IV × 10–14 d	Doxycycline 100 mg PO bid × 14 d Ciprofloxacin 500 mg PO BID × 14 d	
Brucellosis	No human vaccine available	Doxycycline 100 mg/BID PO plus rifampin 600–900 mg/d PO × 6 wk Ofloxacin 400/rifampin 600 mg/d PO × 6 wks	Optimal therapy under dispute.	Trimethoprim-sulfamethoxazole (TMP-SMX) may be substituted for rifampin; however, relapse may reach 30%
Viral encephalitides	VEE DOD TC-3 live attenuated vaccine (IND): 0.5 mL SC × 1 dose VEE DOD C-84 (formalin inactivated TC-83) (IND): 0.5 mL SC for up to 3 h EEE inactivated (IND): 0.5 mL SC at 0 & 28 d WEE inactivated (IND): 0.5 mL SC at 0, 7, and 28 d	Supportive therapy: corticosteroids, analgesics and anticonvulsants prn	NA	TC-83 rectogenic in 20%. No seroconversion in 20%. Only effective against subtypes IA, IB, and IC. C-84 vaccine used for nonresponders to TC-83. EEE and WEE inactivated vaccines are poorly immunogenic; multiple immunizations are required.
Viral hemorrhagic fevers	Yellow fever live attenuated vaccine, single dose then booster q 10 yrs AHF vaccine (x-protective for BHF) (IND) RVF inactivated vaccine (IND)	Ribavarin (CCHF/arenaviruses) 30 mg/kg IV initial dose 16 mg/kg IV q6h × 4 d 8 mg/kg IV q8h × 6 d Passive antibody for AHF, BHF, Lassa fever, and CCHF	Riboflavin (Lassa fever and CCHF)	Aggressive supportive care and management of hypotension very important.
Smallpox	ACAM 2000 vaccine (licensed): 1 dose by scarification	Cidofovir (effective in vitro); animal studies ongoing 5 mg/kg over 1 hr after pretreatment with Probenecid 2 g PO and ILNS IV	Vaccinia immune globulin 100 mg/kg IV (within 3 d of exposure, best within 24 h)	Pre- and postexposure vaccination recommended if >3 years since last vaccine.
Botulism	DOD pentavaient toxoid for serotypes A–E (IND): 0.5 mL deep SC at 0, 2, 12 wk, and 6 mo, then yearly boosters	DOD heptavalent equine despeciated antitoxin for serotypes A-G (IND): 1 vial (10 mL) IV	DOD equine antitoxins (IND)	Skin test for hypersensitivity before equine antitoxin administration

Key: AHF, Argentine hemorrhagic fever; BHF, Bovine hemorrhagic fever; bid, twice a day; CCHF, Crimean-Congo hemorrhagic fever; CDC, Centers for Disease Control and Prevention; DOD, U.S. Department of Defense; EEE, Eastern equine encephalitis; FDA, Food and Drug Administration; IM, intramuscular; IND, investigational new drug; IV, intravenous; NA, not applicable; PCN, penicillin; PO, by mouth; q, every; Rx, prescription; SC, subcutaneous; VEE, Venezuelan equine encephalitis; WEE, Western equine encephalitis.

Source: Medical Management of Biological Casualties Handbook, 7th ed. U.S. Army Medical Research Institute of Infectious Diseases, September 2010.

PEDIATRIC CONSIDERATIONS

I. Challenges

a. Undergoing medical treatment can be emotionally and psychologically difficult for the child (infant through adolescent) and his or her family.

b. Children are not "small adults" and require child-friendly care with adaptation of interventions dependent on maturation of body systems and organ function and the child's age and developmental level (London et al, 2007).

   i. Growth—generally follows a predictable pattern influenced by gender, heredity, environmental factors (such as nutrition), and cultural practices

   ii. Development—each child's maturational pattern is unique; however, the sequence for acquisition of skills is uniform in children, essentially proceeding from the head down and from the center of the body out to the extremities.

c. Special approaches are required to meet the physical, emotional, social, spiritual, and cultural needs of the hospitalized child and his or her family.

   i. Child-sized equipment

   ii. Diversional activities—age-appropriate play rooms, games, arts, recreation

   iii. Learning opportunities—age-appropriate print and visual teaching tools, tutoring during prolonged hospitalization

   iv. Family-centered care—inclusion of all members, as appropriate, with consideration of sociocultural and spiritual factors

II. Developmental Factors Relating to Hospitalization

(Morgan Stanley Children's Hospital of New York Presbyterian, 2008; The Children's Hospital of Philadelphia, n.d.)

a. Infant—birth to 12 months

   i. Just learning to make sense of the world; child can become very unsettled when cared for by multiple or different providers.

   ii. Cannot understand how various procedures and treatments that he or she perceives to "hurt" can actually produce recovery or make them well

   iii. From about age 6 months and older, child can become very afraid if parents leave him or her.

b. Toddler—12 to 36 months

   i. Issues of separation, rather than being ill, can be the major stress for child if required to stay in hospital without parent or familiar caregiver.

   ii. Has no concept or understanding of what is happening when they are ill

   iii. Does not understand time and space so all this can be very frightening for them

c. Preschool—3 to 5 years

   i. Fear of the unknown and being left alone are major concerns.

   ii. Have limited ability to distinguish fantasy from reality

   iii. Tend to misunderstand words they hear, leading to misconceptions

   iv. May view hospitalization as a punishment—fearing needles, body mutilation, or loss of function

d. School-age child—6 to 11 years

   i. Almost all school-age children will have seen and heard about illness and hospitals on TV.

   ii. May have seen people "die" in hospital and know about cancer and other illnesses that can cause children to die

   iii. Need to know what will happen to them, and that they will not die from this illness—may be too frightened to ask about this themselves

   iv. Often misunderstand what they overhear; require opportunities to ask questions

e. Adolescent—12 to 18 years

   i. Understands what causes illness and how it affects the body

   ii. Fears separation from peers and group activities

   iii. Hospitalization represents a loss of control over almost all areas of life, even the most basic aspects—when the teen eats, sleeps, or uses the bathroom, coupled with a loss of privacy at a time when self-consciousness is peaking.

   iv. May express anger or indifference to mask feelings of fear

   v. May feel bothered by frequent examinations by different professionals

   vi. Hospitalization represents a challenge to all teens, especially teens from ethnic, religious, or cultural minority groups.

III. Statistics

a. More than 3 million children in the United States are hospitalized annually, with 3.1 million hospitalized in 2009 (Maternal and Child Health Bureau [MCHB], 2011). *Note:* It has been estimated that chronic health conditions affect 10% to 30% of children. Examples of chronic illnesses include asthma, cystic fibrosis, congenital heart disease, diabetes mellitus, attention-deficit/hyperactivity disorder, and depression. Examples of chronic physical disabilities include developmental delays, hearing or visual impairments, cerebral palsy. Children with chronic health conditions may experience limitations in some activities; frequent pain or discomfort; abnormal growth and development; and more hospitalizations, outpatient visits, and medical treatments (Merck Manuals, 2010).

For additional information concerning pediatric concerns, see Pediatric Pearls (PP) in the following care plans: Appendectomy, Asthma, Brain Infections, Burns, Disaster Considerations, Fractures, Inflammatory Bowel, Pneumonia, Seizure Disorders, Substance Use Disorders, and Sickle Cell Crisis.

GLOSSARY

Development: The qualitative increase in a child's capabilities or function, attainment or mastery of skills.

Growth: Increase in physical size and internal development as measured by multiple factors, such as height, weight, blood pressure, and sexual maturation, as well as the number of words in vocabulary.

Major Theories of Development (London et al, 2007):

Behaviorism: The research of animal behaviorists was applied to children and demonstrated that behaviors can be elicited by positive reinforcement or extinguished by negative reinforcement. Application of theory to hospitalization—repetition of desired behaviors can be encouraged by providing positive reinforcement for child's efforts.

Ecologic theory: Although controversy exists about heredity (nature) versus environment (nurture) and which one has more influence in human development, this theory recognizes the effect of both through mutual interactions between the child and the various levels of the environment (from close to remote) in all of life's settings. Application of theory to hospitalization—use of tool based on this theory to assess child's interface with varied levels of the environment identifies areas of strength that can help with addressing individual challenges or areas that are nonsupportive.

Erikson's Theory of Psychosexual Development: Describes psychosocial stages during eight periods of human life with a particular challenge that is needed for healthy development to occur. Application of theory to hospitalization—interrupts usual support provided by family and peers and adds a situational crisis to the normal developmental crisis experienced by the child.

Freud's Theory of Psychosexual Development: Early childhood experiences form the unconscious motivation for actions in later life. Application of theory to hospitalization—defensive mechanisms, such as regression and repression, may be used by the child to cope with excess anxiety, and the crisis of illness can interfere with normal developmental processes.

Kohlberg's Theory of Moral Development: Using Piaget's cognitive theory as a basis for moral development, three levels of moral reasoning—preconventional, conventional, and postconventional—were identified with associated age ranges. Application of theory to hospitalization—based on stage of development, decisions made by the child may reflect a desire to avoid punishment, to please others, or to present a sense of social responsibility. This provides some direction to care providers as they present information to the child to assist them in the decision-making process.

Piaget's Theory of Cognitive Development: The child's view of the world is influenced largely by age and maturational ability and matures naturally. Application of theory to hospitalization—level of cognitive development and thought processes affects choice of approaches when providing appropriate stimulation and creating teaching plans for the child.

Resiliency Theory: A child's characteristics and how these traits interact with the environment determines his or her resiliency or ability to use healthy responses even in adverse situations. In the face of a crisis, the child and the family have protective characteristics that provide strength and risk factors or characteristics that magnify challenges. Application of theory to hospitalization—providing positive reinforcement for protective characteristics encourages continuation of desired behaviors that can be used to support the period of adjustment and facilitate adaptation to change. Identification of risk factors provides an opportunity to target interventions and teaching activities to assist family and child to deal more effectively with the challenge and increase their resiliency.

Social Learning Theory: Children learn attitudes, beliefs, customs, and values through their social contacts with adults and other children, and they model the behavior they see. Application of theory to hospitalization—the provision of positive role model, such as a peer experiencing a similar situation, facilitates learning and child's cooperation with interventions.

Temperament Theory: The child both influences, and is influenced by, the environment and has innate qualities of personality or certain patterns of temperament that he or she brings to daily life. Application of theory to hospitalization—understanding the child's temperament provides opportunities to alter or manipulate the environment to meet the child's needs and maximize the experience.

Care Setting

Any setting in which nursing contact with children occurs and care is provided.

Client Assessment Database

Data depend on the specific pathology necessitating therapeutic interventions.

Assessment Factors—in addition to routine assessment of current condition or comorbidities

SUBJECTIVE	OBJECTIVE
INDIVIDUAL • Perception of body and its functions in health, illness, and in this situation • Emotional reactions in feeling or sensory terms; for example, client states, "I feel scared." • Food and eating concerns • Sleep patterns • Lifestyle concerns requiring consideration—dietary preferences and problems; sexual identity and activity; beliefs and practices surrounding alcohol, tobacco, and other drugs; other community (e.g., school, religious environment, home of record [e.g., nuclear family, foster care, homeless])	• Age, developmental level, gender • Personality, temperament • Patterns of communication with significant others (SOs) • Behavior when anxious, afraid, impatient, withdrawn, or angry • Emotional response to current treatment or hospitalization • How child experiences illness versus reality of situation
SIGNIFICANT OTHERS • Nuclear family, extended family; peer group, friends • Family developmental cycle • Child's role in family tasks and functions • How are SOs affected by the illness and prognosis?	• Interaction processes within the family
SOCIOECONOMIC	• Social class, value system • Social acceptability of current situation
CULTURAL • Ethnic background, heritage, and residence • Family beliefs regarding caring and curing • Family health-seeking behaviors, illness referral system • Family values related to health and treatment • Cultural factors related to illness in general and to pain response	
DISEASE/CONDITION • Past experience with illness, hospitalization, healthcare systems and providers • Family and child expectations if illness is terminal	• Response of child and family to situation or condition requiring treatment • Nature of condition—acute, chronic, recurrent • Emotional response to current treatments • Availability and use of resources

Nursing Priorities

1. Enhance level of comfort and minimize pain.
2. Reduce anxiety and fear.
3. Provide growth-promoting environment for child and parent(s).
4. Prevent or minimize complications.

Discharge Goals

1. Pain relieved or controlled.
2. Child and family dealing appropriately with current situation.
3. Safe environment maintained.
4. Plan in place to meet needs after discharge.

NURSING DIAGNOSIS: acute/chronic Pain

May Be Related To

Injuring agents—biological, chemical, physical, psychological

Possibly Evidenced By

Verbal/coded reports of pain
Expressive behavior (e.g., restlessness, moaning, crying, irritability)
Changes in appetite; sleep pattern disturbance
Positioning to avoid pain
Changes in vital signs (acute pain)

Desired Outcomes/Evaluation Criteria—Child Will

Pain Level (NOC)

Report or indicate pain is relieved or controlled.
Manifest decreased restlessness and irritability.
Demonstrate age-appropriate blood pressure (BP), pulse, and respiratory rates.

Pain Disruptive Effects (NOC)

Participate in usual activities within level of ability.

ACTIONS/INTERVENTIONS	RATIONALE
Pain Management (NIC)	
Independent	
Perform routine comprehensive pain assessment, including location, characteristics, onset, duration, frequency, quality, and severity using some type of rating scale, such as numbers or visual analog, facial expressions, or color scale.	Assessment of children involves observational skills and may require enlisting the aid of parent or caregiver to clarify cues and verbalizations. Choice of rating scale is dependent on age and developmental level (Suresh, 2009).
Accept child's description of pain, noting precipitating, exacerbating, and relieving factors.	Pain is subjective and cannot be experienced by others. *Note:* In presence of chronic pain situation, use of a pain diary may be appropriate for adolescents (Suresh, 2009).
Investigate changes in frequency or description of pain.	May signal worsening of condition or development of complications.
Observe for guarding, rigidity, crying, and restlessness.	Nonverbal expressions, body movement, and behavioral state may signal pain or changes in pain severity, especially in infants and younger children (Suresh, 2009).
Monitor heart rate, BP using correctly sized cuff, and respiratory rate, noting age-appropriate normals and variations.	Changes in autonomic responses may indicate increased pain before child verbalizes. *Note:* Autonomic responses change with acute pain, not chronic pain. BP may be lower than normal or higher than normal.
Note location and type of surgical incisions or trauma.	Influences degree and severity of pain manifestations.
Provide comfort measures, such as holding, repositioning, back rub, and use of breathing or guided visualization relaxation techniques, as indicated.	Nonpharmacological pain management promotes relaxation; may reduce level of pain and enhance coping.
Identify ways to avoid or minimize pain, such as splinting surgical incisions during coughing, sleeping on a firm mattress, or wearing brace on sprains.	Many factors may reduce pain intensity based on specific situation. Child can quickly learn and use such pain-management techniques, enhancing sense of control as well as comfort.
Encourage sleep and rest periods.	Helps reduce fatigue and enhances coping ability.
Encourage diversional activities such as TV, music, reading, playing computer or table games, and texting friends.	Helps distract child's attention from pain and reduces tension.
Review procedures and expectations and tell child when it will hurt. Provide distraction during painful procedures, such as deep breathing or counting, or looking at something that interests child.	Although the procedure may still be stressful, child will find it easier to handle if he or she knows what to expect and has developed coping strategies.
Encourage expression of feelings about pain.	Can relieve anxiety and help reduce intensity of pain.
Suggest parent and caregiver be with child during procedures, as possible.	Provides comforting presence.
Collaborative	
Collaborate in treatment of underlying conditions or disease process.	Treating cause, when possible, can eliminate pain.
Administer medications, such as opioid and nonsteroidal analgesics, as indicated. Use multiple routes to deliver analgesia, such as oral, nebulized, transdermal, or patient-controlled analgesia (PCA), as indicated by current situation.	Depending on the cause and type of pain, as well as its chronicity, various means of pain management may be needed to overcome or control pain.

NURSING DIAGNOSIS: Anxiety/Fear

May Be Related To

Situational/maturational crises; interpersonal transmission or contagion
Threat to, or change in, health status
Separation from support system in potentially stressful situation—hospitalization, procedures
Innate origin—pain, loss of physical support

Possibly Evidenced By

Apprehensive; distressed; fear
Restlessness; poor eye contact
Changes in vital signs; increased tension; nausea/vomiting
Avoidance or attack behaviors; reports being scared

Desired Outcomes/Evaluation Criteria—Child Will

Anxiety Level [or] Fear Level: Child (NOC)

Appear relaxed and report or demonstrate relief from somatic manifestations of anxiety.
Demonstrate a decrease in somatic complaints and physical symptoms when faced with stressful situations such as impending separation from SO.

Anxiety Self-Control (NOC)

Engage in age-appropriate activities in absence of parent or primary caregiver without fear or distress noted.

ACTIONS/INTERVENTIONS	RATIONALE
Anxiety Reduction (NIC) *Independent*	
Establish an atmosphere of calmness, trust, and genuine positive regard.	Trust and unconditional acceptance are necessary for satisfactory therapeutic relationship. Calmness is important because anxiety is easily transmitted from one person to another, and children are often adept at sensing changes in the moods of adults around them.
Prepare child for activities and procedures. Provide explanations in language appropriate for age. Use terms familiar to child, such as for care activities—"walk" instead of "ambulate"—or procedures—"take a picture" instead of "fluoroscope." Provide opportunity for client to ask questions, observe or touch equipment as appropriate.	Accurate and age-appropriate communication promotes trust and creates an atmosphere where child feels free to ask questions. Based on child's developmental level, tour of facility or surgical suite and observation of "machinery" in action may help reduce concerns regarding the unknown. *Note:* Children may become frightened of things they cannot articulate.
Ensure child of his or her safety and security—listen to child, identify needs, and be available for support.	Strange people and surroundings, changes in routine, and loss of control in situation create anxiety and can be very frightening. Children may believe that situation is punishment for some wrongdoing—imagined or real—on their part. Providing information and being available can be reassuring.
Be honest with child and parents by saying, "Yes, this will hurt and I will help you manage it."	Promotes trust and belief that child will not be left alone to deal with situation.
Refrain from conversations unrelated to child in his or her presence or failing to include child in conversations regarding him or her.	Ignoring the child or talking about, instead of to, the child or allowing child to overhear partial or unrelated conversations may be very stressful and result in child imagining things that are incorrect.
Maintain home routines whenever possible. Encourage child and parents to bring transitional object from home, such as familiar toys, handheld computer games or digital music player, special pillow or blanket, some favorite pictures, or posters, if hospitalized.	Use of age-appropriate object enhances sense of security when child or adolescent is hospitalized or in treatment setting.
Provide consistency of caregivers.	Becoming acquainted with caregiver enhances sense of security, facilitates communication, and lessens anxiety.
Promote child and family contact and interaction. Encourage parents to participate in care planning and care provision.	Family involvement in activities promotes continuity of family unit, provides opportunity to learn and practice new skills, and enhances coping skills.
Emphasize importance of staff and family giving verbal prompts in anticipation of absences. Provide honest information about leaving and returning.	Avoidance of these issues increases the likelihood of anxiety responses when separation occurs.
Help family support child emotionally by being available and active-listening.	Conveys acceptance of child and confidence in ability to cope with situation.
Encourage contact with peers via phone, texting, social network sites, online chats, or visits, as appropriate.	Helps child stay connected with friends and life outside hospital.

ACTIONS/INTERVENTIONS (continued)	RATIONALE (continued)
Provide child with age-appropriate choices, when possible.	Promotes sense of control, demonstrates regard for individual.
Schedule ample time for play and age-appropriate diversions.	Promotes normalcy and helps divert attention from situation.
Use play materials, such as puppets, doll house, doctor/nurse kits, fairy tale stories, clay, coloring book, and so on.	Play therapy enables child to explore conflicts, express fears, and release tension.
Engage in exercise program as appropriate to situation.	Provides physical outlet for energy, releasing tension. May stimulate release of endorphins, decreasing anxiety and enhancing child's ability to deal with illness and situation.
Collaborative	
Administer medications, as indicated.	Mild sedation can be effective in ameliorating symptoms of anxiety and enhancing child's receptiveness to therapeutic regimen.

NURSING DIAGNOSIS: Activity Intolerance [specify level]

May Be Related To

Generalized weakness; bedrest; immobility
Imbalance between oxygen supply/demand

Possibly Evidenced By

Reports fatigue, feeling weak; exertional discomfort or dyspnea
Abnormal heart rate or BP response to activity

Desired Outcomes/Evaluation Criteria—Child Will

Endurance (NOC)

Participate in customary activities at desired level.
Report or display absence of fatigue.

ACTIONS/INTERVENTIONS	RATIONALE
Activity Therapy (NIC)	
Independent	
Note presence of acute or chronic illness (e.g., heart failure, pulmonary disorders, anemias, cancers).	Conditions associated with increased risk of impaired tolerance for activity related to oxygen supply and demand, resulting in weakness and fatigue.
Ascertain child's usual level of activity, taking into account age and developmental level.	Establishes baseline in order to determine needed interventions and to assess progress of recovery.
Determine usual sleep and rest routine and any bedtime rituals or security objects. Plan care with adequate rest periods.	Attempting to maintain usual sleep routines promotes rest and maximizes energy and endurance.
Adjust activities, reducing intensity level or discontinuing activities, as needed. Assist with activities of daily living (ADLs) and promote exercise, as indicated.	Protects child from injury and enhances ability to participate in activity to improve strength.
Promote participation in individually appropriate recreational and diversional activities.	Enhances sense of well-being and expectation of return to usual activities.
Promote optimal mobility, providing safe transport such as wagon, child-size wheelchair, or walker.	Provides normalcy to child, who is not accustomed to inactivity, and will help reduce complications associated with immobility.
Monitor response to activity, including BP, pulse, respiratory rate, skin color, and behavior.	Helps identify and monitor degree of fatigue and potential for complications.
Collaborative	
Collaborate in treatment of underlying condition.	Treating or curing underlying condition can restore child's energy and ability to carry on desired activities.
Provide and monitor response to oxygen administration via appropriate route and effects of medication.	Oxygen may be needed to improve tolerance to activity and treat underlying cause for fatigue. High-flow oxygen via nonrebreather mask is ideal if child can tolerate it. Blow-by oxygen can provide some benefit if child refuses to wear mask.
Refer to physical and occupational therapists.	Helpful to develop activity and exercise programs to meet individual and family needs.

NURSING DIAGNOSIS: risk for delayed Growth and Development

Risk Factors May Include

Chronic illness; infection; frequent otitis media; substance abuse
Economically disadvantaged; malnutrition; maladaptive feeding behaviors
Congenital disorders; multiple gestation; prematurity
Inadequate/late or lack of prenatal care
Behavior disorders; brain damage; lead poisoning; seizures; abuse

Possibly Evidenced By

(Not applicable, presence of signs and symptoms establishes an *actual* diagnosis)

Desired Outcomes/Evaluation Criteria—Child Will

Child Development: [specify age group] (NOC)

Perform motor, social, and/or expressive skills typical of age group within scope of present capabilities.
Demonstrate weight and growth-stabilization or progress toward age-appropriate size.

ACTIONS/INTERVENTIONS	RATIONALE
Development Enhancement: Child [or] Adolescent (NIC)	
Independent	
Determine existing factors or condition(s) that could contribute to growth or development deviation, such as chronic illness, substance use or abuse, familial history of pituitary tumors, Marfan's syndrome, and genetic anomalies.	Plan of care will be based on individual factors present, immediacy of threat, and potential long-term complications. *Note:* Tobacco, alcohol, or other drug use are major healthcare concerns for children.
Determine child's birth weight and length and compare present growth with norms.	Identifies the child's status compared with other children of the same age.
Note chronological age and familial factors, such as body build and stature, stage of sexual maturity. Review expectations for current height and weight percentiles and degree of deviation.	Aids in determining growth expectations.
Measure developmental level using age-appropriate tests, such as the Denver Developmental Screening Test. Note reported losses or alterations in functional level.	Provides comparative baseline and basis for choosing developmentally appropriate interventions.
Determine child's cognitive and perceptual level, such as grade level in school. Note behavioral reaction to environment and stimuli, such as withdrawal or aggression.	Illness or injury can lead to a temporary increase in level of dependency and a decline in functional level. Although this may not be of major concern for the short term, chronic and recurrent conditions may delay acquisition of important developmental milestones.
Note severity and pervasiveness of situation. For example, is the child showing effects of long-term physical or emotional abuse or neglect versus experiencing recent-onset situational disruption or inadequate resources during period of crisis or transition?	Problems existing over a long period may have more severe effects and require longer course of treatment to reverse.
Determine occurrence and frequency of significant stressful events in the child's life, including losses, separation, and environmental changes, such as abandonment, divorce, death of parent or sibling, and relocation.	Lack of resolution or repetition of stressor can have a cumulative effect over time and result in regression in, or deterioration of, functional level.
Discuss nature and effectiveness of parenting and caregiving activities, noting inadequate, inconsistent, unrealistic, or insufficient expectations as well as lack of stimulation, limit setting, or responsiveness.	Assessment of parenting and potential for conflict and negative interaction between parent or caregiver and child identifies interventions needed to maximize care.
Provide parents with information regarding normal growth and development, as appropriate, including pertinent reference materials.	Helps parents understand potential changes in relation to current illness or problem.
Identify realistic goals with child and parents. Discuss actions to take to avoid or minimize preventable complications.	Provides anticipatory guidance. Increases probability of reaching goals and managing situation more effectively. Can enhance sense of control and independence.
Encourage self-care activities, as appropriate, such as feeding, grooming, and playing. Provide privacy when desired and when privacy is safe for child.	Promotes independence and maintenance of self-esteem.
Collaborative	
Assist with therapy to treat or correct underlying conditions, such as Crohn's disease, cardiac problems, or renal disease; endocrine problems, such as hypothyroidism, type 1 diabetes mellitus, or growth hormone abnormalities; and genetic or intrauterine growth retardation, infant feeding problems, or nutritional deficits.	Illness, hospitalization, treatments, and separation from parents and family have a negative effect on physical and psychological growth and development.

ACTIONS/INTERVENTIONS (continued)	RATIONALE (continued)
Include family, nutritionist, physical and occupational therapists, and other specialists in developing plan of care.	Multidisciplinary team involvement increases likelihood of a well-rounded plan of care that meets child's special and varied needs.
Refer to available community resources as appropriate, such as public health programs, medical equipment suppliers, nutritionist, substance abuse program, and specialist in endocrine conditions or genetics.	Although acute situations may be readily resolved with limited support and few ill effects, chronic or recurrent conditions require many resources to maximize growth potential of child and family.
Contact client's school for educational resource or tutor and learning plan, as indicated.	Prevents child from falling behind in studies and provides sense of normalcy during prolonged illness or hospitalization.

NURSING DIAGNOSIS: risk for imbalanced Nutrition: less than body requirements

Risk Factors May Include

Inability to ingest or digest food or absorb nutrients because of biological, psychological, or economic factors

Possibly Evidenced By

(Not applicable, presence of signs and symptoms establishes an *actual* diagnosis)

Desired Outcomes/Evaluation Criteria—Child Will

Nutritional Status (NOC)

Ingest nutritionally adequate diet for age, activity level, and metabolic demands.
Demonstrate stable weight or progressive weight gain toward goal.

ACTIONS/INTERVENTIONS	RATIONALE
Nutrition Management (NIC)	
Independent	
Identify child at risk for malnutrition, such as with intestinal surgery, hypermetabolic states, restricted intake, and/or prior nutritional deficiencies.	Provides opportunity for timely intervention.
Determine ability to chew, swallow, and taste. Note presence of conditions affecting food intake, such as nausea and vomiting; food intolerances or allergies; lactose intolerance, cystic fibrosis, diabetes, inflammatory bowel diseases, or eating disorders (including anorexia and overeating).	These factors can affect specific dietary choices, desire to eat and/or ingestion and digestion of nutrients.
Ascertain child's oral health, noting presence and condition of teeth, impairment of oral mucous membranes (e.g., painful lesions, enlarged tonsils); or problems with facial structures (e.g., facial/jaw trauma, cleft palate, presence of ET tube).	Various conditions of the mouth and facial structures can impair child's ability and desire to ingest food.
Determine child's current nutritional status using age-appropriate measurements, including weight and body build, strength, activity level, and sleep and rest cycles.	Identifies individual nutritional needs and provides comparative baseline.
Auscultate bowel sounds. Note characteristics of stool, including color, amount, and frequency of bowel movements.	Provides information about digestion and bowel function and may affect choice and timing of feeding.
Elicit information from child/parent regarding typical daily food intake, determining foods and beverages normally consumed. Note types of snacks. Discuss eating habits and food preferences—likes and dislikes.	Baseline information to determine adequacy of intake. Knowledge of child's specific likes and dislikes may be helpful in meeting child's nutritional needs during a time when appetite is suppressed or child has no interest in food.
Determine whether infant is breast-fed or formula-fed, and note typical pattern of feedings during a 24-hour period. Note type and amounts of solid foods infant or toddler eats.	Providing usual and typical feedings is important to infant well-being and early growth.
Determine psychological factors and cultural or religious desires or influences on dietary choices.	Dietary beliefs, such as vegetarianism, can affect nutritional intake. Usual ethnic food choices can improve a child's intake when appetite is poor.
Review drug regimen, noting potential side effects and possible interactions with other medications, over-the-counter (OTC) drugs, and herbs.	Timing of medication doses and interaction with certain foods can alter effect of medication or digestion and absorption of nutrients.
Discuss with parent what types of snacks (e.g., candy, other sweets, fruits, and beverages) child eats or drinks.	Identifies what child eats in a typical day, and can provide opportunity for teaching about healthy snacks when that is needed/desired.
Emphasize importance of well-balanced meals. Provide information regarding individual nutritional needs and ways to	Although nutritious intake is important, arguing over food is counterproductive. Providing age-appropriate guidelines to

(continues on page 880)

ACTIONS/INTERVENTIONS (continued) | RATIONALE (continued)

meet these needs within financial constraints. Avoid arguing over food choices.

children as well as to parents or care provider may help them in making healthy choices. *Note:* Childhood obesity with associated long-term physical and psychological effects is a potential concern regardless of current weight.

Clarify caregiver access to and use of resources, such as food stamps, budget counseling, Women, Infants, and Children (WIC) program, community food bank, and/or other appropriate assistance programs.

May be necessary to improve child's intake and/or availability of food to meet nutritional needs.

Collaborative

Establish a nutritional plan (with monitoring, when needed) that meets individual needs incorporating or limiting specific foods.

Certain medical conditions (e.g., diabetes, cancer, gluten allergy, malabsorption syndrome, anorexia) require special dietary considerations to manage symptoms or bring about healing.

Consult dietitian or nutritional team, as indicated.

Helps determine individual nutritional needs and therapeutic diet.

Review laboratory studies, such as serum albumin or prealbumin, transferrin, amino acid profile, iron, blood urea nitrogen (BUN), nitrogen balance studies, glucose, liver function, electrolytes, and total lymphocyte count.

Indicators of nutritional health and effects of nutrients in organ function.

Refer for dental hygiene care, nutritional counseling, or psychiatric or family therapy, as indicated.

May be needed to provide assistance, support, and direction for meeting nutritional needs not only in the present but for achieving long-term goals as well.

Refer to home-care resources when indicated by specific condition or illness.

Assists with initiation and supervision of home nutrition therapy when used.

NURSING DIAGNOSIS: risk for Injury (specify: Trauma, Suffocation, Poisoning)

Risk Factors May Include

Developmental age (physiological, psychosocial); cognitive or emotional difficulties
Disease or injury process; misuse of restraints or safety devices
Chemical (e.g., poisons, pollutants, drugs, pharmaceutical agents, alcohol, nicotine)
Deficient knowledge regarding safety or drug precautions
Immune or autoimmune dysfunction; malnutrition; exposure to nosocomial agents

Possibly Evidenced By

(Not applicable, presence of signs and symptoms establishes an *actual* diagnosis)

Desired Outcomes/Evaluation Criteria—Child Will

Risk Control (NOC)

Be free of injury.

Caregiver/Parent—Will

Verbalize understanding of individual risk factors that contribute to possibility of injury.
Take steps to correct identified risks and protect child from hazards.

ACTIONS/INTERVENTIONS | RATIONALE

Risk Surveillance (NIC)

Independent

Note client's and SO's age, developmental stage level of cognition, decision-making ability.

These factors are critical in assessing safety needs and evaluating client's or caregiver's ability to meet client's needs as discharge planning begins.

Identify individual risk factors in child's healthcare setting, including (1) physical needs (e.g., airway patency, therapeutic use of potentially toxic medications, invasive lines or procedures, exposure to latex products); (2) medical conditions (e.g., impaired cognitive, developmental, psychological, or neurological status); (3) environmental factors (e.g., exposure to safety hazards in healthcare setting [e.g., immobility, use of restraints/braces/casts], home, or community [including violence and substance use])

Provides opportunity to modify environment and eliminate factors that place child at risk.

ACTIONS/INTERVENTIONS (continued)	RATIONALE (continued)
Provide healthcare within a culture of safety (e.g., adherence to nursing standards of care and facility safe-care policies):	Prevents errors resulting in child injury, promotes safety and models safety behaviors to client/SO.
Provide appropriate level of supervision.	Promotes child's well-being and allows for timely intervention, when needed.
Initiate safety precautions as individually appropriate, such as bed in low position, padded side rails, infection precautions, floors clear of hazards, supervised use of mobility aids.	Preventing injuries and complications is a prime responsibility of parents and caregivers.
Have age-appropriate equipment available, including properly sized BP cuff, intravenous (IV) catheters, airway adjuncts, and oxygen mask or hood; suction equipment, ventilator bag, low-flow IV pump, or warming devices.	Prevents treatment-related injuries and ensures availability of age- or size-appropriate life-saving equipment.
Monitor medication administration closely, paying careful attention to allergies, dosage measurements and conversions, side effects, and potential adverse effects. Use pediatric concentrations of medications when available.	Provides for effective therapeutic management, prevents overdose, and reduces risk for toxic reactions.
Note history of latex allergies or dermatitis. Avoid latex products while in facility care and instruct client/SO in ways to avoid recurrent exposure to latex products, including gloves, catheters, and tubing, when client requires those for postdischarge care.	Repeat exposure increases risk of developing sensitivity or serious adverse reactions to latex products.
Review home situation for safety hazards, especially when child has sustained some type of injury related to unsafe home environment.	Provides opportunity for teaching about factors that could promote a safer home environment, or might identify need for more intensive interventions.
Ascertain client and caregiver knowledge of safety needs and injury prevention in child's play and sports setting.	Specific attention needs to be focused on childhood recreational and sports injuries, including impact of repeated concussions, which is often underestimated.
Provide written resources for parent or caregiver and age-appropriate handouts for child, including information about safety issues, such as immunizations, obesity, smoking, substance use, and safer sex practices.	Provides information for later review and self-paced learning.
Encourage parent or caregiver to learn cardiopulmonary resuscitation (CPR) and individually appropriate procedures or emergency interventions and responses, such as carrying an EpiPen.	Being prepared for emergencies promotes confidence for adults and children in their own ability to deal with their situation.
Collaborative	
Refer to home-care assistance, medical supplies, community safety and education programs, and resources, such as Family Effectiveness Training, as indicated.	Can provide additional opportunities for support for child safety, for improving parenting skills, and obtaining necessary equipment.

NURSING DIAGNOSIS: risk for imbalanced Fluid Volume

Risk Factors May Include

Burns; sepsis; rapid loss—hemorrhage, vomiting, diarrhea, fistulas
Rapid or excessive fluid replacement; lack of adequate intake

Possibly Evidenced By

(Not applicable; presence of signs and symptoms establishes an *actual* diagnosis)

Desired Outcomes/Evaluation Criteria—Child Will

Hydration (NOC)

Demonstrate adequate fluid balance as evidenced by stable vital signs, palpable pulses of good quality, normal skin turgor, moist mucous membranes; individually appropriate urinary output; lack of excessive weight fluctuation—loss or gain; and absence of edema.

Parent/Caregiver Will

Risk Control (NOC)

Verbalize understanding of child's fluid needs.
Promote adequate age-appropriate fluid intake.

ACTIONS/INTERVENTIONS	RATIONALE
Fluid Management (NIC)	
Independent	
Note potential sources of fluid loss and intake, presence of conditions such as diabetes or burns, recurrent blood draws, and use of total parenteral nutrition (TPN).	Causative and contributing factors for fluid imbalances.
Note child's age, size, weight, and cognitive abilities.	Affects ability to tolerate fluctuations in fluid level and ability to respond to fluid needs.
Monitor vital signs; color of palms, soles of feet, and mucous membranes; weight; skin turgor; breath sounds; urinary and gastric output; and hemodynamic measurements.	Indicators of hydration status. *Note:* Hypotension indicative of developing shock may not be readily observed in child until very late in the clinical course because of vasoconstriction.
Review child's intake of fluids.	Children often do not take in enough oral fluids to meet hydration needs.
Determine child's normal pattern of elimination and whether child is toilet trained.	Provides information for baseline and comparison. If child is in diapers, output may be determined by weighing diapers.
Determine whether child has problems with urination, such as urine retention, bed-wetting, burning, or holding.	Evaluation of these issues is important for determining cause and treatment of underlying problem.
Note use of drainage devices such as nasogastric (NG) tube or wound drain and use of laxatives, enemas, or suppositories.	May increase fluid and electrolyte losses.
Collaborative	
Administer IV fluids via control device.	Because smaller volumes are administered, close monitoring and regulation is required to prevent fluid overload while correcting fluid balance.
Replace electrolytes, as indicated, by oral route whenever possible.	Replacement solutions formulated for children are often safer and better tolerated when given orally if time and condition allow. *Note:* Child with mild dehydration not caused by trauma may respond well to oral rehydration starting with 5 to 10 mL by mouth every 15 to 20 minutes and increasing according to tolerance.
Monitor laboratory results, such as hemoglobin/hematocrit (Hgb/Hct), BUN, urine osmolality, and specific gravity.	Indicators of adequacy of hydration and effectiveness of therapeutic interventions.
Arrange with laboratory to combine common tests and draw smallest amount of blood that is necessary to perform required studies.	Excessive or repetitive blood draws may markedly reduce Hgb and Hct levels in pediatric client.

NURSING DIAGNOSIS: interrupted Family Processes

May Be Related To
Situational transition and/or crises
Shift in health status of a family member
Modification in family finances or social status

Possibly Evidenced By
Changes in communication patterns or availability for emotional support
Changes in participation in problem-solving
Changes in expressions of conflict within family

Desired Outcomes/Evaluation Criteria—Parent/Caregiver Will

Family Functioning (NOC)
Verbalize positive feelings about parenting abilities.
Be involved in problem-solving solutions for current situation.
Develop skills to deal with present situation.
Strengthen parenting skills.

ACTIONS/INTERVENTIONS	RATIONALE
Family Support (NIC)	
Independent	
Determine existing situation and parental perception of the problems, noting presence of specific factors such as psychiatric or physical illness and disabilities of child or parent.	Identification of the individual factors will aid in focusing interventions and establishing a realistic plan of care.
Identify developmental stage of the family—first child, new infant, school-age or adolescent children, or stepfamily.	These factors affect how family members view current problems and choices of solutions.
Determine cultural and religious influences on parenting and expectations of self and child.	This information is crucial to helping the family identify and develop a treatment plan that meets its specific needs, enhancing likelihood of success.

ACTIONS/INTERVENTIONS (continued)	RATIONALE (continued)
Assess parenting skill level, considering intellectual, emotional, and physical strengths and limitations.	Identifies areas of need for further education, skill training, and factors that might interfere with ability to assimilate new information.
Note attachment behaviors between parent and child(ren), recognizing cultural background. Encourage parent(s) to hold and spend time with child, particularly newborn or infant.	Lack of eye contact and touching may indicate bonding problems. Failure to bond effectively with newborn is thought to affect subsequent parent-child interaction.
Observe interactions between parent(s) and child(ren).	Identifies relationships, communication skills, and feelings about one another.
Note presence and effectiveness of extended family support systems.	Provides role models for parent(s) to help them develop own style of parenting. *Note:* Role models may be negative and/or controlling.
Emphasize positive aspects of situation, maintaining a positive attitude toward parent's capabilities and potential for improving.	Helping parent(s) to feel accepting about self and individual capabilities will promote growth.
Involve all members of the family in learning activities.	Learning new skills is enhanced when everyone is participating and interacting.
Encourage parent(s) to identify positive outlets for meeting own needs, such as going to a movie or out to dinner. Discuss use of home care and respite services, as appropriate.	Parent often believes it is "selfish" to do things for own self, that children are primary. However, parents are important, children are important, and the family is important. As a rule, when parents take care of themselves, their coping abilities are enhanced and they are better parents. *Note:* Siblings also require time with parents to attend to their needs and to have positive interactions.
Discuss issues of stepparenting and ways to achieve positive relationships in a blended family.	Blending two families can be a very demanding task, and preconceived ideas can be counterproductive.
Collaborative	
Refer to resources such as books, classes, and support groups.	Providing information and/or role models can help people learn to negotiate and develop skills for parenting and living together.

NURSING DIAGNOSIS: risk for imbalanced Body Temperature

Risk Factors May Include

Extremes of age or weight; dehydration

Exposure to extremes of environmental temperature

Illness or trauma affecting temperature regulation; altered metabolic rate

Possibly Evidenced By

(Not applicable; presence of signs and symptoms establishes an *actual* diagnosis)

Desired Outcomes/Evaluation Criteria—Child Will

Thermoregulation (NOC)

Regain or maintain appropriate body temperature for age and size.

Parent/Caregiver Will

Risk Control (NOC)

Provide proper environmental controls and safeguards.

ACTIONS/INTERVENTIONS	RATIONALE
Temperature Regulation (NIC)	
Independent	
Note conditions promoting fevers—infection, inflammation, hot environment, and dehydration.	Determines choice of interventions.
Measure and monitor child's temperature, using properly functioning thermometer.	Inaccurate measurement can result in inappropriate treatment.
Discuss variables in temperature measurements for age of child and where temperature is measured.	Knowledge of normal ranges for age of child—newborn through adolescent—is critical to knowing when a fever requires treatment. Temperature may be measured orally, rectally, and at the axillary space, with rectal measurement being on average approximately 1 degree higher than oral, and axillary being 1 degree lower than oral. *Note:* Temperature of 100.4°F

(continues on page 884)

ACTIONS/INTERVENTIONS (continued)	RATIONALE (continued)
	(38°C) or greater in newborns and infants needs immediate attention. For toddlers and older children, temperatures up to 104°F (40°C) may be tolerated unless accompanied by other signs, such as poor color, breathing problems, severe lethargy, headache, or stiff neck (Cincinnati Children's Hospital Medical Center [CCHMC], 2010).
Be aware of heat loss related to age and body mass.	Newborn is more vulnerable to heat loss than older child because of body surface area, higher metabolic rate, and sensitivity to environmental conditions.
Observe for seizure activity. Provide safety precautions, as indicated.	Higher fevers may trigger febrile seizures in susceptible children.
Adjust bedclothes, linens, and environment. Apply cool cloth to head and bathe in lukewarm bath.	Limiting linens and use of room fan can help lower body temperature. *Note:* Use of alcohol sponge bath is contraindicated—can be inhaled or alcohol absorbed through skin (Kids Health, 2013).
Collaborative	
Administer antipyretics, for example, acetaminophen (Tylenol) 10 to 15 mg/kg every 4 hours or ibuprofen (Motrin) 10 to 15 mg/kg every 6 hours, as indicated. Avoid use of aspirin.	Some degree of fever may be useful for fighting infection; however, excessive levels may have adverse effects and require intervention. Aspirin is believed to be associated with the onset of Reye's syndrome (London et al, 2007).

NURSING DIAGNOSIS: risk for ineffective Health Maintenance

Risk Factors May Include

Unachieved developmental tasks
Perceptual or cognitive impairment
Ineffective family coping
Insufficient resources

Possibly Evidenced By

(Not applicable; presence of signs and symptoms establishes an *actual* diagnosis)

Desired Outcomes/Evaluation Criteria—Parent/Caregiver Will

Health-Seeking Behavior (NOC)

Identify necessary health maintenance activities.
Verbalize understanding of factors contributing to current situation.
Develop plan to meet specific needs.

ACTIONS/INTERVENTIONS	RATIONALE
Health System Guidance (NIC)	
Independent	
Explore with parents how child's health status is maintained—nutrition (especially if child is over- or underweight), exercise, sleep and rest, immunization status, and social/environmental issues such as child care setting and homelessness.	Identifies strengths; may reveal problems requiring immediate intervention.
Discuss mother's health status when pregnant, such as exposure to toxic agents, substance use, and complications of pregnancy or birth.	Helps identify issues, such as fetal alcohol syndrome, that may arise in child's future health status.
Ascertain frequency of routine health exams, including eye and dental care, monitoring by primary care provider, and immunizations. Note availability and use of resources. Problem-solve barriers to meeting healthcare needs.	Identifies areas of child's healthcare that may be lacking, and provides parents with information about areas that need to be monitored and care provided to promote optimum health. *Note:* Financial issues, such as being under- or uninsured, having high insurance co-pays, or a lack of transportation may restrict ability to follow through on needed or routine care.
Note desire and level of ability to meet health maintenance needs, as well as self-care ADLs.	Care providers and children who can provide much of their own care may have areas of need, either because of illness or other stressors.
Develop plan with parent or caregiver for child's care.	Allows for incorporating existing strengths or limitations and assistance in adapting and organizing care, as necessary.
Provide time to listen to concerns of parent or caregiver.	Long-term care for chronically ill child or acute care for a child can be very challenging to parent's physical, emotional, and financial resources.

ACTIONS/INTERVENTIONS (continued)	RATIONALE (continued)
Provide anticipatory guidance for periods of wellness, and identify ways parent can adapt when progressive illness or long-term health problems occur.	Information and support is vital for maintaining and managing effective health practices.
Provide for communication and coordination between the healthcare facility team and community healthcare providers.	Promotes continuity of care and continuation of goals.
Monitor adherence to prescribed medical regimen. Determine causes for deviations.	Additional education or problem-solving may be required for success of therapeutic plan.
Provide information about individual healthcare needs. Identify signs and symptoms requiring further evaluation and follow-up.	Provides for prevention of complications and early intervention in times of illness.
Collaborative	
Make referral as needed for community support services such as homemaker, skilled nursing care, well-baby clinic, and respite care.	Provides for child care and parental support in home setting to enhance coping with therapeutic regimen.
Refer to social services, as indicated.	May need assistance with financial, housing, or legal concerns.
Arrange for palliative or hospice services, if needed.	May be indicated when illness is prolonged or terminal.

POTENTIAL CONSIDERATIONS following acute hospitalization (dependent on client's age, physical condition and presence of complications, and family resources).

Refer to primary diagnosis for specific concerns.

- ***ineffective Self-Health Management***—perceived seriousness; economic difficulties; complexity of therapeutic regimen; excessive demands made on family; family patterns of healthcare
- ***delayed Growth and Development***—effects of physical disability; prescribed dependence; environmental or stimulation deficiencies.

FLUID AND ELECTROLYTE IMBALANCES

I. Homeostasis

- **a.** The body is equipped with homeostatic mechanisms to keep the composition and volume of body fluids within narrow limits.
- **b.** Organs involved in this mechanism are kidneys, lungs, heart, blood vessels, adrenal glands, parathyroid glands, and pituitary gland.

II. Composition

- **a.** Body fluid is composed primarily of water and electrolytes and is divided into two types.
  - **i.** Intracellular—within the cells
  - **ii.** Extracellular—interstitial or tissue fluid, intravascular or plasma, and transcellular, such as cerebrospinal or synovial fluids

Related Concerns

All plans of care specific to underlying health condition causing imbalance, such as diabetes mellitus (DM), heart failure (HF), upper gastrointestinal (GI) bleeding, renal failure, and dialysis.

Metabolic acidosis—primary base bicarbonate deficiency, page 450

Metabolic alkalosis—primary base bicarbonate excess, page 455

Respiratory acidosis (primary carbonic acid excess), page 179

Respiratory alkalosis (primary carbonic acid deficit), page 184

Nursing Priorities

1. Restore homeostasis.
2. Prevent or minimize complications.
3. Provide information about condition, prognosis, and treatment needs, as appropriate.

Discharge Goals

1. Homeostasis restored.
2. Free of complications.
3. Condition, prognosis, and treatment needs understood.
4. Plan in place to meet needs after discharge.

Fluid Balance

Note: Because fluid and electrolyte imbalances usually occur in conjunction with other medical conditions, the following information is offered as a reference. The interventions are presented in a general format for inclusion in the primary plan of care.

GLOSSARY

Dehydration: Loss of too much body water, which can affect cellular and organ function.

Fluid balance: State in which the volume of body water and its solutes (electrolytes and nonelectrolytes) are within normal limits and there is normal distribution of fluids within the intracellular and extracellular compartments.

Fluid volume deficit: Imbalance in fluid volume in which there is loss of fluid from the body not compensated for by an adequate intake of water. The major causes are (1) insufficient fluid intake and (2) excessive fluid loss from vomiting; diarrhea; suctioning of gastric contents; or drainage through operative wounds, burns, or fistulae.

Fluid volume excess: Overabundance of water in the interstitial fluid spaces or body cavities (edema) or an excess of fluid within the blood vessels (hypervolemia). Factors that contribute to the accumulation of excess fluid are (1) dilatation of the arteries, as occurs in inflammatory process; (2) reduced effective osmotic pressure, as in hypoproteinemia, lymphatic obstruction, and increased capillary permeability; (3) increased venous pressure, as in congestive heart failure, thrombophlebitis, and cirrhosis of the liver; and (4) retention of sodium due to increased reabsorption of sodium by the renal tubules.

Hypervolemia: Increase in the volume of circulating blood; also known as fluid overload or fluid excess. Excess fluid can accumulate in the intravascular space and/or the interstitial space.

Hypovolemia: Decreased circulating volume in the intravascular compartment; also known as fluid deficit or dehydration. Relative and absolute hypovolemic states can commonly coexist in certain clinical conditions as well. A client who is relatively hypovolemic may have adequate volume; however, it does not remain or exist in the intravascular space. In other words, it is not effective circulating volume. Absolute hypovolemia is considered to be measurable fluid (greater than 500 mL/day).

Interstitial fluid: Extracellular fluid bathing most tissues, excluding the fluid within the lymph and blood vessels.

Intracellular fluid: Portion of total body water with its dissolved solutes within the cell membranes.

Orthopnea: Labored breathing occurring when lying flat.

Osmotic pressure: Pressure produced by a solution in a space divided by a semipermeable membrane due to a differential in the concentrations of solute. The colloid osmotic pressure is influenced by proteins. This is due to the proteins being the only dissolved substance in the plasma and interstitial fluid that do not diffuse readily through the capillary membrane.

Positive fluid balance: Fluid gain is greater than fluid loss, which might suggest a problem with either the renal or cardiovascular system.

HYPERVOLEMIA (EXTRACELLULAR FLUID VOLUME EXCESS)

I. Predisposing or Contributing Factors

a. Excess sodium intake: sodium-containing foods, medications, or fluids (orally/intravenously); excessive or rapid administration of hypertonic or, possibly, isotonic parenteral fluids

b. Hormone imbalance: increased release of antidiuretic hormone (ADH), excessive adrenocorticotropic hormone (ACTH) production, hyperaldosteronism

c. Decreased plasma proteins: chronic liver disease with ascites, major abdominal surgery, malnutrition, or protein depletion

d. Chronic kidney disease, acute renal failure (ARF)

e. Heart failure (HF)

Client Assessment Database

DIAGNOSTIC DIVISION MAY REPORT	MAY EXHIBIT
ACTIVITY/REST • Fatigue • Generalized weakness	
CIRCULATION	• Hypertension, elevated central venous pressure (CVP) • Pulse full and bounding • Tachycardia usually present; bradycardia—late sign of cardiac decompensation • Extra heart sounds (S_3) • Edema variable from dependent to generalized • Neck and peripheral vein distention
ELIMINATION • Decreased urinary output • Diarrhea	• Oliguria

DIAGNOSTIC DIVISION MAY REPORT (continued)	MAY EXHIBIT (continued)
FOOD/FLUID • Anorexia; nausea, vomiting • Thirst—may be absent, especially in elderly	• Abdominal girth increased with visible fluid wave on palpation (ascites) • Sudden weight gain, often in excess of 5% of total body weight • Edema initially dependent; pitting may progress to facial or periorbital, general or anasarca
NEUROSENSORY	• Changes in level of consciousness from lethargy, disorientation, confusion to coma • Aphasia • Muscle twitching, tremors, seizure activity • Hyperreflexia, rigid paralysis—severe hypernatremia
PAIN/DISCOMFORT • Headache • Abdominal cramps	
RESPIRATION • Shortness of breath • Productive cough	• Changes in respiratory pattern • Tachypnea with or without dyspnea, orthopnea • Adventitious breath sounds [rales or crackles]
SAFETY	• Fever • Skin changes in color, temperature, and turgor, such as taut and cool where edematous
TEACHING/LEARNING • Refer to predisposing or contributing factors	
DISCHARGE PLAN CONSIDERATIONS • May require assistance with changes in therapeutic regimen, dietary management ➧ Refer to plan of care concerning underlying medical or surgical condition for possible postdischarge considerations.	

Diagnostic Studies

TEST WHY IT IS DONE	WHAT IT TELLS ME
BLOOD TESTS	
• ***Hematocrit (Hct):*** Measures the proportion of blood that is made up of red blood cells. Normal adult female range is 39% to 47%; normal adult male range is 44% to 52% (Matheny, 2012).	Elevated in dehydration due to hemoconcentration; decreased with fluid overload.
• ***Serum sodium (Na^+):*** Sodium is the body's most abundant extracellular ion. It plays a key role in maintaining fluid balance—where sodium goes, water will follow. Normal adult range is 135 to 145 mEq/L.	Serum sodium may be high, low, or normal, depending on cause for fluid excess and balance of other electrolytes, including intracellular potassium. Because sodium is the only cation to exert significant osmotic pressure, sodium levels are closely linked to both blood volume and blood.
• ***Serum potassium (K^+):*** An essential intracellular ion needed to regulate water balance, levels of acidity, and blood pressure (BP). Normal range is 3.5 to 5.0 mEq/L (Matheny, 2012).	Normal or decreased in fluid overload unless renal damage present. Potassium deficit may occur with kidney dysfunction or diuretic therapy.

(continues on page 888)

Diagnostic Studies (continued)

TEST WHY IT IS DONE (continued)	WHAT IT TELLS ME (continued)
• *Blood urea nitrogen (BUN):* Measures the amount of urea nitrogen in blood; used primarily to evaluate kidney function. Normal range is 10–20 mg/dL (Matheny, 2012).	Normal or decreased in fluid overload unless renal damage present.
• *Plasma proteins:* Plasma proteins (such as albumin) help to transport substances and water throughout the body. Albumin helps maintain intravascular pressure. More than half of the protein in blood serum is albumin. Normal albumin range is 3.6 to 5.5 g/dL (Matheny, 2012).	May be decreased. The most common cause of decreased plasma albumin levels is related to inflammatory processes, including hemodilution, loss of extravascular space, increased consumption by cells locally, and decreased synthesis. Approximately 75% of the total colloid osmotic pressure is related to albumin (Hankins, 2006).
• *Serum glucose:* Type of sugar found in blood. Normal adult fasting range is 70 to 99 mg/dL.	May be elevated if dehydration is result of osmotic diuresis associated with metabolic acidosis.
• *Serum osmolality:* An indirect measurement of the number of particles—sodium, glucose, and urea—in plasma, reflecting fluid balance. Normal range is 280 to 295 mOsm/kg (Matheny, 2012).	Usually unchanged, although hypo-osmolality may occur with hyponatremia.
OTHER DIAGNOSTIC STUDIES	
• *Urine sodium:* Measures the amount of sodium in urine and must be evaluated in association with blood levels. Concentrations may mirror blood levels or be the opposite. Normal values are not fixed; kidneys vary rate of excretion to match dietary intake (Matheny, 2012), but generally range from 15 to 250 mEq/L/day.	The body normally excretes excess sodium; so, the concentration in the urine may be elevated because it is elevated in the blood. It may also be elevated in the urine when the body is losing too much sodium. If blood sodium levels are low due to insufficient intake, then urine concentrations will also be low.
• *Urine specific gravity(SG):* Measures the concentration of particles in urine such as glucose, sodium, and urea. Normal range is 1.003 to 1.035 (Matheny, 2012).	Decreased levels can be associated with fluid excess and such conditions as diabetes insipidus.

NURSING DIAGNOSIS: excess Fluid Volume

May Be Related To
Excess fluid or sodium intake

Compromised regulatory mechanism (e.g., syndrome of inappropriate antidiuretic hormone [SIADH] or decreased plasma proteins as found in conditions such as malnutrition, draining fistulas, organ failure)

[Pharmaceutical agents (e.g., chlorpropamide, tolbutamide, vincristine, triptylines, carbamazepine)]

Possibly Evidenced By
Signs and symptoms noted in database

Outcomes/Evaluation Criteria—Client Will

Fluid Overload Severity (NOC)

Demonstrate stabilized fluid volume as evidenced by balanced intake and output (I&O), vital signs within client's normal range, stable weight, and absence of signs of edema.

Knowledge: Treatment Regimen (NOC)

Verbalize understanding of individual dietary and fluid restrictions.

Demonstrate behaviors to monitor fluid status and prevent or limit recurrence.

ACTIONS/INTERVENTIONS	RATIONALE
Hypervolemia Management (NIC)	
Independent	
Monitor vital signs as well as CVP, if available.	Tachycardia and hypertension are common manifestations. Tachypnea usually present with or without dyspnea. Elevated CVP may be noted before dyspnea and adventitious breath sounds occur. Hypertension may be a primary disorder or occur secondary to other associated conditions such as heart failure (HF).

ACTIONS/INTERVENTIONS (continued)	RATIONALE (continued)
Auscultate lung and heart sounds.	Adventitious sounds (crackles) and extra heart sounds (S_3) are indicative of fluid excess, possibly resulting in rapid development of pulmonary edema.
Assess for presence and location of edema formation.	Edema can be either a cause or a result of various pathological conditions reflecting four competing forces: blood hydrostatic and osmotic pressures and interstitial fluid hydrostatic and osmotic pressures. The dynamic interaction of these four forces allows fluid to shift from one body compartment to another. Edema may be generalized or localized in dependent areas. Elderly clients may develop dependent edema with relatively little excess fluid.
Note presence of neck and peripheral vein distention, along with pitting edema, and dyspnea.	Signs of cardiac decompensation and HF.
Maintain accurate I&O. Note decreased urinary output and positive fluid balance on 24-hour calculations.	Decreased renal perfusion, cardiac insufficiency, and fluid shifts may cause decreased urinary output and edema formation.
Weigh, as indicated. Be alert for acute or sudden weight gain.	One liter of fluid retention equals a weight gain of 1 kilogram (2.2 pounds).
Give oral fluids with caution. If fluids are restricted, set up a 24-hour schedule for fluid intake.	Fluid restrictions, as well as extracellular shifts, can aggravate drying of mucous membranes, and client may desire more fluids than are prudent.
Monitor infusion rate of parenteral fluids closely; administer via control device, as necessary.	Rapid fluid bolus or prolonged excessive administration potentiates volume overload and risk of cardiac decompensation.
Encourage coughing and deep-breathing exercises.	Pulmonary fluid shifts potentiate respiratory complications.
Maintain semi-Fowler's position if dyspnea or ascites is present.	Gravity improves lung expansion by lowering diaphragm and shifting fluid to lower abdominal cavity.
Turn or reposition, and promote early ambulation, where possible. Provide skin care at regular intervals.	Reduces pressure and friction on edematous tissue, which is more prone to breakdown than normal tissue.
Encourage rest periods. Schedule care to provide frequent rest periods.	Limited cardiac reserves result in fatigue and activity intolerance. Rest, particularly lying down, favors diuresis and reduction of edema.
Provide safety precautions as indicated, such as use of side rails, bed in low position, frequent observation, and soft restraints, if required to prevent client injury.	Fluid shifts may cause cerebral edema and changes in mentation, especially in the geriatric population. *Note:* Restraints must be used as infrequently as possible, and be limited to a specified time period with client under close supervision (Dugdale, 2012).
Collaborative	
Assist with identification and treatment of underlying cause.	Refer to listing of predisposing and contributing factors to determine treatment needs.
Monitor laboratory studies, such as sodium, potassium, BUN, and arterial blood gases (ABGs), as indicated.	Extracellular fluid shifts, sodium and water restriction, and renal function all affect serum sodium levels. Potassium deficit may occur with kidney dysfunction or diuretic therapy. BUN may be increased as a result of renal dysfunction. ABGs may reflect metabolic acidosis.
Provide balanced protein, low-sodium diet. Restrict fluids, as indicated.	If serum proteins are low because of malnutrition or gastrointestinal (GI) losses, intake of dietary proteins can enhance colloidal osmotic gradients and promote return of fluid to the vascular space. Restriction of sodium or water decreases extracellular fluid retention.
Administer diuretics: loop diuretic such as furosemide (Lasix), thiazide diuretic such as hydrochlorothiazide (Esidrix), or potassium-sparing diuretic such as triamterene (Direnium), amiloride (Midamore), spironolactone (Aldactone).	To achieve excretion of excess fluid, either a single thiazide diuretic or a combination of agents may be selected, such as thiazide and spironolactone. The combination can be particularly helpful when two drugs have different sites of action, allowing more effective control of fluid excess.
Replace potassium losses, as indicated.	Potassium deficit may occur, especially if client is receiving potassium-wasting diuretic. This can cause lethal cardiac dysrhythmias if untreated.
Prepare for and assist with dialysis or ultrafiltration, if indicated.	May be done to rapidly reduce fluid overload, especially in the presence of severe cardiac or renal failure.

HYPOVOLEMIA (EXTRACELLULAR FLUID VOLUME DEFICIT)

I. Classification (Stevens, 2008)

  a. Absolute: measurable intravascular loss or hemorrhage
  b. Relative: secondary to internal fluid shifts or insensible losses

II. Predisposing or Contributing Factors

  a. Excessive fluid losses: vomiting, gastric suctioning, diarrhea, polyuria, diaphoresis, wounds or burns, intraoperative fluid loss, hemorrhage
  b. Insufficient or decreased fluid intake: preoperative and postoperative nothing-by-mouth (NPO) status
  c. Systemic infections, fever
  d. Intestinal obstruction or fistulas
  e. Pancreatitis, peritonitis, cirrhosis, ascites, adrenal insufficiency
  f. Kidney disease, diabetic ketoacidosis, hyperglycemic hyperosmotic nonketotic coma (HHNC), diabetes insipidus, syndrome of inappropriate antidiuretic hormone (SIADH)

Client Assessment Database

DIAGNOSTIC DIVISION MAY REPORT	MAY EXHIBIT
ACTIVITY/REST • Fatigue • Generalized weakness	
CIRCULATION	• Hypotension, including postural changes • Pulse weak or thready • Tachycardia • Neck veins flattened • Central venous pressure (CVP) decreased
ELIMINATION • Constipation or, occasionally, diarrhea • Abdominal cramps	• Urine volume decreased; oliguria • Dark, concentrated color
FOOD/FLUID • Thirst • Loss of appetite • Nausea and vomiting • Complete, sudden cessation of intake; or prolonged diminished intake of fluids	• Weight loss often exceeding 2% to 8% of total body weight • Abdominal distention • Mucous membranes dry, furrows on tongue, decreased tearing and salivation • Skin dry with poor turgor or pale, moist, clammy (shock)
NEUROSENSORY • Tingling of the extremities • Vertigo, syncope	• Behavior change such as apathy, restlessness, confusion
RESPIRATION	• Tachypnea
SAFETY	• Temperature usually subnormal, although fever may occur
TEACHING/LEARNING • Refer to predisposing or contributing factors • Use, misuse of diuretics	
DISCHARGE PLAN CONSIDERATIONS • May require assistance with changes in therapeutic regimen, dietary management ➧ Refer to plan of care concerning underlying medical or surgical condition for possible considerations after discharge.	

Diagnostic Studies

WHY IT IS DONE	WHAT IT TELLS ME
BLOOD TESTS	
• *Complete blood count (CBC):* Battery of screening tests, which typically includes hemoglobin (Hgb); hematocrit (Hct); red blood cell (RBC) count, morphology, indices, and distribution width index; platelet count and size; and white blood cell (WBC) count and differential.	Hgb, Hct, and RBC count may be increased because of hemoconcentration. These factors will be decreased with hemorrhage.
• *Hgb:* Normal adult female range, 12 to 16 g/dL; normal adult male range, 14 to 18 g/dL.	
• *Hct:* Normal adult female range, 39% to 45%; normal adult male range, 44% to 56% (Matheny 2012).	
• *Serum sodium:* Sodium is the body's most abundant extracellular ion. Normal range is 135 to 145 mEq/L.	May be normal, high, or low.
• *Plasma proteins:* Plasma proteins, such as albumin, help to transport substances and water throughout the body. Albumin helps maintain intravascular pressure. More than half of the protein in blood serum is albumin. Normal albumin range is 3.6 to 5.0 g/dL (Matheny, 2012).	Levels are increased.
• *Blood urea nitrogen (BUN)/creatinine (Cr ratio):* Measurement of ratio of two serum laboratory values—BUN and serum Cr. Normal BUN/Cr ratio is 10 to 20:1.	BUN out of proportion to Cr level is associated with hypovolemia or other causes of diminished renal blood flow. Ratio greater than 20:1 confirms diagnosis of dehydration (Mentes, 2006).
• *Serum lactate:* Measures lactic acid to help detect and evaluate the severity of hypoxia and metabolic acidosis.	Elevated lactate levels may be present with hypoperfusion, as may occur with hypovolemic shock, and signifies ongoing oxygen debt at the tissue and cellular level (Stevens, 2008).
OTHER DIAGNOSTIC STUDIES	
• *Urine sodium:* Measures the amount of sodium in urine and must be evaluated in association with blood levels. Concentrations may mirror blood levels or be the opposite. Normal values are not fixed; kidneys vary rate of excretion to match dietary intake (Matheny, 2012) but generally range from 15 to 250 mEq/L/day.	Usually decreased when losses are from diarrhea and fluid loss or kidney failure. Levels may be higher than normal if sodium intake is excessive or kidneys are not reabsorbing sodium.
• *Urine specific gravity (SG):* Measures concentration of particles to water. Normal range is 1.003 to 1.035 (Matheny, 2012).	Increased with dehydration, water restriction, and conditions causing water loss, such as vomiting, diarrhea, and certain types of kidney failure.

NURSING DIAGNOSIS: deficient Fluid Volume

May Be Related To
Active fluid loss (e.g., hemorrhage, gastric intubation, acute or prolonged diarrhea, abdominal cancer, burns, fistulas, ascites; use of hyperosmotic radiopaque contrast agents)
Failure of regulatory mechanisms (e.g., fever, thermoregulatory response, renal tubule damage)

Possibly Evidenced By
Signs and symptoms noted in client database

Desired Outcomes/Evaluation Criteria—Client Will

Fluid Balance (NOC)
Maintain fluid volume at a functional level as evidenced by individually adequate urinary output with normal specific gravity, stable vital signs, moist mucous membranes, good skin turgor, and prompt capillary refill.

Knowledge: Treatment Regimen (NOC)
Verbalize understanding of causative factors and purpose of therapeutic interventions.
Demonstrate behaviors to monitor and correct deficit, as appropriate.

ACTIONS/INTERVENTIONS	RATIONALE
Hypovolemia Management (NIC)	
Independent	
Note client age, chronic conditions, and medications.	Older adults (who are more likely to have serious and chronic conditions than young people) are at increased risk for dehydration, one of the most frequent causes of hospitalization in adults ages 65 to 75 (Russo, 2012). Additional risk factors for dehydration include female gender, more than four chronic conditions, more than four medications, immobility, and laxative use (Post, 2011).
Monitor vital signs and CVP. Note presence and degree of postural blood pressure (BP) changes. Observe for temperature elevations or fever.	Tachycardia is present along with a varying degree of hypotension, depending on degree of fluid deficit. *Note:* Older adults may not exhibit tachycardia, especially if they're taking medications such as beta-blockers or calcium channel blockers (Wotton, 2008). CVP measurements are useful in determining degree of fluid deficit and response to replacement therapy. Fever increases metabolism and exacerbates fluid loss.
Palpate peripheral pulses; note capillary refill and skin color, turgor, and temperature. Assess mentation.	Conditions that contribute to extracellular fluid deficit can result in inadequate organ perfusion to all areas and may cause circulatory collapse and shock.
Monitor urinary output. Measure or estimate fluid losses from all sources such as gastric losses, wound drainage, and diaphoresis.	Fluid replacement needs are based on correction of current deficits and ongoing losses. A decreased urinary output may indicate insufficient renal perfusion or hypovolemia, or polyuria can be present, requiring more aggressive fluid replacement.
Weigh daily and compare with 24-hour fluid balance. Measure edematous areas such as abdomen and limbs.	Although weight gain and fluid intake greater than output may not accurately reflect intravascular volume, these measurements provide useful data for comparison.
Evaluate client's ability to manage own hydration.	Impaired gag and swallow reflexes, anorexia, nausea, oral discomfort, and changes in level of consciousness (LOC) are among the factors that affect client's ability to replace fluids orally.
Ascertain client's beverage preferences, and set up a 24-hour schedule for fluid intake. Encourage foods with high fluid content.	Relieves thirst and discomfort of dry mucous membranes and augments parenteral replacement. *Note:* Sense of thirst is often diminished in the older adult (Claros, 2008).
Turn frequently, gently massage skin, and protect bony prominences.	Tissues are susceptible to breakdown because of vasoconstriction and increased cellular fragility.
Provide skin and mouth care. Bathe every other day using mild soap. Apply lotion, as indicated.	Skin and mucous membranes are dry with decreased elasticity because of vasoconstriction and reduced intracellular water. Daily bathing may increase dryness.
Provide safety precautions, as indicated, such as use of side rails where appropriate, bed in low position, frequent observation, and soft restraints if required.	Decreased cerebral perfusion frequently results in changes in mentation or altered thought processes, requiring protective measures to prevent client injury. *Note:* The use of restraints may increase agitation and can pose a safety risk.
Investigate reports of sudden or sharp chest pain, dyspnea, cyanosis, increased anxiety, and restlessness.	Hemoconcentration and increased platelet aggregation may result in systemic emboli formation.
Monitor for sudden or marked elevation of BP, restlessness, moist cough, dyspnea, basilar crackles, and frothy sputum.	Too rapid a correction of fluid deficit may compromise the cardiopulmonary system, especially if colloids are used in general fluid replacement.
Collaborative	
Assist with identification and treatment of underlying cause.	Refer to listing of predisposing or contributing factors to determine treatment needs. *Note:* Dehydration is the most common fluid and electrolyte imbalance in older adults (Russo, 2007).
Monitor laboratory studies, as indicated.	Depending on the avenue of fluid loss, differing electrolyte and metabolic imbalances may be present and require correction. For example, use of glucose solutions in clients with underlying glucose intolerance may result in serum glucose elevation and increased urinary water losses.
Administer IV solutions, as indicated, for example:	Choice of fluids is dependent upon client's underlying condition causing hypovolemia and may include blood, blood products, crystalloid or colloid solutions, or combinations of the above.
Isotonic solutions such as 0.9% NaCl (normal saline) and 5% dextrose/water	Crystalloids provide prompt circulatory improvement, although the benefit may be transient because of increased renal clearance.

ACTIONS/INTERVENTIONS (continued)	RATIONALE (continued)
0.45% NaCl (half-normal saline) and lactated Ringer's (LR) solution	As soon as the client is normotensive, a hypotonic solution (0.45% NaCl) may be used to provide both electrolytes and free water for renal excretion of metabolic wastes. *Note:* Buffered crystalloids (LR) are used with caution because they may potentiate the risk of metabolic acidosis.
Colloids such as synthetic plasma expanders (low-molecular-weight dextran [LMW] and high-molecular-weight dextran [HMWD]), plasma protein fraction (human) solution (Plasmanate), human albumin solution, or hetastarch (HES) (Crawford, 2011)	Corrects plasma protein concentration deficits, thereby increasing intravascular osmotic pressure and facilitating return of fluid into vascular compartment.
Whole blood or packed RBC transfusion and autologous collection of blood	Indicated when hypovolemia is related to active blood loss.
Provide tube feedings, including free water, as appropriate.	Enteral replacement can provide proteins and other needed elements in addition to meeting general fluid requirements when swallowing is impaired.

Sodium

I. Function

a. Primarily responsible for osmotic pressure in that compartment

b. Enhances neuromuscular conduction or transmission of impulses and is essential for maintaining acid-base balance

c. Chloride is carried by sodium and will display the same imbalances.

II. Normal Laboratory Values

a. Serum sodium range: 135 to 145 mEq/L

b. Intracellular sodium: 10 mEq/L

c. Serum chloride range: 95 to 105 mEq/L

HYPONATREMIA (SODIUM DEFICIT)

III. Predisposing or Contributing Factors

a. Primary hyponatremia—loss of sodium

i. Heavy sweating (e.g., heat exhaustion), wounds or trauma (hemorrhage), burns, gastric suctioning, vomiting, diarrhea, small-bowel obstruction, peritonitis, salt-wasting renal dysfunction, adrenal insufficiency (Addison's disease)

ii. Lack of sufficient dietary sodium, severe malnutrition, infusion of sodium-free solutions

b. Dilutional hyponatremia—water gains

i. Excessive water intake

ii. Electrolyte-free intravenous (IV) infusion

iii. Water intoxication—psychiatric illness, too aggressive hypotonic IV therapy, tap-water enemas

iv. Gastric irrigations with electrolyte-free solutions

v. Presence of tumors or central nervous system (CNS) disorders predisposing to syndrome of inappropriate antidiuretic hormone (SIADH), heart failure (HF), renal failure, nephrotic syndrome, hepatic cirrhosis, diabetes mellitus (DM), or hyperglycemia

vi. Freshwater near-drowning

vii. Use of certain drugs—hypoglycemia medications, barbiturates, antipsychotics, aminophylline, morphine (may stimulate pituitary gland to secrete excessive amounts of antidiuretic hormone [ADH]), anticonvulsants, some antineoplastic agents, or NSAIDs

Client Assessment Database

Client may be asymptomatic until serum sodium level is less than 125 mEq/L, depending on rapidity of onset.

General

DIVISION MAY REPORT	MAY EXHIBIT
ACTIVITY/REST	
• Malaise • Generalized weakness, faintness • Muscle cramps	

(continues on page 894)

Client Assessment Database (continued)

DIAGNOSTIC DIVISION MAY REPORT (continued)	MAY EXHIBIT (continued)
EGO INTEGRITY	
• Anxiety	• Restlessness, apprehension
FOOD/FLUID	
• Nausea, anorexia • Thirst • Low-sodium diet • Diuretic use	
NEUROSENSORY	
• Headache • Blurred vision • Vertigo	• Loss of coordination • Personality changes • Stupor
TEACHING/LEARNING	
• Refer to predisposing or contributing factors • Use of oral hypoglycemic agent, potent diuretics, NSAIDs, other drugs that impair renal water excretion	
DISCHARGE PLAN CONSIDERATIONS	
• May require assistance with changes in therapeutic regimen, dietary management	
➧ Refer to plan of care concerning underlying medical or surgical condition for possible considerations after discharge.	

Sodium/Water Deficit

Sodium less than 135 mEq/L, urine specific gravity elevated, and serum osmolality normal.

Client Assessment Database

DIAGNOSTIC DIVISION MAY REPORT	MAY EXHIBIT
CIRCULATION	
	• Hypotension • Tachycardia • Peripheral pulses diminished • Pallid, clammy skin
ELIMINATION	
• Abnormal cramping • Diarrhea	• Urinary output decreased
FOOD/FLUID	
• Anorexia • Nausea, vomiting	• Poor skin turgor • Mucous membranes dry, decreased saliva and perspiration • Soft, sunken eyeballs
NEUROSENSORY	
• Dizziness	• Muscle twitching • Lethargy, restlessness, confusion, stupor

DIAGNOSTIC DIVISION MAY REPORT (continued)	MAY EXHIBIT (continued)
RESPIRATION	• Tachypnea
SAFETY	• Skin flushed, dry, hot • Fever

Sodium Deficit/Water Excess

Sodium less than 135 mEq/L, urine specific gravity low, serum osmolality decreased.

Client Assessment Database

DIAGNOSTIC DIVISION MAY REPORT	MAY EXHIBIT
CIRCULATION	• Hypertension • Generalized edema **When Na+ less than 120 mEq/L:** • Hypotension with vasomotor collapse • Rapid, thready pulse • Cold, clammy skin; fingerprinting on sternum • Cyanosis
ELIMINATION	• Urinary output increased
NEUROSENSORY	• Muscle twitching • Restlessness • Changes in mentation—more severe when problem is acute, develops rapidly **When Na+ less than 120 mEq/L:** • Hyporeflexia • Convulsions • Coma
PAIN/DISCOMFORT • Headache • Abdominal cramps	

Diagnostic Studies (depend on associated fluid level)

DIAGNOSTIC DIVISION MAY REPORT	MAY EXHIBIT
BLOOD TESTS • *Serum sodium:* Sodium is the body's most abundant extracellular ion. It plays a key role in maintaining fluid balance—where sodium goes, water will follow. Normal adult range is 135 to 146 mEq/L.	Decreased, less than 135 mEq/L. However, signs and symptoms may not occur until level is less than 120 mEq/L.

(continues on page 896)

DIAGNOSTIC DIVISION MAY REPORT (continued)	MAY EXHIBIT (continued)
• *Serum potassium:* An essential intracellular ion needed to regulate water balance, levels of acidity, and blood pressure (BP). Normal range is 3.5 to 5.5 mEq/L.	May be decreased as the kidneys attempt to conserve sodium at the expense of potassium.
• *Serum chloride/bicarbonate (HCO_3–):* Normal range for chloride is 97 to 110 mEq/L, whereas normal range for HCO_3^- is 18 to 23 mmol/L (Matheny, 2012).	Levels are decreased depending on which ion is lost with the sodium.
• *Serum osmolality:* An indirect measurement of the number of particles (sodium, glucose, and urea) in plasma, reflecting fluid balance. Normal range is 280–295 mOsm/kg (Matheny, 2012).	Commonly low, but may be normal as in pseudohyponatremia, or high as in hyperglycemic hyperosmotic nonketotic coma (HHNC).
• *Hematocrit (Hct):* Volume percentage of red blood cells (RBCs) in whole blood. Normal range for adult female is 39% to 45%; normal adult male range, 44% to 56% (Matheny 2012).	Depends on fluid balance—fluid excess versus dehydration.
OTHER DIAGNOSTIC STUDIES	
• *Urine sodium:* Measures the amount of sodium in urine and must be evaluated in association with blood levels. Concentrations may mirror blood levels or be the opposite. Normal values are not fixed; kidneys vary rate of excretion to match dietary intake (Matheny, 2012) but generally range from 15 to 250 mEq/L/day.	Less than 15 mEq/L indicates renal conservation of sodium due to sodium loss from a nonrenal source, unless sodium-wasting nephropathy is present. Urine sodium greater than 20 mEq/L indicates syndrome of inappropriate antidiuretic hormone (SIADH).
• *Urine osmolality:* Measures concentration of particles to water in urine. Normal range for random specimen is 50 to 1400 mOsm/kg.	Usually low unless SIADH present; in which case, it will exceed serum osmolality.
• *Urine specific gravity:* Measures the concentration of particles in urine such as glucose, sodium, and urea. Normal values range from 1.003 to 1.035 (Matheny, 2012).	May be decreased or increased if SIADH is present.

NURSING DIAGNOSIS: risk for Electrolyte Imbalance

Risk Factors May Include

Vomiting; diarrhea
Renal dysfunction
Treatment-related side effects (e.g., medications, drains)
Excess fluid volume (e.g., water intoxication)

Possibly Evidenced By

(Not applicable, presence of signs and symptoms establishes an *actual* diagnosis)

Desired Outcomes/Evaluation Criteria—Client Will

Electrolyte & Acid/Base Balance (NOC)

Display heart rate, BP, and laboratory results within normal limits (WNL) for client; absence of muscle weakness; and neurological irritability.

ACTIONS/INTERVENTIONS	RATIONALE
Electrolyte Management: Hyponatremia (NIC)	
Independent	
Identify client at risk for hyponatremia and the specific cause such as sodium loss or fluid excess.	Provides clues for early intervention. Hyponatremia is a common imbalance, especially in the elderly, and may range from mild to severe. Severe hyponatremia can cause neurological damage or death if not treated promptly.
Monitor intake and output (I&O). Calculate fluid balance. Weigh daily.	Indicators of fluid balance are important because either fluid excess or deficit may occur with hyponatremia.
Assess level of consciousness (LOC) and neuromuscular response.	Sodium deficit may result in decreased mentation to the point of coma, as well as generalized muscle weakness, cramps, or convulsions.

ACTIONS/INTERVENTIONS (continued)	RATIONALE (continued)
Maintain quiet environment; provide safety and seizure precautions.	Reduces CNS stimulation and risk of injury from neurological complications such as seizures.
Note respiratory rate and depth.	Co-occurring hypochloremia may produce slow and shallow respirations as the body compensates for metabolic alkalosis.
Encourage foods and fluids high in sodium such as milk, meat, eggs, carrots, beets, and celery. Use fruit juices and bouillon instead of plain water.	Unless sodium deficit causes serious symptoms requiring immediate IV replacement, the client may benefit from slower replacement by oral method or removal of previous salt restriction.
Irrigate nasogastric (NG) tube (when used) with normal saline instead of water.	Isotonic irrigation will minimize loss of gastrointestinal (GI) electrolytes.
Observe for signs of circulatory overload, as indicated.	Administration of sodium-containing IV fluids in presence of HF increases risk.
Collaborative	
Assist with treatment of underlying cause.	Refer to listing of predisposing or contributing factors to determine treatment needs.
Monitor serum and urine electrolytes and osmolality.	Evaluates therapy needs and effectiveness.
Provide or restrict fluids, depending on fluid volume status.	In presence of hypovolemia, volume losses are replaced with isotonic saline (e.g., normal saline) or, on occasion, hypertonic solution (3% NaCl) when hyponatremia is life-threatening. In the presence of fluid volume excess, or SIADH, fluid restriction is indicated. *Note:* Too rapid or excessive administration of hypertonic solutions can be lethal.
Administer medications, as indicated, for example:	
Loop diruetics, e.g., furosemide (Lasix)	Effective in reducing fluid excess to correct sodium and water balance.
Sodium chloride	Used to replace deficits in the presence of chronic or ongoing losses.
Potassium chloride	Corrects potassium deficit, especially when diuretic is used.
Vasopressin receptor antagonists, e.g., conivaptan (Vaprisal), tolvaptin (Samsca)	These agents block ADH action and increase water excretion. The potential benefits of these drugs include the predictability of their effect, rapid onset of action, and limited urinary electrolyte excretion (Thomas, 2013).
Demeclocycline (Declomycin).	Useful in treating chronic SIADH, or when severe water restriction may not be tolerated. *Note:* May be contraindicated in clients with liver disease because nephrotoxicity may occur.
Prepare for/assist with dialysis as indicated.	May be done to restore sodium balance without increasing fluid level when hyponatremia is severe or response to diuretic therapy is inadequate.

Sodium (continued)

HYPERNATREMIA (SODIUM EXCESS)

IV. Predisposing or Contributing Factors

a. Excessive water losses: polyuria (as may occur with diabetes insipidus); use of osmotic diuretics (such as mannitol); presence of fever, profuse sweating, vomiting, diarrhea

b. Extracellular fluid volume excesses: renal disease, HF, primary aldosteronism, excessive steroids, Cushing's disease; excessive ingestion or infusion of sodium; salt-water near-drowning

c. Insufficient water intake: administration of tube feedings or high-protein diets with minimal fluid intake, self-medication, "ulcer diet" primarily using half and half or whole milk

Sodium Excess/Water Deficit

Sodium greater than 145 mEq/L and elevated urine specific gravity.

Client Assessment Database

DIAGNOSTIC DIVISION MAY REPORT	MAY EXHIBIT
ACTIVITY/REST • Weakness	• Muscle rigidity, tremors • Generalized weakness
CIRCULATION	• Decreased BP, postural hypotension • Tachycardia **If sodium/water excess—Na+ greater than 145 mEq/L, urine specific gravity decreased:** • Elevated BP, hypertension
ELIMINATION	• Decreased urinary output **If sodium/water excess:** • Polyuria
FOOD/FLUID • Thirst	• Mucous membranes dry, sticky • Tongue dry, swollen, rough **If sodium/water excess:** • Skin pale, moist, taut with pitting edema • Weight gain
NEUROSENSORY	• Irritability, lethargy, coma—depending on rapidness of onset rather than actual serum sodium level • Delusions, hallucinations • Muscle irritability, seizure activity
RESPIRATION	• Dyspnea
TEACHING/LEARNING • Refer to predisposing or contributing factors	
DISCHARGE PLAN CONSIDERATIONS • May require assistance with changes in therapeutic regimen, dietary management ➧ Refer to plan of care concerning underlying medical or surgical condition for possible considerations after discharge.	

Diagnostic Studies

TEST WHY IT IS DONE	WHAT IT TELLS ME
BLOOD TESTS	
• ***Serum sodium:*** Sodium is the body's most abundant extracellular ion. It plays a key role in maintaining fluid balance—where sodium goes, water will follow. Normal adult range is 135 to 146 mEq/L.	Levels are increased. Serum levels greater than 160 mEq/L may be accompanied by severe neurological signs.
• ***Serum chloride:*** Measures the amount of chloride in fluid portion of blood. It works with other electrolytes to maintain fluid and acid-base balance. Normal range for chloride is 97 to 110 mEq/L (Matheny, 2012).	Increased with dehydration and metabolic acidosis. May be lower than normal if SIADH is present.
• ***Serum potassium:*** An essential intracellular ion needed to regulate water balance, levels of acidity, and BP. Normal range is 3.5 to 5.0 mEq/L (Matheny, 2012).	Levels are decreased.
• ***Serum osmolality:*** An indirect measurement of the number of particles (sodium, glucose, and urea) in plasma, reflecting fluid balance. Normal range is 280 to 295 mOsm/kg (Matheny, 2012).	Greater than 295 mOsm/L with dehydration. Is reduced in presence of extracellular fluid excess and less than 200 mOsm/L with excessive polyuria.
• ***Hct:*** Volume percentage of RBCs in whole blood. Normal range for adult female is 39% to 45%; normal adult male range, 44% to 56% (Matheny, 2012).	May be normal or elevated depending on fluid status.
OTHER DIAGNOSTIC STUDIES	
• ***Urine sodium:*** Measures the amount of sodium in urine and must be evaluated in association with blood levels. Concentrations may mirror blood levels or be the opposite. Normal values are not fixed; kidneys vary rate of excretion to match dietary intake (Matheny, 2012) but generally range from 15 to 250 mEq/L/day.	Levels are decreased.
• ***Urine osmolality:*** Measures concentration of particles to water in urine. Normal range for random specimen is 50 to 1400 mOsm/kg.	Levels are elevated.
• ***Urine specific gravity:*** Measures the concentration of particles in urine, such as glucose, sodium, and urea. Normal values range from 1.003 to 1.035 (Matheny, 2012).	Increased with water deficit; decreased when hypernatremia is due to polyuria.

NURSING DIAGNOSIS: risk for Electrolyte Imbalance

Risk Factors May Include

Vomiting, diarrhea
Renal dysfunction; impaired regulatory mechanisms (e.g., diabetes insipidus)
Treatment-related side effects (e.g., osmotic diuretics, high-protein diet)
[Fever, profuse sweating]

Possibly Evidenced By

(Not applicable, presence of signs and symptoms establishes an *actual* diagnosis)

Desired Outcomes/Evaluation Criteria—Client Will

Electrolyte & Acid/Base Balance (NOC)

Display BP, heart rate, and laboratory results WNL for client and absence of neuromuscular irritability and cognitive impairment.

ACTIONS/INTERVENTIONS	RATIONALE
Electrolyte Management: Hypernatremia (NIC)	
Independent	
Monitor BP.	Either hypertension or hypotension may be present depending on the fluid status. Presence of postural hypotension may affect activity tolerance.
Identify client at risk for hypernatremia and likely cause such as water deficit or sodium excess.	Early identification and intervention prevents serious complications associated with this problem.
Note respiratory rate and depth.	Deep, labored respirations with air hunger suggest metabolic acidosis due to hyperchloremia, which can lead to cardiopulmonary arrest if not corrected.
Monitor I&O and urine specific gravity. Weigh daily. Assess presence and location of edema.	These parameters are variable, depending on fluid status, and are indicators of therapy needs and effectiveness.
Evaluate LOC and muscular strength, tone, and movement.	Sodium imbalance may cause changes that vary from confusion and irritability to seizures and coma. In presence of water deficit, rapid rehydration may cause cerebral edema.
Maintain safety and seizure precautions, as indicated, such as bed in low position and use of padded side rails.	Sodium excess and cerebral edema increase risk of convulsions.
Assess skin turgor, color, and temperature and mucous membrane moisture.	Water-deficit hyponatremia manifests by signs of dehydration.
Provide and encourage meticulous skin care and frequent repositioning.	Maintains skin integrity.
Provide frequent oral care. Avoid use of mouthwash that contains alcohol.	Promotes comfort and prevents further drying of mucous membranes.
Offer debilitated client fluids at regular intervals. Give free water to client receiving enteral feedings.	May prevent hypernatremia in client who is unable to perceive or respond to thirst.
Recommend avoidance of foods high in sodium such as canned soups and vegetables, processed foods, snack foods, and condiments.	Reduces risk of sodium-associated complications.
Collaborative	
Assist with identification and treatment of underlying cause.	Refer to listing of predisposing or contributing factors to determine treatment needs.
Monitor serum electrolytes, osmolality, and arterial blood gases (ABGs), as indicated.	Evaluates therapy needs and effectiveness. *Note:* Co-occurring hyperchloremia may cause metabolic acidosis, requiring further intervention.
Increase oral (PO) and IV fluid intake.	Replacement of total body water deficit will gradually restore sodium and water balance.
Restrict sodium intake and administer diuretics as indicated.	Restriction of sodium intake while promoting renal clearance lowers serum sodium levels in the presence of extracellular fluid excess.

Potassium

I. Function

a. Major cation of the intracellular fluid
b. Responsible for maintaining intracellular osmotic pressure
c. Also regulates neuromuscular excitability, aids in maintenance of acid-base balance, synthesis of protein, and metabolism of carbohydrates

II. Normal laboratory values

a. Serum range: 3.5 to 5.0 mEq/L
b. Total body: 42 mEq/L

HYPOKALEMIA (POTASSIUM DEFICIT)

III. Predisposing or Contributing Factors

a. Renal loss: use of potassium-wasting diuretics, diuretic phase of acute tubular necrosis (ATN), healing phase of burns, diabetic acidosis, Cushing's syndrome, nephritis, hypomagnesemia; use of sodium penicillins, amphotericin B, carbenicillin, steroids; licorice abuse
b. Gastrointestinal (GI) loss: profuse vomiting, excessive diarrhea, laxative abuse, prolonged gastric suction, inflammatory bowel disease, fistulas
c. Inadequate dietary intake: anorexia nervosa, starvation, high-sodium diet
d. Shift into cells: total parenteral nutrition (TPN), alkalosis, or excessive secretion or administration of insulin
e. Other: sweat losses (heavily perspiring person acclimated to heat); liver disease

Client Assessment Database

DIAGNOSTIC DIVISION MAY REPORT	MAY EXHIBIT
ACTIVITY/REST • Generalized weakness • Lethargy, fatigue	
CIRCULATION	• Hypotension • Pulses weak or diminished, irregular • Heart sounds distant • Dysrhythmias—premature ventricular contractions (PVCs), ventricular tachycardia, fibrillation
ELIMINATION	• Nocturia, polyuria if factors contributing to hypokalemia include heart failure (HF) or diabetes mellitus (DM) • Bowel sounds diminished, decreased bowel motility, paralytic ileus • Abdominal distention
FOOD/FLUID • Anorexia, nausea, vomiting • Thirst	
NEUROSENSORY • Paresthesias	• Depressed mental state, confusion, apathy, drowsiness, irritability, coma • Hyporeflexia, tetany, paralysis—flaccid quadriparesis
PAIN/DISCOMFORT • Muscle pain, cramps	
RESPIRATION	• Hypoventilation, decreased respiratory depth due to muscle weakness, paralysis of diaphragm • Apnea • Cyanosis
TEACHING/LEARNING • Refer to predisposing or contributing factors • May use or misuse herbal supplements that can cause or exacerbate hypokalemia—aloe, caraway, castor oil, dandelion, elder flower, flaxseed, glycerol, licorice, peppermint oil, psyllium, yarrow	
DISCHARGE PLAN CONSIDERATIONS • May require assistance with changes in therapeutic regimen, dietary management ➧ Refer to plan of care concerning underlying medical or surgical condition for possible considerations after discharge.	

Diagnostic Studies

TEST WHY IT IS DONE	WHAT IT TELLS ME
BLOOD TESTS	
• ***Serum potassium:*** An essential intracellular ion needed to regulate water balance, levels of acidity, and blood pressure (BP). Normal range is 3.5 to 5.0 mEq/L (Matheny, 2012).	Levels are decreased. Hypokalemia can result from two general causes: either from an overall depletion in the body's potassium or from excessive uptake of potassium by muscle from surrounding fluids.
• ***Serum chloride:*** Measures the amount of chloride in the fluid portion of the blood. It works with other electrolytes, such as potassium, sodium, and carbon dioxide, to help keep the proper balance of body fluids and maintain the body's acid-base balance. Normal range for chloride is 97 to 110 mEq/L (Matheny, 2012).	Levels are often decreased. *Note:* Use of diuretics may cause chloride (as well as potassium) depletion.
• ***Serum magnesium:*** An essential intracellular ion needed to regulate water balance, levels of acidity, and BP. Normal range is 1.3 to 2.1 mEq/L (Matheny, 2012).	Hypomagnesemia occurs and exacerbates potassium loss and sodium retention.
• ***Arterial blood gases (ABGs):*** Measures blood acidity and levels of oxygen and carbon dioxide in the blood. Used to determine how well lungs are able to move oxygen into the blood and remove carbon dioxide from the blood.	Imbalances may be noted in pH and bicarbonate.
OTHER DIAGNOSTIC STUDIES	
• ***Electrocardiogram (ECG):*** Record of the electrical activity of the heart.	The following changes can be associated with hypokalemia: low voltage, flat or inverted T wave; appearance of U wave; depressed ST segment; peaked P waves; prolonged QT interval; and ventricular dysrhythmias.

NURSING DIAGNOSIS: risk for Electrolyte Imbalance

Risk Factors May Include

Vomiting; diarrhea; [profuse sweating]
Renal dysfunction; diabetic acidosis
Treatment-related side effects (e.g., diuretics, some antibiotics, TPN)
[Starvation, high-sodium diet]

Possibly Evidenced By

(Not applicable, presence of signs and symptoms establishes an *actual* diagnosis)

Desired Outcomes/Evaluation Criteria—Client Will

Electrolyte & Acid/Base Balance (NOC)

Display heart rhythm and laboratory results within normal limit (WNL) for client and absence of muscle weakness, paresthesias, and cognitive impairment.

ACTIONS/INTERVENTIONS	RATIONALE
Electrolyte Management: Hypokalemia (NIC) ***Independent***	
Monitor heart rate and rhythm.	Changes associated with hypokalemia include abnormalities in both conduction and contractility. Tachycardia may develop as well as potentially life-threatening atrial and ventricular dysrhythmias—PVCs, sinus bradycardia, atrioventricular (AV) blocks, AV dissociation, and ventricular tachycardia.
Monitor respiratory rate, depth, and effort. Encourage cough and deep-breathing exercises; reposition frequently.	Respiratory muscle weakness may proceed to paralysis and eventual respiratory arrest.
Assess level of consciousness (LOC) and neuromuscular function, noting strength, sensation, and movement.	Apathy, drowsiness, irritability, tetany, paresthesias, and coma may occur.
Auscultate bowel sounds, noting absence or change.	Paralytic ileus commonly follows gastric losses through vomiting, gastric suction, or protracted diarrhea.

ACTIONS/INTERVENTIONS (continued)	RATIONALE (continued)
Maintain accurate record of urinary, gastric, and wound losses.	Guide for calculating fluid and potassium replacement needs.
Monitor rate of intravenous (IV) potassium administration using microdrop or pump infusion devices. Check for side effects. Provide ice pack, as indicated.	Ensures controlled delivery of medication to prevent bolus effect and reduce associated discomfort such as burning sensation at IV site. When solution cannot be administered via central vein and slowing rate is not possible or effective, applying ice pack to infusion site may help relieve discomfort.
Encourage intake of foods and fluids high in potassium such as bananas, oranges, dried fruits, red meat, turkey, salmon, leafy vegetables, peas, baked potatoes, tomatoes, winter squash, coffee, colas, and tea. Discuss use of potassium chloride salt substitutes for client receiving long-term diuretics.	Potassium may be replaced and level maintained through the diet when the client is allowed oral food and fluids. Dietary replacement of 40 to 60 mEq/L/day is typically sufficient if no abnormal losses are occurring.
Review drug regimen for potassium-wasting drugs, such as furosemide (Lasix), hydrochlorothiazide (Diamox), some steroids, some laxatives, IV catecholamines, gentamicin (Garamycin), carbenicillin (Geocillin), and amphotericin B (Fungizone).	If alternate agents (e.g., potassium-sparing diuretics such as spirinolactone [Aldactone], triamterene [Dyrenium], amiloride [Midamor]) cannot be administered or when high-dose sodium drugs are administered (e.g., carbenicillin), close monitoring and replacement of potassium are necessary.
Discuss preventable causes of condition such as nutritional choices and the proper use of laxatives.	Provides opportunity for client to prevent recurrence. Also, dietary control is more palatable than oral replacement medications.
Watch for signs of digoxin toxicity when used: reports of nausea, vomiting, blurred vision, increasing atrial dysrhythmias, and heart block.	Low potassium enhances effect of digoxin, slowing cardiac conduction. *Note:* Combined effects of digoxin, diuretics, and hypokalemia may produce lethal dysrhythmias.
Observe for signs of metabolic alkalosis such as hypoventilation, tachycardia, dysrhythmias, tetany, and changes in mentation.	Frequently associated with hypokalemia.
Collaborative	
Assist with treatment of underlying cause.	Refer to listing of predisposing or contributing factors to determine treatment needs. *Note:* Hypokalemia is life-threatening; therefore early detection is crucial.
Monitor laboratory studies, such as the following:	
Serum potassium	Levels should be checked frequently during replacement therapy, especially in the presence of insufficient renal function.
ABGs	Correction of metabolic alkalosis raises serum potassium level and reduces replacement needs. Correction of acidosis drives potassium back into cells, resulting in decreased serum levels and increased replacement needs.
Administer oral and/or IV potassium.	May be required to correct deficiencies when changes in medication, therapy, and/or dietary intake are insufficient. *Note:* Even in severe deficit, parenteral replacement should not exceed 40 mEq every 2 hours. Dietary supplementation may also be used to produce a gradual equilibration if client is able to take oral food and fluids.

Potassium (continued)

HYPERKALEMIA (POTASSIUM EXCESS)

IV. Predisposing or Contributing Factors

- **a.** Potassium retention: decreased renal excretion (e.g., renal disease, acute failure, hypoaldosteronism, Addison's disease), hypovolemia, use of potassium-conserving diuretics—especially when associated with potassium supplements, use of NSAIDs
- **b.** Excessive potassium intake: salt substitutes, drugs containing potassium, improper use of oral potassium supplements, too-rapid IV administration of potassium, massive transfusion of banked blood
- **c.** Shift or release of potassium out of cells: severe catabolism, burns, crush injuries, myocardial infarction (MI), severe hemolysis, rhabdomyolysis, chemotherapy with cytotoxic drugs, respiratory or metabolic acidosis, anoxia, hyperglycemia with insulin deficiency, use of some beta-adrenergic blockers, profound digoxin toxicity
- **d.** Other: use of certain medications such as captopril, heparin, cyclosporine

Client Assessment Database

Data depend on degree of elevation and length of time condition has existed.

DIAGNOSTIC DIVISION MAY REPORT	MAY EXHIBIT
ACTIVITY/REST • Vague muscular weakness	• Restlessness, irritability
CIRCULATION	• Irregular pulse, bradycardia, heart block, asystole
EGO INTEGRITY • Apprehension	
ELIMINATION • Intermittent abdominal cramps • Diarrhea	• Urine volume decreased • Hyperactive bowel sounds
FOOD/FLUID • Nausea, vomiting	
NEUROSENSORY • Paresthesias—often of face, tongue, hands, feet • Slurred speech	• Decreased deep-tendon reflexes • Progressive, ascending flaccid paralysis • Twitching, seizure activity • Apathy, confusion
PAIN/DISCOMFORT • Muscle cramps, pain	
TEACHING/LEARNING • Refer to predisposing or contributing factors	
DISCHARGE PLAN CONSIDERATIONS • May require assistance with changes in therapeutic regimen, dietary management ➧ Refer to plan of care concerning underlying medical or surgical condition for possible considerations after discharge.	

Diagnostic Studies

TEST WHY IT IS DONE	WHAT IT TELLS ME
BLOOD TESTS	
• *Serum potassium:* An essential intracellular ion needed to regulate water balance, levels of acidity, and BP. Normal range is 3.5 to 5.0 mEq/L (Matheny, 2012).	Levels are increased.
• *Serum magnesium:* An essential intracellular ion needed to regulate water balance, levels of acidity, and BP. Normal range is 1.3 to 2.1 mEq/L (Matheny, 2012).	Levels may be elevated if renal failure is present.
OTHER DIAGNOSTIC STUDIES	
• *ECG:* Record of the electrical activity of the heart	In the presence of hyperkalemia, these changes may be seen: T waves tall and peaked or tented; prolonged PR interval; loss of P waves; widening of QRS complex; shortened QT interval and ST segment depression; atrial or ventricular dysrhythmias—bradycardia, atrial arrest, complete heart block, ventricular fibrillation, and cardiac arrest.

NURSING DIAGNOSIS: risk for Electrolyte Imbalance

Risk Factors May Include

Renal dysfunction

Treatment-related side effects (e.g., diuretics, NSAIDs, cytotoxic drugs, medications containing potassium, massive transfusion with banked blood)

Possibly Evidenced By

(Not applicable, presence of signs and symptoms establishes an *actual* diagnosis)

Desired Outcomes/Evaluation Criteria—Client Will

Electrolyte & Acid/Base Balance (NOC)

Display heart rate/rhythm and laboratory results WNL for client and absence of muscle weakness, paresthesias, and cognitive impairment.

ACTIONS/INTERVENTIONS	RATIONALE
Electrolyte Management: Hyperkalemia (NIC)	
Independent	
Identify client at risk or the cause of the hyperkalemia, such as excessive intake of potassium or decreased excretion.	Influences choice of interventions. Early identification and treatment can prevent complication. *Note:* A major cause of hypokalemia is decreased renal excretion.
Instruct client in use of potassium-containing salts or salt substitutes, taking potassium supplements safely.	The client is often able to prevent hyperkalemia through management of supplements, diet, and other medications.
Monitor respiratory rate and depth. Elevate head of bed. Encourage coughing and deep-breathing exercises.	Clients may hypoventilate and retain CO_2, leading to respiratory acidosis. Muscular weakness can affect respiratory muscles and lead to respiratory complications.
Monitor heart rate and rhythm. Be aware that cardiac arrest can occur.	Excess potassium depresses myocardial conduction. Bradycardia can progress to cardiac fibrillation and arrest.
Monitor urinary output.	In kidney failure, potassium is retained because of improper excretion. Potassium should not be given if oliguria or anuria is present.
Assess LOC and neuromuscular function, including movement, strength, and sensation.	Client is usually awake and alert; however, muscular paresthesia, weakness, and flaccid paralysis may occur.
Encourage and assist with range-of-motion (ROM) exercises, as tolerated.	Improves muscular tone and reduces muscle cramps and pain.
Encourage frequent rest periods; assist with care activities, as indicated.	General muscle weakness decreases activity tolerance.
Review drug regimen for medications containing potassium or affecting potassium excretion such as penicillin G, spironolactone (Aldactone), amiloride (Midamor), and hydrochlorothiazide (Dyazide, Maxzide).	Requires regular monitoring of potassium levels and may require alternate drug choices or changes in dosage or frequency.
Identify and discontinue dietary sources of potassium, such as tomatoes, broccoli, orange juice, bananas, bran, chocolate, coffee, tea, eggs, dairy products, and dried fruits, if indicated.	Facilitates reduction of potassium level and may prevent recurrence of hyperkalemia.
Recommend an increase in carbohydrates and fats and foods low in potassium such as canned fruits, refined cereals, and apple or cranberry juice.	Reduces exogenous sources of potassium and prevents catabolic tissue breakdown with release of cellular potassium.
Empasize importance of client's notifying future caregivers when chronic condition potentiates development of hyperkalemia, such as oliguric renal failure.	May help prevent recurrence of hyperkalemia.
Collaborative	
Assist with treatment of underlying cause.	Refer to listing of predisposing and contributing factors to determine treatment needs.
Monitor laboratory results, such as serum potassium and ABGs, as indicated.	Evaluates therapy needs and effectiveness. *Note:* Hypoventilation may result in respiratory acidosis, thereby increasing serum potassium levels.
Discontinue potassium-sparing diuretics, angiotensin-converting enzyme (ACE) inhibitors, angiotensin-receptor blockers (ARBs), and other drugs that inhibit renal potassium excretion (Lederer et al, 2013).	Allows normalization of potassium levels over time.
Administer medications, as indicated, for example:	
Diuretics such as furosemide (Lasix)	Loop or thiazide diuretics promote renal clearance and excretion of potassium.

(continues on page 906)

ACTIONS/INTERVENTIONS (continued)	RATIONALE (continued)
IV glucose with insulin and sodium bicarbonate	Short-term emergency measure to move potassium into the cell, thus reducing toxic serum level. *Note:* Use with caution in presence of HF or hypernatremia.
Calcium chloride or calcium gluconate	Temporary stopgap measure that antagonizes toxic potassium depressant effects on heart and stimulates cardiac contractility. *Note:* Calcium is contraindicated in clients on digoxin because it increases the cardiotonic effects of the drug and may cause dysrhythmias.
Sodium polystyrene sulfonate (Kayexalate, SPS suspension), administered orally, per nasogastric (NG) tube, or rectally	Resin removes potassium by exchanging potassium for sodium or calcium in the GI tract. Sorbitol enhances evacuation. *Note:* Use cautiously in clients with HF and/or edema and in the elderly because it increases sodium and chloride levels. In addition, Kayexalate has been associated with serious gastrointestinal (GI) complications, so should not be used in clients with abnormal bowel function (Lederer et al, 2013).
Provide fresh blood or washed red blood cells (RBCs), if transfusions required.	Fresh blood has less potassium than banked blood because breakdown of older RBCs releases potassium.
Prepare for and assist with dialysis.	May be required when more conservative methods fail or are contraindicated, such as severe HF.

Calcium

I. Function

a. Bone formation and reabsorption
b. Neural transmission and muscle contraction
c. Regulation of enzyme systems
d. Coenzyme in blood coagulation

II. Normal laboratory values

a. Serum: 4.5 to 5.3 mEq/L
b. Total body: 8.5 to 10.5 mg/dL—directly related to the serum albumin, calcium is bound to the protein and must be considered if only total serum readings are available.
c. Ionized: 2.1 to 2.6 mEq/L—physiologically active and clinically important, especially in critically ill clients; altered by changes in pH (affects how much calcium is bound to protein) or increased serum levels of fatty acids, lactate, and bicarbonate

HYPOCALCEMIA (CALCIUM DEFICIT)

III. Predisposing or Contributing factors

a. Primary or surgical hypoparathyroidism, transient hypocalcemia following thyroidectomy; hyperphosphatemia, hypomagnesemia
b. Massive subcutaneous tissue infections, acute pancreatitis, burns, peritonitis, malignancies
c. Excessive gastrointestinal (GI) losses: draining fistula, diarrhea, fat malabsorption syndromes, chronic laxative use (particularly phosphate-containing laxatives and enemas)
d. Extreme stress situations with mobilization and excretion of calcium
e. Diuretic and terminal phase of renal failure
f. Inadequate dietary intake, lack of milk or vitamin D, excessive protein diet
g. Alcoholism: primary effect of ethanol, plus intestinal malabsorption, hypomagnesemia, hypoalbuminemia, and pancreatitis
h. Use of anticonvulsants, antibiotics, corticosteroids; loop diuretics, drugs that lower serum magnesium (e.g., cisplatin, gentamycin)
j. Infusion of citrated blood, calcium-free infusions; rapid infusion of Plasmanate
k. Malignant neoplasms with bone metastases
l. Alkalotic states
m. Decreased ultraviolet exposure

Client Assessment Database

Data depend on duration, severity, and rate of onset of hypocalcemia.

DIAGNOSTIC DIVISION MAY REPORT	MAY EXHIBIT
CIRCULATION	• Hypotension • Pulses weak or decreased, irregular— weak cardiac contraction or premature dysrhythmias

DIAGNOSTIC DIVISION MAY REPORT (continued)	MAY EXHIBIT (continued)
ELIMINATION • Abdominal pain • Diarrhea	• Abdominal distention—paralytic ileus
FOOD/FLUID • Nausea, vomiting	• Difficulty swallowing
HYGIENE	• Coarse, dry skin; alopecia (chronic)
NEUROSENSORY • Numbness and tingling of fingers and toes • Muscle cramps	• Anxiety, confusion, irritability, alteration in mood • Memory impaired • Depression • Hallucinations, psychoses • Muscle spasms—carpopedal and laryngeal • Increased deep-tendon reflexes, tetany • Tonic, clonic seizure activity • Positive Trousseau's (carpopedal spasm that results from ischemia, such as that induced by pressure applied to the upper arm from an inflated blood pressure cuff) and Chvostek's signs (twitching of facial muscles in response to tapping over the area of the facial nerve) (Jesus, 2012).
RESPIRATION	• Labored shallow breathing, stridor—spasm of laryngeal muscles
SAFETY	• Bleeding with no, or minimal, trauma
TEACHING/LEARNING • Refer to predisposing or contributing factors	
DISCHARGE PLAN CONSIDERATIONS • May require assistance with changes in therapeutic regimen, dietary management	
➧ Refer to plan of care concerning underlying medical or surgical condition for possible considerations after discharge.	

Diagnostic Studies

TEST WHY IT IS DONE	WHAT IT TELLS ME
BLOOD TESTS	
• ***Serum calcium:*** Essential mineral for proper functioning of muscles, nerves, and heart. Is required in blood clotting and in formation of bones. Only about 1% of calcium circulates in blood. Normal total calcium ranges from 8.9 to 10.3 mg/dL (Matheny, 2012).	Total calcium is decreased in conditions of low albumin levels, extreme deficiency of dietary calcium caused by malnutrition, and disorders of the kidney. *Note:* A serum calcium level less than 8.5 mg/dL or an ionized calcium level less than 1.0 mmol/L is considered hypocalcemia (Suneja, 2013).
• ***Serum magnesium:*** An essential intracellular ion needed to regulate water balance, levels of acidity, and blood pressure (BP). Normal range is 1.3 to 2.1 mEq/L (Matheny, 2012).	May be decreased—follows calcium.

(continues on page 908)

Diagnostic Studies (continued)

TEST WHY IT IS DONE (continued)	WHAT IT TELLS ME (continued)
• *Serum albumin:* A transport protein, one of the total proteins in blood. More than half of the protein in blood serum is albumin. Normal albumin range is 3.5 to 5.0 g/dL (Matheny, 2012).	A low albumin level causes a deceptively low calcium level due to protein binding. *Note:* Because calcium binds to albumin and only the unbound (free or ionized) calcium is biologically active, the serum level must be adjusted for abnormal albumin levels. For every 1-g/dL drop in serum albumin below 4 g/dL, measured serum calcium decreases by 0.8 mg/dL (Agraharkar, 2012).
• *Bleeding/clotting studies, such as protime (PT) and platelets:* Calcium is an essential part of the clotting mechanism.	Deficit may lead to excessive bleeding.
• *Arterial blood gases (ABGs):* Measures blood acidity and levels of oxygen and carbon dioxide in the blood.	Alkalosis causes surplus bicarbonate to bind with free calcium, impairing function. Acidosis frees calcium, potentiating hypercalcemia.
Other Diagnostic Studies	
• *Electrocardiogram (ECG):* Record of the electrical activity of the heart.	Changes that may be seen with hypocalcemia: prolonged QT interval—characteristic but not necessarily diagnostic. In severe deficiency, T waves may flatten or invert, giving appearance of hypokalemia or myocardial ischemia; ventricular tachycardia may develop.

NURSING DIAGNOSIS: risk for Electrolyte Imbalance

Risk Factors May Include

Diarrhea; [chronic laxative abuse]
Renal dysfunction
Treatment-related side effects (e.g., medications—anticonvulsants, antibiotics, corticosteroids, diuretics)

Possibly Evidenced By

(Not applicable, presence of signs and symptoms establishes an *actual* diagnosis)

Desired Outcomes/Evaluation Criteria—Client Will

Electrolyte & Acid/Base Balance (NOC)

Display heart rhythm and laboratory results within normal limits (WNL) for client and absence of neuromuscular irritability and respiratory impairment.

ACTIONS/INTERVENTIONS	RATIONALE
Electrolyte Management: Hypocalcemia (NIC)	
Independent	
Monitor heart rate and rhythm.	Calcium deficit along with associated hypomagnesemia weakens cardiac muscle contractility.
Assess respiratory rate, rhythm, and effort. Have tracheostomy equipment available.	Laryngeal stridor may develop and result in respiratory arrest.
Observe for neuromuscular irritability, including tetany, or seizure activity. Assess for presence of Chvostek's and Trousseau's signs.	Calcium deficit causes repetitive and uncontrolled nerve transmission, leading to muscle spasms and hyperirritability.
Provide quiet environment and seizure precautions, as appropriate.	Reduces central nervous system (CNS) stimulation and protects client from potential injury.
Encourage relaxation and stress reduction techniques including deep-breathing exercises, guided imagery, and visualization.	Tetany can be potentiated by hyperventilation and stress. *Note:* Direct pressure on the nerves, such as tightening BP cuff, may trigger tetany.
Check for bleeding from any source, such as mucous membranes, puncture sites, wounds, or incisions. Note presence of ecchymosis and petechiae.	Alterations in coagulation can occur as a result of calcium deficiency.
Review client's drug regimen such as use of insulin, mithramycin (Mithracin), parathyroid injection, and digoxin.	Some drugs can lower magnesium levels, affecting calcium level. The effect of digoxin is enhanced by calcium, and, in clients receiving calcium, digoxin intoxication may develop.

ACTIONS/INTERVENTIONS (continued)	RATIONALE (continued)
Discuss use of laxatives and antacids.	Those containing phosphate may negatively affect calcium metabolism.
Review dietary intake of vitamins and fat.	Insufficient ingestion of vitamin D and fat impairs absorption of calcium.
Identify sources to increase calcium and vitamin D in diet such as dairy products, beans, cauliflower, eggs, oranges, pineapples, sardines, and shellfish. Restrict intake of phosphorus such as foods containing barley, bran, whole wheat, rye, liver, nuts, and chocolate.	Vitamin D aids in absorption of calcium from intestinal tract. Phosphorus competes with calcium for intestinal absorption.
Encourage use of calcium-containing antacids if needed, such as Titralac, Dicarbosil, and Tums.	Possible sources for oral replacement to help maintain calcium levels, especially in clients at risk for osteoporosis.
Stress importance of meeting calcium needs.	Adverse effects of long-term deficiency include tooth decay, eczema, cataracts, and osteoporosis.
Collaborative	
Assist with identification and treatment of underlying cause.	Refer to listing of predisposing and contributing factors to determine treatment needs.
Monitor laboratory studies.	Evaluates therapy needs and effectiveness
Administer the following:	
Calcium gluconate, gluceptate, or chloride intravenously (IV)	Provides rapid treatment in acute calcium deficit, especially in presence of tetany or convulsions. *Note:* Calcium chloride is not used as often because it is irritating to the vein and can cause tissue sloughing if it leaks into tissues.
Oral preparations, such as calcium carbonate (Oystercal, Caltrate); calcium citrate (Cal-Citrate)	Indicated to restore and maintain normocalcemia when hypocalcemia is not severe enough to warrant rapid replacement (Suneja, 2012).
Magnesium sulfate IV or orally (PO), if indicated	Hypomagnesemia is a precipitating factor in calcium deficit.
Vitamin D supplement	May be used in combination with calcium therapy to enhance calcium absorption once concomitant phosphate deficiency is corrected.

Calcium (continued)

HYPERCALCEMIA (CALCIUM EXCESS)

IV. Predisposing or Contributing Factors

a. Hyperparathyroidism, hyperthyroidism, multiple myeloma or other malignancies (e.g., cancer of breast, lung), renal disease, skeletal muscle paralysis, parathyroid tumor, sarcoidosis, adrenal insufficiency, tuberculosis (TB)
b. Excessive or prolonged use of vitamins A and D and calcium-containing antacids; prolonged use of thiazide diuretics, theophylline, lithium
c. Multiple fractures, bone tumors, osteoporosis, osteomalacia, prolonged immobilization causing imbalance between the rate of bone formation and resorption
d. Milk-alkali syndrome as a side effect of prolonged milk and antacid self-medication for gastric pain or ulcer
e. Hypophosphatasia, hyperproteinemia
f. Anticancer drugs: tamoxifen, androgens, estrogens

Client Assessment Database

DIAGNOSTIC DIVISION MAY REPORT	MAY EXHIBIT
ACTIVITY/REST	
• General malaise, fatigue, weakness • Lethargy	• Incoordination, ataxia
CIRCULATION	
	• Hypertension • Irregular pulse, dysrhythmias, bradycardia
ELIMINATION	
• Constipation or diarrhea	• Polyuria, nocturia • Kidney stones or calculi

(continues on page 910)

Client Assessment Database (continued)

DIAGNOSTIC DIVISION MAY REPORT (continued)	MAY EXHIBIT (continued)
FOOD/FLUID • Anorexia, nausea, vomiting • Thirst • Abdominal pain	• Poor skin turgor • Dry mucous membranes
NEUROSENSORY • Headache	• Hypotonicity, muscular relaxation, flaccid paralysis • Depressed or absent deep-tendon reflexes • Drowsiness, apathy, confusion, stupor, coma • Paranoia, personality change, inappropriate or bizarre behaviors, psychosis • Decreased attention span, memory loss • Depression • Slurred speech
PAIN/DISCOMFORT • Epigastric, abdominal, deep flank pain • Bone or joint pain	
TEACHING/LEARNING • Refer to predisposing or contributing factors	
DISCHARGE PLAN CONSIDERATIONS • May require assistance with changes in therapeutic regimen, dietary management ➧ Refer to plan of care concerning underlying medical or surgical condition for possible considerations after discharge.	

Diagnostic Studies

TEST WHY IT IS DONE	WHAT IT TELLS ME
BLOOD TESTS	
• ***Serum calcium:*** Essential mineral for proper functioning of muscles, nerves, and heart. It is required in blood clotting and in formation of bones. Only about 1% of calcium circulates in blood. Normal total calcium ranges from 8.9 to 10.3 mg/dL (Matheny, 2012).	Levels are increased.
• ***Serum phosphate:*** Test of trace metal used to help diagnose and evaluate the severity of conditions that affect the GI tract, interfering with the absorption of calcium and magnesium.	Phosphate levels may be low when parathyroid hormone inversely promotes calcium uptake and calcium competes with phosphate for absorption and transport with vitamin D.
OTHER DIAGNOSTIC STUDIES	
• ***Urine calcium:*** Measures amount of calcium passed in urine over 24-hour period.	Levels are increased. Test may be done to determine whether a kidney stone has developed because of high amounts of calcium in the urine. May also be done to check for problems with the parathyroid glands.
• ***X-rays, computed tomography (CT) scan, or magnetic resonance imaging (MRI):*** Helps identify contributing factors or effects of elevated calcium level.	May reveal evidence of bone cavitation, pathological fracture, or osteoporosis, reflecting an imbalance between bone formation and resorption; or urinary calculi associated with hypercalcemia.
• ***ECG:*** Record of the electrical activity of the heart.	Changes seen with hypercalcemia include shortened QT interval and inverted T waves. In severe deficit, QRS may widen, PR interval lengthens, and ventricular prematurities develop.

NURSING DIAGNOSIS: risk for Electrolyte Imbalance

Risk Factors May Include

Renal dysfunction
Treatment-related side effects (e.g., medications—thiazide diuretics, theophylline, lithium, anticancer drugs)
Endocrine dysfunction (e.g., hyperthyroidism, hyperparathyroidism)

Possibly Evidenced By

(Not applicable, presence of signs and symptoms establishes an *actual* diagnosis)

Desired Outcomes/Evaluation Criteria—Client Will

Electrolyte & Acid/Base Balance (NOC)
Display heart rhythm, muscle strength, cognitive status, and laboratory results WNL for client.

ACTIONS/INTERVENTIONS	RATIONALE
Electrolyte Management: Hypercalcemia (NIC)	
Independent	
Monitor cardiac rate and rhythm. Be aware that cardiac arrest can occur in hypercalcemic crisis.	Overstimulation of cardiac muscle occurs with resultant dysrhythmias and ineffective cardiac contraction. Sinus bradycardia, sinus dysrhythmias, wandering pacemaker, and atrioventricular (AV) block may be noted. Hypercalcemia creates a predisposition to cardiac arrest.
Assess level of consciousness and neuromuscular status, including muscle movement, strength, and tone.	Nerve and muscle activity is depressed. Lethargy and fatigue can progress to convulsions or coma.
Monitor intake and output (I&O); calculate fluid balance.	Efforts to correct original condition may result in secondary imbalances and complications.
Encourage fluid intake of 3 to 4 L/day, including sodium-containing fluids (within cardiac tolerance) and use of acid-ash juices, such as cranberry and prune, if kidney stones present or suspected.	Reduces dehydration, encourages urinary flow and clearance of calcium, and reduces risk of stone formation. *Note:* Sodium favors calcium excretion and can be used if not contraindicated by other conditions.
Strain urine if flank pain occurs.	Large amount of calcium present in kidney parenchyma may lead to stone formation.
Auscultate bowel sounds.	Hypotonicity leads to constipation when the smooth muscle tone is inadequate to produce peristalsis.
Maintain bulk in diet.	Constipation may be a problem because of decreased GI tone.
Encourage frequent repositioning and range-of-motion (ROM) and/or muscle-setting exercises with caution. Promote ambulation if client is able.	Muscle activity may reduce calcium shifting from the bones that occurs during immobilization. *Note:* Increased risk for pathological fractures exists because of calcium shifts out of the bones.
Provide safety measures, including gentle handling when moving client.	Reduces risk of injury and pathological fractures.
Review drug regimen, noting use of calcium-elevating drugs, such as heparin, tetracyclines, methicillin, and phenytoin.	May affect drug choice or require reduction in oral sources of calcium.
Identify and restrict sources of calcium intake such as dairy products, eggs, and spinach and calcium-containing antacids such as Titralac, Dicarbosil, and Tums, if indicated.	Foods or drugs containing calcium may need to be limited in chronic conditions causing hypercalcemia.
Collaborative	
Assist with treatment of underlying cause.	Refer to listing of predisposing or contributing factors to determine treatment needs.
Monitor laboratory studies such as calcium, magnesium, and phosphate.	Monitors therapy needs and effectiveness.
Administer isotonic saline and sodium sulfate IV or PO.	Emergency measures in severe hypercalcemia used to dilute extracellular calcium concentration and inhibit tubular reabsorption of calcium, thereby increasing urinary excretion.
Administer medications, as indicated, for example:	
Diuretics, such as furosemide (Lasix)	Diuresis promotes renal excretion of calcium and reduces risks of fluid excess from isotonic saline infusion.
Sodium bicarbonate	Induces alkalosis, thereby reducing the ionized calcium fraction.
Potassium phosphate/sodium acid phosphate (K-Phos, Neutra-Phos)	Rapid-acting agent that induces calcium excretion and inhibits resorption of bone.
Biphosphonates (e.g., pamidronate [Aredia]); etidronate [Didronel])	Used after initial hydration to inhibit bone reabsorption and maintain low serum calcium levels, especially in hypercalcemia of malignancy and Paget disease (Suneja, 2012).

(continues on page 912)

ACTIONS/INTERVENTIONS (continued)	RATIONALE (continued)
Glucocorticoid therapy	Inhibits intestinal absorption of calcium and reduces inflammation and associated stress response that mobilizes calcium from the bone.
Antineoplastic agents (e.g., plicamycin [Mithracin]; gallium nitrate [Ganite]) (Suneja, 2012)	These drugs lower serum calcium by inhibiting inappropriate bone resorption, typically seen in malignancies or hyperparathyroidism.
Antidote/hypercalcemia agents (e.g. calcitonin [Miacalcin, Osteocalcin])	Promotes movement of serum calcium into bones, temporarily reducing serum calcium levels, especially in the presence of increased parathyroid hormone.
Neutra-Phos and Fleet Phospho-Soda.	These drugs bind calcium in the GI tract, promoting excretion.
Prepare for and assist with hemodialysis.	Rapid reduction of serum calcium may be necessary to correct life-threatening situation.

Magnesium

I. Function

- **a.** Influences carbohydrate metabolism, secretion of parathyroid hormone, sodium and potassium transport across the cell membrane, and synthesis of protein and nucleic acid
- **b.** Activates adenosine triphosphate (ATP) and mediates neural transmission within the central nervous system (CNS)
- **c.** Deficit often associated with hypokalemia and promotes intracellular potassium loss and sodium accumulation, altering and exacerbating membrane excitability
- **d.** Normal laboratory value—serum range is 1.3 to 2.1 mEq/L (Matheny, 2012).

HYPOMAGNESEMIA (MAGNESIUM DEFICIT)

II. Predisposing or Contributing Factors

- **a.** Gastrointestinal (GI) losses: biliary or intestinal fistula, surgery (bowel resection, small-bowel bypass); severe, protracted diarrhea, laxative abuse; impaired GI absorption or malabsorption syndrome, gastric or colon cancer, prolonged gastric suction
- **b.** Protein or calorie malnutrition, enteral or parenteral feeding without adequate magnesium replacement
- **c.** Prolonged intravenous (IV) infusion of magnesium-free solutions, multiple transfusions with citrated blood products
- **d.** Chronic alcoholism, alcohol withdrawal, pancreatitis
- **e.** Hyperaldosteronism: primary or secondary (e.g., cirrhosis or heart failure [HF])
- **f.** Toxemia of pregnancy
- **g.** Renal losses: severe renal disease, diuretic phase of acute renal failure (ARF), vigorous and/or prolonged diuresis with mercurial thiazides or loop diuretics, syndrome of inappropriate antidiuretic hormone (SIADH)
- **h.** Drugs that affect magnesium balance: aminoglycosides (gentamicin, tobramycin), antifungals (amphotericin B), chemotherapy agents (cisplatin), antirejection agents (cyclosporine), excessive doses of calcium or vitamin D supplements
- **i.** Diabetic ketoacidosis, malignancies causing hypercalcemic states, severe burns, sepsis, hypothermia, hypoparathyroidism, hypercalcemia, hyperthyroidism

Client Assessment Database

DIAGNOSTIC DIVISION MAY REPORT	MAY EXHIBIT
ACTIVITY/REST	
• Generalized weakness • Insomnia • Vertigo	• Ataxia
CIRCULATION	
	• Tachycardia, dysrhythmias • Hypotension (vasodilation), occasional hypertension
FOOD/FLUID	
• Anorexia, nausea • Diarrhea	

DIAGNOSTIC DIVISION MAY REPORT (continued)	MAY EXHIBIT (continued)
NEUROSENSORY • Paresthesia (legs, feet) • Vertigo	• Nystagmus • Musculoskeletal fasciculations or tremors, neuromuscular irritability or spasticity, spontaneous carpopedal spasms, hyperactive deep tendon reflexes, clonus • Seizure activity, convulsions • Tetany; positive Babinski's, Chvostek's, and Trousseau's signs • Disorientation, apathy, depression, irritability, agitation, hallucinations, psychoses, coma
TEACHING/LEARNING • Refer to predisposing or contributing factors **DISCHARGE PLAN CONSIDERATIONS** • May require assistance with changes in therapeutic regimen, dietary management ➧ Refer to plan of care concerning underlying medical or surgical condition for possible postdischarge considerations.	

Diagnostic Studies

TEST WHY IT IS DONE	WHAT IT TELLS ME
BLOOD TESTS	
• ***Serum magnesium:*** An essential intracellular ion needed to regulate water balance, levels of acidity, and blood pressure (BP). Normal range is 1.3 to 2.1 mEq/L (Matheny, 2012).	Decreased, less than 1.5 mEq/L. Usually symptoms do not appear until level is less than 1 mEq/L.
• ***Calcium:*** Essential mineral for proper functioning of muscles, nerves, and heart. It is required in blood clotting and in formation of bones. Only about 1% of calcium circulates in blood. Normal total calcium ranges from 8.9 to 10.3 mg/dL (Matheny, 2012).	May be decreased unless there is a hypercalcemic condition causing the magnesium deficit.
• ***Potassium:*** An essential intracellular ion needed to regulate water balance, levels of acidity, and BP. Normal range is 3.5 to 5.0 mEq/L (Matheny, 2012).	Decrease associated with severe hypomagnesemia.
OTHER DIAGNOSTIC STUDIES	
• ***Electrocardiogram (ECG):*** Record of the electrical activity of the heart.	Changes associated with hypomagnesemia include prolonged PR and QT intervals, widened QRS complex, ST-segment depression, and T-wave inversion.

NURSING DIAGNOSIS: risk for Electrolyte Imbalance

Risk Factors May Include

Deficient fluid volume
Renal dysfunction
Endocrine dysfunction (e.g., diabetic ketoacidosis, hyperaldosteronism)
Treatment-related side effects (e.g., medications—diuretics, aminoglycosides, antifungals, chemotherapy agents)
[Malnutrition]

(continues on page 914)

NURSING DIAGNOSIS: risk for Electrolyte Imbalance (continued)

Possibly Evidenced By

(Not applicable, presence of signs and symptoms establishes an *actual* diagnosis)

Desired Outcomes/Evaluation Criteria—Client Will

Electrolyte & Acid/Base Balance (NOC)

Display heart rate and rhythm, muscle strength, cognitive status, and laboratory results within normal limits (WNL) for client and absence of neuromuscular irritability.

ACTIONS/INTERVENTIONS	RATIONALE
Electrolyte Management: Hypomagnesemia (NIC)	
Independent	
Monitor cardiac rate and rhythm, noting tachydysrhythmias and characteristic ECG changes.	Magnesium influences sodium and potassium transport across the cell membrane and affects excitability of cardiac tissue.
Monitor for signs of digoxin intoxication when used, including reports of nausea or vomiting and blurred vision; increasing atrial dysrhythmias and heart block.	Magnesium deficit may precipitate digoxin toxicity.
Assess level of consciousness (LOC) and neuromuscular status, noting movement, strength, and reflexes and tone; note presence of Chvostek's and Trousseau's signs.	Confusion, irritability, and psychosis may occur. However, more common manifestations are muscular, including hyperactive deep-tendon reflexes, muscle tremors, spasticity, or generalized tetany.
Monitor status of airway and swallowing.	Laryngeal stridor and dysphagia can occur when depletion is moderate to severe.
Take seizure or safety precautions, such as padded side rails, bed in low position, and frequent observation, as indicated.	Changes in mentation or the development of seizure activity in severe hypomagnesemia increases the risk of client injury.
Provide quiet environment and subdued lighting.	Reduces extraneous stimuli; promotes rest.
Encourage range-of-motion (ROM) exercises, as tolerated.	Reduces deleterious effects of muscle weakness and spasticity.
Place footboard or cradle on bed.	Elevation of linens may reduce spasms.
Auscultate bowel sounds.	Muscle weakness or spasticity may reduce peristalsis and bowel function.
Encourage intake of dairy products, whole grains, green leafy vegetables, meat, and fish.	Provides oral replacement for mild magnesium deficits; may prevent recurrence.
Instruct client in proper use of laxatives and diuretics.	Deficit may be the result of abuse of these drugs.
Observe for signs of magnesium toxicity during replacement therapy—thirst, feeling hot and flushed, diaphoresis, anxiety, drowsiness, hypotension, increased muscular and nervous system irritability, or loss of patellar reflex.	Rapid, excessive IV replacement may lead to toxicity and life-threatening complications.
Collaborative	
Assist with treatment of underlying cause.	Refer to listing of predisposing or contributing factors. *Note:* Studies have shown that chronic alcoholism with malnutrition is the most common cause of hypomagnesemia in the United States.
Monitor laboratory studies such as serum magnesium, calcium, and potassium levels.	Evaluates therapy needs and effectiveness. *Note:* These electrolytes are interrelated, symptoms may be similar, and deficits of more than one may be present.
Administer medications, as indicated, for example:	Treatment for hypomagnesemia depends on the degree of deficiency and the client's clinical symptoms and signs. Therapy can be oral (for mild symptoms) or intravenous (for severe symptoms or for those individuals unable to tolerate oral administration) (Fulop, 2013).
Magnesium sulfate or magnesium chloride IV, monitoring administration closely	IV replacement is preferred in severe deficit because absorption of magnesium from intestinal tract varies inversely with calcium absorption. However, potential for drug interaction with digitalis preparations may lead to increased cardiac dysrhythmias or heart block. *Note:* Calcium gluconate is the antidote should hypermagnesemia be evidenced by depressed deep-tendon reflexes or respiratory depression and hypotension (late sign).
Magnesium oral preparations, e.g., magnesium oxide (Mag-Ox); magnesium gluconate (Mag-G); magnesium chloride (Slow Mag) (Fulop, 2013).	Oral replacement should be given in the asymptomatic client, preferably with a sustained-release preparation, given the ability of magnesium to induce diarrhea.

HYPERMAGNESEMIA (MAGNESIUM EXCESS)

III. Predisposing or Contributing Factors (Fulop et al, 2012)

a. Reduced renal function (e.g., acute processes or age), chronic renal disease or failure, or dialysis with hard water
b. Excessive intake or absorption—too-rapid replacement of magnesium (as in pregnancy-induced hypertension or premature labor), excessive use of magnesium-containing drugs or products, such as Maalox, milk of magnesia, and Epsom salts
c. Untreated diabetic ketoacidosis
d. Hyperparathyroidism, aldosterone deficiency, adrenal insufficiency
e. Extracellular fluid volume depletion (e.g., after diuretic abuse)
f. Saltwater near-drowning, hypothermia, shock
g. Chronic diarrhea; diseases that interfere with gastric absorption

Client Assessment Database

DIAGNOSTIC DIVISION MAY REPORT	MAY EXHIBIT
ACTIVITY/REST • Generalized weakness • Fatigue	• Drowsiness, lethargy, stupor
CIRCULATION	• Hypotension (mild to severe) • Pulses weak, irregular, bradycardia (12–15 mEq/L), cardiac arrest (greater than 25 mEq/L)
FOOD/FLUID • Nausea	
NEUROSENSORY	• Depressed deep-tendon reflexes (7–10 mEq/L) progressing to flaccid paralysis • Decreased LOC, lethargy progressing to coma • Slurred speech
RESPIRATION	• Hypoventilation progressing to apnea (12–15 mEq/L)
SAFETY	• Skin flushing, sweating
TEACHING/LEARNING • Refer to predisposing or contributing factors	
DISCHARGE PLAN CONSIDERATIONS • May require assistance with changes in therapeutic regimen, dietary management ➧ Refer to plan of care concerning underlying medical or surgical condition for possible considerations after discharge.	

Diagnostic Studies

TEST WHY IT IS DONE	WHAT IT TELLS ME
BLOOD TESTS	
• *Serum magnesium:* An essential intracellular ion needed to regulate water balance, levels of acidity, and BP. Normal range is 1.3 to 2.1 mEq/L (Matheny, 2012).	Client is symptomatic when levels are greater than 4 to 6 mEq/L. High levels (>10 mEq/L) result in respiratory depression, coma, and cardiac arrest (Angus, 2012).
OTHER DIAGNOSTIC STUDIES	
• *ECG:* Record of the electrical activity of the heart.	Changes associated with hypermagnesemia include prolonged PR and QT intervals, widened QRS, elevated T waves, development of heart block, and cardiac arrest.

NURSING DIAGNOSIS: risk for Electrolyte Imbalance

Risk Factors May Include

Chronic diarrhea
Renal dysfunction
Treatment-related side effects (e.g., medications containing magnesium, diuretic abuse, dialysis with hard water)
Endocrine dysfunction (diabetic ketoacidosis)

Possibly Evidenced By

(Not applicable, presence of signs and symptoms establishes an *actual* diagnosis)

Desired Outcomes/Evaluation Criteria—Client Will

Electrolyte & Acid/Base Balance (NOC)

Display heart rhythm, muscular strength, cognitive status, and laboratory results WNL for client and absence of respiratory impairment.

ACTIONS/INTERVENTIONS	RATIONALE
Electrolyte Management: Hypermagnesemia (NIC)	
Independent	
Monitor cardiac rate and rhythm.	Bradycardia and heart block may develop, progressing to cardiac arrest as a direct result of hypermagnesemia on cardiac muscle.
Monitor BP.	Hypotension unexplained by other causes is an early sign of toxicity.
Assess LOC and neuromuscular status, including reflexes, muscle tone, movement, and strength.	CNS and neuromuscular depression can cause decreasing level of alertness, progressing to coma, and depressed muscular responses, progressing to flaccid paralysis.
Monitor respiratory rate, depth, and rhythm. Encourage coughing and deep-breathing exercises. Elevate head of bed, as indicated.	Neuromuscular transmissions are blocked by magnesium excess, resulting in respiratory muscular weakness and hypoventilation, which may progress to apnea.
Check patellar reflexes periodically.	Absence of these reflexes suggests magnesium levels about 7 mEq/L or greater. If untreated, cardiac and respiratory arrest can occur.
Encourage increased fluid intake, if appropriate.	Increased hydration enhances magnesium excretion, but fluid intake must be cautious in event of renal or cardiac failure.
Monitor urinary output and 24-hour fluid balance.	Renal failure is the primary contributing factor in hypermagnesemia, and, if it is present, fluid excess can easily occur.
Promote bedrest; assist with personal care activities, as needed.	Flaccid paralysis, lethargy, and decreased mentation can reduce activity tolerance and ability.
Recommend avoidance of magnesium-containing antacids, such as Maalox, Mylanta, Gelusil, and Riopan, in client with renal disease. Caution clients with renal disease to avoid over-the-counter (OTC) drug use without discussing with healthcare provider.	Limits oral intake to help prevent hypermagnesemia.

ACTIONS/INTERVENTIONS (continued)	RATIONALE (continued)
Collaborative	
Assist with treatment of underlying cause.	Refer to listing of predisposing and contributing factors to determine treatment needs. *Note:* Most frequently occurs in clients with advanced renal failure.
Monitor laboratory studies, as indicated.	Evaluates therapy needs and effectiveness.
Administer IV fluids (e.g., Normal Saline, Lactated Ringer's) and thiazide diuretics, as indicated.	Intravenous fluids work by dilution of the extracellular magnesium. Fluids are used with diuretics to promote increased excretion of magnesium by the kidney (Novello, 2012).
Administer 10% calcium chloride or gluconate IV.	Antagonizes action and reverses symptoms of magnesium toxicity to improve neuromuscular function.
Assist with dialysis, as needed.	In the presence of renal disease or failure, dialysis may be needed to lower serum levels.

BIBLIOGRAPHY

CHAPTER 1

Books

American Nurses Association: Code of ethics for nurses. American Nurses Association, Silver Spring, MD, 2001.

American Nurses Association: Nursing scope and standards of practice. American Nurses Association, Silver Spring, MD, 2004.

Jacob, SR: The evolution of professional nursing. In Cheery, B, and Jacob, SR: Contemporary nursing: Issues, trends, and management, ed 6. Elsevier Mosby, St. Louis, 2014.

Lancaster L, and Stillman, D: When generations collide: Who they are. Why they clash. How to solve the generational puzzle at work. Harper Business, New York, 2002.

National Center for Health Statistics. (2007). Health, United States, 2007, with chartbook on trends in the health of Americans. National Center for Health Statistics, Hyattsville, MD, 2007.

Articles

Blegen, MA, Goode, CJ, and Reed, L: Nursing staffing and patient outcomes. Nurs Res 47(1):43–50, 1998.

Buerhaus, PJ: Is a nursing shortage on the way? Nursing98 28(8):34–35, 1998.

Buerhaus, PI, DesRoches, C, Applebaum, S, et al: Are nurses ready for health care reform? A decade of survey research. Nurs Econ 30(6):318–329, 2012.

Desimini, EM, Kennedy, JA, Helsley, MF, et al: Making the case for nurse navigators—. Benefits, outcomes, and return on investment. Oncology Issues 26(5):26–33, 2011.

Dunton, N, Gajewski, B, Taunton, RL, et al: Nurse staffing and patient falls on acute care hospital units. Nurs Outlook 52(1):53–59, 2004.

Erickson, JI, Ditomassi, M, and Adams, JM: Attending registered nurse—An innovative role to manage between the spaces. Nurse Econ 30(5):282–287, 2012.

Gabrielle, S, Jackson, D, and Mannix, J: Older women nurses: Health, ageing concerns, and self care strategies. J Adv Nurs 61(3):316–25, 2008.

Hassmiller, S: Nursing's role in healthcare reform. Am Nurs Today 5(9):68–69, 2010.

Harris, K, and Welton, JM: Guest editorial: Hospital billing and reimbursement: Charging for inpatient nursing care. J Nurs Admin 37(4):164–166, 2007.

Horner, K, Ludman, EJ, McCorkle, R, et al: An oncology nurse program designed to eliminate gaps in early cancer care. Clin J Oncol Nurs 17(1):43–48, 2013.

Keenan, G, Tschannen, D, and Wesley, M: Standardized nursing terminologies can transform practice. JONA 38(3):103–106, 2008.

Keenan, GM, Stocker, JR, Geo-Thomas, AT, et al: The HANDS project: Studying and refining the automated collection of a cross-setting clinical data set. Comp Inform Nurs 20(3):89–100, 2002.

Kohl, BA, Fortino-Mullen, M, Praestgaard, A, et al: Effect of telemedicine on mortality and length of stay in a university ICU. Crit Care Med 35(12):A22, 2007.

Kupperschmidt, BR: Addressing multigenerational conflict: Mutual respect and care fronting a strategy. Online J Issues Nurs 11(2):4, 2006.

Leape, LL, and Berwick, DM: Five years after to err is human: What have we learned? JAMA 293(19):2384–2390, 2005.

Mark, BA, Harless, D, and Berman, WF: Nurse staffing and adverse events in hospitalized children. Policy Polit Nurs Pract 8(2):83–92, 2007.

Matthews, JT: The nursebot project: Developing a personal robotic assistant for frail older adults in the community. Home Health Care Management & Practice 14(5):403–405, 2002.

Needleman, J, Buerhaus, P, Mattke, S, et al: Nurse staffing levels and the quality of care in hospitals. New Eng J Med 346(22):1715–1722, 2002.

Pineau, J, Montemerlo, M, Pollak, M, et al: Towards robotic assistants in nursing homes: Challenges and results. Rob Auton Syst 42(3–4): 271–281, 2003.

Rivera, D, and Halvorson, G: We're in it together. Modern Healthcare 38(11):22, 2008.

Rutherford, MM: Nursing is the room rate. Nurs Econ 30(4):193–199, 206, 2012.

Solovy, A, Hoppszallern, S, and Brown, S: Ten lessons from the top 100; Healthcare most wired. Hosp Health Network 81(7):40–53, 2007.

Yang, KP: Relationships between nurse staffing and client outcomes. J Nurs Res 11(3):149–158, 2003.

Electronic Resources

American Association of Colleges of Nursing (AACN), updated 2012. Nursing shortage. Retrieved July 2013 from **http://www.aacn.nche.edu/media-relations/fact-sheets/nursing-shortage**

American Nurses' Association Health Care Agenda 2005. Retrieved March 2008 from **http://nursingworld.org/MainMenuCategories/HealthcareandPolicyIssues/Reports/HealthCareAgenda.aspx**

Center for American Nurses: Restructuring and redesigning nurses' work environments, 2007 revised. Retrieved March 2008 from **http://www.centerforamericannurses.org/positions/finalworkenviron.pdf**

Economist Intelligence Unit, 2011: Preventive care and health aging: A global perspective. Retrieved June 2013 from **http://digitalresearch.eiu.com/healthyageing/country-profiles/united-states**

Health Information and Management Systems Society (HIMS) and National Committee for Quality Assurance (NCQA): Leveraging health IT to achieve ambulatory quality: The patient-centered medical home (PCMH). Retrieved June 2013 from **http://www.ncqa.org/Portals/0/Public%20Policy/HIMSS_NCQA_PCMH_Factsheet.pdf**

Healthy People 2020—U.S. Department of Health and Human Services Healthy People 2020 Framework, n.d. Retrieved June 2013 from **http://www.healthypeople.gov/2020/Consortium/HP2020Framework.pdf**

Heller, BR, Oros, MT, and Durney-Crowley, J: The future of nursing education: Ten trends to watch, 2011. Retrieved June 2013 from **http://www.nln.org/nlnjournal/infotrends.htm#2**

HHS Secretary Leavitt: 500-Day Plan for improving the health, safety, and well-being of America. Retrieved March 2008 from **www.hhs.gov/500DayPlan**

Hibbard, JH, and Cunningham: How engaged are consumers in their health and health care, and why does it matter? 2008. Research Brief No. 8. Retrieved June 2013 from **http://ualr.edu/seniorjustice/uploads/2008/12/How%20Engaged%20Are%20Consumers%20in%20Their%20Health%20and%20Health%20Care.pdf**

Institute of Medicine (IOM) report: The future of nursing: Leading change, advancing health, 2010. Retrieved June 2013 from **http://www.iom.edu/Reports/2010/The-future-of-nursing-leading-change-advancing-health.aspx**

Park, HK, Hong, HS, Kwon, HJ, et al: A nursing robot system for the elderly and the disabled. Int J of Human-friendly Welfare Robotic Systems 2(4):11–16, 2001. Retrieved April 2008 from **http://web.cecs.pdx.edu/~mperkows/Rehabilitation_Robots/nursing-robot.pdf**

Pollack, ME, Brown, L, Colbry, D, et al: Pearl: A mobile robotic assistant for the elderly, 2002. Retrieved May 2008 from **http://www.eecs.umich.edu/~pollackm/distrib/aaai02wkshp.pdf**

Restuccia, P: The aging nurse project, 2007. Retrieved June 2013 from **http://www.truthaboutnursing.org/news/2007/aug/15_boston_herald.html**

State Health Access Data Assistance Center: The coverage gap: A state-by-state report on access to care. Prepared by University of Minnesota, 2006a. Retrieved March 2008 from **http://www.sph.umn.edu/img/assets/18528/CTUW2006_TheCoverageGap.pdf**

State Health Access Data Assistance Center: Shifting ground: Changes in employer-sponsored health insurance. Prepared by University of Minnesota, 2006b. Retrieved March 2008 from **http://www.sph.umn.edu/img/assets/18528/CTUW2006_ShiftingGround.pdf**

Stokowski, LA: Nurses and the Affordable Care Act: Opportunities and options. Medscape, 2011. Retrieved June 2013 from **http://www.medscape.com/viewarticle/737413**

CHAPTER 2

Books

American Nurses Association: Nursing: Scope and standards of practice. American Nurses Association, Silver Spring, MD, 2004.

American Nurses Association: Nursing: Scope and standards of practice, ed 2. American Nurses Association, Silver Spring, MD, 2010.

American Nurses Association: Nursing's social policy statement. American Nurses Association, Kansas City, MO, 1980.

American Nurses Association: Nursing's social policy statement. American Nurses Association, Washington, DC, 1995.

American Nurses Association: Standards of clinical nursing practice. American Nurses Association, Kansas City, MO, 1991.

Bulechek, GM, Butcher, HK, Dochterman, JM, et al (eds): Nursing Interventions Classification (NIC). Elsevier, St Louis, MO, 2013.

Morehead, S, Johnson, M, Maas, ML, et al (eds): Nursing Outcomes Classification (NOC) Measurement of Health Outcomes. Elsevier, St Louis, MO, 2013.

NANDA-I: Nursing diagnoses: Definitions and classification. NANDA International, Philadelphia, 2007.

Pesut, DJ, and Herman, J: Clinical reasoning, the art and science of critical and creative thinking. Delmar, Albany, NY, 1999.

Shore, LS: Nursing diagnosis: What it is and how to do it: A programmed text. Medical College of Virginia Hospitals, Redmond, VA, 1988.

Articles

Aquilino, ML, and Keenan, G: Having our say: Nursing's standardized nomenclature. Am J Nurs 100(7):33–38, 2000.

Delaney, C, and Maas, M: Reliability of nursing diagnoses documented in a computerized nursing information system. Nurs Diagn 11(3): 121–134, 2000.

CHAPTER 3

Books

Newfield, SA, Hinz, MD, Tilley, DS, et al: Cox's clinical applications of nursing diagnosis. FA Davis, Philadelphia, 2007.

Pesut, DJ, and Herman, J: Clinical reasoning, the art and science of critical and creative thinking. Delmar, Albany, NY, 1999.

Articles

Hickman, JS: A critical assessment of critical thinking in nursing education. Holistic Nurse Practitioner 7(3):36–47, 1993.

Electronic Resources

Paul, R, and Elder, L: The miniature guide to critical thinking concepts and tools. Foundation for Critical Thinking Press, 2008. Retrieved May 2013 from **http://www.criticalthinking.org/pages/defining-critical-thinking/766**

Scriven, M, and Paul, R: Critical thinking as defined by the National Council for Excellence in Critical Thinking. Presented at the 8th Annual International Conference on Critical Thinking and Education Reform, Summer 1987. Retrieved February 2009 from **http://www.criticalthinking.org/aboutCT/define_critical_thinking.cfm**

CHAPTER 4

Books

Deglin, JH, and Vallerand, AH: Davis's drug guide for nurses, ed 13. FA Davis, Philadelphia, 2010.

LeFever Kee, J: Laboratory and diagnostic tests with nursing implications, ed 8. Pearson Prentice Hall, Upper Saddle River, NJ, 2009.

McCance, KL, and Heuther, SE: Pathophysiology: The biologic basis for disease in adults and children, ed 6. Elsevier, New York, 2009.

Smeltzer, S, Bare, BG, Hinkle, JL, et al: Brunner and Suddarth's textbook of medical-surgical nursing, ed 11. Lippincott, Williams & Wilkins, Philadelphia, 2010.

Van Leeuwen, AM, Poelhuis-Leth, D, and Bladh, M: Davis's comprehensive handbook of laboratory and diagnostic tests with nursing implications, ed 5. FA Davis, Philadelphia, 2013.

Williams, SE: Chapter 4: The fourth heart sound. In Walker HK, Hall WD, and Hurst, JW (eds). Clinical methods: The history, physical, and laboratory examinations, ed 3. Boston, Butterworths, 1990.

Wilson, BA, Shannon, MT, Shields, KM, et al: Prentice Hall nurse's drug guide 2009. Pearson Prentice Hall, Upper Saddle River, NJ, 2009.

Articles

Aldrich, D, and Hunt, DP: When can the patient with deep venous thrombosis begin to ambulate? Phys Ther 84(3):268–273, 2004.

Antman, EM, Cohen, M, Bernink, PJ, et al: The TIMI risk score for unstable angina/non-ST elevation MI: A method for prognostication and therapeutic decision making. JAMA 284(7):835–842, 2000.

Balser, JR: Managing arrhythmias after cardiac surgery. AACN News 17(2):10–11, 2000.

Barron, HV, Every, NR, Parsons, LS, et al: The use of intra-aortic balloon counterpulsation in patients with cardiogenic shock complicating acute myocardial infarction: Data from the National Registry of Myocardial Infarction 2. Am Heart J 141(9):933–939, 2001.

Berger, R, et al: B-type natriuretic peptide predicts sudden death in clients with chronic heart failure. Circulation (105):2328–2331, 2002.

Bocchi, EA: Cardiomyoplasty for treatment of heart failure. Eur J Heart Fail 3(4):403–406, 2001.

Bond, EA, et al: The left ventricular assist device. Am J Nurs 103(1): 33–41, 2003.

Braun, LT: Cardiovascular disease: Strategies for risk assessment and modification. J Cardiovas Nurs 21(6)(suppl):S20–S42, 2006.

Braun, LT, and Davidson, MH: Cholesterol-lowering drugs bring benefits to high-risk populations even when LDL is normal. J Cardiovas Nurs 18(1):44–49, 2003.

Cheek, D, and Cesan, A: What's different about heart disease in women? Nursing(8):36–42, 2003.

Cheek, DJ, Grauity, R, Hawkins, J, et al: Oral heart failure medications: An update for home health clinicians. Home Healthcare Nurse 26(10):600–611, 2008.

Chobanian, AV, Bakris, GL, Black, HR, et al: Seventh report of Joint National Committee (JNC) on detection, evaluation, and treatment of high blood pressure. Hypertension 42(6):1206–1252, 2003.

Colwell, CW, and Hardwick, ME: Natural history of venous thromboembolism. Tech Orthop 19:236–239, 2004.

Coughlin, RM: Recognizing ventricular arrhythmias and preventing sudden cardiac death: Be prepared to stop these dangerous arrhythmias. Am Nurse Today 2(5):38–43, 2007.

Coviello, JS, and Nystrom, KV: Obesity and heart failure. J Cardiovasc Nurs 18(5):360–368, 2003.

Craft, J: Eplerenone (Inspra), a new aldosterone antagonist for the treatment of systemic hypertension and heart failure. Proc (Bayl Univ Med Cent) 17(2):217–220, 2004.

Crowther, M, and McCourt, K: Get the edge on deep vein thrombosis. Nurs Manage 35(1):21–29, 2004.

Crowther, M, and McCourt, K: Venous thromboembolism: A guide to prevention and treatment. Nurse Pract 30(8):26–43, 2005.

Cucinelli, C: Minimally invasive coronary artery bypass surgery. Crit Care Nurse 23(1):54, 2000.

Cunningham, C: Managing hospitalized client with heart failure: What you need to know about the new practice guidelines for evaluation, care, and treatment of heart failure clients in the hospital. Am Nurse Today 1(1):44–50, 2006.

Curtis, A: Prophylactic defibrillators for the prevention of sudden cardiac death: The SCD-HeFT Trial. American College of Cardiology Presentation. March 7–10, New Orleans, LA, 2004.

Daly, J, Elliot, D, Cameron-Traub, E, et al: Health status, perceptions of coping and social support immediately after discharge of survivors of acute myocardial infarct. Am J Crit Care 9(1):62–69, 2000.

Day, MW: Recognizing and managing deep vein thrombosis. Nursing 33(5):36–41, 2003.

Dechant, LM: UA/NSTEMI: Are you following the latest guidelines? Nursing 42(9):26–33, 2012.

De Jong, MJ, and Morton, PG: Predictors of atrial dysrhythmias for patients undergoing coronary artery bypass grafting. Am J Crit Care 9(6):388–396, 2000.

Elmer, PJ, Obarzanek, E, Vollmer, WM, et al: Effects of comprehensive lifestyle modification on diet, weight, physical fitness, and blood pressure control: 18-month results of a randomized trial. Ann Intern Med 144(7):485–495, 2006.

Fareed, M, Suri, K, and Qureshi, AI: Prehypertension as a risk factor for cardiovascular diseases. J Cardiovasc Nurs 21(6):478–482, 2006.

Fihn, SD, Gardin, JM, Abrams, J, et al: ACCF/AHA/ACP/AATS/PCNA/SCAI/STS guideline for the diagnosis and management of patients with stable ischemic heart disease. J Am Coll Cardiol 60(24):e44–4164, 2012.

Franks, MJ, and Lawson, L: Body surface mapping improves diagnosis of acute myocardial infarction in the emergency department. Adv Emerg Nurs J 34(1):32–40, 2012.

Fredericks, S, Beanlands, H, Spalding, K, et al: A systematic review. Eur J Cardiovasc Nurs 9(1):30–37, 2010.

Freeman, JJ, and Hedges, C: Cardiac arrest: The effect on the brain. Am J Nurs 103(6):51–55, 2003.

Fuster, V, Ryden, LE, Cannom, DS, et al: ACC/AHA/ESC 2006. Guidelines for the management of patients with atrial fibrillation. Circ 114:e257–e354, 2006.

Futterman, LG, and Lemberg, L: Update on management of acute myocardial infarction: Facilitated percutaneous coronary intervention. Am J Crit Care 9(1):70–76, 2000.

Glassman AH: Depression and cardiovascular comorbidity. Dialogues Clin Neurosci 9(1):9–17, 2007.

Go, AS, Mozaffarian, D, Roger, VL, et al: Heart disease and stroke statistics—2013 update: A report from the American Heart Association. Circ 127:e6–3245, 2013.

Gylys, K, and Gold, M: Acute coronary syndromes—New developments in pharmacological treatment strategies. Crit Care Nurse April (suppl):3–14, 2000.

Hagan, K: LVDAs help mend a broken heart. Nurse Pract 35(6):28–36, 2010.

Heart Failure Society of America: Evaluation of clients for ventricular dysfunction and heart failure. J Card Fail 12(1):e16–e25, 2006.

Heart Failure Society of America. Executive summary: HFSA 2010 comprehensive heart failure practice guideline. J Card Fail 16(6):475–539, 2010.

Heidenreich, PA, Gubins, MA, Fonarow, GC, et al: Cost effectiveness of screening with B-type natriuretic peptide to identify patients with reduced left ventricular ejection fraction. J Am Coll Cardiol 17 43(6):1019–1026, 2004.

Heidenrich, PA, et al: AHA policy statement: Forecasting the future of cardiovascular disease in the United States. Circulation 123(8):933–944, 2011.

Hill, MN, Han, HR, Dennison, CR, et al: Hypertension care and control in underserved urban African American men: Behavioral and physiologic outcomes at 36 months. Am J Hypertens 16:906–913, 2003.

Hu, A, Chow, M, Dao, D, et al: Factors influencing patient knowledge of warfarin therapy after mechanical heart valve replacement. J Cardiovasc Nurs 21(3):169–175, 2006.

Jaffer, AK: An overview of venous thromboembolism: Impact, risk and issues in prophylaxis. Cleve Clin J Med 75(3):S3–S6, 2008.

Jessup, M, Abraham, WT, Casey, DE, et al: 2009 focused update: ACCF/AHA guidelines for the diagnosis and management of heart failure in adults: A report of the American College of Cardiology Foundation/American Heart Association Task Force on Practice Guidelines: Developed in collaboration with the International Society for Heart and Lung Transplantation. Circ 119:1977–2066, 2009.

Jiang, H, Lui, Y, Zhang, Y, et al: Association of plasma brain-derived neurotrophic factor and cardiovascular risk factors and prognosis in angina pectoris. Biochem Biophys Res Commun 415(1):99–103, 2011.

Kahn, K, and Jones, M: Ranolazine in the management of chronic stable angina. Br J Cardiol 18(4):179, 2011.

Kanbay, M, Turgut, F, Karakurt, F, et al: Relation between serum thyroid hormone and "nondipper" circadian blood pressure variability. Kidney Blood Press Res 30(6):416–420, 2007.

Kark, VA: The future of minimally invasive cardiac surgery. OR Nurse 2(1):25–30, 2008.

Katritsis, DG, Siontis, GC, Kastrati, A, et al: Optimal timing of coronary angiography and potential intervention in non-ST-elevation acute coronary syndromes. Eur Heart J 32(1):32–40, 2011.

Kearney, K: Digitalis toxicity. Am J Nurs 100(6):51–52, 2000.

Kehl-Pruett, W: Deep vein thrombosis in hospitalized patients: A review of evidence-based guidelines for prevention. Dimens Crit Care Nurs 25(2):53–59, 2006.

Keib, CN: Mediastinitis following coronary artery bypass graft surgery: Pathogenesis, clinical presentation, risks, and management. J Cardiovasc Nurs 21(6):493–499, 2006.

Kern, LS: Postoperative atrial fibrillation: New directions in prevention and treatment. J Cardiovasc Nurs 19:103–115, 2004.

Khan, NA, McAlister, FA, Campbell, NR, et al: The Canadian recommendations for management of hypertension. Can J Cardiol 20(1):41–54, 2004.

Kocial, NA, Horton, JR, Fonarow, GC, et al: Admission, discharge, or change in B-type natriuretic peptide and long-term outcomes: Data from Organized Program to Initiate Lifesaving Treatment in Hospitalized Patients with Heart Failure (OPTIMIZE-HF) linked to Medicare claims. Circ Heart Fail 4(5):628–636, 2011.

Kumar, A, and Cannon, CP: Acute coronary syndromes: Diagnosis and management, part 1. Mayo Clin Proc 84(10):917–938, 2009.

Marchigiano, G, Riendeau, D, and Morse, CJ: New technology applications: Thrombolysis of acute deep vein thrombosis. Crit Care Nurs Quart 29(4):312–323, 2006.

Matros, E, Aranki, SF, Bayer, LR, et al: Reduction in incidence of deep sternal wound infections: Random or real? J Thorac Caridovasc Surg 139(3):680–685, 2010.

McKhann, GM, Grega, MA, Borowicz, LM, et al: Stroke and encephalopathy after cardiac surgery: An update. Stroke 37:562–571, 2006.

McSweeney, JC, Cody, M, O'Sullivan, P, et al: Women's early warning symptoms of acute myocardial infarction. Circ 108(21):2619–2623, 2003.

Miller, DD, and Shaw, LJ: Coronary artery disease: Diagnostic and prognostic models for reducing patient risk. J Cardiovas Nurs 21(6) (suppl):S2–S16, 2006.

Mosca, L, Benjamin, EJ, Berra, K, et al: Effectiveness-based guidelines for the prevention of cardiovascular disease in women—2011 update: A guideline from the American Heart Association. Circ 123(11):1243–1262, 2011.

Morbidity & Mortality Weekly Report. Centers for Disease Control and Prevention (CDC): Vital signs: Prevalence, treatment, and control of hypertension. United States, 1999–2002 and 2005–2008. MMWR 60(4):103–108, 2011.

Oler A, Whooley MA, Oler J, et al: Adding heparin to aspirin reduces the incidence of myocardial infarction and death in patients with unstable angina. A meta-analysis. JAMA 276(10):811–815, 1996.

Overbaugh, KJ: Acute coronary syndrome. Am J Nurs 109(5):42–52, 2009.

Owens, SG: Nursing management of arrhythmias after cardiac surgery. AACN News 17(2):11–12, 2000.

Pahan, K: Lipid-lowering drugs. Cell Mol Life Sci 63(10): 1165–78, 2006.

Pantilat, SZ, and Steimle, AE: Palliative care for clients with heart failure. JAMA 291:2476–2482, 2004.

Pilote, L, Dasgupta, K, Guru, V, et al: A comprehensive view of sex-specific issues related to cardiovascular disease. CMAJ 176(6): S1–S44, 2007.

Ridker, PM: Clinical application of C-reactive protein for cardiovascular disease detection and prevention. Circ 107:363–369, 2003.

Roger, VL, Go, AS, Lloyd-Jones, DM. et al: Heart disease and stroke statistics—2012 update: A report from the American Heart Association. Circ 125(1):e2–220, 2012.

Saab, R, Stevermer, JL, and Meadows, S: Should patients with acute DVT limit activity? J Fam Pract 59(1):50–52, 2010.

Sakallaris, BR, Halpin, LS, Knapp, M, et al: Same-day transfer of patients to the cardiac telemetry unit after surgery: The rapid after bypass back into telemetry (RABBIT) program. Crit Care Nurse 20(2):50–68, 2000.

Sesso, HD, Buring, JE, Rifai, N, et al: C-reactive protein and the risk of developing hypertension. JAMA 290:2945–2951, 2003.

Siomko, AX: Demystifying cardiac markers. Am J Nurs 100(1):36, 2000.

Skolnik, NS, Beck, JD, and Clark, M: Combination antihypertensive drugs: Recommendations for use. Am Fam Physician 61(10):3049–3056.

Smith, SC, Allen J, Blair, SN, et al: AHA/ACC guidelines for secondary prevention for patients with coronary and other atherosclerotic vascular disease: 2006 update. Circ 113:2363–2372, 2006.

Smith, TW, Butler, VP, Haber, E, et al: Treatment of life-threatening digitalis intoxication with digoxin-specific Fab antibody fragments: Experience in 26 cases. N Engl J Med 307(22):1357–1362, 1982.

Snow, V, Barry, P, Fihn, SD, et al: Evaluation of primary care patients with chronic stable angina: Guidelines from the American College of Physicians. Ann Intern Med 141:57–64, 2004.

Sorensen, ER, Lorme, TB, and Heath, D: Improve cardiac outcomes with TEG. Nurs 2008 Crit Care 1(2):18–24, 2006.

Steinke, EE: Sexual counseling after myocardial infarction. Am J Nurs 100(12):38–43, 2000.

Stockman, J: In too deep: Understanding deep vein thrombosis. Nursing Made Incredibly Easy! 6(2):29–38, 2008.

Suter, PM, Gorski, LA, Hennessey, B, et al: Best practices for heart failure: A focused review. Home Healthc Nurse 30(7):394–405, 2012.

Thadani, U, and Opie, LH: Nitrates for unstable angina. Cardiovasc Drugs Ther Oct 1994;8(5):719–726.

Tomaselli, GF, and Zipes, DG: What causes sudden death in heart failure? Circ Res 95(8):764–763, 2004.

Walke, LM, Gallo, WT, Tinetti, ME, et al: The burden of symptoms among community-dwelling older persons with advanced chronic disease. Arch Int Med 164(21):2321–2324, 2004.

Weitz, JI: Management of venous thromboembolism: Present and future. Circ 31;110(9 Suppl 1):I2, 2004.

Whitman, GR: Nursing-sensitive outcomes in cardiac surgery patients. J Cardiovasc Nurs 19(5):293–298, 2004.

Wingate, S: Caring for persons with advanced heart failure. Home Healthc Nurse 25(8):511–520, 2007.

Woods, A, and Moshang, J: Lowering risks of diabetes, hypertension, and heart disease. Holist Nurs Pract 20(1):5–9, 2006.

Yee, CA: Atrial fibrillation: The ruthless irregular rhythm. Nurs 2008 Crit Care 1(5):30–37, 2006.

Yutsis, P: High blood pressure: Prescription drugs causing more problems than they solve? J Longev 6(1):21, 2000.

Electronic Resources

Abrams, J, and Block, PC: New agent for for chronic angina pectoris, 2007. Retrieved February 2013 from **http://www.medscape.com/viewarticle/553395**

American Heart Association (AHA): Common tests for arrhythmia, 2012. Retrieved February 2013 from **http://www.heart.org/HEARTORG/Conditions/Arrhythmia/SymptomsDiagnosisMonitoringofArrhythmia/Common-Tests-for-Arrhythmia_UCM_301988_Article.jsp**

American Heart Association: What your cholesterol levels mean. Retrieved February 2013 from **http://www.heart.org/HEARTORG/Conditions/Cholesterol/AboutCholesterol/What-Your-Cholesterol-Levels-Mean_UCM_305562_Article.jsp**

Ballard, DJ: Applying appropriateness methods to address overuse while ensuring the delivery of appropriate care: The example of cardiac revascularization. Prescriptions for Excellence in Health Care Spring 2010(8):1–3. Retrieved March 2013 from **http://jdc.jefferson.edu/cgi/viewcontent.cgi?article=1069&context=pehc**

Centers for Disease Control and Prevention (CDC): Heart failure fact sheet, 2012. Retrieved February 2013 from **http://www.cdc.gov/dhdsp/data_statistics/fact_sheets/fs_heart_failure.htm**

Coven, DL, Kalyanasundaram, A, and Shirani, J: Acute coronary syndrome, 2013. Retrieved February 2013 from **http://emedicine.medscape.com/article/1910735-overview**

Fogoros, RN: Beta blockers for angina, 2011. Retrieved February 2013 from **http://heartdisease.about.com/od/coronaryarterydisease/a/betablockers.htm**

Fogoros, RN: Compression ultrasound, 2012. Retrieved February 2012 from **http://heartdisease.about.com/od/lesscommonheartproblems/g/Compression-Ultrasound.htm**

Fogoros, RN: Unstable angina, 2011. Retrieved February 2013 from **http://heartdisease.about.com/cs/coronarydisease/a/unstableangina.htm**

Go, AS, Mozaffarian D, Roger VL, et al: Heart disease and stroke statistics—2013 update: A report from the American Heart Association. Circ 127: e6–e245, 2012. Retrieved March 2013 from **http://circ.ahajournals.org/content/123/8/933.long**

Kaiser, C: DVT/PE treatment enters a new era. MedPage Today, 2013. Retrieved February 2013 from **http://www.medpagetoday.com/Cardiology/VenousThrombosis/36835**

Kochanek, KD, Xu, J, Murphy, SL, et al: Deaths: Final data for 2009. National Vital Statistics Reports 60(3): Dec 29, 2011. Retrieved February 2013 from **http://www.cdc.gov/nchs/data/nvsr/nvsr60/nvsr60_03.pdf**

Lab Tests Online staff: Cardiac biomarkers, 2012. Retrieved February 2013 from **http://labtestsonline.org/understanding/analytes/cardiac-biomarkers/tab/glance**

Lytle, B, and Pettersson, G: Arterial coronary artery bypass grafts, 2013. Retrieved February 2013 from **http://my.clevelandclinic.org/heart/disorders/cad/lytle_arterialcabg.aspx#**

Mayo Clinic Staff: Acute coronary syndrome: Risk factors, 2010. Retrieved February 2013 from **http://www.mayoclinic.com/health/acute-coronary-syndrome/DS01061/DSECTION=risk-factors**

Mayo Clinic Staff: Heart arrhythmias, 2011. Retrieved February 2013 from **http://www.mayoclinic.com/health/heart-arrhythmias/DS00290/DSECTION=risk-factors**

Medline Plus: Prasurge, 2009. Retrieved February 2013 from **http://www.nlm.nih.gov/medlineplus/druginfo/meds/a609027.html**

National Heart, Lung and Blood Institute (NHLBI): 2011 Factbook 4. Disease statistics. Retrieved February 2013 from **http://www.nhlbi.nih.gov/about/factbook/chapter4.htm**

National Heart, Lung, and Blood Institute (NHLB): Factbook fiscal year 2012, #4. Disease statistics. Retrieved March 2013 from **http://www.nhlbi.nih.gov/about/factbook/chapter4.htm**

National Heart, Lung, and Blood Institute (NHLB): What is long QT syndrome, various pages, 2011. Retrieved February 2013 from **http://www.nhlbi.nih.gov/health/health-topics/topics/qt/**

National Heart, Lung and Blood Institute: NHLBI issues new high blood pressure clinical practice guidelines. Article for U.S. Department of Health and Human Services National Institutes of Health (NIH) News website, 2003. Retrieved February 2013 from **http://www.nih.gov/news/pr/may2003/nhlbi-14.htm**

No author listed. High blood pressure drugs and erectile dysfunction. Retrieved February 2013 from **http://www.webmd.com/erectile-dysfunction/medicine-ed**

Pai, M, and Douketis, JD: Patient information: Deep vein thrombosis (DVT) (Beyond the basics), 2013. Retrieved February 2013 from **http://www.uptodate.com/contents/deep-vein-thrombosis-dvt-beyond-the-basics?view=print**

Patel, K, and Chun, LJ: Deep vein thrombosis, 2013. Retrieved February 2013 from **http://emedicine.medscape.com/article/1911303-overview**

Patel, V, and James, PA: Digitalis toxicity, 2011. Retrieved February 2013 from **http://emedicine.medscape.com/article/154336-overview#a0156**

Pfunter, A, Levit, K, and Elixhauser, A: Healthcare Cost and Utilization Project (H_CUP); Statistical brief #133 Components of cost increases for inpatient hospital procedures, 1997–2009, 2012. Retrieved April 2012 from **http://www.hcup-us.ahrq.gov/reports/statbriefs/sb133.pdf**

Rasavong, C: Reliability and validity for Homan's sign for the detection of deep vein thrombosis, 2009. Retrieved February 2013 from **http://www.cyberpt.com/homansign.asp**

Reynolds, MW, et al: A systematic review of the economic burden of chronic angina. AJMC.com, 2004. Retrieved March 2013 from **http://www.ajmc.com/publications/supplement/2004/2004-10-vol10-n11suppl/oct04-1920ps347-s357/1**

Siskin, GP, and Kyung, JC: Inferior vena cava filters, 2011. Retrieved February 2013 from **http://emedicine.medscape.com/article/419796-overview#showall**

Stranges, E, Kowlessar, N, and Elixhauser, A: Components of growth in inpatient hospital costs, 1997–2009, 2011. Retrieved March, 2013 from **http://www.hcup-us.ahrq.gov/reports/statbriefs/sb123.jsp**

Vaughn's Summaries: Human heart drugs summary, 2012. Retrieved February 2013 from **http://www.vaughns-1-pagers.com/medicine/prescription-heart-drugs.htm#topofpage**

Vidt, DG: Thyroid dysfunction and hypertension: What's the connection? The Cleveland Clinic Disease Management Project, 2004. Retrieved February 2013 from **http://www.consultantlive.com/display/article/10162/45704**

Wedro, BC: Heart rhythm disorders, 2013. Retrieved February 2013 from **http://www.medicinenet.com/heart_rhythm_disorders/article.htm**

Zafari, AM, Reddy, SV, Jeroudi, AM, et al: Myocardial Infarction, 2013. Retrieved February 2013 from **http://emedicine.medscape.com/article/155919-overview**

CHAPTER 5

Books

Blair, KA: The aging pulmonary system. In Stanley, M, Blair, KA, and Beare, PG (eds): Gerontological nursing: Promoting successful aging with older adults, ed 3. FA Davis, Philadelphia, 2005.

Centers for Disease Control and Prevention. National Center for Health Statistics. National Hospital Discharge Survey, 1979–2006. 2006 Unpublished Data.

Clochesy, JM: Interventions for critically ill clients with respiratory problems. In Ignatavicius, DD, and Workman, ML (eds): Medical-surgical nursing: Critical thinking for collaborative care, ed 5. Elsevier Saunders, St. Louis, MO, 2006.

Daniels, R, and Nicoll, L: Contemporary medical-surgical nursing, ed 2. Delmar Cengage Learning, Clifton Park, NY, 2012.

DeConti, RC: Carcinomas of the head and neck. In Skeel, RT (ed): Handbook of cancer chemotherapy, ed 6. Lippincott, Williams & Wilkins, Philadelphia, 2003.

Deglin, JH, and Vallerand, AH: Davis's drug guide for nurses, ed 13. FA Davis, Philadelphia, 2010.

Felver, L: Acid-base homeiostasis and imbalances. In Copstead, LEC, and Banasik, JL (eds): Pathophysiology, ed 3. Elsevier Saunders, St. Louis, MO, 2005.

Ferki, SD: Pediatric care plans: Asthma. In Swearingen, PL (ed): All-in-one care planning resource, ed 3. Elsevier/Mosby, St Louis, MO, 2012.

Fink, JG, and Hess, DR: Secretion clearance techniques. In Hess, DR, et al (eds): Respiratory care: Principles and practices. Saunders, Philadelphia, 2002.

Ginsberg, RJ, Vokes, EE, and Rosenzweig, K: Non–small cell lung cancer. In DeVita, VT, Hellman, S, and Rosenberg, SA (eds): Cancer principles and practice of oncology, ed 6. Lippincott-Raven, Philadelphia, 2001.

Hoang, T, and Schiller, J: Carcinoma of the lung. In Skee, R (ed): Handbook of cancer chemotherapy, ed 6. Lippincott, Williams & Wilkins, Philadelphia, 2003.

Kee, JL, Paulanka, BJ, and Polek, C: Handbook of fluid, electrolyte, and acid-base imbalances, ed 3. Delmar, Clifton Park, NY, 2010.

Metheny, N: Fluid and electrolyte balance: Nursing considerations, ed 5. Jones & Bartlett, Sudbury, MA, 2010.

Morton, P, and Fontaine, DK. Critical care nursing: A holistic approach, ed 9. Wolters Kluwer; Lippincott, Williams, & Wilkins, Philadelphia, 2008.

Pagana, KD, and Pagana, TJ: Mosby's manual of diagnostic and laboratory tests, ed 3. Mosby, St. Louis, MO, 2006.

Schumann, L: Respiratory function and alterations in gas exchange. In Copstead, LEC, and Banasik, JL (eds): Pathophysiology, ed 3. Elsevier Saunders, St. Louis, MO, 2005.

Springhouse, PA (ed): Pathophysiology made incredibly easy!, ed 3. Lippincott, Williams & Wilkins, Philadelphia, 2006.

Workman, ML: Interventions for clients with electrolyte imbalances. In Ignatavicius, DD, and Workman, ML (eds): Medical-surgical nursing: Critical thinking for collaborative care, ed. 5. Elsevier Saunders, St. Louis, MO, 2006.

Articles

Astle, SM: Restoring electrolyte balance. RN 68(5):31–34, 2005.

Bale, E, and Berrecloth, R: The obese patient. Anaesthetic issues: Airway and positioning. J Periop Pract 8:294–299, 2010.

Banning, M: Chronic obstructive pulmonary disease: Clinical signs and infections. Br J Nurs 15(16):874–880, 2006.

Bauldoff, GS, and Diaz, PT: Improving outcomes for COPD patients. Am J Primary Care 31(8):26–43, 2006.

Baumann, M, and Noppen, M: Pneumothorax. Respirology 9:157–164, 2004.

Bausewein, C, Farquhar, M, Booth, S, et al: Measurement of breathlessness in advanced disease: A systematic review. Resp Med 101(3): 399–410, 2007.

Beltzan, MA, Scott, AS, Wolkvone, N, et al: Fatigue in COPD: Prevalence and effect on outcomes in pulmonary rehabilitation. Chron Respir Dis 8(12):119–128, 2011.

Benninger, M, and Segreti, J: Is it bacterial or viral? Criteria for distinguishing bacterial and viral infections. Suppl J Fam Prac 3:S5–S11, 2008.

Boyle, AH, and Locke, DC: Update on chronic obstructive pulmonary disease. Medsurg Nurs 13(1):42–48, 2004.

Braman, SS: Asthma and chronic obstructive pulmonary disease in later life. Generations Fall:33–38, 2006.

Brar, NK, and Niederman, MS: Management of community-acquired pneumonia. Ther Adv Resp Dis 5(1):61–78, 2011.

Burman, ME, and Wright, WL: Diagnosis and management of community-acquired pneumonia: Evidence-based practice. J Nurse Pract 10:633–649, 2007.

Burns, SM: Mechanical ventilation of patients with acute respiratory distress syndrome and patents requiring weaning: The evidence guiding practice. Crit Care Nurse 25(4):14–24, 2005.

Burns, SM, Fisher, C, and Tribble, SSE: Multifactor clinical score and outcome of mechanical ventilation weaning trials: Burns Wean Assessment Program. Am J Crit Care 19:431–439, 2010.

Byers, JF, and Sole, ML: Analysis of factors related to the development of ventilator-associated pneumonia: Use of existing databases. Am J Crit Care 9(5):344–349, 2000.

Celli, B, Decramer, M, Leimer, I, et al: Cardiovascular safety of tiotropium in patients with COPD. Chest 137 (1):20–30, 2010.

Centers for Disease Control and Prevention: Guidelines for the investigation of contacts of persons with infectious tuberculosis and guidelines for using the QuantiFERON®-TB Gold test for detecting *Mycobacterium tuberculosis* infection, United States. MMWR 54:RR-15, 2005.

Coleman, PR: Pneumonia in the long-term care setting: Etiology, management, and prevention. J Gerontol Nurs 4:14–23, 2004.

Coughlin, AM, and Parchinsky, C: Go with the flow of chest tube therapy. Nursing 36(3):36–41, 2006.

Corbridge, S, Wilken, L, Kapella, MC, et al: An evidenced-based approach to COPD, Part 1. Am J Nurs 112(3):46–57, 2012.

Covey, ML, and Larson, JL: Beats and breaths: Exercise and COPD. Am J Nurs 104(5):40–43, 2004.

Cox, CE, and Carson, SS: Medical and economic implications of prolonged mechanical ventilation and expedited post-acute care. Semin Respir Crit Care Med 33(4):357–366, 2012.

Cross, S: Managing exacerbations of chronic obstructive pulmonary disease. Br J Nurs 14(11):607–609, 2005.

D'Arcy, Y: Eye on capnography. Men in Nursing 2(2):25–29, 2007.

Dasta, JF, McLaughlin, TP, Mody, SH, et al: Daily cost of an intensive care unit day: The contribution of mechanical ventilation. Crit Care Med 33(6):1266–1271, 2005.

Davis, J, and Finley, J: The breadth of hospital-acquired pneumonia: Nonventilated versus ventilated patients in Pennsylvania. PA Patient Safety Advisory, Sept 9(3):99–105, 2012.

DeVito, DA, Hoffman, LA, Iacono, AT, et al: Pattern and predictors of early rejection after lung transplantation. Am J Crit Care 12:497–507, 2003.

Diacon, AH, Pym, A, Grobusch, M, et al: The diarylquinoline TMC207 for multidrug-resistant tuberculosis. N Engl J Med 360:2397–2405, 2009.

Diehl-Oplinger, L, and Kaminski, MF: Flash pulmonary edema. Nursing 32(7):96, 2002.

Dosanjh, D: Improved diagnostic evaluation of suspected tuberculosis. Ann Intern Med 148(5):325–336, 2008.

Douglas, SL, and Daly, BJ: Caregivers of long-term ventilator patients: Physical and psychological outcomes. Chest 123:1073–1081, 2003.

Eisner, MD, Anthonisen N, Coultas D, et al: An official American Thoracic Society Public Policy Statement: Novel risk factors and the global burden of chronic obstructive pulmonary disease. Am J Respir Crit Care Med 1882(5):693–718, 2010.

Epstein, CD, and Peerless, JR: Weaning readiness and fluid balance in older critically ill surgical patients. Am J Crit Care 15(1):54–64, 2006.

Fahlman, MM, Morgan, AL, McNevin, N, et al: Salivary s-IgA response to training in functionally limited elders. J Aging Phys Act 11:502–515, 2003.

Fay, S, and Narayan, MC: Diagnosis: Tuberculosis. Home Healthc Nurse 24(4):236–246, 2006.

Forastiere, A, Koch, W, Trotti, A, et al: Head and neck cancer. N Engl J Med 345:1890–1900, 2001.

Forey, BA, Thorton, AD, and Lee, PN: Systematic review with meta-analysis of the epidemiological evidence relating smoking to COPD, chronic bronchitis and emphysema. BMC Pulm Med 11:36, 2011.

Funk, GC, Anders, S, and Breyer, MK: Incidence and outcome of weaning from mechanical ventilation according to new categories. Eur Respir J 35:88–94, 2010.

Genuit, T, Bochicchio, G, Napolitano, LM, et al: Prophylactic chlorhexidine oral rinse decreases ventilator associated pneumonia in surgical ICU patients. Surg Infect (Larchmt) 2:5–18, 2001.

Girard, TD, and Bernard, GR: Mechanical ventilation in ARDS. Chest 131:921–929, 2007.

Goldrick, BA, and Goetz, AM: "'Tis the season" for influenza. Nurse Pract 31(12):24–33, 2006.

Gronkiewicz, C, and Brokgren-Okonek, M: Acute exacerbation of COPD. Nursing application of evidence-based guidelines. Crit Care Nurs Q 27(4):336–352, 2004.

Hashibe, M, Boffetta, P, Zaridze, D, et al: Evidence for an important role of alcohol- and aldehyde-metabolizing genes in cancers of the upper aerodigestive tract. Cancer Epidemiol Biomarkers and Prev 15(4): 696–703, 2006.

Hogg, JR, Caccavale, M, Gillen, B, et al: Tube thoracostomy: A review for the interventional radiologist. Semin Intervent Radiol 28(1):39–47, 2011.

Irwin, RS: Introduction to the diagnosis and management of cough: ACCP evidence-based clinical practice guidelines. Chest 29(1 Suppl):255–275, 2006.

Johnson, DB: Follow-up recommendations for chest CT scan reports of incidental pulmonary nodules. Chest 141(1):280–281, 2012.

Kollef, MH, Hamilton, CW, and Ernst, FR: Economic impact of ventilator-associated pneumonia in a large matched cohort. Infect Control Hosp Epidemiol Mar, 33(3):250–256, 2012.

Lorente, L, Lecuona, M, Jimenez, A, et al: Ventilator-associated pneumonia using a heated humidifier or a heat and moisture exchanger: A randomized controlled trial. Crit Care 10:4, 2006.

Lutfiyya, MN, Henley, E, Chang, LF, et al: Diagnosis and treatment of community-acquired pneumonia. Am Fam Physician 73:442–450, 2006.

Mackay, AJ, Donaldson, GC, Patel, AR, et al: Usefulness of the COPD Assessment Test(tm) (CAT) to evaluate severity of COPD exacerbations. Am J Respir Crit Care Med 185(11):1218–1222, 2012.

Mariotto, AB, Yabroff, KR, Shao, Y, et al: Projections of the cost of cancer care in the U.S.: 2010–2020. J Natl Cancer Inst 103(2): 117–128, 2011.

McCool, FD, and Rosen, MJ: Nonpharmacologic airway clearance therapies. Chest 129(1Suppl):250S–259S, 2006.

McEnroe-Ayers, DM, and Lappin, JS: Act fast when your patient has dyspnea. Nursing 34(7):36–41, 2004.

McLean, SE, Jensen, LA, Schroeder, DG, et al: Improving adherence to a mechanical ventilation weaning protocol for critically ill adults: Outcomes after an implementation program. Am J Crit Care 15(3):299–309, 2006.

Muller, AC, and Bell, AE: Diagnostic update: Electrolyte update: Potassium, chloride and magnesium. Nurs Crit Care 3(1):5–7, 2008.

Munro, C, and Grap, MJ: Oral health and care in the intensive care unit: State of science. Am J Crit Care 13(1):25–33, 2004.

Murphy, KR, Cecil, B, and Sarver, NL: Asthma: Helping patients breathe easier. Nurse Pract 29(10):38–55, 2004.

Myrianthefs, PM, Kalafati, M, Samara, I, et al: Nosocomial pneumonia. Crit Care Nurs Q 27(3):241–257, 2004.

Nair, H, Verma, VR, Theodoratou, E, et al: An evaluation of the emerging interventions against Respiratory Syncytial Virus (RSV)-associated acute lower respiratory infections in children. BMC Public Health Apr 13;11 Suppl 3:S30, 2011.

Niel-Weise, BS, Gastmeier, P, Kola, A, et al: An evidence-based recommendation on bed head elevation for mechanically ventilated patients. Crit Care 15(2):R111, 2011.

Nichol, KL, Baken, L, and Nelson, A: Relation between influenza vaccination and outpatient visits, hospitalization, and mortality in elderly persons with chronic lung disease. Ann Intern Med 130:397–403, 1999.

Nsier, S, Makris, C, Mathieu, D, et al: Intensive care unit-acquired infection as a side effect of sedation. Crit Care 14(2):R30, 2010.

Nussbaumer-Ochsner, Y, and Rabe, KF: Systemic manifestations of COPD. Chest 139(1):165–173, 2011.

Orgill, R, Krempl, GA, and Medina, JE: Acute pain management following laryngectomy. Arch Otolaryngol Head Neck Surg 128:829–832, 2002.

Pierce, LNB: Protocols for practice: Applying research at the bedside—traditional and nontraditional modes of mechanical ventilation. Crit Care Nurse 20(1):81–86, 2000.

Pieterman, RM, van Putten, JWG, Meuzelaar, JJ, et al: Preoperative staging of non–small-cell lung cancer with positron-emission tomography. N Engl J Med 343:254–261, 2000.

Polomano, RC, and Farrar, JT: Pain and neuropathy in cancer survivors: Surgery, radiation, and chemotherapy can cause pain; research could improve its detection and treatment. Am J Nurs 106(3, suppl):39–47, 2006.

Prahlow, JA, Prahlow, TJ, and Rakow, RJ: Case study: Asphyxia caused by inspissated oral and nasopharyngeal secretions. Am J Nurs 109(6):38–43, 2009.

Pruitt, B, and Jacobs, M: Best-practice interventions: How can you prevent ventilator-assisted pneumonia? Nursing 2:36–41, 2006.

Qaseem, A, Wilt, TJ, Weinberger, SE, et al: Diagnosis and management of stable chronic obstructive pulmonary disease: A clinical practice guideline update from the American College of Physicians, American College of Chest Physicians, American Thoracic Society, and European Respiratory. Ann Intern Medicine 155(3):179–191, 2011.

Roman, M, Weinstein, A, and Macaluso, S: Primary spontaneous pneumothorax. Medsurg Nurs 12(3):161–169, 2000.

Rose-Ped, AM, Bellm, LA, Epstein, JB, et al: Complications of radiation therapy for head and neck cancers: The patient's perspective. Cancer Nurs 25(6):461–467, 2002.

Scheinhorn, DJ, Hassenpflug, MS, Votto, JJ, et al: Post-ICU mechanical ventilation at 23 long-term care hospitals: A multicenter outcomes study. Chest 131(1):85–93, 2007.

Schleder, B: Taking charge of hospital-acquired pneumonia. Nurse Pract 29(3):50–53, 2004.

Schouchoff, B, and Rodriguez, A: Blunt chest trauma. Top Emerg Med 23(1):1–11, 2001.

Schultz, TR: Community-acquired pneumonia: Hunting the elusive respiratory infection. Nursing Made Incredibly Easy! 1(1):29–34, 2003.

Schultz, TR: On the trail of community-acquired pneumonia. Nurs Manage 34(2):27–31, 2003b.

Sellares, J, Ferro, M, Cano, E, et al: Predictors of prolonged weaning and survival during ventilator weaning in a respiratory ICU. Intensive Care Med 37:775–784, 2011.

Shah, VP, Tunik, MG, and Tsung, JW: Prospective evaluation of point-of-care ultrasonography for the diagnosis of pneumonia in children and young adults. JAMA Pediatr 167(2):119–125, 2013.

Sorce, LR: Respiratory syncytial virus: From primary care to critical care. J Pediatr Health Care 23(2):101–108, 2009.

Stawicki, SP: Mechanical ventilation: Weaning and extubation. OPUS 12 Scientist 1(2):13–16, 2007.

Stuban, SL: Home mechanical ventilation. Am J Nurs 110(5):63–67, 2010.

Sud, S, Sud, M, Friedrich, JO, et al: Effect of mechanical ventilation in the prone position on clinical outcomes in patients with acute hypoxemic respiratory failure: A systematic review and meta-analysis. Can Med Assoc J 178(9):1153–1161, 2008.

Temel, JS, Greer, JA, Muzikansky, A, et al: Early palliative care for patients with metastatic non–small-cell lung cancer. N Engl J Med 363(8):733–742, 2010.

Theron, G, Peter, J, Dheda, K, et al: Xpert MTB/RIF test for tuberculosis.The Lancet 378(9790):481, 2011.

Tomioka, H: Development of new antituberculous agents based on new drug targets and structure—activity relationships. Expert Opinion on Drugs 3(1):21–49, 2008.

Unoki, T, Serita, A, and Grap, MJ: Automatic tube compensation during weaning from mechanical ventilation: Evidence and clinical implications. Crit Care Nurs 28(4):34–42, 2008.

Varkey, JB, Varkey, AB, and Varkey, B: Prophylactic vaccinations in chronic obstructive pulmonary disease: Current status. Curr Opin Pulm Med 15(2):90–99, 2009.

Volpe, DI, Smith, MF, and Sultan, K: Managing pediatric asthma exacerbations in the ED. Am J Nurs 111(2):48–53, 2011.

Electronic Resources

Agency for Healthcare Research and Quality (AHRQ): Exercise-induced bronchoconstriction and asthma: EPC Evidence Reports, 2010. Retrieved December 2012 from **http://www.ahrq.gov/clinic/tp/eibeiatp.htm**

Amanullah, S, and Posner, DH: Ventilator-associated pneumonia: Overview of nosocomial pneumonias, 2011. Retrieved February 2013 from **http://emedicine.medscape.com/article/304836-overview#showall**

American Cancer Society (ACS): Articles concerning lung cancer: Small cell and non-small cell, 2012. Retrieved December 2012 from **http://www.cancer.org/cancer/lungcancer-non-smallcell/index**

American Head and Neck Society: Management of cancer of the head and neck imaging: General guidelines (n.d.). Retrieved February 2013 from **http://www.ahns.info/clinicalresources/docs/imaginggeneral.php**

American Lung Association: Asthma in adults fact sheet, 2012. Retrieved February 2013 from **http://www.lung.org/lung-disease/asthma/resources/facts-and-figures/asthma-in-adults.html**

American Lung Association: Asthma & children fact sheet, 2012. Retrieved February 2013 from **http://www.lung.org/lung-disease/asthma/resources/facts-and-figures/asthma-children-fact-sheet.html**

American Lung Association: Chronic obstructive pulmonary disease (COPD): Fact sheet, 2011. Retrieved December 2012 from **http://www.lung.org/lung-disease/copd/resources/facts-figures/COPD-Fact-Sheet.html**

American Lung Association. Research and Program Services Epidemiology and Statistics Unit: Trends in pneumonia and influenza morbidity and mortality, 2010. Retrieved December 2012 from **http://www.lung.org/finding cures/our research/trend reports.pdf**

American Speech-Language-Hearing Association (ASHA): Speech for people with tracheostomies or ventilators. Information sheet, 1997–2012. Retrieved December 2012 from **http://www.asha.org/public/speech/disorders/tracheostomies.htm**

Amitai, A, and Sinert, D: Ventilator management, 2011. Retrieved December 2012 from **http://emedicine.medscape.com/article/810126-overview**

Atrium Medical Corporation: Product support (n.d.). Retrieved February 2013 from **http://www.atriummed.com/EN/chest_drainage/education.asp**

Bradley, JS, Byinton, CL, and Samir, S, et al: The management of community-acquired pneumonia in infants and children older than 3 months of age: Clinical practice guidelines by the Pediatric Infectious Diseases Society and the Infectious Diseases Society of America, 2011. Retrieved December 2012 from **http://www.idsociety.org/uploadedFiles/IDSA/Guidelines-Patient_Care/PDF_Library/2011%20CAP%20in%20Children.pdf**

Byrd, RP, and Roy, TM: Mechanical ventilation, 2012. Retrieved February 2013 from **http://emedicine.medscape.com/article/304068-overview**

Centers for Disease Control and Prevention (CDC): CDC and healthcare infection control practices: Ventilator-associated pneumonia (VAP) event, 2010. Retrieved January 2012 from **http://www.cdc.gov/nhsn/pdfs/pscmanual/6pscvapcurrent.pdf**

Centers for Disease Control and Prevention CDC). National Center for Health Statistics. Final Vital Statistics Report. Deaths: Final data for 2007, 58(19), 2010. Retrieved December 2012 from **http://www.cdc.gov/nchs/data/nvsr/nvsr58/nvsr58_19.pdf**

Centers for Disease Control and Prevention (CDC): Diseases and conditions, 2012. Retrieved December 2012 from **http://www.cdc.gov/Features/COPDAdults/index.html**

Centers for Disease Control and Prevention (CDC): Human parinfluenza viruses (HPIVs), 2012. Retrieved December 2012 from **http://www.cdc.gov/parainfluenza/about/index.html**

Centers for Disease Control and Prevention (CDC): MMWR National Surveillance for Asthma—United States, 1980–2004, 2007. Retrieved February 2013 from **http://www.cdc.gov/mmwr/preview/mmwrhtml/ss5608a1.htm**

Centers for Disease Control and Prevention (CDC). National Center for Health Statistics: Faststats 2012. Retrieved December 2012 from **http://www.cdc.gov/nchs/fastats/pneumonia.htm**

Centers for Disease Control and Prevention CDC): Pneumonia can be prevented: Vaccines can help, 2012. Retrieved December 2012 from **http://www.cdc.gov/features/pneumonia/**

Centers for Disease Control and Prevention (CDC): Reported tuberculosis in the United States, 2010, Executive Commentary, 2010. Retrieved February 2013 from **http://www.cdc.gov/tb/statistics/reports/2010/**

Centers for Disease Control and Prevention (CDC): Treatment of drug-susceptible tuberculosis disease in persons not infected with HIV, 2012. Retrieved February 2013 from **http://www.cdc.gov/tb/publications/factsheets/treatment/treatmentHIVnegative.htm**

Centers for Disease Control and Prevention (CDC): Updated guidelines for the use of nucleic acid amplification tests in the diagnosis of tuberculosis, MMWR January 16, 2009. Retrieved February 2013 from **http://www.cdc.gov/mmwr/preview/mmwrhtml/mm5801a3.htm**

Elias, A, and Baldini, E: Patient information: Small cell lung cancer (beyond the basics, 2012. Retrieved December 2012 from **http://www.uptodate.com/contents/small-cell-lung-cancer-treatment-beyond-the-basics**

Fayyaz, J, and Lessnau, K-D: Hypoventilation syndromes, 2012. Retrieved December 2012 from **http://emedicine.medscape.com/article/304381-overview**

GlaxoSmithKline: Medication guide: Serevent Diskus (salmetrol xinafoate inhalation powder), 2010. Retrieved December 2012 from **http://www.fda.gov/downloads/Drugs/DrugSafety/ucm089125.pdf**

Global Initiative for COPD (GOLD): Global strategy for the diagnosis, management and prevention of COPD, updated 2011. Retrieved December 2012 from **http://www.goldcopd.org/uploads/users/files/GOLD_Report_2011_Feb21.pdf**

Goodwin, RS: Prevention of aspiration pneumonia: A research-based protocol, 2009. Retrieved December 2012 from **http://www.pspinformation.com/disease/aspiration/pneu.shtml**

Holmquist, L, Russo, A, and Elixhauser, A: Tuberculosis stays in U.S. hospitals, 2006 Healthcare Cost and Utilization Project Statistical Brief #60, October 2008. Retrieved February 2012 from **http://www.hcup-us.ahrq.gov/reports/statbriefs/sb60.pdf**

Imperial College London News Release: New TB test means quicker and easier diagnosis for patients, 2008. Retrieved February 2013 from **http://www3.imperial.ac.uk/newsandeventspggrp/imperialcollege/newssummary/news_7-3-2008-13-34-11?newsid=30474 Kleinschmidt P. (2011)**

Kleinschmidt, P: Chronic obstructive pulmonary disease and emphysema in emergency medicine, 2012. Retrieved December 2012 from **http://emedicine.medscape.com/article/807143-overview**

Lalvani, A: Introduction to the new ELISPOT TB test (T SPOT-TB) and summary of clinical trial results. A presentation given at the John Radcliffe Hospital, Oxford, UK, n.d. Retrieved November 2012 from **http://www.finddiagnostics.org/export/sites/default/resource-centre/presentations/find_oxford_symposium_paris_2005/lalvani.pdf**

Lin, J: Rapid tuberculosis test, 2011. Retrieved February 2013 from **http://emedicine.medscape.com/article/1970954-overview#showall**

Moore, M, Meyers, AD, Alum, M, et al: Head and neck cutaneous squamous cell carcinoma, 2012. Retrieved February 2013 from **http://emedicine.medscape.com/article/1965430-overview**

National Cancer Institute (NCI): Fact sheet: Head and neck cancers, updated 2013. Retrieved February 2013 from **http://www.cancer.gov/cancertopics/factsheet/Sites-Types/head-and-neck#r2**

National Cancer Institute (NCI): Lung cancer, various articles, 2012. Retrieved December 2012 from **http://www.mayoclinic.com/health/lung-cancer/DS00038/DSECTION=treatments-and-drugs**

Parker, LC: Top 10 care essentials for ventilator patients, 2012. Retrieved December 2012 from **http://www.medscape.com/viewarticle/761358_4**

Sawicki, G, and Haver, K: Patient information: Asthma treatment in children (Beyond the Basics), 2012. Retrieved February 2013 from **http://www.uptodate.com/contents/asthma-treatment-in-children-beyond-the-basics**

Schiffman, G: Pneumothorax, 2012. Retrieved December 2012 from **http://www.medicinenet.com/pneumothorax/article.htm**

Schiffman, G: Tuberculosis (TB), 2011. Retrieved February 2013 from **http://www.medicinenet.com/tuberculosis/article.htm**

Sharma, GD, and Gupta, P: Pediatric asthma, 2013. Retrieved February 2013 from **http://emedicine.medscape.com/article/1000997-overview**

Simon, S: Lung cancer also affects nonsmokers, 2011. Retrieved December 2012 from **http://www.cancer.org/cancer/news/lung-cancer-also-affects-nonsmokers**

Steingart, KR, Sohn, H, and Schiller, I: Xpert® MTB/RIF assay for pulmonary tuberculosis and rifampicin resistance in adults, 2012. Retrieved from the Cochrane Library, February 2013, from **http://onlinelibrary.wiley.com/doi/10.1002/14651858.CD009593.pub2/full**

Tejani, NR: Febrile seizures in emergency medicine, 2011. Retrieved February 2013 from **http://emedicine.medscape.com/article/801500-overview#showall**

West, HJ: Patient information: Non–small-cell lung cancer treatment; stage I to III cancer (Beyond the Basics), 2012. Retrieved December 2012 from **http://www.uptodate.com/contents/non-small-cell-lung-cancer-treatment-stage-i-to-iii-cancer-beyond-the-basics**

Williams, ME: The basic geriatric respiratory examination, 2009. Retrieved December 2012 from **http://www.medscape.com/viewarticle/712242**

World Health Organization (WHO): Tuberculosis: Fact sheet, 2013. Retrieved February 2013 from **http://www.who.int/mediacentre/factsheets/fs104/en/**

CHAPTER 6

Books

Abrams, AC, Pennington, SS, and Lammon, CB: Clinical drug therapy: Rationales for nursing practice, ed 8. Lippincott, Williams and Wilkins, Philadelphia, 2007.

Deglin, JH, and Vallerand, AH: Davis's drug guide for nurses, ed 13. FA Davis, Philadelphia, 2010.

Ferri, F: Ferri's best test: A practical guide to clinical laboratory medicine and diagnostic imaging, ed 2. Mosby Elsevier, Philadelphia, 2010.

Finkelstein, EA, Corso, PS, and Miller, TR: The incidence and economic burden of injuries in the United States. Oxford University Press, New York, 2006.

Granacher, RP, Jr: Traumatic brain injury: Methods for clinical and forensic neuropsychiatric assessment. CRC Press, Boca Raton, FL, 2003.

Hamilton, BB, Granger, CV, Sherwin, FS, et al: A uniform national data system for medical rehabilitation. In Fuhrer, MJ (ed): Rehabilitation outcomes: Analysis and measurement. Brookes, Baltimore, MD, 1987.

Hausman, KA: Interventions for clients with problems of the central nervous system. In Ignatavicius, DD, and Workman, ML (eds): Medical-surgical nursing: Critical thinking for collaborative care, ed 5. Elsevier Saunders, St. Louis, MO, 2006.

LWW: Professional guide to pathophysiology, ed 3. Lippincott, Williams and Wilkins, Philadelphia, 2011.

National Multiple Sclerosis Society: Recommendations regarding corticosteroids in the management of multiple sclerosis: Expert opinion paper. New York, 2008.

Nettina, SM: Lippincott manual of nursing practice, ed 8. Lippincott, Williams and Wilkins, Philadelphia, 2006.

Pagana, K, and Pagana, T: Mosby's diagnostic and laboratory test reference, ed 10. Elsevier Mosby, St. Louis, 2011.

Rönnbäck, L, and Johansson, B: Long-lasting mental fatigue after recovery from meningitis or encephalitis—A disabling disorder hypothetically related to dysfunction in the supporting sytems of the brain. In Olisah, V (ed): Essential notes in psychiatry. Intech, Sweden, 2012.

Smeltzer, SS, Bare, BG, Hinkle, JL, et al: Brunner and Suddarth's textbook of medical-surgical nursing, ed 11. Lippincott, Williams and Wilkins, Philadelphia, 2008.

Springhouse, PA: Handbook of diseases, ed 3. Lippincott, Williams and Wilkins, Philadelphia, 2003.

Van Leeuwen, AM, Kranpitz, TR, and Smith, L: Davis's comprehensive handbook of laboratory tests with nursing implications, ed 2. FA Davis, Philadelphia, 2006.

Articles

Albert, HB, Kjaer, P, and Jensen, TS: Modic changes, possible causes and relation to low back pain. Med Hypotheses 70(2):361–368, 2008.

Aref, AA, and Schmitt, BP: Open-angle glaucoma: Tips for earlier detection and treatment selection. J Fam Pract 54(2):117–125, 2005.

Aschenbrenner, DS: Drug watch: New drug treats partial seizures. Am J Nurs 111(10):23, 2011.

Balague, F, and Dudler, J: An overview of conservative treatment for lower back pain. Int J Clin Rheumatol 6(3):281–290, 2011.

Bay, E, and McLean, SA: Mild traumatic brain injury: An update for advanced practice nurses. J Neurosci Nurs 39(1):43–51, 2007.

Bazarian, J, McClung, J, Shah, M, et al: Mild traumatic brain injury in the United States, 1998–2000. Brain Injury 19(2):85–91, 2005.

Berg, PJ, Smallfield, S, and Svien, L: An investigation of depression and fatigue post West Nile virus infection. S D Med, 63(4):127–129, 2010.

Bonner, SM: My aching back: Relieving the pain of herniated disk. Nursing Made Incredibly Easy! 6(1):19–30, 2008.

Brandt, JD, Gordon, MO, and Kass, MA: Central corneal thickness in the ocular hypertension treatment study (OHTS). Opthalmology 108(10): 1779–1788, 2001.

Brethour, MK, Nystrom, KV, Broughton, S, et al: Controversies in acute stroke treatment. AACN Advanced Crit Care 23(2):158–172, 2012.

Brodkey, MB, Ben-Zacharia, AB, and Reardon, JD: Living well with multiple sclerosis. Am J Nurs 111(7):40–48, 2011.

Chipman, JG, Taylor, JH, Thorson, M, et al. Kinetic therapy beds are associated with more complications in patients with thoracolumbar spinal column injuries. Surg Infect (Larchmt) 7(6):513–518, 2006.

Cortese, I, Chaudhry, V, So, YT, et al. Evidence-based guideline update: Plasmapheresis in neurologic disorders: Report of the Therapeutics and Technology Assessment Subcommittee of the American Academy of Neurology. Neurology 76(3):294–300, 2011.

Cottrell, DA, Kremenchutzky, M, Rice, GP, et al: The natural history of multiple sclerosis: A geographically based study. 5. The clinical features and natural history of primary progressive multiple sclerosis. Brain 122(Pt 5):625–639, 1999.

Crimlisk, JT, and Grande, MM: Neurologic assessment for the acute medical surgical nurse. Orthop Nurs 23(1):3–9, 2004.

de Kruijk, J, Leffers, P, Menheere, P, et al: Prediction of post-traumatic complaints after mild traumatic brain injury: Early symptoms and biochemical markers. J Neurol Neurosurg Psych 73:727–732, 2002.

Dryden, T, Baskwill, A, and Preyde, M: Massage therapy for the orthopaedic patient: A review. Orthop Nurs 23(5):327–332, 2004.

Edwards, RR, Doleys, DM, Fillingim, RB, et al: Ethnic differences in pain tolerance: Clinical implications in a chronic pain population. Psychosom Med 63:316–323, 2001.

Fagley, MU: Taking charge of seizure activity. Nursing 37(9):42–47, 2007.

Fazekas, F, Offenbacher, H, Fuchs, S, et al: Criteria for an increased specificity of MRI interpretation in elderly subjects with suspected multiple sclerosis. Neurology 38(12):1822–1825, 1988.

Fonte, N, and Moore, KN: Urological care of the spinal cord-injured patient. J Wound Ostomy and Continence Nurs 35(3):323–331, 2008.

Franges, EZ: A sudden storm: Caring for seizure patients. LPN 2009: 28–36, 2006.

French, DD, Campbell, RR, Sabharwal, S, et al: Health care costs for patients with spinal cord injury in the Veterans Health Administration. J Spinal Cord Med 30(5):477–481, 2007.

Galvin, TJ: Dysphagia: Going down and staying down. Am J Nurs 101(1):37–42, 2001.

Gray, M: Urinary retention: Management in the acute care setting. Am J Nur 100(8):36–43, 2000.

Harvey, J: Countering "brain attacks." Nurs Manage 35(8):27–32, 2004.

Hilton, L: We've got your back: Recovery from spinal cord injuries starts with the first hours of critical care. NurseWeek Mountain West January 10:12, 2005.

Huff, JS, and Fountain, NB: Pathophysiology and definitions of seizures and status epilepticus. Emerg Med Clin North Am 29(1):1–13, 2011.

Kase, CS, and Kurth, T: Prevention of intracerebral hemorrhage recurrence. Continuum (Mineappolis, MN) 17(6 Secondary Stroke Prevention):1304–1317, 2011.

Kennedy, MS: News: Growing older, seeing less: Blindness and visual impairment are on the rise in older Americans. Am J Nurs 104 (7):21, 2004.

Kolk, A, Handschel, J, and Drescher, W: Current trends and future perspectives of bone substitute materials—From space holders to innovative biomaterials. J Craniomaxillofac Surg 40(8):706–718, 2012.

Kowing, D, and Kester, E: Keep an eye out for glaucoma. Nurse Pract 32(7):18–23, 2007.

Kurtzke, JF. Rating neurological impairment in multiple sclerosis: An expanded disability scale. Neurology 33:1444–1452, 1983.

Larsson, G, Raty, LKA, Sterrin, B, et al: Epilepsy patients' conceptions of epilepsy as a phenomenon. J Neuroscience Nurs 41(4):201–210, 2009.

Lawes, R: Uncovering the layers of meningitis and encephalitis. Nursing Made Incredibly Easy! 5(4):26–35, 2007.

Lee, S, Lee, JH, Choi, WC, et al: Anterior minimally invasive approaches for the cervical spine. Orthop Clin North Am 38(3):327–337, 2007.

Lemke, DM: Sympathetic storming after severe traumatic brain injury. Crit Care Nurse 27(1):30–37, 2007.

Manchikanti, L, Staats, S, Singh, V, et al: Evidence-based practice guidelines for interventional techniques in the management of chronic spinal pain. Pain Physician 6:3–81, 2003.

Martin, BI, Deyo, RA, and Mirza, SK: Expenditures and health status among adults with back and neck problems. JAMA 299(6):656–674, 2008.

Matthews, C, Miller, L, and Mott, M: Getting ahead of acute meningitis and encephalitis. Nursing 37(11):36–39, 2007.

McCarberg, BH: Acute back pain: Benefits and risks of current treatments. Curr Med Res Opin 26(1):79–90, 2010.

Meyer, K, Helmick, K, Doncevik, S, et al: Severe and penetrating traumatic brain injury in the context of war. J Trauma Nurs 15(4):185–189, 2008.

Morrison, K: Improving the care of stroke patients. Using an evidence-based quality improvement initiative enhances outcomes for stroke patients. Am Nurse Today 38–43, 2007.

Nayduch, DA: Back to basics: Identifying and managing acute spinal cord injury. Nursing 40(9):24–31, 2010.

Noe, KH: Seizures: Diagnosis and management in the outpatient setting. Semin Neurol 31(1):54–64, 2011.

Phillips, RA: Treating carotid artery stenosis to prevent stroke. Nursing Made Incredibly Easy! 5(1):40–48, 2007.

Quigley, HA, and Broman, AT: The number of people with glaucoma worldwide in 2010 and 2020. Br J Opthalmol 90:262–267, 2006.

Reddy, L, and Santoni, C: Heads up on cerebral bleeds. Nursing 36(5, ED Insider):4–9, 2006.

Reder, AT, Goodin, DS, Ebers, GC, et al: Clinical outcomes and cause of death for interferon beta-1b versus placebo, 21 years following randomization. Neurology 2012:P04 (Meeting Abstracts), 129, 2012.

Rein, DB, Zhang, P, Wirth, KE, et al: The economic burden of major adult visual disorders in the United Stated. Arch Ophthalmol 124(12):1754–1760, 2006.

Rothke, SE, and Michael, E: Integrating the head injury team. Rehab Manage 13(2):38–40, 96, 2000.

Rutherford, EE, Tarplett, LJ, Davies, EM, et al: Radiographics 27, 1737–1749, 2007.

Sadovnick, AD, Ebers, GC, Wilson, RW, et al: Life expectancy in patients attending multiple sclerosis clinics. Neurology 42(5):991–994, 1992.

Santillo, VM, and Lowe, FC: Cranberry juice for the prevention and treatment of urinary tract infections. Drugs Today (Barc) 43(1):47–54, 2007.

Santoni-Reddy, LC: Heads up on cerebral bleeds. Nursing Made Incredibly Easy! 2(3):8–16, 2004.

Sauerbeck, LR: Primary stroke prevention. Am J Nurs 106(11):40–49, 2006.

Schmidt, H, Heimann, B, Djukic, M, et al: Neuropsychological sequelae of bacterial and viral meningitis. Brain 129(2):333–345, 2006.

Secrest, JA: Transformation of the relationship: The experience of primary support persons of stroke survivors. Rehab Nurs 25(3):93–99, 2000.

Stuifbergen, AK, and Harrison, TC: Complementary and alternative therapy use in persons with multiple sclerosis. Rehab Nurs 28:141–147, 158, 2003.

Sullivan, MP, and Sharts-Hopko, NC: Preventing the downward spiral: Osteoporosis and MS. Am J Nurs 100(8):26–32, 2000.

Teasell, RW, Arnold, JM, Krassioukov, A, et al: Cardiovascular consequences of loss of supraspinal control of the sympathetic nervous system after spinal cord injury. Arch Phys Med Rehab 4:81, 2000.

Thigpen, MC, Whitney, CG, Messonnier, NE, et al: Bacterial meningitis in the United States, 1998–2007. N Engl J Med 364:2016–2025, 2011.

Trembly, A: Stroke care in the 21st century. Nurs Manage 41(6):30–36, 2010.

Tunkel, AR, Hartman, BJ, Kaplan, SL, et al: Practice guidelines for the management of bacterial meningitis. Clin Infect Dis 39(9):1264–1284, 2004.

Turkoski, BB: Glaucoma and glaucoma medications. Orthopaedic Nursing 31(1):37–41, 2012.

Turner, JA, et al: Chronic pain associated with spinal cord injuries: A community survey. Arch Phys Med Rehabil (82):501–508, 2001.

Tyler, KL: Herpes simplex virus infections of the central nervous system: Encephalitis and meningitis, including Mollaret's. Herpes 11(Suppl 2): 57A–64A, 2004.

Vignes, JR, De Seze, M, Sesay, M, et al [Translated]: Anterior sacral root stimulation with dorsal rhizotomy (Brindley technique)]. Neurochirurgie 49(2–3 Pt 2):383–394, 2003.

Weeks, SK, Hubbartt, E, and Michaels, TK: Keys to bowel success. Rehab Nurs 25(2):66–69, 2000.

Weir, NU: An update on cardioembolic stroke. Postgraduate Med J 84: 133–142, 2008.

Winkelman, C: Effect of backrest position on intracranial and cerebral perfusion pressure in traumatically brain-injured adults. Am J Crit Care 9(6):373–380, 2000.

Wong, FW: Prevention of secondary brain injury. Crit Care Nurse 20(5):18–27, 2000.

Zink, EK, and McQuillan, K: Managing traumatic brain injury. Nursing 35(9):36–43, 2005.

Electronic Resources

Agency for Healthcare Research and Quality (AHRQ): Early acute management in adults with spinal cord injury: A clinical practice guideline for health-care professionals, 2008. Retrieved January 2013 from **http://guideline.gov/content.aspx?id=14281**

American Academy of Orthopaedic Surgeons: Bone-graft substitutes: Facts, fictions & applications, 2008. Retrieved January 2013 from **http://www.aatb.org/aatb/files/ccLibraryFiles/Filename/000000000101/AAOSbonegraftsubstitutes.pdf**

American Association of Neurological Surgeons (AANS): Gunshot wound head trauma, 2011. Retrieved January 2013 from **http://www.aans.org/en/Patient%20Information/Conditions%20and%20Treatments/Gunshot%20Wound%20Head%20Trauma.aspx**

American Spinal Injury Association (ASIA): International standards for neurological classification of spinal cord injury, n.d. Retrieved January 2013 from **http://www.asia-spinalinjury.org/elearning/ISNCSCI_Exam_Sheet_r4.pdf#search="impairment scale"**

American Stroke Association: Impact of stroke: Stroke statistics, 2012. Retrieved January 2013 from **http://www.strokeassociation.org/STROKEORG/AboutStroke/Impact-of-Stroke-Stroke-statistics_UCM_310728_Article.jsp**

Bakshi, R. Fatigue and multiple sclerosis: A review, 2003. Retrieved January 2013 from **http://www.medscape.com/viewarticle/462361**

Balentine, JR, and Shiel, WC: Encephalits and meningitis, 2012. Retrieved August 2012 from **http://www.medicinenet.com/encephalitis_and_meningitis/article.htm**

Barrett, AM, and John, ST: Spatial neglect, 2012. Retrieved January 2012 from **http://emedicine.medscape.com/article/1136474-overview**

Bitan, FD: Motion preservation and spine surgery, various pages, 2013. Retrieved January 2013 from **http://www.bitanmd.com/procedures/mpo.php**

Benaroch, R (reviewer): Epilepsy in children, 2012. Retrieved March 2013 from **http://www.webmd.com/epilepsy/epilepsy-children**

Brown University: Glaucoma, 2007. Retrieved January 2013 from **http://biomed.brown.edu/Courses/BI108/2006-108websites/group02glaucoma/glaucoma.html**

Campagnolo, DI: Autonomic dysreflexia in spinal cord injury, 2011. Retrieved January 2013 from **http://emedicine.medscape.com/article/322809-overview**

Cavazos, JE, and Lum, F: Seizures and epilepsy, 2012. Retrieved January 2012 from **http://emedicine.medscape.com/article/1184846-overview**

Centers for Disease Control and Prevention (CDC): Encephalitis or meningitis, arboviral (includes Californa serogroup, Eastern equine, St Louis, Western equine, West Nile, Powassan): 2001 case definition, 2011. Retrieved August 2012 from **http://www.cdc.gov/osels/ph_surveillance/nndss/casedef/encephalitiscurrent.htm**

Centers for Disease Control and Prevention (CDC): Fact sheet: Viral meningitis, 2009. Retrieved August 2012 from **http://www.cdc.gov/ncidod/dvbid/arbor/arbofact.htm**

Centers for Disease Control and Prevention (CDC): Facts about traumatic brain injury, 2006. Retrieved January 2013 from **http://www.cdc.gov/traumaticbraininjury/tbi_ed.html**

Centers for Disease Control and Prevention (CDC): Meningococcal: Who needs to be vaccinated?, 2011. Retrieved January 2013 from **http://www.cdc.gov/vaccines/vpd-vac/mening/who-vaccinate.htm**

Centers for Disease Control and Prevention (CDC): West Nile Virus: Clinical description, 2004. Retrieved August 2012 from **http://www.cdc.gov/ncidod/dvbid/westnile/clinicians/clindesc.htm**

Center for Injury Prevention and Control (CDC): Traumatic brain injury in the United States: Emergency department visits, hospitalizations, and deaths, 2002–2006, 2010. Retrieved January 2013 from **http://www.cdc.gov/traumaticbraininjury/tbi_ed.html**

Centre for Neuro Skills: TBI resource guide. Various articles concerning brain injury, 2006. Retrieved January 2013 from **http://www.neuroskills.com/brain-injury/brain-function.php**

Congressional Research Service. U.S. Military Casualty Statistics: Operation New Dawn, Operation Iraqi Freedom, and Operation Enduring Freedom, 2010. Retrieved January 2013 from **http://www.fas.org/sgp/crs/natsec/RS22452.pdf**

Coronado, VG, Thurman, DJ, Greenspan, AI, et al: MMWR: Surveillance for traumatic brain injury—related deaths—United States, 1997–2007, 2011. Retrieved January 2013 from **http://www.cdc.gov/mmwr/preview/mmwrhtml/ss6005a1.htm?s_cid=ss6005a1_w**

Cruz-Flores, S, and Chaisam, T: Stroke anticoagulation and prophylaxis, 2011. Retrieved January 2013 from **http://emedicine.medscape.com/article/1160021-overview#aw2aab6b3**

Epilepsy Foundation: Epilepsy stats and facts, 2009. Retrieved March 2013 from **http://www.epilepsy.com/node/986825**

Epilepsy Foundation: Seizure dogs, n.d. Retrieved March 2013 from **http://www.epilepsyfoundation.org/livingwithepilepsy/healthandwellness/Seizure-Dogs.cfm**

Epilepsy Foundation: What is epilepsy: Incidence and prevalence, 2012. Retrieved October 2012 from **http://www.epilepsyfoundation.org/resources/**

Epilepsy Foundation: Various pages, 2012. Retrieved March 2013 from **http://www.epilepsyfoundation.org/aboutepilepsy/causes/index.cfm**

Epilepsy Society: Medications for adults, n.d. Retrieved January 2013 from **http://www.epilepsysociety.org.uk/aboutepilepsy/treatment/medicationforadults**

Fox, RJ: Multiple sclerosis. Cleveland Clinic Disease Management Project, 2011. Retrieved January 2013 from **http://www.clevelandclinicmeded.com/medicalpubs/diseasemanagement/neurology/multiple_sclerosis/**

Fruedenthal, J, Pascotto, A, Sacca, SC, et al: Glaucoma, complications and management of glaucoma filtering, 2012. Retrieved January 2013 from **http://emedicine.medscape.com/article/1207755-overview**

Glaucoma Research Foundation: Treating glaucoma, various pages, n.d. Retrieved January 2013 from **http://www.glaucoma.org/glaucoma/**

Holmquist, L, Russo, CA, and Elixhauser, A: Meningitis-related hospitalizations in the United States, 2006. Statistical Brief #57. July 2008. Retrieved April 2013 from **http://hcup-us.ahrq.gov/reports/statbriefs/sb57.jsp**

Horn, J, and Felter, RA: Pediatric meningitis and encephalitis, 2012. Retrieved August 2012 from **http://emedicine.medscape.com/article/802760-overview**

Lab Tests online: Various pages, updated 2012. Retrieved August 2012 from **http://labtestsonline.org/understanding/conditions/meningitis/**

Lettieri, CJ: Neurotrauma: Management of acute head injuries, 2006. Retrieved January 2013 from **http://www.medscape.com/viewarticle/542508_4**

Liebeskind, DS, Kirshner, HS, Nassisi, D, et al: Hemorrhagic stroke in emergency medicine, 2011. Retrieved January 2013 from **http://emedicine.medscape.com/article/1916662-overview**

Lowes, R: FDA approvals: Combo meningitis vaccine for infants. CME article for medscape, 2012. Retrieved August 2012 from **http://www.medscape.org/viewarticle/766119**

Luzzio, C, and Dangond, F: Multiple sclerosis, 2012. Retrieved January 2013 from **http://emedicine.medscape.com/article/1146199-overview**

Mann, S: Approach to the child with a seizure, 2011. Retrieved March 2013 from **http://learnpediatrics.com/body-systems/nervous-syste/approach-to-the-child-with-a-seizure/**

Medicinenet staff: Treatment for epilepsy, 2009. Retrieved January 2013 from **http://www.medicinenet.com/epilepsy_treatment/article.htm**

Miami Childrens Hospital: In-depth reports: Seizure/Epilepsy, 2010. Retrieved February 2013 from **http://www.mch.com/page/EN/4819/In-Depth-Reports/Epilepsy.aspx**

Muller, ML: Pediatric bacterial meningitis, 2012. Retrieved July 2013 from **http://emedicine.medscape.com/article/961497-overview**

National Center for Health Statistics: Health, United States, 2006, with chartbook on trends in the health of Americans. Hyattsville, MD, 86. Retrieved February 2013 from **http://www.cdc.gov/nchs/data/hus/hus06.pdf**

National Heart, Lung and Blood Institute (NHLBI): 4. Disease statistics, 2008. Retrieved January 2013 from **http://www.nhlbi.nih.gov/about/factbook/chapter4.htm**

National Institutes of Health: Stroke scale, 2003. Retrieved January 2013 from **http://www.ninds.nih.gov/doctors/NIH_Stroke_Scale.pdf**

National Institute of Neurological Disorders and Stroke (NINDS): ASIA spinal impairment scale, 2012. Retrieved January 2012 from **http://www.ninds.nih.gov/disorders/sci/detail_sci.htm**

National Institute of Neurological Disorders and Stroke (NINDS): Low back pain fact sheet, 2012. Retrieved January 2013 from **http://www.ninds.nih.gov/disorders/backpain/detail_backpain.htm**

National Institute for Neurological Disorders and Stroke (NINDS): Multiple sclerosis: Hope through research, 2012. Retrieved January 2013 from **http://www.ninds.nih.gov/disorders/multiple_sclerosis/detail_multiple_sclerosis.htm#210763215**

National Institute for Neurological Disorders and Stroke (NINDS): Seizures and epilepsy: Hope through research, updated 2012. Retrieved January 2013 from **http://www.ninds.nih.gov/disorders/epilepsy/detail_epilepsy.htm**

National Institute for Neurological Disorders and Stroke (NINDS): Spinal cord injury: Hope through research, updated 2012. Retrieved January 2013 from **http://www.ninds.nih.gov/disorders/sci/detail_sci.htm**

National Institute for Neurological Disorders and Stroke (NINDS): Traumatic brain injury: Hope through research, 2012. Retrieved January 2013 from **http://www.ninds.nih.gov/disorders/tbi/detail_tbi.htm#193663218**

National MS Society: Various pages, n.d. Retrieved January 2013 from **http://www.nationalmssociety.org/about-multiple-sclerosis/what-we-know-about-ms/faqs-about-ms/index.aspx#howmany**

National Spinal Cord Injury Statistical Center (NSCISC): Facts and figures at a glance, updated 2012. Retrieved January 2013 from **https://www.nscisc.uab.edu/PublicDocuments/fact_figures_docs/Facts%202012%20Feb%20Final.pdf**

Perina, DG: Mechanical back pain, 2012. Retrieved January 2012 from **http://emedicine.medscape.com/article/822462-overview**

Rashbaum, RF: Types of back pain, 1999–2013. Retrieved January 2013 from **http://www.spine-health.com/conditions/chronic-pain/types-back-pain**

Razonable, RR, and Keathing, BA: Meningitis. Medscape article, 2012. Retrieved August 2012 from **http://emedicine.medscape.com/article/232915-overview**

Ritter-Lang, K, and Clavel, P: Artificial disc replacement (ADR) surgery. Public information, various pages, n.d. Retrieved January 2013 from **http://www.betterdiscreplacement.com/about/index.asp**

ScienceDaily, Rush University Medical Center: Cost effectiveness of spinal surgery analyzed, December 29, 2008. Retrieved April, 2013, from **http://www.sciencedaily.com/releases/2008/12/081229200744.htm**

Sen, S: Blood dyscrasias and stroke, 2011. Retrieved January 2013 from **http://emedicine.medscape.com/article/1160261-overview#aw2aab6c13**

Senelick, R (reviewer): Epilepsy Health Center—Drugs for children with epilepsy, 2012. Retrieved March 2013 **from http://www.webmd.com/epilepsy/medicines-for-children-with-epilepsy**

Singh, NN, Uppal, G, and Thomas, FP: Meningitis in HIV. Medscape article, 2011. Retrieved August 2012 from h**ttp://emedicine.medscape.com/article/1952165-overview**

Springhouse: Nurse's 3-minute clinical reference, ed 2. Lippincott, Williams and Wilkins, Philadelphia, PA, 2008. Retrieved September 2012 from **http://www.r2library.com/Resource/Title/1582556709**

Statistic Brain: Multiple sclerosis statistics, 2012. Retrieved January 2012 from **http://www.statisticbrain.com/multiple-sclerosis-statistics/**

Tejani, NR: Febrile seizures in emergency medicine, 2011. Retrieved February, 2013 from **http://emedicine.medscape.com/article/801500-overview#showall**

Ullrich, PF: Common causes of back pain, 2001. Retrieved January 2013 from **http://www.spine-health.com/conditions/back-pain/common-causes-back-pain-and-neck-pain**

Wedro, B: Transient ischemic attack (mini-stroke), 2010. Retrieved January 2012 from **http://www.emedicinehealth.com/transient_ischemic_attack_mini-stroke/article_em.htm**

CHAPTER 7

Books

Beyer, PL: Inflammatory bowel diseases section of medical nutrition therapy for lower gastrointestinal tract disorders. In Mahan, LK, and Escott-Stump, S (eds): Krause's food and nutrition therapy, ed 12. Saunders Elsevier, Philadelphia, 2008.

Black, P: Holistic stoma care. London. Harcourt Publishers, 2000.

Boehmke, MM: Interventions for clients with inflammatory intestinal disorders. In Ignatavicius, DD, and Workman, ML (eds): Medical-surgical nursing: Critical thinking for collaborative care. Elsevier Saunders, St. Louis, MO, 2006.

Fauci, A: Harrison's manual of medicine, ed 17. McGraw-Hill, New York, 2009.

Gibbs, JR: Interventions for clients with stomach disorders. In Copstead, LEC, and Banasik, JL (eds): Pathophysiology, ed 3. Elsevier Saunders, St. Louis, MO, 2005.

Mettina, S: Manual of nursing practice, ed 8. Lippincott, Williams & Wilkins, Philadelphia, 2006.

Sartin, JS: Alterations in function of the gallbladder and exocrine pancreas. In Copstead, LEC, and Banasik, JL (eds): Pathophysiology, ed 3. Elsevier Saunders, St. Louis, MO, 2005a.

Sartin, JS: Gastrointestinal disorders. In Copstead, LEC, and Banasik, JL (eds): Pathophysiology, ed 3. Elsevier Saunders, St. Louis, MO, 2005b.

Swearingen, P: Manual of medical-surgical nursing care: Nursing interventions and collaborative management. Mosby, St. Louis, MO, 2003.

Pamphlets

American Autoimmune Related Disease Association (AARDA): The cost of autoimmune disease: The latest front in the war on healthcare spending. Author, Eastpoint, MI, 2011.

Everhart, JE (ed): The burden of digestive diseases in the United States. US Department of Health and Human Services, Public Health Service, National Institutes of Health, National Institute of Diabetes and Digestive and Kidney Diseases, Washington, DC, US Government Printing Office, 2008; NIH Publication No. 09-6443.

Rooney, D: Colostomy irrigation: A personal account of managing a colostomy. The Phoenix, pp 1–5, A publication of the United States Ostomy Association (USOA), 2007.

Washuta, L: Basic colostomy care. Colostomy new patient guide. In The Phoenix, pp 26–33, A publication of the United States Ostomy Associaten (USOA), 2010.

Articles

Alloo, J, Gerstle, T, Shiliansky, J, et al: Appendicitis in children less than 3 years of age, a 28-year review. Pediatr Surg Int 17(2):777–779, 2004.

Bae, J, Park, J, Yang, H, et al: Nutritional status of gastric cancer patients after total gastrectomy. World J Surg 22(3):254–261, 1998.

Bildozola, M, Kravetz, D, Argonz, J, et al: Efficacy of octreotide and sclerotherapy in the treatment of acute variceal bleeding in cirrhotic patients. A prospective, multicentric, and randomized clinical trial. Scand J Gastroenterol 35(4):419–425, 2000.

Borwell, B: Stoma management and palliative care. JCN 25(4):4–10, 2011.

Bosshardt, TL: Outcomes of ostomy procedures in patients aged 70 years and older. Arch Surg 138(10):1077–1082, 2003.

Boyer, TD, and Haskal, ZJ: The role of transjugular intrahepatic portosystemic shunt (TIPS) in the management of portal hypertension: Update 2009. Hepatology 51(1):306, 2010.

Bozetti, F, Ravera, E, Cozzaglio, L, et al: Comparison of nutritional status after total or subtotal gastrectomy. Nutrition 6(5):371–375, 1990.

Butler, DL: Early postoperative complications following ostomy surgery: A review. J Wound Ostomy Continence Nurs 38(5):513–519, 2009.

Chen, GZ, and Freeman, ML: Management of upper gastrointestinal bleeding emergencies: Evidence-based medicine and practical considerations. World J Emerg Med 2(1):5–12, 2011.

Cheng, HC, and Sheu, BS: Intravenous proton pump inhibitors for peptic ulcer bleeding: Clinical benefits and limits. World J Gastrointest Endosc 16; 3(3):49–56, 2011.

Day, MW: Fight back against inflammatory bowel disease. Nursing 38(11):34–40, 2008.

de Bartoli, N, Leonardi, G, Ciancia, E, et al: *Helicobacter pylori* eradication: A randomized prospective study of triple therapy versus triple therapy plus lactoferrin and probiotics. Am J Gastroenterol 102:951–956, 2007.

Dorman, C: Ostomy basics. RN 72(7):22–27, 2009.

Garcia-Tsao, G, Sanyal, AJ, Grace, ND, et al: Prevention and management of gastroesophageal varices and variceal hemorrhage in cirrhosis. Hepatology 46(3):922–938, 2007.

Gracey, D, and McClure, MJ: The impact of ultrasound in suspected acute appendicitis. Clin Radiol 62(6):573–578, 2007.

Hanauer, SB: Inflammatory bowel disease: Epidemiology, pathogenesis, and therapeutic opportunities. Inflamm Bowel Dis (12):Suppl 1:S3–S9, 2006.

Hegab, AM, and Luketic, VA: Bleeding esophageal varices. How to treat this dreaded complication of portal hypertension. Postgrad Med 109(2):75–89, 2001.

Huang, J-Q, Sridhar, S, and Hunt, RH: Role of *Helicobacter pylori* infection and non-steroidal antiinflammatory drugs in peptic ulcer disease: A metaanalysis. Lancet 359:14–22, 2002.

Huffman, JL, and Schenker, S: Acute acalculous cholecystitis—A review. Clin Gastroenterol Hepatol 8(1):15–22, 2010.

Kane, SV: Systematic review: Adherence issues in the treatment of ulcerative colitis. Aliment Pharmacol Ther 23(5):577–585, 2006.

Keane, WF, Bailie, GR, Boeschoten, E, et al: Adult peritoneal dialysis-related peritonitis treatment recommendations: 2000 update. Peri Dial Int 20(4):396–411, 2000.

Krishnamoorthi, R, Ramarajan, N, Barth, RA, et al: Effectiveness of a staged US and CT protocol for the diagnosis of pediatric appendicitis: Reducing radiation exposure in the age of ALARA. Radiology 259(1): 231–239, 2011.

Layke, JC, and Lopez, PP: Gastric cancer: Diagnosis and treatment. Am Fam Phys 69(5):1133–1140, 2004.

Levitzky, BE, and Wassef, WY: Endoscopic management in the bariatric surgical patient. Curr Opin Gastroenterol 26(6):632–639, 2010.

Lewis, JD, Gelfand, JM, Troxel, AB, et al: Immunosuppressant medications and mortality in inflammatory bowel disease. Am J Gastroenterol 103:1428–1435, 2008.

Movius, M: What's causing the gut pain? RN 69(7):25–30, 2006.

Nance, ML, Adamson, WT, and Hendricks, HL: Appendicitis in the young child continuing diagnostic challenge. Pediatr Emerg Care 16(3): 160–162, 2000.

Pontieri-Lewis, V. Basics of ostomy care. Medsurg Nurs 15(4):199–202, 2004.

Radigan, AE: Post-gastrectomy: Managing the nutrition fall-out. Practical Gastroenterol (June):63–74, 2004.

Ringhofer, J: Meeting the needs of your ostomy patient. RN 68(8):37–41, 2005.

Sands, BE, Cuffari, C, Katz, J, et al: Guidelines for immunizations in patients with inflammatory bowel disease. Inflamm Bowel Dis 10(5):677–692, 2004.

Smith, GD: The management of acute upper gastrointestinal bleeding. Nurs Times 100(26):40, 2004.

Smith, MM: Variceal hemorrhage from esophageal varices associated with alcoholic liver disease. AM J Nurs 110(2):32–39, 2010.

Wei, B, Qi, CL, Chen, TF, et al: Laparoscopic versus open appendectomy for acute appendicitis: A metaanalysis. Surg Endosc 25(4):1199–1208, 2011.

Yeh, C, Wu, S, Liao, C, et al: Laparoscopic appendectomyfor acute appendicitis is more favorable for patients with comorbidities, the elderly, and those with complicated appendicitis: A nationwide population-based study. Surg Endosc 25(9):2932–2942, 2011.

Yokoyama, S, Takifuji, K, Hotta, T, et al: C-reactive protein is an independent surgical indication marker for appendicitis: A retrospective study. World J Emerg Surg 4(36):1186–1749, 2009.

Electronic Resources

Allen, JI, Dassopoulas, T, Brill, JV, et al: Adult inflammatory bowel disease: Physician performance measures set. Retrieved March 2013 from **http://www.gastro.org/practice/quality-initiatives/IBD_Measures.pdf**

American Cancer Society (ACS): Cancer facts and figures, 2012. Retrieved March 2013 from **http://www.cancer.org/acs/groups/content/@epidemiologysurveilance/documents/document/acspc-031941.pdf**

American Cancer Society (ACS): Surgery for stomach cancer, 2012. Retrieved March 2013 from **http://www.cancer.org/cancer/stomachcancer/overviewguide/stomach-cancer-overview-treating-surgery**

American Society for Gastrointestinal Endoscopy (ASGE): Sclerosing agents for use in GI endoscopy, 2007. Retrieved March 2013 from **http://www.asge.org/assets/0/71312/71314/C705B082-84EB-4549-96B4-1C21FE67C463.pdf**

Anand, BS, Bank, S, Qureshii, WA, et al: Peptic ulcer disease medication, 2012. Retrieved March 2013 from **http://emedicine.medscape.com/article/181753-medication#4**

Antipuesto, DJ: T-tube care, 2010. Retrieved March 2013 from **http://nursingcrib.com/demo-checklist/t-tube-care/**

Bloom, AA, Amin, Z, Anand, BS, et al: Cholecystitis, 2011. Retrieved March 2013 from **http://emedicine.medscape.com/article/171886-overview**

Cabebe, EC, Mehta, VK, and Fisher, G: Gastric cancer, 2013. Retrieved March 2013 from **http://emedicine.medscape.com/article/278744-treatment**

Centers for Disease Control and Prevention (CDC): Inflammatory bowel disease (IBD), 2012. Retrieved March 2013 from **http://www.cdc.gov/ibd/**

Cerulli, MA, and Iqbal, S: Upper gastrointestinal bleeding, 2013. Retrieved March 2013 from **http://emedicine.medscape.com/article/187857-overview#showall**

Cleveland Clinic Staff: ERCP (Endoscopic Retrograde Cholangiopancreatography), 2009. Retrieved March 2013 from **http://my.clevelandclinic.org/services/endoscopic_retrograde_cholangiopancreatography/hic_ercp_endoscopic_retrograde_cholangiopancreatog.aspx**

Craig, S, Incesu, L, and Taylor, CR: Appendicitis clinical presentation, 2012. Retrieved January 2013 from **http://emedicine.medscape.com/article/773895-clinical#showall**

Crohn's & Colitis Foundation of America (CCFA). What are Crohn's and colitis? 2013. Retrieved March 2013 from **http://www.ccfa.org/what-are-crohns-and-colitis/what-is-ulcerative-colitis/types-of-ulcerative-colitis.html**

Daley, BJ, Long, C, Lapolitano, LM, et al: Peritonitis and abdominal sepsis, 2011. Retrieved March 2013 from **http://emedicine.medscape.com/article/180234-overview**

Denson, L, Moyer, S, and Ballard, E: Evidence-based care guideline for management of pediatric moderate/severe inflammatory bowel disease, 2007. Retrieved March 2013 from **http://www.cincinnatichildrens.org/assets/0/78/1067/2709/2777/2793/9199/488d3bf6-5f6b-47ca-b263-9805277ba18b.pdf**

Digestive Diseases Information Clearing House (NDDIC): Digestive diseases statistics in the United States, 2012. Retrieved March 2013 from **http://digestive.niddk.nih.gov/statistics/statistics.aspx#2**

Franz, JF, and Wright, KD: Colostomy. In Gale encyclopedia of surgery: A guide for patients and caregivers, 2004. Retrieved March 2013 from **http://www.encyclopedia.com/topic/Colostomy.aspx**

Gutman, N: Colostomy guide, 2011. Retrieved March 2013 from **http://www.ostomy.org/ostomy_info/pubs/ColostomyGuide.pdf**

HCUP: Hospitalizations for gastrointestinal bleeding in 1998 and 2006, 2008. Retrieved March 2013 from **http://www.hcup-us.ahrq.gov/reports/statbriefs/sb65.jsp**

Heuman, DM, Mihas, AA, and Allen, J: Cholelithiasis, 2011. Retrieved March 2013 from **http://emedicine.medscape.com/article/175667-overview#showall**

International Association for the Study of Pain: Pain, 2012. Retrieved December 2012 from **http://www.iasp-pain.org/Content/NavigationMenu/GeneralResourceLinks/PainDefinitions/default.htm#Pain**

Jamidar, PA, and Kinzel, JE: Endoscopic sphincterotomy, 2011. Retrieved March 2013 from **http://emedicine.medscape.com/article/1891681-overview#a1**

Janssen Biotech Staff: Pediatric Crohn's disease, 2011. Retrieved March 2013 from **http://www.livingwithcrohnsdisease.com/livingwithcrohnsdisease/pediatric_crohns/index.html**

Kehler, A: 10 Tips on how to calm down peptic ulcer pain, 2008. Retrieved March 2013 from **http://www.healblog.net/10-advices-on-how-to-calm-down-peptic-ulcer-pain**

Khan, AN, Patankar, TA, Krishna, TA, et al: Acute cholecystitis imaging, 2011. Retrieved March 2013 from **http://emedicine.medscape.com/article/365698-overview#a21**

Kim, J: Management and prevention of upper GI bleed in gastroenterology and nutrition. American College of Clinical Pharmacology (n.d.). Retrieved March 2013 from **http://www.accp.com/docs/bookstore/psap/p7b11sample01.pdf**

Kolecki, P, and Menckhoff, CR: Hypovolemic shock, 2012. Retrieved March 2013 from **http://emedicine.medscape.com/article/760145-overview**

LWW: Evidence-based nursing guide to disease management, Lippincott William & Wilkins, Philadelphia, 2009. Retrieved December 2012 from **http://www.r2library.com/Resource/Title/0781788269**

Springhouse: Nurse's 3-minute clinical reference, ed 2. Lippincott, Williams & Wilkins, Philadelphia, 2008. Retrieved December 2012 from **http://www.r2library.com/Resource/Title/1582556709**

Marks, JW, and Lee, DL: Capsule endoscopy (wireless capsule endoscopy), 2008. Retrieved March 2013 from **http://www.medicinenet.com/capsule_endoscopy/article.htm**

Mayo Clinic Staff: Crohn's disease, 2011. Retrieved March 2013 from **http://www.mayoclinic.com/health/crohns-disease/DS00104/DSECTION=symptoms**

Mayo Clinic Staff: Dumping syndrome: Treatment and drugs. 2013. Retrieved March 2013 from **http://www.mayoclinic.com/health/dumping-syndrome/DS00715/DSECTION=treatments-and-drugs**

Mazotti, MV, and Minkes, RK: Pediatric appendectomy, 2011. Retrieved April 2013 from **http://emedicine.medscape.com/article/933825-overview#a1**

Minkes, RK, Bechtel, KA, Billmire DF, et al: Pediatric appendicitis, 2011. Retrieved April 2013 from **http://emedicine.medscape.com/article/926795-overview**

Naiditch, JA: Acute appendicitis in children, 2011. Retrieved April 2013 from **http://www2.luriechildrens.org/ce/online/article.aspx?articleID=256**

Naqesh-Bandi, N, Moir, JAG, and McCaslin, JE: A prospective study of cholecystectomy in district general hospital settings with literature review, 2011. Retrieved March 2013 from **http://archive.ispub.com/journal/the-internet-journal-of-surgery/volume-26-number-2/a-prospective-study-of-cholecystectomy-in-district-general-hospital-settings-with-literature-review.html**

National Cancer Institute: SEER STAT Fact Sheets: Stomach cancer 2012. Retrieved March 2013 from **http://seer.cancer.gov/statfacts/html/stomach.html**

National Institute of Diabetes and Digestive and Kidney Diseases (NIDDK): Appendicitis, 2008. Retrieved January 2013 from **http://digestive.niddk.nih.gov/ddiseases/pubs/appendicitis/index.aspx**

National Institute of Diabetes and Digestive and Kidney Diseases (NIDDK): Gallstones: Number and age-adjusted rates of deaths and years of potential life lost (to age 75) by age, race, and sex in the United States, 2004. Retrieved March 2013 from **http://www2.niddk.nih.gov/NR/rdonlyres/B60FA826-0A38-4773-86F7-9402C81C50EA/0/BurdenDD_ch22_Jan2009.pdf**

National Digestive Diseases Information Clearinghouse (NDDIC): NSAIDs and peptic ulcers, 2012. Retrieved March 2013 from **http://digestive.niddk.nih.gov/ddiseases/pubs/nsaids/#4**

No author listed: A guide to sex with an ostomy, 2010. Retrieved March 2013 from **http://www.ostomyguide.com/a-guide-to-sex-with-an-ostomy/**

Peralta, R, Nepolitano, LM, Jacocks, A, et al: Surgical approach to peritonitis and abdominal sepsis, 2011. Retrieved March 2013 from **http://emedicine.medscape.com/article/1952823-overview#showall**

Seibert, A: The five types of Crohn's disease, 2011. Retrieved March 2013 from **http://www.webmd.com/ibd-crohns-disease/crohns-disease/5-types-crohns-disease**

Simon, H (reviewer): Gallstones and gallbladder disease-surgery, 2009. Retrieved March 2013 from **http://www.umm.edu/patiented/articles/what_surgical_procedures_gallstones_gallbladder_disease__000010_8.htm**

Stephens, M, Rosh, JR, Richardson, MD, et al: A case-based monograph: Optimizing therapeutic safety in children and young adults with IBD, 2010. Retrieved March 2013 from **http://www.naspghan.org/user-assets/Documents/pdf/CDHNF%20Old%20Site/CME%20Case-Based%20Monograph%20&%20Podcast%20Series/Optimiz-ingTherapeuticSafety_ChildrenandYoungAdultsIBD.pdf**

Tan, J, File, T, Salata, R, et al: Expert guide to infectious diseases, ed 2· 2008. Retrieved December 2012 from **http://www.r2library.com/Resource/Title/1930513852**

U.S. Department of Health and Human Services: Deaths: Final data for 2009. National Vital Statistics Report, 60(3):1–117, 2011. Retrieved January 2013 from **http://www.cdc.gov/nchs/products/nvsr.htm#vol60**

Varma, MK, Allen, AW, and Sawyer, MAJ: Upper gastrointestinal bleeding: Imaging, 2011. Retrieved March 2013 from **http://emedicine.medscape.com/article/417980-overview**

Wax, A (reviewer): Colostomy irrigation, 2012. Retrieved March 2013 from **http://www.webmd.com/colorectal-cancer/colostomy-irrigation**

Westhoff, JL, and Holt, KR: Gastrointestinal bleeding: An evidence-based ED approach to risk stratification, 2004. Retrieved March 2013 from **http://www.ebmedicine.net/topics.php?paction=showTopic&topic_id=75**

Wolf, J: Inflammatory bowel disease fact sheet, 2009. Retrieved March 2013 from **http://womenshealth.gov/publications/our-publications/fact-sheet/inflammatory-bowel-disease.cfm#a**

CHAPTER 8

Books

Bernal-Mizrachi, E, and Bernal-Mizrachi, C: Diabetes mellitus and related disorders. In Green, GB, et al (eds): The Washington manual of medical therapeutics, ed 31. Lippincott, Williams & Wilkins, St. Louis, MO, 2004.

Cash, J, and Glass, C: Family practice guidelines, ed 2. Springer, New York, 2011.

Clutter, WE: Endocrine diseases: Hyperthyroidism. In Green, GB, et al (eds): The Washington manual of medical therapeutics, ed. 31. Lippincott, Williams & Wilkins, St. Louis, MO, 2004.

Daniels, R, and Nicoll, L: Contemporary medical-surgical nursing, ed 2. Delmar Cengage Learning, Clifton Park, NY, 2012.

Fauci, A: Harrison's manual of medicine, ed 17. Mcgraw-Hill, New York, 2009.

Felver, L: Acid-base homeostasis and imbalances. In Copstead, LEC, and Banasik, JL (eds): Pathophysiology, ed 3. Elsevier Saunders, St. Louis, MO, 2005.

Foster, J, and Prevost, S: Advanced practice nursing of adults in acute care. FA Davis, Philadelphia, 2012.

Ignatavicius, DD: Interventions with clients with problems of the biliary system and pancreas. In Ignatavicius, DD, and Workman, ML (eds): Medical-surgical nursing: Critical thinking for collaborative care, ed 5. Elsevier Saunders, St. Louis, MO, 2006.

Klein, S: Nutrition support. In Green, GB, et al (eds): The Washington manual of medical therapeutics, ed 31. Lippincott, Williams & Wilkins, St. Louis, MO, 2004.

LeFever Kee, J: Laboratory and diagnostic tests with nursing implications, ed 7. Prentice Hall, Upper Saddle River, NJ, 2005.

Lemone, P, and Burke, K: Medical surgical nursing: Critical thinking in client care, ed 4. Prentice Hall, Upper Saddle River, NJ, 2008.

Lewis, SL, et al: Medical surgical nursing: Assessment and management of clinical problems, ed 7. Mosby Elsevier, St. Louis, MO, 2007.

Murphy, MB: Interventions for clients with liver problems. In Ignatavicius, DD, and Workman, ML (eds): Medical-surgical nursing: Critical thinking for collaborative care, ed 5. Elsevier Saunders, St. Louis, MO, 2006.

Pagana, K, and Pagana, T: Mosby's diagnostic and laboratory test reference, ed 10. Mosby, St. Louis, MO, 2011.

Springhouse (ed): Fluids and electrolytes made incredibly easy! Lippincott, Williams & Wilkins, Philadelphia, 2007.

Springhouse (ed): Pathophysiology made incredibly easy!, ed 3. Lippincott, Williams & Wilkins, Philadelphia, 2005.

Townsend, M: Psychiatric mental health nursing: Concepts of care in evidence-based practice, ed 5. FA Davis, Philadelphia, 2006.

Venes, D, Biderman, A, and Taber, CW (eds): Taber's cyclopedic medical dictionary, ed 20. FA Davis, Philadelphia, 2005.

Articles

Agaba, EA, Shamsedeen, H, Gentles, CV, et al: Laparoscopic vs open gastric bypass in the management of morbid obesity: A 7-year retrospective study of 1,364 patients from a single center. Obes Surg 18(11):1359–1363, 2008.

American Diabetes Association: American Diabetes Association's 2004 position statement: Diagnosis and classification of diabetes mellitus. Diabetes Care 27(Suppl 1):S5–S10, 2004a.

American Diabetes Association: Summary of revisions for the 2004 clinical practice recommendations. Diabetes Care 27(Suppl 1):S3, 2004b.

American Diabetes Association: Standards of medical care in diabetes—2007. Diabetes Care 30(Suppl 1):S4–S41, 2007.

American Heart Association (AHA). Heart disease and stroke statistics—2013 update. Circ 127(e6–e245), 2012.

Allison, DB, Fontaine, KR, Manson, JE, et al: Annual deaths attributable to obesity in the United States. JAMA 282(16):1530–1538, 1999.

Astle, SM: Restoring electrolyte balance. RN 68(5):34–39, 2005.

Bahn, RS, Burch, HB, Cooper, DS, et al: Hyperthyroidism and other causes of thyrotoxicosis: Management guidelines of the American Thyroid Association and American Association of Clinical Endocrinologists (ATA/AACE). Endocr Pract 17(3):457–520, 2011.

Beauchamp-Johnson, BM: Scale down bariatric surgery's risks. Men in Nurs 1(3):20–26, 2006.

Benton, MJ, Whyte, MD, and Dyal, BW: Scarpenic obesity: Strategies for management. Am J Nurs 111(12):38–44, 2011.

Black, JM, Gray, M, Bliss, DZ, et al: Incontinence-associated dermatitis and intertriginous dermatitis: A consensus. J Wound Ostomy Continence Nurs 38(4):359–370, 2011.

Blackett, A, Gallagher, S, Dugan, S, et al: Caring for persons with bariatric health care issues: A primer for the WOC nurse. J Wound Ostomy Continence Nurs 38(2):133–138, 2011.

Blackwood, HS: Obesity: A rapidly expanding challenge. Nurs Manage 35(5):27–35, 2004.

Boisvert, JA, and Harrell, WA: Ethnicity and spirituality as risk factors for eating disorder symptomatology in men. Int J Men's Health 11(1):36, 2012.

Bonnel, AR, Bunchorntavakul, C, and Reddy, KR: Immune dysfunction and infections in patients with cirrhosis. Clin Gastroenterol Hepatol 9(9):727–738, 2011.

Booker, KJ, Niedringhaus, L, Eden, B, et al: Comparison of 2 methods of managing gastric residual volumes from feeding tubes. Am J Crit Care 9(5):318–324, 2000.

Borzio, M, Salerno, F, Piantoni, L, et al: Bacterial infection in patients with advanced cirrhosis: A multicentre prospective study. Dig Liver Dis 33(1):41–48, 2001.

Bouldin, M, et al: The effect of obesity surgery and obesity comorbidity. Am J Med Sci 331(4):183–193, 2006.

Bunevicius, R, and Prang, AJ: Psychiatric manifestations of Graves' hyperthyroidism: Pathophysiology and treatment options. CNS Drugs 20(11):897–909, 2006.

Burkey, SH, van Heerden, JA, Thompson, GB, et al: Reexploration for symptomatic hematomas after cervical exploration. Surgery 130(6):914–920, 2001.

Cammon, SA, and Hackshaw, HS: Are we starving our patients? Am J Nurs 100(5):43–46, 2000.

Cheung, DS, Maygers, J, Khouri-Stevens, Z, et al: Failure modes and effects analysis: Minimizing harm to our bariatric patients. Bariatr Nurs Surg Patient Care 1(2):107–114, 2006.

Coelho, GM, Soares, EA, and Ribeiro, BG: Are female athletes at increased risk for disordered eating and its complications? Appetite 55(3):379–338, 2010.

Cole, L: Unraveling the mystery of acute pancreatitis. Dimen Crit Care Nurs 21(3):86–89, 2002.

Corbell, CF, and Cook, D: Diabetes ABCs: Do you know them, get them, improve them? Home Healthc Nurse 22(7):452–459, 2004.

Crawford, A, and Harris, H: Thyroid imbalances: Dealing with disorderly conduct. Nursing 42(11):44–50, 2012.

Crow, SJ, Peterson, CB, Swanson, SA, et al: Increased mortality in bulimia nervosa and other eating disorders. Am J Psychiatr 166:1342–1346, 2009.

Davidson, JE, Kruse, MW, Cox, DH, et al: Critical care of the morbidly obese. Crit Care Nurse Q 26(2):105–116, 2003.

Demaria, EF, Pate, V, Warthen, M, et al: Baseline data from American Society for Metabolic and Bariatric Surgery-designated Bariatric Surgery Centers of Excellence using the Bariatric Outcomes Longitudinal Database. Surg Obes Rel Dis 6(4):347–355, 2010.

Deshpande, AD, Harris-Hayes, M, and Schootman, M: Epidemiology of diabetes and diabetes-related complications. Phys Ther 88(11):1254–1264, 2008.

Dixon, JB: Obesity and diabetes: The impact of bariatric surgery on type-2 diabetes. World J Surg 33(10):2014–2021, 2009.

Dudek, SG: Malnutrition in hospitals: Who's assessing what patients eat? Am J Nurs 100(4):36, 2000.

Durston, S: The ABCs—and more—of hepatitis. Nursing Made Incredibly Easy! 2(4):22–32, 2004.

Elisha, S, Boytim, M, Bordi, S, et al: Anesthesia case management for thyroidectomy. AANA J 78(2):151–160, 2010.

Fairburn, CG, Cooper, Z, Doll, HA, et al: Transdiagnostic cognitive-behavioral therapy for patients with eating disorders: A two-site trial with 60-week follow-up. Am J Psychiatry 166(3):311–319, 2009.

Farooqi, IS, and O'Rahilly, S: Genetic factors in human obesity. Obesity Reviews 2007 8(Suppl 1):37–40, 2007.

Favoretti, F, Ashton, D, Busetto, L, et al: The gastric band: First-choice procedure for obesity surgery. World J Surg 33(10):2039–2048, 2009.

Fisher, JN: Management of thyrotoxicosis. South Med J 95(5):493–505, 2002.

Funnell, MM, and Barlage, DL: Saying a mouthful about oral diabetes drugs. Nursing2000 30(11):34, 2000.

Funnell, MM, and Kruger, DF: Type 2 diabetes: Treat to target. Nurs Pract 29(1):11–13, 2004.

Gagnon, LE, and Karwacki Sheff, EJ: Outcomes and complications after bariatric surgery. Am J Nurs 112(9):26–36, 2012.

Gallagher, S: Taking the weight off with bariatric surgery. Nursing 34(3):58–64, 2004.

Gammage, MD., Parle, JV, Holder, RL, et al: Association between serum free thyroxine concentration and atrial fibrillation. Arch Int Med 167:928–934, 2007.

Garcia-Tsao, G: Current management of the complications of cirrhosis and portal hypertension: Variceal hemorrhage, ascites, and spontaneous bacterial peritonitis. Gastroenterology 120(3):726–748, 2001.

Garcia-Tsao, G, Lim, J, and Members of the Veterans Affairs Hepatitis C Resource Center Program: Management and treatment of patients with cirrhosis and portal hypertension: Recommendations from the Department of Veterans Affairs Hepatitis C Resource Center Program and the National Hepatitis C Program. Am J Gastroenterol 104(7):1802–1829, 2009.

Goldfield, GS, Blouin, AG, and Woodside, B: Body image, binge eating and bulimia nervosa in male body builders. Can J Psychiatry 51(3):160–168, 2006.

Gopalan, S, and Khanna, S: Enteral nutrition delivery technique. Curr Opin Clin Nutr Metab Care 6(3):313–317, 2003.

Greenleaf, C, Petrie, T, Reel, J, et al: Psychosocial risk factors of bulimic symptomology among female athletes. JCSP 4(3):177–190, 2010.

Heathcote, EJ: Management of primary biliary cirrhosis. Hepatology 31(4):1005–1022, 2000.

Heidelbaugh, JJ, and Bruderly, M: Cirrhosis and chronic liver failure: Part I. Diagnosis and evaluation. Am Fam Physician 74:765–774, 2006.

Hermann, M, Hellebart, C, and Freissmuth, M: Neuromonitoring in thyroid surgery: Prospective evaluation of intraoperative electrophysiological responses for the prediction of recurrent laryngeal nerve injury. Ann Surg 240(1):9–17, 2004.

Iscoe, KE, et al: Efficacy of continuous real-time blood glucose monitoring during and after prolonged high-intensity cycling exercise: Spinning with a continuous glucose monitoring system. Diabetes Technol Ther 8(6):627–635, 2006.

Jorgensen, RA: Nonalcoholic fatty liver disease. Gastroenterol Nurs 26(4):150–154, 2003.
Leininger, SM: The role of nutrition in wound healing. Crit Care Nurse 25(1):13–21, 2002.
Levy, P, Fried, M, Santini, F, et al: The comparative effects of bariatric surgery on weight and type 2 diabetes. Obes Surg 17(9):1248–1256, 2007.
Livingston, EH. The incidence of bariatric surgery has plateaued in the U.S. Am J Surg 200(3):378–385, 2010.
Longitudinal Assessment of Bariatric Surgery Consortium (LABS), et al: Perioperative safety in the longitudinal assessment of bariatric surgery. N Engl J Med 361(5):445–454, 2009.
McInnis, KJ: Diet, exercise, and the challenge of combating obesity in primary care. J Cardiovas Nurs 18(2):93–100, 2003.
Molinaro, RJ. Diabetes cases on the rise: Current diagnosis guidelines and research efforts for a cure. MLO Med Lab Obs 43(2):8, 10, 12, 2011.
Morrissey, AT, Chau, J, Yunker, WK, et al: Comparison of drain versus no drain thyroidectomy: Randomized prospective clinical trial. J Otolaryngol Head Neck Surg 37(1):43–47, 2008.
Moy, J, Pomp, A, Dakin, G, et al: Laparoscopic sleeve gastrectomy for morbid obesity. Am J Surg 196:56–59, 2008.
Murphy, K: The skinny on eating disorders. Nursing Made Incredibly Easy! 5(3):40–48, 2007.
Nardi, M, Tognana, G, Schiavo, G, et al: Nutritional support in liver cirrhosis. Nutr Ther Metab 27(4):155–163, 2009.
No author listed: Comparing psychotherapies for bulimia. Harv Ment Health Lett 17(99):8, 2001.
Noble, KA: Name that tube. Nursing2003 33(3):56–62, 2003.
Olohan, K, and Zappitelli, D: The insulin pump. Am J Nurs 103(4):48–56, 2003.
Olson, RS: An update in diabetes management. Rehab Nurs 25(5):177–184, 2000.
Orbanic, S: Understanding bulimia, signs, symptoms and the human experience. Am J Nurs 101(3):35, 2001.
Padula, CA, et al: Enteral feedings: What the evidence says. Am J Nurs 104(7):62–69, 2004.
Peeples, M, and Seley, JJ: Diabetes care: The need for change. Am J Nurs 107(6 Suppl):13–19, 2007.
Petrie, TA, Greenleaf, C, Carter, JE, et al: Psychosocial correlates of disordered eating among male collegiate athletes. JCSP 1(4):157, 2007.
Powers, J, et al: Bedside placement of small-bowel feeding tubes in the intensive care unit. Crit Care Nurse 23(1):1624, 2003.
Reiber, GE, Lipsky, BA, and Gibbons, GW: The burden of diabetic foot ulcers. Am J Surg 176(Suppl 2A):5–10, 1998.
Rose, C: The role of nurses in caring for the eating disordered patient. HealthReach [newsletter], Denver Health Medical Center, 2001.
Ruggiero, FP, and Fred GF: Outcomes in reoperative thyroid cancer. Otolaryngol Clin North Am 41(6):1261–1268, 2008.
Runyon, BA: AASLD practice guidelines: Management of adult patients with ascites due to cirrhosis: An update. Hepatology 49(6):2087–2107, 2009.
Salemeh, JR: Bariatric surgery: Past and present. Am J Med Sci 331(4):194–200, 2006.
Scemons, D: Are you up-to-date on diabetes medications? Nursing2007 37(7):45–49, 2007.
Schantz, S: Child and adolescent obesity, BMI and the school nurse's role. NASN Newsletter 7:22–24, 2007.
Simmons, S: A delicate balance: Detecting thyroid disease. Nursing, 40(7):22–29, 2010.
Simmons-Holcomb, S: An update on hepatitis. Dimen Crit Care Nurs 21(5):170–177, 2002.
Speranza, M, et al: Predictive value of alexithymia in patients with eating disorders: A 3-year prospective study. J Psychosom Res 63(4):365–371, 2007.
Sundgot-Borgen, J, and Torstveit, MK: Aspects of disordered eating continuum in elite high-intensity sports. Scand J Med Sci Sports 20(Suppl 2):112–121, 2010.
Torstveit, MK, and Sundgot-Borgen, J: The female athlete triad exists in both elite athletes and controls. Med Science Sport Exerc 37(9):1449–1459, 2005.
Trus, TL, Pope, GD, and Finlayson, SR: National trends in utilization and outcomes of bariatric surgery. Surg Endosc 19(5):616–620, 2005.
Vairman, M, Nagibin, A, Hagag, P, et al: Subtotal and near total versus total thyroidectomy for the management of multinodular goiter. World J Surg, 32(7):1546–1551, 2008.
Verna, EC, and Brown, RS: Hepatitis C virus and liver transplantation. Clin Liver Dis 10(4):19–40, 2006.
Vink, T, Hinney, A, van Elberg, AA, et al: Association between an agouti-related protein gene polymorphism and anorexia nervosa. Mol Psychiatry 6(3):325–328, 2001.
Wasley, A, Grytdal, S, Gallagher, K, et al: Surveillance for acute viral hepatitis—United States, 2006. MMWR Surveill Summ 57(2):1–24, 2008.
Whitcomb, DC, Yadav, D, Adam, S, et al: Multicenter approach to recurrent acute and chronic pancreatitis in the United States: The North American Pancreatitis Study 2 (NAPS2). Pancreatology 8(4–5):520–531, 2008.
Xu, J, Kochanek, KD, Murphy, SL, et al: Deaths: Final data for 2007. National Vital Statistics 58(19):1–73, 2010.
Yee, HS, Chang, ME, Pocha, C, et al: Update on the management and treatment of hepatitis C virus infection: Recommendations from the Department of Veterans Affairs Hepatitis C Resource Center Program and the National Hepatitis C Program office. Am J Gastroenterol 107(5):669–689, 2012.

Electronic Resources

Adair, JD, and Ellsmere, JC: Complications of bariatric surgery, 2013. Retrieved March 2013 from paid Web site **http://www.uptodate.com/contents/complications-of-bariatric-surgery**
American Association of Diabetes Educators (AADE): Insulin pump therapy: Guidelines for successful outcomes, 2009. Retrieved March 2013 from **http://www.diabeteseducator.org/export/sites/aade/_resources/pdf/Insulin_Pump_White_Paper.pdf**
American Diabetes Association (ADA): Diabetes basics, 2013. Retrieved March 2013 from **http://www.diabetes.org/diabetes-basics/**
American Diabetes Association (ADA): Diabetes statistics, updated 2013. Retrieved March 2013 from **http://www.diabetes.org/diabetes-basics/diabetes-statistics/?print=t**
American Liver Foundation (ALA): Liver transplant, 2012. Retrieved March 2013 from **http://www.liverfoundation.org/abouttheliver/info/transplant/**
Anorexia Nervosa and Associated Disorders (ANAD): Eating disorders statistics, 2013. Retrieved March 2013 from **http://www.anad.org/get-information/about-eating-disorders/eating-disorders-statistics/**
Bedinghaus, T: Graves' disease, 2008. Retrieved March 2013 from **http://vision.about.com/od/eyediseases/a/Graves_Disease.htm**
Bernstein, BE: Pediatric anorexia nervosa, 2012. Retrieved March 13 from **http://emedicine.medscape.com/article/912187-overview#showall**
Brandis, K: Acid-base physiology. Chapters 5 and 7, 2006, update 2008. Retrieved April 2013 from **http://www.anaesthesiamcq.com/AcidBaseBook/ABindex.php**
Buggs, AM: Viral hepatitis, 2012. Retrieved March 2013 from **http://emedicine.medscape.com/article/775507-overview**
Centers for Disease Control and Prevention, (CDC): Adult obesity facts, 2012. Retrieved March 2013 from **http://www.cdc.gov/obesity/data/adult.html#baseline**
Centers for Disease Control and Prevention (CDC): Chronic liver disease or cirrhosis, 2009. Retrieved March 2013 from **http://www.cdc.gov/nchs/fastats/liverdis.htm**
Centers for Disease Control and Prevention (CDC): National diabetes fact sheet, 2011. Retrieved March 2013 from **www.cdc.gov/diabetes/pubs/pdf/ndfs_2011.pdf**
Centers for Disease Control and Prevention (CDC): NCHS data brief, no 82 (2012). Prevalence of obesity in the United States, 2009–2010. Retrieved March 2013 from **http://www.cdc.gov/nchs/data/databriefs/db82.pdf**
Centers for Disease Control and Prevention (CDC): Viral hepatitis statistics and surveillance, 2012. Retrieved March 2013 from **http://www.cdc.gov/hepatitis/Statistics**
Chakraborty, KM, and Basu, D: Management of anorexia and bulimia nervosa: An evidence-based review, 2010. Retrieved February 2013 from

http://www.questia.com/library/1G1-230841988/management-of-anorexia-and-bulimia-nervosa-an-evidence-based

Colquitt, JL, Picot, J, Loveman, E, et al: Surgery for obesity. Cochrane Database of Systematic Reviews, 2009. Retrieved March 2013 from **http://summaries.cochrane.org/CD003641/weight-loss-surgery-for-obesity**

Daniel, C: Chronic hepatitis nutrition, 2008. Retrieved March 2013 from **http://hepatitis.about.com/od/lifestyle/a/NutritionHep.htm**

Dhringa, JK, and Raval, T: Minimally invasive surgery of the thyroid, 2011. Retrieved March 2013 from **http://emedicine.medscape.com/article/1298816-overview#showall**

Diaz, JJ, Pousman, R, Mills, B, et al: Critical care nutrition practice management guidelines, 2004. Retrieved April 2013 from **http://www.mc.vanderbilt.edu/surgery/trauma/Protocols/nutrition-protocol.pdf**

Fallon, LF: Thyroidectomy. Encycopedia of surgery: A guide for patients and caregivers, 2004. Retrieved March 2013 from **http://www.encyclopedia.com/topic/Thyroidectomy.aspx**

Flagel, KM, Williamson, DF, and Pamuk, ER: Estimating deaths attributable to obesity in the United States, 2004. Retrieved March 2013 from **http://www.ncbi.nlm.nih.gov/pmc/articles/PMC1448478/**

Gardner, TB, and Berk, BS: Acute pancreatitis, 2013. Retrieved April 2013 from **http://emedicine.medscape.com/article/181364-overview#showall**

Gibson, MC: Anorexia nervosa pathophysiology, 2012. Retrieved February 2013 from **http://www.wikidoc.org/index.php/Anorexia_nervosa_pathophysiology**

Gilroy, RK, Wu, GY, and Talavera, F: Hepatitis A, 2012. Retrieved March 2013 from **http://emedicine.medscape.com/article/177484-overview**

Hamdy, O, Citkowitz, E, Uwaifo, GI, et al: Obesity, 2013. Retrieved March 2013 from **http://emedicine.medscape.com/article/123702-overview**

Hep B Foundation: Approved drugs for adults, 2012. Retrieved March 2013 from **http://www.hepb.org/patients/hepatitis_b_treatment.htm#**

Hoyert, DL, and Xu, J: Deaths: Preliminary data for 2011. National Vital Statistics Report [NVSR]. 61(6):3–4. Retrieved March 2013 from **http://www.cdc.gov/nchs/data/nvsr/nvsr61/nvsr61_06.pdf**

Huffman, JL, Obideen, K, and Wehbi, M: Chronic pancreatitis, 2012. Retrieved April 2013 from **http://emedicine.medscape.com/article/181554-overview**

Joint Commission on Accreditation of Healthcare Organizations (JCAHO): Standards: Environment of care list of standards TX.4, updated April 2002. Retrieved April 2013 from **http://www.nyspi.org/jcho/NYSPI/nutritionsrv/nsmission.htm**

Kaye, WH: Atypicals in the treatment of anorexia nervosa. (No date), Retrieved March 2013 from **http://www.medscape.org/viewarticle/479929_4**

Labtestsonline: Acute viral hepatitis panel, last review 2010. Retrieved March 2013 from **http://labtestsonline.org/understanding/analytes/hepatitis-panel/tab/test**

LWW: Nurse's 3-minute clinical reference, ed 2. Philadelphia: Lippincott, Williams & Wilkins, 2008. Retrieved January 22, 2013 from **http://www.r2library.com/Resource/Title/1582556709**

Mears, E: Nutritional assessment: An opportunity for laboratorians to improve health care. Clinical Laboratory News, 2005. Retrieved April 2013 from **http://www.aacc.org/publications/cln/series/2005/Documents/nutrition_assessJune2005.pdf**

Medical College of Georgia: Robots preclude neck incision for thyroid surgery, 2010. Retrieved March 2013 from **http://www.sciencedaily.com /releases/2010/07/100706112607.htm**

Mehler, PS, Winkleman, AB, Anderson, DM, et al: Nutritional rehabilitation: Practical guidelines for refeeding the anorectic patient, 2010. Retrieved April 2013 from **http://www.hindawi.com/journals/jnume/2010/625782/**

National Association for Weight Loss Surgery (NAWLS): Weight loss surgery statistics and definitions, 2005–2012. Retrieved May 2013 from **http://www.nawls.com/public/102.cfm?sd=2**

National Diabetes Information Clearinghouse (NDIC), What I need to know about diabetes medicines, 2011. Retrieved March 2013 from **http://diabetes.niddk.nih.gov/dm/pubs/medicines_ez/insert_C.aspx**

National Heart, Lung and Blood Institute: What are overweight and obesity? Diseases and conditions index, 2012. Retrieved March 2013 from **http://www.nhlbi.nih.gov/health/health-topics/topics/obe/**

National Institute of Diabetes and Digestive and Kidney Disorders (NIDDK): What I need to know about Hepatitis C. NIH publication 07-4230, n.d. Retrieved March 2013 from **http://digestive.niddk.nih.gov/ddiseases/pubs/hepc_ez/hepc_508.pdf**

Nazario, B: Oral diabetes medications, 2011. Retrieved March 2013 from **http://diabetes.webmd.com/guide/oral-medicine-pills-treat-diabetes**

No author listed: Pathophysiology of obesity, 2012. Retrieved March 2013 from **http://www.obesityeducationnetwork.com/pathophysiology**

No author listed: What are eating disorders? The alliance for eating disorder awareness, 2013. Retrieved February 2013 from **http://www.allianceforeatingdisorders.com/what-are-eating-disorders**

Ogunyemi, DA: Autoimmune thyroid disease and pregnancy, 2012. Retrieved March 2013 from **http://emedicine.medscape.com/article/261913-overview#showall**

OPTN/SRTR Annual data report 2011. Liver. Retrieved March 2013 from **http://srtr.transplant.hrsa.gov/annual_reports/2011/pdf/03_%20liver_12.pdf**

Polin, BS: Ketoacidosis: A diabetes complication, 2012. Retrieved March 2013 from **http://www.diabeticlifestyle.com/type-1-diabetes/ketoacidosis-diabetes-complication**

Pyrsopoulos, NT, and Reddy, KR: Primary biliary cirrhosis, 2013. Retrieved April 2013 from **http://emedicine.medscape.com/article/171117-overview**

Quigley, P, and Moreno, MA: Pediatric bulimia, 2011. Retrieved March 2013 from **http://emedicine.medscape.com/article/913721-overview**

Radar, J: Eating disorders and men, 2011. Retrieved February 2013 from **http://eatingdisorderstreatment.com/eating-disorders-and-men/**

Raghavan, RA, Bensson, HA, Hamdy, O, et al: Diabetic ketoacidosis treatment & management, 2012. Retrieved March 2013 from **http://emedicine.medscape.com/article/118361-treatment#showall**

Ross, DS: Iodine in the treatment of hyperthyroidism, 2012. Retrieved March 2013 from **http://www.uptodate.com/contents/radioiodine-in-the-treatment-of-hyperthyroidism**

Schraga, ED: Hyperthyroidism, thyroid storm, and Graves' disease in emergency medicine, 2008, 2012. Retrieved March 2013 from **http://emedicine.medscape.com/article/767130-overview**

Shah, R, and Fields, JM: Ascites treatment & management, 2012. Retrieved March 2013 from **http://emedicine.medscape.com/article/170907-treatment#showall**

Stevens, T, and Conwell, D: Chronic pancreatitis. Cleveland Clinic Disease Management Project, 2010. Retrieved March 2013 from **http://www.clevelandclinicmeded.com/medicalpubs/diseasemanagement/gastroenterology/acute-pancreatitis/**

Sun, GH, DeMonner, S, and Davis, MM: Epidemiological and economic trends in inpatient and outpatient thyroidectomy in the United States, 1996–2006. Thyroid, 2012. Retrieved March 2013 from **http://online.liebertpub.com/doi/abs/10.1089/thy.2012.0218?journalCode=thy**

Thomas, CP, and Hamawi, K: Metabolic acidosis, 2013. Retrieved April 2013 from **http://emedicine.medscape.com/article/242975-overview#showall**

Thompson, EG, and Tavakkolizadeh, A: Biliopancreatic diversion and biliopancreatic diversion with duodenal switch, 2011. Retrieved March 2013 from **http://www.webmd.com/diet/weight-loss-surgery/biliopancreatic-diversion-1920**

Tortorice, J: Total parenteral nutrition, 2007. Retrieved April 2013 from **http://www.ceufast.com/courses/viewcourse.asp?id=180**

Waldrop, R, and Brenner, BE: Emergent management of anorexia nervosa, 2011. Retrieved February 2013 from **http://emedicine.medscape.com/article/805152-overview**

Wolf, DC: Cirrhosis, 2012. Retrieved March 2013 from **http://emedicine.medscape.com/article/185856-overview**

World Health Organization (WHO): Fact sheet. Obesity and overweight, 2013. Retrieved March 2013 from **http://www.who.int/mediacentre/factsheets/fs311/en/**

Yaseen, S, and Thomas, C: Metabolic alkalosis, 2011. Retrieved April 2013 from **http://emedicine.medscape.com/article/243160-overview**

Zhoa, Y, and Encinosa, W: An update on hospitalizations for eating disorders, 1999 to 2009. AHRQ Healthcare Cost and Utilization Project (HCUP); Statistical Brief #120, 2011. Retrieved February 2013 from **http://www.hcup-us.ahrq.gov/reports/statbriefs/sb120.pdf**

CHAPTER 9

Books

American Academy of Pediatrics: Scheduling immunizations. In Red Book for PDA: Report of the Committee on Infectious Diseases. American Academy of Pediatrics, Committee on Infectious Diseases, ed 26. Elk Grove Village, IL, 2003.

Beers, MK (ed): The Merck manual of diagnosis and therapy, ed 11. Merck Research Laboratories, West Point, PA, 2006.

Evens, A, and Tallman, M: Acute leukemias. In Skeel, RT (ed): Handbook of cancer chemotherapy, ed 6. Lippincott, Williams & Wilkins, Philadelphia, 2003.

Foster, J, and Prevost, S: Advanced practice nursing of adults in acute care. FA Davis, Philadelphia, 2012.

Iltano, JK, and Taoka, KN: ONS core curriculum for oncology nursing, ed 4. Elsevier Saunders, Philadelphia, 2005.

Johnston, L: Sexuality. In Johnson, L (ed): Non-Hodgkin's lymphomas: Making sense of diagnosis, treatment, and options. O'Reilly Media (no location given), 1999.

Katz, A: Breaking the silence on cancer and sexuality: A handbook for healthcare providers. Oncology Nursing Society, Philadelphia, 2006.

Lippincott, Williams & Wilkins (contributors): Professional guide to pathophysiology, ed 3. Lippincott, Williams & Wilkins, Philadelphia, 2010.

Stein, R, Morgan, D, and Greer, J: Hodgkin's disease and non-Hodgkin's lymphoma. In Skeel, RT (ed): Handbook of cancer chemotherapy, ed 6. Lippincott, Williams & Wilkins, Philadelphia, 2003.

Visovsky, C: Interventions for clients with hematologic problems. In Ignatavicius, DD, and Workman, ML (eds): Medical-surgical nursing: Critical thinking for collaborative care, ed 5. Elsevier Saunders, St. Louis, MO, 2006.

Articles

American Academy of Pediatrics, Committee on Infectious Diseases: Policy statement: Recommendations for the prevention of pneumococcal infections, including the use of pneumococcal conjugate vaccine (Prevnar), pneumococcal polysaccharide vaccine, and antibiotic prophylaxis. Pediatrics 2000;106(2 Pt 1):362–366.

Basile, J: Clinical considerations and practical recommendations for the primary care practitioner in the management of anemia of chronic kidney disease. South Med J 100(12):1200–1207, 2007.

Bernard, AW, Yasin, Z, and Venkat, A: Acute chest syndrome of sickle cell disease. Hosp Physician 43(1):13–18, 2007.

Brousseau, DC, Panepinto, JA, Minner, M, et al: The number of people with sickle-cell disease in the United States: National and state estimates. Am J Hematol 85(1):77–78, 2009.

Cerrato, PL: Complementary therapies: Diet and herbs for BPH? RN 63(2):63–64, 2000.

Corwin, H, and Krantz, S: Anemia of the critically ill: Acute anemia of chronic disease. Crit Care Med 29(9):S199–S200, 2001.

Creary, M, Williamson, D, and Kulkarni, R: Sickle cell disease: Current activities, public health implications, and future directions. J Women's Health 16(5):575–582, 2007.

Cushman, M, Cantrell, RA, McClure, LA, et al: Estimated 10-year stroke risk by region and race in the United States: Geographic and racial differences in stroke risk. Ann Neurol 64(5):507–513, 2008.

Dahoui, HA, Hayek, MN, Nietert, PJ, et al: Pulmonary hypertension in children and young adults with sickle cell disease: Evidence for familial clustering. Pediatr Blood Cancer 54(3):398–402, 2010.

Druker, BJ, Guilhot, F, O'Brien, SG: Five-year follow-up of patients receiving imatinib for chronic myeloid leukemia. N Engl J Med 355(23):2408–2417, 2006.

Ellison, AM: Sickle cell disease advice on handling emergencies. Contemporary Pediatrics 29(9):18–27, 2012.

Harel, S, Ferme, C, and Poirot, C: Management of fertility in patients treated for Hodgkin's lymphoma. Haematol 96(11):1692–1699, 2010.

Hebbar, AK, and Gibson, MV: Recognizing and managing anemia of chronic disease. Patient Care 40(11):36–40, 2006.

Held-Warmkessel, J: How to prevent and manage tumor-lysis syndrome. Nursing 40(2):26–31, 2010.

Jordan, K, Sippel, C, and Schmoll, H-J: Guidelines for antiemetic treatment of chemotherapy-induced nausea and vomiting: Past, present, and future recommendations. Oncologist 12(9):1143–1150, 2007.

Klepin, HD, and Balducci, L: Acute myelogenous leukemia in older adults. Oncologist 14(3):222–232, 2009.

Knight, K, Wade, S, and Balducci, L: Prevalence and outcomes of anemia in cancer: A systematic review of the literature. Am J Med 116 (Suppl 7A):11S–26S, 2004.

Kosits, C, and Callaghan, M: Rituximab: A new monoclonal antibody therapy for non-Hodgkin's lymphoma. Oncol Nurs Forum 27(1):51, 2000.

Maples, BL, and Hagemann, TM: Treatment of priapism in pediatric patients with sickle cell disease. Am J Health Syst Pharm 61(4):355–363, 2004.

Meier, ER, and Miller, JL: Sickle cell disease in children. Drugs 72(7): 895–906, 2012.

Mohanty, D, Mukherjee, MB, and Colah, RB: Iron deficiency anaemia in sickle cell disorders in India. Indian J Med Res 127:366–369, 2008.

Mullen, E: Hodgkin lymphoma: An update. J Nurse Pract 3(6):393–403, 2007.

Pack-Mabien, A, and Haynes, J: A primary care provider's guide to preventive and acute care management of adults and children with sickle cell disease. J Am Acad Nurse Pract 21(5):250–257, 2009.

Phillips, RM: The mystery of leukemia in older adults. Nursing Made Incredibly Easy! 10(1):39–45, 2012.

Rogers, B: Looking at lymphoma and leukemia. Nursing 35(7):56–63, 2005.

Rogers, GM, Becker, PS, Blinder M, et al: Cancer- and chemotherapy-induced anemia. J Natl Compr Canc Netw 10(5):628–653, 2012.

Roy, C, Weinstein, D, and Andrews, N: 2002 E. Mead Johnson award for research in pediatrics lecture: The molecular biology of the anemia of chronic disease: A hypothesis. Pediat Res 53(3):507–512, 2003.

Sherbenou, D, and Druker, B: Applying the discovery of the Philadelphia chromosome. J Clin Invest 117(8):2067–2074, 2007.

Steinberg, MH, Barton, F, Castro, O, et al: Effect of hydroxyurea on mortality and morbidity in adult sickle cell anemia: Risks and benefits up to 9 years of treatment. JAMA 289(13):1645–1651, 2003.

Stremick, K, and Gallagher, E: Malignant lymphomas. Am J Nurs 4(Suppl):18–22, 2000.

Verduzco, LA, and Nathan, DG: Sickle cell disease and stroke. Am Fam Physician 61(5):1349–1356, 2000.

Vichinsky, EP, Neumayr, LD, Earles, AN, et al: Causes and outcomes of the acute chest syndrome in sickle cell disease. National Acute Chest Syndrome Study Group. N Engl J Med 342(25):1855–1865, 2000.

Yale, SH, Nagib, N, and Guthrie, T: Approach to the vaso-occlusive crisis in adults with sickle cell disease. Am Fam Physician 61(5):1349–1356, 2000.

Yusuf, HR, Lloyd-Puryear, MA, Grant, AM, et al: Sickle cell disease. The need for a public health agenda. Am J Prev Med 41(6S4):S376–S383, 2011.

Electronic Resources

American Cancer Society (ACS): Cancer facts and figures, 2013. Retrieved March 2013 from **http://www.cancer.org/acs/groups/content/@epidemiologysurveilance/documents/document/acspc-036845.pdf**

American Cancer Society (ACS): What happens after treatment for Hodgkin Disease?, 2012. Retrieved April 2013 from **http://www.cancer.org/cancer/hodgkindisease/detailedguide/hodgkin-disease-after-follow-up**

Cancer Treatment Centers of America (CTCA): Cancers we treat: Various pages, 2012. Retrieved April 2013 from **http://www.cancercenter.com/cancer-type.cfm**

Dunleavy, KM, Kass, E, and Wilson, W: Lymphoma of the head and neck, 2012. Retrieved April 2012 from **http://emedicine.medscape.com/article/854110-overview**

Ellison, AM: Sickle cell disease. Advice on handling emergencies. Contemporary Pediatrics 29(9):18–27, 2012. Retrieved January 2013 from **www.ebscohost.com**

Hoyert, DL, and Xu, J: Deaths: Preliminary data for 2011. National Vital Statistics Report [NVSR] 61(6):3–4. Retrieved March 2013 from **http://www.cdc.gov/nchs/data/nvsr/nvsr61/nvsr61_06.pdf**

Hu, W: Leukemia, 2012. Retrieved April 2013 from **http://www.emedicinehealth.com/leukemia/article_em.htm**

Iron Disorders Institute: Iron overload with anemia, 2009. Retrieved from **http://www.irondisorders.org/iron-overload-with-anemia**

Leukemia and Lymphoma Society (LLS): Facts 2012. Retrieved March 2013 from **http://www.lls.org/content/nationalcontent/resourcecenter/freeeducationmaterials/generalcancer/pdf/facts.pdf**

Leukemia and Lymphoma Society (LLS): Hodgkin and Non Hodgkin lymphoma. In Facts, Spring 2013. Retrieved April 2013 from **http://www.lls.org/content/nationalcontent/resourcecenter/freeeducationmaterials/generalcancer/pdf/facts.pdf**

LWW: Nurse's 3-Minute Clinical Reference, ed 2. Lippincott, Williams & Wilkins, Philadelphia, 2008. Retrieved January 2013 from **http://www.r2library.com/Resource/Title/1582556709**

Lymphoma Research Foundation: About lymphoma: Various pages, including Non-Hodgkin lymphoma (NHL), 2012. Retrieved April 2013 from **http://www.lymphoma.org/site/pp.asp?c=bkLTKaOQLmK8E&b=6296735**

Maakaron, JE, Taher, A, and Conrad, ME: Anemia, 2011. Retrieved April 2013 from **http://emedicine.medscape.com/article/198475-overview#showall**

Maakaron, JE, Taher, A, and Woermann, UJ: Sickle cell anemia, 2013. Retrieved April 2013 from **http://emedicine.medscape.com/article/205926-overview**

Nabili, ST: Anemia, 2012. Retrieved April 2013 from **http://www.emedicinehealth.com/anemia/article_em.htm**

National Cancer Institute: Chronic lymphocytic leukemia treatment (PDQ®): Various pages, 2013. Retrieved April 2013 from **http://www.cancer.gov/cancertopics/pdq/treatment/CLL/healthprofessional**

National Cancer Institute: The cost of cancer, 2011. Retrieved April 2013 from **http://www.cancer.gov/aboutnci/servingpeople/cancer-statistics/costofcancer**

National Cancer Institute: Fatigue. PDQ®, 2013. Retrieved April 2013 from **http://www.cancer.gov/cancertopics/pdq/supportivecare/fatigue/HealthProfessional/page1**

National Heart, Lung, and Blood Institute (NHLBI) Morbidity and Mortality: 2012 chart book on cardiovascular, liver and blood diseases, 2012. Retrieved March 2013 from **http://www.nhlbi.nih.gov/resources/docs/2012_ChartBook_508.pdf**

National Hospital Discharge Survey 2009: Table: Average length of stay and days of care—Number and rate of discharges by first-listed diagnostic categories. Retrieved April 2013 from **http://www.cdc.gov/nchs/data/nhds/2average/2009ave2_firstlist.pdf**

National Institutes of Health (NIH): National Heart, Lung and Blood Institute: What is anemia? updated 2012. Retrieved April 2013 from **http://www.nhlbi.nih.gov/health/health-topics/topics/anemia/**

Raj, AB, and Bertolone, S: Sickle cell anemia, n.d. Retrieved January 2013 from **http://img.medscape.com/pi/android/medscapeapp//html/A958614-business.html**

ReutersHealth: Sickle cell disease healthcare costs high in U.S., 2009. Retrieved April 2013 from **http://www.reuters.com/article/2009/07/03/us-sickle-cell-idUSTRE5623EL20090703**

Rxlist: Aranesp, 2012. Retrieved April 2013 from **http://www.rxlist.com/aranesp-drug.htm**

Schrier, SL, Steensma, DP, and Loprinzi, CL: Role of erythropoiesis-stimulating agents in the treatment of anemia in patients with cancer, 2013. Retrieved April 2013 from paid site: **http://www.uptodate.com/contents/role-of-erythropoiesis-stimulating-agents-in-the-treatment-of-anemia-in-patients-with-cancer?source=see_link#H7**

Seiter, K: Acute myelogenous leukemia, 2012. Retrieved April 2013 from **http://emedicine.medscape.com/article/197802-overview**

SwierzewskI, SJ: Leukemia types, acute myelogenous leukemia (AML), chronic myelogenous leukemia (CML), 1999, update 2012. Retrieved April 2013 from **http://www.healthcommunities.com/leukemia/types.shtml**

Thompson, G: Splenic sequestration and sickle cell disease, 2010. Retrieved April 2013 from **http://www.webmd.com/a-to-z-guides/splenic-sequestration-and-sickle-cell-disease**

CHAPTER 10

Books

Bernhard, JD: Itch: Mechanisms and management of pruritus. McGraw-Hill, New York, 1994.

Caputi, LJ: Interventions for male clients with reproductive problems. In Ignatavicius, DD, and Workman, ML (eds): Medical-surgical nursing: Critical thinking for collaborative care, ed 5. Elsevier Saunders, St. Louis, MO, 2006.

Choka, KP: Renal failure. In Copstead, LEC, and Banasik, JL (eds): Pathophysiology, ed 3. Elsevier Saunders, St. Louis, MO, 2005.

Doenges, ME, Moorhouse, MF, and Murr, AC: Nurse's pocket guide diagnoses, prioritized interventions and rationales, ed 13. FA Davis, Philadelphia, 2013.

Fulgham, PF, and Bishoff, JT: Urinary tract imaging: Basic principles. In Wein, AJ (ed): Campbell-Walsh urology, ed 10. Saunders Elsevier, Philadelphia, 2011.

Karch, AM: Lippincott's nursing drug guide. Lippincott, Williams & Wilkins, Ambler, PA, 2008.

Lacharity, LA: Interventions for clients with acute and chronic renal failure. In Ignatavicius, DD, and Workman, ML (eds): Medical-surgical nursing: Critical thinking for collaborative care, ed 5. Elsevier Saunders, St. Louis, MO, 2006.

National Institutes of Health (NIH): Urostomy and continent urinary diversion. Publication no. 06–5629. Washington, DC, May 2006.

Porth, CM: Essentials of pathophysiology: Concepts of altered health states, ed 2. Lippincott, Williams & Wilkins, Philadelphia, 2007.

Springhouse (ed): Emergency nursing made incredibly easy! Lippincott, Williams & Wilkins, Ambler, PA, 2007.

Springhouse (ed): Pathophysiology made incredibly easy! Lippincott, Williams & Wilkins, Philadelphia, 2005.

Wei, JT, Calhoun, EA, and Jacobsen, SJ: Benign prostatic hyperplasia. In Litwin, MS, and Saigal, CS (eds): Urologic diseases in America. National Institutes for Health. NIH publication 07-5512:43–67, Washington, DC, 2007.

Winkleman, C: Interventions for clients with urinary problems. In Ignatavicius, DD, and Workman, ML (eds): Medical-surgical nursing: Critical thinking for collaborative care, ed 5. Elsevier Saunders, St. Louis, MO, 2006.

Wolfson, AB, et al: Clinical practice of emergency medicine, ed 4. Lippincott, Williams & Wilkins, Philadelphia, 2005.

Articles

Ali, B, and Gray-Vickery, P: Limiting the damage from acute kidney injury. Nursing 41(3):22–31, 2011.

Bak, GP: Teaching ostomy patients to regain their independence. Am Nurse Today 3(3):30–34, 2008.

Bent, S, Kane, C, Shinohara, K, et al: Saw palmetto for benign prostatic hyperplasia. N Engl J Med 354(6):557–566, 2006.

Burrows-Hudson, S: Chronic kidney disease: An overview. Am J Nurs 105(2):40–49, 2005.

Calabrese, DA: Prostate cancer in older men. Urol Nurs 24(4):258–264, 2004.

Cartin-Ceba, R, Kashiouris, M, Plataki, M, et al: Risk factors of development of acute kidney injury in critically ill patients: A systematic review and meta-analysis of observational studies. Crit Care Res Pract, vol. 2012, Article ID 691013, 15 pages, 2012, 10.1155/2012/691013

Centers for Disease Control and Prevention (CDC): Acute kidney injury associated with synthetic cannabinoid use—multiple states, 2012. MMWR 62(6):93–98, 2013.

Cheung, CM, Ponnusamy, A, and Anderton, JG: Management of acute renal failure in the elderly: A clinician's guide. Drugs Aging 25(6):455–476, 2008.

Chung, SH, Lindholm, B, and Lee, HB: Influence of initial nutritional status on continuous ambulatory peritoneal dialysis patient survival. Perit Dial Int 20(1):19–26, 2000.

Colwell, JC, Goldberg, M, and Carmel, J: The state of the standard diversion. J Wound Ostomy Continence Nurs 28(1):6–17, 2001.
Corbello, J, and Rosner, MH: Intradialytic total parenteral nutrition (IDPN): Evidence-based recommendations. Practical Gastroenterol April:14–28, 2009.
Davison, BJ, Moore, KN, MacMillian, H, et al: Client evaluation of a discharge program following a radical prostatectomy. Urol Nurs 24(6):483–489, 2004.
Finkelstein, VA, and Goldfarb, DS: Strategies for preventing calcium oxalate stones. CMAJ 174(10):1407–1409, 2006.
Gilchrist, K: Benign prostatic hyperplasia: Is it a precursor to prostatic cancer? Nurse Pract 29(6):30–37, 2004.
Goldberg, R, and Dennen, P. Long-term outcomes of acute kidney injury. Adv Chronic Kidney Dis 15(3):297–307, 2008.
Goodman, ED, and Ballou, MB: Perceived barriers and motivators to exercise in hemodialysis patients. Nephrol Nurs J 31(1):23–29, 2004.
Herdiman, O, Johnson, L, Lawrentschuk, N, et al: Orthotopic bladder substitution (neobladder) indications, patient selection, preoperative education, and counseling. J Wound Ostomy Continence Nurs 40(1):73–82, 2013.
Holcomb, SS: Evaluating chronic kidney disease risk. Nurse Pract 30(4):12–25, 2005.
How, PP, and Lau, AH: Malnutrition in patients undergoing hemodialysis: Is intradialytic parenteral nutrition the answer? Pharmacotherapy 24(12);1748–1758, 2004.
Litwin, MS, and Saigal, CS (eds): Urologic diseases in America. U.S. Department of Health and Human Service, Public Health Service, National Institutes of Health, National Institute of Diabetes and Digestive and Kidney Diseases. NIH Publication No. 12-7865. U.S. Government Printing Office, Washington, DC, 2012.
McGlynn, B, Al-Saffar, N, Begg, H, et al: Management of urinary incontinence following radical prostatectomy. Urol Nurs 24(6):475–482, 2004.
Mehta, RL, Kellam, JA, Shah, SV, et al: Acute Kidney Injury Network: Report of an initiative to improve outcomes in acute kidney injury. Crit Care 11(2):R31, 2007.
Miller, NL, and Lingeman, JE: Management of kidney stones. BMJ 334(7591):468–472, 2007.
Mills, RD, and Studer, UE: Metabolic consequences of continent urinary diversion. J Urol 161:1057–1066, 1999.
Mountokalakis, TD: Magnesium metabolism in chronic renal failure. Magnes Res 3(2):121–127, 1990.
National Kidney Foundation: Clinical practice guidelines for nutrition in chronic renal failure. Am J Kidney Dis 35(6 Suppl 2):S1–S140, 2000.
Neal, RH, and Keister, D: What's best for your patient with BPH? J Fam Pract 58(5):241–247, 2009.
Nikken, JJ, and Krestin, GP: MRI of the kidney—state of the art. Eur Radiol November, 17(11): 2780–2793, 2007.
Parsons, JK, Mougey, J, Lambert, L, et al: Lower urinary tract symptoms and the risk of falls in older men. J Urol 179(suppl):140; Abstract 394, 2008.
Paton, M: CRRT: Help for acute renal failure. Nursing Made Incredibly Easy! 5(5):28–38, 2007.
Pieper, B, et al: Discharge information needs of patients after surgery. J Wound, Ostomy, Continence Nurs 33(3):281–290, 2006.
Perl, J, and Chan, CT: Sleep apnea in peritoneal dialysis: Nocturnal versus continuous ambulatory treatment. Nat Clin Pract Nephrol 3(2):72–73, 2007.
Polzien, G: Chronic kidney disease and kidney failure important numbers to know. Home Health Nurs 25(10):655–660, 2007.
Pupim, LB, Flakoll, PJ, and Brouillette, JR: Intradialytic parenteral nutrition improves protein and energy homeostasis in chronic hemodialysis patients. J Clin Invest 110(4):483–492, 2002.
Rosner, MH: Acute kidney injury in the elderly: Pathogenesis, diagnosis and therapy. Aging Health 5(5):635–646, 2009.
Scales, SC, Smith, AC, Hanley, JM, et al: Prevalence of kidney stones in the United States. Eur Urol 62(1):160–165, 2012.
Sexena, R, and West, C: Peritoneal dialysis: A primary care perspective. Am Board Fam Med 19(4):380–389, 2006.
Silverman, SG, Leyendecker, JR, and Amis, ES: What is the current role of CT urography and MR urography in the evaluation of the urinary tract? Radiology 250(2):209–223, 2009.
Thurairaja, R, Burkhard, FC, and Studer UE: The orthotopic neobladder. BJU Int 102(9 Pt B):1307–1313, 2008.
Wei, JT, Calhoun, E, and Jacobson, SJ: Urologic diseases in America project: Benign prostatic hyperplasia. J Urology 179(5 Suppl):S75–S80, 2008.
Wojcik, M, and Dennison, D: Photoselective vaporization of the prostate in ambulatory surgery. AORN J 83(2):330, 2006.
Xue, JL, Daniels, F, Star, RA, et al: Incidence and mortality of acute renal failure in Medicare beneficiaries, 1992 to 2001. J Am Soc Nephrol 17(4):1135–1142, 2006.

Electronic Resources

Advanced Renal Education Program: Mortality trends in peritoneal dialysis and hemodialysis, 2011. Retrieved April 2013 from **http://www.advancedrenaleducation.com/peritonealdialysis/clinicaloutcomes/clinicaloutcomesofpdandhd**
Alper, AB, Senava, RG, and Young, BA: Uremia, 2012. Retrieved April 2012 from **http://emedicine.medscape.com/article/245296-overview#showall**
American Cancer Society (ACS): Cancer facts & figures 2013. Bladder cancer: Statistics. Retrieved April 2013 from **http://www.cancer.net/cancer-types/bladder-cancer/statistics**
American Cancer Society (ACS): Urostomy: A guide, revised 2011. Retrieved April 2013 from **http://www.cancer.org/acs/groups/cid/documents/webcontent/002931-pdf.pdf**
American Urological Association Education and Research, Inc.: AUA guideline on the management of benign prostatic hyperplasia: Diagnosis and treatment recommendations, updated 2010. Retrieved April 2013 from **http://www.auanet.org/content/guidelines-and-quality-care/clinical-guidelines/main-reports/bph-management/chap_1_GuidelineManagementof(BPH).pdf**
Centers for Disease Control and Prevention (CDC): FastStats2009: National hospital discharge survey: 2009 table, procedures by selected patient characteristics—number by procedure category and age. Retrieved March 2013 from **http://www.cdc.gov/nchs/fastats/prostate.htm**
Costa, JA, and Kreder, K: Urinary diversions and neobladders, 2012. Retrieved April 2013 from **http://emedicine.medscape.com/article/451882-overview#showall**
Deters, LA, Costabile, RA, and Leveille, RJ: Benign prostatic hypertrophy, 2013. Retrieved April 2013 from **http://emedicine.medscape.com/article/437359-overview#showall**
Fathallah-Shaykh, S, and Neiberger, R: Uric acid stones, 2013. Retrieved April 2013 from **http://emedicine.medscape.com/article/983759-overview#showall**
Gonzalez-Parra, E, Gracia-Iguacel, C, Egido, J, et al: Phosphorus and nutrition in chronic kidney disease, 2012. Retrieved April 2013 from **http://www.hindawi.com/journals/ijn/2012/597605/#B12**
Guilli, LF, Mori, A, Ettaher, AF, et al: Open prostatectomy. Surgery encyclopedia: A guide for patients and caregivers, n.d. Retrieved April 2013 from **http://www.surgeryencyclopedia.com/La-Pa/Open-Prostatectomy.html**
Hoyert, D, and Xu, J: Deaths: Preliminary data for 2011. National Vital Statistics Report (NVSR) 6(1):18, 2012. Retrieved March 2013 from **http://www.cdc.gov/nchs/data/nvsr/nvsr61/nvsr61_06.pdf**
Hudson, K: Acute renal failure. Nursing CE course, n.d. Retrieved April 2013 from **http://dynamicnursingeducation.com/class.php?class_id=131&pid=18**
Kontamwar, A: Complications of peritoneal dialysis. Slide presentation for Renal Consultants, Inc., 2011. Retrieved April 2013 from **http://www.slideshare.net/kenar78/complications-of-peritoneal-dialysis**
Lewington, A, and Kanagasundaram, S: Acute kidney injury (guidelines), 2011. Retrieved April 2013 from **http://www.renal.org/clinical/guidelinessection/AcuteKidneyInjury.aspx**
Mailloux, LU, and Henrich, WL: Patient survival and maintenance dialysis, 2013. Retrieved April 2013 from paid site: **http://www.uptodate.com/contents/patient-survival-and-maintenance-dialysis#H1**

Milenkovic, M, Russo, A, and Elixhauser, A: Hospital stays for prostate cancer, 2004. AHRQ Healthcare cost and utilization project. Statistical brief #30, 2007. Retrieved April 2013 from **http://www.hcup-us.ahrq.gov/reports/statbriefs/sb30.jsp**

Miles, BJ, Khera, M, Colen, JS, et al: Simple prostatectomy, 2011. Retrieved April 2013 from **http://emedicine.medscape.com/article/445996-overview**

National Cancer Institute (NCI): The cost of cancer, 2011. Retrieved April 2013 from **http://www.cancer.gov/aboutnci/servingpeople/cancer-statistics/costofcancer**

National Cancer Institute (NCI): Surveillance Epidemiology and End Results (SEER) 2012: SEER stat fact sheets: Bladder. Retrieved March 2013 from **http://seer.cancer.gov/statfacts/html/urinb.html**

National Cancer Institute (NCI): Tracking the rise of robotic surgery for prostate cancer. National Cancer Bulletin 8(16):2011. Retrieved March 2013 from **http://www.cancer.gov/ncicancerbulletin/080911/page4**

National Institutes of Health: Fact sheet: Chronic kidney disease and kidney failure, 2013. Retrieved April 2013 from **http://report.nih.gov/nihfactsheets/ViewFactSheet.aspx?csid=34**

National Institutes of Health: Kidney failure: Choosing a treatment that's right for you, 2010. Retrieved April 2013 from **http://kidney.niddk.nih.gov/kudiseases/pubs/choosingtreatment/**

National Kidney Foundation: Kidney Disease Outcome Quality Initiative (KDOQI). KDOQI clinical practice guidelines for chronic kidney disease: Evaluation, classification, and stratification, 2002. Retrieved April 2013 from **http://www.kidney.org/professionals/kdoqi/guidelines_ckd/p1_exec.htm**

National Kidney Foundation: Fact sheets 2013. Retrieved March 2013 from **http://www.kidney.org/news/newsroom/factsheets/CKD-A-Growing-Problem.cfm**

National Kidney and Urologic Diseases Information Clearinghouse (NKUDIC): Eat right to feel right on hemodialysis, update 2012. Retrieved April 2013 from **http://kidney.niddk.nih.gov/kudiseases/pubs/eatright/**

National Kidney and Urologic Diseases Information Clearinghouse (NKUDIC): Hemodialysis dose and adequacy, 2009. Retrieved April 2013 from **http://kidney.niddk.nih.gov/kudiseases/pubs/hemodialysisdose/index.aspx**

National Kidney and Urologic Diseases Information Clearinghouse (NKUDIC): Kidney disease statistics for the United States, 2012. Retrieved April 2013 from **http://kidney.niddk.nih.gov/KUDiseases/pubs/kustats/index.aspx**

National Kidney And Urologic Diseases Information Clearinghouse (NKUDIC): Kidney disease statistics for the United States, 2012. Retrieved March 2013 from **http://kidney.niddk.nih.gov/kudiseases/pubs/kustats/ku_diseases_stats_508.pdf**

National Kidney and Urologic Diseases Information Clearing House (NKUDIC): Kidney stones in adults, 2013. Retrieved April 2013 from **http://kidney.niddk.nih.gov/kudiseases/pubs/stonesadults/**

National Kidney and Urologic Diseases Information Clearinghouse (NKUDIC): Treatment methods for kidney failure: Hemodialysis, 2010. Retrieved April 2013 from **http://kidney.niddk.nih.gov/kudiseases/pubs/hemodialysis/index.aspx**

National Kidney and Urologic Diseases Information Clearinghouse (NKUDIC): Treatment methods for kidney failure: Peritoneal dialysis, 2010. Retrieved April 2013 from **http://kidney.niddk.nih.gov/kudiseases/pubs/peritoneal/**

Peacock, PR, and Sinert, RH: Management of acute complications of acute renal failure, 2011. Retrieved April 2013 from **http://emedicine.medscape.com/article/777845-overview**

Pradeep, A, and Batuman, V: Chronic kidney disease, 2013. Retrieved April 2013 from **http://emedicine.medscape.com/article/238798-overview**

Prostatehealthcures.com: Prostate disease statistics, 2006–2013. Retrieved April 2013 from **http://www.prostatehealthcures.com/prostate-cat/prostate-statistics**

Schmidt, M: Non-cancerous causes of elevated PSA, 2009. Retrieved April 2013 from **http://prostatecancer.about.com/od/symptomsanddiagnosis/a/psacauses.htm**

Sofocleous, CT, Cerveira, J, Cooper, SG, et al: Dialysis fistulas, 2011. Retrieved April 2013 from **http://emedicine.medscape.com/article/419393-overview#showall**

Suracusano, S, Ciciliato, S, and Visalli, F: Current trends in urinary diversion in men, 2012. Retrieved April 2013 from **http://cdn.intechopen.com/pdfs/27330/InTech-Current_trends_in_urinary_diversion_in_men.pdf**

Urology Care Foundation: Continent urinary diversion, 2011. Retrieved April 2013 from **http://www.urologyhealth.org/urology/index.cfm?article=106**

U.S. Renal Data System (USRDS): 2012 Annual data report: Atlas of chronic kidney disease and end-stage renal disease in the United States. National Institutes of Health, National Institute of Diabetes and Digestive and Kidney Diseases, Bethesda, MD, 2012. Retrieved March 2013 from **http://www.usrds.org/reference.aspx**

Wedro, BC: Kidney stones, 2010. Retrieved April 2013 from **http://www.emedicinehealth.com/kidney_stones/article_em.htm**

Wolf, JS, Howes, DS, Craig, S, et al: Nephrolithiasis, 2013. Retrieved April 2013 from **http://emedicine.medscape.com/article/437096-overview#showall**

Workeneh, BT, Agraharkar, M, and Gupta, R: Acute kidney injury, 2013. Retrieved April 2013 from **http://emedicine.medscape.com/article/243492-overview**

CHAPTER 11

Books

American Cancer Society (ACS): Breast cancer facts and figures 2011–2012. American Cancer Society, Atlanta, GA, 2011.

Bland, KI, and Copeland, EM: The breast: Comprehensive management of benign and malignant disease. Vols 1 and 2, ed 4. Saunders Elsevier, Philadelphia, 2009.

Mohamed, I, and Skeel, RT: Carcinoma of the breast. In Skeel, RT (ed): Handbook for cancer chemotherapy, ed 6. Lippincott, Williams & Wilkins, Philadelphia, 2003.

Winer, EP, Morrow, M, Osborne, CK, et al: Malignant tumors of the breast. In DeVita, VT, Hellman, S, and Rosenberg, SA (eds): Cancer: Principles and practice of oncology. Lippincott, Williams & Wilkins, Philadelphia, 2001.

Articles

Augustus, CE: Beliefs and perspectives of African American women who have had hysterectomies. J Transcul Nurs 13(4):296–302, 2002.

Bunde, M, et al: On-line hysterectomy support: Characteristics of website experience. Cyberpsychol Behav 10(1):80–85, 2007.

Buren, JM, and Linton, C: The role of exercise in treating lymphedema. Rehab Manage 13(6):26–31, 2000.

Downs-Holmes, C, and Silverman, P: Breast cancer: Overview & updates. Nurse Pract 36(12):20–26, 2011.

Ely, S, and Vioral, AN: Breast cancer overview. Plast Surg Nurs 27(3):128–133, 2007.

Greenlee, RT, Murray, T, Bolden, S, et al: Cancer statistics, 2000. CA Cancer J Clin 50(1):7–33, 2000.

Katz, A: Sexuality after hysterectomy: A review of the literature and discussion of nursing roles. J Adv Nurs 42(3):297–303, 2003.

Ligibel, JA, Giobbe-Hurder, A, Olenzcuk, D, et al: Impact of a mixed strength and endurance exercise intervention on insulin levels in breast cancer survivors. J Clin Oncol 26(6):907–912, 2008.

Lo, SS, Mumby, PB, Norton, J, et al: Prospective multicenter study of the impact of the 21-gene recurrence score assay on medical oncologist and patient adjuvant breast cancer treatment selection. J Clin Oncol 28(10):1671–1676, 2010.

Mamounas, EP, Tang, G, Fisher, B, et al: Association between the 21-gene recurrence score assay and risk of locoregional recurrence in node-negative, estrogen receptor-positive breast cancer: Results from NSABP B-14 and NSABP B-20. J Clin Oncol 28(10):1677–1683, 2010.

Moreria, V: Hysterectomy: Nursing the physical and emotional wounds. Nurs Times 96(20):41–42, 2000.

Risser, N, and Murphy, M: Literature review: Women's health care: Sexual function after hysterectomy. Nurs Pract 29(2):49, 2004.

Thomas, S, and Greifzu, SP: Oncology today: Breast cancer. RN 63(4):40–45, 2000a.
Thomas, S, and Greifzu, SP: Oncology today: Breast reconstruction. RN 63(4):45–47, 2000b.
Walling, AD: Laparoscopic vs. abdominal hysterectomy: A comparison. Am Family Phys 70(8):1570–1575, 2004.
Warren, A, Brorson, H, Barud, SJ, et al: Lymphedema: A comprehensive review. Ann Plast Surg 59(4):464–472, 2007.

Electronic Resources

American College of Obstetricians and Gynecologists: Hysterectomy, 2011. Retrieved April 2013 from **http://www.acog.org/~/media/For%20Patients/faq008.pdf?dmc=1&ts=20130424T1346545747**
Bauers, D: Emotional effects of having a hysterectomy in your 30's, 2010. Retrieved April 2013 from **http://www.helium.com/items/1874487-how-can-having-a-hysterectomy-women-in-their-thirties**
Cancer Action Network: Cancer and Medicare—A chartbook, 2009. Retrieved April 2013 from **http://www.allhealth.org/briefingmaterials/CancerandMedicareChartbookFinalfulldocumentMarch11-1412.pdf**
Cancer Treatment Centers of America (CTCA): Types of breast cancer, 2012. Retrieved April 2013 from **http://www.cancercenter.com/breast-cancer/types.cfm**
Centers for Disease Control and Prevention (CDC): Hysterectomy in the United States, 2000–2004, 2008. Retrieved April 2013 from **http://www.cdc.gov/reproductivehealth/womensrh/00-04-FS_Hysterectomy.htm**
Encyclopedia of Surgery: Hysterectomy, n.d. Retrieved April 2013 from **http://www.surgeryencyclopedia.com/Fi-La/Hysterectomy.html**
Gor, HB: Hysterectomy, 2012 Retrieved April 2013 from **http://emedicine.medscape.com/article/267273-overview**
Mayo Clinic: Mastectomy, 2011. Retrieved April 2013 from **http://www.mayoclinic.com/health/mastectomy/MY00943**
National Cancer Institute (NCI): Breast cancer, 2013: Retrieved March 2013 from **http://www.cancer.gov/cancertopics/types/breast**
National Cancer Institute (NCI): Breast cancer. Various articles, including statistics, 2012. Retrieved April 2013 from **http://www.cancer.gov/cancertopics/wyntk/breast/page6**
National Cancer Institute (NCI): The cost of cancer, 2011. Retrieved April 2013 from **http://www.cancer.gov/aboutnci/servingpeople/cancer-statistics/costofcancer**
National Comprehensive Cancer Network (NCCN): Breast cancer treatment guidelines for patients, 2011. Retrieved April 2013 from **http://www.nccn.com/cancer-guidelines.html**
National Guideline Clearinghouse: Breast cancer screening: A national clinical guideline, 2011. Retrieved April 2013 from **http://guideline.gov/content.aspx?id=34275**
National Women's Health Network (NWHN): Hysterectomy: Fact sheets, 2005. Retrieved April 2013 from **http://nwhn.org/hysterectomy**
New York Presbyterian: Lymphedema following mastectomy, 2008. Retrieved April 2013 from **http://nyp.org/health/breast-lymph.html**
Pfunter, A, Levit, K, and Elixhauser, A: Healthcare Cost and Utilization Project (H_CUP); Statistical brief #133: Components of cost increases for inpatient hospital procedures, 1997–2009, 2012. Retrieved April 2012 from **http://www.hcup-us.ahrq.gov/reports/statbriefs/sb133.pdf**
Surgery.com: Hysterectomy: Morbidity and mortality, 2009. **http://www.surgery.com/procedure/hysterectomy/morbidity-mortality**
Todd, N: Surgical menopause: Should you take estrogen after your hysterectomy? 2012. Retrieved April 2013 from **http://women.webmd.com/surgical-menopause-estrogen-after-hysterectomy**

CHAPTER 12

Books

Margolis, DJ, Malay, DS, Hoffstad, OJ, et al: Incidence of diabetic foot ulcer and lower extremity amputation among medicare beneficiaries, 2006–2008. In Data Points Publication Series [Internet]. Rockville (MD): Agency for Healthcare Research and Quality (US), 2011.
Weinstein, SL, and Buckwalter, JA: Turek's orthopaedics principles and their applications, ed 6. Philadelphia, Lippincott, Williams, & Wilkins. 2005.

Articles

Aulivola, B, Hile, CN, Hamdan, AD, et al: Major lower extremity amputation: Outcome of a modern series. Arch Surg 139(4):395–399, 2004.
Bailey, J: Getting a fix on orthopedic care. Nursing 33(6):58–63, 2003.
Bradley, JB, Slauterbeck, J, and Benjamin, JB: Fracture patterns and mechanisms in pedestrian motor vehicle trauma: The ipsilateral dyad. J OrthopTrauma 6(3):279–282, 1992.
Cho, TJ, Gerstenfeld, C, and Einhorn, TA: Differential temporal expression of members of the transforming growth factor β superfamily during murine fracture healing. J Bone Miner Res 17(3):513–520, 2002.
D'Arcy, Y, and Tovornik, M: How to control pain and improve functionality after total joint replacement surgery. Nursing 6(Suppl Therapy Insider):2–5, 2007.
Dillingham, TR, Pezzin, LE, and Shore, AD: Reamputation, mortality, and health care costs among persons with dysvascular lower-limb amputations. Arch Phys Med Rehabil 86(3):480–486, 2005.
Frost, HM: The biology of fracture healing. An overview for clinicians. Part I. Clin Orthop Relat Res (248):283–293, 1989.
Frakes, M, and Evans, T: Major pelvic fractures. Crit Care Nurse 24(2):24–30, 2004.
Inderjeeth, CA, Glennon, D, and Petta, A: Study of osteoporosis awareness, investigation and treatment of patients discharged from a tertiary public teaching hospital. Intern Med 36(9):547–555, 2006.
Iverson, MD: Rehabilitation interventions for pain and disability in osteoarthritis: A review of interventions including exercise, manual techniques, and assistive devices. Orthop Nurs 31(2):103–108, 2012.
Matielo, MF, Presti, C, Casella, IB, et al: Incidence of ipsilateral postoperative deep venous thrombosis in the amputated lower extremity of patients with peripheral obstructive arterial disease. J Vasc Surg 48(6):1514–1519, 2008.
Matsuda, K, Nozawa, M, Katsube, S, et al: Activation of fibrinolysis by reinfusion of unwashed salvaged blood after total knee arthroplasty. Transfus Apher Sci 42:33–37, 2010.
Nowygrod, R, Egorova, N, Greco, G, et al: Trends, complications, and mortality in peripheral vascular surgery. J Vasc Surg 43(2):205–216, 2006.
Peacock, JM, Keo, HH, Duval, S, et al: The incidence and health economic burden of ischemic amputation in Minnesota, 2005–2008. Preventing Chronic Disease: Public Health Research, Practice, and Policy 8(6):1–8, 2011.
Prvu-Bettger, J, Bates, B, Bidelspach, D, et al: Short- and long-term prognosis among veterans with neurological disorders and subsequent lower-extremity amputation. Neuroepidemiology 32(1):4–10, 2009.
Smeltzer, MD: Making a point about open fractures. Nursing 40(4):24–30, 2010.
Walsh, C: Breaking bad: What you need to know about femur fractures. OR Nurse 5(1):30–38, 2011.
Wilson, T: Advanced prosthetic devices aid amputees. Disabled Am Veterans (DAV) Magazine (November/December), 2004.
Ziegler-Graham, K, Mackenzie, EJ, Ephraim, PL, et al: Estimating the prevalence of limb loss in the United States: 2005 to 2050. Arch Phys Med Rehabil 89(3):422–429, 2008.

Pamphlet

Margolis, DJ, Malay, DS, Hoffstad, OJ, et al: Incidence of diabetic foot ulcer and lower extremity amputation among medicare beneficiaries, 2006–2008. In Data Points Publication Series [Internet]. Rockville (MD): Agency for Healthcare Research and Quality (US), 2011.

Electronic Resources

American Academy of Orthopedic Surgeons (AAOS): Fractures (broken bones), 2012. Retrieved May 2013 from **http://orthoinfo.aaos.org/topic.cfm?topic=A00139**
Amputation Coalition. Limb Loss Resource Center: Resources by amputation level, 2012. Retrieved 2012 from **http://amputee-coalition.org/limb-loss-resource-center/resources-by-amputation-level/**

Buckley, R, and Panaro, CDA: General principles of fracture care. 2012, Retrieved May 2013 from **http://emedicine.medscape.com/article/1270717-overview#showall**

Budd, L: Pediatric fractures, 2012. Retrieved May 2013 from **http://learnpediatrics.com/body-systems/musculoskeletal-system/pediatric-fractures/**

The Burden of Musculoskeletal Diseases in the United States, (BMUS) Joint Project, 2008: Prevalence, societal and economic cost. Retrieved March 2013 from **http://www.boneandjointburden.org/pdfs/BMUS_chpt4_arthritis.pdf**

Centers for Disease Control and Prevention (CDC): National Hospital Discharge Survey: 2010 table, Procedures by selected patient characteristics—Number by procedure category and age, 2010. Retrieved May 2013 from **http://www.cdc.gov/nchs/fastats/insurg.htm**

Clontz, AS, Annonio, D, and Walker, L: Trauma nursing: Amputation, 2004. Retrieved May 2013 from **http://www.modernmedicine.com/modern-medicine/news/trauma-nursing-amputation**

Cram, P, Lu, X, Kates, SL, et al: Total knee arthroplasty volume, utilization, and outcomes among medicare beneficiaries, 1991–2010. JAMA; 308(12):1227–1236, 2012. Retrieved April 2013 from **http://www.sciencedaily.com/releases/2012/09/120925171450.htm**

Ertl, JP, and Ertl, W: Amputations of the lower extremity, 2012. Retrieved May 2013 from **http://emedicine.medscape.com/article/1232102-overview**

Fragomen, AT, and Rozbruch, SR: The mechanics of external fixation, 2007. **http://www.kidsfractures.com/**

Goel, K: Study outlines risk factors for poor outcome, mortality following hip fracture—Mortality and morbidity—Trauma & injuries, 2013. Retrieved May 2013 from **http://www.health.am/ab/more/outcome-mortality-following-hip-fracture/#ixzz2SG93Y9mq**

Goff, BJ, Mccann, TD, Mody, RM, et al: Medical issues in the care of the combat amputee, 2009. Retrieved May 2013 from **https://ke.army.mil/bordeninstitute/published_volumes/amputee/ccachapter10.pdf**

Huffington Post: U.S. wounded in Iraq, Afghanistan includes more than 1,500 amputees, 2012. Retrieved May 2013 from **http://www.huffingtonpost.com/2012/11/07/iraq-afghanistan-amputees_n_2089911.html**

Jackson, DW: Tips and pearls: Minimizing blood transfusion following primary total knee replacement, 2010. Retrieved May 2013 from **http://www.healio.com/orthopedics/hip/news/print/orthopedics-today/%7B311e17c7-da5a-4aaf-b34e-5252ea55bf56%7D/tips-and-pearls-minimizing-blood-transfusion-following-primary-totalknee-replacement**

Jagminas, L: Compartment pressure measurement, 2011. Retrieved May 2013 from **http://emedicine.medscape.com/article/140002-overview**

Kalapatapu, V: Lower extremity amputation, 2012. Retrieved May 2013 from paid site **http://www.uptodate.com/contents/lower-extremity-amputation**

Kidsfractures.com: Various pages, 2011. Retrieved May 2013 from **http://www.kidsfractures.com/**

Kirkland, L: Fat embolism, 2013. Retrieved May 2013 from **http://emedicine.medscape.com/article/460524-overview**

Kirshner, S, and Laborde, JM: Gait analysis after amputation, 2011. Retrieved May 2013 from **http://emedicine.medscape.com/article/1237638-overview**

Liu, SS, Della Valle, AG, Besculides, AC, et al: Trends in mortality, complications, and demographics for primary hip arthroplasty in the United States, 2009. Retrieved May 2013 from **http://www.ncbi.nlm.nih.gov/pmc/articles/PMC2903109/**

Mahar, P: Pediatric orthopedic emergencies (PowerPoint presentation at The Children's Hospital, University of Colorado Health Sciences), 2011. Retrieved May 2013 from **http://www.rockymtncme.com/sites/rockymtncme.com/UserFiles/Pediatric%20Ortho%20Emergencies%20P_%20MAHAR.pdf**

National Health Statistics Report: National Hospital Discharge Survey: 2007 Summary, 2007. Retrieved May 2013 from **http://www.cdc.gov/nchs/data/nhsr/nhsr029.pdf**

National Limb Loss Information Center (NLLIC): Fact Sheet: Pain management and the amputee, updated 2008. Retrieved May 2013 from **http://www.amputee-coalition.org/easyread/fact_sheets/painmgmt-ez.html**

National Limb Loss Information Center (NLLIC) Staff: Wound care: Preventing infection. Amputee Coalition of America Fact Sheet revised 2009. Retrieved May 2013 from **http://www.amputee-coalition.org/fact_sheets/woundcare.pdf**

Rasul, AT, and Wright, J: Total joint replacement rehabilitation, 2012. Retrieved May 2013 from **http://emedicine.medscape.com/article/320061-overview**

Schuch, CM: Consumer guide for amputees: A guide to lower limb prosthetics: Part 1—Prosthetic designs: Basic concepts. inMotion: a Publication of the Amputee Coalition of America, updated 2008. Retrieved May 2013 from **http://www.amputee-coalition.org/inmotion/mar_apr_98/pros_primer/page1.html**

Shiel, WC: Total hip replacement, 2012. Retrieved May 2013 from **http://www.emedicinehealth.com/total_hip_replacement/article_em.htm**

Wedro, B: Compartment syndrome, 2010. Retrieved May 2012 from **http://www.medicinenet.com/compartment_syndrome/article.htm**

CHAPTER 13

Books

Benjamin, D, and Herndon, DN: Special considerations of age: The pediatric burned patient. In Herndon, DN (ed): Total burn care, ed 2. Saunders, London, 2002.

Green, TL: Principles and practices of rehabilitation. In Smeltzer, SC, Bare, BG, Hinkle, JL, et al (eds): Brunner & Suddarth's textbook of medical-surgical nursing, ed 12. Wolters Kluwer/Lippincott, Williams & Wilkins, Philadelphia, 2010.

Hartford, CE, and Kealey, GP: Care of outpatient burns. In Herndon, DN, and Jones, JH (eds): Total burn care, ed 3. WB Saunders, Philadelphia, 2007.

Stotts, NA: Nutritional assessment and support. In Bryant, RA, and Nix, DP (eds): Acute & chronic wounds: Current management concepts, ed 4. Elsevier, St. Louis, MO, 2012.

Articles

Abbade, LP, and Lastória, S: Venous ulcer: Epidemiology, physiopathology, diagnosis and treatment. Int J Dermatol 44(6):449–456, 2005.

Alexander, G, Saldanha, J, Ebrahim, MK, et al: Is routine admission chest radiograph of any clinical value in non-intensive care burn patients without inhalation injury? Burns 29(5):499–500, 2003.

Ayello, AE, Burrell, RE, Goodman, L, et al: Special considerations in wound bed preparation 2011: An update. Adv Skn Wound Care 24(9):415–436, 2011.

Brem, H, Sheehan, P, Rosenberg, H, et al: Evidence-based protocol for diabetic foot ulcers. J Plast Reconstr Surg 117:193S–209S, 2006.

Connor-Ballard, PA: Understanding and managing burn pain: Part 2. Am J Nurs 109(5):54–62, 2009.

Dale, BA, and Wright, DH: Say goodbye to wet-to-dry wound care dressings: Changing the culture of wound care management within your agency. Home Healthc Nurse 29(7):429–440, 2011.

Demling, RH, and DeSanti, L: Closure of partial-thickness facial burns with a bioactive skin substitute in the major burn population decreases the cost of care and improves outcome. Wounds 14(6):230–234, 2002.

DeSanti, L: Pathophysiology and current management of burn injury. Adv Skin Wound Care 18(6):323–332, 2005.

Fogg, E: Best treatment of non-healing and problematic wounds. JAAPA 22(8):46–48, 2009.

Fong, J, Wood, F, and Fowler, B: A silver coated dressing reduces the incidence of early burn wound cellulitis and associated costs of inpatient treatment: Comparative patient care audits. Burns 31(15):562–567, 2005.

Hedman, TL, Evans, EM, Richard, RL, et al: Incidence and severity of combat hand burns after all army activity message. J Trauma 64(2Suppl):S169–172, 2008.

Hettiaratchy, S, and Dziewulski, P: Pathophysiology and types of burns. BMJ 328:1427–1429, 2004.

Jeschke, MG, Mlcak, RP, Finnerty, CC, et al: Burn size determines the inflammatory and hypermetabolic response. Crit Care 11(4):R90, 2007.
Johnson, RM, and Richard, R: Partial-thickness burns: Identification and management. Adv Skin Wound Care 16(4):178–186, 2003.
Jones, I, Currie, L, and Martin, R: A guide to biological skin substitutes. Br J Plast Surg 55(3):185–193, 2002.
Keast, DH, Bowering, CK, Evans, AW, et al: MEASURE: A proposed assessment framework for developing best practice recommendations for wound assessment. Wound Repair Regen 12(3 Suppl):S1–S17, 2004.
Maguire, S, Moynihan, S, Mann, M, et al: A systematic review of the features that indicate intentional scalds in children. Burns 34(8):1072–1081, 2008.
McBride, JW, Labrosse, KR, McCoy, HG, et al: Is serum creatine kinase-MB in electrically injured patients predictive of myocardial injury? JAMA 255(6):764–768, 1986.
Merrell, SW, Saffle, JR, Sullivan, JJ, et al: Fluid resuscitation in thermally injured children. Am J Surg 15(6):664–669, 1986.
Morgan, ED, Bledsoe, SC, and Barker, J: Ambulatory management of burns. Am Fam Physician 62(9):2015–2026, 2000.
Nemeth, KA, Harrison, MB, Graham, ID, et al: Understanding venous leg ulcer pain: Results of a longitudinal study. Ostomy Wound Management 50(1):34–36, 2004.
Park-Lee, EY, and Decker, FH: Comparison of home health and hospice agencies by organizational characteristics and services provided: United States 2007. National Health Statistics Report, No 30, 2007.
Peck, MD, and Priolo-Kapel, D: Child abuse by burning: A review of the literature and an algorithm for medical investigations. J Trauma 53(5):1013–1022, 2002.
Pham, C, Greenwood, J, Cleland, H, et al: Bioengineered skin substitutes for the management of burns: A systematic review. Burns 33(8):946–957, 2007.
Pham, TN, Cancio, LC, and Gibran, NS: American Burn Association practice guidelines, burn shock resuscitation. J Burn Care Res 29(1):257–266, 2008.
Rayner, R: Effects of cigarette smoking on cutaneous wound healing. Prim Intent 14:100–102, 104, 2006.
Reed, JL, and Pomerantz, WJ: Emergency management of pediatric burns. Pediatr Emerg Care 21(2):118–129, 2005.
Singer, AJ, and Thode, H:. National analgesia prescribing patterns in emergency department patients with burns. J Burn Care Rehabil 23(6):361–365, 2002.
Sullivan, SR, Friedrich, JB, Engrav, LH, et al: "Opioid creep" is real and may be the cause of "fluid creep." Burns 30(6):583–590, 2004.
Tang, JC, Vivas, A, Kirsner, RS, et al: Atypical ulcers: Wound biopsy results from a university wound pathology service. Ostomy Wound Manage 58(6):20–29, 2012.
Tomkins, KL, and Holland AJ: Electrical burn injuries in children. J Paediatr Child Health 44(12):727–730, 2008.
Toon, MH, Maybauer, DM, and Arceneaux, LL: Children with burn injuries—Assessment of trauma, neglect, violence and abuse. J Inj Violence Res 3(2):98–110, 2011.
Wiebelhaus, P, and Hansen, SL: What you should know about managing burn emergencies. Nursing 31(1):36–41, 2001.
Wiechman, SA, and Patterson, DR: ABC of burns: Psychosocial aspects of burn injuries. BMJ 329(7462):391–393, 2003.
Williams, FN, Herndon, DN, Hawkins, HK, et al: The leading causes of death after burn injury in a single pediatric burn center. Crit Care 13(6):183, 2009.
Woo, K, Sibbald, G. Fogh, K, et al: Assessment and management of persistent (chronic) and total wound pain. Int Wound J 5(2):205–215, 2008.

Electronic Resources

American Burn Association (ABA): Burn incidence and treatment in the United States: 2012 Fact Sheet, 2012. Retrieved March 2013 from **http://www.ameriburn.org/resources_factsheet**
Burn Injury online.com: Burn injury deaths, 2011. Retrieved May 2013 from **http://www.burninjuryonline.com/burn-injury-deaths/**
Centers for Disease Control and Prevention: Fire deaths and injuries: Fact sheet, 2011. Retrieved May 2013 from **http://www.cdc.gov/HomeandRecreationalSafety/Fire-Prevention/fires-factsheet.html**
Cunha, J: Thermal (heat or fire) burns, 2007. Retrieved May 2013 from **http://www.emedicinehealth.com/thermal_heat_or_fire_burns/article_em.htm**
Daley, BJ: Wound care, 2013. Retrieved May 2013 from **http://emedicine.medscape.com/article/194018-overview#showall**
Edlich, RF, Drake, DB, and Long, WB: Thermal burns, 2010. Retrieved May 2013 from **http://emedicine.medscape.com/article/1278244-overview**
Enoch, S, and Price, P: Cellular, molecular and biochemical differences in the pathophysiology of healing between acute wounds, chronic wounds and wounds in the aged, 2004. Retrieved May 2013 from **http://www.worldwidewounds.com/2004/august/Enoch/Pathophysiology-Of-Healing.html**
European Pressure Ulcer Advisory Panel and National Pressure Ulcer Advisory Panel (EPUAP/NPUAP): Prevention and treatment of pressure ulcers: Quick reference guide. National Pressure Ulcer Advisory Panel, Washington, DC, 2009. Retrieved May 2013 from **http://www.npuap.org/wp-content/uploads/2012/02/Final_Quick_Prevention_for_web_2010.pdf**
Granger, JP, Estrada, CM, and Abramo, TJ: An evidence-based approach to pediatric burns, 2009. Retrieved May 2013 from **http://www.ebmedicine.net/topics.php?paction=showTopic&topic_id=186**
Mirsaidi, N: U.S. Food and Drug Administration Medical Devices—Negative pressure wound therapy: Use with caution, update 2012. Retrieved May 2013 from **http://www.fda.gov/MedicalDevices/Safety/AlertsandNotices/TipsandArticlesonDeviceSafety/ucm225038.htm**
National Institute of Health and Clinical Excellence (NICE): Surgical site infection: Prevention and treatment of surgical site infection (CG74), 2008. Retrieved May 2013 from **http://www.nice.org/uk/guidance/CG74/NiceGuidance/pdf/English**
National Pressure Ulcer Advisory Panel (NPUAD):. NPUAP pressure ulcer stages/categories, 2007. Retrieved May 2013 from **http://www.npuap.org/resources/educational-and-clinical-resources/npuap-pressure-ulcer-stagescategories/**
Salcido, R, Popescu, A, Potter, PJ, et al: Pressure ulcers and wound care, 2012. Retrieved May 2013 from **http://emedicine.medscape.com/article/319284-overview**
Serebrisky, D, Nazarian, EB, and Connolly, H: Inhalation injury, 2012. Retrieved May 2013 from **http://emedicine.medscape.com/article/1002413-overview**
U.S. Food and Drug Administration (FDA): Medical devices. Epicel® cultured epidermal autograft (CEA)-H990002, 2013. Retrieved May 2013 from **http://www.fda.gov/MedicalDevices/ProductsandMedicalProcedures/DeviceApprovalsandClearances/Recently-ApprovedDevices/ucm074878.htm**

CHAPTER 14

Books

Abrams, AC, Pennington, SS, and Lammon, CB: Clinical drug therapy: Rationales for nursing practice, ed 8. Lippincott, Williams and Wilkins, Philadelphia, 2007.
Bulechek, GM, Butcher, HK, and Dochterman, JM (eds): Nursing Interventions Classification (NIC), ed 5. Mosby/Elsevier, St. Louis, MO, 2008.
Deglin, JH, and Vallerand, AH: Davis's drug guide for nurses, ed 13. FA Davis, Philadelphia, 2010.
Durham, JD, and Lashley, FR (eds): The person with HIV/AIDS, ed 4. Springer Publishing Company, New York, 2010.
Flynn, JA, and Johnson, T: The Johns Hopkins white papers: Arthritis. Stuart Jordon, Baltimore, MD, 2008.
Herdman, TH (ed): NANDA International Nursing Diagnoses: Definitions & classifications, 2012–2014. Wiley-Blackwell, Oxford, UK, 2012.
Moorhead, S, Johnson, M, Maas, M, et al (eds): Nursing Outcomes Classification (NOC), ed 4. Mosby/Elsevier, St. Louis, MO, 2008.
Nettina, SM: Lippincott manual of nursing practice, ed 8. Lippincott, Williams and Wilkins, Ambler, PA, 2006.
Sampson, JG: Interventions for clients with HIV/AIDS and other immunodeficiencies. In Ignatavicius, DD, and Workman, ML

(eds): Medical-surgical nursing: Critical thinking for collaborative care, ed 5. Elsevier Saunders, St. Louis, MO, 2006.

Smeltzer, SS, Bare, BG, Hinkle, JL, et al: Brunner and Suddarth's textbook of medical-surgical nursing, ed 11. Lippincott, Williams and Wilkins, Philadelphia, 2008.

Van Leeuwen, AM, Kranptiz, TR, and Smith, L: Davis's comprehensive handbook of laboratory and diagnostic tests with nursing implications, ed 2. FA Davis, Philadelphia, 2006.

Workman, ML: Concepts of inflammation and the immune response. In Ignatavicius, DD, and Workman, ML (eds): Medical-surgical nursing: Critical thinking for collaborative care, ed 5. Elsevier Saunders, St. Louis, MO, 2006.

Articles

Abuedo, MA: Regulations, technology guide multivisceral transplant success. OR Nurse 1(7):24–29, 2007.

Arhens, T: Sepsis: Stopping an insidious killer. Am Nurse Today 2(1): 36–39, 2007.

Bosek, M, and Shaner-McRae, H: Ethics in practice: Hand hygiene as standard practice: Do the rules apply to all healthcare professionals? JONA's Healthc Law, Ethics, and Regul 12(4):101–105, 2010.

Braun, L, Cooper, LM, Malatestinic, WN, et al: A sepsis review: Epidemiology, economics, and disease characteristics. Dimens Crit Care Nurs 22 (3):117–124, 2003.

Bruce, ML, and Peck, B: New rheumatoid arthritis treatments. Holistic Nurs Pract 19(5):197–204, 2005.

Clancy, RL, McCabe, S, Pierce, JD, et al: Biomarkers: An important clinical assessment tool. Am J Nurs 112(9):52–58, 2012.

Coe, PF: Managing pulmonary hypertension in heart transplantation: Meeting the challenge. Crit Care Nurse 20(2):22–28, 2000.

Dew, MA, DiMartini, AF, De Vito, D, et al: Rates and risk factors for non-adherence to the medical regimen after adult solid organ transplantation. Transplantation 83(7):858–873, 2007.

Frank-Bader, M, Beltran, K, and Dojlidko, D: Improving transplant discharge education using a structured teaching approach. Prog Transplant 21(4):332–339, 2011.

Gebo, KA, Fleishman, JA, Conviser, R, et al: HIV Research Network. Contemporary costs of HIV healthcare in the HAART era. AIDS 24(17):2705–2715, 2010.

Graudal, NA, Jurik, AG, de Carvalho, A, et al: Radiographic progression in rheumatoid arthritis: A long-term prospective study of 109 patients. Arthritis and Rheumatism 41(8):1470–1480, 1998.

Greenwald, JL, Burstein, GR, Pincus, J, et al: A rapid review of Rapid HIV Antibody Tests. Curr Infect Dis Rep 8:125–131, 2006.

Helmick, CG, Felson, DT, Lawrence, RC, et al: Estimates of the prevalence of arthritis and other rheumatic conditions in the United States. Part I. Arthritis Rheum 58(1):15–25, 2008.

Jones, SG: A step-by-step approach to HIV/AIDS. Nurse Pract 31(6):26–39, 2006.

Johnson, M, Kaehler, B, Lecy, B, et al: Patient safety: Tips for successful hand hygiene. Nursing 41(11):18–20, 2011.

Kaplan, JE, Benson, C, and Holmes, KK: Guidelines for prevention and treatment of opportunistic infections in HIV-infected adults and adolescents. MMWR Recommendations and Reports, April 10, 2009/58(RR04):1–198, 2009.

Kleinpell, RM: Stop severe sepsis in its tracks. Nursing2008 1(1):20–26, 2006.

Kurz, JM, and Cavanaugh, JC: A qualitative study of stress and coping strategies used by well spouses of lung transplant candidates. Families, Systems, & Health 19(2):181–197, 2001.

Latto, C: An overview of sepsis. Dimensions of Crit Care 27(5):195–200, 2008.

Lucey, MR, Terrault, N, Ojo, N, et al: Long-term management of the successful adult liver transplant: 2012 practice guideline by the American Association for the Study of Liver Diseases and the American Society of Transplantation. Liver Transpl 19(1):3–26, 2013.

Mallard, VJ, et al: Increasing knowledge of sexually transmitted infection risk. Nurse Pract 32(2):26–32, 2007.

Martin, F, and Taylor, GP: The safety of highly active antiretroviral therapy for the HIV-positive pregnant mother and her baby: Is "the more the merrier"? J Antimicrob Chemother 64(5):895–900, 2009.

O'Grady, JG, Asderakis, A, Bradley, R, et al: Multidisciplinary insights into optimizing adherence after solid organ transplantation. Transplantation 89(5):627–632, 2010.

Ojo, AO, Held, PJ, Port, FK, et al: Chronic renal failure after transplantation of a nonrenal organ. N Engl J Med 349(10):931–940, 2003.

Parimon, T, Madtes, DK, Au, DH, et al: Pretransplant lung function, respiratory failure, and mortality after stem cell transplant. Am J Respir Crit Care Med 172(3):384–390, 2005.

Pierrakos, C, and Vincent, J-L: Sepis biomarkers: A revew. Crit Care 14(1):R15, 2010.

Rayl, J: Home health care of the post-transplant patient. Adv Nurses 2(12):25–35, 2000.

Ress, B: AIDS/HIV—Caring for patients with HIV disease in the millennium. Crit Care Nurse 21(1):69–76, 2001.

Sacks, JJ, Helmick, CG, and Langmaid, G: Deaths from arthritis and other rheumatic conditions, United States, 1979–1998. J Rheumatol 31(9):1823–1828, 2004.

Singh, JA, Furst, DE, and Bharat, A: 2012 Update of the 2008 American College of Rheumatology Recommendations for the use of disease-modifying antirheumatic drugs and biologic agents in the treatment of rheumatoid arthritis. Arthritis Care Res 64(5):625–639, 2012.

Snyder, SR, Kivlehan, SM, and Collopy, KT: Managing sepsis in the adult patient. EMS World 41(5):36–45, 2012.

Soong, J, and Soni, M: Sepsis: Recognition and treatment. Clin Med 12(3):276–280, 2012.

Sullivan, DM, and Schoonover-Shoffner, K: Sorting through the stem cell hype. J Christian Nurs 24(4):182–189, 2007.

Swam, A, Daley, AM, and Crowley, A: Contraceptive counseling for adolescents with HIV. Nurse Pract 32(5):38–45, 2007.

Symmons, DP, and Gabriel, SE: Epidemiology of CVD in rheumatic disease, with a focus on RA and SLE. Nat Rev Rheumatol 7(7):399–408, 2011.

Veitz, A: Managing the side effects of chemotherapy. Adv Nurses 2(14): 11–13, 2000.

Webb, A, and Norton, M: Clinical assessment of symptom-focused health-related quality of life in HIV/AIDS. JANAC 15(2):67–81, 2004.

Wood, S, and Lavieri, MC: What you need to know about sepsis. Nursing2007 37(3):46–51, 2007.

Xu, J, Kochanek, K., Murphy, S, et al: Deaths: Final data for 2007. National Vital Statistics Report 58(19):12–13, 2010.

Electronic Resources

AIDSMEDS: Currently approved drugs for HIV: A comparative chart, 2012. Retrieved June 2013 from **http://www.aidsmeds.com/articles/DrugChart_10632.shtml**

Arthritis Foundation: Rheumatoid arthritis fact sheet, 2008. Retrieved March 2013 from **http://www.arthritis.org/files/images/newsroom/media kits/Rheumatoid_Arthritis_Fact_Sheet.pdf**

Avert Staff: HIV types, subtypes, groups and strains, n.d. Retrieved June 2013 from **http://www.avert.org/hiv-types.htmNov**

Bentley, TS, and Hanson, SG: 2011 U.S. organ and tissue transplant cost estimates and discussion. Milliman Research Report, 2011. Retrieved May 2013 from **http://publications.milliman.com/research/health-rr/pdfs/2011-us-organ-tissue.pdf**

Bingham, C: RA pathophysiology, 2012. Retrieved June 2013 from **http://www.hopkinsarthritis.org/arthritis-info/rheumatoid-arthritis/ra-pathophysiology-2/**

Burdette, SD, Parilo, M, and Kaplan, LJ: Systemic inflammatory response syndrome, 2012. Retrieved April 2013 from **http://emedicine.medscape.com/article/168943-overview**

Centers for Disease Control and Prevention (CDC): MMWR recommendations and reports. Appendix A, AIDS-defining conditions, December 5, 2008. Retrieved June 2013 from **http://www.cdc.gov/mmWR/preview/mmwrhtml/ rr5710a2.htm**

Centers for Disease Control and Prevention (CDC): Injury prevention and control: Data and statistics (WISQARS). Leading causes of death,

2012. Retrieved March 2013 from **http://webappa.cdc.gov/cgi-bin/broker.exe**

Centers for Disease Control and Prevention (CDC): Living with HIV/AIDS, 2007. Retrieved June 2013 from **http://www.cdc.gov/hiv/resources/brochures/livingwithhiv.htm#q3**

Centers for Disease Control and Prevention (CDC): Rheumatoid arthritis, 2011. Retrieved June 2013 from **http://www.cdc.gov/arthritis/basics/rheumatoid.htm**

Centers for Disease Control and Prevention (CDC): HIV surveillance report 2010; Vol 22. Diagnoses of HIV infection and AIDS in the U.S. & dependent areas. Available at **http://www.cdc.gov/hiv/surveillance/resources/reports/2010report/pdf/2010_HIV_Surveillance_Report_vol_22.pdf#Page=21**

Centers for Disease Control and Prevention (CDC): HIV surveillance report; Vol 23. Diagnoses of HIV infection and AIDS in the United States and dependent areas, 2011. HIV prevalence estimate, 2011. Retrieved March 2013 from **http://www.cdc.gov/hiv/topics/surveillance/basic.htm#hivest**

Centers for Disease Control and Prevention (CDC): MMWR vital signs. HIV prevention through care and treatment—U.S. Dec 2, 2011/60, 1518–1623. Retrieved from **http://www.cdc.gov/mmwr/preview/mmwrhtml/mm6047a4.htm?s_cid=mm6047a4_w**

Centers for Disease Control and Prevention (CDC): MMWR. Recommendations and reports. April 10, 2009/Vol 58. Guidelines for prevention and treatment of opportunistic infections in HIV-infected adults and adolescents. Recommendations from the CDC, The National Institutes of Health, and the HIV Medicine Association of the Infectious Diseases Society of America. Retrieved June 2013 from **http://www.cdc.gov/mmwr/pdf/rr/rr58e324.pdf**

Cunha, BA: Bacterial sepsis, 2012. Retrieved April 2013 from **http://emedicine.medscape.com/article/234587-overview**

Fox, JE, Tobias, CR, Bachman, SS, et al: Increasing access to oral healthcare for people living with HIV/AIDS in the U.S.: Baseline evaluation results of the innovations in oral health care initiative. Public Health Reports 127 (supplement 2):6, 2012. Retrieved April 2013 from **http://www.publichealthreports.org/issuecontents.cfm?Volume=127&Issue=8**

Guillen, S, Black, M, Thomas, G, et al: Liver transplant, 2005. Retrieved June 2013 from **http://www.emedicinehealth.com/liver_transplant/article_em.htm**

Hall, M, Williams, S, DeFrances, C, et al: Inpatient care for septicemia or sepsis: A challenge for patients and hospitals. Centers for Disease Control (CDC) NCHS Data Brief 62:2, 2011. Retrieved March 2013 from **http://www.cdc.gov/nchs/data/databriefs/db62.pdf**

Health and Human Services (HHS) Panel on Antiretroviral Guidelines for Adults and Adolescents—A Working Group of the Office of AIDS Research Advisory Council (OARAC): Guidelines for the use of antiretroviral agents in HIV-1-infected adults and adolescents, update 2013. Retrieved June 2013 from **http://aidsinfo.nih.gov/contentfiles/lvguidelines/adultandadolescentgl.pdf**

Health Resources and Services Administration (HRSA), U.S. Department of Health & Human Services: Organ Procurement and Transplantion Network (OPTA). Data reports, 2013. Retrieved March 2013 from **http://optn.transplant.hrsa.gov/**

Health24: Symptoms and phases of HIV infection & AIDS, updated 2012. Retrieved June 2013 from **http://www.health24.com/Medical/HIV-AIDS/Symptoms-and-diseases-associated/Symptoms-and-phases-of-HIV-infection-Aids-20120721**

Hoyert, D, and Xu, J: Deaths: Preliminary data for 2011. National Vital Statistics Report (NVSS), 6(1):18, 2012. Retrieved March 2013 from **http://www.cdc.gov/nchs/data/nvsr/nvsr61/nvsr61_06.pdf**

Kaiser Family Foundation (KFF): HIV/AIDS policy fact sheet: Medicaid and HIV/AIDS, 2013. Retrieved April 2013 from **http://kff.org/hivaids/fact-sheet/medicaid-and-hivaids/**

Kaiser Family Foundation (KKF): U.S. global health policy fact sheet; The global HIV/AIDS epidemic, 2012. Retrieved March 2013 from **http://www.kff.org/hivaids/upload/3030-17.pdf**

Khamsi, R: Drug-resistant HIV battled in a new way, 2007. Retrieved June 2013 from **http://www.newscientist.com/article/dn10893-drugresistant-hiv-battled-in-a-new-way.html**

Mink, S, and Sharma, S: Septic shock, 2012. Retrieved May 2013 from **http://emedicine.medscape.com/article/168402-overview**

National Institute of Arthritis and Musculoskeletal and Skin Disease: Rheumatoid arthritis, updated 2009. Retrieved June 2013 from **http://www.niams.nih.gov/Health_Info/Rheumatic_Disease/default.asp**

National Institutes of Health. AIDS Info. Panel on Treatment of HIV-Infected Pregnant Women and Prevention of Perinatal Transmission: Recommendations for use of antiretroviral drugs in pregnant HIV-1-infected women for maternal health and interventions to reduce perinatal HIV transmission in the United States, 2012. Retrieved June 2013 from **http://aidsinfo.nih.gov/contentfiles/lvguidelines/perinatalgl.pdf**

New York Times: Rheumatoid arthritis in-depth report, 1998–2008. Retrieved June 2013 from **http://health.nytimes.com/health/guides/disease/rheumatoid-arthritis/print.html**

Organ Procurement and Transplantation Network (OPTA): Data reports, 2013. Retrieved March 2013 from **http://optn.transplant.hrsa.gov/**

Powderly, WG: Opportunistic infections—Diminishing returns, 2001. Retrieved June 2013 from **http://www.medscape.org/viewarticle/420623**

Ruffing, V, and Bingham, CO: Rheumatoid arthritis signs and symptoms, 2012. Retrieved June 2013 from **http://www.hopkinsarthritis.org/arthritis-info/rheumatoid-arthritis/ra-symptoms/**

San Francisco AIDS Foundation: The stages of HIV disease, 2008. Retrieved June 2013 from **http://www.thebody.com/content/art2506.html?getPage=1**

Schmidt, GA, and Mandel, J: Evaluation and management of severe sepsis and septic shock in adults, 2013. Retrieved May 2013 from paid site. **http://www.uptodate.com/contents/evaluation-and-management-of-severe-sepsis-and-septic-shock-in-adults**

Sharma, S, and Unruh, H: History of adult transplantation, 2006. Retrieved June 2013 from **http://www.eglobalmed.com/opt/MedicalStudent-dotcom/www.emedicine.com/med/topic3497.htm**

Temprano, KK, and Smith, HR: Rheumatoid arthritis, 2013. Retrieved June 2013 from **http://emedicine.medscape.com/article/331715-overview**

Twyman, T: Tissue matching for transplants, 2003. Retrieved June 2013 from **http://genome.wellcome.ac.uk/doc_wtd020937.html**

U.S. Department of Health and Human Services: OPTN/SRTR annual report: Survival rate data tables, 2011, 2012. Retrieved June 2013 from **http://srtr.transplant.hrsa.gov/annual_reports/2011/pdf/2011_SRTR_ADR.pdf**

UnitedHealth Group: 2012 Transplant review guidelines: Solid organ and stem cell transplantation including selected references for organ transplantation and pediatric heart disease, 2012. Retrieved June 2013 from **https://www.unitedhealthcareonline.com/ccmcontent/ProviderII/UHC/en-US/Assets/ProviderStaticFiles/ProviderStaticFilesPdf/Tools%20and%20Resources/Policies%20and%20Protocols/Medical%20Policies/Clinical%20Guidelines/Transplant_Review_Guidelines.pdf**

United Nations Programme on HIV/AIDS and World Health Organization: AIDS epidemic update, December 2007. Retrieved June 2013 from **http://data.unaids.org/pub/epislides/2007/2007_epiupdate_en.pdf**

U.S. Food and Drug Adminstration (FDA): Approved rapid HIV antibody screening tests, February 2008. Retrieved June 2013 from **http://www.cdc.gov/hiv/topics/testing/rapid/rt-comparison.htm**

U.S. Food and Drug Adminstration (FDA): Vaccines, blood and biologics: OraQuick In-Home HIV Test, 2012. Retrieved June 2013 from **http://www.fda.gov/BiologicsBloodVaccines/BloodBloodProducts/ApprovedProducts/PremarketApprovalsPMAs/ucm310436.htm**

World Health Organization (WHO): HIV transmission through breastfeeding: A review of available evidence, update 2007. Retrieved June 2013 from **http://whqlibdoc.who.int/publications/2008/9789241596596_eng.pdf**

World Health Organization (WHO): Time to act. Save a million lives by 2015. Prevent and treat tuberculosis among people living with HIV [Brochure], 2011. Retrieved June 2013 from **http://www.who.int/tb/challenges/hiv/tbhiv_brochure_singles.pdf**

CHAPTER 15

Books

American Psychiatric Association: Diagnosis and Statistical Manual of Mental Disorders, ed 5. Arlington, VA, 2013.

Association of PeriOperative Registered Nurses (AORN). Perioperative standards and recommended practices, 2011 ed. AORN, Inc., Denver, CO, 2011, p 367.

Deglin, JH, and Vallerand, AH: Davis's drug guide for nurses, ed 13. FA Davis, Philadelphia, 2010.

Doenges, M, Townsend, M, and Moorhouse, M: Psychiatric nursing care plans, ed 3. FA Davis, Philadelphia, 1998.

Erickson, E: Childhood and society, ed 2. WW Norton, New York, 1963.

Feldman, D, and Lasher, SA: The end-of-life handbook: A compassionate guide to connecting with and caring for a dying loved one. New Harbinger Publications, Oakland, CA, 2008.

Glaser, BG, and Strauss, AL: Time for dying. Aldine, Chicago, 1968.

Gordon, T: Parent effectiveness training: The proven program for raising responsible children, ed 30. Three Rivers Press, New York, 2000.

Hartung, J, and Galvin, M: Energy psychology and EMDR: Combining forces to optimize treatment. WW Norton, New York, 2003.

Hausman, KA: Interventions for clients with problems of the central nervous system. In Ignatavicius, DD, and Workman, ML (eds): Medical-surgical nursing: Critical thinking for collaborative care, ed 5. Elsevier Saunders, St. Louis, MO, 2006.

James, M, and Jongeward, D: Born to win: Transactional analysis with gestalt experiments. Perseus Publishing, Cambridge, MA, 1996.

Kowalak, J, and Hughes, AS: Handbook of signs and symptoms, ed 2. Lippincott, Williams & Wilkins, Springhouse, PA, 2002.

Krieger, D: Therapeutic touch: Using the hands to help or heal. Simon & Schuster, New York, 1998.

London, ML: Maternal & child nursing care, ed 2. Pearson Prentice Hall, Upper Saddle River, NJ, 2007.

Matheny, NM: Fluid and electrolyte balance, ed 5. Nursing considerations. Jones & Bartlett Learning, Sudbury, MA, 2012.

Nelson-Marsh, JD: Chronic disorders of neurologic function. In Copstead, LEC, and Banasik, JL (eds): Pathophysiology, ed 3. Elsevier Saunders, St. Louis, MO, 2005.

Ortner, N: The tapping solution: A revolutionary system for stress-free living. Hay House, New York, 2013.

Skeel, R (ed): Handbook of cancer chemotherapy, ed 6. Lippincott, Williams & Wilkins, Philadelphia, 2003.

Theander, S: Outcome and prognosis in anorexia nervosa and bulimia. In Szmukler, GI, et al (eds): Anorexia nervosa and bulimic disorders. Pergamon, London, 1985.

Townsend, MC: Psychiatric mental health nursing concepts of care. In Evidence-based practice, ed 7. FA Davis, Philadelphia, 2012.

University of Missouri: Handbook of disabilities, substance abuse. Product of RECP7 and Curators of the University of Missouri, Columbia, 2006.

U.S. Department of Health and Human Services: Results from the 2006 National Survey on Drug Use and Health: National findings. DHHS publication (SMA) 07-4293. U.S. Department of Health and Human Services, Substance Abuse and Mental Health Services Administration. Office of Applied Studies, Rockville, MD, September 2007, p 69.

Venes, D (ed): Taber's cyclopedic medical dictionary, ed 20. FA Davis, Philadelphia, 2005.

Young, B, Flamm, JA, and Graham, RM: Improved options for better care: The role of new HIV-1 protease inhibitors. A Continuing Education Monograph, March 2004.

Articles

Aiello-Laws, LB: Assessing the risk for suicide in patients with cancer. Clin J Oncol Nurs 14(6):687–691, 2010.

Ali, S, Nathani, M, Jabeen, S, et al: Alcohol: The lubricant to suicidality. Innovat ClinNeurosci 10(1):20–29, 2013.

Allen, CH: Providing compassionate end-of-life care. Nursing Made Incredibly Easy! 6(4):46–53, 2008.

Amella, EJ: Presentation of illness in older adults. Am J of Nurs 104(10):40–51, 2004.

Arima, K, Uéda, K, Sunohara, N, et al: NACP/alpha-synuclein immunoreactivity in fibrillary components of neuronal and oligodendroglial cytoplasmic inclusions in the pontine nuclei in multiple system atrophy. Acta Neuropathol Nov;96(5):439–444, 1998.

Barry, M: How growth factors help chronic wounds heal. Nursing2000 30(5):52–53, 2000.

Bayard, M, et al: Alcohol withdrawal syndrome. Am Fam Physician 69(6):1443–50, 2004.

Bednarski, D, Burns, J, and Doughty, D: Discharge information needs of patients after surgery. J Wound Ostomy Continence Nurs 33(3):281–289, 2006.

Bjoro, K, and Herr, K: Assessment of pain in the nonverbal or cognitively impaired older adult. Clin Geriatr Med 24(2):237–262, 2008.

Bowles, KH, Holland, DE, and Mistaen, P: Problems and unmet needs of patients discharged home to self-care. Prof Case Manag 16(5): 240–250, 2011.

Boyle, K, Nance, J, and Passau-Buck, S: Post-hospitalization concerns of medical-surgical patients. Appl Nurs Res 5(3):122–126, 1992.

Bridgman, A: Understanding the neurobiological basis of drug abuse: Comorbidity in schizophrenia. Psychiatric Times 30(2):12–14, 2013.

Brown, JK: A systematic review of the evidence on symptom management of cancer related anorexia. Oncol Nurs Forum 29(3):517–532, 2002.

Burton, J: Alcohol withdrawal syndrome. Nurses Nurturing Nurses 19(5):7–12, 2010.

Charles, V, and Weaver, TA: Qualitative study of illicit and non-prescribed drug use amongst people with psychotic disorders. J MentHealth 19(1):99–106, 2010.

Claros, E, and Collins, M: Recognizing the face of dehydration. Nursing 41(8):26–31, 2008.

Claros, E, and Sharma, M: The relationship between emotional intelligence and abuse of alcohol, marijuana, and tobacco among college students. J Alcohol Drug Addiction 56(1):8–37, 2012.

Cravens, DD, and Zweig, S: Urinary catheter management. Am Fam Physician 61(2):369–376, 2000.

Creechan, T: Combining mechanical ventilation with hospice care in the home: Death with dignity. Crit Care Nurse 20(3):49, 2000.

Crews, FT: Immune function genes, genetics, and the neurobiology of addiction. Alcohol Research: Current Reviews 34(3):355–361, 2011.

Criddle, L: Critical care extra: A pinch of salt: Therapy should be on slow restoration of the serum sodium level. Am J Nurs 106(10):72CC–72DD, 2006.

Daly, M, Kermode, S, and Reilly, D: Evaluation of clinical practice improvement programs for nurses for the management of alcohol withdrawal in hospitals. Contemp Nurse 31(2):98–107, 2009.

Daniels, SM: Improved care for surgical patients. OR Nurse 2008 1(7): 18–22, 2008.

Davies, NJ: Alcohol misuse in adolescents. Nursing Standard 26(42): 43–48, 2012.

Davis, C: Emergency assessment bay for patients. Cancer Nursing Practice 12(1):14–17, 2013.

Deering, CG, and Jennings, D: Communicating with children and adolescents. Am J Nurs 102 (3):34, 2002.

DiMaria-Ghalili, RA, and Amella, E: Nutrition in older adults. Am J Nurs 105(3):50, 2005.

Doenges, ME, Moorhouse, MF, and Murr, AC: Nurse's pocket guide: Diagnoses, prioritized interventions and rationales, ed 13. FA Davis, Philadelphia, 2013.

Donnelly, G, Kent-Wilkinson, A, and Rush, A: The alcohol dependent patient in the hospital: Challenges for nursing. MedSurg Nursing 21(1):9–16, 2012.

Drake, K: SCIP core measures: Deep impact. Nurs Manage 42(5):24–30, 2011.

Egan, KA, and Arnold, RL: Grief and bereavement care. Am J Nurs 103(9):42–52, 2003.

Ewing, JA: Detecting alcoholism: The CAGE questionnaire. JAMA 252:1905–1907, 1984.

Frangou, C: Glucose control reduces post-op infections. Anesthesiology News 34(7):7, 2008.
Furman, J: Taking a holistic approach to the dying time. Nursing 30(6):46, 2000.
Gallagher, PF, O'Mahony, D, and Quigley, EM: Management of chronic constipation in the elderly. Drugs Aging 25(10):807–821, 2008.
Garcia, A: State laws regulating prescribing of controlled substances: Balancing the public health problems of chronic pain and prescription painkiller abuse and overdose. J Law, MedEthics 41(Suppl 1):42–45, 2013.
Ginsberg, DA, Phillips, SE, Wallace, J, et al: Evaluating and managing constipation in the elderly. Urol Nurs 27(3):191–200, 2007.
Granholm, E, Morris, S, Galasko, D, et al: Tropicamide effects on pupil size and pupillary light reflexes in Alzheimer's and Parkinson's disease. Int J Psychophysiol 47:95–115, 2003.
Gray-Vickery, P: Combating abuse, part 1: Protecting the older adult. Nursing30 (7):34–38, 2000.
Hankins, J: The role of albumin in fluid and electrolyte balance. J Infusion Nursing 29(5):260–265, 2006.
Haroun, MD. Dry skin in the elderly. Geriatr Aging 6(21):41–44, 2003.
Hawkins, JD, Kosterman, R, Catalano, R., et al: Effects of social development intervention in childhood 15 years later. Arch Pediatr Adolesc Med 162(12):1133–1141, 2008.
Henderson-Martin, B: No more surprises: Screening patients for alcohol abuse. Am J Nurs 100(9):26–32, 2000.
Henkel, GE: Nutrition basics for LTC. Caring for the Ages 5(1):12–22, 2004.
Hopkinson, J, Fenlon, DR, and Foster, CL: Outcomes of a nurse-delivered psychosocial intervention for weight and eating-related distress in family carers of patients with advanced cancer. Int J Palliat Nurs 19(3):116–123, 2013.
Hopkinson, JB, MacDonald, J, Wright, DNM, et al: The prevalence of concern about weight loss and change in eating habits in people with advanced cancer. J Pain Symptom Manage 32(4):322–333, 2006.
Horn, LB: Reducing the risk of falls in the elderly. Rehab Manage 13(5):36–38/96, 2000.
Horneber, M, Fischer, I, Dimeo, F, et al: Cancer-related fatigue: Epidemiology, pathogenesis, diagnosis, and treatment. Dtsch Ärztebl Int 109(9):161–172, 2012.
Jesus, JE, and Landry, A: Chvostek's and Trousseau's signs. N Engl J Med 13:367, 2012.
Kearney, K: Hyperkalemia. Am J Nurs 100(1):55–56, 2000.
Kiecolt-Glaser, JK, McGuire, L, Robles, TF, et al: Emotions, morbidity, and mortality: New perspectives from psychoneuroimmunology. Annu Rev Psychol 53:83–107, 2002.
Kiecolt-Glaser, JK, and Glaser, R: Psychoneuroimmuneology and cancer: Fact or fiction? Eur J Cancer 35(11):1603–1607, 1999.
Kirckhoff, KT, Spuhler, V, Walker, L, et al: Intensive care nurses' experiences with end-of-life care. Am J Crit Care 9(1):36, 2000.
Lagman, RL, Davis, MP, LeGrand, SB, et al: Common symptoms in advanced cancer. Surg Clin North Am 85(2):237–255, 2005.
Leadbeater, M: The role of a community palliative care specialist nurse team in caring for people with metastatic breast cancer. Int J Palliat Nurs 19(2):93–97, 2013.
Lee, RD: Polypharmacy: A case report and new protocol for management. J Am Board Fam Pract 11(2):140–144, 1998.
Liberto, LA, and Fornili, KS: Managing pain in opioid-dependent patients in general hospital settings. MedSurg Nursing 22(1):33–37, 2013.
López, F, Bargo, G, Luis, R, et al: Alcoholic ketoacidosis and reversible neurological complications due to hypophosphatemia. Nutri Hospital 27(3):936–939, 2012.
Lussier-Cushing, M, Repper-DeLisi, J, Mitchel, MT, et al: Is your medical/surgical patient withdrawing from alcohol? Nursing 37(10):50–55, 2007.
Mattson, N, Zetterberg, H, Hansson, O, et al: CSF biomarkers and incipient Alzheimer disease in patients with mild cognitive impairment. JAMA 302(4):385–393, 2009.
Mazanec, P, and Tyler, MK: Cultural considerations in end-of-life care. Am J Nurs 103(3):50–57, 2003.
McHugh, ME, Miller-Saultz, D, Wuhrman, E, et al: Interventional pain management in the palliative care patient. Int J Palliat Nurs 18(9), 426–433, 2012.
McInally, W, and Cruickshank, S: Transition from child to adult services for young people with cancer. Nurs Child Young People 25(1):14–18, 2013.
McPeake, J: Assessing alcohol-related attendance at emergency departments. Emergency Nurse 20(9):26–30, 2013.
Mentes, J: Oral hydration in older adults: Greater awareness is needed in preventing, recognizing, and treating dehydration. Am J Nurs 106(6):40–49, 2006.
Miller, J: Potassium in the balance: Understanding hyperkalemia and hypokalemia. LPN2007 2(5):42–49, 2006.
Munoz, C, and Hilgenberg, C: Ethnopharmacology. Am J Nurs 105(8): 40–48, 2005.
Nayduch, DA: Back to basics: Identifying and managing acute spinal cord injury. Nursing 40(9):24–31, 2010.
Nelson, K, Walsh, D, Abdullah, O, et al: Common complications of advanced cancer. Semin Oncol 27(1):34–44, 2000.
Nevius, KS, and D'Arcy, Y: Decrease recovery time with proper pain management. OR Nurse 2008 2(4):34–39, 2008.
de Nijs, EJM, Ros, W, and Gripdonck, MH: Nursing intervention for fatigue during the treatment for cancer. Cancer Nursing 31(3):191–206, 2008.
No author listed: Treatment of alcoholism—Part II. Harvard Mental Health Lett 16(12):1, 2000.
No author listed: Disaster and trauma. Harvard Mental Health Lett 18(7):1–5, 2002.
Panke, JT: Difficulties in managing pain at the end of life. Am J Nurs 102(7):26–33, 2002.
Park-Lee, E, Sengupta, M, Bercovitz, A, et al: Oldest old long-term care recipients: Findings from the National Center for Health Statistics' Long-Term Care Surveys. Research on Aging 35(3):296–321, 2013.
Patel, CT, Kinsey, GC, Koperski-Moen, KJ, et al: Vacuum-assisted wound closure. Am J Nurs 100(12):45–48, 2000.
Phillips, J: Prescription drug abuse: Problem, policies, and implications. Nurs Outlook 61(2):78–84, 2013.
Pitorak, EF: Care at the time of death. Am J Nurs 103(7):42–52, 2003.
Portenoy, RK, and Itri, LM: Cancer-related fatigue: Guidelines for evaluation and management. Oncologist 4(1):1–10, 1999.
Rentz, CA: Alzheimer's disease: An elusive thief. Nurs Manage 39(6):33–37, 2008.
Riddle, E, Bush, J, Tittle, M, et al: Alcohol withdrawal: Development of a standing order set. Crit Care Nurse 30(3):38–47, 2010.
Sachse, DS: Emergency: Delirium tremens. Am J Nurs 100(5):41–42, 2000.
Salati, DS: Caring for a sick child in a nonpediatric setting. Nursing 34(4):54–61, 2004.
Santos, EM, Edwards, QT, Floria-Santos, M, et al: Integration of genomics in cancer care. J Nurs Scholarsh 45(1):43–51, 2013.
Sartor, CE, Waldon, M, Duncan, AE, et al: Childhood sexual abuse and early substance use in adolescent girls: The role of familial influences. Addiction 108(5):993–1000, 2013.
Scanlon, C: Ethical concerns in end-of-life care. Am J Nurs 103(1):48–53, 2003.
Schiffman, RF: Drug and substance use in adolescents. MCN, Am J Maternal/Child Nurs 29(1):21–27, 2004.
Schmidt, C, Bernaix, L, Koski, A, et al: Hospitalized children's perceptions of nurses and nurse behaviors. MCN, Am J of Maternal/Child Nurs 32(6):336–342, 2007.
Schmidt, TC: New eye on diagnostics: Assessing a sodium and fluid imbalance. Nursing 30(1):18, 2000.
Sharer, J: Tackling sundowning in a patient with Alzheimer's disease. MedSurg Nurs 17(1):27–30, 2008.
Sheehan, DK, and Schirm, V: End-of-life care of older adults. Am J Nurs 103(11):48–57, 2003.
Solomon, PR, Hirschcoff, A, Kelly, B, et al: A 7-minute neurocognitive screening battery highly sensitive to Alzheimer's disease. Arch Neurol 55(3):349–355, 1998.
Sprigle, S: Prescribing pressure ulcer treatment. Rehab Manage 13(5): 72–77, 2000.

Springer, R: The Surgical Care Improvement Project—Focusing on infection control. Plast Surg Nurs 27(3):163–167, 2007.

Stasser, F, Binswanger, J, Cerney, T, et al: Fighting a losing battle: Eating-related distress of men with advanced cancer and their female partners. A mixed-methods study. Palliat Med 21(2):129–137, 2007.

Stewart, KB, and Richards, AB: Recognizing and managing your patient's alcohol abuse. Nursing2000 30(2):56–59, 2000.

Stevens, WJ: Fluid balance and resuscitation: Critical aspects of ICU care. Nursing2008 Critical Care 3(2):12–21, 2008.

Stockdell, R, and Amella, EJ: How to try this: The Edinburgh Feeding Evaluation in Dementia Scale. Am J Nurs 108(8):46–54, 2008.

Sullivan, T, Harrold, K, Bell, K, et al: Benefits of attending nurse-led prechemotherapy group sessions. Cancer Nursing Practice 12(1): 27–31, 2013.

Suter, PM, Rogers, J, and Strack, C: Hospice & palliative pare: Artificial nutrition for the terminally ill: A reasoned approach. Home Healthc Nurse 26(1):23–29, 2008.

Taur, FM, Chai, S, Chen, MB, et al: Evaluating the suicide risk-screening scale used by general nurses on patients with chronic obstructive pulmonary disease and lung cancer: A questionnaire survey. J Clin Nurs 21(3–4):398–407, 2013.

Taylor, C, Cummings, R, and McGilly, C: Holistic needs assessment following colorectal cancer treatment. Gastrointestinal Nursing 10(9):42–49, 2012.

Tetrault, JM, and Fiellin, DA: Current and potential pharmacological treatment options for maintenance therapy in opioid-dependent individuals. Drugs 72(2):217–228, 2012.

Trahan, M, Khang, SW, Fisher, AB, et al: Behavior-analytic research on dementia in older adults. JAARA 44(3):687–691, 2011.

Tsai, Y, Tsai, M, Lin, Y, et al: Facilitators and barriers to intervening for problem alcohol use.. J Adv Nurs 66(7):1459–1468, 2010.

USAMRIID: Medical management of biological casualties handbook, ed 7. Fort Detrick, MD, September, 2011.

van Kasteren, ME, Mannien, J, Ott, A, et al: Antibiotic prophylaxis and the risk of surgical site infections following total hip arthroplasty: Timely administration is the most important factor. Clin Inf Dis 44(7):921–992, 2007.

Vassallo, BM: The spiritual aspects of dying at home. Holistic Nurs Pract 15(2):19–29, 2001.

Virani, R, and Sofer, D: Improving the quality of end-of-life care. Am J Nurs 103(5):52–60, 2003.

Winters, KC, and Arria, A: Adolescent brain development and drugs. Prev Res 18(2):21–24, 2011.

Wotton, K, Crannitch, K, and Munt, R: Prevalence, risk factors and strategies to prevent dehydration in older adults. Contemp Nurse 31(1):44–56, 2008.

Zambroski, CH: Hospice as an alternative model of care for older patients with end-stage heart failure. J Cardiovasc Nurs 19(1):76–85, 2004.

Ziere, G, Dieleman, JP, Hofman, A, et al: Polypharmacy and falls in the middle age and elderly population. Br J Clin Pharmacol 61(2):218–223, 2006.

Pamphlets

Forest Pharmaceuticals: Understanding and living with Alzheimer's disease, your guide to treatment and help. Treatment options and expectations. In it Together series, 2007.

Johnston, LD, O'Malley, PM, and Bachman, JG: Monitoring the future national survey results on drug use, 1975–2002. Vol 1: Secondary school students. National Institute on Drug Abuse, Bethesda, MD, 2002.

The Mayo Clinic: Pain-pill addiction: What's the risk? Mayo Foundation for Medical Education and Research, June 2006.

No author listed: The family matters: Substance abuse and the American family. The National Center on Addiction and Substance Abuse at Columbia University, New York, 2005.

No author listed: What does America think about addiction prevention and treatment? Robert Wood Johnson Foundation, Princeton, NJ, 2007.

Russo, A, Wier, LM, and Elixhauser, A: Hospital utilization among near-elderly adults, ages 55 to 64 years: Health Cost and Utilization Project (HCUP). Statistical Brief #79. Agency for Health Care Policy and Research (U.S.), Rockville, MD, 2007.

Electronic Resources

Agraharkar, M, Dellinger, OD, and Gangakhedkar, AK: Hypercalcemia, 2012. Retrieved June 2013 from **http://emedicine.medscape.com/article/240681-overview**

Alvarez, N: Alzheimer disease in Down syndrome, 2012. Retrieved June 2013 from **http://emedicine.medscape.com/article/1136117-overview**

Alzheimer's Association: Alzheimer's disease medications fact sheet, 2012. Retrieved June 2013 from **http://www.nia.nih.gov/print/alzheimers/publication/alzheimers-disease-medications-fact-sheet**

Alzheimer's Association: Latest facts and figures report, 2013. Retrieved March 2013 from **http://www.alz.org/downloads/facts_figures_2013.pdf**

Alzheimer's Association: 2013 Alzheimer's disease facts and figures. Retrieved March 2013 from **http://www.alz.org/downloads/facts_figures_2013.pdf**

Alzheimer's Foundation of America: About Alzheimer's: Definition, 2013. Retrieved June 2013 from **http://www.alzfdn.org/AboutAlzheimers/definition.html**

American Academy of Child and Adolescent Psychiatry: Teens: Alcohol and other drugs, 2012. Retrieved June 2013 from **http://www.aacap.org/cs/root/facts_for_families/teens_alcohol_and_other_drugs**

American Academy of Pediatrics (AAP): Pediatric terrorism and disaster preparedness: A resource for pediatricians. In Foltin, GL, Schonfeld, DJ, and Shannon, MW (eds): AHRQ publication 06(07)-0056. Agency for Healthcare Research and Quality, Rockville, MD, 2006. Retrieved May 2013 from **http://archive.ahrq.gov/research/pedprep/**

American Cancer Society (ACS): Cancer facts & figures 2013. Retrieved March 2013 from **http://www.cancer.org/acs/groups/content/@epidemiologysurveilance/documents/document/acspc-036845.pdf**

American Cancer Society (ACS). Testing biopsy and cytology specimens for cancer. Revised 2013. Retrieved Oct 2013 from **http://www.cancer.org/treatment/understandingyourdiagnosis/examsandtestdescriptions/testingbiopsyandcytologyspecimensforcancer/testing-biopsy-and-cytology-specimens-for-cancer-special-studies**

Anandarajah, G, and Hight, E: Spirituality and medical practice: Using the HOPE questions as a practical tool for spiritual assessment, 2001. Retrieved June 2013 from **http://www.aafp.org/afp/2001/0101/p81.html**

Anderson, HS: Alzheimer's disease, 2013. Retrieved June 2013 from **http://emedicine.medscape.com/article/1134817-overview**

Angus, ZS: Symptoms of hypermagnesemia, 2012. Retrieved June 2013 from paid site. **http://www.uptodate.com/contents/symptoms-of-hypermagnesemia**

Balentine, JR, and Doerr, S: Alcohol intoxication, 2013. Retrieved June 2013 from **http://www.emedicinehealth.com/alcohol_intoxication/article_em.htm**

Benetti, G: Familial Alzheimer's disease, 2012. Retrieved June 2013 from **http://www.alzheimer-europe.org/Dementia/Other-forms-of-dementia/Neuro-Degenerative-Diseases/Familial-Alzheimer-s-disease#fragment-1**

Bright Focus Foundation: Alzheimer's prevention and risk factors, 2013. Retrieved June 2013 from **http://www.brightfocus.org/alzheimers/about/risk/**

Brymer, M, Jacob, A, Layne, C, et al: (National Child Traumatic Stress Network and National Center for PTSD): Psychological first aid—Field operations guide, ed 2, 2006. Retrieved May 2013 from **http://www.nctsn.org/nctsn_assets/pdfs/pfa/2/PsyFirstAid.pdf**

Burns, MJ, Price, JB, and Lekawa, ME: Delirium tremens, updated 2013. Retrieved June 2013 from **http://www.emedicinehealth.com/alcohol_intoxication/article_em.htm**

Casciani, J: Sensory loss in older adults—Taste, smell and touch–Behavioral approaches for caregivers, 2008. Retrieved June 2013 from **http://ezinearticles.com/?Sensory-Loss-in-Older-Adults---Taste,-Smell-and-Touch---Behavioral-Approaches-for-Caregivers&id=1099819**

Center for Behavioral Health Statistics and Quality (CBHSQ), Substance Abuse and Mental Health Services Administration (SAMHSA), U.S.

Department of Health and Human Services (HHS): Results from the 2010 National Survey on Drug Use and Health. Summary of National Findings. Retrieved June 2013 from **http://oas.samhsa.gov/NSDUH/2k10NSDUH/2k10Results.htm**

Centers for Disease Control and Prevention (CDC): Adults having five or more alcoholic beverages in 1 day, 2010. Retrieved June 2013 from **http://www.cdc.gov/features/ds5drinks1day/**

Centers for Disease Control and Prevention (CDC): Cancer: FastStats, 2010. Retrieved June 2013 from **http://www.cdc.gov/nchs/fastats/cancer.htm**

Centers for Disease Control and Prevention (CDC): CDC reports excessive alcohol consumption cost the U.S. $224 billion in 2006, 2011. Retrieved March 2013 from **http://www.cdc.gov/media/releases/2011/p1017_alcohol_consumption.html**

Centers for Disease Control and Prevention (CDC): Coping with a traumatic event: Information for health professionals, reviewed 2013. Retrieved May 2013 from **http://www.bt.cdc.gov/masscasualties/copingpro.asp**

Centers for Disease Control and Prevention (CDC): Fact sheets: Alcohol use and health, 2012. Retrieved March 2013 from **http://www.cdc.gov/alcohol/fact-sheets/alcohol-use.htm**

Centers for Disease Control and Prevention (CDC): FastStats: Leading causes of death, 2012. Retrieved March 2013 from **http://www.cdc.gov/nchs/fastats/lcod.htm**

Centers for Disease Control and Prevention (CDC): FastStats: 2004 Nursing home survey, 2006. Retrieved March 2013 from **http://www.cdc.gov/nchs/fastats/nursingh.htm**

Centers for Disease Control and Prevention (CDC): Web-based Injury Statistics Query and Reporting System (WISQARS): Injury prevention and control: Data & statistics, 2012. Retrieved June 2013 from **www.cdc.gov/injury/wisqars/index.html**

The Children's Hospital of Philadelphia: Preparing your child for a hospital experience. [Portal to age-specific sites], 1996–2013. Retrieved June 2013 from **http://www.chop.edu/visitors/before-your-visit/preparing-your-child.html**

Cincinnati Children's Hospital Medical Center: Evidenced-based clinical practice guidelines for fever of uncertain source in children 2 to 36 months of age, updated 2010. Retrieved June 2013 from **http://www.guidelines.gov/content.aspx?id=24529**

Cunha, BA: Nursing home acquired pneumonia, 2013. Retrieved June 2013 from **http://emedicine.medscape.com/article/234916-overview**

Department of Veterans Affairs and Department of Defense (VA/DoD): Clinical practice guidelines for the management of post-traumatic stress, Washington, DC, 2004, 2010. Retrieved May 2013 from **http://www.healthquality.va.gov/PTSD-FULL-2010c.pdf**

Dowling-Castronovo, A, and Bradway, C: Urinary incontinence—Nursing standards of practice protocol, updated 2012. Retrieved June 2013 from **http://consultgerirn.org/topics/urinary_incontinence/want_to_know_more#item_8**

Dryden-Edwards, R: Club drugs, 2012. Retrieved June 2013 from **http://www.emedicinehealth.com/club_drugs/page16_em.htm#authors_and_editors**

Dugdale, DC: Use of restraints, 2012. Retrieved June 2013 from **http://www.nlm.nih.gov/medlineplus/ency/patientinstructions/000450.htm**

Emanuel, L, Ferris, FD, von Gunten, CF, et al: The last hours of living: Practical advice for clinicians, update 2012. Retrieved June 2013 from **http://www.medscape.org/viewarticle/716874**

EMDR Institute Inc: A brief description of EMDR, 2004. Retrieved May 2013 from **http://www.emdrnetwork.org/description.html**

Evesham, F: Therapeutic and non-therapeutic communication, 2011. Retrieved June 2013 from **http://www.livestrong.com/article/188795-therapeutic-and-non-therapeutic-communication/?utm_source=dontgo2&utm_medium=a1**

Family Caregiver Alliance: Selected long-term care statistics, 2005. Retrieved June 2013 from **http://www.caregiver.org/caregiver/jsp/content_node.jsp?nodeid=440**

Fulop, T, and Agarwal, M: Hypomagnesemia, 2013. Retrieved June 2013 from **http://emedicine.medscape.com/article/2038394-overview**

Fulop, T, Agraharkar, M, Workeneh, BT, et al: Hypermagnesemia, 2012. Retrieved June 2013 from **http://emedicine.medscape.com/article/246489-overview**

Girgis, A, Johnson, C, Currow, D, et al: Palliative care needs assessment guidelines, 2006. Retrieved June 2013 from **http://www.caresearch.com.au/caresearch/Portals/0/Documents/WhatisPalliativeCare/NationalProgram/PallCareNeedsAssessmentGde.pdf**

Healthwise Staff: Guided imagery, 2011. Retrieved June 2013 from **http://www.webmd.com/balance/guided-imagery**

Hoyert, D, and Xu, J: Deaths: Preliminary data for 2011, National Vital Statistics Report (NVSS) 6(1):18, 2012. Retrieved March 2013 from **http://www.cdc.gov/nchs/data/nvsr/nvsr61/nvsr61_06.pdf**

Kids Health for Parents: Fever and taking your child's temperature, reviewed 2013. Retrieved June 2013 from **http://kidshealth.org/parent/general/body/fever.html#**

Lederer, E, Alsauskas, ZC, Mackelaite, L, et al: Hyperkalemia, 2013. Retrieved June 2013 from **http://emedicine.medscape.com/article/240903-overview**

Lewy Body Dementia Association: What is LBD? 2012. Retrieved June 2013 from **http://www.lbda.org/node/7**

Lohmann, RC: Bath salts—the new designer drug, 2012. Retrieved June 2013 from **http://www.psychologytoday.com/blog/teen-angst/201206/bath-salts-the-new-designer-drug**

Lunney, J: Trajectories of dying: There's more than one way to go. Science and Theology Seminar, Oak Ridge, TN, 2007. Retrieved June 2013 from **http://fumcor.org/clientimages/33585/science_theology/lunneytn21007.pdf**

MA Youth Alcohol Prevention Task Force: Underage drinking in MA, 2002. Retrieved June 2013 from **http://files.hria.org/files/SA1017.pdf**

Malloy, P, Virani, RM, Kelly, K, et al: End-of-life care: Improving communication skills to enhance palliative care. Top Adv Nurs Pract eJournal, 2008. Retrieved June 2013 from **http://www.medscape.org/viewarticle/574420**

Marsh, GC, and Nelson, CW: Handcuffed: Alzheimer's and dementia: A report of the Alzheimer's Challenging Behaviors Task Force, 2010. Retrieved June 2013 from **http://www.alz.org/sewi/documents/alzheimers_report_handcuffed(2).pdf**

Mayo Clinic Staff: Lewy body dementia, 2013. Retrieved June 2013 from **http://www.mayoclinic.com/health/lewy-body-dementia/DS00795**

Mayo Clinic Staff: Vascular dementia, 2011. Retrieved June 2013 from **http://www.mayoclinic.com/health/vascular-dementia/DS00934/DSECTION=risk-factors**

McKeown, NJ, and West, PL: Withdrawal syndromes, 2012. Retrieved June 2013 from **http://emedicine.medscape.com/article/819502-overviewMedical College of Georgia: Antibody detection in Alzheimer's may improve diagnosis, treatment**

MedPac: Report to the Congress: Medicare payment policy, chapter 11, hospice services, March 2012. Retrieved March 2013 from **http://www.medpac.gov/chapters/Mar12_Ch11.pdf**

Merck Manuals: Children with chronic health conditions, 2010. Retrieved June 2013 from **http://www.merckmanuals.com/professional/pediatrics/caring_for_sick_children_and_their_families/children_with_chronic_health_conditions.html**

MetLife Insurance Co: Market survey of long-term care costs, 2012. Retrieved March 2013 from **https://www.metlife.com/mmi/research/2012-market-survey-long-term-care-costs.html#keyfindings**

Morgan Stanley Children's Hospital of New York Presbyterian: Preparing a child for surgery, update 2008. [Portal to age-specific sites.] Retrieved June 2013 from **http://childrensnyp.org/mschony/surgery-prephub.html**

National Cancer Institute, National Institutes of Health (NIH): The cost of cancer, 2011. Retrieved March 2013 from **http://www.cancer.gov/aboutnci/servingpeople/cancer-statistics/costofcancer**

National Hospice and Palliative Care Organization (NHPCO): NHPCO facts and figures: Hospice care in America, 2012 ed. Retrieved March 2013 from **http://www.nhpco.org/sites/default/files/public/Statistics_Research/2012_Facts_Figures.pdf**

National Institute on Aging (NIA) Alzheimer's Disease Education and Referral Center: Treatment, 2010. Retrieved June 2013 from **http://www.nia.nih.gov/alzheimers/publication/alzheimers-disease-medications-fact-sheet**

National Institute on Alcohol Abuse and Alcoholism (NIAAA) Division of Epidemiology and Prevention Research Alcohol Epidemiologic Data System: Trends in alcohol-related morbidity among short-stay community hospital discharges, United States, 1979–2007, 2010. Retrieved June 2013 from **http://pubs.niaaa.nih.gov/publications/surveillance89/HDS07.pdf**

National Institute on Drug Abuse (NIDA): DrugFacts: High school and youth trends, 2012. Retrieved June 2013 from **http://www.drugabuse.gov/publications/drugfacts/high-school-youth-trends**

National Institute for Drug Abuse (NIDA): Drugs of abuse (various monographs, dated from 2009–2013). Retrieved June 2013 from **http://www.drugabuse.gov/drugs-abuse**

National Institute for Drug Abuse (NIDA): Research Report Series. Prescription Drugs: Abuse and Addiction, 2010. Retrieved June 2013 from **http://www.drugabuse.gov/sites/default/files/rrprescription.pdf**

National Institute for Drug Abuse (NIDA): Trends and statistics, 2012. Retrieved March 2013 from **http://www.drugabuse.gov/related-topics/trends-statistics#costs**

National Institute for Drug Abuse (NIDA) for Teens: Facts on drugs, various pages, 2012. Retrieved June 2013 from **http://teens.drugabuse.gov/drug-facts/inhalants**

Neergard, L: One in three seniors dies with dementia, report finds, 2013. Retrieved June 2013 from **http://www.nbcnews.com/health/one-three-seniors-dies-dementia-report-finds-1C8942964?franchiseSlug=healthmain**

Novello, NP, and Blumstein, HA: Hypermagnesemia in emergency medicine, 2012. Retrieved June 2013 from **http://emedicine.medscape.com/article/766604-overview**

Otto, MA: REM sleep problems predict Parkinson's, Lewy body dementia, 2013. Retrieved June 2013 from **http://www.internalmedicinenews. com/index**

Post, TW, and Rose, BD: Clinical manifestations and diagnosis of volume depletion in adults, 2011. Retrieved June 2013 from **http://www.uptodate.com/contents/clinical-manifestations-and-diagnosis-of-volume**

QualityNet Specifications Manual: Benchmark of care reports, 2011. Retrieved June 2013 from **http://www.qualitynet.org/dcs/ContentServer?c=Page&pagename=QnetPublic%2FPage%2FQnetTier2&cid=1228768205213**

Robinson, RG, and Krishnan, KR: Depression and the medically ill. In Davis, KL, Charney, D, Coyle, JT, et al (eds): Neuropsychopharmacology: The fifth generation of progress. American College of Pharmacology, 2002. Retrieved June 2013 from **http://www.acnp.org/Docs/G5/CH81_1179-1186.pdf**

Stewart, K, Grabowski, D, and Lakdawalla, D. National Institutes of Health (NIH). 2009. Annual expenditures for nursing home care: Public and private payer price growth, 1977–2004. Retrieved March 2013 from **http://www.ncbi.nlm.nih.gov/pmc/articles/PMC2763425**

Substance Abuse and Mental Health Services Administration (SAMHSA): The Drug Abuse Warning Network (DAWN) Report, 2013. Retrieved March 2013 from **http://www.samhsa.gov/data/2k13/DAWN127/sr127-DAWN-highlights.htm**

Suneja, M, and Muster, HA: Hypocalcemia, 2013. Retrieved June 2013 from **http://emedicine.medscape.com/article/241893-treatment#showall**

Suresh, S: Chronic pain management in children and adolescents, 2009. Retrieved June 2013 from **http://archive.is/SKFVA**

Tales, A, Jefferis, J, Taylor, J-P, et al (reviewers): Sight, perception, and hallucinations in dementia, 2012. Retrieved June 2013 from **http://www.alzheimers.org.uk/site/scripts/download_info.php?fileID=1837**

Thomas, A: Depression and physical illness, 2005. 2010. Retrieved June 2013 from **http://www.netdoctor.co.uk/diseases/depression/depressionandphysicalillness_000601.htm**

Thomas, CP, and Fraer, M: Syndrome of inappropriate antidiuretic hormone secretion, 2013. Retrieved June 2013 from **http://emedicine.medscape.com/article/246650-overview**

Umscheid, C, Gould, C, and Pegues, DA: 2009 Guideline for preventing catheter-associated urinary tract infections. Retrieved June 2013 from **http://www.cdc.gov/hicpac/pdf/cauti/cautiguideline2009final.pdf**

U.S. Department of Health and Human Services (HHS), National Clearinghouse for Long Term Care Information: Costs of care, 2010. Retrieved March 2013 from **http://www.longtermcare.gov/LTC/Main_Site/Paying/Costs/Index.aspx**

U.S. Department of Health and Human Services (HHS), Health Resources and Services Administration, Maternal and Child Health Bureau: Child health USA, 2011 Hospitalization. Retrieved March 2013 from **http://mchb.hrsa.gov/chusa11/hstat/hsc/pages/211h.html**

U.S. Department of Justice (DOJ) National Drug Intelligence Center: The economic impact of illicit drug use on American society, 2011. Retrieved March 2013 from **http://www.justice.gov/archive/ndic/pubs44/44731/44731p.pdf**

U.S. Department of Veterans Affairs, National Center for PTSD: PTSD and problems with alcohol use, updated 2011. Retrieved May 2013 from **http://www.ptsd.va.gov/public/pages/ptsd-alcohol-use.asp**

U.S. Department of Veterans Affairs, National Center for PTSD: Treatment of PTSD, updated 2013. Retrieved May 2013 from **http://www.ptsd.va.gov/public/pages/treatment-ptsd.asp**

Wedro, B: Electrolytes. Various pages, 2010. Retrieved June 2013 from **http://www.emedicinehealth.com/electrolytes/article_em.htm**

World Health Organization (WHO): Definition of palliative care, 2002. Retrieved June 2013 from **http://www.who.int/cancer/palliative/definition/en/**

Presentations

Lewis, MM: End of life care in long term care settings. Presentation: End of Life Care and Bereavement, National Geropsychology Conference, University of Colorado at Colorado Springs, 2008.

Otis-Green, S: Building your legacy: Making moments matter. Presentation: End of Life Care and Bereavement, National Geropsychology Conference, University of Colorado at Colorado Springs, 2008a.

Otis-Green, S: Grief and bereavement care. Presentation: End of Life Care and Bereavement, National Geropsychology Conference, University of Colorado at Colorado Springs, 2008b.

INDEX OF NURSING DIAGNOSES

L

M

N

O

P

R

S

T

U

V